D1032327

A Practical Approach to Occupational and Environmental Medicine

Third Edition

A Practical Approach to Occupational and Environmental Medicine

Third Edition

Editor-in-Chief

Robert J. McCunney, M.D., M.P.H., M.S.
Research Scientist
Department of Biological Engineering
Massachusetts Institute of Technology
Cambridge
Clinical Associate
Pulmonary Unit
Massachusetts General Hospital
Harvard Medical School
Boston, Massachusetts
Past President
American College of Occupational and Environmental Medicine

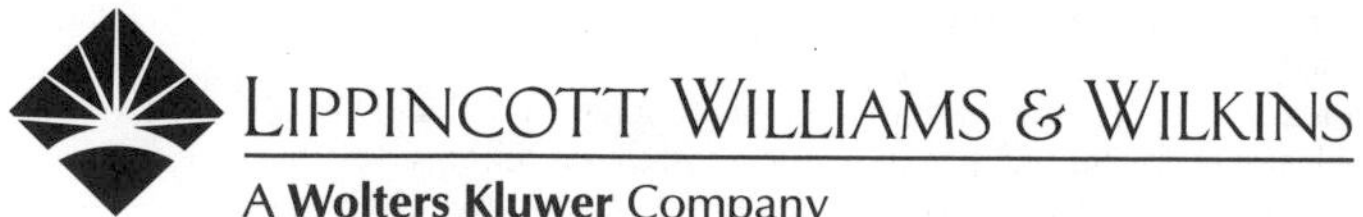

LIPPINCOTT WILLIAMS & WILKINS
A **Wolters Kluwer** Company
Philadelphia • Baltimore • New York • London
Buenos Aires • Hong Kong • Sydney • Tokyo

Acquisitions Editor: Hal Pollard
Developmental Editor: Stacey L. Baze
Production Editor: Thomas Boyce
Manufacturing Manager: Colin Warnock
Cover Designer: Catherine Lau Hunt
Compositor: Lippincott Williams & Wilkins Desktop Division
Printer: Maple Press

530 Walnut Street
Philadelphia, PA 19106 USA
LWW.com

Printed in the USA

Library of Congress Cataloging-in-Publication Data

A practical approach to occupational and environmental medicine / editor-in-chief, Robert J. McCunney ; editor, Paul P. Rountree ; associate editors, Cheryl S. Barbanel ...[SC]
[et al.].— 3rd ed.
p. ; cm.
Includes bibliographical references and index.
ISBN 0-7817-3674-9
1. Medicine, Industrial—Handbooks, manuals, etc. 2. Environmental health—Handbooks, manuals, etc. 3. Environmentally induced diseases—Handbooks, manuals, etc. I. Title: Occupational and environmental medicine. II. McCunney, Robert J.
[DNLM: 1. Occupational Diseases—Handbooks. 2. Occupational Health Services—Handbooks. 3. Environmental Exposure—Handbooks. 4. Environmental Medicine—methods—Handbooks. WA 39 H2356 2003]
RC963 .H34 2003
616.9′803—dc21

2002040640

Care has been taken to confirm the accuracy of the information presented and to describe generally accepted practices. However, the authors, editors, and publisher are not responsible for errors or omissions or for any consequences from application of the information in this book and make no warranty, expressed or implied, with respect to the currency, completeness, or accuracy of the contents of the publication. Application of this information in a particular situation remains the professional responsibility of the practitioner.

The authors, editors, and publisher have exerted every effort to ensure that drug selection and dosage set forth in this text are in accordance with current recommendations and practice at the time of publication. However, in view of ongoing research, changes in government regulations, and the constant flow of information relating to drug therapy and drug reactions, the reader is urged to check the package insert for each drug for any change in indications and dosage and for added warnings and precautions. This is particularly important when the recommended agent is a new or infrequently employed drug.

Some drugs and medical devices presented in this publication have Food and Drug Administration (FDA) clearance for limited use in restricted research settings. It is the responsibility of the health care provider to ascertain the FDA status of each drug or device planned for use in their clinical practice.

10 9 8 7 6 5 4 3 2 1

To the best family an overworked physician can have:
My wife, Mal, my son, Robby, and my daughter, Kelsey

Associate Editors

Editor

Paul P. Rountree, M.D.
Occupational and Environmental Medicine
Occupational Health Sciences
University of Texas Center at Tyler
Tyler, Texas

Associate Editors

Cheryl S. Barbanel, M.D., M.P.H., F.A.C.O.E.M.
Director
Boston University Occupational Health Center
Chief, Occupational and Environmental Medicine
Boston Medical Center
Boston, Massachusetts

Jonathan B. Borak, M.D., D.A.B.T.
Associate Clinical Professor of Internal Medicine
Yale University School of Medicine
President
Jonathan Borak & Company, Inc.
New Haven, Connecticut

William B. Bunn, M.D., J.D., M.P.H.
Vice President
Health, Safety, and Productivity
International Truck and Engine Corporation
Warrenville, Illinois

Philip Harber, M.D., M.P.H.
Professor of Family Medicine
Chief, Division of Occupational and Environmental Medicine
University of California, Los Angeles
Los Angeles, California

Jeffrey L. Levin, M.D., M.S.P.H.
Professor and Chairman
Occupational Health Sciences
University of Texas Center at Tyler
Tyler, Texas

Contents

Part II. Occupationally Related Disorders

Part III. Evaluating a Hazard and Work Environments

Part IV. Environmental Medicine

Appendix

Contributing Authors

Donald Accetta, M.D.
President, Allergy and Asthma Care PC, Taunton, Massachusetts
29. Allergy and Immunology

L. Kristian Arnold, M.D., F.A.C.E.P.
Department of Emergency Medicine, Boston Medical Center, Boston, Massachusetts
55. Emergency Response to Environmental Incidents
56. Occupational Medicine Aspects of Terrorism

Amy J. Behrman, M.D.
Medical Director, Occupational Medicine, Department of Emergency Medicine, University of Pennsylvania Health System, Philadelphia, Pennsylvania
36. The Human Genome Project and Occupational Medicine Practice

Bernard R. Blais, M.D., F.A.A.O., F.A.C.O.E.M., F.A.C.S.
Blais Consulting, Ltd., Clifton Park, New York
34. Occupational Ophthalmology

Jonathan B. Borak, M.D., D.A.B.T.
Associate Clinical Professor of Internal Medicine, Yale University School of Medicine; President, Jonathan Borak & Company, Inc., New Haven, Connecticut
39. Toxicology
43. Ergonomics
54. Medical Aspects of Environmental Emergencies

Reid T. Boswell, M.D.
Occupational Health and Rehabilitation, Inc., Wilmington, Massachusetts
22. Musculoskeletal Disorders

William Boucher, M.D., M.P.H.
President, Fortune Rocks Consultants, Biddeford, Maine
7. The Independent Medical Evaluation

Christopher R. Brigham, M.D., M.M.S.
Brigham & Associates, Inc., Portland, Maine
7. The Independent Medical Evaluation

William B. Bunn, M.D., J.D., M.P.H.
Vice President, Health, Safety, and Productivity, International Truck and Engine Corporation, Warrenville, Illinois
17. International Occupational Medicine
50. Environmental Medicine: The Regulatory Issues
51. International Environmental Health
57. The Environmental, Health, and Safety Audit
58. Environmental Risk Assessment

Wayne N. Burton, M.D.
Corporate Medical Director, Bank One, Chicago, Illinois
11. Health and Productivity

Kenneth H. Chase, M.D., F.A.C.O.E.M.
President, Washington Occupational Health Associates, Inc., Washington, D.C.
42. Risk Assessment in the Workplace

Chang-Ming Joseph Chern, M.D., M.P.H.
Neurological Institute, Veterans General Hospital–Taipei, Taipei, Taiwan (ROC)
25. Neurotoxic Disorders

Craig Conlon, M.D.
Pacific Occupational Medical Association, Agoura Hills, California
41. Occupational Medical Surveillance

Barry A. Cooper, M.H.A.
Vice President, Occupational Health Strategies, Inc., Arlington, Virginia
16. Computers and Informatics in Occupational Medicine Practice

Alain Couturier, M.D., M.S.
Executive Medical Director, Global OEM Solutions LLC, Lincoln, Rhode Island
31. Infectious Disease

Alan M. Ducatman, M.D.
Director, Institute of Occupational and Environmental Health, West Virginia University School of Medicine, Morgantown, West Virginia
52. Clinical Environmental Medicine

Dee W. Edington, Ph.D.
Health Management Research Center, University of Michigan, Ann Arbor, Michigan
11. Health and Productivity

Edward A. Emmett, M.D., M.S.
Professor, Department of Occupational Medicine, University of Pennsylvania, Philadelphia, Pennsylvania
15. Educational Opportunities
27. Occupational Skin Diseases

Alan L. Engelberg, M.D., M.P.H.
HealthLine Corporate Health Services, St. Louis, Missouri
7. The Independent Medical Evaluation

Nancy English, M.D.
SmithKline Beecham, Philadelphia, Pennsylvania
Appendix B. Government and Regulatory Agencies

Jack E. Farnham, M.D.
Assistant Professor of Medicine, Occupational Medicine Division, University of Texas Health Center at Tyler, Tyler, Texas
29. Allergy and Immunology

Robert G. Feldman, M.D.
Professor and Chairman of Neurology, Department of Neurology, Boston University School of Medicine, Boston, Massachusetts
25. Neurotoxic Disorders

Jean Spencer Felton, M.D.
Clinical Professor, Department of Medicine, University of California, Irvine, Mendocino, California
46. The Construction Industry: Its Occupational Health and Safety Experience and Needs
Appendix C. A History of the American College of Occupational and Environmental Medicine and the Growth of a Specialty

Daniel E. Forman, M.D.
Assistant Professor of Medicine, Boston University School of Medicine; Director, Cardiovascular Services, Boston Healthnet Services, Boston Medical Center, Boston, Massachusetts
24. Cardiovascular Disorders

Arthur Frank, M.D.
Drexel University School of Public Health, Philadelphia, Pennsylvania
23. Occupational Cancers

David O. Freedman, M.D.
Division of Geographic Medicine, University of Alabama at Birmingham, Birmingham, Alabama
13. Principles of Travel Medicine

David H. Garabrant, M.D., M.P.H.
Department of Environmental Health Sciences, School of Public Health, University of Michigan, Ann Arbor, Michigan
47. Health Risk Communication

Stuart Gitlow, M.D.
26 Glen Drive, Providence, Rhode Island
28. Psychiatric Aspects of Occupational Medicine

Rose H. Goldman, M.D., M.P.H.
Assistant Professor of Medicine, Harvard Medical School; Director, Occupational and Environmental Medicine, Cambridge Hospital, Cambridge, Massachusetts
20. Suspecting Occupational Disease: The Clinician's Role

Ian A. Greaves, M.B., B.S.
Associate Dean for Research, School of Public Health, University of Minnesota, Minneapolis, Minnesota
21. Occupational Pulmonary Disease

William W. Greaves, M.D., M.S.P.H.
MPH Programs and Division of Public Health, Health Policy Institute, Medical College of Wisconsin, Milwaukee, Wisconsin
48. Reproductive Hazards

Judith Green-McKenzie, M.D., M.P.H.
Director of Clinical Practice and Associate Residency Director, Department of Emergency Medicine, Division of Occupational Medicine, University of Pennsylvania Health System, Phildelphia, Pennsylvania
36. The Human Genome Project and Occupational Medicine Practice

Tee L. Guidotti, M.D.
Department of Environmental and Occupational Health, School of Public Health and Health Services, The George Washington University, Washington, D.C.
49. Environmental Health

David M. Gute, Ph.D., M.P.H.
Department of Civil and Environmental Engineering, Tufts University, Medford, Massachusetts
60. Accessing Environmental Data

Nortin M. Hadler, M.D, F.A.C.P., F.A.C.R., F.A.C.O.E.M.
Professor of Medicine and Microbiology/Immunology, Department of Medicine, University of North Carolina School of Medicine, Chapel Hill, North Carolina
30. Arm Pain in the Workplace

Ridgway M. Hall, Jr., LL.B.
Attorney, Crowell & Moring, Washington, D.C.
57. The Environmental, Health, and Safety Audit

Philip Harber, M.D., M.P.H.
Professor of Family Medicine, Chief, Division of Occupational and Environmental Medicine, University of California, Los Angeles, California
41. Occupational Medical Surveillance

Jeffrey S. Harris, M.D., M.P.H.
President, Jeff Harris & Associates, Inc., Mill Valley, California
14. Economics of Occupational Medicine
18. Workers' Compensation

Myron C. Harrison, M.D., M.P.H.
Senior Health Advisor, Safety, Health, & Environmental Policies, Exxon Mobil Corporation, Irving, Texas
38. Workplace Safety

Natalie P. Hartenbaum, M.D., M.P.H.
Chief Medical Officer, Occumedix, Maple Glen, Pennsylvania
45. Fitness for Duty in the Transportation Industry

James A. Hathaway, M.D., M.P.H.
Corporate Medical Director, Rhodia, Inc., Cranbury, New Jersey
3. Role of Regulatory Agencies

Donald S. Herip, M.D., M.P.H.
Medical Director, Naval Hospital, Pensacola, Florida
13. Principles of Travel Medicine

Jessica Herzstein, M.D., M.P.H.
Chief Medical Officer, Global Health and Wellness, Air Products & Chemicals, Inc., Allentown, Pennsylvania
51. International Environmental Health

Peter J. Holland, M.D.
President, Boca Raton Psychiatric Group, Boca Raton, Florida
28. Psychiatric Aspects of Occupational Medicine

Marilyn V. Howarth, M.D.
Occupational and Environmental Consultant Services, University of Pennsylvania Medical Center, Philadelphia, Pennsylvania
44. Medical Center Occupational Health

Jeffrey G. Jones, M.D., M.P.H.
Director, Travel Medicine, St. Francis Occupational Health Center, Indianapolis, Indiana
13. Principles of Travel Medicine

Todd D. Kissam, B.A.
Occupational Health Strategies, Inc., Charlottesville, Virginia
16. Computers and Informatics in Occupational Medicine Practice

Frank H. Leone, M.B.A., M.P.H.
President, Ryan Associates, Santa Barbara, California
8. The Physician Working with the Business Community

Loren Lipworth, Sc.D.
International Epidemiology Institute, Ltd., Rockville, Maryland
40. Epidemiology and Biostatistics

Molly J. McCauley, M.P.H., R.N.
Employee Health Services, Hoffman-LaRoche, Nutley, New Jersey
12. Health Promotion

Roger O. McClellan, D.V.M., D.A.B.V.T., D.A.B.T., F.A.T.S.
President Emeritus, Chemical Industry Institute of Toxicology, Research Triangle Park, North Carolina; Advisor, Toxicology and Human Health Risk Analysis, Albuquerque, New Mexico
58. Environmental Risk Assessment

James P. McCunney, M.S., C.I.H.
Safety and Health Administrator, Boeing Company, Seattle, Washington
37. Industrial Hygiene

Robert J. McCunney, M.D., M.P.H.
Massachusetts Institute of Technology, Cambridge; Massachusetts General Hospital, Boston, Massachusetts
1. Occupational Medical Services
12. Health Promotion
22. Musculoskeletal Disorders
41. Occupational Medical Surveillance

Junius C. McElveen, Jr., J.D.
Partner, Jones, Day, Reaves & Pogue, Washington, D.C.
2. Legal and Ethical Issues

Joseph K. McLaughlin, Ph.D.
President, International Epidemiology Institute, Ltd., Rockville, Maryland
40. Epidemiology and Biostatistics

Robert K. McLellan, M.D.
Medical Director, Center for Occupational and Environmental Health, Exeter Hospital, Inc., Exeter, New Hampshire
53. Indoor Environmental Quality

John D. Meyer, M.D., M.P.H.
Division of Occupational Medicine, University of Connecticut, Farmington, Connecticut
26. Noise-induced Hearing Loss

J. Steven Moore, M.D., M.P.H., C.I.H., C.P.E.
Department of Environmental and Occupational Health, School of Rural Public Health, Texas A&M University Health Science Center, Bryan, Texas
43. Ergonomics

Ross S. Myerson, M.D., M.P.H., F.A.C.O.E.M.
Myerson Associates, Silver Spring, Maryland
32. Hepatic Disorders

J. Torey Nalbone, M.D.
Assistant Professor, Department of Occupational Health Sciences; Associate Director, Environmental Science Graduate Program, University of Texas at Tyler, Tyler, Texas
37. Industrial Hygiene

Claudia O'Brien
Attorney, Latham & Watkins, Washington, D.C.
50. Environmental Medicine: The Regulatory Issues

Sadhna Paralkar, M.B., M.P.H.
Manager, Clinical Management and Disability, International Truck and Engine Corporation, Warrenville, Illinois
17. International Occupational Medicine

William B. Patterson, M.D., M.P.H.
Occupational Health and Rehabilitation, Wilmington, Massachusetts
4. Establishing an Occupational Health Program

Kent W. Peterson, M.D., F.A.C.O.E.M.
President, Occupational Health Strategies, Inc., Charlottesville, Virginia
5. Understanding the Americans with Disabilities Act
9. Drug Testing in the Occupational Setting
16. Computers and Informatics in Occupational Medicine Practice

Richard C. Pleus, Ph.D.
Senior Toxicologist and Principal, Intertox, Seattle, Washington
39. Toxicology

D. Gary Rischitelli, M.D., J.D., M.P.H., F.A.C.O.E.M.
Center for Research on Occupational and Environmental Toxicology, Oregon Health and Science University, Portland, Oregon
5. Understanding the Americans with Disabilities Act

Bonnie Rogers, Dr.P.H., C.O.H.N.-S., L.N.C.C., F.A.A.N.
Director and Associate Professor of Occupational Health Nursing, School of Public Health, University of North Carolina at Chapel Hill, Chapel Hill, North Carolina
6. Occupational Health Nursing: Roles and Practice

Stacy R. Rose, M.S.
College of Engineering, Texas A&M University, College Station, Texas
43. Ergonomics

Victor S. Roth, M.D., M.P.H.
Clinical Assistant Professor, University of Michigan Health System, Division of Occupational Medicine and Urgent Care; Clinical Assistant Professor, Department of Environmental Health Sciences, The University of Michigan School of Public Health, Ann Arbor, Michigan
47. Health Risk Communication

Paul P. Rountree, M.D., F.A.C.O.E.M.
Associate Professor, Department of Occupational and Environmental Medicine, University of Texas Health Center at Tyler, Tyler, Texas
24. Cardiovascular Disorders

Mark Russi, M.D., M.P.H.
Associate Professor of Medicine and Public Health, Yale University School of Medicine; Director of Occupational Health, Yale–New Haven Hospital, New Haven, Connecticut
44. Medical Center Occupational Health

Dennis Schultz, M.D.
Concentra, Brookfield, Wisconsin
10. Accreditation of Occupational Health Services

Peter G. Shields, M.D.
Professor of Medicine and Oncology, Georgetown University Medical School; Associate Director for Cancer Control and Population Sciences, Director, Cancer Genetics and Epidemiology, Lombardi Cancer Center, Georgetown University Medical Center, Washington, D.C.
35. Use of Molecular Genetics in Occupational Medicine

Jack Shih, P.E., Q.E.P.
Manager, Environmental Affairs, International Truck and Engine Corporation, Warrenville, Illinois
50. Environmental Medicine: The Regulatory Issues

Thomas J. Slavin, M.S., M.B.A.
Manager, Occupational Safety and Health, International Truck and Engine Corporation, Warrenville, Illinois
57. The Environmental, Health, and Safety Audit

Kevin Soden, M.D., M.P.H.
Corporate Medical Director, Celanese Acetate Corporation, Charlotte, North Carolina
48. Reproductive Hazards

Weimin Song
Department of Environmental Health, Fudan University, Shanghai, People's Republic of China
49. Environmental Health

Larry M. Starr, Ph.D.
Coordinator, Organizational Development and Leadership Program, Department of Psychology, Philadelphia College of Osteopathic Medicine, Philadelphia, Pennsylvania
Appendix A. First Aid Supplies in the Occupational Setting

David J. Tollerud, M.D., M.P.H.
Director, Center for Environmental and Occupational Health, School of Public Health, MCP Hahnemann University, Philadelphia, Pennsylvania
15. Educational Opportunities

Melissa D. Tonn, M.D., M.B.A., M.P.H.
Chief Medical Officer, OccMD Group, P.A., Dallas, Texas
19. Health Care Management

Thomas J. Tredici, M.D., F.A.A.O.
Department of Ophthalmology, Brooks Air Force Base, San Antonio, Texas
34. Occupational Ophthalmology

Craig F. Turet, J.D.
Attorney, Duane, Morris & Heckscher, LLP, Philadelphia, Pennsylvania
47. Health Risk Communication

Peter A. Valberg, Ph.D.
Gradient Corporation, Cambridge, Massachusetts
59. Ambient Particulates and Health Effects

Erin K. Walline, M.S.
College of Engineering, Texas A&M University, College Station, Texas
43. Ergonomics

John Whysner, M.D., Ph.D., D.A.B.T.
Vice President, Washington Occupational Health Associates, Inc., Sleepy Hollow, New York
42. Risk Assessment in the Workplace

John Williams, Sr., M.D., F.A.A.O., F.A.C.O.E.M.
Chairman, Department of Ophthalmology, Marshfield Clinic, Marshfield, Wisconsin
34. Occupational Ophthalmology

William E. Wright, M.D., M.S.P.H.
Medical Director, Core, Inc., McLean, Virginia
33. Case Report: Discovery of Occupational Disease

Foreword

It's hard to believe that eight years have passed since the publication of the second edition of *A Practical Approach to Occupational and Environmental Medicine*. At that time, I had noted that the field had expanded significantly from occupational medicine to include environmental medicine as well, leading to a significant expansion in the book also. Over the last eight years, the trend has continued unabated.

The scope of the field of occupational and environmental medicine continues to encompass additional areas, and in each area the fund of knowledge grows inexorably. This new edition of *A Practical Approach to Occupational and Environmental Medicine* is again expanded in an attempt to keep pace. There are new areas of the book that represent logical foreseeable extensions, areas that we were barely aware of at the time of the previous edition, and areas that have been thrust upon us in totally unexpected (and unwelcome) ways. Chapters on additional organ systems affected by occupational or environmental exposures (hepatic disorders, eye disorders) were a logical and necessary addition. The recognition of the important and unique health hazards of certain industries warranting separate chapters (agriculture, transportation, high technology, construction) is entirely apropos. The Human Genome Project is completed ahead of schedule and will transform the way in which all medicine is practiced, with significant implications for society in general. There will be special challenges from it for occupational and environmental medicine—as we learn to identify the genetic susceptibilities for work-related and non-work-related disorders, we must remain steadfast in using this knowledge to benefit the worker or individual. We are rediscovering old concepts—that worker productivity is intimately connected to worker health, so our efforts to improve worker health do not just benefit the worker, but they also benefit the industry, the economy, and the country. This lesson has world-wide implications for improving the global economy, particularly in developing countries. Unfortunately, we must also learn to cope with new public health emergencies, including chemical, nuclear, and biological terrorism, but fortunately because of our experience in dealing with hazardous exposures, we are well prepared to make important contributions to this effort. Finally, for all areas, old and new, we must be able to communicate effectively; health risk communication is vital if we are to translate our knowledge into actions that will prevent disease.

This edition clearly demonstrates the difficulty for the expert in occupational and environmental medicine, let alone the non-expert practitioner, to keep abreast of all the relevant areas in the field. This is why *A Practical Approach to Occupational and Environmental Medicine* will continue to serve as a useful reference and an invaluable resource for anyone interested in the health of workers, communities, or the entire planet.

Paul W. Brandt-Rauf, Sc.D., M.D., Dr.P.H.
Professor and Chairman
Department of Environmental Health Sciences
The Mailman School of Public Health
Columbia University
New York

Preface

Since the publication of the first edition of this text in 1987, Occupational and Environmental Medicine has gained a firm place in the delivery of healthcare. Hospitals, businesses, and group practices have recognized the specialty for its unique contributions to the prevention of disease and the promotion of health. The third edition of this text amply reflects the breadth and depth of the field. Topics as diverse as the human genome and molecular genetics now attract the attention of astute occupational health professionals as due updates on the treatment of musculoskeletal disorders. In furthering a theme introduced in the second edition, environmental medicine topics are well addressed in this new edition as well.

This book contains 60 chapters that are organized into major sections. The first section addresses the milieu of occupational health practice, including the type of services provided and the corresponding issues associated with the delivery of occupational health care. The second section focuses on occupational diseases by organ system, along with the use of scientific methods to enhance diagnostic accuracy and to aid in prevention. The third section provides principles in evaluating a potential hazard or a work environment. The tools of the trade, as it were—ranging from industrial hygiene and epidemiology to toxicology—are described in detail to enable a reader to apply the principles to various work settings. Specific chapters have been devoted to hospitals, transportation, and construction because of their widespread role in the life of the majority of occupational health professionals worldwide. Space considerations limited our ability to provide detailed descriptions of other industries; however, the principles addressed in this section can be applied to virtually any occupational setting. The environmental section in this new edition builds upon the success of the second edition in providing a global overview, a regulatory and clinical perspective, and an update on environmental risk assessment.

As most general literature has reflected, our lives have been changed as a result of the tragedy of September 11th, 2001. This book reflects, in part, an aspect of that change by including a new chapter on Occupational Health Aspects of Terrorism.

Undoubtedly, a book of this nature will not include every aspect of occupational health practice. Topics for the new edition were selected based on a number of meetings held among the associate editors and me. Decisions were largely based on topics from earlier editions, new publications, and observations at various professional meetings, among others. Ultimately, what becomes included in a new edition is essentially a matter of judgment, consistent with the focus of this book, which, in this case, is practical application of the science.

As with the second edition, this edition serves as the basis of the Occupational Medicine Self Assessment Review (OMSAR) of the American College of Occupational & Environmental Medicine (ACOEM). Physicians who complete the OMSAR can receive CME credits for their efforts.

Like the previous two editions, this version has undergone extensive peer review. In fact, all chapters were reviewed by at least two of the editors before final acceptance for publication. It is hoped that this rigorous oversight will enhance the value of the book for our readers.

The work involved in overseeing this new edition demanded a considerable amount of time that needed to be borrowed from other commitments at work and at home. Inevitably, nights and weekends were used to complete a review, develop a new chapter, or address the publisher's timelines in some way or another. To my employer, MIT, I am grateful for the support. To my family, I am appreciative of the time and encouragement you provided. To my associate editors, I appreciate the suggestions for chapter topics and authors, but most importantly, the rigorous scientific reviews you performed, which undoubtedly enhance the quality of the text. To Max Lum from NIOSH, I appreciate your efforts in coordinating the inclusion of the CD-ROM on the Health Effects of Common Substances, with this book.

Three others deserve special mention in providing the support that I needed to publish this text. My editors at Lippincott Williams & Wilkins, including Hal Pollard and Stacey Baze, and finally my colleague and friend, Paul Rountree, who served as editor.

Like the first two editions, it is my pleasure to donate the royalties from the sale of this text to ACOEM's Research and Education Fund. As a firm supporter of both research and education in furthering our field, I am proud to make this small step for the benefit of the specialty of occupational and environmental medicine. On behalf of the editors and many others who helped in developing this text, I hope you appreciate our efforts. We would value your comments.

Robert J. McCunney, M.D., M.P.H., M.S.
January 2003

Acknowledgments

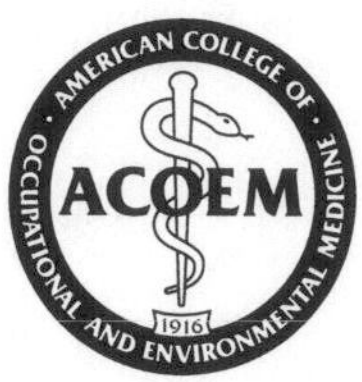

The following members of the Publications Committee of the American College of Occupational and Environmental Medicine participated in the peer review process of various sections of this book. Their insights and suggestions played a major role in improving the quality of the final effort. All of the reviewers contributed chapters to the text as well.

Cheryl S. Barbanel, M.D., M.P.H., F.A.C.O.E.M.
Jonathan B. Borak, M.D., D.A.B.T.
William B. Bunn, M.D., J.D., M.P.H.
Philip Harber, M.D., M.P.H.
Jeffrey L. Levin, M.D., M.S.P.H.
Paul P. Rountree, M.D.

Royalties from the sale and distribution of this book benefit the Samuel E. Bacon Research and Education Fund of the American College of Occupational and Environmental Medicine.

American College of Occupational and Environmental Medicine Code of Ethical Conduct

This code establishes standards of professional ethical conduct with which each member of the American College of Occupational and Environmental Medicine (ACOEM) is expected to comply. These standards are intended to guide occupational and environmental medicine physicians in their relationships with: the individuals they serve; employers and worker's representatives; colleagues in the health professions; the public and all levels of government, including the judiciary.

Physicians should:

1. Accord the highest priority to the health and safety of individuals in both the workplace and the environment;
2. Practice on a scientific basis with integrity and strive to acquire and maintain adequate knowledge and expertise upon which to render professional service;
3. Relate honestly and ethically in all professional relationships;
4. Strive to expand and disseminate medical knowledge and participate in ethical research efforts as appropriate;
5. Keep confidential all individual medical information, releasing such information only when required to do so by law or overriding public health considerations, or to other physicians according to accepted medical practice, or to others at the request of the individual;
6. Recognize that employers may be entitled to counsel about an individual's medical work fitness, but not to diagnoses or specific details, except in compliance with the law or other regulations;
7. Communicate to individuals and/or groups any significant observations and recommendations concerning their health and/or safety; and
8. Recognize those medical impairments in oneself and others, including chemical dependency or abusive personal practices, which interfere with one's ability to follow the above principles, and take appropriate treatment measures.

1
Occupational Medical Services

Robert J. McCunney

The range of services provided by a physician who practices occupational medicine depends largely on the *setting* of the practice. Since the last edition, the range of settings has expanded, although the thrust of occupational health services continues to be delivered from a clinical base. To be most effective, occupational medicine practitioners also work with other professionals such as epidemiologists, toxicologists, and industrial hygienists. In fact, a *team* approach to controlling occupational illnesses and injuries is usually most effective. This chapter provides an introduction to the *range of occupational medical services* provided by physicians who deliver health care to the working population.

Although occupational medicine has been a distinct discipline within the American Board of Preventive Medicine since 1954, a considerable shortage of well-trained and certified specialists in this field continues to exist. In large part, this shortage is due to a deficiency of postgraduate training positions. Since the late 1970s, Educational Resource Centers established by the National Institute for Occupational Safety and Health (NIOSH) and other institutions, such as hospitals (1), have been instrumental in educating physicians in the discipline of occupational medicine. More recently, additional residency programs have been established. As of 2002, institutions sponsored 37 graduate training programs in occupational medicine. In addition, "mini-residency" programs and other educational opportunities such as those established by the American College of Occupational and Environmental Medicine have furthered the growth and influence of the specialty. These endeavors, however, have not yet substantially increased the number of trained physicians appropriate for the provision of quality occupational medical services.

The shortage of occupational medicine specialists combined with wider awareness of occupational and environmental hazards creates an opportunity for the primary care physician (2). One needs only to read a daily newspaper to find topics such as the air pollution and asthma, contamination of the water supply, and cancer in certain groups of workers. Educated workers and consumers offer further challenges to the physician to become abreast of these and other issues and to develop protocols for the evaluation and prevention of occupationally related illnesses (3).

HISTORY OF OCCUPATIONAL MEDICINE

Occupational medicine can be traced back to antiquity. Observations related to increased rates of illnesses and mortality among miners date back to Roman times; however, explanations for this phenomenon were often attributed to the fact that workers were slaves and thus of a more feeble constitution. It was not until the late 17th century, when an Italian physician published *Disease and Occupations,* that physicians were formally urged to pay attention to the role of one's work in the development of certain illnesses (4). Throughout the two centuries after Dr. Ramazzini's book appeared, periodic reports described illnesses associated with a variety of substances including asbestos and radiation, among others (5).

In the first part of the 20th century, a rising number of employee-directed suits against employers for work-related injuries prompted the development of workers' compensation statutes (6). The workers' compensation system essentially established a no-fault insurance program such that any injured worker would be guaranteed compensation for medical bills, time lost from work, and permanent impairment or death. In turn, employers were granted immunity from further legal action by workers for work-related illnesses or injuries.

In 1916, the Industrial Medical Association, the forerunner of the American College of Occupational and Environmental Medicine, was formed. The group was composed primarily of surgeons who had developed a strong interest and expertise in the treatment of work-related injuries. Most forms of occupational medicine practice at that time focused on injury care and management. Little, if any, recognition was given to hazardous substances such as silica or asbestos, although the U.S. Public Health Service began to conduct work-site surveys during this period.

Clinical activities associated with treating work-related injuries were referred to as *industrial medicine.* As physicians became more concerned with *preventing* work-related injuries and illnesses, the medical discipline became known as *occupational medicine.* Eventually, the area of knowledge and expertise associated with delivering health care to the working population began to recognize the importance of scientific principles of other disciplines in the prevention of disease. Toxicology, epidemiology, industrial hygiene, and ergonomics, for example, became integral elements of the education of the well-trained occupational physician.

In 1946, the American Academy of Occupational Medicine was founded to foster the growth and development of the formally educated occupational physician; its founding led to occupational medicine becoming a distinct medical specialty in 1954, under the auspices of the American Board of Preventative Medicine. The American Academy eventually merged with the American Occupational Medical Association to form the American College of Occupational Medicine, which eventually added "Environmental" to its title.

Throughout the first four to five decades since the establishment of the workers' compensation laws, occupational health services were primarily delivered in corporate settings and in some cases from the private physician's office. Larger corporations with a sufficient number of employees could economically justify onsite facilities, especially if the work situations warranted immediate medical care. During this period, however, the needs of small businesses for occupational medical services appeared to have been overlooked. A relatively unknown fact is that over 90% of business in the United States *and the world* have 100 or fewer employees. It is rarely economically feasible for these enterprises to provide anything other than meager health care and, in some cases, at best first aid.

To meet the need for providing occupational health services to small businesses, a number of approaches can be effective. An entire medical facility can provide occupational health services to a range of small businesses within a certain geographic area. Alternatively, occupational health services can be delivered from the private physician's office or by the physician making periodic visits to the local business facility.

OCCUPATIONAL HEALTH SERVICES

What does one *do* in occupational medicine? The occupational physician lacks the trademark associ-

TABLE 1.1. *Occupational and environmental health programs: essential components*

Health evaluation of employees
Preplacement
Medical surveillance
After illness or injury
Diagnosis and treatment of occupational and environmental injuries or illnesses, including rehabilitation
Emergency treatment of nonoccupational injury or illness
Education of employees and jobs of potential occupational hazards
Implementation of programs for personal protective equipment
Evaluation, inspection, and abatement of workplace hazards
Toxicologic assessments, including advice on chemical substances that have not had adequate toxicologic testing
Biostatistics and epidemiology assessments
Maintenance of occupational medical records
Immunization against possible occupational infections
Medical interpretation and participation in governmental health and safety regulations
Periodic evaluation of the occupational or environmental health program
Disaster preparedness: planning for the workplace and community; local emergency planning committees
Assistance in rehabilitation of alcohol- and drug-dependent employees or those with emotional disorders

Adapted from Scope of occupational and environmental health programs and practices: report of the Occupational Medical Practice Committee of the American College of Occupational and Environmental Medicine. *J Occup Med* 1992;34:436.

ated with other specialties, such as the electrocardiogram of the cardiologist, the bronchoscope of the pulmonary specialist, or the scalpel of the surgeon. Occupational health services, in their broadest sense, can include the range of health care delivered to working populations. Although any definition is likely to be arbitrary, the following description of occupational health services is designed mainly for the primary care physician who may provide such services at a local plant, as part of a private practice or multispecialty group, or at an occupational health center designed for small business. Residents and other health care professionals such as physician assistants and nurse practitioners also find many of these services within their realm of expertise. These services should be considered essential in primary occupational health care. Clinicians are advised that business professionals responsible for overseeing the delivery of these services expect knowledge and understanding in these areas. The physician in turn is advised to become familiar with the scientific principles of occupational medicine practice through the educational programs that are widely available.

The scope of services provided in an occupational medicine practice setting varies depending on a variety of factors. To help set a framework of consistency, the American College of Occupational and Environmental Medicine published guidelines regarding essential and elective components (Tables 1.1 and 1.2). Guidelines for the staffing, type of facilities, and equipment appropriate for an occupational health service have been proposed (7).

TABLE 1.2. *Elective components of occupational and environmental health programs*

Palliative treatment of nonoccupational disorders
Management of nonoccupational conditions prescribed and monitored by personal physicians
Assistance and control of illness-related job absenteeism
Assistance and evaluation of personal health care
Immunizations against nonoccupational infectious diseases
Health education and counseling
Termination and retirement administration
Participation in and planning and assessing of the quality of employee health benefits
Participation in research efforts (27)

Adapted from Scope of occupational and environmental health programs and practices: report of the Occupational Medical Practice Committee of the American College of Occupational and Environmental Medicine. *J Occup Med* 1992;34:436.

CLINICAL SERVICES

Preplacement Evaluation

Preplacement evaluations (PPE), formerly known as the preemployment physical, are an essential part of occupational health programs. The purpose of a preplacement evaluation is to ensure that the person examined does not have any medical condition that may be aggravated by the job duties or that may affect the health and safety of others. Although this category is reasonably broad, the physician should recognize that the primary obligation is to the patient's health and to evaluate such situations accordingly. The critical determinants in this decision-making process are the person's health and the job itself. Incumbent on physicians conducting preplacement examinations is a thorough understanding of the job duties and the *work environment* (see Chapter 4 for discussion of the work-site visit).

Preplacement evaluations can also be of value in complying with certain Occupational Safety and Health Administration (OSHA) standards and in serving as a baseline for health improvement programs. For example, the OSHA standard for occupational exposure to asbestos requires that workers undergo a chest film and pulmonary function studies prior to job assignment. Health promotion and wellness programs often include baseline examinations and routine ancillary testing; results are used to screen for certain illnesses, promote more healthful behavior, and serve as a frame of reference to evaluate the effectiveness of certain interventions.

The decision regarding the need for and content of preplacement evaluations depends on the nature of the industry and the particular job. In some cases, however, in particular when workers are exposed to substances regulated by OSHA standards, such evaluations are legally mandated. Other situations that call for mandatory preplacement examinations include the transportation industry, for example, the Interstate Commerce Commission (ICC) and the Federal Aviation Administration (FAA) (see Chapter 45 in this text related to the transportation industry).

The type of testing to be conducted at a preplacement examination depends on the job for which the worker is being considered. For example, in workers who paint with isocyanates, pulmonary function testing prior to assignment can help to assess the person's breathing capacity and capability of safely wearing a respirator. This examination can also serve as a baseline on which to compare future evaluations that are part of a medical surveillance program.

The physician is urged to exercise restraint, however, in recommending the type of ancillary testing (e.g., laboratory, x-ray) that should be included in a preplacement evaluation. Attention needs to be directed to the effectiveness of the ancillary procedure used as a screening tool to uncover unrecognized illness or as a "predictor" of future occupational illness or injury. Indiscriminate testing can divert resources away from programs of potentially greater benefit as well as cause needless alarm and greater expense in evaluating the inevitable false-positive results. Arbitrary use of certain tests can also be considered discriminatory, legally unsound, and of limited medical utility. Random use of low back films to "predict" future back disorders falls under this category. In light of the Americans with Disabilities Act, physicians are likely to be called on to ensure that testing is job specific and has some pertinence in evaluating a person's fitness for duty. With the completion of the sequencing of the human genome, the use of genetic tests in employment settings will attract the attention of practitioners (see Chapter 36 on the Human Genome). At this time (2002), such tests have been employed only in research settings, in which defined protocols and privacy safeguards have been developed. Ethical issues are likely to arise with the use of genetic tests (8).

Name: ______________________ Employer: ______________________
Address: ______________________ Occupation: ______________________
______________________ Age: ______ Date of birth: ____________
Phone: ______________________ SS#: ______________________

Person to contact in case of medical emergency: ______________________
Relationship to you: ______________ Phone number: ______________

Are you allergic to any medications? Yes No
If *Yes,* what medications are you allergic to: ______________________
Do you have a family physician? Yes No Do you have health insurance? Yes No
Physician's name: ______________ Name of insurance: ______________
Address ______________________ Membership #: ______________
______________________ Subscriber: ______________

I authorize this medical facility, its physicians and health care professionals, to provide treatment, examinations, and/or evaluations, etc. as deemed necessary, and in accordance with sound medical procedures.

Signature: ______________________ Date: ______________________

Release of Information to Employer

(The section below applies to patients being treated <u>or</u> examined for work-related illness and injury, and for those patients undergoing preplacement, fitness for duty, and return to work evaluations.)

The answers that I give are true to the best of my knowledge. The information shall be used to determine whether: (a) I am capable of performing the job requirements of the position for which I am being considered; or (b) I am able to return to work after an illness or work-related injury. Medical information related to this evaluation will pertain only to my ability to perform essential job functions. Specific diagnostic information will not be released, in accordance with the Code of Ethical Conduct of the American College of Occupational and Environmental Medicine. Medical records will not be released to any party, without my consent, except in the context of workers' compensation, when information related <u>only</u> to a specific injury or illness can be transmitted. <u>Other information will be held strictly confidential.</u>

Signature: ______________________ Date: ______________________

FIG. 1.1. Sample medical treatment authorization form.

The physician conducting a preplacement evaluation has an obligation to the business enterprise to report functional limitations and corresponding accommodations that may be necessary for the applicant to work. Although the criteria used to define health conditions that fall under this category may be blurred at times, the physician should strive to be recognized as impartial in these often-difficult settings. Ideally, the patient should be advised as to what information will be released to the employer, and the physician should pay heed to *medical confidentiality* on non–work-related illnesses (9,10). As part of the PPE process, it is advisable that a person undergoing the evaluation sign an appropriate release form that allows the physician to discuss pertinent medical findings with the business (Fig. 1.1).

To communicate effectively with the business enterprise, it is advisable to have a simple form that notifies a designated person that an examination has taken place and that the person is either medically suitable with or without certain restrictions or not medically suitable. Medical records should be kept on site at the medical facility, and not released to the business unless an on-site medical office is maintained and supervised by a registered nurse or physician who has responsibility for the ethical maintenance of the records.

A protocol to follow up abnormalities noted during PPEs can be helpful. During PPEs, people may exhibit abnormalities such as idiopathic hematuria, mild hypertension, and other conditions that will not interfere with work ability but warrant some medical follow-up (11). Ideally, these people should be apprised of the abnormal findings and referred to their personal physician for diagnostic and therapeutic care. The occupational health program will most likely need to develop referral patterns, however, because as much as 40% of the workforce in some areas lack a primary care physician.

Work-related Injuries

The physician who provides primary occupational health care is likely to encounter a variety of minor injuries ranging from cuts and lacerations to strains and burns, treatment of which is well within the expertise of the primary care clinician. According to workers' compensation statutes, the injured worker may have the right to choose the *site and provider of medical care,* although businesses often establish relationships with designated medical facilities or physicians to provide occupational health services. These regulations, however, may have variations among the states.

The physician is advised to be aware of *recurring* clinical events such as injuries from one type of machinery or certain tasks such as lifting or repetitive motion activities. Businesses are required to record work-related injuries, periodic review of which can stimulate the search for preventive measures (OSHA 300 log; see Chapter 2).

Return to Work Evaluation

Following a worker's lengthy absence from work, many businesses request a medical evaluation before the worker may resume job duties. Such examinations are conducted on workers who have missed a prescribed amount of time as a result of a non–work-related or work-related disorder. The respective time periods and disorders (e.g., lumbar disc disease, coronary artery disease, tendonitis) covered by return-to-work policies vary among organizations. Sound clinical judgment coupled with an understanding of the needs of both the business and the worker is essential. More time away from work is not always in the best interest of the worker's health.

The purpose of these examinations is to ensure proper placement of the worker to prevent future injury and illness. The focus of these examinations should be on the patient's health. In turn, the decision related to ability to work is based on whether the worker's health will be adversely affected by the work duties. In some cases, it may be appropriate to recommend alternative or modified duty assignments for a certain period of time. All decisions regarding work capabilities, however, should be based on a thorough review of the job history. Physicians performing such examinations are advised to request suitable job descriptions and become generally familiar with the work site. A brief report is recommended.

Periodic Examinations

Certain occupations, such as those regulated by the ICC and FAA, require periodic medical evaluations for licensing purposes. Other occupations come under the auspices of OSHA, which has established standards for periodic medical evaluations of workers exposed to materials such as asbestos and lead (12). In some cases, such as the ICC examinations, guidelines are strict and adherence is mandatory.

Another type of periodic examination is the so-called preventive medicine examination. Over the past few years, the effectiveness of periodic medical evaluations has been evaluated by a variety of professional groups, including the American Cancer Society, American College of Physicians, and Council on Scientific Affairs of the American Medical Association. These reviews were in turn assessed by the U.S. Preventive Services Task Force, which published a monograph that evaluated the effectiveness of 169 interventions (13). The pace and need for developing screening interventions, however, has proceeded unabated with concern about the use of prostatic specific antigen for prostatic cancer and genetic biomarkers for ovarian and breast cancer. The thrust of the respective reviews is that most annual physicals and other periodic medical evaluations include more ancillary services (laboratory and x-ray) than are necessary to ensure good health. Moreover, these reports indicate that more attention should be directed toward lifestyle issues such as diet, exercise, and smoking habits to prevent illness. Physicians asked to provide these types of examinations are encouraged to review the recent guidelines, which are periodically updated; a third edition is expected to be released shortly.

Health Assessments

Since up to a third of the workforce may not have a primary care physician, it is likely that individuals evaluated for occupational health purposes may return for care of routine illness. These illnesses—often described as "episodic"—range from influenza to pharyngitis and sunburn. Following an initial evaluation and treatment, it is often appropriate for the occupational health center to refer these patients to primary care physicians or to appropriate specialists for follow-up care, especially for chronic ailments such as hypertension, asthma, or allergic disorders.

The occupational physician may also be requested to conduct evaluations regarding an individual's work capabilities. Although the factors involved in these decisions are often complicated, the focus should always be on the worker's health. Physicians, however, may hear counterbalancing opinions about whether the business wants the person back at work or whether the person actually wants to return to work. If the physician always focuses on health with attention to the job duties, however, some of the inherent difficulties in making these decisions will be minimized. If the physician believes that a certain job will *more than likely* aggravate the medical condition or impede recovery, an alternative assignment should be recommended if suitable accommodations are not feasible. The ultimate decision regarding placement rests with the organization; the physician's role is to serve as a consultant and to render a *medical* opinion.

The clinician may also be asked to conduct a *disability evaluation* of a worker who does not appear medically able to return to a particular position. In these settings, it is advisable to employ standard guidelines such as the American Medical Association's guidelines to the evaluation of permanent impairment (see Chapter 7). The physician should appreciate that in most situations the medical opinion concerns *impairment,* that is, an objective impairment in some physiologic function; *disability* is a far more complex concept, with medical considerations representing only part of the entire picture, along with educational and vocational factors.

The full assessment of disability, in addition to the medical evaluation, also incorporates a review of social factors, such as education, occupational experiences, and training capabilities. A person with emphysema, for example, may demonstrate severe pulmonary impairment that disables him from working as a material handler but does not disable him from working as an accountant. The term *impairment* connotes a measurable deficit in physiologic functioning (e.g., decrease in lung function, abnormal hearing, reduced motion of a joint), whereas *disability* refers to how the medical impairment affects work capabilities and other life activities.

Ancillary Services

As a result of wider awareness of the health implications of certain jobs, industries, and materials, occupational physicians are often called on to conduct more detailed evaluations. These reviews necessitate supportive diagnostic information, such as radiographic examinations, laboratory testing, and at times reviews of industrial hygiene sampling data. A proper coordination of these efforts can help provide quality care while preventing illness and injury.

Ancillary services refer to laboratory and related procedures conducted as part of clinical evaluations. The type and level of ancillary services administered depend on the practice setting and the local medical community. In the provision of occupational health services to small businesses, however, the following equipment is considered essential: (a) an audiometric booth and audiometer, (b) a well-functioning and calibrated spirometer, and (c) a vision screener. Optional services include laboratory, x-ray, and physical therapy; however, the appropriateness of including these services on-site varies, especially if readily available nearby. In some cases, it may be suitable to employ referral services.

According to the OSHA Hearing Standard, as many as 10 million Americans may be exposed at work to excessive noise, at levels that damage their hearing. Numerous industries have the potential to produce noise-induced hearing loss. Consequently, physicians providing occupational health services are urged to have an audiometric booth and audiometer on site or to have access to such. Many PPEs require an audiometric evaluation prior to job assignment.

A well-functioning spirometer is a critical component of an occupational health program, and NIOSH has established guidelines for the training of technicians in its proper use. Many OSHA standards, especially those concerning asbestos and cotton, require periodic pulmonary function testing, which is often performed in the context of determining medical suitability for wearing a respirator. There are no specific guidelines for the type of examination to perform, and discretion is left to the examining physician. By convention, however, most occupational physicians administer a questionnaire and pulmonary function testing at a minimum. Other settings, such as hazardous waste work, may warrant detailed evaluations that include an exercise electrocardiogram, usually as a result of the need to wear potentially bulky, cumbersome protective equipment in hot environments that pose a risk of heat stress. The level of pulmonary function below which a person should not be advised to wear a respirator is subject to opinion. In general, however, results below 70% of the forced expiratory volume in the first second of the test (FEV_1) warrant a careful review.

Since people rarely undergo routine eye examinations, a properly functioning vision testing machine is strongly recommended (as opposed to the standard Snellen chart). Many periodic examinations such as ICC and FAA examinations require vision screening and adherence to strict guidelines. The importance of good vision in an effective safety program should not be overlooked. As a result of eye fatigue and strain among video display terminal (VDT) operators, periodic vision screening has been recommended in some settings. A directive in the European Community requires periodic eye examinations of those who use VDTs for designated periods of time.

Optional services include laboratory, x-ray, and physical therapy. Customarily, it is not practical, even for an occupational health center, to have complete on-site laboratory services. The decision to employ laboratory services depends on many factors, including the type of specimen to be analyzed, as well as volume of testing and cost-effectiveness. The physician who provides occupational health services, however, should be aware that some medical monitoring and toxicologic analyses for substances such as mercury, trichloroethanol, and lead are not routinely performed at most hospitals and laboratories. Thus, the physician needs to be sure that the laboratory chosen to provide such services is appropriately qualified. Quality control, proficiency, and pricing can vary widely. For measurement of blood lead levels, however, the Centers for Disease Control periodically evaluate laboratories according to defined criteria. With the increased interest demonstrated in the value of biomarkers in the diagnosis of occupational illness, a quality reference laboratory becomes an important service in the delivery of occupational medical services (14).

For occupational health programs that treat work-related injuries, it is essential to have access to radiology facilities. Often it is worthwhile to have x-ray facilities on site for proper assessment of injuries, illnesses, or medical surveillance examinations. If on-site facilities are not available, provisions should be made for local referral.

Physical therapy can also play an instrumental role in promoting prompt and efficient recovery from work-related injuries. In some cases, on-site services can be economically justified.

Practitioners are advised to become aware of various regulations, involved in the delivery of health care, including provisions of the Clinical Laboratory Improvement Act (CLIA).

Nonclinical Activities

Educational activities are an essential component of an occupational health service. The physician will likely be asked to give presentations on a variety of health-related topics to both manager and worker groups. For example, a discussion on causes, prevention, and treatment of back pain can help managers understand why injured workers need sufficient time away from the job for effective treatment and that modified assignments may be needed on return to work. Other topics of interest include occupational risks associated with acquired immunodeficiency syndrome (AIDS), urinary screening for abused drugs, and the role of smoking policies. The physician may also be asked to discuss with worker groups the value of medical surveillance examinations or how to interpret health-related information on material safety data sheets (see Chapter 2 on Hazard Communication Standard).

The physician providing occupational health care is often viewed as a *health consultant* to the business.

Thus, the physician may be asked to recommend first-aid protocols, hazard control programs, or back education seminars. It is not realistic to expect the physician to be even remotely involved in all of these activities; however, he or she is encouraged to become aware of available resources and to assist in the review of programs. Working with and supervising the efforts of other health care professionals such as nurses, physician assistants, and physical therapists can help expand the physician's role. As corporations become more accountable for the health of their employees, occupational physicians are being called on to address many of the nonclinical health issues associated with operating a business. Serving as an advisor on epidemiology, toxicology, or health policy is a notable example.

Work-site policies related to health issues, such as annual examinations, cigarette smoking, or health promotion programs, may need to be developed. In some cases, a local business facility may be part of a larger corporation that has established guidelines for specific occupational health issues. In other cases, unions associated with particular occupations have issued guidelines and prepared information that may be of assistance to the clinician.

The communication of health information to groups of people, especially workers, has become an increasingly important role for occupational health professionals. Examples include educational sessions related to results of research studies.

Health Promotion Activities

The definition of health promotion is considerably broad and includes virtually any type of preventive medicine activity designed to *educate people regarding the role of lifestyle* in promoting health and to facilitate behavior change. Typically considered under this heading are smoking cessation, weight reduction, stress management, fitness, and hypertension and cancer screening. Because of rising health care costs and greater awareness of the public regarding the role of prevention, the clinician is likely to be faced with questions such as whether the local business facility should institute a health promotion program and may be asked to design its components. It is unrealistic to expect the physician to be involved in the administration and planning of these activities; however, an advisory role to ensure that all activities are conducted in accordance with current medical standards is recommended. In addition, this text includes chapters devoted to health promotion (Chapter 12) and health and productivity (Chapter 11), areas of emerging importance in occupational health. A recent review critiqued the cost-effectiveness of health promotion programs at the workplace (15).

REFERRAL PATTERNS

The provision of primary occupational health services requires occasional referrals to a certified occupational medicine physician; other medical specialists, such as orthopedic surgeons and neurologists; and other occupational health professionals, such as industrial hygienists.

Occupational Medicine Physician

Although fewer than 1,000 practicing physicians are board certified in occupational medicine, it is wise for the clinician to investigate within the local community whether such a physician may be available as a consultant. Information related to occupational physicians can be obtained through the directory of the American College of Occupational and Environmental Medicine *(www.acoem.org)*. The clinician is urged to be aware of the complicated nature of many occupational medical problems, and is advised to seek appropriate advice on medical surveillance of substances not covered by OSHA standards and in evaluating the work-relatedness of certain illnesses. For some substances, such as asbestos or lead, OSHA has established standards that define medical guidelines on the type of testing to be performed and measures to be followed based on the results. In other cases, however, especially in work settings where exposure may occur to untested substances or to materials with unusual health risks, further consultation is suggested. These settings may require more industrial hygiene assessments, including air-level measurements in addition to toxicology testing, before appropriate advice can be given.

Because of wider awareness of occupational illnesses, a clinician is likely to encounter patients concerned as to whether a particular health condition may be due to exposure to an occupational or environmental substance. At times, these decisions can be straightforward, such as evaluating lead intoxication in a pistol shooter or pleural abnormalities in a sheet metal worker who spent 30 years working with asbestos. In other cases the decision can be considerably complicated by either insufficient medical information regarding the toxicity of a substance or inadequate information regarding working conditions. Most occupational illnesses, however, are originally recognized by astute clinicians. When an unusual occupational illness is suspected, appropriate consultation with a trained and experienced occupational physician is suggested.

Local Medical Specialists

The clinician is advised to be active in the local medical community. Specific needs for specialists include orthopedic surgeons, general surgeons, otolaryngologists (particularly as part of the OSHA hearing standard), pulmonary specialists, neurologists (to conduct nerve conduction studies and neuropsychiatric testing), and psychiatrists or psychotherapists. In provision of occupational health services, these specialists are likely to be called on routinely. Consequently, it is strongly advised that a good working professional relationship be established to enhance communication between the clinician and the specialist. It is important that the specialist be sensitive to the need for prompt scheduling and a complete and timely report. Unfortunately, not all physicians are willing to meet these specific needs of an occupational health service.

Other Professionals

The occupational physician occasionally requires the services of other professionals such as industrial hygienists, audiologists, or physical therapists (26). Professional ties with these individuals can help the clinician provide quality occupational health care.

A wide array of government agencies such as NIOSH and OSHA provide educational information related to the workplace and environmental substances. Other organizations such as the American College of Occupational and Environmental Medicine, American Conference of Governmental Industrial Hygienists, and other professional societies publish material related to occupational health that may be of benefit to the physician.

DELIVERY OF OCCUPATIONAL MEDICAL SERVICES

Today, occupational medical services are delivered from a variety of perspectives, most commonly by the primary care clinician, although hospitals have become more assertive in the past decade. Occupational health centers have also been developed to provide health services to a range of small businesses in the immediate geographic area of the facility. In some cases, freestanding health centers have incorporated occupational medical services as part of their program. Unions and corporations have also sponsored health care clinics.

Determining the Need for Occupational Medical Services

The goals of an occupational health service include the following:

1. To protect people at work from health and safety hazards
2. To protect the local environment
3. To facilitate safe placement of workers according to their physical, mental, and emotional capacities
4. To assure adequate medical care and rehabilitation of the occupationally ill and injured
5. To assist in measures related to personal health maintenance

In deciding the economic feasibility of an occupational health center, a number of factors need to be considered (Table 1.3). The type and diversity of the business community should be reviewed, since some types of industries require more health care than others. Business groups can be categorized by the number of workers, the location of the medical facility, and the type of industry. It is usually worthwhile to assess competitors providing occupational health services in the geographic region under consideration for the occupational health program. Based on this review, one can determine the type of medical services that may

TABLE 1.3. *Factors in establishing need for occupational medical services for small businesses*

Determine:

1. The number of *businesses* in the service area and categorize by
   a. Number of employees
   b. Geographic concentration
   c. Type of industry (SIC code may be helpful)
2. Level of local *competition,* i.e., presence of other group practices or occupational health programs providing occupational health care
3. *Types* of occupational medical services in *demand* by the local business community (i.e., workers' compensation, preplacement examinations, treatment of work-related injuries)
4. Cost analysis, including marketing, equipment, staff, and operating expenses

SIC, Standard Industrial Classification.

be required, such as PPEs, treatment of injuries, or more complicated occupational medical consultations. The expectations of the business and labor community should also be considered. Finally, after careful evaluation of the market area and costs involved in equipment and staff, a decision can be made.

In the establishment of an occupational health service, professionals knowledgeable in marketing, accounting, and management will be valuable aids in the success of the venture. The quality of the medical staff, however, is crucial, especially regarding training and experience in occupational medicine. Careful attention should be directed toward the type of staff that is employed, including the cost-effectiveness of medical care providers, such as physician assistants and nurse practitioners (13). Organizations or physicians considering establishing an occupational health program should be aware of the code of ethical conduct of the American College of Occupational and Environmental Medicine *(www.acoem.org)*.

Once a decision is made to develop an occupational health service, one should have realistic expectations for when the facility can become self-supporting. Appropriate business counseling regarding fee schedules, equipment, and staffing costs is advisable. Policies and procedures, as well as appropriate forms for PPEs and treatment of work-related injuries need to be developed. Guidelines for referrals to local physicians are essential.

A well-run program depends on *effective communication* between the business facility and the physician. In providing occupational health services, the physician is advised that the primary responsibility is always to the patient and that the physician should not be viewed as an advocate of the company but instead as an impartial professional concerned primarily with the worker's health. Proper communication, however, requires strict attention to medical confidentiality (see Chapter 2 for further discussion on this complex issue).

Once an occupational health center has been established or a physician has decided to incorporate occupational medical services into his or her practice, a visit to the business is essential. Such a visit can enable the physician to become acquainted with the nature of the enterprise and with respective work responsibilities. This knowledge enhances the physician's ability to make effective determinations as to whether someone can handle a job duty in light of existing health or whether work-site modifications are necessary. During this visit, the physician can become familiar with the expectations of the organization and the personnel responsible for occupational health. Inevitably, this contact person will play a major role in the effectiveness of the occupational health services. One visit, however, is hardly adequate to become familiar with the intricacies of many jobs (Chapter 4 discusses issues the physician can address during a plant visit).

An occupational health center ideally should provide fundamental clinical services, such as PPEs and treatment of work-related injuries. Other types of services, such as health promotion, educational seminars, and screening programs, will likely be requested as the business gains confidence in the capabilities of the physician and/or organization providing basic care.

The considerations described refer to an occupational health center or physicians who provide occupational health services as part of their practice. These physicians are encouraged to become aware of other types of occupational health care delivery, such as corporate and union settings and hospitals.

Corporate-sponsored Health Care Delivery

Corporations assumed a role in providing occupational health services shortly after the institution of the workers' compensation statutes. Sears Roebuck, for example, and some insurance companies were some of the first to institute preemployment examinations, as they were known at that time. Because some corporations or businesses employed a large number of people, it was economically feasible to deliver health care on site. Episodic illnesses and minor injuries, for example, could be more promptly and accurately treated. Similarly, in the event of a more serious injury, prompt medical treatment was close at hand. Corporate-sponsored health care delivery later evolved into more comprehensive programs that also included treatment of non–work-related illnesses. Most recently, however, corporations have tended to reduce their commitment to on-site programs and instead have looked to local physicians for provision of these services. Staffing and medical equipment used at an on-site corporate facility will parallel that necessary at an occupational health center. The trend for businesses to contract occupational health services continued through the late 1980s, but has begun to stabilize. In some settings, for example, it is cost-effective to deliver services on site (16). Nonetheless, this decline in corporate-sponsored services was reflected in a study of positions available in corporate occupational medicine (17).

Many corporations employ professionals skilled in fields related to occupational medicine, including epidemiology, toxicology, and industrial hygiene. The clinician is urged to contact the parent corporation when providing occupational health services for a subsidiary plant or division. Valuable information and policy guidelines can often be obtained from corporate staff.

Many corporate offices also oversee and provide guidance to international locations (18). In some European facilities, recommendations from the International Labor Organization (ILO) are used as a standard of experience for occupational health services (19). A recent survey of occupational health services in Europe, however, indicated a disparity in the type and range of services in various countries (20). Provision of trend-related medical advice is often carried out by occupational health professionals (21).

Union-sponsored Occupational Health Care

Although few medical facilities sponsored by unions actually deliver health care, unions have been active in various aspects of occupational health. Other union efforts related to occupational health have been directed toward the collective bargaining process, lobbying local legislators, and preparation of educational material for union members.

With respect to occupational health, labor has identified three main goals (22): (a) to prevent disease by ensuring a safe work environment, (b) to notify and treat workers when prevention has failed, and (c) to compensate workers and families when disease takes its toll. Some unions have implemented educational programs directed toward preventing occupational illness. The patient may be able to obtain valuable information that can be of assistance to the physician in evaluating an illness. Union groups may also have access to medical information related to products used at a particular business. Unfortunately, because of the adversarial nature of many labor and management dealings, the physician may be inadvertently thrust into a conflict. To enhance effectiveness, however, it is critical that the physician *maintain neutrality* and make decisions based on health. Table 1.4 outlines questions that a physician might ask either management or the union regarding occupational health care.

Hospital-based Occupational Health Programs

Although most hospitals have had some type of employee health service for many years, hospitals have been marketing occupational health services to the local business community with vigor since the mid- to late 1980s. These types of programs have varied considerably, such as provision of services through the emergency department or through a separate department within the hospital or by a group of hospital staff physicians who provide some type of clinical occupational health services. Some hospitals have developed independent subsidiaries off-site to provide health care to the small-business community. Guidelines presented for the establishment of an independent occupational health center are applicable to hospital programs as well.

University-based Teaching Centers

Few university-based residency training centers for occupational medicine exist in the United States; at last count there were only 37. Some hospitals, however, have developed sections of occupational medicine within departments of internal or community medicine, or at a school of public health.

TABLE 1.4. *Local union health and safety involvement*

Does a joint union/management health and safety committee exist at the plant?
Is there a shop floor committee with health and safety interests?
Does the union conduct training for its members in health and safety, and if it does, are materials available for the health care providers?
Are there grievance procedures for health and safety?
Do collective bargaining agreements pertain to health and safety issues?
How does the union help its members in handling compensation claims?
How does the union handle its relationship with the Occupational Safety and Health Administration?
Does the union have a working relationship with a local clinic for occupational health programs?
What is the local union's involvement in substance abuse, rehabilitation, and/or employee assistance programs?
Do joint union/company health screening programs exist for non–work-related problems, such as blood pressure, cholesterol, diabetes, and glaucoma detection?
Some unions have educational arrangements with local physicians to educate members on general health topics. Does such exist in your area?
Does the local union have available medical consultants through their international affiliation?

These centers often can be of value to the clinician as a place to refer people with more complex occupational medical problems. In addition, some occupational medical sections at universities are educational resource centers (ERCs) funded by NIOSH for graduate training in occupational medicine. These ERCs also provide educational programs related to occupational medicine for physicians and other health professionals.

Because of the need for well-trained occupational physicians, the clinician who provides occupational medical services can be instrumental in the educational process. University programs may sponsor students or house staff at appropriate health care centers, where the student of occupational medicine can gain valuable practical experience.

The university-based center can channel a patient to the appropriate specialist, such as physicians skilled in occupational lung disease, dermatology, or neurology. University programs also have access to consultants in toxicology, audiology, and industrial hygiene. Since research activities are a major emphasis of university programs, opportunities may exist for an occupational health program to coparticipate in certain ventures.

SUMMARY

Occupational health services will continue to be an integral part of any organization's mission, values, and operation responsibilities. For occupational health professionals, the challenge is to continue to demonstrate both value and effectiveness in the prevention of occupational illnesses and injuries. In the immediate future, considerable opportunities will exist to demonstrate the role of occupational health services in improving productivity (23). Additional challenges include the integration of occupational health with preventative services (24). Performance and quality measurement are additional demands of occupational health services in demonstrating the value of their contributions to the success of the organization for which services are provided (25–27).

ACKNOWLEDGMENTS

I acknowledge Dr. Robert Neparstek for his assistance in this revision of this chapter.

REFERENCES

1. McCunney RJ, Couturier AC. Where do occupational medicine residency programs fit in the institution? *J Occup Med* 1993;35:889.
2. Warshaw LJ. Toward the year 2000: challenges to the occupational physician. *J Occup Med* 1990;32:524.
3. Walsh DC. The vanguard and the rearguard: occupational medicine revisits its future. *J Occup Med* 1988; 30:124.
4. Ramazzini B. Diseases of workers. Translated by WC Wright. From *DeMorbis Artificum. Diatriba,* 1713. New York: Hafner, 1964.
5. Raffle PAB, et al. *Hunter's diseases of occupations,* 2nd ed. Boston: Little, Brown, 1988.
6. Felton JS. 200 years of occupational medicine in the U.S. *J Occup Med* 1976;18:809.
7. Reith LU. The occupational health service: staffing, facilities, and equipment. *AAOHN J* 2000;48:395–403.
8. McCunney RJ. Ethical issues of genetic testing in the workplace. *State Art Rev* 2002 (in press).
9. McCunney RJ. Medical records and confidentiality. *J Occup Med* 1984;26:790.
10. McCunney RJ. Preserving confidentiality in occupational medical practice. *Am Fam Physician* 1996;53(5): 1751–1756.
11. McCunney RJ. A hospital-based occupational health program. *J Occup Med* 1984;26:375.
12. McCunney RJ. Medical surveillance: the role of the family physician. *Am Fam Physician* 2001;63: 2339–2340.
13. US Preventive Services Task Force. *Guide to clinical preventive services,* 2nd ed. Baltimore: Williams & Wilkins, 1996.
14. McCunney RJ. Use of biomarkers in occupational medicine. In: Mendelsohn, Mohr, Peeters, eds. *Biomarkers: medical and workplace applications.* Washington, DC: John Henry Press, 1998:377–386.
15. Pelletier R. A review and analysis of the clinical and cost effectiveness studies of comprehensive health promotion and disease management programs at the worksite: 1998–2000 update. *Am J Health Promot* 2001;16: 107.
16. Anstadt G, et al. The business planning process applied to an in-house corporate occupational medicine unit. *J Occup Med* 1991;33:354.
17. Ducatman AM. Career options of occupational physicians. *J Occup Med* 1988;30:776.
18. Bunn WB, McCunney RJ. Corporate occupational health services in the USA. In: *Encyclopedia of occupational health and safety,* 4th ed. Geneva: International Labor Office, 1998:16.35–16.38.
19. Bratveit M, McCormick D, Moen BE. Activity profiles of the occupational health services in a multinational company. *Occup Med* 2001;51:168–173.
20. Nicholson PJ. Occupational health in the European Union. *Occup Med* 2002;52:80–84.
21. Prince TS, Spengler SE, Collins TR. Corporate travel medicine: benefit analysis of on-site services. *J Travel Med* 2001;8:163–167.
22. Parsons M. Seminars in occupational medicine—the role of occupational medicine. *Prospectives from Labor* 1986(March);1(1):18–26.
23. McCunney RJ. Health and productivity: a role for occupational health. *J Occup Environ Med* 2001:1–56.
24. Rudolph L, Deitchman S. Integrating occupational health services and occupational prevention services. *Am J Ind Med* 2001;40:307–318.
25. Pransky G, Benjamin K, Dembe AE. Performance and quality measurement in occupational health services:

current status and agenda for further research. *Am J Ind Med* 2001;40:295–306.
26. Masson GK. The "value case" for investments in occupational health. *Occup Med* 2001;51:496–500.
27. Deitchman S, Dembe AE, Himmelstein J. Advent of occupational health services research. *Am J Ind Med* 2001;40:291–294.

Other General Texts

International Labor Organization encyclopedia, 4th ed. Geneva, ILO: 1996.

The Occupational and Environmental Medicine Report. Available from OEM Health Information, 55 Tozer Road, Beverly, MA 01915, Tel. (508) 921-7300. This monthly report, published since 1987, includes critical reviews of articles pertinent to occupational medicine practice by a board of directors from hospitals, corporations, academia, and government.

Rom WN. *Environmental and occupational medicine,* 3rd ed. Philadelphia: Lippincott Williams & Wilkins, 1998. The most comprehensive text in the field. This edition includes 129 chapters that address specific toxins in detail. The text is especially strong in occupational pulmonary disorders.

Scope of occupational and environmental health programs and practice. Report of the Occupational Medical Practice Committee of the American College of Occupational and Environmental Medicine. *J Occup Med* 1992; 34:436.

2

Legal and Ethical Issues

Junius C. McElveen, Jr.

The practice of occupational medicine is likely to present the practitioner with legal, ethical, and regulatory issues not customarily a part of clinical medicine. It is necessary, therefore, for occupational medicine practitioners to develop a working knowledge of topics such as workers' compensation, medical record confidentiality, the Occupational Safety and Health Administration's (OSHA) Hazard Communication Standard, the Americans with Disabilities Act, and toxic torts in order to practice effectively. This chapter presents the essentials of these issues along with practical guidelines to enhance the delivery of occupational health care.

WORKERS' COMPENSATION LAW

History

Until the early years of the 20th century, an employee who was injured at his or her place of employment had but one remedy—a lawsuit against the employer. To recover damages, the employee had to prove that the employer had failed to act as a reasonable person would have (i.e., had been negligent), and that the employer's negligence had resulted in injury to the employee. Both parties disliked this system. Employers objected to the costliness of the lawsuits. Employees did not like the fact that certain defenses the employers could raise might bar their recovery completely. For example, if a jury found the employee's lack of care had contributed to the injury (contributory negligence), the employee, by law, was not entitled to recover any damages at all. Similarly, if the jury determined the employee had knowingly and voluntarily assumed the risk of the kind of work that resulted in the injury (assumption of the risk), the employee was barred from any recovery. Finally, if the employee had been injured by a co-employee (the co-employee doctrine), the employee could not get damages.

Therefore, in the early 20th century, employers and employees in the various states began to make a deal. That deal was known as workers' compensation. The workers' compensation statutes varied a bit from state to state (each state has its own workers' compensation law), but each was composed of several compromises:

1. Employees gave up their right to sue employers at common law and agreed to accept a certain sum of money per week for their inability to work as a result of work-related injuries. They agreed to accept this compensation as their *exclusive remedy* against the employer.
2. Employers give up their right to assert the defenses of contributory negligence, assumption of the risk, and the co-employee doctrine, and agreed to give injured employees a certain sum of money per week if they were unable to work as a result of work-related injuries. Thus, payment would be made *regardless of fault*.
3. Payment would be automatic unless disputes arose. The disputes over issues of work-relatedness, amounts of entitlement, timeliness of claim, etc., would (generally) be *resolved administratively,* rather than by courts.
4. Payments would be made only for disability (i.e., inability to work). There would be no damages recoverable for pain and suffering. Additionally, no damages would be allowed as a punishment for the employer (punitive damages).

Thus, although the monetary recovery for employees (usually 66% of their weekly wage) would generally not be as much as they might recover at common law, the recovery would be substantially more certain, since fault was no longer an issue. Moreover, since matters were determined administratively, recovery would presumably be quicker.

At first, most of the state workers' compensation systems covered only work-related traumatic injuries. Illness and disease coverage were added later. When disease coverage was added, it was generally grafted onto statutory schemes designed to compensate for traumatic injuries. Therefore, a disease or illness would be considered work related ("occupational") if it satisfied the prerequisites for injury coverage: that is, if it "arose out of and in the course of employment." However, the effort to treat diseases like traumatic injuries was fraught with problems. Unlike traumatic injuries, diseases do not generally manifest themselves immediately after exposure. Many have long latency periods. By the time a disease occurred, the employee might have had a large number of different jobs and exposures. He or she might not even be working. In addition, proof of causation is not as easy with diseases as with most traumatic injuries. Furthermore, the period of time during which a claim could be filed, known as the "statute of limitations," was generally only 1 or 2 years, depending on the state, and often was held to run from the date on which the last exposure occurred. For a disease with a long latency period, such as certain types of cancer, a worker might be barred from even filing a claim. In some states, statutes even forbade the filing of a claim after 5 years from the last exposure.

Because some of these procedural rules led to very unfair results, and because of the difficulties in determining what an occupational disease was, many states gradually revised their workers' compensation laws to address these issues.

With regard to statutes of limitation, most states have now adopted the so-called discovery rule. A claim is timely if it is filed within a certain number of years after the claimant becomes, or should have become, aware of the disease and its potential work-relatedness. Almost all states have eliminated the requirement that a claim be filed within a certain number of years after exposure. However, as noted, workers' compensation law is state law, and occupational health professionals must be familiar with the law of the state in which they practice.

Regarding the determination of whether a disease is work related, some states passed laws that actually created lists of diseases that would be deemed to be occupational diseases (1). Those diseases listed in the statute were compensable, and those not listed were not compensable. The unfairness of this concept soon became apparent, and most states developed more general concepts of *compensability*.

Two lines of authority developed. The first held that a disease was compensable if a work-related "accident" aggravated or accelerated the underlying disease (2). Thus, if a myocardial infarction occurred at work and the employee could show that some work-related stress contributed to precipitate the myocardial infarction, the employee's disability was compensable, even though the underlying disease process—coronary artery disease—was not work related. Gradually, many courts have abolished the requirement that such a special stress occur. Now, in a number of states, if a doctor is prepared to testify that ordinary working conditions aggravated a non–work-related condition, the disability produced by the disease will be compensable.

The second line of authority held that a disease would be compensable if the employee's occupation put him or her at a greater risk of getting the disease than that of the general public. Thus, diseases caused by hazardous substances at the workplace, to which the employee had greater exposure than did the general public, were compensable, but so-called ordinary diseases of life, for which everyone ran the same risk, were not compensable. As one court said, "Such [occupational] disease is not the equivalent of a disease resulting from the general risks and hazards common to every individual regardless of the employment in which he is engaged" (3). Following this rationale, workers' compensation boards began to award compensation for lead colic in painters, ear trouble in telephone operators, and phosphorus poisoning in fireworks manufacturing employees, because they were "injuries or diseases common to workers in those particular trades" (4). However, state boards were still reluctant to extend coverage to most infectious diseases and cancers, which were considered ordinary diseases of life, in the sense that both workers and nonworkers got them.

Despite the state boards' initial reluctance, that barrier has also fallen in most states in recent years. The first incursion into "ordinary diseases of life" was a line of cases in which those ordinary diseases were found compensable if they occurred under unusual circumstances. Thus, for example, an employee on a ship who contracted meningitis after being required to work with numerous passengers who had meningitis was compensated through the workers' compensation system (5). This approach has now evolved to the extent that, in many jurisdictions, a disease is considered occupationally related if epidemiologic studies demonstrate a statistically significantly elevated risk of contracting that disease in those who are engaged in the occupation (6).

Psychological or psychiatric problems arising from work stress may also be compensable under these rationales. For example, just as some tribunals have found heart attacks and strokes (even those not occurring on the job) to be covered by workers' compensation if it could be shown that workplace stress or exertion materially contributed to the progression of cardiovascular disease (7), a number of courts recently have awarded workers' compensation for mental stress and anguish if triggered by a significant employment incident. The Supreme Court of Texas, for example, held that workers' compensation was the only available remedy to a woman who suffered mental anguish as a result of the stillbirth of a child after an accident at work. The employee had not been physically injured, and thus was not entitled to workers' compensation, but the court viewed the stillbirth and the resultant emotional distress as part and parcel of the workplace accident (8).

Courts, however, have not gone so far as to award compensation for mental stress or simple upset attributable to the general work environment. Some specific precipitating incident must have occurred, and the claimed mental problem must be clearly causally related to the incident (9). Moreover, some states have legislatively excluded from coverage minor mental upset without any accompanying injury (10), and mental disorders stemming from an employer's bona fide disciplinary or termination decisions (11).

Workers' compensation boards in some jurisdictions have taken the view that cumulative trauma disorders (CTDs) or repetitive stress injuries occur so frequently in the general population that they should be classified as ordinary diseases of life. However, other jurisdictions, such as Missouri, have found CTDs compensable if the employee had an exposure at work greater than or different from that of the general public, and if a recognizable link is established through expert testimony between the disorder and some distinctive feature of the employee's job that was common to all jobs of that type (12). In other words, if some excessively forceful and repetitious motion is a requirement of the job, and if medical evidence attributes the disorder to that motion, to a reasonable degree of medical certainty, the disorder would be compensable in those states.

Exceptions to the Exclusivity of Workers' Compensation

In recent years, some courts have created rather significant exceptions to the rule that the exclusive remedy of an employee for workplace injuries and illnesses is workers' compensation. The reasons for these exceptions are quite complex, but occupational medicine practitioners should be aware of these exceptions, including the exception that an occupational physician may have potential liability even when performing services in the context of a work-related injury or disease.

Intentional Tort Exception

A number of states have long had one major exception to the workers' compensation exclusive remedy doctrine. Workers' compensation is not the employee's exclusive remedy if the injury was caused by a deliberate and intentional act of the employer (the so-called intentional tort exception). For many years, this exception to the exclusivity rule was narrowly construed; only situations in which an employer actually assaulted an employee were customarily included. In recent years, however, the exception has been interpreted more broadly, particularly in cases alleging occupational disease. In 1980, for example, the California Supreme Court held that an employee could sue the employer at common law for aggravation of an occupational disease if the employee could prove that the employer knew of the presence of the disease, and failed to tell the employee, and the disease was exacerbated as a result (13). In the California case, the employee had asbestosis. The court held that the employee could not sue for asbestosis because that disorder was covered under workers' compensation. This was true even if the infliction of the disorder was intentional. However, once the employer knew of the employee's asbestosis, the employer had a responsibility to inform the affected worker. Intentional failure to meet this obligation allowed the employee to file a suit under common law. The California Supreme Court also put the burden of proof on the employer to differentiate impairment caused by the disease and impairment caused by aggravation of the disease. To the extent the employer could not do so, it would be liable for the whole disease.

The New Jersey Supreme Court also held that damages for aggravation of an occupational disease could be recovered at common law:

> An employer's fraudulent concealment of diseases already developed is not one of the risks an employee should have to assume. Such intentionally deceitful action goes beyond the bargain struck by the Compensation Act (14).

In the New Jersey case, however, the court also permitted the plaintiffs to sue physicians who allegedly knew of the presence of the disease and fraudulently concealed that fact from the employees. As the court pointed out, the problems of proving such allegations could be substantial. Nonetheless, a physician should be aware of the importance, medically, ethically and legally, of advising an employee of abnormal findings noted during an evaluation.

There has also been a notable, if not yet widespread, expansion of the exceptions to workers' compensation as an exclusive remedy, to allow civil action against employers for egregious workplace conduct resulting in emotional distress. For instance, a Pennsylvania decision allowed an employee to pursue a claim against his employer for alleged emotional distress caused by racial harassment by coworkers. Such a claim was found not to be preempted by the Pennsylvania Workers' Compensation Act (15).

Similarly, the California Supreme Court held that an employer's conduct in allegedly accusing its employee of gross misconduct before finally firing him so "exceeded the normal risks of the employment relationship" that it was not entitled to insulation from civil liability. The court allowed the employee's claim for severe emotional distress, but carefully noted that emotional distress caused by everyday management decisions (hiring, firing, demotion, criticism) would be covered exclusively by workers' compensation (16).

Following these sorts of decisions, some legislatures have amended their workers' compensation laws to narrow the "intentional tort" exception to the workers' compensation laws.

Dual Capacity Doctrine

A few states permit actions against corporations or co-employees, such as medical personnel, for violation of a concept called the dual capacity doctrine. This doctrine provides that an employee may sue under common law if the employee is injured as a result of some action of the employer that occurs when the employer and employee stand in some relationship other than the employer–employee relationship. For example, in a California case, a chiropractor's receptionist sought treatment from the chiropractor for a back disorder. The chiropractor's treatment was allegedly negligent because it made the employee's back worse. The California Supreme Court held that the injury (to the employee) arose as a result of the doctor–patient relationship, not the employer–employee relationship. Because the injury arose in this context, the employee could sue the chiropractor (17).

Similarly, an Ohio court held that an allegation that a company physician's failure to inform an employee that he had silicosis was a case that could proceed under common law because of the dual capacity doctrine. The court stated that once the employer got into the medical examination business, it took on obligations to the employee over and above those duties it had as the employer (18).

Obligations of the Occupational Physician

The *potential for liability* is another reason, in addition to good medical and ethical practice, for being completely candid with the employee regarding a suspected occupational disorder. If further testing is necessary, the employer should be consulted, as that testing may be covered under workers' compensation rather than other insurance. As soon as an occupational condition is identified, the employer and the appropriate state workers' compensation agency should be notified (19).

Health care professionals have been sued for malpractice or negligence in a number of states by individuals who have been either employees of the same employer (i.e., co-employees) or employees of a company for which the health care professional was doing contract work. The allegations of malpractice and negligence have covered a wide range of conduct. In some states, courts have held that the exclusive remedy provisions of the state's workers' compensation law bar a lawsuit against the health care professional. Here, the employee's exclusive remedy is workers' compensation (20). Other courts have held, in a variety of circumstances, that health care professionals can be sued outside the compensation system.

In the New Jersey Supreme Court case, discussed above, the court held that company physicians could be sued outside the compensation system based on employee allegations that the physicians knew the employees had an occupational disease, and did not tell the employees about the disease (21). In that case the employees alleged that the employer's physicians had diagnosed asbestosis, based on chest x-ray findings, but had fraudulently failed to tell the employees.

Similarly, some courts have said that when a physical examination or some type of testing, such as drug or alcohol testing, is a condition of future or continued employment, that examination creates a physician–patient relationship between the examiner and the employee. That relationship imposes a duty to conduct the required tests and diagnose the results thereof in a nonnegligent manner. However, it should be noted that courts have not held any testing laboratories liable if their sole function is to obtain samples, test them, and report the results, if the work was done nonnegligently.

OSHA'S HAZARD COMMUNICATION STANDARD

In the 1980s, OSHA enacted a rule mandating that employees be provided with information about the chemical exposures they receive, or may receive, in the workplace and how those exposures may affect their health. OSHA's rule is known as the Hazard Communication Standard (HCS) (22). The HCS covers all employers covered by the Occupational Safety and Health (OSH) Act. In addition, many states have right-to-know laws that require manufacturers and users of chemicals to provide information on chemical hazards to the public (23).

Generally, the HCS requires the following:

1. Containers in the workplace that contain hazardous chemicals must be labeled with the chemical's identity, appropriate hazard warnings, and the identity of the manufacturer, importer, or other responsible party.
2. Employees must be *trained* about the hazards of chemicals to which they are or may be exposed.
3. *Material Safety Data Sheets* (MSDS), which set out in considerable detail the hazards of specific chemicals, must be made available to employees who may be exposed to those chemicals. Table 2.1 is a listing of the information MSDSs must contain.

In taking a complete occupational history of an employee who presents with signs or symptoms that might be consistent with occupational disorder, it may be very helpful to find out from the employee what type of information was conveyed in the employee's hazardous chemical training program and what warnings are on containers of materials with which the employee frequently works. However, the most valuable information to the practicing physician may be that contained on the MSDS. Although MSDSs contain an enormous amount of information (Table 2.1), some of it may be incomplete. Therefore, the physician may find it necessary to conduct a separate literature review.

With regard to MSDSs, the HCS does permit manufacturers to assert that the identities of certain chemicals are *trade secret*. However, under certain circumstances, treating physicians and other health professionals can obtain that information, as follows: (a) If a treating physician determines a *medical emergency* exists and the chemical identity of a trade-secret–protected hazardous chemical is necessary for proper treatment, the physician can obtain that information immediately from the manufacturer, importer, or employer who asserts the trade secret (telephone numbers, for example, are listed on the MSDS). However, the manufacturer or other party asserting the trade secret may obtain a statement of need and a con-

TABLE 2.1. *Information provided on Material Safety Data Sheets (MSDSs)*

The *label identity* of the chemical
The chemical and common names including synonyms
If the substance is a *mixture* that has been tested as a whole to determine its hazards, the chemical and common names of the ingredients that contribute to the known hazards
If the substance is a mixture that has *not* been tested as a whole, the chemical and common names of all ingredients that have been determined to be health hazards and that constitute 1% or more of the mixture (or 0.1% or more, if the hazard is a carcinogen)
The chemical and common names of all ingredients that have been determined to present a physical hazard
The physical and chemical characteristics of the chemical
The physical hazards of the chemical
The health hazards of the chemical, including signs and symptoms of exposure, and any medical conditions that can be aggravated by exposure to the chemical
The primary routes of exposure
The Occupational Safety and Health Administration (OSHA) Permissible Exposure Limit, the American Conference of Governmental Industrial Hygienists (ACGIH) Threshold Limit Value, or any other recommended exposure limit
Whether the substance is listed on the National Toxicology Program's Annual List of Carcinogens or has been found to be a potential carcinogen by the International Agency for Research on Cancer or OSHA
Known precautions for safe handling and use
Applicable control measures
The date of preparation of the latest MSDS or its latest change
The name, address, and telephone number of the manufacturer, importer, employer, or other responsible party preparing or distributing the MSDS, who can provide additional information on the hazardous chemical and appropriate emergency procedures

fidentiality agreement as soon as circumstances permit. (b) In *nonemergency situations,* physicians, industrial hygienists, toxicologists, or epidemiologists providing medical or other occupational health services to employees may obtain trade secret information, if certain prerequisites are met, if a need for the actual chemical identity is shown to be necessary, and if a guarantee of confidentiality is set out (24).

Right to Know Laws

Under the 1986 amendments reauthorizing the Superfund Act [Superfund Amendments and Reauthorization Act (SARA)], and Environmental Protection Agency (EPA) regulations implementing those amendments, companies that maintain inventories of certain hazardous chemicals at levels above defined reportable thresholds are required to provide certain information about those chemicals to various government entities and to the public. Those requirements include that companies that are required by OSHA's HCS to prepare MSDSs must furnish those MSDSs, or lists of chemicals that are required to have MSDSs, to Local Emergency Planning Committees, State Emergency Response Commissions, and local fire departments. Any citizen who requests that information from the state or local authorities is entitled to receive it, with certain trade secret exceptions (25).

OCCUPATIONAL SAFETY AND HEALTH AND OTHER RECORD-KEEPING AND REPORTING REQUIREMENTS

OSHA Requirements

History

The OSH Act of 1970 and regulations promulgated under the Act require that occupational injuries and illnesses be recorded and reported (26). Although the obligation to generate these records is restricted to *employers of 11 or more employees* in certain Standard Industrial Classification (SIC) codes, except under very limited circumstances (27), physicians should always be aware of the requirements because they may be called on to determine if a condition is work related and how it should be recorded or reported.

On January 19, 2001, OSHA revised the Occupational Injury and Illness Recording and Reporting Requirements, which are contained in 29 C.F.R. Part 1904 (28). Those revisions took effect on January 1, 2002, and replaced the requirements set out in Part 1904. These revisions also replaced a very large body of guidance, which had been issued—by OSHA and by the Bureau of Labor Statistics (BLS)—over the last 30 years (29).

There has never been much question regarding the recordability of a large majority of the injuries or illnesses that occurred at the workplace. However, almost as soon as OSHA's original record-keeping requirements were published in 1971, OSHA began to receive complaints that the regulations did not provide adequate guidance for employers regarding the recordability of certain conditions (30). Indeed, as early as 1972, the BLS published supplemental instructions to the record-keeping forms. That publication was revised and reissued in 1973, 1975, and 1978. In 1986, after a public comment period, the BLS replaced the earlier publications with a new document entitled "Recordkeeping Guidelines for Occupational Injuries and Illnesses." Among other things, these Guidelines attempted to provide clearer definitions of the type of cases to be recorded, introduced a number of exceptions to the general geographic presumption that injuries and illnesses that occurred "on premises" were work related, and updated lists that distinguished medical treatment and first aid (31). However, even in light of those attempted clarifications, questions persisted about record-keeping issues, and, since 1986, OSHA has issued many letters of interpretation, attempting to clarify various record-keeping issues, as they applied to particular cases (32). Finally, as noted above, on January 19, 2001, OSHA issued very substantial revisions to its original 1971 regulations. Although it is beyond the scope of this chapter to analyze each and every change to OSHA's record-keeping regulations, some of the major issues addressed in those revisions are discussed below.

Summary of the New Regulations

Work-relatedness

The threshold question for determining if an injury or illness should be recorded, is, and always has been, determining whether the injury or illness is work related. If an injury or illness is not work related, it is not recordable. If it is work related, it is recordable if it resulted in death, days away from work, job restriction or transfer, medical treatment beyond first aid, or loss of consciousness. Work-related injuries and illnesses are also recordable if they are significant injuries or illnesses, as defined by the regulations, if they are needle-stick or sharps injuries, if the illness is tuberculosis, or if the case involves medical removal under OSHA standards. Each of these situations will be discussed briefly.

In the original record-keeping regulations, an injury or illness was considered to be work related if work caused or contributed to the injury or illness, or aggravated a preexisting condition (33). All injuries and illnesses that occurred on the employer's premises were presumed to be work related, with three exceptions:

1. Cases that occurred in a parking lot or a recreational facility;
2. Cases that occurred when the employee was present on the employer's premises as a member of the general public;
3. Cases in which symptoms started at work, but were the result of a non–work-related injury or illness.

Under the new regulations, an injury or illness is considered to be work related if work caused or contributed to the injury or illness or *significantly* aggravated a preexisting condition (34) (emphasis added). The new regulations add several more exceptions to the presumption of work relatedness if the injury or illness occurs at the employer's workplace:

1. If the injury or illness occurs while the employee is engaged in voluntary participation in a wellness program or in a medical, fitness or recreational activity, such as a blood donation, a physical exam, a flu shot, an exercise class, or a sports activity (the emphasis here is clearly on "voluntary");
2. If the injury or illness occurs while the employee is eating, drinking, or preparing food or beverages for personal consumption, whether brought in from outside or bought from the employer;
3. If the injury occurs as the result of intentionally self-inflicted wounds;
4. If the injury or illness occurs as the result of personal grooming, or self-medication for a non–work-related condition;
5. If the illness is a common cold or the flu; and
6. If the injury or illness is solely the result of the employee doing personal tasks at the employer's establishment, outside of the employee's assigned working hours (35).

Even though these additional exceptions to work-relatedness were intended to address the many questions raised by employers prior to the revisions to the record-keeping regulations regarding when an injury or illness should be considered work related and thus recordable, the question still remains: If an illness or injury occurs in the workplace and is not subject to one of the exceptions, is it recordable? The answer is: Perhaps not. In the rule making, OSHA rejected a suggestion that an injury or illness be considered work related if the worker ever experienced a workplace event or exposure that had any possibility of playing a role in the case. It also rejected suggestions that, to be work related, work must be "primarily" or "significantly" responsible for the injury or illness (36). So, there is still a gray area.

Distinction Between Injuries and Illnesses Eliminated

The original record-keeping rules mandated that all work-related illnesses, no matter how severe, be recorded. However, injuries were required to be recorded only if they resulted in days away from work, restricted work, transfer to another job, medical treatment beyond first aid, or loss of consciousness. The basis for this distinction was the language of Section 8(c)(2) of the OSH Act itself, which addressed the exclusion of minor injuries but said nothing about minor illnesses (37).

However, the new rules eliminate this distinction between injuries and illnesses, for recordability purposes, and state that any case (injury or illness) is recordable only if it results in death, days away from work, job restriction or transfer, medical treatment beyond first aid, or loss of consciousness (38).

Significant Injury or Illness

An injury or illness is recordable, under the new rules, if the case is a "significant" injury or illness, diagnosed by a physician or other licensed health care professional (39). Those injuries and illnesses are defined in the regulations to include cancer, any chronic, irreversible disease, a fractured or cracked bone, and a punctured eardrum. They are recorded if they are work related, no matter if anything is done for those conditions or not (40).

Work at Home

The revised regulations also address cases that may be recordable, if they arise from work at home. According to the revised rules, the key to potential recordability of an injury or illness that occurs while the employee is working at home is whether the case is directly related to performance of work, rather than to the home environment. For example, according to the revised rules, if an employee injured his or her foot by dropping a box of work papers on it, that would establish the requisite work-relatedness. However, if the employee tripped over the dog, on the way to answer the phone, an injury that resulted from that incident would not be work related, even if the call was a call about work (41).

First Aid

Many questions were raised, prior to revisions to the record-keeping regulations, about what constituted first aid and what constituted medical treatment. The new regulations attempt to address all those questions by setting out a list of 14 first-aid treatments. Any treatment that is not listed is not first aid. Those 14 treatments are as follows:

1. Using a nonprescription drug at nonprescription strength (if it is used at prescription strength, it is medical treatment);
2. Administering tetanus immunizations (any other immunizations, such as hepatitis B or rabies, are medical treatment);
3. Cleaning, flushing, or soaking wounds on the surface of the skin;
4. Using wound coverings such as Band-Aids, gauze pads, etc.; or using butterfly bandages or Steri-Strips (other wound closing devices, such as sutures, staples, etc., are considered medical treatment);
5. Using hot or cold therapy;
6. Using any nonrigid means of support, such as elastic bandages, wraps, nonrigid back belts, etc.;
7. Using temporary immobilization devices while transporting an accident victim;
8. Drilling a fingernail or toenail to relieve pressure, or draining fluid from a blister;
9. Using eye patches;
10. Removing foreign bodies from the eye using only irrigation or a cotton swab;
11. Removing splinters or foreign material from areas other than the eye by irrigation, tweezers, cotton swabs, or other simple means;
12. Using finger guards;
13. Using massage (physical therapy or chiropractic treatment are medical treatment); and
14. Drinking fluids for relief of heat stress (42).

There are no other procedures that are considered first aid by OSHA for record-keeping purposes. Therefore, any administration of oxygen, intravenous saline, or glucose, and any physical therapy, formerly considered first aid, are not now considered first aid. As well, the preamble to the new regulations points out that any issuance of a prescription for a prescription medication is medical treatment, whether the prescription is used or not (under the old rules, one dose of a prescription medicine was considered first aid; it is no longer) (43). In addition, any recommendation for any form of medical treatment is considered medical treatment, even if the recommendation is not followed (44).

Job Restrictions or Transfer

The revised regulations change the prior requirements with respect to what constitutes job restrictions or transfer. With regard to restricted work activities, employers were previously required to record any case that involved restricted work, even if the restriction occurred only on the day the injury or illness occurred. Now, if a work restriction is limited to the day of the injury or illness, and if no other recordability criteria are met, the case is not recordable (45). Under the old rules, the definition of restricted work was any situation in which (a) the employee was assigned to another job on a temporary basis, (b) the employee worked at a permanent job less than full time, or (c) the employee worked at his or her permanently assigned job but could not perform all of his or her routine duties. Routine duties were defined to include any activity the employee would be expected to perform even once during the course of a year. Under the new rule, routine duties are redefined to include only duties that he or she would have performed at least once a week before the injury or illness (46).

Privacy Issues

Several previously unresolved privacy issues have also been addressed in the revised regulations. One of the privacy issues that is addressed is that of the recordability of mental illness. The new regulations provide that mental illness, including workplace stress cases, are no longer recordable unless the employee submits a medical opinion that he or she has work-related mental illness (47).

As well, employees names are not entered in the OSHA log of work-related illnesses or injuries, if they are "privacy concern cases." Instead, these names are entered in a confidential log (48). These cases include the following:

1. Any injury or illness to an intimate body part or a part of the reproductive system;
2. Any injury or illness due to a sexual assault;
3. Voluntarily reported mental illness;
4. HIV, hepatitis, or tuberculosis;
5. Injuries due to needle-sticks and sharps; and
6. Any illnesses that the employee independently and voluntarily requests not be entered on the log (49).

Under these provisions, in order to protect the privacy of employees, the employer may modify the description of the injury or illness, to some extent (50).

Generation and Posting of Records

The new regulations make some modifications in the records that must be generated and change the requirements for the posting and retention of others. Under the old rules, employers were required to maintain two forms: the OSHA 200, Log and Summary of Occupational Injuries and Illnesses, and the OSHA 101, Supplementary Record of Occupational Injuries and Illnesses. Now, up to four forms are required: (a) the OSHA 300 (formerly the log portion of the OSHA 200); (b) the OSHA 300-A (formerly the Annual Summary portion of the OSHA 200); (c) the OSHA 301, Injury and Illness Incident Report (formerly the OSHA 101, Supplementary Record); and (d) the Confidential List of employees who experience injuries or illnesses classified as privacy concern cases. The Annual Summary (Form 300-A) must now be posted from February through April, not just during the month of February, as the old rule required (51). Finally, a company executive must certify the accuracy of the Annual Summary (52).

These changes to the record-keeping requirements make the defense of OSHA record-keeping citations more difficult. Under the old system, courts had held that the BLS guidelines were not entitled to the deference usually accorded to agency regulations, because they weren't agency regulations. Letter interpretations of those guidelines had even less claim to deference. Now, the rules have been subject to notice and comment, and they have been published in the Federal Register. There is a substantial risk that violations of the rules, as now written, will be characterized as willful violations. It should also be pointed out that record-keeping violations that are "failure to record" violations are considered continuing violations; that is, if an injury or illness that OSHA thinks should have been recorded is not recorded, a violation exists, as far as OSHA is concerned, until that injury or illness is recorded.

Workers' Compensation Law Requirements

Each state's workers' compensation statute imposes certain reporting requirements for all physicians who treat occupational injuries and illnesses. It is imperative that all physicians be familiar with the reporting requirements of the workers' compensation laws of the states in which they practice. What the employer actually knows, however, often depends on what is related by the treating physician. In the case of work-related injuries and illnesses, the physician is entitled to be paid by the employer or the employer's workers' compensation insurance carrier. However, in some states, failure to file an attending physician's report within a certain period of time may excuse the employer's obligation to pay the treating physician's bill.

MEDICAL AND EXPOSURE RECORD ACCESS

Occupational physicians may be asked to provide the medical records of an employee who has been treated; they, or persons under their supervision, may also be asked to provide information regarding actual, or potential, employee exposures to chemicals or physical agents. There are two important considerations in a request of this sort: the confidentiality expectations of the employee and the rights of the employer. There are also two types of laws to consider: federal and state. The federal law is OSHA's Standard on Access to Employee Exposure and Medical Records; the state laws are those statutory or case law pronouncements regarding who can examine medical records and under what circumstances. These rules will be considered separately.

Federal Law: OSHA's Medical and Exposure Record Access Standard

Who Is Covered?

By its terms, OSHA's Record Access Standard "applies to each general industry, maritime, and construction employer who makes, maintains, contracts for, or has access to employee exposure or medical records, or analyses thereof, pertaining to employees exposed to 'toxic substances' or 'harmful agents'" (as those terms are defined in the standard, and discussed below.) It also "applies to all employee exposure and medical records, and analyses thereof, made or maintained in any manner, including on an in-house or contractual (e.g., fee-for-service) basis" (53).

General Provisions

Under the Record Access Standard, any employer who has employees exposed to "toxic substances" or "harmful physical agents," and who has, or has access to, medical or exposure records, must provide the employee (or his or her authorized representative) access to his or her medical and exposure records (absent special circumstances) within 15 working days of a request. The employer may require that requester (employee or representative) to provide information that may be necessary to locate or identify the records being requested (e.g., dates and locations of employment). The employer must provide to the requesting employee, or his or her designated representative, either (a) a copy of the employee's record, at the employer's expense; (b) the necessary copying facilities, supplied at the employer's expense, so the employee can make copies of the record; or (c) temporary custody of the record, so that the employee can make copies. This provision applies to all present and former employees exposed to toxic substances or harmful physical agents.

Upon commencement of employment, and at least annually thereafter, employers must advise their employers of their medical and exposure record access rights.

All records (with exceptions set out in the standard) must be retained for the duration of the employee's employment plus 30 years, in the case of medical records, or 30 years, in the case of exposure records, and all analyses using medical records must be retained for 30 years (unless another OSHA standard directs otherwise). The length of this retention period is justified, according to OSHA, because of the extremely long latency periods of some occupational diseases.

Definitions of "Toxic Substances" and "Harmful Physical Agents"

As noted above, the event that triggers coverage by this OSHA Standard is employee exposure to "toxic substances" or "harmful physical agents," which, under the Record Access Standard, include chemical substances, biologic agents, and physical stress (noise, heat, cold, vibration, repetitive motion, ionizing and nonionizing radiation, hypo- and hyperbaric pressure), that:

1. are listed in the latest edition of the National Institute for Occupational Safety and Health (NIOSH) Registry of Toxic Effects of Chemical Substances;
2. have yielded evidence of an *acute or chronic health hazard* in human, animal, or other biologic testing conducted by, or known to, the employer; or
3. are the subject of an MSDS kept by, or known to the employer, indicating that the material may pose a hazard to human health.

When records are provided, employers may delete trade secret information from medical (and exposure) records, to the extent they disclose manufacturing processes or the percentage of chemical substances in mixtures. However, the employee must be notified that the deletions have been made, and the employer must provide effective alternative information about when and where the exposure occurred. In addition, the employer may not withhold chemical names or levels of exposure, although it may obtain a confidentiality agreement (54).

Medical Records

What Constitutes a Medical Record?

OSHA's Record Access Standard defines medical records to include, but not necessarily be limited to, medical and employment questionnaires or histories; results of all medical examinations, laboratory tests, and biologic monitoring; medical opinions, diagnoses, progress notes, and recommendations; descriptions of treatments and prescriptions; and employee medical complaints. Health insurance records are also covered, if they are accessible to the employer by employee name, social security number, or "other personal identifier."

There are four specific *exemptions* from coverage. First, physical specimens, such as blood or urine, that are routinely discarded are not required to be kept (although the written results of such tests are). Second, health insurance records, to the extent they are not accessible by personal identifier, are not part of the medical records. Third, records created solely in preparation for litigation, which are privileged from discovery under the applicable rules of procedure, are not covered. Finally, records regarding employee alcohol, drug abuse, or personal counseling programs are not covered if they are maintained separate and apart from the employee's medical program and its records (55). Given the highly sensitive nature of some of these latter records and the high public visibility these cases may receive, it is prudent to keep records related to alcohol and substance abuse separate. Failure to do so may result in a lawsuit by the employee whose records are divulged.

Who Can Review Medical Records and Under What Circumstances?

Any current or former employee can always request to see his or her medical record, and that request does not have to be in writing. Under the Record Access Standard, the employee can also name a "designated representative" to obtain medical record information. That representative may be a collective bargaining representative, physician, attorney, family member, fellow employee, or anyone else.

However, to obtain access to medical records, any of these designated representatives *must have the written consent of the employee*. That written consent need not be in any particular form, but it must contain the following (56):

1. The name and signature of the employee authorizing the release of medical information;
2. The date of the authorization (because any authorizations expire after 1 year);
3. The name of the organization or individual authorized to release the information;
4. The name of the designated representative to whom the information is authorized to be released;
5. A general description of the purpose for the release of the medical information;
6. The date or condition on which the release will expire, if less than a year.

When Can Access to Medical Records Be Refused?

There is one circumstance under which a physician for the employer may prohibit an employee from seeing his or her medical record. If the physician believes that direct employee access to a record concerning a terminal illness or a psychiatric condition of that employee could be detrimental to the employee's health, the employer may refuse to show these records to the employee. However, the records must be shown to the employee's authorized representative.

Exposure Records

What Constitutes an Exposure Record?

Exposure records are broadly defined as "records containing exposure information concerning the employee's workplace or working conditions" and "exposure records pertaining to workplaces or working conditions to which the employee is being assigned or transferred." Exposure records include (a) *environmental (workplace) monitoring* or measuring, including personal, area, grab, wipe, or other forms of sampling, including collection and analytic methodologies, calculations, and other background data relevant to interpretation; (b) *biologic monitoring* results that directly assess the absorption of a substance or agent by a body system; and (c) Material Safety Data Sheets. Since exposure records may not be available for all employees, the standard provides that an employee can review other "exposure records [of employees]...with past or present job duties or working conditions related to or similar to those of the employee." Similarly, records of exposure measurements made in particular work sites, but not tied to any specific employee, would also be obtainable.

Who Can Review Exposure Records and Under What Circumstances?

Current or former employees may request to see their exposure records. Exposure records may also be obtained by designated representatives. However, with regard to exposure records, a collective bargaining representative of the employee is automatically deemed to be a "designated representative," and, without written employee authorization, is entitled to review exposure records, after a written request to the employer (57).

Analyses Using Exposure or Medical Records

Employees and their designated representatives are also entitled, by the Record Access Standard, to review any *analysis* using employee exposure or medical records. This term *analysis* is defined as

> Any compilation of data, [or] any statistical study based...in part on information collected from...employee exposure or medical records; [and] information...from health insurance records, [if] the analysis has been reported to the employer....

This portion of the rule also permits collective bargaining representatives to examine analyses without obtaining specific employee written consent. However, if the analyses contain any information by which individual employees can be identified, the employer must remove that information before it is turned over (58).

State Laws

State laws regarding the availability of medical records are basically of two types. The first is statute or case law that sets out a physician's obligations to disclose medical record information. All physicians should familiarize themselves with any pertinent state law regarding who can obtain medical records and when they may be obtained. These laws, in the main, are designed for purposes of setting out the conditions under which patients themselves may obtain their records.

The other type of state law is that found in the workers' compensation statutes. Generally, those laws provide that if an employee has made his or her physical condition an issue in a workers' compensation proceeding, that employee's medical records are discoverable by the parties to that proceeding. However, to be on the safe side, physicians should (a) make sure they know what the law of their particular state provides, and (b) in a compensation proceeding, insist on a *subpoena* setting out the style of the case and precisely the types of records requested.

Confidentiality

As noted, OSHA's Record Access Standard and certain state laws provide that, under certain specified circumstances, patients, their representatives, and opposing parties in litigation can get medical records. Two other situations in which the physician might be asked for medical information should be addressed.

The first situation is when records are requested by a state or federal agency, investigating worker health or attempting, in some way, to cope with a public health problem. In the public health context, courts have been very reluctant to interfere with a state's efforts to deal with a perceived problem. For example, the United States Supreme Court upheld the right of New York State to require that a copy of any prescription for a narcotic drug be sent to the state health department. The Court held that state public health concerns outweighed privacy considerations (59).

Insofar as federal agencies are concerned, the most commonly litigated issue has involved a request by NIOSH for employee medical information to conduct studies regarding potential health hazards in the workplace. Courts have routinely permitted NIOSH to obtain this information pursuant to a subpoena (60). However, one court of appeals has held that, to prevent unwanted invasions of privacy, NIOSH should notify employees that their records will be examined after a certain period of time has elapsed, unless the employee requests that the record not be reviewed (61).

The second situation occurs when an employer wants information about an employee's medical condition. This request for information may arise in several contexts: (a) in conjunction with a preplacement or periodic physical examination, (b) in connection with workers' compensation, and (c) not in conjunction with anything in particular, to the physician's knowledge.

With regard to preplacement or periodic examinations, physicians should be aware of the Code of Ethical Conduct of the American College of Occupational and Environmental Medicine (ACOEM), originally adopted in 1976 and updated in 1994: "Employers are entitled to counsel about the medical fitness of individuals in relation to work, but are not entitled to diagnoses or details of a specific nature." Thus, under this section and without a release from the employee, physicians may advise employers, for example, that an employee should not work in high places because of possible dizziness but would not convey information about the etiology of the dizziness if the dizziness is not work related. As to non–work-related conditions that would have no effect on the ability to do the job, the physician should not convey those to the employer at all. If the employee wants the employer's insurance to pay the medical bill, however, as a practical matter a release will be required by the employer or insurance company to process appropriate payments.

As to work-related disorders, the situation is somewhat different. State workers' compensation statutes *mandate* reporting of work-related disorders, and the employer is *obliged* to know what the employee's condition is, so as to protect him or her from further exposure and not violate any necessary restrictions. Again, as a practical matter, the information contained on most state workers' compensation Attending Physician Reports will suffice to provide the employer with the necessary information.

Finally, an employer may request information on an employee's health status for *no apparent reason*. OSHA's rule-making on the Record Access Standard revealed that OSHA believed that management access to employee medical records might be much more extensive than the ACOEM Code of Ethical Conduct permits. OSHA, however, has specifically declined to issue specific rules limiting management access to records (62). However, a physician who provides such information may be open to a malpractice suit by the employee whose records are so disclosed. In the absence of one of the permissible situations outlined above, the physician is advised not to release medical information without the employee's consent.

THE AMERICANS WITH DISABILITIES ACT

History

Some practitioners of occupational medicine have had to concern themselves with the legal ramifications of disabilities in the workplace since at least 1973, when the Rehabilitation Act of 1973 banned disability discrimination by federal contractors. Since

1990, when the Americans with Disabilities Act (ADA) was enacted, all occupational physicians have had to deal with those issues. (See Chapter 5 for a comprehensive discussion of the ADA.)

The ADA is intentionally worded very broadly, and even though the Equal Employment Opportunity Commission (EEOC), charged with issuing regulations and enforcing the Act, has issued detailed guidelines, many of the ADA's provisions have not been fully explicated. The EEOC and others have acknowledged that clarification of the ADA's specific requirements will only come as courts interpret the Act on a case-by-case basis. However, we can look to the language of the Act itself and some of the EEOC's regulations and interpretations for a basic understanding of the ADA's methods and objectives.

Structure of the ADA

Under the ADA a "disability" is (a) a physical or mental impairment that substantially limits one or more of the major life activities of an individual, (b) a record of such an impairment, or (c) a situation in which an individual is regarded as having such an impairment. The thrust of the ADA (relevant to employers) is that employees or job applicants with such disabilities may not be discriminated against in any aspect of the employment relationship if that employee or applicant is "qualified" for the job. A disabled person is "qualified" if, with "reasonable accommodation" he or she can perform the "essential functions" of the job as well as one who is not disabled.

Notably, a person is disabled, even if not presently impaired, if he or she "has a record of such impairment" or "is regarded as having" a disability. The first phrase covers those who have been misclassified as having a disability, or who were impaired but have at least temporarily recovered (63). The second phrase covers those who are not actually impaired in the major life activities, but are nevertheless viewed and treated by others as being impaired (64).

The EEOC sets out three factors, to which others may be added, to assess whether a job function is essential. The function may be essential if (a) the position exists specifically to perform that function, (b) only a limited number of employees can perform the function, and/or (c) the function is highly specialized and the person is hired specifically for his or her expertise in performing that function (65). Evidence considered in assessing whether a job function is essential includes, among other things, (a) the employer's judgment as to what is essential, (b) the amount of time spent on the particular function, (c) written job descriptions, and (d) the consequences of not requiring the employee to perform the function (66). A more fact-specific, case-by-case determination can hardly be imagined.

Once the essential functions are determined, the employees or applicants may not be treated differently due to their disability, if any "reasonable accommodation" will enable them to do the job. An accommodation is necessarily reasonable if it does not impose on the employer an "undue hardship." An accommodation must be effective, but it need not be the best available accommodation (67). Reasonable accommodations include making work facilities physically accessible, and acquiring or modifying equipment. It might even require steps such as hiring readers for blind employees or interpreters for deaf employees (68).

An "undue hardship" is "action requiring significant difficulty or expense." The EEOC elaborates by explaining an undue hardship as an accommodation that would (a) be unduly costly, (b) be extensive, (c) be substantial, (d) be disruptive, or (e) fundamentally alter the nature or operation of the business (69). In analyzing the financial burden of an accommodation, the cost of accommodation is not compared to the value of the position being accommodated (i.e., employee's salary) but is analyzed in light of the employer's entire financial resources (70).

Impairments that "Substantially Limit" Major Life Activities

For a number of years, two of the most hotly contested issues in ADA litigation centered on what type of impairments constitute disabilities under the ADA, and what "substantially limits a major life activity." A major life activity is exemplified in the EEOC rules by such things as caring for oneself, seeing, hearing, speaking, walking, learning, and working (71). The EEOC regulations also say that a major life activity is "substantially limited" if, due to disability, the person cannot perform that activity, or cannot perform it as well as or as easily as the average person in the general population (72).

In 2002, the United States Supreme Court held that, if an employee claims disability, under the ADA, by virtue of inability to perform manual tasks (one of the categories of potential disability set out in the EEOC's regulations), that employee must establish that he or she is unable to perform the variety of tasks central to most people's daily lives, not just the tasks associated with his or her specific job. In that case, the employee's job required her to engage in repetitive activity with her hands and arms at or above shoulder level for extended periods of time. The employee, who had carpal tunnel syndrome, thoracic outlet compression, and tendinitis, was not able to do that type of work. However, the Court held that the manual tasks unique to any particular job are not necessarily important parts of most people's lives, and specifically concluded that the employment-related manual tasks that the employee could not perform in the case before the Court were not the sorts of manual tasks that are an important part of most people's daily lives (73).

The U.S. Supreme Court also held, in 1999, that, in determining whether a person has an impairment that substantially limits a major life activity, or is "regarded as" having such an impairment, it is necessary to take into consideration any measures used by that person to mitigate the impairment. These measures would include such things as eyeglasses and medications (74). In this context, the Court said that people are not limited in the major life activity of working, if their otherwise bad vision is correctable by glasses or contact lenses, or their hypertension is controlled by medication, even if they don't qualify for certain jobs that impose very stringent requirements (such as the job of international airline pilot) (75).

The ADA's Impact on Medical Examinations

Of special note to medical practitioners is the ADA's impact on employment-related medical examinations. The ADA prohibits such examinations before an offer of employment is made. Examinations are allowed only after an offer is made, and the offer may be conditioned on passing the examination. However, the same examination must be given to all entering employees in the same job classification, and the information derived therefrom may not be used to discriminate against the disabled applicant.

The "Direct Threat to Others" Exception

The practitioner may also be called on to assess whether an applicant should be rejected as posing a "direct threat" to others "that cannot be eliminated by reasonable accommodation." This is an issue in situations in which the disability is, or is related to, an infectious disease. The regulations emphasize that the "direct threat" determination must be an individualized assessment, relying on the most current medical knowledge and the best available objective evidence (76). The risk must be evaluated in terms of its duration, and the likelihood, imminence, and severity of the potential harm (77).

TOXIC TORTS

Background

Toxic tort cases are lawsuits brought by those who claim that exposure to toxic substance caused their illness or disease. Normally, but not always (see the exception to workers' compensation exclusivity for intentional torts), workers' compensation is the sole remedy for employees allegedly harmed by exposure to toxic substances at the workplace. However, workers may sue third-party manufacturers or suppliers of chemicals (e.g., asbestos) for their injuries. As well, some employees have brought lawsuits on behalf of their children, who, they contend, suffered birth defects as a result of the parent's exposure to toxic substances in the workplace. Courts in many jurisdictions have held that such suits are not barred by workers' compensation. Consumers of products (e.g., pharmaceuticals such as diethylstilbestrol) and those exposed to allegedly toxic waste in the environment (e.g., at a Superfund site) can also bring a civil suit.

Theories of Law

Toxic tort lawsuits can be brought under many different legal theories, including (a) negligence (lack of reasonable care by defendant), (b) strict liability (defendant liable for his or her abnormally dangerous activity or defective and unreasonably dangerous product), (c) breach of express or implied warranty, and even (d) intentional misconduct (defendant knew that injury was substantially certain to flow from his or her act or omission).

Analysis

Most peculiar to toxic tort suits are the types of damages that are recoverable by plaintiffs. In addition to the usual damages for medical expenses, lost earning capacity, and pain and suffering, plaintiffs who claim exposure to toxins may, in some states, seek damages for future risk of illness, fear of future illness, or the cost of medical surveillance.

Plaintiffs who claim future risk of injury are arguing that their exposure to a toxic agent has increased their risk of a particular illness (or illnesses) associated with such exposure. It is very difficult to prove that a future illness will probably occur absent some present injury or symptoms. Thus, most courts allow recovery for increased risk only if there is some present manifestation of the deleterious effects of the exposure. Even if such is the case, plaintiffs still must prove, usually with expert testimony, that the possible future illness is produced by exposure to the toxin, and that the illness is likely to occur some time in the future.

Closely related to increased risk of future illness is fear of future illness. Here, as in a claim for infliction of emotional distress, the claimant is claiming psychic injury damages for worry and anxiety (78). Courts that allow such a claim require that the fear be "reasonable." This requirement is sometimes met when there is a sufficiently rational causal relationship between the toxin and the disease. In a number of cases, courts have held that the chance of contracting the disease need not be greater than 50% to justify a reasonable fear. Thus, even where a plaintiff's claim for increased risk fails, he or she might still recover for fear. Even here, in the great majority of cases that have permitted this cause of action, some physical injury or some physical manifestation of the fear must be shown in order to prove the genuineness of the fear (79). However, courts have, on occasion, allowed corroborative medical and psychological testimony to substitute for actual injury. A few courts have found a reasonable fear based only on proof of exposure to the toxin (80).

Medical surveillance suits seek recovery of expenses of future medical examinations and tests, for purposes of monitoring the plaintiff's health and facilitating early diagnosis and treatment of disease that may result from exposure to toxic substances. Some courts that have considered such suits have allowed surveillance costs to be recovered if expert testimony establishes a reasonable probability that the plaintiff will contract a particular disease in the future. In the absence of a present injury. However, most courts have not ruled for the plaintiffs.

REFERENCES

1. 1920 N.Y. Laws Ch. 538 [codified as amended at N.Y. Workmen's Comp. Law [3(2)] (McKinney 1965 and Suppl. 1982)].
2. *Southern Shipping Co. v. Lawson,* 5 F. Suppl. 321 (S.D. Fla. 1933) (heavy labor resulted in rupture of preexisting aortic aneurysm; death held to be compensable).
3. *Chausse v. Lowe,* 35 F. Supp. 1011, 1014 (E.D.N.Y. 1938) [quoting *Goldberg v. 954 Marcy Corp.*, 276 N.Y. 313, 12 N.E.2d 311 (1938)].
4. *Ivancik v. Wright Aeronautical Corp.,* 68 F. Supp. 270, 273 (D.N.J. 1946) [quoting *Bollinger v. Wagaraw Building Supply Co.*, 122 N.J.L. 512, 6 A.2d 396 (1939)].
5. *Todd Dry Docks v. Marshall,* 61 F.2d 671 (9th Cir. 1932).
6. *Dower v. General Dynamics Corp.,* 14 Ben. Rev. Bd. Serv. (MB) 342 (1981) (rectal cancer allegedly potentiated by asbestos exposure); *Compton v. Pennsylvania Avenue Golf Service Center,* 14 Ben. Rev. Bd. Serv. (MB) 472 (1981) (leukemia allegedly caused by exposure to benzene).
7. *Ryan v. Connor,* 503 N.E.2d 1379 (Ohio 1986).
8. *Witty v. American General Capital Distrib., Inc.,* 727 S.W.2d 503 (Tex. 1987).
9. *Sparks v. Tulane Med. Ctr. Hosp. & Clinic,* 546 So. 2d 138 (La. 1989). [The Louisiana legislature amended its workers compensation statue. The *Sparks* court held that claimant's burden of proof was by a preponderance of evidence. The legislature required the mental injury to be the result of a sudden unexpected and extraordinary stress related to the employment, and it changed claimant's burden to clear and convincing evidence; *see Lewis v. Beauregard Mem. Hosp., 649 S.2d 655 (1994); Barnes v. City of Cincinnati, 590 N.E.2d 294 (Ohio Ct. App. 1990)].*
10. Fla. Stat. Ann. § 440.02(1).
11. Maine Rev. Stat. Ann., title 39-A, § 102.
12. *Prater v. Thorngate, Ltd.*, 761 S.W.2d 226 (Mo. Ct. App. 1988).
13. *Johns-Manville Products Corp. v. Contra Costa Superior Court,* 165 Cal. Rptr. 858, 612 P.2d 948 (1980).
14. *Millison v. E.I. duPont de Nemours & Co.,* 501 A.2d 505, 516 (N.J. 1985), *appeal after remand,* 545 A.2d 213 (N.J. Super. Ct. 1988), *aff'd,* 558 A.2d 461 (N.J. 1989); *see also Mabee v. Borden, Inc.,* 720 A.2d 342 (N.J. Super. Ct. 1998); *but see Crippen v. Central Jersey Concrete Pipe Co.,* 775 A.2d 716 (N.J. Super. Ct. App. Div. 2001).
15. *Price v. Philadelphia Electric Co.,* 790 F. Supp. 97 (E.D. Pa. 1992).
16. *Livitsanos v. Superior Court,* 2 Cal. 4th 744 (1992).
17. *Duprey v. Shane,* 39 Cal. 2d 781, 249 P.2d 8 (1952).
18. *Delamotte v. Unitcast Div. Of Midland Ross Corp.,* 411 N.E.2d 814, 818 (Ohio Ct. App. 1978).
19. Billauer BF. The legal liability of the occupational health professional. *J Occup Med* 1985;27:185.
20. *Abbott v. Gould, Inc.,* 443 N.W.2d 591 (Neb. 1989).
21. *Millison v. E.I. DuPont de Nemours & Co.,* 501 A.2d 505 (N.J. 1985), *appeal after remand,* 545 A.2d 213 (N.J. Super. Cto. 1988), aff'd, 558 A.2d 461 (N.J. 1989); *see also Mabee v. Borden, Inc.,* 720 A.2d 342 (N.J. Super. Ct. 1998); *but see Crippen v. Central Jersey Concrete Pipe Co.,* 775 A.2d 716 (N.J. Super. Ct. App. Div. 2001).
22. 29 C.F.R. § 1910.1200.
23. *Gade v. Nat'l Solid Wastes Mgmt. Ass'n* 505 U.S. 88 (1992); *New Jersey State Chamber of Commerce v. Hughey,* 774 F.2d 587 (3d Cir. 1985); *Mfr. Ass'n of Tri-County v. Knepper,* 801 F.2d 130 (3d Cir. 1986); *Ohio Mfr. Ass'n v. City of Akron,* 801 F.2d 824 (6th Cir. 1986).
24. 29 C.F.R. § 1910.1200(i).
25. Superfund Amendments and Reauthorization Act of 1986, Emergency Planning and Community Right-to-Know Act (EPCRA) (Pub. L. No. 99-499) H 311-312; *see also* 52 Fed. Reg. 38, 344; 40 C.F.R. §§ 370.20;370.21;370.30.
26. 29 U.S.C. § 651 *et seq.* and 29 C.F.R. Part 1904.
27. 42 Fed. Reg. 38, 568 (July 29, 1977). Chapter 1.
28. 66 Fed. Reg. 5916-6135 (Jan. 19, 2001).
29. 66 Fed. Reg. 5921. Occupational Safety and Health Administration. A brief guide to recordkeeping requirements for occupational injuries and illnesses (OMB No. 1220-0029), Apr. 1986.

30. 66 Fed. Reg. 5919.
31. 66 Fed. Reg. 5919.
32. 66 Fed. Reg. 5919.
33. 29 C.F.R. Part 1904.5(a). (2000.)
34. 29 C.F.R. Part 1904.5(a). (2002.)
35. 29 C.F.R. Part 1904.5(b)(2).
36. 66 Fed. Reg. 5948.
37. 29 U.S.C. § 662 (c)(2).
38. 29 C.F.R. Part 1904.7(a).
39. 66 Fed. Reg. 6126.
40. 29 C.F.R. Part 1904.7(b)(7).
41. 29 C.F.R. Part 1904.5(b)(7).
42. 29 C.F.R. Part 1904.7(b)(5)(ii).
43. 66 Fed. Reg. 5987.
44. 29 C.F.R. Part 1904.7(b)(5)(v).
45. 29 C.F.R. Part 1904.7(b)(4)(iii); *see also* 66 Fed. Reg. 6084.
46. 29 C.F.R. Part 1904.7(b)(4)(i) and (ii).
47. 29 C.F.R. Part 1904.5(b)(2)(ix).
48. 29 C.F.R. Part 1904.29(b)(6).
49. 29 C.F.R. Part 1904.29(b)(7).
50. 29 C.F.R. Part 1904.29(b)(9).
51. 29 C.F.R. Part 1904.32(b)(6).
52. 29 C.F.R. Part 1904.32(b)(3&4).
53. 29 C.F.R. 1910.1020(b), (c), (e), and (f).
54. 29 C.F.R. 1910.1020(c) and (f).
55. 29 C.F.R. 1910.1020(b) and (c).
56. 29 C.F.R. 1910.1020(c) and (e).
57. 29 C.F.R. 1910.1020(c) and (e).
58. 29 C.F.R. 1910.20(c)(2) and (e).
59. *Whalen v. Roe,* 429 U.S. 589 (1977).
60. *General Motors Corp. v. Director,* NIOSH, 9 OSHC (BNA) 1139 (6th Cir. 1980).
61. *United States v. Westinghouse,* 8 OSHC (BNA) 2131 (3d Cir. 1980).
62. 45 Fed. Reg. 35, 243 (1980).
63. 56 Fed. Reg. 35, 725 (July 26, 1991) ("Regulations"), Section 1630.2(k).
64. Regulations, Section 1630.2(1).
65. Regulations, Section 1630-2(n)(2).
66. Regulations, Section 1360.2(n)(3).
67. *EEOC Technical Assistance Manual* (TAM) (1992) III-3-5.
68. Regulations, Section 1630.2(o)(2).
69. Appendix to Regulations, 56 Fed. Reg. 35,744.
70. TAM III-15.
71. Regulations, Section 1630.2(i); TAM.
72. Regulations, Section 1630.2Q)(1).
73. *Toyota Motor Manufacturing, Kentucky, Inc. v. Williams* 534 U.S. 184; 151 L. Ed.2d 615 (2002).
74. *Sutton v. United Airlines, Inc.,* 527 U.S. 471 (1999) (eyeglasses); *Murphy v. United Parcel Service Inc.*, 527 U.S. 516 (1999) (high blood pressure medicine); *see also Albertson's Inc. v. Kirkingburg* 527 U.S. 555 (1999) (monocular vision).
75. *Sutton, supra,* note 82, at 475–476, 488.
76. Regulations, Section 1630.2(r).
77. *Ibid.*
78. *Jackson v. Johns-Manville Sales Corp.,* 781 F.2d 394 (5th Cir. 1986).
79. Payton *v. Abbott Lab.,* 437 N.E.2d 171 (Mass. 1982).
80. In re *Moorenovich,* 634 F. Supp. 634 (D. Me. 1986).

3

Role of Regulatory Agencies

James A. Hathaway

Governmental activity continues to have a very significant influence on the practice of medicine in the United States. This is especially true regarding reimbursement for services provided through governmental programs such as Medicare and Medicaid. In the occupational arena, physicians in many specialties are affected by state workers' compensation regulations that set fees and prescribe rules for independent medical examiners. Additional governmental regulations are anticipated as pressure for federal legislation regarding privacy of medical records increases. Concerns regarding this issue have been heightened by the increased use of computerized medical records and their distribution electronically.

The delivery of occupational and environmental health services, however, has a unique background with respect to governmental activity. Not only do issues such as workers' compensation statutes affect the practitioner, but also regulations established by federal and state agencies have a direct effect on the practice of occupational and environmental medicine. In particular, the Occupational Safety and Health Administration (OSHA), the National Institute for Occupational Safety and Health (NIOSH), and the Environmental Protection Agency (EPA) all carry out activities that directly affect the practice of occupational and environmental medicine in some capacity. OSHA standards, NIOSH research activities, and certain EPA regulations should become familiar topics for physicians who provide occupational and environmental health care. This chapter provides an overview of the activities of these and other agencies that have the most significant impact on practitioners providing occupational and environmental health services.

It is not the purpose of this chapter to review the history of the regulatory agencies or to discuss in detail the philosophy behind their stated lofty objectives. Whether the agencies are accomplishing their goals or doing so efficiently and effectively will also not be covered even though this is often a topic of debate. Interested individuals are referred to textbooks that have chapters on these topics (1,2). How these agencies affect the day-to-day practice of occupational medicine in either a clinical or administrative setting and what a practitioner should know are the foci of this chapter.

Agencies that focus mainly on worker health and safety and those that have primarily an environmental focus are discussed. Government agencies seem to be particularly fond of acronyms, and an occupational medicine practitioner would be wise to develop at least a passing knowledge of this alphabet soup (Table 3.1).

OCCUPATIONAL SAFETY AND HEALTH ADMINISTRATION

The Occupational Safety and Health Administration is mandated to ensure safe and healthy working conditions for employees. OSHA has legislative authority to accomplish this mission by setting health and safety standards, enforcing these standards through workplace inspections, and assisting employers in solving work-site problems by offering consultation. Of all the regulatory agencies that affect the practice of occupational medicine, OSHA has the greatest impact. Some states have taken advantage of an option in the Occupational Safety and Health (OSH) Act to establish and administer their own state OSHA plan. Standards promulgated by these states are usually identical to the federal OSHA standards but in some cases may be more stringent. The OSH Act does not cover federal, state, or local municipal employees or work sites covered by concurrent legislation. However, executive branches of the federal government are expected to have equivalent regula-

TABLE 3.1. *Federal agencies with rules that affect the practice of occupational and environmental medicine*

Occupational Safety and Health Administration (OSHA)
National Institute for Occupational Safety and Health (NIOSH)
National Institute of Environmental Health Sciences (NIEHS)
National Toxicology Program (NTP)
Mine Safety and Health Administration (MSHA)
Nuclear Regulatory Commission (NRC)
Department of Transportation (DOT)
Federal Aviation Administration (FAA)
Federal Railroad Administration (FRA)
Federal Highway Administration (FHA)
U.S. Coast Guard (USCG)
Research and Special Programs Administration (RSPA)
Equal Employment Opportunity Commission (EEOC)
Environmental Protection Agency (EPA)
Agency for Toxic Substances and Disease Registry (ATSDR)

tions, and most state-run programs cover state and local municipal employees.

The OSHA standards that have the greatest potential impact on physicians who provide occupational health services are listed in Tables 3.2 and 3.3. The numerical reference in the tables refers to the specific section(s) of Title 29 of the Code of Federal Regulations (CFR), which provide more detailed information.

Occupational Injuries and Illnesses

Recording of occupational injuries and illnesses is the responsibility of the employer. In some cases, determining whether an injury is work related, and therefore recordable, is difficult. With illnesses, the determination of work-relatedness is even more problematic. Physicians are frequently asked to assist with this determination. Dermatitis and cumulative trauma disorders are examples of conditions that are often controversial regarding work-relatedness. Physicians can assist by making a definitive diagnosis and then weighing the probable impact of workplace and other exposure factors to make a decision as to whether or not the condition is work related. Injuries and illnesses in the past were recorded on *OSHA Form 200* by the employer. In 2001 OSHA required a change to a new OSHA 300 log.

Access to Employee Medical Records

Physicians practicing occupational medicine may expect to be asked to maintain medical records for their employer or client. In general, these records must be maintained for the duration of a person's employment plus 30 years. This time period is much longer than that typically required for non–work-related, inactive patient files. OSHA also requires that medical records be released to designated representatives, including the employee, on presentation of signed consent. Compliance with such requests is required within 15 working days (4).

Occupational Noise Exposure

This OSHA standard requires annual audiograms for employees exposed to noise of 85 dB or higher on a daily time-weighted average (TWA) basis. The hearing level thresholds are compared each year to the baseline audiogram. Audiograms that show a standard threshold shift (STS), which is defined as an

TABLE 3.2. *OSHA standards that impact occupational medicine*

Section title	Section no.[a]
Log and Summary of Occupational Injuries and Illnesses	1904.2
Access to Employee Exposure and Medical Records	1910.20
Occupational Noise Exposure	1910.95
Hazardous Waste Operations and Emergency Response	1910.120
Respiratory Protection	1910.134
Medical Services and First Aid	1910.151
Fire Brigades	1910.156
Commercial Diving Operations	1910.401–1910.441
Air Contaminants and Chemical Specific Standards[b]	1910.1000 and following
Bloodborne pathogens	1910.1030
Hazard Communication	1910.1200
Occupational Exposure to Hazardous Chemicals in Laboratories	1910.1450

[a]From Title 29 of the Code of Federal Regulations.

[b]See Table 3.3 for details.

TABLE 3.3. *OSHA chemical specific standards*

Section no.[a]	Chemical
1910.1001	Asbestos
1910.1003	4-Nitrobiphenyl
1910.1004	α-Naphthylamine
1910.1006	Methyl chlormethyl ether
1910.1007	3,3′-Dichlorobenzidine (and its salts)
1910.1008	bis-Chloromethyl ether
1910.1009	β-Naphylamine
1910.1010	Benzidine
1910.1011	4-Aminodiphenyl
1910.1012	Ethyleneimine
1910.1013	β-Propiolactone
1910.1014	2-Acetylaminofluorene
1910.1015	2-Dimethylaminoazobenzene
1910.1016	*N*-Nitrosodimethylamine
1910.1017	Vinyl chloride
1910.1018	Inorganic arsenic
1910.1025	Lead
1910.1027	Cadmium
1910.1028	Benzene
1910.1029	Coke oven emissions
1910.1043	Cotton dust
1910.1044	1,2-dibromo 3-chloropropane
1910.1045	Acrylonitrile
1910.1047	Ethylene oxide
1910.1048	Formaldehyde
1910.1050	Methylene dianiline
1910.1051	1,3-Butadiene
1910.1052	Methylene chloride

[a]From Title 29 of the Code of Federal Regulations.

age-adjusted decrease of 10 dB or greater in either ear averaged for the frequencies of 2,000, 3,000, and 4,000 Hz, must be reviewed by an audiologist or physician to determine the need for further evaluation. Employers frequently expect physicians practicing occupational medicine to perform these evaluations and provide medical direction for their hearing conservation program. One controversial area is recordability of work-related hearing loss. In previous OSHA field directives, a work-related change in hearing of 25 dB averaged over the frequencies of 2,000, 3,000, and 4,000 Hz was recorded on the OSHA Form 300 as a disorder due to repeated trauma. In 2002, OSHA revised the criteria for recording work-related hearing loss. Beginning in January, 2003, employers will be required to record 10-decibel shifts from the employee's initial hearing test when they also result in an overall hearing level of 25 decibels (see Chapter 26 for more details).

Physical Fitness Evaluations

Several OSHA standards, including those for hazardous waste operations and emergency response, respiratory protection, and some chemical-specific standards, require the employee to have a medical examination or evaluation to determine physical fitness to perform certain jobs, or to wear specific personal protective equipment (e.g., respirators). Two other standards, fire brigades and commercial diving operations, do *not* require examinations unless the employee has a specific medical condition; however, the need for examinations is implied due to the strenuous physical activities.

Few of these standards specify *details* of the medical examination, which are left to the discretion of the examining physician. Employers may specify requirements, and additional guidance can be found in Chapter 41. Physicians should request authorization for additional tests from employers if the tests are clinically appropriate.

In 1999 OSHA revised the standard for respiratory protection modifying the requirements for medical evaluations. A mandatory Respirator Medical Evaluation Questionnaire, found in Appendix C of CFR 1910.134, can be used in lieu of a medical examination. If certain questions are answered positively, then a medical examination is required. Otherwise, the questionnaire is all that is required. Alternately, the mandatory questionnaire is not required if a medical examination that covers the same information is performed initially. A physician or other licensed health care professional can perform the evaluation of the questionnaire and any related examination. The American College of Occupational and Environmental Medicine argued unsuccessfully that only a licensed physician should perform these evaluations and examinations.

In general, the OSHA standards require the physician to furnish the employer a *written opinion* on whether the employee has any medical conditions that would place the employee at increased risk of impairment from the work or use of protective equipment. The physician must provide in writing any limitations on the employee's assigned work. The employee should be informed of any conditions that require further examination or treatment and be referred to private physicians, as necessary. The written opinion should not reveal to the employer specific findings or diagnoses unrelated to the occupational exposure.

Medical Services and First Aid

This standard requires employers to ensure ready availability of medical personnel for advice and consultation on matters of plant health. It is common practice for employers to develop agreements with physicians or clinics to obtain this advice and to have a resource for treatment of injuries or illnesses and for medical examinations.

The standard also requires that a physician approve first-aid supplies for the work site. Many employers have the physician visit the site annually and sign the list of approved first-aid supplies.

Chemical-specific Standards

There are detailed individual standards for 28 chemicals. Each of these standards includes a section on medical surveillance. In all standards, medical examinations are required if certain conditions are met. These conditions typically refer to airborne exposure levels above a designated concentration [usually 50% of the permissible exposure limits (PEL)] or dermal exposure to material containing the substance at a level above 0.1% or 1.0% by weight or volume. (See Chapter 41 for a detailed description on the methods used to determine the need for medical examinations.)

With the exception of the carcinogen standards (1910.1003–1910.1016), most OSHA regulations include detailed requirements for specific examinations and tests. The asbestos standard (1910.1001) even includes a required medical history form. All the standards include a provision that additional tests can be performed at the option of the examining physician. More recent standards include an appendix on medical surveillance that provides additional information in determining the type of additional tests that may be useful in specific situations.

In addition to the specified requirements of OSHA standards, several administrative procedures affect the physician performing the examinations. For example, the employer must furnish the physician with a copy of the standard, a description of the employee's duties as they relate to exposure, information on the employee's level of exposure, a description of personal protective equipment used, and information from previous medical examinations. After completion of the medical surveillance examination, the physician must furnish a *written opinion* as to whether the employee has any detected condition that would put him/her at increased risk of material health impairment. Also required is a statement that the employee is fit to wear a respirator or other protective equipment or whether there are limitations in using such equipment.

Some of the more recent standards also include provisions for *medical removal protection* and multiple physician review [e.g., lead in general industry (1910.1025) and methylene dianiline (MDA) (1910.1050)]. In some cases, the criteria for medical removal may be straightforward. In lead exposure (1910.1025), for example, temporary removal from exposure is required if the average of the last three blood tests for lead is greater than 50 μg/100 g whole blood and the last test is over 40 μg/100 g whole blood. In other cases, greater discretion is given the physician. An abnormal liver function test in someone exposed to MDA requires medical removal if the abnormal results are believed due to MDA or if the abnormal results are not due to MDA, but the physician believes MDA exposure may exacerbate the condition. MDA causes cholestasis, which results in elevated alkaline phosphatase and bilirubin levels. Usually no hepatocellular damage occurs. In contrast, nonoccupational conditions such as viral infections or alcohol abuse cause hepatocellular damage with elevated levels of alanine aminotransferase [ALT (serum glutamic-pyruvic transaminase, SGPT)] and aspartate aminotransferase [AST (serum glutamic-oxaloacetic transaminase, SGOT)]. There is no experimental evidence or clinical experience to know whether MDA exposure would exacerbate viral or alcoholic hepatitis. Therefore, one can imagine that physicians may have differences of opinion regarding the risk of MDA exacerbating hepatocellular damage, which could trigger the multiple physician review provisions of the standard. Future standards will likely incorporate medical removal protection and multiple physician review.

In addition to the 28 chemical-specific standards, over 600 other chemicals have an OSHA-specified PEL. In 1989, OSHA made the regulations more stringent when they revised downward the airborne exposure limit for many of these chemicals. In 1992, a circuit court of appeals invalidated those revisions. At the time this chapter was written, there were no requirements for medical surveillance for these other chemicals. However, OSHA is considering an expedited mechanism to introduce several standards at one time. If such standards are adopted in the future, they will probably require medical examinations if exposure is above an action level (most likely 50% of the PEL).

Blood-borne Pathogens

OSHA's standard on blood-borne pathogens is directed primarily at the health care industry, but also affects blood processing and research activities using human blood or other bodily fluids, as well as any employer that has designated first-aid responders.

Physicians who practice occupational medicine may be asked to assist employers in drafting written exposure control plans, in conducting training, and particularly in reviewing exposure incidents and providing counseling and advice. (See Chapter 44 for a detailed description of this standard.)

Hazard Communication

The Hazard Communication Standard requires manufacturers and distributors of chemicals to draft *Material Safety Data Sheets* (MSDSs) that include detailed information on the product. Of particular interest to the physician are sections on health hazards and first aid. In addition, many companies also include a section on notes to physicians. The MSDS can be a very useful reference to determine the ingredients of a chemical mixture and to learn summary information on toxicity and expected effects of overexposure. First-aid recommendations and, in some cases, specific medical treatment information are also available. Information regarding carcinogenicity is also provided where relevant. The MSDS includes a phone number for the manufacturer/distributor who can be a source of more detailed information. In some cases, because of trade secret concerns, the identity of all ingredients may not be listed on the MSDS. In an emergency, a treating physician or nurse can request immediate disclosures of the chemical identity of the ingredients. The health care professional can and probably will be required to sign a confidentiality agreement as soon as possible after such a request. In nonemergency situations, similar information can be requested in writing if a legitimate health concern is stated. A signed confidentiality agreement may be required by the manufacturer/distributor.

Occupational Exposure to Hazardous Chemicals in Laboratories

This standard requires employers to furnish medical examinations if employees develop signs or symptoms related to exposure to chemicals in the laboratory, or if they have routine exposures above the action level of a regulated chemical (see Chemical-Specific Standards, above) or following an accidental overexposure from a spill, leak, explosion, or similar occurrence. The content of the examination is left to the discretion of the physician but should be based on the known toxic effects of the chemical(s) of concern. There are similar administrative requirements for written opinions, and related functions as found in Chemical-Specific Standards, above.

Ergonomics

OSHA proposed an ergonomics standard in 1999, which Congress prevented from moving forward in the rule-making process. In 2000, OSHA reintroduced this proposed standard. The standard was rescinded in 2001 (for more information, the reader is referred to Chapter 43).

NATIONAL INSTITUTE FOR OCCUPATIONAL SAFETY AND HEALTH

The National Institute for Occupational Safety and Health (NIOSH) is the research agency created by the OSH Act passed in 1970. In 1973, under the auspices of the former Department of Health, Education, and Welfare (now Health and Human Services), NIOSH became part of the Centers for Disease Control (CDC). In addition to its Atlanta headquarters, it has regional offices in Boston, Massachusetts, and Denver, Colorado, and research facilities in Morgantown, West Virginia, and Cincinnati, Ohio. The institute is mandated to protect the health and safety of workers by conducting research on workplace hazards. In addition to its responsibilities designated under the OSH Act, NIOSH has responsibilities legislated by the Federal Mine Safety and Health Act, the Public Health Service Act, the Toxic Substance Control Act, the Clean Air Act, the Superfund legislation, and for certifying respirators.

NIOSH plays an important role in providing information pertinent to the development of OSHA standards. Before making specific recommendations, NIOSH performs research and conducts a literature review of human and animal literature and other test systems. This information is assembled into a criteria document that OSHA often uses as a basis for its standards. This document contains information on hazards, material use, and control measures. The NIOSH paper on labeling hazardous chemicals, for example, formed the basis of the Hazard Communication Standard promulgated by OSHA in October 1985. NIOSH has more recently established the National Occupational Research Agenda (NORA) to lay out its plans and priorities for research activities in the near term.

Health Hazard Evaluations

At either employee or employer request, NIOSH may conduct a health hazard evaluation (HHE), which includes an industrial hygiene study and appropriate medical evaluation of an occupational health problem.

Training and Publications

The majority of the training and educational services provided by NIOSH are conducted at 15 educational resource centers (ERCs), which were established in 1977 because of the shortage of occupational health professionals. A variety of programs are offered, including occupational medicine residencies and graduate school training in occupational nursing, industrial hygiene, and safety. Physicians who desire training in occupational disease epidemiology may enroll in a 2-year program administered by NIOSH in conjunction with the CDC in the Epidemic Intelligence Service.

NIOSH publishes its findings in a variety of scientific journals and government publications including the CDC's *Morbidity and Mortality Weekly Report* (see Further Information, below). It also maintains a library, several databases, and a publication office to respond to inquiries about occupational safety and health concerns.

The physician can use several NIOSH publications when evaluating a patient who may have been exposed to a hazardous substance. Additional sources of information include the criteria documents and current intelligence bulletins (CIBs), which describe new scientific information about occupational hazards. A CIB may discuss a previously unrecognized hazard or report that a known hazard is more or less dangerous than previously considered.

Although NIOSH makes its own publications available to the public, it does not perform literature reviews for inquiring health personnel.

NATIONAL INSTITUTE OF ENVIRONMENTAL HEALTH SCIENCES

The National Institute of Environmental Health Sciences (NIEHS) conducts research on public health issues related to the environment. That research is often designed to provide information to the EPA to support its regulations.

One activity within the NIEHS is the National Toxicology Program (NTP). Toxicologic research is conducted within this program and historically has been focused on evaluating the potential of chemicals to cause cancer. The NTP is also required by Congress to issue a biennial report on carcinogens (5). Known or potential carcinogens identified in this report are required by OSHA to be identified on product labels and MSDSs.

MINE SAFETY AND HEALTH ADMINISTRATION

The Mine Safety and Health Administration (MSHA) was established by the Federal Mine Safety and Health Act of 1977. Its purpose is similar to that of OSHA except it covers only workers in the mining industry. Rules issued by MSHA are found in Title 30 of the CFR. Many of the standards promulgated by MSHA are similar to those issued by OSHA. In addition, there are regulations specific to the mining industry. For example, *health and safety training* is mandated for all new miners, and refresher teaching is required annually. All underground mines are inspected four times a year and all surface mines twice a year. NIOSH develops health standards for MSHA, but only advises OSHA concerning health standards. In general, health standards under MSHA place requirements on physicians regarding medical examinations that are similar to OSHA standards.

NUCLEAR REGULATORY COMMISSION

The Nuclear Regulatory Commission (NRC) has primary responsibility for regulating hazards from ionizing radiation, including x-rays, gamma rays, and radioactive material that can be taken into the body. Regulations issued by the NRC are found in Title 10 of the CFR. Part 20 covers radiation protection programs and occupational dose limits. Section 20.1703 requires that a physician determine a worker's ability to wear a respirator every 12 months. This is in contrast to OSHA's standard in which longer time intervals are acceptable.

Enforcement of NRC regulations is usually delegated to state departments of health. Medical examination requirements are typically included in the facility's operating license. Physicians providing services to employers with an NRC license should follow appropriate requirements. In addition, they should review potential exposures to radionucleotides. Specific biologic monitoring may be possible using whole-body counting or assaying urine samples for radioactivity. External radiation hazards are monitored with personal dosimeters. The results of such monitoring should be reviewed by the physician and explained to the employee.

DEPARTMENT OF TRANSPORTATION

Several Department of Transportation (DOT) agencies have issued regulations of potential interest to the physician practicing occupational medicine. These agencies include the Federal Aviation Administration (FAA) (pilots), the Federal Railroad Administration (FRA) (locomotive engineers), the Federal Highway Administration (FHA) (interstate commercial drivers), the U.S. Coast Guard (barge operations and unloading, etc.), and the Research and Special Programs Administration (RSPA) (pipeline workers). All of these agencies have issued regulations dealing with drug and alcohol testing (see Chapter 9).

Federal Aviation Administration

Title 14 of the CFR, part 67, includes the medical standards and certification requirements of the FAA. These standards are very detailed regarding medical or physical conditions that disqualify airmen and pilots. The standards also include qualifications regarding who can perform medical examinations. A physician who wants to examine pilots under these standards must become an aviation medical examiner approved by the FAA.

Federal Railroad Administration

Medical fitness requirements for railroad locomotive engineers are found in Title 49 of the CFR, section 240.119 related to substance abuse disorders, and section 240.121 covering vision and hearing acuity. Section 240.119 details specific conditions and time periods for return to service following alcohol or drug abuse. Section 240.121 details visual acuity and hearing threshold levels required for one to be certified as a locomotive engineer. After appropriate medical evaluation, a physician may conclude that someone can safety operate a locomotive despite not meeting the visual and hearing thresholds and may condition that certification on special instructions.

Federal Highway Administration

Truck drivers in interstate commerce must meet the physical qualifications required by the FHA. Sections 391.41 to 391.49 of Title 49, CFR, detail the specific examinations and criteria required to be used when examining interstate truck drivers. Physicians performing these examinations must carefully follow these rules.

EQUAL EMPLOYMENT OPPORTUNITY COMMISSION

The Equal Employment Opportunity Commission (EEOC) is charged with enforcing the Americans with Disabilities Act. This act and the EEOC regulations in Title 29 of the CFR, Part 1630, affect the practice of occupational medicine in three major areas. These regulations establish federal laws regarding the confidentiality of occupational medical records. They limit mandatory examinations and tests of employees to those that are job related. They also require "reasonable" accommodation of applicants or employees with medical impairments. Physicians who practice occupational medicine must have knowledge of employees' work assignments and the physical requirements of essential job functions to properly advise employers regarding the placement of persons with impairments (see Chapter 5).

ENVIRONMENTAL PROTECTION AGENCY

The EPA was established by presidential order in 1970. It is responsible for implementation of numerous acts of Congress promulgated to protect the environment. Although these laws should be of general interest to physicians in occupational medicine, most do not have a significant impact on the day-to-day activities of most physicians in the field. However, it is worth noting that standards related to the quality of air and water are increasingly being based on *health effects* rather than engineering technology. Cleanup criteria at hazardous waste sites are also based on potential health effects in addition to technical feasibility. Some physicians in occupational medicine may serve as consultants to government agencies or to private companies in coordinating and/or evaluating risk assessments related to proposed ambient air and water standards or cleanup criteria. Other physicians practicing clinical occupational medicine may be asked questions concerning such standards by their patients or by citizens in their community. While it is not necessary for most occupational physicians to have detailed knowledge of the specifics of environmental laws and regulations, it is desirable for them to become more knowledgeable concerning the concepts and process of *risk assessment* (see Chapters 42 and 58). The EPA also performs risk assessments for many specific chemicals. They are stored in a database called the Integrated Risk Information System (IRIS). This information is available on-line (see Further Information, below).

Several issues related to the risk assessment process have recently become the focus of attention by the EPA. These include an initiative that resulted in voluntary action by industry to perform toxicity screening tests on over 1,000 high production chemicals. Another includes activity related to chemicals that may have the potential to affect endocrine function. A third relates to children's health issues, especially those where children may be more susceptible than adults to the adverse health effects of chemicals.

Pressure from Environmental Defense, the environmental activist organization, resulted in the EPA sponsoring an initiative where manufacturers of high production volume (more than one million pounds per year) chemicals were encouraged to volunteer to review the available toxicity information on their products. If insufficient information was available, the manufacturers would agree to conduct the testing. Some of these reviews and testing will be conducted under EPA sponsorship. Some will also be conducted under sponsorship of the International Association of Chemical Industries (ICCA) so that there will be participation from manufacturers in Europe and Asia-Pacific. Activities under ICCA sponsorship will also require exposure estimation and/or measurement. Risk assessments will likely be performed using this exposure information and the hazard information derived from the testing. Exposure assessment and subsequent risk assessment is anticipated with the EPA-sponsored program, even though it is not formally required. Physicians practicing either environmental or occupational medicine will likely be asked questions regarding the risk of chemicals.

Recent concern with the potential for some chemicals to interfere with endocrine function has led the EPA to propose a voluntary testing program for what is called potential "endocrine disruption." Most chemicals have not been specifically tested for these effects, and there is debate whether traditional toxicity testing is adequate to identify these effects. Testing will produce information on the hazard of endocrine disruption. Exposure measurements and/or estimation will lead to risk assessments.

It is known that children are different from adults in how they metabolize some chemicals. They also have a higher intake of food per body weight than adults and eat different types of food. In some cases it is known that children are more susceptible than adults to adverse health effects. In a limited number of cases the reverse is true. For most chemicals there is insufficient information to provide a definitive answer to the question, Are children at greater risk from a similar exposure dose (e.g., mg/kg) than adults? In the absence of additional information, children are assumed to be ten times more susceptible. This rebuttal assumption will likely lead to additional testing to demonstrate whether children are really more susceptible than adults from exposure to specific chemicals. When it is demonstrated that there is no difference or a smaller difference than tenfold, the allowable exposure to children would be increased. This could be important to manufacturers of chemicals that are intentionally released to the environment, such as pesticides.

Physicians who practice occupational medicine should become familiar with two provisions of one of the environmental laws, the Toxic Substance Control Act (TSCA). Section 8(c) of this act requires manufacturers or users of a specific chemical to keep a record of any allegation of a heretofore-unknown adverse health effect. The purpose of these records is similar to that of adverse reaction reports for pharmaceuticals. If a company sees several similar reports, further investigation is warranted. Physicians practicing occupational medicine will often be the first to learn of a purported relationship between exposure to a substance and an adverse health effect. If it is a previously unknown effect, they should notify the manufacturer or user of the chemical or encourage the patient to do so.

Section 8(e) of TSCA requires manufacturers, producers, and users of chemicals to report to the EPA new information that reasonably supports the conclusion that the chemical or mixture presents a substantial risk of injury to health or the environment. Such information is often discovered during toxicity testing but may also be developed from investigations of 8(c) allegations. Occasionally, clinical information from a single case may be strong enough to warrant reporting. Section 8(e) reports are publicly available. This allows other users of the same substance to become informed so that they can take action to prevent adverse health effects. Early recognition of unrecognized health effects is an important role of the physician. Physicians learning of such effects should be encouraged to report new information to companies so that the TSCA 8(c) and 8(e) provisions work effectively.

AGENCY FOR TOXIC SUBSTANCES AND DISEASE REGISTRY

The Agency for Toxic Substances and Disease Registry (ATSDR) is a Public Health Service Agency created in 1980 under the Superfund legislation to implement the health-related activities of the Comprehensive Environmental Response, Compensation, and Liability Act (CERCLA). ATSDR is primarily concerned with the potential adverse health effects associated with environmental exposure to toxic substances. ATSDR's mission is to support activities designed to protect the public from the adverse health consequences of toxic chemical exposure. Specific responsibilities include health consultations at Resource Conservation Recovery Act sites and at hazardous chemical spills, such as an overturned railway car filled with toxic gases. Part of its mission is to conduct research about the health effects of toxic materials identified at these locations.

ATSDR is mandated to establish a disease and exposure registry to provide an information base of health effects of toxic substances. It also provides continuing education training for physicians through case studies in environmental medicine. In addition, it has developed medical management guidelines for treatment of some chemical overexposures.

REFERENCES

1. Felton JS. *Occupational medical management.* Boston: Little, Brown, 1990.
2. Rom WN, et al. *Environmental and occupational medicine,* 2nd ed. Boston: Little, Brown, 1992.
3. U.S. Department of Labor, Bureau of Labor Statistics. *Recordkeeping guidelines for occupational injuries and illnesses* (OMB No. 1220-0029). September 1986.
4. Doyle JR. Access to medical record standard. *Occup Env Med Rep* 1989;3:53.
5. *9th Report on Carcinogens, National Toxicology Program,* 9th ed. 2000. U.S. Department of Health and Human Services, Research Triangle Park, NC.

FURTHER INFORMATION

See the federal regulation that pertains to the agency of interest. The title and part or section is referenced in the text as the agency is discussed.

Morbidity and Mortality Weekly Report is published by the Massachusetts Medical Society, P.O. Box 9120, Waltham, MA 02254-9120.

Potentially useful Web sites to find out more information on regulatory and related agencies are as follows:

OSHA—*http://www.osha.gov*
NIOSH—*http://www.cdc.govnioshhomepage*
NIEHS—*http://www.niehs.nih.gov*
NTP—*http://ntp-server.niehs.nih.gov*
EPA—*http://www.epa.gov*
IRIS—*http://www.epa.goviris*
ATSDR—*http://www.atsdr.cdc.govatsdrhome*
Code of Federal Regulations—
http://www.access.gpo.govnavacfrindex

APPENDIX: AN OVERVIEW OF OSHA REGULATIONS

B. Hoffman

The OSHA regulations are contained in Title 29 of the Code of Regulations, part 1910 (29 CFR 1910). This part is divided into subparts A to Z, sections 1 to 1500.

Subpart A contains sections 1 to 7 under the title "General." It cites the references and applicability of the regulations, and defines the procedures established to appeal or amend them. This subpart has had one major change since its promulgation, which is the addition of 29 CFR 1910.7, titled "Definition and Requirements for a Nationally Recognized Testing Laboratory" (NRTL). It allows the establishment of privately owned NRTLs to test and certify OSH equipment of various kinds, similar to the way Underwriters Laboratory tests and certifies electrical equipment.

Subpart B contains sections 11 to 19 under the title "Adoption and Extension of Established Federal Standards." It deals with the construction and maritime trades. **Subpart C,** section 20, is titled "Access to Employee Exposure and Medical Records," and is very important to occupational physicians and industrial hygienists. **Subpart D** contains sections 21 to 32 under the heading "Walking and Working Surfaces." It deals with ladder safety, floor and wall openings, scaffolding, and fall protection. None of these three subparts has been the subject of major revisions.

Subpart E contains sections 35 to 40 under the title "Means of Egress." Major changes have been proposed for this subpart in the form of a new Confined Spaces regulation working its way through the process.

Subpart F, sections 66 to 70, deals with "Powered Platforms, Manlifts, and Vehicle-mounted Work Platforms." **Subpart G** contains sections 94 to 100, titled "Occupational Health and Environmental Control." It includes ventilation, noise exposures, and ionizing and nonionizing radiation exposures. There are no major changes in these subparts.

Subpart H, sections 101 to 120, deals with "Hazardous Materials." It gives specific instructions for the use and handling of specific materials, such as acetylene, hydrogen, oxygen, nitrous oxide, flammable and combustible materials, explosives, anhydrous ammonia, and hazardous waste operations and emergency response (HAZWOPs and ER; thus this section is sometimes referred to as "hazwoper"). This last regulation, 29 CFR 1910.120, HAZOPs and ER, is a major addition to the OSHA regulations, and is of concern to every industry or individual whose activities are affected by these regulations. It sets requirements for training of individuals involved in HAZOPs and in ER, and sets minimum requirements for safe operations of these activities. This subpart also contains section 29 CFR 1910.119, "Process Safety Management of Highly Hazardous Chemicals." This section defines a list of chemicals for which greatly extended written procedures and risk analysis documentation are required, and is a major addition to the OSHA regulations.

Subpart I, sections 132 to 140, deals with "Personal Protective Equipment." It covers general requirements, and eye and face, respiratory, head, foot, and electrical protective devices and measures. Significant changes to the respiratory protection standard were made in 1999.

Subpart J, containing sections 141 to 150, is titled "General Environmental Controls." It deals with sanitation, temporary labor camps, non-water carriage disposal problems, safety color codes for marking physical hazards, specifications for accident prevention signs and tags, and lock-out/tag-out regulations for energy sources. This last section, 29 CFR 1910.147, lock-out/tag-out, is a major revision.

Subpart K, sections 151 to 153, deals with "Medical Services and First Aid," and is of concern to occupational physicians. **Subpart L,** sections 155 to 165, deals with "Fire Protections." **Subpart M,** sections 166 to 171, is titled "Compressed Gas and Compressed Air Equipment." **Subpart N,** sections 176 to 190, deals with "Materials Handling and Storage." It covers servicing of wheel rims, powered industrial truck operations, crane operations, crawler locomotive operations, derricks, helicopters, and slings. These subparts have had fairly frequent changes, but no major revisions.

Subpart O contains sections 211 to 222 under the title "Machinery and Machine Guarding." **Subpart P,** sections 241 to 247, is titled "Hand and Portable Power Tools and Other Hand-held Equipment." **Subpart Q** contains sections 251 to 257 under the heading "Welding, Cutting and Brazing." **Subpart R** contains sections 261 to 275, and is titled "Special Industries." It contains regulations of operations in selected industries, including pulp, paper, pulpwood logging, agricultural operations, telecommunications, and grain handling facilities. There have been no major changes in any of these subparts.

Subpart S contains sections 301 to 399, under the heading "Electrical." It has had continual small changes since its promulgation, but no major changes. **Subpart T,** sections 401 to 441, is titled "Commercial Diving Operations." It is a special case, and has little application to most occupational health specialists. No major changes have occurred here, either.

Subparts U to **Y** are not used. These subparts are set aside for future regulations.

Subpart Z contains sections 1000 to 1500 and is titled "Toxic and Hazardous Substances." These are the sections in which all of the specific PELs and specific procedures for selected toxic materials are listed. This subpart has been the site for most of the changes in OSHA regulations, and includes one former and three recent major revisions. The oldest major revision is 29 CFR 1910.1200, the OSHA Hazard Communication Standard. When it was first promulgated, it was subjected to lengthy court challenges before finally being accepted. The first recent revision in subpart Z was the PEL update, in which OSHA attempted to change over 600 PEL values at one time. Previous PEL changes had been tackled one by one, and numbered only about 24 in the first 20 years of OSHA's existence. The PEL update was successfully challenged in court. There have been only two new chemical specific standards since the last edition of this book. OSHA has indicated it would like to set up a mechanism to issue several new standards at the same time. As of the publication of this edition, such a process had not been put in place.

The second recent revision was 29 CFR 1910.1450, titled "Occupational Exposure to Hazardous Chemicals in Laboratories." This section did not face major court challenges, since it supersedes existing provisions of the hazard communication regulations for laboratories, and is thus really a modification of OSHA's previous regulations. The final recent major change is section 29 CFR 1910.1030, titled "Bloodborne Pathogens." This section applies to every person or organization in which any person might be occupationally exposed to human blood or body fluids, such as emergency response teams, first-aid workers, and medical aid personnel.

4

Establishing an Occupational Health Program

William B. Patterson

Occupational health services are a core need of every business. Even in apparently low-risk occupations, employers are fiscally and legally responsible for injuries and illnesses that are caused or aggravated by the workplace. At the other extreme, certain industries are highly regulated and must spend considerable administrative resources and money in the effective management of their occupational safety and health risks. The first and most important variable affecting workplace health and safety is the attitude and skill set that employers bring to management of this responsibility. Some employers leave medical care of their injured workers to community-based, nonspecialist practitioners and let their workers' compensation insurer manage everything else. Large, regulated industries, especially those with hazardous work environments, often have sophisticated and extensive occupational safety and health programs.

The second key variable affecting the types of occupational health programs available to employers is the local population base and economic environment. Sparsely populated areas may have significant occupational health hazards, such as agriculture or a particular local industry, but there may not be a sufficient industrial base to support a comprehensive, specialized occupational health program. The occupational health needs of local employers will be met by local practitioners, who may find economic opportunity, intellectual challenge, and professional satisfaction in developing their skills in occupational and environmental medicine. In contrast, large industrial cities often support a wide variety of occupational health programs, including hospital-based programs, independent consultants, and clinic networks.

The third key variable influencing the development of occupational health programs is the philosophy and mission of the program sponsor(s). For example, a hospital may wish to establish an occupational health program primarily to strengthen its ties to local employers and industries. They may wish to ensure that the hospital-sponsored Health Maintenance Organization (HMO) is offered to local employees, to increase the likelihood of donations, or to attract downstream revenue in the form of emergency room visits, x-ray utilization, and operations. Academic occupational health programs may be interested primarily in complex and challenging cases of occupational disease and less interested in the provision of routine occupational health services, such as Department of Transportation (DOT) physicals and the treatment of back injuries. Such programs may be engaged in the education of occupational medicine or primary care residents and attached to schools of public health, and they can serve as an excellent resource for the evaluation of complex occupational health cases. Other occupational health programs include independent, union-based clinics, clinic networks, and various specialized delivery systems.

In all but the smallest occupational health program, there are several commonalties, which are reviewed in this chapter. These include the importance of a multidisciplinary team of health professionals and other support personnel, the value of managing the program with sound business practices, and the importance of providing services based on good medicine and consistent with the many legal constraints governing occupational health services.

This chapter provides an overview of occupational health programs for those wishing an introduction to the field. More detailed references are available (1). It is not meant to substitute for the business or administrative expertise necessary to manage a program, but we hope it will be helpful to those seeking an overview of the various occupational programs common in the United States. This chapter's context and framework also will be helpful to experienced occupational health practitioners.

PLANNING AN OCCUPATIONAL HEALTH PROGRAM

The first task facing an organization wishing to establish an occupational health program is to consider the goals, mission, and culture of the organization itself. The second critical task is to assess community needs or expectations of occupational health services. This may be accomplished in several ways, ranging from a sophisticated analysis of Dunn and Bradstreet employment and industrial data to checking the Yellow Pages for listings of occupational health physicians and programs. Employers considering establishing their own occupational health programs generally look at the regulations pertaining to their industry, the size of the workforce, their hazards, and their injury rate.

When the goals of the program have been decided and the community environment assessed, a business plan or economic analysis should be developed. Too often, occupational health programs are begun with unrealistic expectations regarding the volume of business, the likelihood of growth, or the level of profitability. For community-based physicians considering integrating some occupational medicine into their practices, factors to consider include the need to incorporate new knowledge into their practice and local competitive factors. In some states, mandated fees for workers' compensation reimbursement may limit profitability and economic viability of the program. In others, employer control over treatment of work-related conditions may facilitate practice growth.

TYPES OF PROGRAMS

Hospitals and health care organizations often see occupational health as a natural service to provide to the community. Further, they have their own occupational health needs (2). In their early stages, programs are sometimes associated with primary care clinics, residency training programs, or emergency rooms. Hospitals have a number of natural advantages in establishing occupational health programs, including their experience in the delivery of health services, the availability of ancillary services (such as x-ray, pulmonary function testing, hearing testing, and laboratory testing), their reputation, and access to multiple medical specialties. Already established ties with local businesses may aid in marketing and generating leads for new clients.

There are, however, several disadvantages faced by hospital organizations in the efficient delivery of occupational health services, each of which must be addressed in order for the program to operate successfully. Often, the most important challenge is philosophical: a commitment to client service being a cornerstone of successful occupational health programs. The flexibility and responsiveness required by an effective occupational health program is often difficult to execute in the hospital culture. An average occupational health clinic may gross $1–2 million in annual revenue, making it quite small in comparison to the total hospital budget. Decisions affecting the program are often made slowly, the administration may be distracted by larger problems, and the hospital community as a whole may not value the occupational health program mission. Additional problems facing hospitals include integrating the very different data management needs of an occupational health program with their own computer system, the need for competitive pricing, and the expectation of employers for frequent and effective communication. While these challenges have been overcome by many hospital-based programs, a good understanding of these obstacles and an organized plan to address them increase the likelihood of success.

Occupational health services may also be delivered by physicians who have established their own programs. These offices may have been spun-off from a hospital and be operated by a physician or be the result of a deliberate start-up. Strengths of the private practice model include the flexibility and autonomy available to the physician-manager, the ability to offer highly customized or specialized services to local employers, and the financial advantages that accrue from ownership. Challenges faced by physicians owning and operating small occupational health programs include competition from larger occupational health programs and the need for additional business expertise and resources, which may be difficult to obtain for small practitioners. When such a practice reaches about $1.5 million in annual revenue, it often needs a substantially higher level of business and administrative support than is available to physician-owners.

One major trend in the delivery of occupational health services is the growth of for-profit or privately held occupational health networks. Ranging in size from 3 to 300 offices, such networks are playing an increasing role in the delivery of occupational health services in the United States. Large, multisite networks have substantial advantages over other occupational health programs in depth of resources. There are certain economies of scale (information technology, purchasing, administration) which aid such networks in competition with other providers of occupational health services. By leveraging sales and marketing across regions, such networks can gain significant market share in selected communities. Professional collegiality may also be promoted if there are established procedures to engage providers in the company as a whole, a useful strategy since occupational medicine practice can feel quite isolating for physicians. The challenges facing large networks include balancing necessary standardization with local autonomy, balancing bottom-line pressures with quality of care and with working conditions, and identifying ways to work cooperatively with local health organizations.

Historically, a disproportionate number of occupational and environmental medicine (OEM) physicians were employed by public corporations. Changes in American business practice have substantially reduced this number, but large employers often operate on-site employee occupational health programs, which vary greatly in complexity. A manufacturing plant of several hundred workers or a municipality may employ a part-time nurse in a small office, while a plant of several thousand employees using hazardous technologies or substances may have a full occupational health department with a physician and other OEM professionals and support staff. Employers providing occupational health services on-site see advantages in provider knowledge of the workplace, in ongoing relationships with employees, and in improved access to care, resulting in reduced time away from work for injured employees. Employer-based programs are also more likely to provide an extended range of health services, including health promotion, disease management, and absentee monitoring (3) (see Chapters 11 and 12). In contrast, employers who have reduced their investment in on-site services have pointed out that establishing and managing occupational health services is outside the scope of their core business and better left to vendors of occupational health services. With an emphasis on the bottom line and difficulty in accurately calculating the cost-effectiveness of an occupational health program, continued investment in on-site services may prove difficult for corporate managers.

When employers outsource their occupational health programs, they may turn to any of the types of vendors described above. A corporation outside a municipal area may hire a local primary care physician on a part-time basis who has expressed interest in and spent some time studying OEM. Multinational corporations may contract with large vendors of occupational health services, while small to medium-sized employers near cities are more likely to contract with local occupational health programs for staffing and support.

This discussion has covered some of the more common occupational health programs, but there are many others. Unions have played an important role in the history of occupational health and safety in the United States (4,5). In the early 1900s, many important organizing battles were fought over safe working conditions. One hundred years later, many unions have paid less attention to occupational health and safety, focusing their energies on job security, salary, and benefits. Nevertheless, union supported occupational health programs have an important place in selected locations in delivering occupational health services to their members. Some unions hire OEM physicians on a consultative basis to ensure that government standards are met and that scientific research is interpreted appropriately or to aid in lobbying for stronger regulatory protection in the workplace.

A number of universities have established internal occupational health programs, primarily to meet the needs of the parent institution. Other occupational health programs focus exclusively on the management of specialty occupational health services such as service to federal agencies, managing surveillance programs, or providing legal and high-level technical support for complex cases. A detailed description of such programs is outside the scope of this chapter, but OEM physicians should appreciate the large number of career options available to them.

BUSINESS RELATIONSHIPS

At the core of every occupational health program is a relationship between the client and the health care professional. In primary care practice, the physician almost always assumes an ethical obligation to advocate for the patient. Occupational medicine is different. Inevitably there are pulls on the provider from several directions, including the opinion hoped for by the employer, the expectation of medical treatment from the employee, the goal of profitability by the program manager, and the requirement to comply with existing government regulations. Unfortunately, the history of occupational medicine has been stained by episodes when occupational physicians withheld information or treatment regarding workplace hazards from their patients or the public (6–8). Conflicts of this nature still occur (9–12).

Ethically, occupational health professionals must be on constant guard in the management of their relationships with their clients (13,14). Several core behaviors are critical to supporting ethical occupational health practice. These include ensuring that opinions rest upon sound science, being up to date regarding regulatory and legal constraints, having honest insight regarding the degree to which the provider may be subject to various influences, practicing and discussing dilemmas with other occupational health professionals, and adhering to codes of occupational health ethics (see Chapter 2).

For most community-based occupational health programs, formal contracts with clients are not necessary. Contracts written by lawyers are often complicated and constraining. Many occupational health programs providing services to hundreds of clients find it administratively burdensome and unnecessary to have separate contracts with each client. Contracts are more typically used when an occupational health program is providing a large dollar volume of services to a major employer or working with a government agency. Individual physicians providing contract medical services to a large corporation should expect to sign a contract or a professional service agreement.

Even in the absence of contracts, occupational health programs should ensure that any agreements regarding the types and prices of services, the nature and means of communication, and lines of authority are made clear at the beginning of a business relationship. Too often, in the eagerness to grow an occupational health program, insufficient attention is paid to the details of agreements, generating friction and dissatisfaction in the early stages of the relationship.

Employers utilizing occupational health services in the community generally do not expect those services to be exclusive. While the occupational health program may wish to have 100% of the client's occupational health business, employers often use another occupational health program for reasons such as hours of operation or specialized services. Exclusivity of service is generally earned and should not be expected by occupational health programs.

Several key relationship variables influence how occupational health services are delivered, whether by a community-based primary care physician or a large network of occupational health providers managing a comprehensive medical surveillance program. First, the influence of the occupational health professional on the client's health and safety program varies greatly. For example, in a corporation with a strong commitment to occupational and environmental health and safety, a senior occupational physician may wield considerable influence, and the occupational health program may be fully integrated into the operations of the company. In the community, an occupational health provider may be kept at arm's length by company health and safety personnel, limiting the OEM professional's involvement to simply treating injuries and performing basic examinations. OEM professionals providing services must be prepared for a range of relationships and effectiveness with their clients.

A second key variable that affects the relationship between the OEM physician and the employer/client is the flow of information. This may vary from free and complete to limited and incomplete. Access to the workplace in the form of a workplace walk-through (see below) should be considered basic information. Many Occupational Safety and Health Administration (OSHA) standards (e.g., asbestos, hazard communication, respiratory protection) require that the employer provide certain information to the occupational health professional. Unfortunately, too often employers do not comply with this part of relevant OSHA standards. Under the OSHA Access to Medical Records Standard (1910.1020), occupational physicians have a right of access to information regarding employee exposures, information that may be necessary for the proper evaluation of an occupational health problem. OEM physicians and professionals should advocate appropriately for the free flow of information necessary to effectively manage patients, evaluate workers, comply with government regulations, and work with employees and employers to prevent occupational injuries and illnesses.

Ultimate responsibility for health and safety in the workplace rests with the employer, not the OEM physician. This responsibility is recognized under the Americans with Disabilities Act (ADA) (see Chapter 5) (15), OSHA standards, workers' compensation laws (see Chapter 18) (16), and employment laws. Despite this, OEM physicians may have the opportunity to assume considerable responsibility for health and safety in selected workplaces, based on their own skills, leadership ability, and the culture of the employer.

THE TEAMS

In perhaps no other specialty of medicine is the physician interacting so freely with individuals of so many job titles, with varied expertise and responsibility. This section reviews the key team members of both the occupational health program and the client with whom the program must interact. Good verbal and written communication skills are key to the management of the relationships among team members and between teams. Programs with well-trained, clinically competent physicians have sometimes foundered due to arrogance, lack of responsiveness, or ineffective communication by the occupational health provider.

The Program Team

The physician in the occupational health program is primarily responsible for delivering and supervising clinical services. In addition, an unappreciated responsibility of the OEM physician is to oversee the provision of specialty testing, such as pulmonary function and audiograms. These and other ancillary tests often have standards or regulations [e.g., American Thoracic Society pulmonary function standards (17), and Council for Accreditation in Occupational Hearing Conservation (CAOHC) hearing standards (18)] of which non-OEM professionals may be unaware. The OEM physician may or may not become involved in the management of other business aspects of the program, depending on the size of the program, the personal skills and interests of the physician, and the parent organization. Physicians may also supervise on-site occupational health nurses (19).

Most occupational health programs have an operations manager, who is responsible for staffing, patient and paper flow, scheduling, and all the routine operations necessary to run an office. As a program expands, additional individuals may be hired to assume responsibility for specific functions, such as billing.

Another basic component of most occupational health programs is sales and marketing (20). In smaller programs, this function is often delegated to a nurse or a clinical staff member with an interest in outreach and communication. In larger occupational health programs, sales professionals will usually assume this responsibility.

Occupational health programs employ various clinical staff to perform the routine functions of the medical office. Unlike most medical practices, such staff are usually cross-trained in everything from urine and drug collection and pulmonary function testing to phlebotomy and basic wound management. Such cross-training may be constrained by local or state regulation (e.g., taking x-rays), but it may serve as a source of career satisfaction for clinical personnel seeking work variety and responsibility.

Management of the "back-office staff" represents an important component of a successful occupational health program. Some hospital programs delivering high-quality clinical services have failed because billing and collections were not managed efficiently. Other functions that may be necessary depending on the size of the program and scope of services include bookkeeping, care coordinators, and secretarial support.

Most community-based occupational medicine programs place a strong focus on early return to work and reduced disability time and costs for injured or ill workers. In achieving these goals, there is often a close relationship between the delivery of clinical occupational health services and rehabilitation services. In some cases, the rehabilitation program may be owned and operated by the same corporate parent (e.g., hospitals, large networks). In other situations, the occupational provider may have a close but noncontractual relationship with a local vendor of rehabilitation services. In certain cases, state regulations or laws may govern these relationships.

The Employer Team

A good relationship with the employer representatives responsible for occupational health and safety is useful for the occupational health physician. The most important variable is the person who is ultimately responsible for occupational health and safety at the employer's site(s). In some cases, it may be a senior vice president, who takes an active interest and provides effective leadership in health and safety. Among other employers, the responsible person may be a lower level office manager, with or without any training or interest in the field. The more sophisticated and committed the client manager is to an effective occupational health and safety program, the more effective and satisfying the working relationship with the occupational program is likely to be.

In some companies, occupational health and safety is assigned to the human resources (HR) function. More commonly, occupational health and safety is either within manufacturing or a separate department of environmental health and safety. The number of health and safety professionals on-site varies greatly based on the size of the employer, ranging from none to over 25, a sophisticated, multidisciplinary department in a small site of 5–10 specialists. Larger employers may have industrial hygiene professionals, safety engineers, and occupational health nurses, all of whom will interact with the provider of the occupational health services.

Employees are an important and underutilized resource for health and safety in the workplace. The degree to which employers successfully engage their employees in an ongoing manner in a commitment to a safe workplace will have a large influence on both employee attitude toward health and safety and the frequency and severity of occupational incidents. There is increasing evidence regarding the value of safety committees, and OSHA may be promulgating a safety committee standard in the near future.

Many employers have access to Employee Assistance Programs (EAPs) (see Chapter 28), which are a valuable resource for employees with emotional or social difficulties, whether related to work or to their situation outside of work. It is very helpful to the OEM professional to have an awareness of the mental health resources available to employees and to develop a working relationship with those mental health professionals.

In summary, a working knowledge of the employer's occupational and environmental health and safety team greatly facilitates the effective delivery of occupational health services. A commitment to relationship building between the occupational health program and the employer's health and safety team will increase access to information, trust in clinical decision making, and the likelihood that prevention recommendations will be followed.

OCCUPATIONAL MEDICINE AS A PUBLIC HEALTH DISCIPLINE

The practice of occupational and environmental medicine is at its core a field within preventive medicine. Board-certified OEM physicians are trained in the various disciplines of public health, which are often unfamiliar to other practicing physicians. These include health law (see Chapter 2), health systems (see Chapter 19), toxicology (see Chapter 39), health statistics, epidemiology (see Chapter 40), and the delivery of health promotion services to large groups (see Chapter 12). Corporations of varying sizes may have substantial commitments to the maintenance of a healthy workforce and have a serious interest in the prevention of work-related morbidity, reducing absenteeism, and improving worker productivity.

Theoretically, most occupational health injuries and illnesses are preventable (21). Unfortunately, injuries described by Ramazzini in his classic text of 1777 (22) are still recognized today. Occupational health programs and providers should have a good working knowledge of the basic principles of prevention and should advocate preventive measures in the workplaces where they provide services.

Public health professionals classify prevention as having three components: primary, secondary, and tertiary. *Primary prevention* is any intervention that identifies and attempts to reduce risk factors for disease or injury in the workplace. In clinical practice, immunization against infectious disease would represent a primary prevention. *Secondary prevention* refers to the early detection of disease, allowing intervention before symptoms or complications appear. The goal is to reverse, halt, or retard the progression of a disorder. The detection of cervical cancer by periodic testing is an example of secondary prevention in clinical practice. *Tertiary prevention* refers to efforts to minimize the effect of disease and disability by effective treatment, thereby altering disease progression, reducing the likelihood of complications, and preventing further morbidity. In the clinical setting, effective management of arthritis with a multidisciplinary program would qualify as tertiary prevention. Effective occupational health programs integrate all three types of prevention in their consultation to clients and their delivery of occupational health services. OEM physicians should recognize that there is both an important scientific foundation and many legal requirements that support the development and implementation of prevention programs.

PRIMARY PREVENTION PROGRAMS

The National Institute of Occupational Safety and Health (NIOSH) has defined a hierarchy of controls aimed at preventing work-related injuries and illnesses (Table 4.1). Although the effectiveness of control decreases as the employer moves down the list, most effective occupational health programs use all of these measures. An informed occupational health professional may play an important role in advising the employer regarding the seriousness of the hazards and the availability of preventive measures. Substitution of a toxic substance in the workplace by a safer one or of a physically hazardous operation by automation may dramatically reduce the risk of injury or illness in the workplace. While the design and operation of engineering controls are usually not the responsibility of the OEM physician, occupational health and safety professionals are in an ideal position to interpret industrial hygiene reports regarding exposures and to advise companies regarding the health implications and risks of the measured exposures. With an understanding of human factors, ergonomics, and the physiologic workload of protective equipment, OEM professionals play an important role in implementing all the preventive measures in NIOSH's hierarchy.

An unrecognized basic primary prevention measure is the safety committee. Safety committees typi-

TABLE 4.1. *Hierarchy of controls*

Substitution
Enclosure
Engineering controls
Personal protective equipment
Administrative controls

cally include employees with different responsibilities and from multiple levels within the organization. While OEM physicians in the community often do not sit on safety committees of their clients, occupational health programs based in hospitals or universities often have the OEM physician as a key player in the organization's safety committee. Some safety committees, unfortunately, are no more than generators of written policies, but an effective safety committee can successfully engage employees at all levels of the organization in a commitment to a healthy and safe workplace.

Based on the toxic substances used in a workplace, industrial hygiene monitoring may be an important primary preventive measure. In certain situations, OSHA mandates periodic monitoring of hazardous substances in an effort to keep exposures to employees at levels unlikely to cause disease. The OEM physician, by review of Material Safety Data Sheets (MSDSs) and chemical processes, may identify other potentially hazardous substances, exposure to which should be measured on a routine basis (see Chapter 2).

Another way in which the OEM physician serves primary prevention is to provide information to employees and employers regarding health hazards and their control. In some cases, this may include participating in the employer's hazard communication program, such as counseling individual workers regarding the importance of safe work practices or the proper use of personal protective equipment in order to prevent toxic exposures.

There has been increasing interest in programs designed to effectively match workers to their job. Historically, examiners sometimes applied arbitrary and unjustified criteria in the preplacement evaluation process, thereby excluding individuals who would have been able to safely perform their job. To protect workers from inappropriate, unscientific discrimination, the Americans with Disabilities Act (ADA) was passed in 1990. It is described in greater detail in Chapter 5, and all physicians practicing occupational health medicine should have a working knowledge of this important law.

The first step in establishing whether potential employees are capable of performing the job for which they are being considered is to develop a job description. A *functional job description* outlines the job requirements, including exposures to biologic, chemical, and physical hazards. The specific physical tasks that the employee must perform are an important component of the functional job description. The functional job description can then be used by the occupational health professional to develop an appropriate testing protocol to ensure that the prospective employee is medically qualified to perform the essential functions of the proposed job or to determine any accommodations to essential job functions that may be indicated.

SECONDARY PREVENTION PROGRAMS

Secondary prevention programs in the workplace are designed to detect occupational injuries or illnesses at an early stage, before the worker has developed symptoms or a complication. As in the case of primary prevention, secondary prevention programs typically involve several professional disciplines.

Medical surveillance is the systematic evaluation of employees to monitor for the early occurrence of disease or to detect biomarkers of exposures (see Chapter 41). Occupational physicians play an important role in selecting the conditions for which surveillance will be performed, defining the surveillance protocol (23), and communicating results to employees.

There is increasing interest in health promotion and disease prevention programs in the workplace. As data have accumulated documenting the cost-effectiveness of these programs (24–26), more employers have begun implementing programs designed to reduce and prevent absenteeism, control health insurance costs, and improve worker productivity. The occupational physician may play an important role in the design and implementation of such programs, which may include health risk appraisals, individualized counseling for employees with multiple risk factors or high-risk diseases, or screening in the workplace for non–work-related medical conditions (see Chapter 11).

TERTIARY PREVENTION AND CLINICAL CARE

Tertiary prevention involves the clinical management of workers who are injured or ill and appropriate rehabilitation (vocational and physical) to maximize their work capacity, minimize the effects of disease, and improve their long-term outcome. A full-range of clinical services falls under this category, from first aid for a bruise to comprehensive rehabilitation for major trauma.

There are several aspects to the delivery of clinical occupational health services that are different from the delivery of clinical services outside the occupational health setting, some of which are nonintuitive for providers who have not been trained in OEM. In the workers' compensation system (see Chapter 18) the employer is directly responsible for the bill, has a legal right of access to information regarding the case, and has an expectation that the employee will return to work as promptly and as completely as possible. This legal protection for the employer may be unsettling to physicians without OEM experience. However, there is good evidence that the longer patients stay out of work for any reason, the less likely they are to return to work (27). Therefore, it is in the economic interest of the employer, and it is in the physical and personal interest of the employee to seek prompt and effective treatment and to return to work as quickly as possible.

There have been many changes in effective management of work-related injuries in recent years. Whereas formerly, bed rest was believed to be helpful for back injuries, it has now been demonstrated that bed rest is ineffective and perhaps counterproductive (28). Whereas community-based physicians are often counseled not to see patients too frequently, most occupational health programs see their patients on a weekly basis in order to effectively monitor therapy and home exercise, response to medication, activities of daily living (ADL), and safe assignment to restricted work. Since the costs to employers of indemnity payments (partial wage replacement under workers' compensation) are much higher than the costs of medical services, employers are almost always happy to have their employees seen more frequently in order to get the patient back to work, thereby reducing indemnity and total costs to the employer.

Another difference between primary care practice and occupational health practice is the management of information. While most physicians appropriately take confidentiality quite seriously, employers have a legal right to information regarding the work-related condition. Occupational health physicians should be careful to communicate only details of the work-related condition to the employer and to maintain as confidential other medical information that is gathered as part of the routine history taking and that may be sensitive and confidential.

Injured or ill workers often assume that the primary loyalty of the occupational health physician is to the employer, but attitudes vary depending on past experience, the provider's reputation, and the attitudes of the employer. Alternatively, workers may assume that the occupational health provider will advocate for them no matter what and that everything they say will be confidential. The effective OEM physician should always offer an independent opinion, carefully evaluating each case on its merit and recommending treatment or restrictions that are consistent with the clinical case. Providers must avoid either being too sympathetic to workers who may ask for excessive time away for work or too eager to please their employer-client who may inappropriately push people to return to full duty too quickly.

Another aspect of occupational medicine practice that is different from primary care practice is that the OEM physician's clinical care will be audited and evaluated by many people, health professionals and administrators. This may seem invasive, but the OEM physician must recognize the legal obligation of the employer to ensure compliance with government regulations and the fiduciary responsibility of the insurance company to the employer for quality care. Among those who may be auditing physician charts/records are reviewers for accurate completion of DOT forms, case managers, claims adjusters, other physicians, the patients and their advisors, union members, lawyers, and government representatives. OEM physicians should document their care and communication based on the assumption that whatever they put down will be reviewed by others.

Conscientious occupational health programs will also develop an internal audit system in order to ensure quality of care to injured or ill workers and compliance with applicable regulations. Hospital-based occupational health programs are often included in the inspections conducted by the Joint Commission on Accreditation of Healthcare Organizations (JCAHO) and are subject to many standards, while non–hospital-based programs usually do not participate. There may be state standards that pertain to occupational health programs, and the Commission on Accreditation of Rehabilitation Facilities (CARF) promulgates standards for physical therapy and rehabilitation. The Association of Occupational and Environmental Clinics (AOEC) has a well-defined set of criteria for clinic membership that include internal audit and an inspection program (29). For a clinic to be a part of the AOEC network, it must meet these standards and pass a peer-reviewed inspection by other OEM professionals. Quality improvement is a basic responsibility of program management that is aimed at ensuring the quality of care delivered and the continuous education and improvement of the providers within the program.

Managing communication is an important responsibility of every occupational health program. Protocols and policies must be developed to manage the tremendous flow of information back and forth between employer and provider. These should include consent forms, protection of confidential medical information, documentation of verbal telephone conversations, and policies regarding electronic transmission of patient information. The Health Insurance Privacy and Accountability Act (HIPAA) of 1996 sets standards regarding electronic transmission of identifiable patient information (30). Occupational health programs should be sure that their policies are consistent with this federal act. Employee training regarding the management of communication is also important, to guard against the inadvertent release of confidential medical information.

One important consideration is the professionalism with which employers manage the information internally. Some employers are conscientious, restricting access to medical information and carefully guarding confidential information. Others are less aware of this potential problem, delegating sensitive medical issues to untrained staff. The occupational health professional can play an important role in the education of employers and their representatives in the proper management of medical information. Since employers have a legal right to information regarding workers' compensation, details regarding work-related injuries may circulate among appropriate employer personnel and their vendors of insurance and disability management services. Sometimes employers fail to appreciate the difference between workers' compensation medical information and other medical information that may be inappropriately transmitted while performing fitness for duty or other examinations. Occupational health providers should take care to minimize the medical information that is transmitted to employers, focusing on an accurate description of a person's capabilities, ability to perform job functions, and recommended restrictions or other administrative controls.

THE WORKPLACE WALK-THROUGH

Occupational physicians require certain data in order to provide effective occupational health services. Just as cardiologists expect an electrocardiogram (ECG) and pulmonologists expect a pulmonary function test, knowledge of the workplace is a fundamental responsibility of occupational health providers (31).

In delivering occupational health services to a new client, efforts should be made to obtain information regarding the workplace. Often, an informal walk-through, a review of appropriate MSDSs, and an orientation to the health and safety program is sufficient for the provider to adequately provide occupational health services to the employees. Generally, such a walk-through will take 1 to 2 hours and be part of the orientation of the new client to the occupational health program and of the provider to the workplace. Such a walk-through will be especially helpful in establishing the relationship between the provider and the injured employee. It facilitates medical care when employees from the company arrive and the provider is able to say, "I have been to your workplace and understand your job." In some cases, a workplace walk-through is less helpful, particularly for common industries with which the provider already has experience. For example, a provider who has toured several nursing homes or trucking terminals may not need to tour each new client in these industries. Nevertheless, efforts should be made, usually by a personal meeting or discussion with the client representative, to determine what factors particular to that employer are relevant to the delivery of effective occupational health services.

Some employers have useful job descriptions, industrial hygiene reports, and loss-control reports. Occupational health programs should encourage employers to share such information with the occupational health provider. It is often unrealistic to maintain records of job descriptions in large programs that have hundreds of clients, but efforts should be made to obtain detailed job descriptions when necessary for the evaluation of individual cases.

THE COMPREHENSIVE WORKPLACE WALK-THROUGH

In selected situations, it is helpful for the occupational health provider to perform a comprehensive workplace walk-through. This will generally be performed when providing comprehensive services to large employers with multiple hazards or when an employer wishes to implement a more comprehensive health and safety program. In other situations, the employer may want a detailed provider review of a specific hazard or process in the workplace. The role of the occupational physician is to bring a public health and preventive orientation to the evaluation of the workplace, identifying potential hazards in a comprehensive way and recommending appropriate preventive measures.

PRE–WALK-THROUGH PREPARATION

Before conducting a workplace walk-through, there are several steps that the OEM physician should take. First, the physician should identify the contact person and reach a good understanding of the goals of the walk-through and its timing. For example, if the walk-through will take several hours, it is a good idea for the employer to set aside that time and not expect that it will take only one hour. Additionally, it is a good idea to let the employer know ahead of time that the provider expects to speak to employees in an open-ended and nonthreatening way. Further, it is very important to be sure that the walk-through is scheduled at a time that will allow the physician to observe normal work practices and activities in the workplace. In selected situations, this may mean scheduling the walk-through very early in the morning (e.g., trucking terminals). The provider should ask whether special clothing, footwear, or personal protective equipment will be necessary. The provider may also wish to request permission to photograph selected workplace processes or hazards, either for educational purposes or for orientation of other providers.

A pre–walk-through telephone conference allows the provider to gather basic information regarding the likely exposures and industrial processes that will be seen and regulations that cover the workplace. The provider can then use this information to familiarize him- or herself with the health hazards associated with these exposures and industrial processes and the regulations themselves (32–35). The provider may ask for copies of any industrial hygiene or inspection reports to review ahead of time. If the occupational health program information system allows, it is helpful to review the services and types of injuries that have been provided to an existing client. Such pre–walk-through preparation will be extremely valuable to the provider in making observations in the workplace, questioning employer representatives, and promoting confidence in the provider's knowledge base and expertise.

OPENING CONFERENCE

A comprehensive walk-through generally begins with an opening conference. This allows the provider to obtain an overview of the company, its structure and administration, its existing occupational health and safety programs, and its identified problem areas. Employer representatives who typically will be present at such a conference include those who are responsible for health and safety, human resources, and (sometimes) maintenance and engineering. It is always desirable to have representatives of employees present as well, and providers should ask for such representation. At the opening conference, the provider can ask about the types of injuries the company is experiencing, applicable OSHA standards, and other pertinent regulations and laws.

Additional information pertinent to the opening conference includes the history of the plant and parent company. For example, changes in materials or work processes may mean that past exposures (e.g., asbestos, heavy metals, PCBs) may have put exposed workers at risk of current or future illness. The history of personal protective equipment availability and use may be helpful, since workers may not have been protected from noise or other hazards. The demographics of workers should also be explored, including the number of workers, the sex ratio, the primary language, educational background, turnover, and shift work. All of these factors influence the risk of injury or illness and the selection of health and safety educational programs, and will help the provider to understand the workers themselves.

The health and safety services of the employer should be reviewed. These include the organization of health and safety responsibility, the workers' compensation insurance carrier, substance abuse testing programs, emergency procedures, training and education of employees, and the various health and safety programs for that workplace. It is desirable to review the company's OSHA 300 log to get a better idea of injury patterns and company familiarity with OSHA record-keeping requirements.

THE WALK-THROUGH

It is generally best to perform a walk-through beginning at incoming shipping and receiving and following the natural manufacturing or other processes in the workplace. This gives the occupational health physician an understanding of the actual processes that occur. During a walk-through it is important to speak to workers, as they will often have their own ideas regarding health and safety hazards or potential preventive measures. This will also initiate a relationship between the physician and the workers and will give the physician an indication of the workers' understanding of their job and potential hazards and their attitude toward their work and safety. Appropriate questions for workers might include the following: What kind of hazards are there in your particular job? What measures do you take to keep yourself safe? What kind of preventive measures do you think might be helpful in this workplace?

In performing the walk-through, the occupational health professional should pay attention to the following four general categories of risk: the task, the environment in which the task is being performed, the equipment that is being used, and the worker (Table 4.2). In viewing the *task,* the provider should carefully look at worker factors such as body position and pos-

TABLE 4.2. *Workplace walk-through checklist*

I. The task
1. Is work performed in shifts?
2. Are hours of work reasonable?
3. Are adequate rest periods provided and used?
4. How much overtime is worked? Is it required?
5. Are tasks rigidly paced?
6. Do workers have any input in work design?
7. Are changes in work procedures explained to workers?
8. Are extended periods of heavy work required?
9. Is there any visual strain?

A. Physical demands
1. How much lifting, pulling, pushing is required?
2. What is the frequency of the physical task?
3. What are the locations of the physical actions?
4. Are unusual or uncomfortable working positions required?
5. Are workers required or induced to work at excessive speeds?
6. Can work be performed while following all safety rules?
7. Are workers thoroughly trained?
8. Is training available in their languages?
9. Is work done sitting, standing, or walking or is there a combination of positions?

B. Mental demands
1. Are directions easy to follow?
2. Are frequent decisions necessary?
3. Are lengthy periods of concentration required?
4. Are there rest periods during monitoring or inspection tasks?
5. Is the work pace too fast?
6. Does the job create boredom?
7. Are social interactions possible?
8. Does the worker have a sense of control over the work?
9. How are labor management relations?

II. The environment
1. Is adequate space for working available?
2. Is the workstation comfortable to use or does it require unusual positions, straining, or stretching?
3. Is a clear path of egress provided for emergency escape and are exits well marked?
4. Are working surfaces slippery or unnecessarily hard?
5. Are there protruding objects (handles, knobs, materials, etc.)?
6. Are there any blind corners?
7. Is the work space safe from materials handling equipment, such as trucks and cranes?
8. Is the work space located in an unnecessarily hot, cold, drafty, noisy, or contaminated area?
9. Is the temperature comfortable?
10. Are there temperature extremes experienced?
11. Is the relative humidity comfortable?
12. Is there adequate general ventilation?
13. Are all ventilation, heating, and cooling devices working properly?
14. Is the lighting appropriate for the work?
15. Is the housekeeping effective?

III. The equipment
1. Is equipment or machinery difficult to operate?
2. Are controls hard to reach?
3. Does movement of controls require excessive effort?
4. Can controls be moved without placing hands, wrists, arms, or body in unusual positions?
5. Are controls on materials handling equipment compatible with operator characteristics?
6. Are gauges and instruments easy to read and understand?
7. Are the characteristics of hand controls compatible with the forces required to operate them (shape, size, surface), and are forces acceptable?
8. Are emergency shut-offs accessible from locations where an operator might get caught?
9. Are lockouts provided and are they foolproof?
10. Are the functions of all controls labeled or readily apparent?
11. Are the functions of controls logical and compatible with operator stereotypes or expectancies?
12. Are chairs or stools comfortable?
13. Are they adjustable for proper height?
14. Are appropriate backrests provided?
15. Is there adequate space for legs and feet?

TABLE 4.2. *Continued*

16. Are working surfaces of the proper height so as not to cause unnecessary reaching, bending, stretching, etc.?
17. Do working surfaces cause glare?
18. Are foot pedals used to operate equipment?
19. Are foot pedals guarded?
20. Are foot pedals used by standing operators?
21. Are all guards and safety devices in use and in good working condition?
22. Do they interfere with operation or maintenance in any way?
23. Does equipment vibrate or cause excessive noise?
24. Is mobile equipment stable?
25. Does material handling equipment allow unobstructed vision in all necessary directions?
26. Are containers used and are size, height, and weight satisfactory?
27. Are any parts of the body exposed to continuous or repeated motions of equipment?

A. Hand tools
1. Are tools easy to hold?
2. Are tools too heavy?
3. Are there sharp edges?
4. Are there pinch points?
5. Is use of tool difficult (e.g., hard to squeeze, twist, slippery, etc.)?
6. Does tool vibrate?
7. Are power tools noisy?
8. Does use require unusual or uncomfortable hand, wrist, arm, shoulder, or body position?
9. Are tools maintained properly?
10. Is there a selection of tools?

B. Personal protective equipment (PPE)
1. Is personal protective equipment provided?
2. Is personal protective equipment adequate, comfortable, and effective?
3. Are personal protective devices required?
4. Are devices selected or fitted properly?
5. Are they comfortable or are they causing added irritation?
6. Are they properly maintained?
7. Do protective devices obscure vision or create other hazards themselves?
8. Do protective devices produce false sense of confidence?
9. Are there written policies and procedures regarding PPE use? Is PPE training effective?
10. Is there good compliance with PPE use?

IV. The worker
1. How many workers are there?
2. What is the age distribution of the workforce?
3. What languages do the workers speak?
4. What is the turnover rate?
5. What educational background do the workers have?
6. What is the physical condition of the workforce?
7. What medical problems are common in the workforce?
8. What psychosocial resources are available to workers in the workplace?
9 What psychosocial resources are available to workers in the community?
10. Is the workforce unionized?

ture. What kind of movements are required by the worker? Observation of the physical effort may include measuring or observing the force required, the direction of the movements (forward, backward, etc.), the location (floor to waist or above shoulder-level), the frequency (once per hour or once per minute), and the duration (sustained for several minutes or intermittent).

Understanding of the task itself should include such aspects of work practices as productivity expectations, variation in physical demands during the day, and how the job is compensated. For example, is there a quota system or an incentive system? Incentive pay for productivity may increase the risk of cumulative-trauma disorders by promoting continuous, sustained exertion by employees.

In evaluating the *environment,* the OEM professional should review workplace conditions such as temperature, ventilation, labeling, vessels and pipes, housekeeping, sanitary facilities, and lighting. The degree of crowding, the ambient noise, and the general appearance of the workplace are all relevant to safety and the likelihood of injuries or illnesses. For example, an increase in the ambient noise can stimulate the sympathetic nervous system and increase the likelihood of accidents. There is evidence that a reduction in general noise level is accompanied by a reduction in accidents (36,37). Poor housekeeping may increase the risk of accidents by the presence of oil or water on the floor and the persistence of trip and fall hazards. Signage and labeling, chemical storage, emergency preparations and equipment such as eye-wash stations, automatic emergency defibrillators (AEDs), and first aid and fire equipment can be check and evaluated for working order, suitability, and location.

Providers should remember that environmental conditions may vary over the course of a year. A manufacturing process that generates considerable heat (e.g., chemical manufacturing) may provide a comfortable work environment in the winter or spring but entail a risk of heat stress in the summer. A loading dock where substantial materials handling takes place may also entail a risk of heat stress in the summer. Similarly, an unheated warehouse may be comfortable in the summer but quite cold in the winter. Long exposure to heat or cold is each associated with specific health risks, which may be prevented by specific measures.

The *equipment* with which employees work includes their own equipment, other machines, and the ventilation system. There are many design aspects to hand tools with which the OEM physician should become familiar. These include size and composition of the handle, tool automation (automatic screw drivers), torque control, and hand-tool suspension. Hand tools should be inspected for such aspects as ergonomic fit, appropriate use for the job, and maintenance (Table 4.2). For example, the design of the hand tool influences its position of use. The shape and composition of the handle influence the comfort of use and the likelihood that the prolonged use of this tool will increase the risk of cumulated-trauma disorder. At employer sites that use hand tools extensively, there should be a well-developed program of tool selection, and employees should be offered options depending on their own demographics and preferences.

Machinery can be inspected for ergonomics, effectiveness, and maintenance. The presence and effectiveness of safety devices for the machines should be carefully reviewed. Modern machine design has dramatically reduced the risk of major traumatic injuries (power presses and cutting devices), but these safety devices must not be bypassed or modified, and workers must be carefully educated in their use and effectiveness. In many environments, machines themselves are ventilated.

The four basic components of a local ventilation system are *hoods* to capture a contaminant, *ducts* to carry the contaminant away, *filters* to clean the air before it is discharged or recirculated, and *fans* to power the system. OEM health providers should have a good working knowledge of how a ventilation system works and potential problems (38). Unfortunately, ventilation systems in workplaces are not always properly designed to control the health hazard. For example, the hood may not effectively capture the contaminant because it is not close enough or encapsulating enough of the process. A duct system may not be properly balanced or maintained. The cleaning devices may be inappropriately selected for the specific contaminant or not changed frequently enough. Finally, fans may lack sufficient power to carry the contaminant through the duct system. An effective occupational safety and health program should have a well-designed program to monitor the effectiveness of a local ventilation system, and the OEM provider should ask enough questions to ensure that the program is effective.

Dilution ventilation is the general exhaust of air from a workplace and the replacement of an appropriate portion with outside, fresh air. The purpose of general ventilation is to maintain comfort for workers by controlling humidity, removing unpleasant odors, and maintaining a comfortable ambient temperature. A portion of air in every general ventilation system is recirculated to control the costs of conditioning the air. An insufficient supply of "makeup" air from the outside may contribute to the buildup of carbon dioxide, nonspecific irritants, or identifiable contaminants in the workplace. Dilution ventilation is appropriate to control by-products of the work processes (e.g., smoke) only if these products are not toxic and are present at very low levels. Care must be taken to ensure that the exhaust of the general ventilation is not close to any intake air vents on the outside of the building.

The workplace walk-through provides the opportunity for OEM professionals to directly observe the workers. When providers see only injured workers or those with other problems in the clinic, their attitude toward a workplace may be affected by selection bias. A walk-through gives the provider a feel for the workforce as a whole. By observing the age, apparent physical condition, and other demographics of the workforce, the provider may be able to advise the employer regarding other interventions such as health promotion programs and screening programs. Speaking to the workers during a walk-through can be very enlightening with respect to worker attitude toward health and safety, their knowledge of the hazards, and their feelings about work.

AFTER THE WALK-THROUGH

After a comprehensive walk-through, the provider should always send the employer a written report that documents the provider's observations and recommendations and helps guide the employer in improving the health and safety of the workplace. This report should generally begin with a summary statement, identifying the major manufacturing processes, the important occupational health hazards, and suggested preventive measures.

The body of the report should contain more detailed discussions of each hazard identified (Table 4.3), the rationale for preventive measures, and suggestions for preventive measures. The hierarchy of controls (Table 4.1) should be used. In all cases, worker education and training should be part of the recommended preventive measures (39).

The OEM provider should generally supply additional resources to the employer to support the report's recommendations. For example, the OSHA standard inspection procedures and interpretations applicable for a specific hazard are readily available on the OSHA Web site (40). The Public Health Statements of the Agency for Toxic Substances and Disease Registry (ATSDR) Toxicological Profiles (41) may be provided to employers for use in employee education. Finally, the provider should convey the findings to other staff of the occupational health program. This aids providers in their understanding of the workplace, the operations staff in their efficient delivery of services, and the sales staff in identifying additional opportunities.

CONCLUSION

Occupational morbidity and mortality is an important public health problem in the United States. The delivery of high-quality occupational health services to workers can be a satisfying career or a meaningful portion of a medical practice. The vast majority of injured or ill workers appreciate high-quality medical care and are interested in prompt recovery and return to work. An effective occupational health program plays an important public health role in both treating injured and ill workers and in preventing injuries and illnesses from occurring. Whether the occupational health program is a large clinic or part of a primary care practice, the basic principles of high-quality medical care, effective communication and management, and a commitment to prevention form the foundation of success.

TABLE 4.3. *Hazard analysis*

What is the exposure?
What are the sources of the exposure?
What is the nature of the exposure: frequency, amount, pure, contaminated?
What control measures are present?
How effective are the control measures?
What are the ambient environmental conditions that affect exposure?
What is the interaction of the worker with the exposure?
What preventive measures are recommended?

ACKNOWLEDGMENTS

The author acknowledges the administrative support of Joan Giacomozzi in preparation of this chapter.

REFERENCES

1. Moser R Jr. *Effective management of occupational and environmental health and safety programs: a practical guide,* 2nd ed. Beverly Farms, MA: OEM Press, 1999.
2. McCunney RJ. *Medical center occupational health and safety.* Philadelphia: Lippincott Williams & Wilkins, 1999.
3. Harris JS, et al. *Integrated health management: the key role of occupational medicine in managed care, disability management, productivity, prevention, and integrated delivery systems.* Beverly Farms, MA: OEM Press, 1998.
4. Abrams HK. A short history of occupational health. *J Public Health Policy* 2001;22:34–80.
5. Derickson A. The United Mine Workers of America and the recognition of occupational respiratory diseases, 1902–1968. *Am J Public Health* 1991;81:781–789.
6. Tweedale G. Science or public relations?: the inside story of the Asbestos Research Council, 1957–1990. *Am J Ind Med* 2000;38:723–734.
7. Lilienfeld DE. The silence: the asbestos industry and early occupational cancer research—a case study. *Am J Public Health* 1991;81:791–800.
8. Bayer R, ed. *The health and safety of workers.* New York: Oxford University Press, 1988.
9. Kern DG. The unexpected result of an investigation of an outbreak of occupational health lung disease. *Int J Occup Environ Health* 1998;4:19–32.
10. Shuchman M. Secrecy in science: the flock worker's lung investigation. *Ann Intern Med* 1998;129:341–344.
11. Davidoff F. New disease, old story (editorial). *Ann Intern Med* 1998;129:327–328.
12. Kern DG. Confidentiality agreements and scientific independence. *Med Decis Making* 1998;4:239.
13. Rest KM, Patterson WB. Ethics and moral reasoning in occupational health. *Semin Occup Med* 1986;1:49–57.
14. Brodkin AC, Frumkin H, Kirkland KH, et al. AOEC position paper on the organizational code for ethical conduct. *J Occup Environ Med* 1996;38:869–881.
15. Goren WD. *Understanding the Americans with Disabilities Act.* Chicago: American Bar Association, 2000.
16. Menzel NN. *Workers' comp management from A to Z,* 2nd ed. Beverly Farms, MA: OEM Press, 1998.
17. American Thoracic Society. Standardization of spirometry. *Am J Respir Crit Care Med* 1995;152:1107–1136.
18. Suter A. *Hearing conservation manual,* 3rd ed. El-

dridge, IA: Council for Accreditation in Occupational Hearing Conservation, 1993.
19. Rogers B, et al. *Occupational health nursing guidelines for primary clinical conditions,* 2nd ed. Beverly Farms, MA: OEM Press, 1996.
20. Leone FH. *A comprehensive guide to occupational health sales and marketing,* 2nd ed. Santa Barbara, CA: Ryan Associates, 1998.
21. Weeks JL, Levy BS, Wagner GR, ed. *Preventing occupational disease and injury.* Washington, DC: American Public Health Association, 1991.
22. Ramazzini B. *Diseases of workers.* Chicago: University of Chicago Press, 1940.
23. Lauwerys RR, Hoet P. *Industrial chemical exposure guidelines for biological monitoring,* 3rd ed. Boca Raton, FL: Lewis Publishers, 2001.
24. Pelliter KR. A review and analysis of the clinical and cost-effectiveness studies of comprehensive health promotion and disease management programs at the worksite: 1998–2000 update. *Am J Health Promot* 2001;16:107–116.
25. Aldana SG. Financial impact of health promotion programs: a comprehensive review of the literature. *Am J Health Promot* 2001;15:296–320.
26. Golaszewski T. Shining lights: studies that have most influenced the understanding of health promotion's financial impact. *Am J Health Promot* 2001;15:332–340.
27. Bigos S, Bowyer O, Braen G, et al. *Acute low back problems in adults.* Clinical Practice Guideline No. 14. AHCPR Pub. No. 95-0642. Rockville, MD: Agency for Health Care Policy and Research, Public Health Service, U.S. Department of Health and Human Services, December, 1994.
28. Bigos S, Bowyer O, Braen G, et al. *Acute low back problems in adults.* Clinical Practice Guideline No. 14. AHCPR Pub. No. 95-0642. Rockville, MD: Agency for Health Care Policy and Research, Public Health Service, U.S. Department of Health and Human Services, December, 1994.
29. The Association of Occupational Environmental Clinics. 1010 Vermont Avenue, NW, #513, Washington, DC 20005.
30. 45 CFR 164. Security and Privacy.
31. Kornberg JP. *The workplace walk-through.* Boca Raton, FL: Lewis Publishers, 1992.
32. Burgess WA. *Recognition of health hazards in industry: a review of materials and processes.* New York: John Wiley & Sons, 1995.
33. DiNardi SR. *The occupational environment—its evaluation and control.* Fairfax, VA: American Industrial Hygiene Association (AIHA), 1997.
34. Sullivan JB, Krieger G. *Clinical environmental health and toxic exposures,* 2nd ed. Philadelphia: Lippincott Williams & Wilkins, 2001.
35. Wald PH. *Physical and biological hazards of the workplace,* 2nd ed. New York: Wiley-Interscience, 2002.
36. Cohen A. The influence of a company hearing conservation program on extra-auditory problems in workers. *J Safety Res* 1976;8:146–162.
37. Schmidt JW, Roster LH, Pearson RG. Impact of an industrial hearing conservation program on occupational injuries for males and females. *J Acoust Soc Am* 1980;67[suppl 1]:S59.
38. Burgess WA. *Recognition of health hazards in industry: a review of materials and processes.* New York: John Wiley & Sons, 1995.
39. Wallerstein N, Rubenstein HL. *Teaching about job hazards: a guide for workers and their health providers.* Washington, DC: American Public Health Association, 1993.
40. *www.osha.gov.*
41. *www.atsdr.cdc.gov.*

5

Understanding the Americans with Disabilities Act

Kent W. Peterson and D. Gary Rischitelli

In 1990, the U.S. Congress enacted Public Law 101-336, the most far-reaching civil rights legislation in recent history with the following words:

> The Congress finds that...some 43,000,000 Americans have one or more physical or mental disabilities, and this number is increasing as the population as a whole is growing older;...historically, society has tended to isolate and segregate individuals with disabilities, and, despite some improvements, such forms of discrimination against individuals with disabilities continue to be a serious and pervasive social problem;...the continuing existence of unfair and unnecessary discrimination and prejudice denies people with disabilities the opportunity to compete on a equal basis and to pursue those opportunities for which our free society is justifiably famous, and costs the United States billions of dollars in unnecessary expenses resulting from dependency and nonproductivity" (1).
>
> The Americans with Disabilities Act of 1990 (PL101-336)
>
> July 26, 1990

Eleven years later, President George W. Bush reflected on the accomplishments of the Americans with Disabilities Act as follows:

> Eleven years ago today, people from across America gathered to celebrate the signing of the Americans with Disabilities Act of 1990 (ADA), one of the Nation's most important civil rights laws since the Civil Rights Act of 1964. The ADA opened up the true promise of America to people with disabilities who, for far too long, have found impediments to getting an education, getting a job, or just getting around...
>
> Much has been accomplished in the past 11 years. Attitudes are changing and barriers are coming down all across America. Employers now provide a range of "accommodations" to ensure that employees with disabilities can keep their place in the wage-earning world, resulting in unprecedented economic opportunities...
>
> In fact, the message of the ADA is being heard all around the world. Over 40 countries, from Australia to Uganda, now have laws prohibiting discrimination against people with disabilities—many of them inspired by the ADA...
>
> The Americans with Disabilities Act was an unprecedented step forward in promoting freedom, independence, and dignity for millions of our people. On this, the 11th anniversary of the Americans with Disabilities Act, I remain committed to tearing down the remaining barriers to equality that face Americans with disabilities today" (2).

The Americans with Disabilities Act (ADA) is intended to bring those with physical and mental disabilities into the mainstream of American society. The ADA provided yet another measure of federal protection against improper discrimination in the workplace. Previously, the Equal Pay Act of 1963 had prohibited gender-based discrimination in pay for substantially equal work (3). Title VII of the Civil Rights Act of 1964 prohibited employment discrimination based on race, color, religion, sex, or national origin (4), and the Age Discrimination in Employment Act (ADEA) of 1967 prohibited discrimination against workers who are 40 years of age or older (5).

The ADA filled an important gap by providing protection to individuals with disabilities in the private sector and in state and local governments. Employees of the federal government and employees of federal contractors had already been afforded similar protection under the Rehabilitation Act of 1973 (6), and the ADA built upon many provisions of Section 503 and 504 of the Rehabilitation Act.

The subsequent Civil Rights Act of 1991 made major changes in the federal laws against employment discrimination. Enacted in part to reverse several Supreme Court decisions that limited the rights of persons protected by these laws, this Act also provided additional protections, such as authorizing compensatory and punitive damages in cases of intentional discrimination, and providing attorneys' fees and the possibility of jury trials. The U.S. Equal Employment Opportunity Commission (EEOC) enforces all of these laws *(http://www.eeoc.gov)*.

Under Title VII, the ADA, and the ADEA, it is illegal to discriminate in any aspect of employment including hiring and firing; compensation, assignment, or classification of employees; transfer, promotion, layoff, or recall; job advertisements; recruitment; testing; use of company facilities; training and apprenticeship programs; fringe benefits; pay, retirement plans, and disability leave; or other terms and conditions of employment.

Prohibited discriminatory practices under these laws also include harassment on the basis of race, color, religion, sex, national origin, disability, or age; retaliation against an individual for filing a charge of discrimination, participating in an investigation, or opposing discriminatory practices; employment decisions based on stereotypes or assumptions about the abilities, traits, or performance of individuals of a certain sex, race, age, religion, or ethnic group, or individuals with disabilities; and denying employment opportunities to a person because of marriage to, or association with, an individual of a particular race, religion, national origin, or an individual with a disability.

The "relief" or remedies available for employment discrimination, whether caused by intentional acts or by practices that have a discriminatory effect, may include back pay, hiring, promotion, reinstatement, front pay, reasonable accommodation, or other actions that will place individuals in the same circumstances or with the same benefits that they would have received in the absence of discrimination. Remedies also may include payment of attorneys' fees, expert witness fees, and court costs. Under most EEOC-enforced laws, compensatory and punitive damages also may be available where intentional discrimination is found. Punitive damages are not available against the federal, state, or local governments.

The employer also may be required to take corrective or preventive actions to cure the source of the identified discrimination and minimize the chance of its recurrence, as well as discontinue the specific discriminatory practices involved in the case.

BASIC ADA PROVISIONS

The ADA addresses four areas: Title I covers employment; Title II covers access to public services; Title III deals with public accommodations and services operated by private entities, including hospitals and medical clinics; and Title IV covers telecommunications. This chapter primarily focuses on Title I employment provisions as they affect employee health and safety.

The employment provisions of the ADA apply to all private employers, state and local governments, and educational institutions that employ 15 or more individuals. The law also covers private and public employment agencies, labor organizations, and joint labor–management committees controlling apprenticeship and training. In addition to the ADA, many states have disability discrimination laws that may have even broader application to smaller employers or organizations.

The federal government is covered by Sections 501 and 505 of the Rehabilitation Act of 1973, which incorporates the requirements of the ADA. However, different procedures are used for processing complaints of federal discrimination.

Discrimination is prohibited in recruitment, advertising, job application procedures, hiring, upgrading, promotion, transfer, layoff, termination, and return from layoff or rehiring. Discrimination pertains to pay rates or other compensation, job assignments, job classifications, organizational structure, position descriptions, lines of progression, seniority lists, leaves of absence, sick or other leave, fringe benefits, training, and social or recreational programs.

Discrimination means not making a reasonable accommodation to a known physical or mental limitation of an otherwise qualified individual with a disability. Unless the disability and the required accommodation are obvious, the duty to accommodate must first be initiated by a request from the applicant or employee. The examining health professional can play a significant role in helping to initiate or facilitate this process both with the employer and with appropriate vocational rehabilitation professionals.

It is helpful to distinguish between the responsibilities of individuals, of management, and of health professionals in this process. The individual applicant or employee must make the employer aware of a "hidden" disability and request a reasonable accommodation. Management is responsible for making employment decisions and must face the legal consequences. As a result, the health professional becomes an expert advisor, responsible for providing management with sufficient information to make its own decision and thus be accountable. A health professional may function in multiple roles: as a company agent and member of a management team, as a contract physician or nurse, or as a private treating physician or other health professional. The health professional may find him/herself with multiple duties and responsibilities: obtaining, interpreting, and holding confidential medical information; communicating with personal physicians and consultant specialists; and negotiating or mediating between worker and employer. The ADA forces occupational health professionals to sharpen their awareness of these overlapping and sometimes conflicting roles.

The ADA does not override other health and safety requirements established by other federal laws. This allows certain blanket exclusions to remain (e.g., Department of Transportation Federal Motor Carrier Safety Administration driver qualification criteria). If a standard is required by another law, the employer does not need to show that it is job related or consistent with business necessity. However, the employer still has an obligation to determine whether a reasonable accommodation is possible. When the ADA conflicts with health and safety provisions of state and local laws, the situation is less clear.

In preparing for Title I implementation, the EEOC prepared detailed regulations (7), interpretive guidance, and an extensive technical assistance manual (8). Subsequent cases in the federal courts have conflicted with some interpretations by the EEOC, leading to additional interpretive statements and revisions of previously published guidelines. Impending cases currently under review in the U.S. Supreme Court will further refine or even reverse previous practices under the ADA. Readers are cautioned to stay abreast of recent developments under the ADA, many of which can be easily be accessed through government Web sites (e.g., *http://www.eeoc.gov; http://www.supremecourtus.gov)*.

KEY CONCEPTS, TERMS, AND DEFINITIONS

Terminology is instructive about the evolution of thinking in our society. The term *handicapped* (allegedly taken from beggars with caps in hand) yielded to *disabled* (those lacking certain abilities) and, more recently, to individuals with *disabilities*. Speaking of the handicapped or the disabled creates a label with a sense of inherent limitation. The current term emphasizes the person first and only secondarily any disability that he or she might have. It also reflects the ADA's strong emphasis on considering each individual situation on a case-by-case basis.

Distinctions among pathology, impairment, functional limitation, and disability are fundamental to an understanding of the social and employment context of disability. *Pathology* is an interruption or interference with normal bodily processes or structures. It occurs at a structural level within cells and tissues. *Impairment* is the loss and/or abnormality of mental, emotional, physiologic, or anatomic structure or function. It includes all losses or abnormalities including pain, not just those attributable to active pathology. It occurs at an organ system level. *Functional limitation* is a restriction or lack of ability to perform an action or activity in the manner or within the range considered normal. Functional limitation results from impairment. It occurs at the level of action or activity performance of the whole person or organism. *Disability* is the inability or limitation in performing socially defined activities and roles expected of individuals within a social and physical environment. It occurs on a societal level, i.e., in the performance of tasks within the social and cultural context.

The relationship among impairment, functional limitation, and disability varies enormously from individual to individual, based on biologic, psychological, social, environmental, lifestyle, and cultural factors. Some employees with apparently minimal impairment appear to have severe functional limitations and to be disabled. Conversely, many individuals with major impairments and limitations experience minimal disability.

The ADA prohibits discrimination on the basis of disability in all employment practices. To interpret and implement the ADA, it is critical to understand several important ADA definitions to know who is protected by the law and what constitutes illegal discrimination. The following definitions have been issued by the EEOC:

Individual with a Disability

An individual with a disability under the ADA is a person who (a) has a physical or mental impairment that substantially limits one or more major life activities, (b) has a record of such an impairment, or (c) is regarded as having such an impairment. Major life activities are activities that an average person can perform with little or no difficulty such as walking, breathing, seeing, hearing, speaking, learning, and working.

Qualified Individual with a Disability

A qualified employee or applicant with a disability is someone who satisfies skill, experience, education, and other job-related requirements of the position held or desired, and who, with or without reasonable accommodation, can perform the essential functions of that position.

Reasonable Accommodation

Reasonable accommodation may include, but is not limited to, making existing facilities used by employees readily accessible to and usable by persons with disabilities; job restructuring; modification of work schedules; providing additional unpaid leave; reassignment to a vacant position; acquiring or modifying equipment or devices; adjusting or modifying examinations, training materials, or policies; and providing qualified readers or interpreters. Reasonable accommodation may be necessary to apply for a job, to perform job functions, or to enjoy the benefits and privileges of employment that are enjoyed by people without disabilities. An employer is not required to lower quality or production standards to make an accommodation. An employer generally is not obligated to provide personal use items such as eyeglasses or hearing aids.

Undue Hardship

An employer is required to make a reasonable accommodation to a qualified individual with a disability unless doing so would impose an undue hardship on the operation of the employer's business. Undue hardship means an action that requires significant difficulty or expense when considered in relation to factors such as a business's size, financial resources, and the nature and structure of its operation.

Prohibited Inquiries and Examinations

Before making an offer of employment, an employer may not ask job applicants about the existence, nature, or severity of a disability. Applicants may be asked about their ability to perform job functions. A job offer may be conditioned on the results of a medical examination, but only if the examination is required for all entering employees in the same job category. Medical examinations of employees must be job related and consistent with business necessity.

Other key definitions are set forth in Table 5.1.

The ADA's tripartite definition of disability takes into account not only current actual disability but also the powerful potential for discrimination against those with a past history of impairment (e.g., addiction, back pain, cancer) or who become inappropriately labeled as disabled (e.g., being treated as if one were HIV positive or using illicit drugs).

Courts continue to refine the definition of disability under the ADA. For example, a recent series of cases from the U.S. Supreme Court severely curtailed the ADA's broad definition of disability by stating that disability had to be evaluated in light of any potential mitigating interventions such as visual or hearing aids, prosthetics, medications, or other medical treatments (9).

Similarly, the U.S. Supreme Court also recently reiterated that merely submitting evidence of a medical diagnosis of impairment is insufficient to establish that one has a disability for the purposes of the ADA. Because of the wide individual variation in response to impairment, disability is defined in terms of its effect on the person's major life activities. A substantial limitation of a major life activity means that an individual's activities are restricted "to a large degree" or in a "considerable way." Major life activities must in fact be "major" and are therefore activities "that are of central importance to most people's daily lives" (10).

Determining what is a disability under the ADA for employment purposes is largely a managerial, not a medical, decision. Health professionals make technical medical judgments about pathology, impairment, and functional limitation within a framework of generally accepted medical principles and practice (11). Established medical diagnostic criteria such as the AMA's *Guides to the Evaluation of Permanent Impairment* are intended to bring objectivity and uniformity to the process (12). The technical medical information must then be applied to the human resource management process. The ADA places clear responsibility upon management to make appropriate decisions about disability, direct threat to the health of the individual or others, and reasonable accommodation, taking into consideration information provided by the applicant/employee, occupational health professionals, personal physicians, rehabilitation specialists, psychologists, and others.

Provision of Reasonable Accommodation

Employers are required to provide reasonable accommodation to qualified individuals with disabilities who are employees or applicants for employment,

TABLE 5.1. *Definitions from the Americans with Disabilities Act (ADA)*

Disability (with respect to an individual):
- A physical or mental impairment that substantially limits one or more of the major life activities of such individual;
- A record of such an impairment; or
- Being regarded as having an impairment.

Physical or mental impairment:
- Any physiological disorder, or condition, cosmetic disfigurement, or anatomic loss affecting one or more the following body systems: neurologic, musculoskeletal, special sense organs, respiratory (including speech organs), cardiovascular, reproductive, digestive, genitourinary, hemic and lymphatic, skin and endocrine; or
- Any mental or psychological disorder, such as mental retardation, organic brain syndrome, emotional or mental illness, and specific learning disabilities.

Major life activities:
- Functions such as caring for oneself, performing manual tasks, walking, seeing, hearing, speaking, breathing, learning, and working.

Substantially limits:
- Unable to perform a major life activity that the average person in the general population can perform; or
- Significantly restricted as to the condition, manner or duration under which an individual can perform a particular major life activity as compared to the average person in the general population.

Qualified individual with a disability:
- An individual with a disability who satisfies the requisite skill, experience, education and other job-related requirements of the employment position such individual holds or desires, and who, with or without reasonable accommodation, can perform the essential functions of such position.

Reasonable accommodation:
- Modifications or adjustments
  - To a job application process that enable a qualified applicant with a disability to be considered for the position; or
  - To the work environment, or to the manner or circumstances under which the position held or desired is customarily performed, that enable a qualified individual with a disability to perform the essential functions of that position; or
  - That enable a covered entity's employee with a disability to enjoy equal benefits and privileges of employment as are enjoyed by its other similarly situated employees without disabilities.

Direct threat:
- A significant risk of substantial harm to the health or safety of the individual or others that cannot be eliminated or reduced by reasonable accommodation. The determination that an individual poses a "direct threat" shall be based on an individualized assessment of the individual's present ability to safety perform the essential functions of the job. This assessment shall be based on a reasonable medical judgment that relies on the most current medical knowledge and/or on the best available objective evidence. In determining whether an individual would pose a "direct threat," the factors to be considered include:
  - The duration of the risk;
  - The nature and severity of the potential harm;
  - The likelihood that the potential harm will occur; and
  - The imminence of the potential harm.

From Equal Employment Opportunities for Individuals with Disabilities. Equal Employment Opportunity Commission; Final Rule. *Federal Register* 1991 (July 26);56(144):35735–35736.

unless doing so would cause an undue hardship for the employer. According to the EEOC, "An accommodation is any change in the work environment or in the way things are customarily done that enables an individual with a disability to enjoy equal employment opportunities." There are three categories of reasonable accommodations:

> (i) modifications or adjustments to a job application process that enable a qualified applicant with a disability to be considered for the position such qualified applicant desires; or
>
> (ii) modifications or adjustments to the work environment, or to the manner or circumstances under which the position held or desired is customarily performed, that enable a qualified individual with a disability to perform the essential functions of that position; or
>
> (iii) modifications or adjustments that enable a covered entity's employee with a disability to enjoy equal benefits and privileges of employment as are enjoyed by its other similarly situated employees without disabilities (13).

Part-time, full-time, temporary, and probationary workers are entitled to reasonable accommodation, but the individual with a disability must first request an accommodation. In some situations, a family member, friend, health professional, or other representative may request the accommodation on behalf of the worker. This request does not obligate the employer to provide the requested accommodation. It is, instead, the first step in a process of information exchange between the individual and the employer.

The employer and the worker must cooperatively identify the nature of the disability and what the worker needs to be reasonably accommodated. The worker does not have to specify the precise accommodation required, but should be able to describe the barriers encountered in performing the essential functions of the job, and the employer may ask the individual relevant questions that will permit an informed decision about the request. Suggestions from the individual with a disability are particularly valuable in determining the type of reasonable accommodation needed. Where the individual or the employer is not familiar with possible accommodations, there are extensive public and private resources to help the employer identify reasonable accommodations, such as the Job Accommodation Network (see Further Information, below).

When the disability and/or the need for accommodation is not obvious, the employer may ask the individual for reasonable documentation about his/her disability and functional limitations. The employer may ask the employee for information describing the impairment; the nature, severity, and duration of the impairment; the activity or activities that the impairment limits; and the extent to which the impairment limits the employee's ability to perform the activity or activities. An employer cannot ask for documentation when (a) both the disability and the need for reasonable accommodation are obvious, or (b) the individual has already provided the employer with sufficient information to substantiate that s/he has an ADA disability and needs the reasonable accommodation requested (13).

The reasonable accommodation process never requires the employer to eliminate an essential job function, i.e., a fundamental duty of the position. If a disabled individual is unable to perform the essential functions, even with reasonable accommodation, s/he is not an otherwise "qualified" individual with a disability. An employer is also not required to lower production standards (quality or quantity), but an employer may have to provide reasonable accommodation to enable an employee with a disability to meet the production standard.

A proposed employment modification, restriction, or adjustment satisfies the ADA's reasonable accommodation obligation if it is effective, i.e., it enables the individual to perform the essential functions of the position. If there are two possible reasonable accommodations, the employer may choose the less expensive or less burdensome accommodation. The employer may choose among many reasonable accommodations as long as the chosen accommodation is effective. Thus, as part of the accommodative process, the employer may offer alternative suggestions for reasonable accommodations and evaluate their effectiveness in removing workplace barriers for the individual with a disability.

The only statutory limits on an employer's obligation to provide reasonable accommodation is that no such change or modification is required if it would cause undue hardship on the employer. Undue hardship addresses the technical, financial, or other limitations on an employer's ability to provide reasonable accommodation. Undue hardship means significant difficulty or expense when evaluated in light of the resources and circumstances of a particular employer. Undue hardship refers not only to financial difficulty, but also to accommodations that are unduly extensive, substantial, or disruptive, or those that would fundamentally alter the nature or operation of the business.

Direct Threat to Oneself or Others

The ADA allows employers to refuse to hire or to terminate an individual who constitutes a "direct threat" to the health or safety of the individual or others that cannot be eliminated or reduced by reasonable accommodation. The EEOC went beyond Congress's provision for threats only to others; it allows exclusion for a direct threat to oneself, but only at a very high level of risk. This difference in interpretation is scheduled for review by the U.S. Supreme Court in 2002 (14).

The employer must show a "significant risk of substantial harm" (i.e., a high probability of serious injury). It is not enough to conclude that an individual is simply at some increased risk compared to other workers, or that the worker may have posed a direct threat in the past or may do so at some uncertain time in the future. To prove that a direct threat exists, the specific risk must be identified and evaluated based on four factors:

1. the duration of risk
2. the nature and severity of potential harm
3. the likelihood that the potential harm will occur
4. the imminence of the potential harm

The assessment of risk must be based on objective medical or other evidence related to a particular individual. It cannot be based on blanket exclusions or stereotypes about the nature or effect of a particular disability. The regulations specifically call for reasonable medical judgment that relies on the most current medical knowledge and/or best available objective advice. Often this means reviewing past medical records, requesting additional testing, obtaining specialty consultations, and reviewing published medical literature. Failure to do so prospectively may create significant liability for the employer if the decision is subsequently challenged and appears to be arbitrary, ill-informed, or hasty.

Even if a significant risk of substantial harm can be demonstrated, the employer must determine whether a reasonable accommodation can reduce the risk to below the level of a direct threat. Decisions must be made on a case-by-case basis, looking at the specific risk posed by each individual, information provided by the individual, the person's experience in previous similar positions, and opinions of physicians, rehabilitation counselors, physical therapists, and other professionals.

IMPACT OF ADA ON OCCUPATIONAL HEALTH PRACTICE

The ADA impacts many occupational health policies and procedures, and the role of the occupational health professional in general. Table 5.2 highlights some ways in which prior practices have been affected by the ADA. Fortunately, many employers and occupational health services providers long ago adopted the approach required under the ADA, for example by operating under Sections 503/504 of the Rehabilitation Act of 1973. However, compliance with the ADA demands a more sophisticated approach to occupational health services delivery.

Occupational medical examinations are performed for many purposes, including employment entrance and periodic health evaluation, medical screening and surveillance, symptomatic evaluation and fitness for duty, impairment and disability evaluation, and return to work (15). Title I of the ADA substantially limits an employer's ability to make disability-related inquiries or require medical examinations preoffer, postoffer, and during employment. At the first stage (prior to an offer of employment), the ADA prohibits all disability-related inquiries and medical examinations, even if they are related to the job. At the second stage (after an applicant is given a conditional job offer, but before s/he starts work), an employer may make disability-related inquiries and conduct medical examinations, regardless of whether they are related to the job, as long as it does so for all entering employees in the same job category. At the third stage (after employment begins), an employer may make disability-related inquiries and require medical examinations only if they are job-related and consistent with business necessity (16).

A "disability-related inquiry" is a question (or series of questions) that is likely to elicit information about a disability. A "medical examination" is a procedure or test that seeks information about an individual's physical or mental impairments or health. The EEOC lists the following factors to be considered in determining whether a test (or procedure) is a medical examination: (a) whether the test is administered by a health care professional; (b) whether the test is interpreted by a health care professional; (c) whether the test is designed to reveal an impairment or physical or mental health; (d) whether the test is invasive; (e) whether the test measures an employee's performance of a task or measures his/her physiologic responses to performing the task; (f) whether the test normally is given in a medical setting; and (g) whether medical equipment is used (16).

Fitness for duty must be individually determined, taking into consideration the nature of the individual's disability and the nature of the individual's job. Medical fitness and risk evaluation can best be achieved by the examiner's having intimate familiarity with the essential job functions, frequency, and importance of job tasks/demands, and workplace environment (e.g., exposures, use of personal protective equipment, emergency procedures). This familiarity can be gained through extremely clear written descriptions (Figs. 5.1–5.3) walk-through inspections, or videotapes. Although the ADA requires employers to distinguish between essential and marginal job functions, they are not required to have detailed written job descriptions. Furthermore, employment job descriptions often do not specify functional job requirements in a level of detail required for an optimal medical examination.

Employment Entrance Examinations

As stated above, the ADA prohibits preoffer, preemployment medical "inquiries" (e.g., health histories), medical "examinations," and other medical information gathering (e.g., workers' compensation claims) until after a job offer has been made. In doing so, Congress wanted to prohibit employers from using medical information to discriminate against those who might have a silent disability or more likely incur higher health benefit costs, e.g., those with diabetes, cancer, heart disease, epilepsy, or mental ill-

TABLE 5.2. *Influence of the ADA on employee medical examinations*

	Traditional approach	ADA approach
Employment application	Inquires into medical conditions/ disabilities	Inquires only regarding ability to perform essential functions
Drug testing	Preoffer	Preoffer (not considered a medical test)
Agility or strength testing	Preoffer	Preoffer (not considered a medical test)
Applicant medical examination	Preoffer preemployment; no restrictions	Postoffer preplacement; no restrictions
Job information received by medical examiner	Job title, possibly job description	Essential job functions, likely detailed information on job, environment, etc.
Medical criteria	Blanket restrictions permitted	Individual consideration on case-by-case basis
Medical information reported back	Qualified/not qualified; specific job restrictions	Functional abilities and limitations with/without reasonable accommodation; detailed information re: "direct threat"
Confidentiality of medical information	Often kept in personnel files	Separate files, with restricted access
Medical information provided to supervisor	No legal restrictions; guideline is ACOEM Code of Ethical Practices	Work abilities/limitations; recommended reasonable accommodations
Employer medical standards for job eligibility	Employer dependent: for some, all employees must be 100% functional	Employees must perform essential functions with reasonable accommodation
Return to work practices	Employer dependent: for some, no light duty; all employees must be 100% functional	Light duty not required; reasonable accommodation encouraged
Mandated current employee exams	No restrictions	By mandate (e.g., OSHA) or by business necessity but related to essential job functions
Voluntary exams	No restrictions	No restrictions

ACOEM, American College of Occupational and Environmental Medicine.

ness. They also wanted applicants to know when they were being rejected for medical reasons. Thus, job application forms may not inquire about current or past medical conditions, limitations, or disabilities; they may inquire only about current ability to perform the essential job functions.

Employers may ask about an applicant's ability to perform specific job function or even ask applicants to describe or demonstrate how they would do it. Employers may also ask applicants if they require reasonable accommodation to complete the hiring process. If an employer reasonably believes that an applicant needs reasonable accommodation because of an obvious disability or from a disability that the applicant has voluntarily disclosed, an employer may ask questions about the need for accommodation. Employers may also describe attendance requirements, ask if an applicant can meet those requirements, and even ask questions about the applicant's prior attendance record. Employers may not, however, inquire as to the prior use of sick leave, a history of job-related injuries, or prior workers' compensation claims (17).

An employer may condition a job offer upon satisfactorily completing a postoffer medical examination, as long as this is required of all other entering employees in the same job category. Employers are permitted, however, to require examination of some but not all job titles or categories of work. For example, an employer may choose to require employment entrance examinations for materials handling or security personnel while foregoing examinations for clerical or administrative positions.

Of note, strength testing and agility tests are not considered to be medical procedures; therefore, they may be required prior to a job offer. Employers may require applicants to take job-related strength, agility, and other tests, work simulations, or even demon-

Job title: ____________________

1. Description (essential functions):

2. Physical demands (see attached requirements):

Body part most affected	Type of stress (force/repetitive/ awkward position)	Priority

Environment: noise/heat/cold/vibration

3. Chemical, biologic, psychological hazards:

Personal protective eqipment:

4. Previous health problems from employees in same/similar jobs:

Information source: ____WC data ____ employer ____ employee

5. Emergency and unusual situations or risks:

6. Accommodations available/previously made for job:

7. A regulatory standard: ____ Dept. of Transportation
____ Respirator
____ OSHA for noise
____ OSHA for chemical substance ____________
____ Other ____________

8. Medical examination for this job:

____ Basic hx/exam	____ Back fitness
____ Hand/arm fitness	____ Hearing
____ Vision	____ Respirator
____ Aerobic fitness	

____ Special (test or system) ____________

Information provided by: ____________

Date: ____________

FIG. 5.1. Information requested from employer. (Adapted from Pransky GS. Presentation materials. In: Peterson KW, Cooper BA, eds. *Americans with Disabilities Act handbook.* Arlington Heights, IL: American College of Occupational and Environmental Medicine, 1992.)

Body Part	Effort Level	Continuous Effort Time	Efforts/ Minute	Priority
Neck/ Shoulders	___	___	___	___
Back	___	___	___	___
Arm/Elbow	___	___	___	___
Wrists/hand fingers	___	___	___	___
Legs/knees	___	___	___	___
Ankles/feet	___	___	___	___

KEY:

Effort Categories	Continuous Effort Time Categories	Efforts/Minute Categories
1 = Light	1 = < 6 seconds	1 = < 1/minute
2 = Moderate	2 = 6-20 seconds	2 = 1-5/minute
3 = Heavy	3 = > 20 seconds	3 = > 5/minute

Priority for Change/Relative Risk

Moderate:	High:	Very High:
123	223	323
132	313	331
213	321	332
222	322	333
231		
232		
312		

FIG. 5.2. Ergonomic job analysis.

strate their ability to perform essential job functions through an actual job trial. However, if an employer measures an applicant's physiologic or biologic response to performance (e.g., blood pressure and heart rate), this would constitute a medical examination under the ADA (17).

The postoffer, prehire medical examination is a unique opportunity for employers, because it is the only time that a comprehensive medical history, physical examination, and battery of tests may be performed without restriction. Questions may be asked about previous illness and injuries and workers' compensation claims. Thus, a complete baseline of health information can be collected for future comparison. Although the scope of the medical examination is not limited to functional assessment of job capabilities, any assessment that concludes that an individual cannot perform essential functions without accommodation needs to be well documented. If the individual is rejected from the job, the employer must be able to demonstrate that the reasons were job related and necessary for the business, and that no reasonable accommodation was possible. Individuals may be disqualified because they pose a direct threat to themselves or others (see above), but if they can currently perform essential job duties, they may not be rejected because of speculation that the disability will cause a future injury. Note: The ADA legislation did does not describe "threat to self" as a part of the direct threat exclusion. The EEOC, as well as traditional occupational medical ethics and practice, have included "threat to self" as a legitimate reason to exclude workers if the risk cannot be removed through reasonable accommodation. This issue is currently scheduled for review in the United States Supreme Court (18).

Because all employees within a job category must be treated the same, if one has a medical inquiry, all

Please place an "X" in the box that best describes current job activities

WORK TASKS	NEVER	OCCASIONAL 0.33%	FREQUENT 34-66%	CONSTANT 67-100%	JOB RESPONSIBILITIES
SITTING					
STANDING					
WALKING					
CLIMBING					
STAIRS					
RAMPS					
LADDERS/ POLES					
BENDING					
SQUATTING					
LIFTING					
VERY LIGHT (<10lb)					
LIGHT (10-19lb)					
MEDIUM (20-49lb)					
HEAVY (50-99lb)					
VERY HEAVY (100lb)					
PUSHING					
PULLING					
TWISTING					
REACHING FORWARD					
REACHING OVERHEAD					
KNEELING					
CRAWLING					
HAND TASKS (BOTH HANDS)					
RIGHT HAND					
LEFT HAND					
TOOLS/ EQUIPMENT					
TEMPERATURE (HOT)					
TEMPERATURE (COLD)					
HIGH NOISE					
VIBRATION					

ARE MODIFICATIONS AVAILABLE? TEMPORARY: ☐ YES ☐ NO PERMANENT: ☐ YES; ☐ NO

FIG. 5.3. Physical demand requirements.

must have some kind of medical inquiry. If one has a medical exam, all must have some kind of medical exam. However, the inquiries or exams do not have to be identical. Therefore, hierarchical or branching screening questions can be used, e.g., "Do you or have you ever had any problems with back pain that restricted your activity?" An examiner may go into detail for those who answer affirmatively. Similarly, positive screening tests may be followed by more definitive ones on a case-by-case basis.

Examinations of Current Employees

Occupational physicians should be aware that the ADA places severe restrictions on employee disability-related inquiries and medical examinations. Unless required by other federal laws, disability-related inquiries or examinations of current employees must be job related and necessary for business. Generally, a disability-related inquiry or medical examination of an employee meets these criteria when an employer "has a reasonable belief, based on objective evidence, that: (1) an employee's ability to perform essential job functions will be impaired by a medical condition; or (2) an employee will pose a direct threat due to a medical condition." Disability-related inquiries and medical examinations that follow up on a request for reasonable accommodation when the disability or need for accommodation is not known or obvious also may be job related and consistent with business necessity. In addition, periodic medical examinations and other monitoring under specific circumstances may be job related and consistent with business necessity.

Sometimes this standard may be met when an employer knows about a particular employee's medical condition, has observed performance problems, and reasonably can attribute the problems to the medical condition. An employer also may be given reliable information by a credible third party that an employee has a relevant health problem, or the employer may observe symptoms indicating that an employee may have a health problem that could impair his/her ability to perform essential job functions or could pose a direct threat.

Individuals may be considered employees by the EEOC even if they are not actually employed by the covered entity. An individual is considered an employee if the entity controls the means and manner of his/her work performance. Where more than one entity controls the means and manner of how an individual's work is done, the individual is an employee of each entity. Therefore, temporary or leased employees are considered employees of both the staffing agency and the organization where they are working for purposes of ADA coverage. Undocumented workers are protected by the ADA as well, even if their employment is illegal under U.S. immigration law.

An employer must treat a current employee who applies for a new position within the same entity as an applicant. The employer, therefore, is prohibited from asking disability-related questions or requiring a medical examination before making the individual a conditional offer of the new position. Further, where a current supervisor has medical information regarding an employee who is applying for a new job, that supervisor may not disclose that information to the person interviewing the employee for the new job or to the supervisor of that job.

After an offer for the new position has been extended, the employer may ask the individual disability-related questions or require a medical examination. If an employer withdraws the offer based on medical information (i.e., screens the employee out because of a disability), it must show that the reason for doing so was job related and consistent with business necessity.

A current employee is not considered an applicant, however, when he/she is noncompetitively entitled to the other position (e.g., because of seniority or satisfactory performance in his/her current position). An individual who is temporarily assigned to another position and then returns to his/her regular job also is not treated as an applicant.

When evaluating a current employee's ability to safely perform the essential functions of the job, the employer may require the employee to provide documentation that she or he has a qualifying disability and needs the reasonable accommodation that has been requested. The employer may not, however, request unrelated medical information. This means simply that, in most circumstances, an employer cannot ask for an employee's entire medical record because it is likely to contain information unrelated to the disability at issue and the need for accommodation.

The EEOC will consider the worker's documentation sufficient if it (a) describes the nature, severity, and duration of the employee's impairment, the activity or activities that the impairment limits, and the extent to which the impairment limits the employee's ability to perform the activity or activities; and, (b) substantiates why the requested reasonable accommodation is needed.

Any determination that an employee poses a direct threat must follow a careful individualized assessment of that employee's present ability to safely perform the essential functions of the job. Ethical practice in occupational medicine (and the EEOC) requires that this assessment must be based "on a reasonable medical judgment that relies on the most current medical knowledge and/or the best objective medical evidence." The employer does have the right to have the employee examined by a physician of its choice "who has expertise in the employee's specific condition and can provide medical information that allows the employer to determine the effects of the condition on the employee's ability to perform his/her job." The examination, however, must be limited to "determining whether the employee can perform his/her job without posing a direct threat, with or without reasonable accommodation" (16).

The EEOC cautions employers, however, about relying solely on the opinion of their own health care professional where that opinion is contradicted by documentation from the employee's own treating physician (if that physician is knowledgeable about the employee's medical condition and job functions, and/or other objective evidence). The EEOC advises employers who encounter conflicting medical information to consider:

> (1) the area of expertise of each medical professional who has provided information; (2) the kind of information each person providing documentation has about the job's essential functions and the work environment in which they are performed; (3) whether a particular opinion is based on speculation or on current, objectively verifiable information about the risks associated with a particular condition; and (4) whether the medical opinion is contradicted by information known to or observed by the employer (e.g., information about the employee's actual experience in the job in question or in previous similar jobs).

Clearly, the direct threat domain is one where the appropriately trained and qualified occupational physician can perform an invaluable role in the evaluation process. One of the most important functions in that role is facilitating the exchange of information regarding medical findings, job tasks, and exposures among the parties (worker, personal physician, and employer). The occupational physician plays a key role as educator, mediator, and technical expert.

The EEOC recognizes that an employer may be required to make disability-related inquiries or require employees to submit to medical examinations that are mandated or governed by another federal agencies such as the U.S. Department of Transportation regulations, the Occupational Safety and Health Act, the Federal Mine Health and Safety Act, and other federal statutes that require employees who may be exposed to toxic or hazardous substances to be medically monitored at specific intervals. These inquiries or examinations, however, must be limited to fulfilling the intended purposes of the authorizing agency.

Employers are permitted to make disability-related inquiries or conduct medical examinations as part of a voluntary wellness programs as long as they are truly voluntary (employer neither requires participation nor penalizes employers who do not participate), and any medical records acquired as part of the wellness program are kept confidential and separate from personnel records.

Confidentiality of Medical Information

The ADA directly addresses the confidentiality of employment-related medical records (19,20).

Specifically, it calls for information obtained from medical inquiries or medical examinations to be collected and maintained on separate forms, and these confidential medical records are to be maintained by the employer in locked cabinets, separate from personnel files and accessible only to designated persons. Access to this confidential medical information is limited to five situations: (a) informing supervisors and managers about necessary work restrictions and accommodations; (b) informing first aid and safety personnel, as necessary, if a disability might require emergency treatment (e.g., limited mobility, epilepsy or diabetes); (c) providing government officials investigating compliance with relevant information on request; (d) providing relevant information to state workers' compensation offices, second-injury funds, or to workers' compensation insurers in accordance with state workers' compensation laws; and (e) administering insurance programs such as employee health, disability, or life.

The applicant/employee should sign a medical release authorizing the dissemination of certain medical information. Note that Fig. 5.4 contains a signature line for the individual to confirm knowledge of the information being provided to the employer. Such safeguards help protect the physician against charges of inappropriate release of medical information. For risk management purposes, most medical societies now recommend that a physician not release any medical information, even in the presence of a subpoena, without a signed release from the patient.

Under the ADA, sharing of medical information about people with disabilities differs sharply from the traditional view of medical confidentiality, outlined in the American College of Occupational and Environmental Medicine's (ACOEM) Code of Ethical Conduct for Physicians Providing Occupational Medical Services (21). The ADA requires health professionals to share sufficient information for employers to make management decisions about the presence of a disability, a "direct threat" to health or safety, and reasonable accommodation (see ADA Information Flow, below). This information, however, must be limited to a "need to know" basis and should be conveyed without revealing specific medical data or diagnoses whenever possible.

Evaluating Impairment and Fitness for Duty

Because the ADA opened the employment examination to direct legal scrutiny, occupational health professionals must be prepared to have their recommendations challenged. Yet the content, scope, tests, procedures, etc., of preplacement examinations were in the past arbitrarily adopted by the company or a

Employee name ______________________________ Date ____________
Employer ____
Job title ____

My evaluation of this employee indicates:

____ 1. No medical contraindication to performing this job without accommodation.

____ 2. No medical contraindication to performing this job, with the following recommended accommodations, or job training:

____

____

____ 3. Based upon probability of substantial harm, this employee could pose a *direct threat* to self or others. Please refer to the attached information on the extent of the threat and accommodations that may significantly decrease the threat.

____ 4. Further testing is required to fully evaluate ability or risk.

____ 5. Medical hold: waiting for additional data. Reevaluate on ____ / ____ / ____ .

Comments: ____

____

If 2, 3, or 4 is checked, please call me to discuss this further, including recommendations for other information that may aid in accommodations or clarification of risk.

Any attached information on medical conditions should be treated as confidential medical information, in accordance with the Americans with Disabilities Act, with distribution only as needed.

______________________ ______________________
Employee signature Physician signature

FIG. 5.4. Report of preplacement medical evaluation. (Adapted from Pransky GS. Presentation materials. In: Peterson KW, Cooper BA, eds. *Americans with Disabilities Act handbook.* Arlington Heights, IL: American College of Occupational and Environmental Medicine, 1992.)

contract physician without any peer review. Most of the protocols were never made public and might be questioned as discriminatory, unfair, biased, incompetent, and not pertinent to the job. If litigation develops, they will be made public.

The health professional must consider each individual situation through a rigorous, logical process. First, is the employer or entity covered by the ADA? Second, does the individual in question have a disability as defined by the ADA? Third, does the disability create workplace limitations? Fourth, how do the individual's abilities and limitations relate to the essential job functions? Fifth, would a reasonable accommodation make it possible for the person to perform the essential job functions without causing a direct threat to health and safety? And sixth, what information needs to be conveyed to the employer to facilitate an appropriate decision?

The medical examiner should not be lured into making employment decisions or determining whether a reasonable accommodation can be made. The occupational health professional should advise the employer about only two things: (a) an individual's functional abilities and limitations in relation to functional job requirements, i.e., can this person currently perform this specific job, with or without an accommodation; and (b) whether the individual meets the employer's overall health and safety requirements, i.e., whether the individual can perform the job without posing a "direct threat" to the health or safety of him/herself or others.

The ADA does not permit blanket exclusions from certain categories of jobs (e.g., medical standards that exclude all those with diabetes, epilepsy, hypertension, or a learning disorder). Each individual's situation must be considered on its own merits. For example, an epileptic may not have had a seizure for more than 10 years, or may have a distinct aura prior to attacks that allows adequate time to deal with safety threats. The best predictor of job performance is most often past job performance.

Drug and Alcohol Abuse

Employees and applicants currently engaging in the illegal use of drugs are not protected by the ADA when an employer acts on the basis of such use. Tests for illegal use of drugs are not considered medical examinations, and therefore are not subject to the ADA's restrictions on medical examinations. These provisions do not apply to alcohol, which is a legal drug. Employers may hold individuals who are illegally using drugs and individuals with alcoholism to the same standards of performance as other employees. Individuals with current alcoholism or a past history of alcohol or drug abuse may meet one of the three prongs of the definition of disability and thus be eligible for protection under the ADA. Current illegal drug users are not protected. The ADA, however, specifies that employers may ensure that the workplace is free from illegal drug use and the use of alcohol, and they may comply with other federal drug and alcohol laws. Employers may require employees not to be under the influence of drugs or alcohol at work, prohibit the use of illegal drugs and alcohol in the workplace, require employees to submit to drug testing, discharge or deny employment to current users of illegal drugs, and hold illegal drug users and alcoholics to the same performance standards as other employees.

Testing for illegal drugs is not considered a medical test under the ADA. Therefore, tests for illicit drugs may still be conducted at the preemployment stage. However, the medical review officer (MRO) who reviews drug test results must be sensitive to confidentiality concerns. This is most salient when an MRO interview with the person tested reveals use of legitimately prescribed medications (22).

Testing for illegal drugs under the ADA encompasses a broader schedule of drugs than those covered by the Department of Health and Human Services drug testing regulations, and includes any drug that is unlawful under the five schedules of the Controlled Substances Act. Any follow-up inquiry regarding the use of these medications prior to an offer of employment would be a prohibited medical inquiry. Alternatively, refusing to hire the individual who is legitimately using the medication may itself constitute wrongful discrimination and could disqualify excellent candidates. For this reason, the EEOC has recommended informally that employers arrange drug testing so that any medical inquiry associated with drug testing be conducted after a conditional job offer has been made. The Department of Transportation (DOT) considers the MRO function to be an integral part of mandatory drug testing, thus excluded from coverage under the ADA (23).

The ADA does provide limited protection to alcoholics and former drug users who have the disability of addiction. The critical distinction for illegal drug users is between current and former use. Current drug use is defined as "use recently enough to justify an employer's reasonable belief that involvement with drugs is an ongoing problem." The time is not limited by days or weeks, but must be determined on a case-by-case basis. Former users of illegal drugs are protected if they (a) have completed a supervised rehabilitation program; this can include self help programs, such as Narcotics Anonymous; (b) are participating in a drug rehabilitation program and are not currently using drugs illegally; or (c) were erroneously regarded as using illegal drugs. A positive drug test, however, is considered de facto evidence of current drug use.

The EEOC considers alcohol testing of any kind to be a medical examination and therefore must follow a conditional offer of employment. Alcoholics, while having a disability and being entitled to a reasonable accommodation, may be disciplined or discharged where alcohol use adversely affects job performance or conduct to the extent that the person is no longer "qualified" for the job. Once again, the same performance standard must be applied to other employees in the same position. Employers are not required to provide alcohol/drug rehabilitation as a reasonable accommodation.

The law is silent with regard to prescriptions drugs. Thus, there is a large gap in coverage regarding misuse of and addiction to drugs not included in the Controlled Substances Act and use of prescription drugs that can affect work performance as well as the safety of the individual and/or others.

Emotional and Mental Disabilities

The highly stigmatized area of mental health was scrutinized very carefully by Congress in passing the ADA. Mental illnesses were carefully reviewed; nowhere else were symptoms or diagnoses included or excluded with the same degree of specificity. Kleptomania, pyromania, compulsive gambling, transvestism, homosexuality, bisexuality, pedophilia, and other disorders were specifically excluded from protection by the ADA. Conditions found to be impairments under Section 504 of the Rehabilitation Act of 1973 include autism, cerebral palsy, chronic fatigue, dyslexia, learning disabilities, and mental retardation. Borderline cerebral palsy, and acrophobia without an effect on work performance were among those excluded.

The ADA rule defines mental impairment to include "any mental or psychological disorder, such as...emotional or mental illness." Examples of emotional or mental illness include major depression, bipolar disorder, anxiety disorders (which include panic disorder, obsessive-compulsive disorder, and posttraumatic stress disorder), schizophrenia, and personality disorders. The current edition of the American Psychiatric Association's *Diagnostic and Statistical Manual of Mental Disorders* (DSM-IV) is relevant for identifying these disorders (24). The ADA's definition of mental or psychological disorder is very broad, especially given the prevalence of psychological problems in the general population. Repeated studies cite 20% to 25% of the population showing significant emotional symptoms (25). Depression is astonishingly prevalent. Further, an estimated 10% to 15% of the workforce is alcohol or drug dependent or impaired, with an even greater number having used illegal substances regularly in the past.

Not all conditions listed in the DSM-IV, however, are disabilities or even impairments for purposes of the ADA. For example, the DSM-IV lists several conditions, such as use of illegal drugs (see above) that Congress expressly excluded from the ADA's definition of disability. The DSM-IV also includes conditions that are not mental disorders but for which people may seek treatment (for example, problems with a spouse or child). Because these conditions are not disorders, they are not impairments under the ADA.

These findings help to validate the ADA's philosophy of considering every individual on a case-by-case basis. The EEOC Enforcement Guidance on the Americans with Disabilities Act and Psychiatric Disabilities (26) provides some helpful guidance. For example, traits or behaviors are not, in themselves, mental impairments. Stress, in itself, is not automatically considered a mental impairment. Stress, however, may be shown to be related to a mental or physical impairment. Similarly, traits like irritability, chronic lateness, and poor judgment are not, in themselves, mental impairments, although they may be linked to mental impairments.

Even if a condition is an impairment, it is not automatically a disability. To rise to the level of a disability, an impairment must "substantially limit" one or more major life activities of the individual and must be evaluated in light of any mitigating measures such as medication or therapy.

Some elements of cognitive and psychological functioning can be assessed using validated psychometric testing techniques. Unfortunately, psychological and neurobehavioral assessment tools alone are not very good in terms of their ability to predict successful employment. An extensive literature review by Anthony and Janson (27) showed that for severely psychiatrically impaired individuals, symptoms, diagnosis, intelligence, aptitude, and personality tests are all poor predictors of future work performance. There is no correlation between symptoms and functional skills. The best demographic predictor is prior employment history; the best clinical predictors are ratings of adjustment in sheltered job sites or workshops. A significant predictor is the ability to get along or function socially with others. The best paper and pencil test predictors are ego strength or self-concept in the role as worker.

Perhaps the best means of evaluating workers with a mental or psychiatric condition is a global assessment of their condition and abilities in light of a carefully prepared functional job description. Functional job descriptions can include a number of attributes in the psychological and social realm. These include the ability to do the following:

- maintain concentration over time
- screen out external stimuli
- manage time effectively
- relate to others beyond giving and receiving simple instructions
- handle intense interpersonal contacts
- influence people, e.g., negotiate
- accept and respond appropriately to negative feedback
- comprehend and follow instructions
- perform simple and repetitive tasks
- perform complex or varied tasks
- handle multiple simultaneous tasks
- make decisions without immediate supervision
- evaluate and make appropriate generalizations
- maintain work pace appropriate to work load
- accept and carry out responsibility for direction, planning, control over others

Many reasonable accommodations can address mental health issues. Examples in five categories are contained in Table 5.3.

TABLE 5.3. *Examples of reasonable accommodations to emotional and mental disabilities*

Modification of the supervisory process
Put work requests in writing
Train supervisors to give positive feedback, as well as criticism, especially in light of the sensitive emotional antennae of those with mental illness
Allow worker to appraise own performance before getting criticism
Written agreement between worker and supervisor of how crises will be handled (e.g., if become insensitive, manic, alienate others, or work performance slips)
Individualized job training (for those with anxiety or learning disabilities)
Job modification
Work at home
Eliminate marginal job functions that cause problems (e.g., greeting people or handling switchboard during lunch)
Modified work schedule (e.g., to attend therapy sessions)
Job sharing or part-time work
Use of sick leave for emotional or cognitive reasons (mental health days)
Changing policies
Advance unpaid sick leave during treatment
Allow water or soda to be used by cashier with dry mouth
Physical environment changes
Reducing stimuli, e.g., noise, light, vibration, activity
Enclosing an office
Human assistance
Use of a job coach
Peer counselor/advocate as needed
Supervisor available to meet with employee

Communicable Diseases

Some specific communicable diseases, such as tuberculosis or HIV infection, are disabilities for the purposes of the ADA (28). The employer can limit the activities of such individuals only if it can demonstrate that the contagious disease constitutes a significant risk to the health or safety of others that cannot be eliminated by reasonable accommodation.

The EEOC, for example, permits food service industry employers to remove an individual with a contagious disease or infection from a food-handling position if the disease can be spread from a food-handling position, and if the employer cannot take other measures (e.g., gloves or masks) to prevent the problem (29).

Health Insurance Benefits

The 1991 EEOC regulations provided a limited exemption that allowed a covered entity to sponsor a benefit plan based on underwriting risks, as long as risks were classified or administered in accordance with state law. Interpretive guidance indicated that the purpose was to permit development of plans in accordance with accepted principles of risk assessment. The ADA provisions were not intended to disrupt the current nature of insurance underwriting or practices. However, a qualified applicant or employee with a disability cannot be denied access to the insurance process or given different terms or conditions of insurance based on disability alone, if the disability does not pose increased risks. One practical implication is that many employers have instituted surcharges or longer periods of exclusion from insurance coverage for preexisting conditions. The insurance provisions include arrangements with insurance companies, HMOs, third-party administrators, and stop-loss carriers.

Enforcement guidelines released in June 1993 (30) identify four basic ADA requirements: (a) disability-based insurance distinction are permitted only if the employer-provided health insurance plan is bona fide and if the distinctions are not being used as a subterfuge for purposes of evading the Act; (b) decisions about the employment of an individual with a disability cannot be motivated by concerns about the impact of the individual's disability on the employer's health plan; (c) employees with disabilities must be accorded equal access to whatever health insurance the employer provides to employees without disabilities; and (d) an employer cannot make an employment decision about any person, whether or not that person has a disability, based on concerns about the impact on the health plan of the disability of someone with whom that person has a relationship.

A gray area is the extent to which the ADA may limit risk-rated benefit and other financial health incentive programs, such as programs that offer reduced deductibles or co-payments to those who voluntarily participate in health programs, or who have healthier risk factors such as blood pressure, cholesterol, weight, or cardiovascular fitness.

ADA INFORMATION FLOW

Another useful way to review the ADA is in terms of the flow of information among the various participants. First, information needs to be obtained about the applicant or employee, the job and the work environment. Ideally, this includes job title, job description broken down into essential and nonessential functions, job assessment, job analysis, physical job demands, environmental demands, psychological and social requirements, information about the work environment, and even the availability of emergency and other medical services. This information can be conveyed in writing (Fig. 5.1.) or through discussion with supervisor/employer, workplace walk-through inspections, videotaping of the workplace, job analysis, or sophisticated ergonomic analyses.

Second, data are collected from the medical examination: the medical history inquiry, general physical examination, laboratory and other tests, individualized assessment tests or procedures, and specialized information from personal physicians, occupational therapists, rehabilitation specialists, or other providers.

Third is the analysis of impairment (not disability), i.e., what the individual can or cannot do, increased risk that might impose a direct threat to oneself or others, and recommended accommodations.

The fourth step is communication from the health professional to the employer. Information sharing can range from quite restricted to full disclosure. For example, the health professional can limit information provided to whether the applicant/employee is able to perform key functions, identification of work restrictions, recommended accommodations, or notification of potential direct threat. This reflects the attitude of sharing with the employer on a need-to-know basis. An example of a suitable communication form is contained in Fig. 5.4. Additional information is often best shared through an iterative dialogue between management and medical advisor, a process that is encouraged by the ADA.

At the level of "full disclosure," the health professional may need to release medical history, diagnoses, and/or all medical information (e.g., to support a "direct threat" decision or workers' compensation hearing). It may also be necessary to document that a medical opinion reflects "the most current available medical knowledge," a standard to which the ADA explicitly holds the employer for "direct threat" exclusions. The health professional should reinforce that the information must be kept confidential and used on a need-to-know basis (e.g., by a first-aid personnel). Preferably, the receiving entity has another medical or nursing professional who can receive, interpret, and protect this information from improper use or disclosure. Ultimately the ADA places the responsibility for the use or misuse of this information on the organization. Physicians, however, cannot fully avoid liability since other statutory or common law requirements may exist and the physician must act in good faith and with due care.

SUMMARY

The ADA has forced a rethinking of issues and procedures in many areas of occupational medical practice. These included the need to overtly distinguish between essential and nonessential job functions and for health professionals to share previously confidential medical information with employers, who are charged with making reasonable accommodations and determining if individuals represent a direct threat to themselves or others. In addition, the ADA prohibited preemployment medical examinations, allowing them only after a bona fide job offer has been made, and even then, only when all applicants within that job category are required to have a medical examination. For current employees, examinations can be required only when mandated by statue (such as OSHA) or when job related and consistent with business necessity. They must be limited to determining the ability to perform essential job functions. If conducted on a voluntary basis, blood pressure or cholesterol screening, health risk appraisal, periodic medical examinations, and other wellness programs are permitted.

There is a complex interplay of federal, state, and local laws that protect employees rights and privileges in employment. The ADA is an important part of this mosaic but it must be reconciled with employers' duties and responsibilities under other laws and regulations. Occupational health professionals must become familiar with the basic provisions of these other laws in order to play their important role in the implementation of these laws in a way that protects workers' rights and maximizes employer and employee productivity.

The ADA offers the occupational health professional the challenge and the opportunity to serve as internal or external consultants to employers and workers. Experienced clinicians can evaluate individuals with disabilities and advise the employer regarding the potential impacts and possible accommodations accordingly. Another role is helping the employer to interpret physician reports, obtain additional relevant information, review medical literature, facilitate communication, and mediate disputes. Because the ADA is deceptively complex in its nuances for the employer to administer, occupational health professionals can play an invaluable educational and consultative role.

REFERENCES

1. Findings and Purposes, section 2, 42 U.S. Code 12101. The Americans with Disabilities Act of 1990, as amended. In: *Appendix A: a technical assistance manual on the employment provisions (Title I) of the Americans with Disabilities Act.* Washington, DC: Equal Employment Opportunity Commission, January 1992.
2. George W. Bush. Press release. Washington, DC: The White House, July 26, 2001.
3. Equal Pay Act of 1963 (Pub. L. 88-38) (EPA), as amended, appears in Volume 29 of the United States Code, at section 206(d). The EPA, which is part of the Fair Labor Standards Act (FLSA) of 1938, as amended, and which is administered and enforced by the EEOC, prohibits sex-based wage discrimination between men and women in the same establishment who are performing under similar working conditions.
4. Title VII of the Civil Rights Act of 1964 (Pub. L. 88-352) (Title VII), as amended, appears in Volume 42 of the United States Code, beginning at section 2000e. Title VII prohibits employment discrimination based on race, color, religion, sex, and national origin.
5. Age Discrimination in Employment Act (ADEA) of 1967 (Pub. L. 90-202), as amended, appears in Volume 29 of the United States Code, beginning at section 621. The ADEA prohibits employment discrimination against persons 40 years of age or older. The Older Workers Benefit Protection Act (Pub. L. 101-433) amends several sections of the ADEA. In addition, section 115 of the Civil Rights Act of 1991 (P.L. 102-166) amends section 7(e) of the ADEA (29 U. S.C. 626(e)).
6. Sections 501 and 505 of the Rehabilitation Act of 1973 (Pub. L. 93-112) (Rehab. Act), as amended, appear in volume 29 of the United States Code, beginning at section 791. Section 501 prohibits employment discrimination against individuals with disabilities in the federal sector. Section 505 contains provisions governing remedies and attorney's fees under Section 501. Relevant definitions that apply to sections 501 and 505 precede these sections. Section 512 of the Americans with Disabilities Act (ADA) of 1990 (Pub. L. 101-336) amends definitions applicable to the Rehab. Act. The Rehabilitation Act Amendments of 1992 (Pub. L. 102-559) further amends the definition of "individual with a disability" and Section 501. In addition, section 102 of the Civil Rights Act (CRA) of 1991 (Pub. L. 102-166) amends the Revised Statutes by adding a new section following section 1977 (42 U.S.C. 1981), to provide for the recovery of compensatory and punitive damages in cases of intentional violations of Title VII, the Americans with Disabilities Act of 1990, and section 501 of the Rehabilitation Act of 1973.
7. Equal Employment Opportunities for Individuals with Disabilities. Equal Employment Opportunity Commission; Final Rule. *Federal Register* 1991 (July 26);56 (144):35726–35753.
8. *A technical assistance manual on the employment provisions (Title I) of the Americans With Disabilities Act.* Washington, DC: Equal Employment Opportunity Commission, January 1992. Appendix B contains the Interpretive Guidance published earlier by EEOC.
9. *Sutton v. United Airlines, Inc.,* United States Supreme Court No. 97-1943 (June 22, 1999); *Murphy v. United Parcel Service,* United States Supreme Court No. 97-1992 (June 22, 1999).
10. *Toyota Motor Manufacturing, Kentucky, Inc. v. Williams,* United States Supreme Court No. 00-1089 (Slip Opinion).
11. Smith GM. The role of the occupational medicine physician in the management of industrial injury. In: Mayer TG, Mooney V, Gatchel RJ, eds. *Contemporary conservative care for painful spinal disorders*. Philadelphia: Lea & Febiger, 1991:191–201.
12. Cocchiarella L, ed. *Guides to the evaluation of permanent impairment,* 5th ed. Chicago: American Medical Association, 2000.
13. EEOC Enforcement Guidance: Reasonable Accommodation and Undue Hardship Under the Americans with Disabilities Act. United States Equal Employment Opportunity Commission. March 1, 1999 *(http://www.eeoc.govdocsaccommodation.html)*.
14. *Chevron U.S.A. Inc. v. Echazabal.* See Brief Amici Curiae for the American College of Occupational and Environmental Medicine, the Western Occupational and Environmental Association, and the California Society of Industrial Medicine and Surgery.
15. Himmelstein JS. Worker fitness and risk evaluations in context. In: Himmelstein JS, Pransky GS, eds. Worker fitness and risk evaluations. *Occup Med State Art Rev* 1988;3(2):169–178.
16. EEOC Enforcement Guidance: Disability-related inquiries and medical examinations of employees under the Americans with Disabilities Act (ADA). United States Equal Employment Opportunity Commission. July 27, 2000 *(http://www.eeoc.govdocsguidance-inquiries.html)*.
17. ADA Enforcement Guidance: Preemployment disability-related questions and medical examinations. United States Equal Employment Opportunity Commission. October 10, 1995 *(http://www.eeoc.govdocspreemp.html)*.
18. *Chevron U.S.A. Inc. v. Echazabal.* See Brief Amici Curiae for the American College of Occupational and Environmental Medicine, the Western Occupational and Environmental Association, and the California Society of Industrial Medicine and Surgery.
19. Occupational physicians should also be familiar with OSHA regulations governing the collection, use, and storage of employee medical and exposure records. See Access to employee medical and exposure records (29 CFR 1910.1020). United States Occupational Safety and Health Administration.

20. Rischitelli DG. Confidentiality of medical information in the workplace. *J Occup Environ Med* 1995;37: 583–593.
21. Rischitelli DG. Position paper on the confidentiality of medical information in the workplace. American College of Occupational and Environmental Medicine. Arlington Heights, IL: 1994. (Reprinted in *J Occup Environ Med* 1995;37:594–596.)
22. Rischitelli DG. Avoiding discriminatory drug testing practices under the Americans with Disabilities Act. *J Legal Med* 1993;14:597–615.
23. Office of the Secretary, U.S. Department of Transportation. *Federal Register* 2000(December 19);(65) 79462; *Federal Register* 2001(August 9);(65)41944.
24. American Psychiatric Association. *Diagnostic and statistical manual of mental disorders,* 4th ed. Washington, DC: American Psychiatric Association, 1999.
25. Robbins DB. Psychiatric conditions in worker fitness and risk evaluation. In: Himmelstein JS, Pransky GS, eds. Worker fitness and risk evaluations. *Occup Med State Art Rev* 1988;3(2):309–321.
26. EEOC Enforcement Guidance on the Americans with Disabilities Act and Psychiatric Disabilities. United States Equal Employment Opportunity Commission. March 27, 1997 *(http://www.eeoc.govdocspsych.html)*.
27. Anthony WA, Jansen MA. Predicting the vocational capacity of the chronically mentally ill: research and policy implications. *Am Psychol* 1984;39(5):537–544.
28. *Bragdon v. Abbot.* United States Supreme Court No. 97-156 (June 25, 1998).
29. Diseases Transmitted Through the Food Supply. Centers for Disease Control, Department of Health and Human Services. *Federal Register* 1991(August 16);56(159): 40,397–399. This is contained in Appendix C of the EEOC's ADA Technical Assistance Manual, referenced above.

FURTHER INFORMATION

Equal Employment Opportunities for Individuals with Disabilities. Equal Employment Opportunity Commission; Final Rule. *Federal Register* 1991(July 26);56(144): 35726–35753. This contains the basic EEOC Title I Regulations and Interpretive Guidance in 27 pages. This material is reprinted as Appendix B of the ADA Technical Assistance Manual, cited below.

A technical assistance manual on the employment provisions (Title I) of the Americans with Disabilities Act. Washington, DC: Equal Employment Opportunity Commission, (800-669-EEOC voice; 800-800-3302 TDD), January 1992. Detailed but highly readable manual provides an excellent overview, filled with illustrative case study examples. See Chapters VI, Medical Examinations and Inquiries; VIII, Drug and Alcohol Testing; and IX, Workers' Compensation and Work-Related Injury. Appendix B contains the EEOC Title I Regulations and Interpretive Guidance cited above. A Resource Directory (second volume) describes and provides contact information for hundreds federal agency and national nongovernmental technical assistance resources, as well as regional and state locations of federal programs.

EEOC Enforcement Guidance documents have been released on various subjects pertinent to occupational medical practice from 1995 to 2000 and are quite useful. Some of these are cited as references to this chapter. Available from Equal Employment Opportunity Commission, Washington, DC (800-669-EEOC voice; 800-800-3302 TDD) *(http://www.eeoc.govdocsguidance-inquiries.html)*.

Job Accommodation Network, P.O. Box 6123, 809 Allen Hall, Morgantown, WV 26506-6123 (800-526-7234 provides accommodation assistance for Out of State Voice/TDD) (800-526-4698 provides accommodation assistance for In State Voice/TDD) (800-ADA-WORK provides ADA information for voice/TDD) (800-DIAL-JAN provides ADA information for computer modem). Provides free consultant service, funded by the President's Committee on Employment of People with Disabilities, to individuals, health professionals, and employers on customized job and work-site accommodations. Provides individualized searches for workplace accommodations based on the job's functional requirements, the individual's functional limitations, and environmental and other factors.

Fasman ZD. *What business must know about the ADA: 1993 compliance guide.* Washington, DC: U.S. Chamber of Commerce (800-638-6582), 88 pages. This little guide provides a concise, readable summary of provisions under Title I employment and Title III public accommodations and services operated by private entities. Intended for employers, it includes case examples and "helpful hints."

Pimentel RK, Bell CG, Smith GM, et al. *The workers' compensation–ADA connection.* Chatsworth, CA: Milt Wright & Associates, 1993. Subtitled "Supervisory Tools for Workers' Compensation Cost Containment that Reduce ADA Liability," this concise guide includes section on management communication with physicians, identifying "red flag" ADA workers' compensation issues, and fraud and the malingerer. It also explores the often overlapping relationship between obligations for workers' compensation and ADA compliance.

6

Occupational Health Nursing: Roles and Practice

Bonnie Rogers

The scope of occupational health nursing practice has expanded significantly in recent decades. In addition to the provision of direct care of occupational illnesses/injuries as well as worker/workplace surveillance, increasing emphasis is being placed on providing health promotion and wellness education programs, case management, disease and injury prevention services, management and administration, primary care, and research (1,2). This chapter explores the contemporary domains of occupational health nursing practice and examines related strategies aimed at providing and protecting worker health. A historical perspective, which follows, is helpful in providing the context for the practice framework.

HISTORICAL PERSPECTIVES

Historically, nursing care to worker populations, then referred to as industrial nursing, began in the late 19th century. In 1888, a group of coal miners employed Betty Moulder, a graduate of Blockley Hospital School of Nursing in Philadelphia, to care for ailing miners and their families (3–6). However, little else is known about her or the services rendered.

Ada Mayo Stewart, hired in 1895 by the Vermont Marble Company in Rutland, Vermont, is often credited as being the first industrial nurse (4,7,8). Miss Stewart, whose primary mode of transportation was a bicycle, visited sick employees in their homes, provided emergency care, taught habits for healthy living, and taught mothers about child care. She learned much about the customs and methods of caring for the sick in the native countries of the workers and their families. Miss Stewart also gave talks on health and hygiene to schoolchildren initially at the request of the schoolteacher, a personal friend, but also because child health care was considered extremely important by the company's president (7,9).

In the early 1900s, employee health services proliferated rapidly throughout the United States as awareness grew that the provision of health services at the work site resulted in a more productive workforce, decreased illnesses and injuries, and reduced absenteeism. At that time, working conditions in many factories were deplorable and deteriorated even further in the face of an industrial ethic that placed property rights above human rights. The proponents of this ethic maintained that industrial accidents were inevitable and were simply the cost of progress (10). This type of attitude was not supported by the public; thus, safeguards for workers were encouraged, which resulted in the institution of the workers' compensation system.

During the first half of the 20th century, interest in industrial nursing expanded, state professional nursing societies were established, and specialty education courses in occupational health were instituted. With the advent of World War II, industries grew and the demand for nursing services increased dramatically, with a reported 4,000 industrial nurses employed (11). With a sufficient number of nurses to support a national association, the American Association of Industrial Nursing (AAIN) was established in 1942 to improve industrial nursing practice and education and increase interdisciplinary collaborative efforts (3).

In the late 1960s and early 1970s, several laws that were designed to protect worker health and safety were enacted [e.g., Federal Coal Mine Safety and Health Act, 1969; Occupational Safety and Health (OSH) Act, 1970; Toxic Substances Control Act, 1976]. This legislation resulted in an increased need for occupational health nurses at the work site. In addition, the passage of the OSH Act of 1970 provided a new stimulus to prepare occupational health professionals in advanced practice areas as well as for education and research.

As the nurse's role in industry expanded and evolved, the AAIN changed its name to the American Association of Occupational Health Nurses (AAOHN) in 1977 to better reflect the broad scope of practice of the occupational health nurse. The 1980s witnessed the expansion of the role of the occupational health nurse with more involvement in clinical management and health promotion, administration and policy development, cost containment, research, and regulatory monitoring. Several standards were promulgated to protect workers from unwarranted exposures (e.g., Hazard Communication Standard, 1983), and in 1988, the Occupational Safety and Health Administration (OSHA) hired the first occupational health nurse consultant to provide technical assistance in standards development, field consultation, and occupational health nursing expertise. In 1993, the Office of Occupational Health Nursing was established within the agency.

In 1990, AAOHN published its first occupational health nursing research priorities, updated in 1999, which provide the direction for occupational health nursing research (Fig. 6.1) (12). The AAOHN Foundation was established in 1998 to support education and research funding initiatives.

OCCUPATIONAL HEALTH NURSING ROLES AND PRACTICE

In light of population trends, economic demands, and regulatory mandates, more emphasis will likely be placed on primary care delivery at the work site, case management, disability management, and possibly extended care to families. Occupational health nurses need to enhance their skills in cost management and research as well as identify health problems/hazards to determine means for health improvement and enhancement within a cost-effective framework. However, it should be noted that the management, monitoring, and surveillance of work-related illnesses and injuries must remain a priority (13).

Approximately 30,000 nurses are practicing in the occupational health field in the United States (i.e., 1.5% to 2% of the total nursing population). About 60% of these 30,000 nurses work alone, making decisions regarding health and safety issues, influencing policy in health and safety, and planning and implementing a myriad of health programs. The majority of nurses practicing in occupational health are prepared

1. Effectiveness of primary health care delivery at the worksite.
2. Effectiveness of health promotion nursing intervention strategies.
3. Methods for handling complex ethical issues related to occupational health (e.g., ADA, FMLA, confidentiality of employees health records, truth telling).
4. Strategies that minimize work-related health outcomes (e.g., respiratory disease).
5. Health effects resulting from chemical exposures in the workplace.
6. Occupational hazards of healthcare workers (e.g., latex allergy, bloodborne pathogens).
7. Factors that influence workers' rehabilitation and return to work.
8. Effectiveness of ergonomic strategies to reduce worker injury and illness.
9. Effectiveness of case management approaches in occupational illness or injury.
10. Evaluation of critical pathways to effectively improve workers' health and safety and to enhance maximum recovery and safe return to work.
11. Effects of shift work on workers' health and safety.
12. Strategies for increasing compliance with or motivating workers to use personal protective equipment.

It is interesting to note two-thirds of the previous research priorities remained in this group of new priorities. This clearly reflects the need for ongoing research in those areas (i.e., primary care, health promotion, ethics, chemical exposures, healthcare hazards, outcome management, ergonomics, return to work).

FIG. 6.1. Research priorities in occupational health nursing.

at the baccalaureate level and have been practicing in the field of occupational health for at least 10 years (14).

Occupational health nursing practice is grounded in the principles that guide public health practice, that is, examining population trends in health, illness, and injury in order to protect the health of individuals (13). Individual care is provided to ill and injured workers; however, emphasis is on providing programs and services to maintain, improve, and protect the health of the workforce.

The occupational health nurse is often the only health care professional at the work site, and as such has the primary responsibility for the management of worker health and safety with consideration to ethical, cultural, spiritual, and corporate beliefs. This heritage of independence in practice often is not shared by other nursing colleagues in acute care settings. In addition, interdependent functioning with other professionals and groups is integral to occupational health nursing practice and enhances the health care provided at the work site. The nurse collaborates with other disciplines to help management recognize the economic and human benefits of occupational health programs, thereby maximizing worker productivity by promoting employee mental and physical well-being while ensuring cost-effectiveness.

ROLES

As most nurses employed by industry practice alone, they often assume multiple roles such as clinician, manager, and consultant. This is contrasted with a multinurse unit where responsibilities are usually more clearly differentiated, wherein the occupational health nurse may be hired specifically as a clinician, health services manager, or health promotion specialist.

Seven major roles are identified in the practice of occupational health nursing: clinician/practitioner, administrator, educator, health promotion specialist, case manager, researcher, and consultant (15). The clinician/practitioner is primarily responsible for delivering direct care to employees in the management of illnesses and injuries and in the promotion of health. The administrator manages human and operational resources and provides overall direction for accomplishing the goals and objectives of the occupational health service. As an educator in the work setting, the nurse teaches individuals or groups of workers. As a case manager, the occupational health nurse coordinates health care services for the employee from the onset of injury or illness to a safe return to work or an optimal alternative. The health promotion specialist has primary responsibility for the overall management of the health promotion program including the development of a comprehensive program that meets the needs of the workforce population within the context of supporting organizational business objectives for a healthy workforce and work environment. These initiatives might include exercise, nutrition, or smoking cessation programs. As a researcher, the occupational health nurse may conduct or participate in scientific investigations. As a consultant, the nurse provides advice and recommendations related to occupational health nursing practice. Here is an in-depth discussion of these seven roles:

1. The occupational health nurse clinician/practitioner applies the nursing process (i.e., assessment, diagnosis, planning, implementation, and evaluation) in providing nursing care for occupational and nonoccupational health problems, and develops health promotion, protection, and prevention programs and strategies based on worker needs and health hazards. Depending on the knowledge, training, and experience as well as legal scope of practice, the occupational health nurse clinician/practitioner generally performs the following major activities:
    - Assesses the work environment for actual and/or potential health hazards;
    - Collects data about the health status of the worker through an occupational health history, physical assessment, and appropriate laboratory measurements;
    - Develops a diagnosis to formulate a plan of nursing care in collaboration with the employee and other health care professionals, as appropriate;
    - Records health data and maintains accurate employee health records;
    - Provides health promotion and disease prevention interventions (e.g., immunization, respiratory protection, hypertension screening, hearing conservation programs);
    - Provides first aid and primary care;
    - Provides counseling for worker health problems; and
    - Develops liaison relationships with community health care providers and organizations for worker health enhancement (e.g., referral to private providers and agencies such as American Lung Association (ALA), American Heart Association (AHA), and employee assistance programs).

2. The occupational health nurse administrator provides direction for the planning, implementation, and evaluation of occupational health services. To accomplish this task, the administrator must collaborate with others and facilitate interpersonal relationships for the smooth running of the organizational unit. The occupational health nurse administrator generally performs the following major activities:
   - Assesses the health needs of the workforce to plan and develop cost-effective health services;
   - Defines goals and objectives for the occupational health service;
   - Determines resources, such as facilities, staff, and operating expenses, necessary to accomplish unit goals, and develops an appropriate, realistic budget;
   - Determines policies and procedures aimed to foster goal attainment and work performance;
   - Provides leadership in the management and evaluation of human and operational resources;
   - Provides opportunities for enhancement of professional growth;
   - Provides quality management through quality process and assurance techniques (e.g., efficiency and outcome audits, peer review);
   - Participates in strategic planning; and
   - Evaluates effectiveness of services and programs.
3. The role of the occupational health nurse educator is usually described in relation to formal academic and continuing education functions within academic institutions (this role will not be discussed here within this context). In the occupational health setting, the educator role is usually coupled with the role of the clinician. Health education is provided often during a health assessment or visit to the occupational health unit, and to groups in informal group meetings (e.g., lunch) or more formal training sessions. As a work-site health educator, the occupational health nurse generally performs the following major activities:
   - Assesses the needs of the workforce with respect to health information and educational interventions;
   - Develops, implements, and evaluates health promotion and education programs and materials;
   - Acts as a liaison to community agencies in establishing networks for health education and promotion resources; and
   - Provides current information to all workers regarding health issues, trends, and factors that influence health behaviors and impact health outcomes.
4. As a health promotion specialist, the occupational health nurse designs, implements, and evaluates work-site health promotion programs with a goal of improving the overall health status and productivity of the workforce, and reducing health care costs. The nurse manages a multilevel wide-ranging health promotion program that is integrated into the corporate business objectives. The programs may address an awareness level, focus on lifestyle or behavior change programs, and/or encompass environments that encourage healthy lifestyles. Specific functions of the occupational health nurse health promotion specialist generally include the following:
   - Uses appropriate data sources to assess and target health promotion program needs for the workforce;
   - Develops, monitors, and implements the goals and strategies for the health promotion program;
   - Develops primary, secondary, and tertiary prevention programs;
   - Assists employees, dependents, and communities to modify health risk behaviors; and
   - Conducts ongoing evaluation of the specific activities as well as the overall health promotion program integrating cost-containment and cost-effectiveness aspects.
5. The occupational health nurse case manager may have case management as one of several job responsibilities, or an occupational health nurse working in a multinurse setting or employed by a case management firm may have case management as the primary job function. The case manager establishes a provider network, recommends treatment plans that assure quality and efficacy while controlling costs, monitors outcomes, and maintains communication among all involved. While case management services may be limited to occupational injury or illness, they can include nonoccupational injury or illness as well. Services typically begin at the onset of injury or illness and continue until the individual returns to work or achieves an optimum level of functioning. Specific functions of the occupational health nurse case manager generally include the following:
   - Determines the need for case management intervention;
   - Establishes criteria to identify workers who would benefit from case management services;

- Identifies goals, objectives, and actions as part of a comprehensive case management plan in collaboration with the worker and other health care providers;
- Develops and conducts an evaluation process for the case management program; and
- Monitors, documents, and evaluates the quality of individual worker outcomes and makes adjustments as necessary.

6. The occupational health nurse researcher works to increase the knowledge base in occupational health nursing practice to improve the health of the workforce and the working conditions. In the occupational health setting, the nurse may function in several capacities, ranging from identification of trends in illness and injury that may provoke an investigation, to participation in data collection activities, or in the actual design and implementation of a research study. The role the occupational health nurse plays in research depends on the knowledge and skills necessary to carry out the functions. Collaboration with others involved in research is key to a successful project. The occupational health nurse who functions as a researcher generally engages in the following major activities:
   - Identifies researchable questions as related to occupational health and safety or health promotion;
   - Participates with others in the conduct of research; and
   - Disseminates research findings into practice.
7. The occupational health nurse consultant serves as a resource to management and members of the occupational health and safety team. Often, this role is performed by a nurse not employed by the organization; however, a corporate or regional occupational health nurse who works within the organizational structure may provide consultation to nurses and other health care professionals within the company. A nurse consultant may provide services such as developing policies and procedures, record systems, job descriptions, or for hazard evaluation and worker job analysis. The occupational health nurse consultant generally performs the following major activities:
   - Provides advice about the scope and development of occupational health services and programs;
   - Serves as a resource to management on occupational health nursing issues, quality assurance, and the legal scope of practice;
   - Advises occupational health nurses, management, and other health care professionals about trends in health care and the regulatory impact; and
   - Serves as a resource for information and professional networking.

In addition to these roles, an occupational health nurse may function in such diverse roles as academician, policy maker in governmental agencies, disability/claims specialist, or lobbyist, among others.

SCOPE OF OCCUPATIONAL HEALTH NURSING PRACTICE

The definition of occupational health nursing has evolved over time, reflecting the changing role of the occupational health nurse. The AAOHN provides this definition:

> Occupational and environmental health nursing is the specialty practice that focuses on the promotion, prevention, and restoration of health within the context of a safe and healthy environment. It includes the prevention of adverse health effects from occupational and environmental health hazards. It provides for and delivers occupational and environmental health and safety services to workers, worker populations, and community groups. Occupational and environmental health nursing is an autonomous specialty, and nurses make independent nursing judgments in providing health care services (14).

PREVENTION FOUNDATION

Prevention is the cornerstone of occupational health nursing practice (9). Within a framework of prevention, the primary goals of occupational health nursing practice are the following:

- Promote, maintain, and restore the physical and psychosocial well-being of the workers in order to enhance optimal functioning;
- Protect the worker from hazards that may occur as a result of the work experience;
- Encourage and participate in a company culture supportive of health; and
- Collaborate with workers, management, and other disciplines and health care professionals to ensure a safe and healthful work environment.

The occupational health nurse practices at all levels of prevention with an emphasis on cost containment while preserving and improving quality health services (9,16). Primary prevention is aimed at health promotion and protection; secondary prevention focuses on early diagnosis, detection, treatment, and dis-

TABLE 6.1. *Examples of occupational health nursing practice activities within prevention framework*

Primary prevention	Secondary prevention	Tertiary prevention
Immunizations	Health assessment and surveillance	Work hardening
Wellness programs	Preplacement/periodic examinations	Rehabilitation
Nutrition education	Screening programs, i.e., high blood pressure	Disability management
Exercise fitness programs		

ability limitation; and tertiary prevention focuses on rehabilitation (17). Examples of occupational health nursing activities within the prevention framework are shown in Table 6.1 and briefly described here:

The occupational health nurse uses a variety of primary prevention methods with one-on-one interaction as an important strategy for evaluating risk reduction behavior for individuals. The occupational health nurse has daily contact with numerous employees for many reasons (e.g., assessment and treatment of episodic illness or injury and health surveillance); therefore, this is an important method of promoting health. The phrase "seize the moment" aptly describes the opportunity that exists with every employee encounter.

For overall health promotion, the nurse may plan, implement, and evaluate a health fair, which is a multifaceted health promotion strategy that usually includes a number of community health resources to provide expertise on a wide range of health issues and community services. As part of an overall health and wellness strategy, the occupational health nurse may negotiate with the employer for an on-site fitness center or area with fitness equipment; if cost or space is prohibitive, the employer may choose to partially subsidize membership at a local fitness center (18).

Types of nonoccupational programs included in the area of primary prevention are cardiovascular health, cancer awareness, personal safety, immunization, prenatal and postpartum health, accident prevention, retirement health, stress management, and relaxation techniques. Occupational health programs could include topics such as emergency response, first aid and cardiopulmonary resuscitation training, right-to-know training, immunization programs for international business travelers, prevention of back injury through knowledge of proper lifting techniques, ergonomics, and other programs targeted to the specific hazards identified in the workplace (18–20).

Secondary prevention efforts provided by the occupational health nurse include preplacement, periodic, and job transfer evaluations to ensure that the worker is being placed or is continuing to work in a job that is safe for that worker (21). The preplacement evaluation is performed before the worker begins employment in a new company or is placed in a different job. The evaluation is a baseline examination that consists of a medical history, an occupational health history, and a physical assessment that should target the type of work that the employee will be performing such as lifting or sand blasting.

Periodic assessments usually occur at a regular interval (e.g., annual and biannual) and are based on specific protocols for those exposed to substances or irritants such as lead, asbestos, noise, or various chemicals. Examinations of individuals transferring to other jobs are critical to document any changes in health that may have occurred while the employee was working in a specific area or with a specific process. The occupational health nurse can offer health screenings that are designed for early detection of disease with relative ease and at minimal cost. Screenings may focus on vision, cancer, cholesterol, hypertension, diabetes, TB, and pulmonary function. Other types of screening may be contracted with a vendor who uses mobile equipment to provide screenings such as mammography.

On a tertiary level, the occupational health nurse plays a key role in the rehabilitation and restoration of the worker to an optimal level of functioning. Strategies include case management, negotiation of workplace accommodations, and counseling and support for workers who will continue to be affected by chronic disease (22).

Knowledge of the workplace, the ability to negotiate with the employer for appropriate accommodations, early intervention, and comprehensive case management skills have been and will continue to be essential for the disabled employee's successful return to work. The process of returning an individual to work begins with the onset of injury or illness (1).

The occupational health nurse can monitor and support the health of employees returning to work continuing to experience adverse health effects of chronic disease. For example, the employee who is returning to work after sustaining a myocardial infarction may have blood pressure monitored on a routine basis. Counseling regarding adjustment to normal work life and support for behavior modification (e.g., smoking cessation) may also be provided (23).

PRACTICE AND PROGRAM INFLUENCES

As the nurse practices in the occupational health setting, the ultimate goal is to improve, maintain, and restore the health of the worker. There are many factors that impact on this goal, including external and internal or work-setting influences of which the occupational health nurse must have full knowledge and understanding.

Factors external to the organization play a major role in the type and methods of care delivered. How the organization reacts to and handles these factors has a significant impact on health-related costs, programs, and outcomes.

External influences include the following:

- Economic constraints, decreased profits, more costly health care delivery methods, and costs related to health insurance premiums and workers' compensation claims;
- Sociocultural characteristics of the population, reflected in the workforce, such as aging workforce, more women, increased diversity, literacy, more chronic disease;
- Legislation that requires implementation of regulations for workplace health and safety changes and monitoring for compliance, which may also result in increased costs related to programs, controls, resources, and administrative practices (e.g., Americans with Disabilities Act, ADA); and
- Advances in technology related to new work processes/hazards requiring more professional/technical knowledge and skills.

Factors within the work setting itself play a major role in support for health and safety programs, the type and degree of exposure to health hazards in the environment, and the overall view of health and safety at the work site. These factors affect trends in illness and injury at work and the health of the worker population.

Internal influences include the following:

- The workforce, including its size, composition, and demographics, health status, and projected needs;
- The type of work and work processes, related hazards, and monitoring and control systems to prevent and reduce exposure risk;
- The corporate culture, mission, and philosophy with respect to fostering the health of the workforce and control of workplace hazards;
- The allocation of human and capital resources to accomplish the occupational health and safety goals;
- The collaborative interdisciplinary functioning necessary to conduct occupational health and safety programs, assessments, surveillance activities, and research;
- The data/information resources needed to provide best practice and eliminate/reduce hazards in the work environment; and
- The goals of the occupational health unit to support quality program outcomes and productive workers.

The scope of practice of occupational health nursing, depicted in Fig. 6.2, is broad and is directed toward achievement of the following cost-effective health promotion and protection goals:

1. Worker/workplace hazard assessment and surveillance: To determine worker health status, the occupational health nurse may perform assessments, examinations, monitoring, and surveillance activities such as occupational health histories, and preplacement, periodic, and special assessments. Hazard detection and surveillance of the workplace is critical to identify hazards harmful to worker health. Familiarity with the work and work processes and the ability to conduct a comprehensive walk-through assessment including observation of work practices and use of personal protective equipment is critical to accurate hazard detection. Illnesses or injuries on the job are associated with exposures related to the following categories (9):
   a. Biologic/infectious hazards: infectious/biologic agents, such as bacteria, viruses, fungi, or parasites, that may be transmitted via contact with infected patients or contaminated body secretions/fluids.
   b. Chemical hazards: various forms of chemicals that are potentially toxic or irritating to the body system, including medications, solutions, and gases.
   c. Enviromechanical hazards: factors encountered in the work environment that cause or potentiate accidents, injuries/illnesses (e.g., cumulative trauma disorders), strain, or discomfort (e.g., poor equipment or lifting devices, slippery floors).
   d. Physical hazards: agents within the work environment, such as radiation, electricity, extreme temperatures, and noise that can cause tissue trauma.
   e. Psychosocial hazards: factors and situations encountered or associated with one's job or

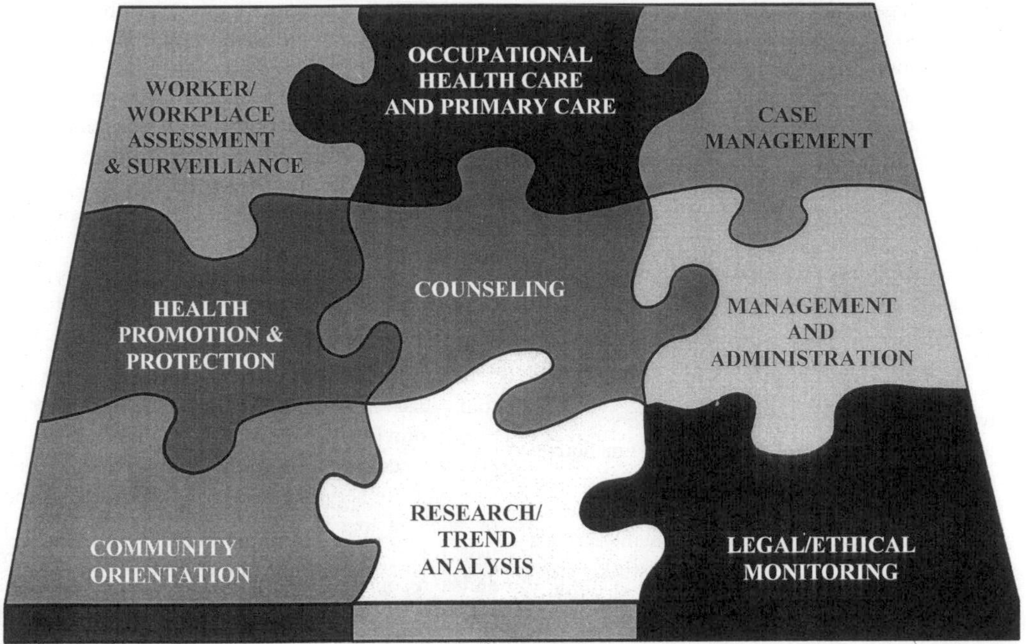

FIG. 6.2. Occupational health nursing practice.

work environment that create or potentiate stress, emotional strain, and/or interpersonal problems.

2. Occupational health care and primary care: Health care is provided to workers for work-related illnesses or injuries and episodic and nonoccupational illnesses and injuries. Primary care for nonoccupational health conditions usually includes, for example, care for emergencies, minor and chronic health problems, such as upper respiratory infections or blood pressure monitoring, including appropriate referral and follow-up.
3. Case management: Case management is an integral component of occupational health care management involving conditions that may be occupational in origin (e.g., from an exposure) or nonoccupational in origin (e.g., cardiovascular disease). Coordination and management of cost-effective quality health care services from the onset of illness or injury to return to work or optimal recovery are key. Early intervention and evaluation of outcomes, including cost savings, are essential components that provide for immediate problem identification and engage the worker in care planning from the beginning of the illness/injury to recovery. Early intervention helps prevent fragmented and delayed care by engaging appropriate health care providers at the beginning of care rather than later after complications may have developed. Case management requires knowledge of all factors that have an impact on worker health, including financial, spiritual, and cultural issues, and intense follow-up.
4. Health promotion/protection: These activities are aimed at increasing awareness and knowledge about occupational toxic exposures, lifestyle risk factors associated with health and illness (e.g., smoking, nutrition), changing attitudes and behaviors to improve health, and increasing self-responsibility for health. Supporting a philosophy of illness prevention is important to health enhancement and improvement. In addition to the activities described above, program planning and management of health promotion and special health programs include regulatory programs (e.g., hearing conservation, respiratory protection); screening programs for early detection (e.g., hypertension, mammography); rehabilitation and disability management programs including return to work; and employee assistance programs for workers' mental health needs and for performance related problems.
5. Counseling: Counseling is an integral component of the nurse's practice and one in which the nurse is particularly skilled. Counseling about physical and psychosocial health-related problems, family

dynamics, parenting, coping, and grief associated with a loss are but a few examples of counseling interventions. The type of care provided should be guided by nursing protocols or guidelines in accordance with state legal requirements.

6. Administration and management: Administration of the occupational health service involves goal setting, policy development planning, and budgeting. The occupational health nurse is often responsible for the effective and efficient management of the occupational health service. Establishment of criteria to measure goal achievement is a necessary component. Quality assurance, including record audits and attention to quality process activities (e.g., identifying quality indicators and barriers), are important to improving the functioning of the occupational health service.
7. Community orientation: The occupational health nurse should collaborate with community groups and organizations to develop a network of resources. For example, agencies such as the American Heart Association, American Lung Association, or American Cancer Association can offer valuable materials, information, and expertise to help with health programs and/or referrals. In addition, working with health departments, hospitals, and community providers can be mutually beneficial to the company and worker.
8. Research: The foundation for practice is based on soundly conducted research. The occupational health nurse is in a key position to examine relationships between exposures, the work environment, and the health or illness of the worker. Once data are generated and analyzed, results can be used to improve current practice or develop new techniques and methods, such as for counseling and health education strategies to reduce risk and improve worker health.
9. Legal/ethical practice: The occupational health nurse must be familiar with the laws that govern the occupational health and safety of workers (e.g., OSH Act, Hazard Communication Standard, ADA) and to recommend or develop programs to meet requirements. The occupational health nurse must be cognizant of the state nurse practice acts, standards for occupational and environmental health nursing practice, and ethical practice parameters. The Code of Ethics from the AAOHN provides guidance for ethical decision making and addresses the following areas:
   - Provision of nondiscriminatory health care in the work environment with regard to human dignity;
   - Collaboration with other health professionals/agencies to meet the needs of the workforce;
   - Protection of employee's right to privacy and protection of confidential information;
   - Provision of quality care and monitoring of unethical/illegal actions;
   - Acceptance of accountability for health care actions;
   - Maintenance of individual competence; and
   - Participation in knowledge-building activities such as research.

While many occupational health nurses practice in traditional manufacturing industry settings, other nurses provide services to workers in hospitals, government, construction sites, and university settings. The types of services and programs provided depend on such factors as the composition and size of the workforce, potential and actual workplace hazards, and a recognized need for occupational health and safety. Thus, the number and mix of occupational health nurses at a given work site is determined by not only the size of the workforce but also the relative type and severity of potential workplace hazards, trends in occupational illness and injuries, regulatory mandated programs, and provision of nonoccupational health services and health promotion and screening programs.

Organizational needs should determine the type of nurse recruited for an occupational health nursing position; that is, the nurse's skills, knowledge, and training should be commensurate with the job requirements. Resources such as the AAOHN professional society, state and local professional occupational health nursing constituent groups, occupational health nursing consultants, and academic institutions that offer occupational health nursing programs may be potential contact sources for employers.

CONCLUSION

The occupational health nurse often functions in a variety of roles, depending on the needs of the workforce and resources available to expand services and programs. The occupational health nurse is an integral part of the occupational health and safety team and is often the primary health care provider at the work site.

The role of the occupational health nurse has expanded considerably in recent decades, with greater emphasis on advanced clinical skills, management, case management, health promotion, cost-containment skills, and regulatory monitoring. The occupational health nurse will continue to assume a major role in the management of occupational health services with increased emphasis on policy making and expansion of research skills to better identify and define occupational health problems in order to improve worker health.

REFERENCES

1. Rogers B. Occupational health nursing expertise: planning for the future of occupational health nursing. *AAOHN J* 1998;46:497–503.
2. Rogers B. Occupational health nursing practice, education, and research: challenge for the future. *AAOHN J* 1990;38:536–543.
3. American Association of Industrial Nurses. *The nurse in industry.* New York: Author, 1976.
4. Markolf AS. Industrial nursing begins in Vermont. *Public Health Nurs* 1945;37:125–129.
5. McGrath BJ. Fifty years of industrial nursing. *Public Health Nurs* 1945;37:119–124.
6. Wright FS. *Industrial nursing.* New York: Macmillan, 1919.
7. Felton J. The genesis of American occupational health nursing: part I. *Occup Health Nurs* 1985;33:615–621.
8. Rogers B. Perspectives in occupational health nursing. *AAOHN J* 1988;36:151–155.
9. Rogers B. *Occupational health nursing: concepts and practice.* New York: WB Saunders, 2001.
10. LaDou J. *Occupational health law.* New York: Marcel Decker, 1981.
11. Brown ML. *Occupational health nursing.* New York: Macmillan, 1981.
12. Rogers B, Agnew J, Pompeii L. Occupational health nursing research priorities. *AAOHN J* 1999;47: 493–500.
13. Harper A. *The health of populations.* New York: Springer, 1986.
14. American Association of Occupational Health Nurses. Standards of Occupational and Environmental Health Nursing Practice. Atlanta: Author, 1999.
15. Randolph SA. Occupational health nursing roles. In: Rogers B, ed. *Occupational health nursing: concepts and practice.* Philadelphia: WB Saunders, 2001.
16. Wachs J, Parker-Conrad J. Occupational health nursing in 1990 and the coming decade. *Appl Occup Environ Hyg* 1990;5:200–203.
17. Leavell HR, Clark EG. *Preventative medicine for the doctor in his community: an epidemiologic approach.* New York: McGraw-Hill, 1965.
18. Blix A. Integrating occupational health protection and health promotion: theory and program application. *AAOHN J* 1999;47:168–174.
19. Dille JH. A worksite influenza immunization program: impact on lost work days, health care utilization, and health care spending. *AAOHN J* 1999;47:301–309.
20. Sorrenson G, et al. The effects of a health promotion-health protection intervention on behavior change: the WellWorks study. *Am Public Health* 1998;88:1685–1690.
21. Meservy D, et al. Health surveillance: effective components of a successful program. *AAOHN J* 1997;45: 500–511.
22. Pergola T, et al. Case management services for injured workers: providers' perspectives. *AAOHN J* 1999;47: 397–404.
23. Perry MC. REACH: an alternative early to work program. *AAOHN J* 1996;44:294–299.
24. Babbitz M. The practice of occupational health nursing in the U.S. *Occup Health Nurs* 1983;31:23–25.

7
The Independent Medical Evaluation

Christopher R. Brigham, William Boucher, and Alan L. Engelberg

The evaluation of work-related injury and illness requires clarification of physical, behavioral, psychosocial, vocational, and legal issues (1,2). Occupational medicine physicians, therefore, must be knowledgeable about the terminology and systems involved (3,4). Physicians participate in this arena through clinical care, case consultation, and performance of independent medical evaluations (IMEs). This chapter discusses the role and context of IMEs in the provision of occupational medicine services.

IMEs are examinations performed by a physician not involved in the person's care for the purpose of clarifying medical and job issues. Occupational medicine physicians are often the most appropriate specialists to evaluate work-related injuries and to determine whether work-site accommodations may be necessary for certain medical disorders.

IMEs are performed to provide information for case management and for evidence in hearings and other legal proceedings (5). IMEs are a component of all workers' compensation statutes, although the specifics vary by state. IMEs also are used in clarifying liability (personal injury) and disability. Insurers, third-party administrators, employers, and attorneys usually request IMEs. States may impose limitations on the number of examinations an injured person may have, and may specify qualifications for evaluating physicians. IMEs may also have different roles, dependent on the context of the evaluation. For example, in some states, examinations performed by an agreed upon examiner or requested directly by the court or commission may be given particular credence.

The physician who performs the IME is not involved in a treating capacity. No direct clinical management is provided and the fee is paid by the party requesting the examination. The information obtained is presented to the client in a written report. The physician must be impartial and unbiased in performing the assessment. Ethics and moral character must be without question.

Assessments are often requested because of a lack of medical information or conflict on specific matters, especially regarding the cause of the condition and a person's ability to work. The physician makes a careful assessment and addresses the issues raised by the referring sources. The assessment process must be precise and detailed, and assure that conclusions are valid, reliable, defensible, and useful. Many assessments undergo legal scrutiny, and the physician must be able to support the conclusions in deposition or testimony.

The examinee is not necessarily a willing participant, and may present with more dysfunctional behavior than is usually encountered in a typical treatment setting. The assessments, therefore, are more challenging and require greater patience. A thorough assessment of chronic pain associated with a musculoskeletal disorder, for example, may require 2 hours or longer of the physician's time. The use of other staff, structured assessment protocols, and software reduces the time needed to conduct a thorough evaluation.

The performance of these assessments requires specific skills in addition to clinical acumen. The physician must have not only a strong clinical background, but also an appreciation of the biomedical, emotional, and vocational aspects of injury and illness. Credentials should be solid; this is not an arena for an inexperienced physician or someone who is unable to support conclusions if challenged.

IMEs are a valuable component of case assessment and management. Unfortunately, many IMEs are inadequate, superficial, and biased, and do not address specific questions. However, a physician who provides a thorough, detailed IME delivers a valued, needed service. The performance of these assessments is challenging because of the intense effort involved and the complexity of the workers' compensation and legal systems.

Depending on the complexity of the case and the tools used in the process, comprehensive IMEs may require up to several hours of physician time, with approximately 2 hours of that time spent with the examinee. It is best to schedule an IME at a time separate from other clinical visits. Because of the challenges involved, it is difficult to devote all one's effort to performing IMEs; they are best approached as one component of a practice in occupational medicine. Physicians with some clinical, consulting, or teaching involvement are considered to be more credible than those who only perform IMEs.

CHALLENGES IN INDEPENDENT MEDICAL EVALUATIONS

Key issues associated with an IME differ from clinical consultations in role and focus. The most common issues are diagnosis, causation, prognosis, maximal medical improvement, permanent impairment, appropriateness of care, and recommendations. Typically, the client requesting the examination poses specific questions. The occupational physician should recognize the importance of addressing these issues in both the performance of an IME and the preparation of a report. An example of a typical referral letter is shown in Fig. 7.1.

Dear:

Thank you for agreeing to see Employee X, an employee of ABC Company, for an independent medical evaluation.

(Provide a short medical history here)

Under separate cover you will receive copies of medical documentation that we have on file, and a description of the employee's job.

Taking this short history and the medical documentation into account, in conjunction with your own thorough evaluation, please answer the following questions:

1. Does the employee have the diagnosis of XXXXX?
2. Does the employee's medical condition preclude travel to and from work? Does it preclude being at work for a full work week (40 hours/week)?
3. Is there a medical reason to believe that the employee is likely to experience injury, harm, or aggravation of the medical condition by performing or attempting to perform the tasks of (title of job)? If so, what is the time-frame within which this injury or harm is likely to occur?
4. Does the employee's medical condition preclude the assignment of the tasks and duties of (title of job)? If so, what tasks, and for what medical reasons? Is there a medical reason to believe that the employee is likely to experience sudden or subtle incapacitation from performing such tasks, and if so, to what degree?
5. If you recognize any restrictions for the employee because of a substantial harm to the employee, what measures should ABC Company consider in identifying accommodations to eliminate the need for the restrictions?

Please send the results of your independent medical evaluation to me at

(address here)

If you have any questions, please feel free to call me at.

Thank you.

Sincerely,

FIG. 7.1. Example of a referral letter.

DIAGNOSES

Clinical impressions include not only the primary illness or injury, but also other conditions that need further evaluation. It is useful to prepare a problem list of clinical diagnoses, particularly other pertinent conditions that contribute to the patient's functional status. It is helpful to present the problem list in relative order of significance, and to number each problem. Standard classification of diagnoses is useful, such as the *International Classification of Diseases (ICD-9)* (6) and, for psychiatric illness, the *Diagnostic and Statistical Manual of Mental Disorders* (7).

Pain, pathology, impairment, residual functional capacity, and disability are separate concepts. *Pain,* especially chronic pain, may not be associated with significant physical pathology (8,9). *Pathology* may be present without symptoms or dysfunction. *Impairment* is a measurable decrement in some physiologic function, whereas *disability* considers not only the physical or mental impairment but also the social, psychological, or vocational factors associated with a person's ability to work (10–12). Functional limitations are manifestations of impairment (13). Factors relating to each of these issues should be identified in the problem list.

The significance of medical problems should be discussed, such as the relationship between the extent of symptoms (subjective complaints) and signs (objective findings). It is necessary to identify which problems are acute and which are chronic or degenerative in nature. Problems that predated an injury and may relate to current dysfunction directly or indirectly must be determined, since this information is used in assessing causal relationship. Psychosocial problems, health behaviors, and the examinee's perceptions/values are often more predictive of the future than is the physical condition.

Chronic pain, the most common problem seen in the performance of IMEs, may be not a symptom of an underlying acute somatic injury but rather a multidimensional biopsychosocial phenomenon (14–16). A multiaxial assessment of biomedical, psychosocial, and behavioral-functional issues is necessary (17–19).

CAUSAL RELATIONSHIP

Causation is a critical issue in work-related and liability cases. A work-related problem is defined as one that "arose out of and during the course of employment" (20). With an acute injury such as a fracture, this determination may be simple. In many workers' compensation cases, however, the process is far more complex, particularly with preexisting, chronic conditions and environmental exposures.

The physician must establish *causation* to a reasonable degree of medical *probability,* which implies that it is more probable than not (i.e., there is more than a 50% probability) that a certain condition arose out of or in the course of work duties. *Possibility* implies less than a 50% likelihood. Stating that a problem is work related implies that, based on the available information, to a reasonable degree of medical certainty, work activities caused the problem. States may vary in the definition of causation, particularly for cumulative trauma disorders and preexisting conditions.

Causation can be ultimate or proximate (21). Ultimate causation refers to the initial factor that leads to the effect. Proximate cause is the factor that immediately or closely precedes the effect.

A medical condition may be the result of one or multiple factors. *Apportionment* refers to the extent to which a condition is related to each of the multiple factors. For example, a worker may have sustained an injury with one employer, then returned to work and sustained a similar injury with another employer. In reviewing the case, it may be necessary to apportion current dysfunction between the two parties. It also may be necessary to apportion responsibility between work- and non–work-related conditions. Assigning apportionment depends largely on clinical judgment, since the science supporting apportionment is in its infancy.

Unique causation occurs when a condition is due to a specific cause, for example, asbestosis. Multifactorial causation, where there are several possible causes, and therefore the apportionment that goes with it, is more common.

Work activities may influence underlying problems. An *aggravation* implies a long-standing effect due to an event, resulting in a worsening, hastening, or deterioration of the condition. An *exacerbation* is a temporary increase in symptoms from the condition. Thus, an aggravation has an ongoing substantial impact on the physical condition, whereas an exacerbation results in a *flare* of symptoms, without a significant change in the underlying pathology.

The evaluator needs to scrutinize the specifics of the case and compare this information to the known pathogenesis of a condition. This analytic process requires careful assessment of the diagnoses, mechanism of injury, preexisting status, and clinical history.

CASE EXAMPLES

The following case examples illustrate some complexities of causation analysis.

Case 1

A 51-year-old man sustained a low back injury as a result of a lifting episode. He developed an acute onset of radicular pain and is found to have a herniated nucleus pulposus. His physician treats him with prolonged bed rest and high-dose steroids, and eventually he undergoes a diskectomy. Later he complains of hip pain, and aseptic necrosis of the hip is diagnosed. He undergoes a total hip replacement, and during the associated hospitalization a pulmonary embolism develops.

Each event would be causally related to the injury at work, since each situation either directly or indirectly resulted in the next one. If there were a break in the chain of events, causation would not be present. For example, if the avascular necrosis had not been caused by the steroids but by alcoholism, the complications would not be causally related, unless it was shown that the alcohol consumption resulted from his injury.

Case 2

A 40-year-old obese woman with hypothyroidism developed a right carpal tunnel syndrome. Her treating physician believes that this disorder is associated with her work as a cashier. Nerve conduction studies are positive on the right, and she undergoes a carpal tunnel release. One year later, similar problems develop on the left, and her treating physician states that these problems must be due to the fact that she now uses her left arm rather than her right.

Careful assessment revealed that this patient did not make significant use of the left hand, and analysis of her previous job as a cashier showed that her work was in a convenience store, with only occasional use of the cash register. It is more probable that her carpal tunnel syndrome was due not to her work activities but to her risk factors of obesity and hypothyroidism. The evaluator therefore concluded that her left carpal tunnel problem was not related to work activities.

Case 3

A 50-year-old woman diagnosed as having "overuse syndrome" is seen for further assessment, which reveals that she has upper and lower body complaints that are symmetric. She has 12 of 18 possible painful tender points, consistent with a diagnosis of fibromyalgia.

The evaluator finds that although the work activities resulted in temporary exacerbation of her symptoms, there is inadequate evidence to conclude that fibromyalgia was caused by these activities.

Case 4

A 41-year-old man sustained a low back muscular strain while lifting at work. Magnetic resonance imaging (MRI) reveals degenerative disc disease with bulging. There is no evidence, however, that his episode of low back pain is related to the degenerative disease. He improves and returns to his usual work activities. One year later, while lifting at home, he has another episode of acute back pain, this time with a radicular component. A herniated nucleus pulposus is diagnosed.

The initial work-related injury was muscular in origin. The degenerative disc disease predated the injury, although this was not known until the imaging study was performed. There is no evidence that the soft tissue injury aggravated the degenerative disc disease. The herniation a year later was unrelated to the initial muscle injury. It was concluded, to a reasonable degree of medical probability, that the subsequent problems were not causally related to the work-related lifting injury.

Prognosis

The physician may need to identify the outlook for a problem, that is, the predicted time of recovery. This opinion is based on a careful clinical assessment that compares the results with the natural history of the problem. Influencing factors are also identified. This information is used in case management to establish the case's financial reserves, which are the predicted expenses for medical care and lost wages. Analysis is influenced largely by concurrent problems. The relative role of each of these factors in determining the clinical prognosis should be identified.

Case 5

A 41-year-old physician fell on the ice and sustained comminuted scapular and thoracic fractures. She is in excellent health, motivated, and unable to afford any work absence.

Although the injury itself is significant, her motivation and the sedentary nature of her job suggest that the prognosis for full recovery and employability is good.

Case 6

A 31-year-old, obese deconditioned woman with a history of prolonged disability associated with carpal tunnel syndrome and a postural disturbance developed a myofascial pain syndrome involving her trapezius. She left school in the eighth grade, did not receive a general equivalency diploma (GED), and has a disabled spouse. She is dissatisfied with her work and supervisor, and angry with her employer about being injured.

The prognosis for the physical problem alone would be good; however, the prognosis for full successful return to work is not as hopeful.

MAXIMUM MEDICAL IMPROVEMENT

Maximal medical improvement is a phrase used to indicate when further recovery and restoration of function can no longer be anticipated to a reasonable degree of medical probability. This assessment implies that a condition is permanent and static. Considerations include whether the current or proposed treatment will result in functional improvement, if surgery has occurred recently, and whether enough time has passed for the process to be stable.

PERMANENT IMPAIRMENT

Often a physician is asked to conduct an *impairment evaluation* as part of the assessment. To physicians who are not independent medical evaluators, an impairment evaluation and an independent assessment may seem synonymous, but they are not (22). The basic philosophies have been detailed in the American Medical Association's *Guides to the Evaluation of Permanent Impairment* (the *Guides*) (23), which is the most widely used and accepted reference for evaluating permanent impairment. The *Guides* distinguishes between an *impairment* evaluation and a *disability* evaluation. According to the *Guides, impairment* is "the loss of, the loss of use of, or a derangement of any body part, system or function" and *disability* is "the limiting loss of the capacity to meet personal, social or occupational demands, or to meet statutory or regulatory requirements." Impairment is considered permanent when it has reached maximum medical improvement (MMI), meaning it is well stabilized and unlikely to change substantially in the next year with or without medical treatment.

Impairment is a measurable decrement in health status evaluated by medical means; disability is the gap between what a person can do and what he or she needs to do, partly because of a diminished health status. Disability is assessed by the consideration of nonmedical issues, such as the person's educational and vocational skills, experience, age, and, in workers' compensation cases, potential for future loss of wages. Assessing education, vocation, and potential for future loss of wages is not a skill most physicians possess, and thus the medical role usually is limited to evaluating impairment, not disability (24).

The *Guides* emphasizes objective assessment, necessitating a medical evaluation. Impairment may lead to functional limitations or the inability to perform activities of daily living (ADLs) and reflects a change from normal or preexisting status. Some chapters place a greater emphasis on either anatomic loss or functional loss. *Anatomic loss* refers to measurable loss of a body structure or organ system, whereas *functional loss* refers to change in function. *Normal* refers to a range or zone that represents healthy functioning; it varies with age, gender, and other factors. Normal is defined from either an individual or a population perspective, depending on the preinjury or preillness information that is available and the physician's clinical judgment.

Impairment criteria are designed to "provide a standardized method for physicians to use to determine medical impairment" and "were developed from scientific evidence as cited and from consensus of chapters authors or of medical specialty societies" (23, p. 4).

Impairment percentages in the fifth edition of the *Guides* are largely unchanged from those in the fourth because the majority of ratings are currently accepted, there are limited scientific data to support changes, and ratings should not be changed arbitrarily. However, some percentages have been changed for greater scientific accuracy or to achieve consistency. Among the most significant changes are impairment ratings of the spine, now only done at MMI, and the assessment of impairment for pain.

Ratings vary from 0% to 100% for whole-person permanent impairment. A 0% whole-person rating implies no organ or body system functional consequences and no limitation on the performance of common ADLs. A 90% to 100% whole-person rating again reflects very severe organ or body system impairment and requires the individual to be fully dependent on others for self-care, approaching death. Most impairments are not added; rather they are combined, so that multiple impairments are equal to or less than the sum of all the individual impairment values. The process of combining reflects that when considering two impairments the combined impairment is equal to the first impairment plus the second impairment as it relates to the remaining portion of the whole person that is unimpaired.

Subjective complaints such as fatigue or pain, when not accompanied by demonstrable organ dysfunction, clinical signs, or other independent, measurable abnormalities, are generally not ratable. However, a significant change with the fifth edition is that pain may be ratable if there is an underlying organic cause, providing up to 3% whole-person permanent impairment in certain circumstances. Disorders that are not ratable include fibromyalgia, chronic fatigue syndrome, and multiple chemical sensitivity.

In some workers' compensation jurisdictions, either by law, regulation, or administrative practice, a formula is used whereby the impairment rating becomes the primary piece of information from which a compensation level is established. This situation is unfortunate because an impairment evaluation can only document a person's health status at a point in time, and not the impact on functioning in society or employability. The impairment evaluation does not determine if a person may meet "personal, social or occupational demands." However, the *Guides* states it is "appropriate for a physician [to be] knowledgeable about the work activities of the patient to discuss the specific activities the worker can and cannot do, given the permanent impairment."

WORK CAPACITY

Work capacity is a primary issue in many IMEs. Judgments of work capability are formed by the patient's report, clinical condition, and measurements of functional performance. Individuals may provide information on their capabilities, particularly if symptom magnification is absent. Certain clinical conditions suggest specific restrictions. For example, in a patient with low back pain, the amount of lifting, bending, sitting, and certain body postures may need to be altered. Cumulative trauma disorders suggest the need for low-repetition, low-force tasks and an ergonomic assessment.

Functional performance assessments are more accurate determinations of ability, if the assessment is valid and reliable and relates to particular job tasks (25). Caution should be exercised because various methodologies are available. A structured protocol is essential. It is customary to express work capacity following parameters in the *Dictionary of Occupational Titles* of the United States Department of Labor, which are based primarily on lifting requirements (Table 7.1).

The examining physician should estimate capacities as carefully as possible, including the number of hours of work per day, based on endurance and tolerance for sitting, standing, and walking. Estimates of lifting and carrying capabilities are noted for specific frequencies. Guidelines should be provided for the

TABLE 7.1. *Dictionary of occupational titles work demands*

Category	Lifting occasionally (lb)	Lifting frequently (lb)
Sedentary	10	5
Light	20	10
Moderate	50	25
Heavy	100	50
Very heavy	150	75

From U.S. Department of Labor. *Dictionary of Occupational Titles,* 4th ed. Washington, DC: Department of Labor, 1991.

frequency and *duration of tasks* such as bending, crouching, squatting, pushing/pulling, climbing stairs, climbing ladders, reaching above shoulder level, lifting above shoulder level, balancing, and working on uneven ground or at heights.

These capacities are compared with the functional requirements of the job, obtained from job descriptions, videotapes, or direct observations. Specific assessments of work capacity based only on a clinical evaluation may be difficult. As a result, a functional performance assessment may be particularly helpful when incorporated into the IME.

Disability durations that provide the length of disability typically associated with a diagnosis or disorder may also provide very valuable insight to how much and how long of an impact a problem may have on functional ability (26).

APPROPRIATENESS OF CARE

Many IMEs call for a review of the appropriateness of clinical management, which should be based on the specifics of the case and not be reflective of bias against a certain discipline or approach. This review can include issues of unnecessary and/or omitted diagnostic evaluation, and inappropriate, excessive, and/or omitted treatment. The need for repeated imaging studies should be assessed. Areas of possible inappropriate treatment may include, for example, use of prolonged bed rest and immobilization, protracted passive physical therapy or manipulation, repeated surgery, and use of narcotic analgesics. A beneficial approach that is sometimes neglected includes the physician's involvement in functional restoration that addresses behavioral issues and focus on return to work. The details of the evaluation should be compared to the accepted standards of care for the problem. For example, manipulative therapy can be compared against standards set forth by the Rand Expert

Panel (27), the Mercy Center Consensus Conference (28), and the North American Spine Society's Ad Hoc Committee on Diagnostic and Therapeutic Procedures (29).

Specific recommendations on further diagnostic studies, treatment, or other aspects of the case may be sought. If further testing or treatment is not needed, the physician should so state. It may be appropriate to recommend obtaining missing records.

CONDUCTING AN EVALUATION AND PREPARING A REPORT

The IME process should address the issues posed by the referral source. The assessment consists of three phases: preevaluation, evaluation, and postevaluation. The use of structured questionnaires and inventories, and software with report templates facilitates this procedure. The physician may want to include ancillary staff members in this process to make the most efficient use of time.

Preevaluation

A request for an IME should specify issues to be addressed and background demographic, clinical, and claims information. The referral source (or the examiners office) needs to identify the party responsible for notifying the person to be examined. Often this responsibility is assumed by the requesting party, often by certified letter. The client should forward records before the examination. Since records may be poorly organized and incomplete, a clerical staff member can organize the records in advance; medical records should be separated from other information in the file and be organized chronologically. Reports of consultants and results of laboratory tests and surgical procedures can be tagged. It is important to review the medical records before the evaluation and to read correspondence from the client, so that the evaluation can be structured to answer specific questions. The examinee may be asked to complete a questionnaire before the evaluation, to facilitate the interview. Pain and functional inventories are particularly helpful in identifying behavioral and psychological components related to an illness or injury.

Evaluation

At the beginning of the visit, the physician should explain the nature of the evaluation and that an independent evaluation will be conducted, but that no treatment will be provided. There is no patient–physician relationship, and a report will be sent to the requesting client. The person should sign a release, stating, for example:

> I understand that the purpose of the examination is for an evaluation only, and that no treatment will be provided. I further understand that the client requesting and paying for the assessment will receive a report. I realize that no physician–patient relationship is established during the course of this assessment.

Key Components of the Evaluation

History

The history, organized in sections (Table 7.2), usually commences with a detailed review of the injury or illness, including the reported mechanism, symptoms at the time, and events immediately thereafter. These comments are compared to other medical records for consistency. The mechanism of injury is important in deciding causal relationship.

The history includes relevant *preexisting conditions* and prior injuries. The patient's baseline is established to determine the framework for examining the effect of the referenced condition. For example, in

TABLE 7.2. *Preparation of the independent medical evaluation (IME) report*

- Background
- History
  - Preexisting status
  - Injury
  - Clinical history
    - Chronology
    - Providers
    - Studies
    - Treatment
  - Current status
    - Complaints
    - Functional reports
    - Perceptions
  - Occupational history
  - Psychosocial history
  - Past medical history
  - Review of systems
  - Family history
- Pain inventories
- Examination
  - Behavioral
  - Structural
  - Regional
- Conclusions
  - Diagnosis
  - Prognosis
  - Recommendations
  - Work status

a patient with a preexisting low back problem, a subsequent event may result in an exacerbation or an aggravation of the condition. If records are available, they should be reviewed to determine the accuracy of the history. Other work- or liability-related incidents should be determined. This information may be particularly significant from a behavioral standpoint. For example, a history of multiple claims or claims associated with significant disability or large monetary settlement may warrant concern.

The *chronology* of events from the time of injury through the present is examined. The pattern of the condition is determined, and the specifics of providers, opinions of other consultants, results of diagnostic studies, and treatment approaches are reviewed. It should be determined whether the complaints are consistent over time, if the symptoms are supported by objective findings, and if the clinical management has been appropriate. The results of various diagnostic studies are examined to clarify the diagnoses and determine whether the evaluations were appropriate. The treatment and corresponding results are detailed and compared with the customary therapeutic approach. Failure of the patient to have any response to multiple treatment modalities suggests a chronic pain syndrome.

The current status is explored in detail, with attention directed to the examinee's primary concern. Most often the complaint is pain, and therefore the location, pattern, and nature of the pain, as well as aggravating/relieving factors, are defined. Associated symptoms such as numbness, tingling, weakness, morning stiffness, and other physiologic difficulties are assessed. It is important to identify not only positives but negatives as well. Anxiety, discouragement, depression, and sleep disturbance are referenced.

The person's perceived *functional status* is documented to clarify both capacity and behavioral issues. Tolerances for sitting, standing, walking, lifting, and carrying, and the ability to carry out a variety of tasks associated with ADLs are noted. In a patient with symptom magnification, inconsistencies may be present.

The examinee's *perceptions* are useful in understanding the personal experience with the medical problem. Several questions can be asked to clarify these issues. For example, "What do you think is causing your problem?" "What do you think will happen in the future?" "How satisfied are you with your medical care, employer, insurer, and the workers' compensation system?" "What is your primary goal?"

A thorough *occupational history* begins with a detailed description of the job at the time of injury, and includes not only physical characteristics but also issues of job satisfaction. For toxicology cases, a detailed review of exposures at the current and previous jobs is required, noting the possibility of latent illness. The course of events from the injury to the present, relative to disability, is explored. If the patient is not working, the involvement of vocational rehabilitation, possibilities for work in the future, and the patient's plans for the future are defined. If the patient is working, the details of this position are explored. It should be identified whether work restrictions have been imposed, along with their rationale. It should be determined if there has been a functional performance assessment; if so, the results should be scrutinized. The patient's previous work experiences, educational background, and future work plans should be defined.

A *psychological history* should be directed to the family unit, activities on a usual day, recreational activities, and changes in the household since the injury. Smoking, alcohol use, and use of recreational drugs are documented. One should attempt to clarify reinforcements for disability, such as changes in roles of other family members.

The complete medical history concludes with a traditional past medical history that notes medical and surgical procedures, medications and allergies, review of systems, and family history.

Examination

The meticulous history is followed by a physical examination including a behavioral assessment and a detailed examination of the involved area(s). The behavioral assessment commences when the patient is greeted. Pain behavior and inconsistencies should be documented. A structural examination focuses on posture, body position, and body movements.

Regional examinations should ensure reliability and ideally reproducibility of positive, negative, and nonphysiologic findings (30,31). For example, in a patient with low back pain, the examination should note gait, structure of the back (lordotic curves, pelvic symmetry, surgical scars), palpatory findings (localized tenderness, spasm, trigger points), and range of motion, among others. Range of motion of the spine should be determined using an inclinometer that measures cervical, thoracic, and lumbosacral angles. A neurologic examination includes, among others, sensory assessment, motor evaluation (strength and atrophy), and straight-leg raising both sitting and supine. Specific maneuvers also should be performed, for example, to determine sacroiliac problems, piriformis syndrome, somatic dysfunction syndrome, and problems that may be masquerading as low back pain. The assessment also should look for nonphysiologic (Waddell) findings of symptom magnification (see Chapter 22).

Pain and Disability Inventories

Psychological and behavioral factors must be considered in a disability assessment (32). A number of self-report, interview, and behavioral inventories have been developed to assess pain and disability (33). The self-report instruments have both comprehensive and brief formats. It is useful to include them in an IME to assess the behavioral and psychosocial aspects.

The self-report instruments assess disability in patients with chronic pain. The Multidimensional Pain Inventory (MPI) was designed specifically for patients with chronic pain (34). Another comprehensive measure of disability is the Sickness Impact Profile (SIP), which was designed as a generic measure of disability associated with any chronic illness (35). The Oswestry Disability Questionnaire (36) and the Roland Disability Questionnaire (37) were developed to assess changes in functional limitations associated with treatment for back pain. Another brief instrument is the Pain Disability Index (38), which measures changes in role functions associated with chronic pain. The Functional Assessment Screening Questionnaire (39) and the Functional Interference Estimate Scale (40) assess both functional limitations and role interference associated with chronic pain. Several interview measures also have been developed, but these have not been researched as intensively as the self-report measures. The Minnesota Pain Inventory is a useful screening test designed to assist in the diagnosis of patients with chronic pain complaints and to clarify the extent of exaggerating pain behavior (41). Pain drawings have been widely used to assess pain distribution and symptom magnification (42,43).

Distress and disability are associated; factors include personality, emotion, cognition, education, and attention/concentration deficits. The Minnesota Multiphasic Personality Inventory (MMPI) assesses personality factors and disability in individuals with chronic pain (44). Depression is common in chronic pain syndromes (45). Several scales have been used to rate depression, including the Center for Epidemiologic Studies–Depressed Mood Scale (CES-D), Zung Depressive Inventory, and Beck Depressive Inventory. Coping responses and attitudes/beliefs affect perception of disability. Attitudes (feelings about a subject) and beliefs (information about a subject) should be clarified when evaluating a patient with chronic pain. The concept of illness behavior refers to the different ways individuals perceive, evaluate, and respond to their symptoms. These have been studied in terms of the overt behaviors that patients use to communicate pain and pain behaviors.

The use of these inventories assists the evaluator in identifying the behavioral and psychosocial issues. The selection of inventories requires assessment of their intended use, appropriateness for the population being evaluated, validity and reliability of the instruments, and feasibility of administration and scoring.

Referral sources, as well as many physicians, may be unfamiliar with the utility of these tools and therefore may not request them in an assessment. Since these inventories require little time to administer and score and provide such useful information, it is suggested that they be included in the IME of a patient with chronic pain.

Diagnostic Studies

Radiographic films brought by the examinee (or supplied by the client) are reviewed at the visit. The findings are compared with those of the reviewing radiologist. Additional studies may be recommended to the referring source; however, they should not be obtained without approval from the referral source to avoid conflicts regarding fiscal responsibilities for the testing.

At the conclusion of the evaluation, it may be appropriate to discuss findings with the examinee, although some referral sources prefer that the examiner withhold certain opinions until the completion of the report.

Postevaluation

The evaluation should address the specific issues requested by the referring source. If the questions are not clear or have not been asked, then the physician should contact the client to determine what questions need to be answered. The physician may need to support the findings in a legal setting, such as in a deposition or in testimony. As a result, unsupported conclusions, emotional statements, or comments that may suggest libel of the examinee or involved doctors should be avoided.

IMEs are usually performed during a single visit, although the examinee may be seen at a future date, often 1 or 2 years later. The follow-up examination may be called by the client because of the availability of medical information missing at the time of the visit or a change in medical status or working conditions.

REPORTS

Reports should be organized and detailed, and present the information obtained during the evaluation. The available medical records, the patient's behavior and quality as a historian, individuals accompanying the examinee, and the context of the assessment should be described. The history, physical examination findings, results of pain inventories, and interpretation of radiographic studies follow.

Although the appendix includes an example of a report that is a thorough, detailed analysis that may be required in certain settings, occupational physicians are also called on to prepare brief reports related to fitness for duty, focused second opinions, or back-to-work evaluations. In these settings brevity is essential, as long as key information is presented. For example, a party requesting such an evaluation may be primarily interested in a person's ability to work or the need for additional medical care. Too often, physicians do not understand medical confidentiality in the context of workers' compensation (which is less strict than in the more common physician–patient relationship) and, as a result, employers and adjudicators may not receive adequate information to which they are entitled.

REFERENCES

1. Aronoff GM. Chronic pain and the disability epidemic. *Clin J Pain* 1991;7:330.
2. Turk DC, Rudy TE, Steig RL. The disability determination dilemma: toward a multi-axial solution. *Pain* 1988; 3:217.
3. Brigham CR. Independent medical evaluations and disability assessment. *OEM Rep* 1992;6:5.
4. Brigham CR. Medical analysis of workers' compensation claims. *Workers' Comp Monthly* 1990;11:1,18.
5. Tompkins N. Independent medical examinations: the how, when, and why of this useful process. *OSHA Compl Adv* 1992;215:7.
6. World Health Organization. *International Classification of Diseases* (9th revision ICD-9). Hyattsville: World Health Organization Collaborating Center, 1991.
7. American Psychiatric Association. *Diagnostic and statistical manual of mental disorders (DSM-IV)*. Washington, DC: American Psychiatric Association, 1994.
8. Loesser JD. What is chronic pain? *Theor Med* 1991;12: 213.
9. Spektor S. Chronic pain and pain-related disabilities. *J Disabil* 1990;1:98.
10. Ryley JF, Aherm DK, Follick MJ. Chronic pain and functional impairment: assessing beliefs about their relationship. *Arch Phys Med Rehabil* 1988;69:579.
11. Brena SF, Spektar S. Systematic assessment of impairment and residual functional capacity in pain-impaired patients. *J Back Musculoskel Rehabil* 1993;3:6.
12. Vasudevan SV. The relationship between pain and disability: an overview of the problem. *J Disabil* 1991;2: 44.
13. Vasudevan SV. Impairment, disability, and functional capacity assessment. In: Turk DC, Melzack R. *Handbook of pain assessment*. New York: Guilford Press, 1992.
14. American Medical Association. Pain and impairment. Appendix B in *AMA guides to the evaluation of permanent impairment,* 3rd ed. Chicago: American Medical Association, 1991.
15. Loesser JD. What is chronic pain? *Theor Med* 1991;12: 213.
16. Melzack R. *Pain measurement and assessment*. New York: Raven Press, 1983.
17. Turk DC. Evaluation of pain and disability. *J Disabil* 1991;2:24.
18. Turk DC, Rudy TE, Steig RL. The disability determination dilemma: toward a multi-axial solution. *Pain* 1988; 3:217.
19. Turk DC, Melzack R. *Handbook of pain assessment*. New York: Guilford Press, 1992.
20. Larson A. *The law of workmen's compensation*. New York: Matthew Bender, 1982.
21. Balsam A. Evaluation of disability under Workers' Compensation. In: Balsam A, Zabin AP, eds. *Disability handbook*. New York: Shepard's/McGraw-Hill, 1990.
22. Frymoyer JW, Haldeman S, Andersson GBJ. Impairment rating—the United States perspective. In: Pope MH, et al., eds. *Occupational low back pain: assessment, treatment, and prevention.* St. Louis: Mosby Year Book, 1991.
23. American Medical Association. *Guides to the evaluation of permanent impairment,* 5th ed. Chicago: American Medical Association, 2000.
24. Babitsky S, Sewall HD. *Understanding the AMA Guides in Workers' Compensation.* Colorado Springs: Wiley Law Publications, 1992.
25. Engelberg AL, Matheson LN. Impairment, disability, and function capacity. In: Rom WM, ed. *Environmental and occupational medicine,* 3rd ed. Philadelphia: Lippincott-Raven, 1998.
26. Reed P. *The medical disability advisor.* Boulder, CO: Reed Group, 2001.
27. Shekelle PG, et al. *The appropriateness of spinal manipulation for low back pain.* Santa Monica, CA: Rand, 1992.
28. *Mercy Center Consensus Conference*. Rockville, MD: Aspen, 1992.
29. North American Spine Society's Ad Hoc Committee on Diagnostic and therapeutic Procedures. Common diagnostic and therapeutic procedures of the lumbosacral spine. *Spine* 1991;16(10).
30. Waddell G, et al. Objective clinical evaluation of physical impairment in chronic low back pain. *Spine* 1992;17:617.
31. Harris JS, Brigham CR. Low back pain: impact, causes, work relatedness, diagnosis, and therapy. *OEM Rep* 1990;4:84.
32. Institute of Medicine Committee on Pain, Disability, and Chronic Illness Behavior. In: Osterweis M, Kleinman A, Mechanic D, eds. *Pain and disability: clinical, behavioral, and public policy perspectives.* Washington, DC: National Academy Press, 1987.
33. Tait RC. Psychological factors in the assessment of disability among patients with chronic pain. *J Back Musculoskel Rehabil* 1993;3:20.
34. Kerns RD, Turk DC, Ruby TE. The West Haven–Yale

Multidimensional Pain Inventory (WHYMPI). *Pain* 1985; 23:345.
35. Bergner M, et al. The sickness impact profile: development and final revision of a health status measure. *Med Care* 1981;19:787.
36. Fairbanks JC, et al. The Oswestry low back pain disability questionnaire. *Physiotherapy* 1980;66:271.
37. Roland M, Morris R. A study of the natural history of back pain. Part I: Development of a reliable and sensitive measure of disability in low back pain. *Spine* 1983; 8:141.
38. Pollard CA. Preliminary validity study of the Pain Disability Index. *Percept Mot Skills* 1984;59:974.
39. Millard RW. The Functional Assessment Screening Questionnaire: application for evaluating pain-related disability. *Arch Phys Med Rehabil* 1989;70:303.
40. Toomey TC, et al. Assessment of functional impairment in chronic pain patients: description of a scale and relation to other pain measures. *Proceedings of the VIth World Congress on Pain,* Adelaide, Australia, April 1990.
41. Hendler N, et al. A preoperative screening test for chronic back pain patients. *Psychosomatics* 1979;20: 801.
42. Ransford AO, Carson DC, Mooney V. The pain drawing as an aid to the psychologic evaluation of patients with low-back pain. *Spine* 1976;1:127.
43. McNeill TW, Sinkora G, Leavitt F. Psychological classification of low-back pain patients: a prognostic tool. *Spine* 1986;11:955.
44. Love AW, Peck CL. The MMPI and psychological factors in chronic low back pain: a review. *Pain* 1987;28:1.
45. Romano JM, Turner JA. Chronic pain and depression: does the evidence support a relationship? *Psych Bull* 1985;97:18.

8

The Physician Working with the Business Community

Frank H. Leone

OVERVIEW—INTO THE NEW MILLENNIUM

Opportunities for physicians to work closely with the business community are virtually limitless as we enter the new millennium. The opportunities range from affiliations with hospital-based occupational health programs to roles with national for-profit clinic networks, to roles as private consultants to industry. Physicians are finding that occupational medicine is a highly evolutionary specialty with a captive audience—millions of working Americans whose health, safety, and livelihoods are at stake. We live in an era in which there is an increasing emphasis on primary care, employers are becoming the leading gatekeepers of the health care system in the United States, and partnerships and networking are replacing the traditional private practice concept of medicine.

Close associations with employers are becoming a paramount positioning strategy for both physicians and medical centers as the private sector assumes greater influence in directing health care funding and service delivery. Well-conceived occupational health programs and delivery systems represent extraordinary opportunities for physicians, clinics, and hospitals with the ability to position themselves to flow with the currents of change.

The emerging provider–employer partnership is not limited to contracting and government mandate. As the United States becomes oriented toward the prevention of deleterious health and safety habits that result in injuries and illnesses, the workplace will become the optimal setting for the provision of training, health monitoring, and management of acute and chronic conditions.

Several characteristics of the current environment are worthy of attention:

- Competition for the health care dollar is increasing markedly with health systems, hospitals, and physician groups actively competing with one another in most markets.
- Technologically advanced communication tools such as the Internet, audionet conferencing, and telemedicine are providing health practitioners of all stripes with heretofore-unimaginable opportunities to communicate directly with the workplace.
- National concern and fears about terrorist-related activities have spawned a critical new calling for occupational medicine physicians to advise employers on biologic and chemical risks, associated mental health issues, and plans for emergency preparedness.

THE CHANGING OCCUPATIONAL HEALTH ENVIRONMENT

As a result of global activities, occupational health is in the throes of a significant shift away from injury management and a move toward provision of health-related consultations. This information-brokering approach is not associated with traditional care. Employers, especially smaller ones, will require more assistance from occupational health professionals in regulatory, mental health, policy, and medical areas.

Physicians should be aware of several significant changes in the regulatory environment. The deregulatory fervor of the 20th century has diminished and is being replaced by an emphasis on public health regulation. Initiatives that affect occupational health practices include the Americans with Disabilities Act, the Drug Free Workplace Act, and the Occupational Safety and Health Administration (OSHA) blood-borne pathogens standard. As additional regulatory reforms take effect, employers will seek the counsel of qualified occupational medicine practitioners. In addition, recent changes in state occupational health and safety law and proposed federal reforms suggest a more prevention-minded health and safety effort at the workplace that stresses planning, education, and collaboration. Here, too, opportunities for the savvy occupational medicine practitioner are likely to abound. It is important to be aware, however, that employers are getting more sophisticated in their understanding of occupational medicine and their expectations of quality service. As financial pressures increase, employers are becoming more selective; they are relying more on professionals with specialty training, as opposed to general physicians.

Health care cost control leads the agenda for many employers who recognize that partnerships with providers, especially physicians, are an essential ingredient for addressing the complex occupational and environmental health issues facing business today. In fact, a growing awareness and sensitivity to environmental issues is a driving factor in many corporate decisions. An increasingly intense effort from the public to address environmental exposures and health issues at the workplace is likely.

Perhaps the most profound change in the practice of medicine is the decline of fee-for-service reimbursement to a variety of managed care arrangements. Indeed, the workers' compensation system is under enormous financial pressure and is easing away from its former fee-for-service base toward preferred provider organizations and related arrangements between employers and providers. The new century may see the end of the fee-for-service era in workers' compensation. Reimbursement for workers' compensation–related medical care is becoming more tightly controlled and will ultimately force providers and employers to become more prevention oriented.

THE CHANGING PHYSICIAN ROLE

The practice of medicine in the United States appears poised for a significant change in which physicians are evaluated less on clinical expertise than on their ability to address broader community health care concerns. Accordingly, prevention is likely to assume a more pronounced role, both in reducing workplace exposures and in using the workplace as a forum for health education. At its best, occupational medicine is a preventive discipline—and the time for prevention is upon us. The successful physician of the 21st century will be as adept at organizational dynamics, consumer education, entrepreneurship, and marketing as at the clinical practice of medicine. Occupational medicine necessitates the ability to work as part of a team, deal with multiple constituencies (e.g., employers, workers, insurance carriers), and show leadership.

Occupational medicine physicians need to pay attention to their own responses and feelings and constantly strive for objectivity and consistency. They must also learn to appreciate the pressures under which client companies operate without compromising patient care. In the absence of a more genuine effort by physicians to establish long-term relationships with employers in their market, other providers are certain to fill the void.

The traditional physician–hospital relationship is also changing. Some version of the community care concept is likely to be developed either by necessity or mandate. Physicians are becoming hospital employees in increasing numbers; hospital and medical groups are forming joint ventures, and both groups are recognizing that collaborative arrangements may be the best way to address the broad opportunities in ambulatory care. One example of a common collaborative venture is the Physician-Hospital Organization, an entrepreneurial company dedicated to marketing and developing the hospital and its medical staff. Hospitals and physicians who work as business partners can be significant players in a competitive market (2).

AN OVERVIEW OF PHYSICIAN OPPORTUNITIES

The trained occupational medicine physician has the option of selecting from a variety of practice settings, each of which offers unique advantages and opportunities.

Opportunities with Hospital-based or Hospital-affiliated Programs

The prevalence growth of hospital-based or hospital-affiliated occupational health programs has been dramatic. In the late 1980s, with the advent of the prospective payment system, many hospitals recognized occupational health as a prudent diversification strategy and entered the market in large numbers. In the past, injury care and other occupational health-related services were loosely provided out of hospital emergency departments. Today, injury care is bundled with other services to create a well-defined product line.

By 2002, an estimated 1,500 or more hospitals of the approximately 7,000 in the United States had dedicated programs that provided occupational medical services for employers. Although a small number of programs are still based in emergency departments, freestanding clinics within the hospital, freestanding ambulatory care locations, and networks of clinics are the most common delivery models.

Furthermore, hospital-affiliated programs have matured and are expanding services to include screening, education, and rehabilitation services along with injury management, mental health, and other core services. A hospital base provides several advantages in the competitive occupational health market:

- Hospitals possess a breadth of services to offer a comprehensive approach in one setting.
- Hospitals typically have the financial resources to withstand a development period that may last 12 to 18 months.
- Hospitals can profit from existing personnel in management, finance, and marketing to offer immediate support for a program.

The physician/medical director is a critical part of the hospital-affiliated program team. Given the chronic undersupply of trained occupational medicine physicians, compensation and negotiation leverage is frequently favorable for the physician. Compensation for medical directors is becoming more creative and ranges from direct salary, to salary plus incentive, to salary plus fee for service.

A hospital setting is especially attractive for the physician who thrives on a team atmosphere and is interested in environmental as well as clinical challenges.

Freestanding Occupational Health Clinics

Freestanding occupational health clinics—with no formal ties to a hospital—grew at a breathless pace during the late 1980s and early 1990s. Although still common, many of these clinics were acquired by national or regional for-profit occupational health clinic networks. In some cases, these clinics include ambulatory care in addition to occupational medicine.

Both the freestanding occupational health clinic model and the for-profit networks tend to provide the physician with greater autonomy and give employers an impression of greater efficiency, easier access, and less cost than services provided by hospitals. Many primary care physicians have sought to increase their patient base by offering occupational medicine services as an adjunct to an existing primary care practice.

As employers become more prudent users of occupational health services, physicians will need to broaden their services and become better acquainted with the workplace. The era of the freestanding injury care mill that lacked an appreciation of the gamut of occupational health responsibilities has thankfully slipped away.

Consulting

The shortage of physicians with training in occupational medicine provides yet a third practice option–that of a consultant. The well-trained occupational medicine physician can provide consultative services to provider groups and to employers. Physicians may be part-time employees, consultants under contract with a specified hourly rate, or receive a fee-for-service payment or a retainer that covers an agreed-upon amount of services.

Numerous hospitals or clinics are actively seeking physicians to help develop a program and/or serve as a part-time medical director. The occupational medicine physician with administrative and managerial expertise has appealing opportunities in many settings, and is especially attractive to institutional providers such as hospitals and medical centers. Likewise, opportunities to work directly with employers are considerable, such as dealing with one or more employers on a part-time basis. The more compelling opportunity, however, may be to develop a relatively narrow niche of expertise and provide replicable services to large numbers of employers. Examples include medical surveillance, educational training, health and safety policy and program development, and regulatory compliance. Cost-containment activities such as workers' compensation loss control and managed care are increasingly discussed with occupational medicine consultants. Another avenue of opportunity in occupational medicine consulting is the workers' compensation insurance industry, as Dr. Joseph LaDou of the Division of Occupational and Environmental Medicine, University of California at San Francisco Medical School, wrote in a commentary on the occupational medicine consultant (3).

The physician serving as a consultant must know how to package and market the services. There are a number of ways to do this:

1. Maintain and publicize a narrow scope of services. A highly specialized consultant in virtually any field is invariably better positioned than the generalist. The physician consultant should define the service (or series of services) to be pro-

vided rather than present him- or herself as the occupational medicine consultant for all causes.

2. Think in terms of general workplace health and safety. To deal effectively with the business community, the occupational medicine specialist must evaluate each discrete issue in terms of the overall health and safety of the workplace. Employers will generally be receptive to this approach.
3. Publicize services in terms of benefits rather than features. Employers want to know whether the services are in their best interest. High-quality care coupled with sensitivity to cost and implications on business operations will demonstrate the benefit.

The occupational health physician should emphasize the following to prospective clients:

1. One-stop shopping: Employers are increasingly attracted to programs with a broad range of services that can be provided in one setting, especially by a single physician. If available, the physician should emphasize such a package.
2. A partnership concept: Employers envision their future partnership with health care providers as being considerably closer than it is today. The physician should be seen as a partner in preventing occupational injuries and illnesses.
3. Training: Employers are increasingly recognizing the value of training in occupational medicine, and in some cases put a premium on it. The physician should emphasize certification and special training in occupational medicine to potential clients.

WHAT THE ASTUTE PHYSICIAN CAN DO NOW

In a dynamic field replete with opportunity, a physician may wonder where to start. There are six key elements to developing a profile that will allow the physician to prosper financially and make a real difference when working with the business community:

1. Gain a basic foundation in occupational medicine: Many physicians offer little more than basic work injury care under the guise of occupational medicine. The discipline is far too complex for such a narrow approach. Physicians must establish a strong foundation in the field through formal education in occupational medicine residency or short courses, other educational opportunities, and the plethora of texts and journals that cover the field. For physicians in practice, it is usually not feasible to enroll in a formal residency program. Nonetheless, programs such as the core curriculum of the American College of Occupational and Environmental Medicine can be invaluable in providing a framework for advanced education. In addition, accredited academic course work can be conducted through offsite computer programs. The Medical College of Wisconsin's Department of Preventive Medicine is a notable example. (See Chapter 15 for educational opportunities for the physician entering the field of occupational medicine.)
2. Be prepared to address the occupational medicine continuum: To provide optimal services to the business community, the physician must embrace the entire occupational medicine continuum, i.e., prevention, acute injury treatment, and the return-to-work process. Prevention should extend directly to the workplace in order to develop a healthier and safer environment and a more trusting relationship between management and labor. The physician must be willing to visit workplaces, communicate by telephone frequently with appropriate parties, and view injury and disease in terms of cause as well as cure. Prevention should include health education of the workforce and counseling during screening examinations and treatment for injuries or illnesses. On the other side of the care continuum, the occupational physician should master the basic tenets of occupational rehabilitation and strive to effect close referral protocols to quality rehabilitation providers.
3. Remain abreast of regulatory measures: As regulations governing occupational heath and safety evolve, so will the role of occupational medicine specialists who must keep abreast of the changes and be prepared to help in implementing the regulations.
4. Associate interventions in terms of health care cost containment: The evolving partnership between occupational medicine physicians and the business community is contingent upon the awareness of cost control associated with preventive and clinical services. This daunting task can be tackled by developing systems for tracking costs and quantifying cost containment. Several basic parameters such as changes in lost workdays associated with workplace injuries, employee absenteeism, group health, and workers' compensation premiums provide objective data. Softer assessments of employee morale, job satisfaction, and productivity can also add valuable information regarding cost containment efforts.

5. Be an educator: Inadequate training and education contributes to most workplace health and safety problems. The successful occupational medicine practitioner must recognize the value of educating employers, workers, and professional colleagues, and take every opportunity to teach others. An effective educator is also a good listener. To practice effectively, the occupational medicine physician must heed the concerns of both employers and workers.
6. Be prepared to play multiple roles: The modern occupational medicine physician is at once an educator, clinician, consultant, and visionary. Although this is a seemingly disparate array of skills, many physicians may find these requirements invigorating.

THE OCCUPATIONAL MEDICINE PHYSICIAN OF THE FUTURE

Change in the nation's health care system and the role of its practitioners is inevitable. In my view, the occupational medicine physician will be in the mainstream of the practice of medicine in the 21st century. The employer–health care organization interface is the centerpiece of this evolution. This relationship addresses two central issues: control of the nation's substantial health care costs and the need to continually improve productivity for American business to maintain a competitive edge in an increasingly global economy.

The emergence of the employer as a key figure in the changing health care delivery system paradigm reform and as a gatekeeper and financial supporter of the health care system presents an extraordinary opportunity to the physician with training and expertise in occupational medicine. Opportunities abound in provider-based and corporate-based programs, and, increasingly, in private consulting. The supply of physicians with specialty training continues to fall short of demand; given the magnitude of this shortfall, it is unlikely to abate in the foreseeable future. There is much to motivate the physician to join the ranks of a growing and highly evolutionary specialty that places a premium on prevention by recognizing the workplace as a perfect venue to address the nation's health through the reduction of workplace health and safety hazards and the practice of genuine preventive medicine. Occupational medicine appears poised to become a key medical specialty of the 21st century.

REFERENCES

1. McCunney RJ, Boswell R, Harzbecker J. Environmental health in the journals. *Environ Res* 1992;59:114–124.
2. Reece R, Coombes D. Clinical corner. *VISIONS, National Association of Occupational Health Professionals* 1993(Jan./Feb.);3(4):14–15.
3. LaDou J. Occupational medicine consultant. *Am J Ind Med* 1991;19:257–266.

9

Drug Testing in the Occupational Setting

Kent W. Peterson

Employee drug testing has grown dramatically during the last two decades. In 1980, drug testing was confined to the military, nuclear power industry, and a few other employers. Now, almost every Fortune 500 company prohibits illegal drug use on or off the job and requires some form of drug or alcohol testing, a trend that has spread to medium and smaller employers. More than 8 million transportation workers are subject to drug testing under federal Department of Transportation (DOT) requirements, including all drivers who are required to hold a commercial driver's license. More than 30 million drug tests are performed annually, including over 10 million that are federally regulated under the authority of the DOT, the Department of Defense, or other federal agency, and 20 million in the non–federally regulated private sector (1).

This chapter reviews the growth of work-site drug testing; the nature and magnitude of heavy alcohol and illicit drug use in the United States; the basics of workplace drug testing; federally regulated vs. non–federally regulated testing models; components of the federal drug-free workplace procedures for urine collection, laboratory analysis for drugs and specimen validity and review, interpretation and reporting of laboratory results by medical review officers (MROs); the role of substance abuse professionals; federal alcohol testing regulations in the transportation industry; and current technical and legal issues.

Two basic forms of drug testing reflect two different purposes: *deterrence vs. fitness for duty*. Federally mandated drug testing for most federal and private sector employees was initiated to deter workers from using illicit drugs. Other components of the federal Drug-Free Workplace Program include a written policy restricting possession and use of illicit drugs and alcohol, employee education, supervisor training, and rehabilitation or some other form of employee assistance. Fitness-for-duty programs, such as those in the nuclear power industry, are quite different, requiring directly witnessed urine collection, on-site testing, and the ability to remove an individual from safety-sensitive duties pending the confirmation of a positive screening test.

GROWTH OF WORK-SITE DRUG TESTING

The extraordinary growth of drug testing is due to many factors. Most essential was the technologic breakthrough of simple, inexpensive immunoassay urine screening tests in the 1960s. Because sensitive immunoassay tests produced some false positives due to cross-reactivity with other substances, testing using this method alone adversely affected some of those tested, with consequent litigation. A two-test quality standard evolved during the 1980s, with a more specific test—gas chromatography/mass spectrometry (GC/MS)—being required to confirm positive screening test results. GC/MS has become the "gold standard" for forensic drug testing and is required in all federally mandated and most private-sector programs.

In the 1970s, the U.S. military successfully reduced the prevalence of drug use by introducing a random testing program with urine collection under direct observation. In the 1980s, large corporate employers began drug testing (2). In response, the American College of Occupational and Environmental Medicine (ACOEM) offered guidance to private employers and occupational health professionals by issuing in 1986 "Drug Screening in the Workplace: Ethical Guidelines," later updated in 1991 (see Appendix) (3). These guidelines became a standard of practice among private employers.

Drug testing of public sector employees was shaped by the 1986 Executive Order 12564 (4) and

Public Law 100-71 (5), which commissioned the Department of Health and Human Services (DHHS) to develop technical procedures for drug testing. These Mandatory Guidelines for Federal Workplace Drug Testing Programs were first published in 1988 (6). The mandatory guidelines outlined the framework for more extensive regulations published by DOT (7), the Department of Defense (DOD), the Department of Energy (DOE) (8), and other federal agencies. Landmark decisions by the U.S. Supreme Court validated that properly conducted drug testing programs, including random testing, were lawful for private and public sector employees working in security and safety-sensitive positions (9,10).

The Bureau of Labor Statistics (BLS) and the National Institute for Drug Abuse (NIDA) have tracked the growth of drug programs in industry. For example, BLS compared companies with more than 250 employees to those with fewer than 50 employees. In 1990 larger employers were much more likely to have written policies (74% vs. 12%), sponsor employee assistance programs (EAPs) (79% vs. 9%), and to conduct drug testing (46% vs. 3%) (11). A 1995 survey of 1,200 companies by the American Management Association showed that 77.7% conducted drug testing, 75% offered EAPs, 47% offered drug-related education to employees, and 45% had supervisor training on drug abuse (12). Surveys by the Substance Abuse and Mental Health Services Administration (SAMHSA) show that this differs widely by occupational category, being highest among protective services, transportation and material moving, and extractive and precision production, and lowest in construction, sales, and the food and beverage industry (13).

WHAT IS THE "DRUG PROBLEM" BEING ADDRESSED?

Substance abuse in the U.S. includes unauthorized or inappropriate use of controlled substances, prescription drugs, alcohol, and tobacco. To date, drug testing has focused largely on illicit drugs. SAMHSA's National Household Survey on Drug Abuse is the best source of data on the prevalence of drug use in the U.S. (14,15). In 1999, 14.8 million Americans ages 12 and over used one or more illicit drugs during the previous month, a decrease of 41% from 1979. Of the 26 million people who in 1997 reported using marijuana, 6.4 million used it once a week or more frequently, 10.2 million used it monthly, and 9.3 million used it occasionally. In 1999, 1.5 million people reported having used cocaine in the last month, 11.2 million used marijuana in the last month, and 13.3 million were heavy drinkers (five or more drinks on five or more occasions in the past month). Although the prevalence of illicit drug use has dropped over a decade, these figures are still high. Prevalence of frequent cocaine use has not changed, and recidivism after rehabilitation for illicit drug abuse is high compared to those treated for alcoholism.

Drugs in the workplace are a concern because 77% of current illicit drug users over the age of 18 are employed; 6.5% of full-time and 8.6% of part-time employees report current illicit drug use. Seven percent of employees are heavy drinkers, and there is a 30% overlap between employees who are heavy drinkers and those who use illicit drugs. Illicit drug use is particularly prevalent among employees aged 18 to 25, and higher among males than females and in those with less formal education and lower personal income (Table 9.1). The reported percentage of substance use is higher than the rate of positive urine drug screens, as shown in Fig. 9.1. Reasons for this discrepancy include (a) the ability to dilute urine by drinking fluids immediately upon notice of needing to provide a specimen; (b) urine substitution or adulteration with a variety of substances; and (c) recreational users who abstain from drug use when they believe drug tests will be scheduled, especially if they get word of an upcoming random drug test. Illicit drug use crosses all industries, being highest in construction, wholesale, and retail trades (15.4%, 13.6%, and 12.2%, respectively, of full-time employees aged 18 to 34). Interestingly, the transportation industry clusters in the middle of other industries, with the prevalence of illicit drug use having dropped substantially over the last decade, presumably in response to the DOT-mandated testing (16).

Illicit drug use among employees is associated with higher rates of absenteeism, accidental injury, involuntary separation, medical care usage, and health care costs. For example, in a study of U.S. Postal Service applicants, those who screened positive for drugs had 66% higher absenteeism, 77% greater likelihood of being fired, 143% more EAP referrals, and 26% higher medical claims over a 3.3-year period than those who screened negative (17). Even though supervisors did not know the results of employment drug tests, disciplinary action for problems of attendance, performance, and conduct was almost twice as high for those with positive tests. In a study of Georgia Power employees, hours of absenteeism for those testing positive for drugs was 165, compared to 91 for those treated for drug abuse, 73

TABLE 9.1. *Current illicit drug and heavy alcohol use among full-time U.S. employees by demographic characteristics, 1994 and 1997, as percent*

	Illicit drugs		Heavy alcohol	
	1994	1997	1994	1997
Age				
18–25	12.4	13.5	13.6	11.7
26–34	8.6	7.2	8.9	7.9
35–49	5.4	6.3	6.3	6.3
Gender				
Male	9.3	9.8	11.9	11.1
Female	5.2	4.6	3.3	2.5
Race				
Caucasian (non-Hispanic)	8.3	8.5	8.9	8.1
Black	6.5	6.2	5.2	4.4
Hispanic	5.6	5.2	8.8	9.8
Education				
<High school	9.7	11.2	13.2	14.7
High school graduate	8.3	7.9	10.0	7.1
Some college	7.5	8.7	8.3	7.3
College graduate	6.1	5.2	4.7	5.8
Personal income				
<$9,000	13.3	14.5	9.3	9.1
$9,000–19,999	9.5	8.6	10.8	9.4
$20,000–39,999	6.2	6.7	7.1	7.3
$40,000–74,999	4.1	6.7	8.1	8.1
$75,000+	12.1	9.3	5.7	2.1

From U.S. Department of Health and Human Services, Substance Abuse and Mental Health Services Administration, Office of Applied Studies. *Worker Drug Use and Workplace Policies and Programs: Results from the 1994 and 1997 National Household Survey on Drug Abuse,* Table 2.1. Washington, DC: Department of Health and Human Services, 1999.

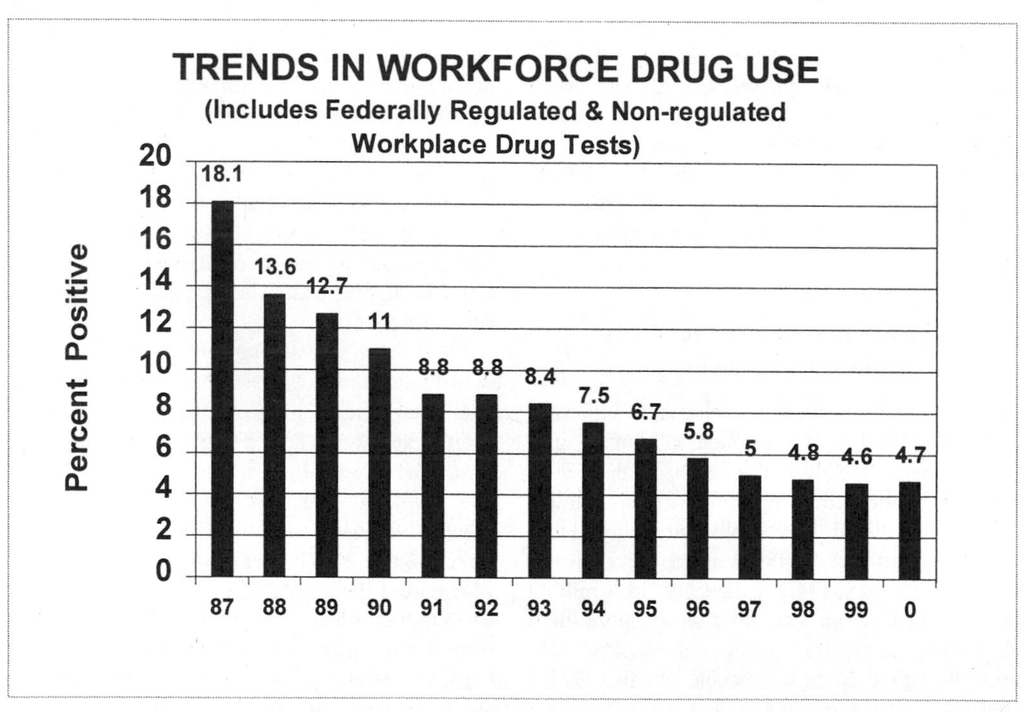

FIG. 9.1. Percentage of substance use and rates of positive urine drug screens. (From Quest Diagnostics, Inc. Drug Testing Index as reported by the U.S. Department of Health and Human Services, Substance and Mental Health Services Administration, 2002.)

for those treated for alcohol, and 41 for the average worker (18). Annual general medical benefit costs were $1,314 for those testing positive for drugs, $1,347 for those treated for drugs, and $842 for those treated for alcohol, in contrast to $590 for the average worker. SAMHSA's 1997 household survey on drug and alcohol abuse showed that current illicit drug users are more likely to have had three or more employers in the past year (9.3% vs. 4.3% for non–current drug users), skipped one or more days of work in the past month (12.9% vs. 5.0%), and been fired in the past year (2.3% vs. 1.2%). This same pattern is true for those reporting heavy alcohol use, and those individuals also reported more likelihood of having workplace accidents (8.5% of current heavy drinkers vs. 5.3% not heavy drinkers).

FEDERALLY REGULATED VS. NON–FEDERALLY REGULATED DRUG TESTING MODELS

There are two divergent worlds of drug testing. In the non–federally regulated private sector, a wide spectrum of approaches is found. For example, a single urine specimen may be tested for panels of two to 20 different drugs; custody and control forms may include the employee's name and list prescription drugs taken within the last 2 weeks. Urine may be analyzed at any laboratory, cutoff levels may be specified by the employer, and results may go directly to the employer, without medical review. Because of concerns about the quality and appropriateness of some company drug testing programs, Congress has considered legislation that would establish a federal standard for all workplace drug testing in the U.S. However more than half of all states regulate some aspect of workplace drug testing. In addition, drug testing is also affected by industry standards, collective-bargaining union agreements, and medical practice acts.

Federally regulated drug testing is governed by the DHHS, DOT, DOD, DOE, and other agencies. DOT regulations are particularly important because they currently affect over 8.2 million Americans in six commercial transportation sectors:

- Aviation (Federal Aviation Administration, FAA)
- Interstate trucking (Federal Motor Carrier Safety Administration, FMCSA)
- Maritime (U.S. Coast Guard, USCG)
- Mass transit (Federal Transit Authority, FTA)
- Pipelines (Research and Special Programs Administration, RSPA)
- Railroads (Federal Railway Administration, FRA)

Federal regulations contain detailed procedures for alcohol testing and urine specimen collection, completion of custody and control forms, analysis of urine specimens by DHHS-certified laboratories for only five specified illicit drugs (amphetamines, cocaine, marijuana, opiates, and PCP—the "DHHS-5" or "SAMHSA-5"), mandatory reporting of all results to an MRO for review and interpretation, reporting of results to the employer, referrals to substance abuse professionals, confidentiality, record keeping, and statistical reporting.

The DHHS and DOT regulations clearly represent the standard of practice, i.e., a "gold standard." The remainder of this chapter summarizes these detailed federal drug testing procedures (19). Those conducting urine collection and medical review are urged to carefully review federal regulations and participate in training offered by federal agencies or by professional societies such as the ACOEM.

Frequently, there is confusion about the relationship of DOT drug testing to DOT physical examinations required of certain transportation workers, e.g., pilots and truck drivers (20). A few years ago, drug testing was included as part of scheduled biennial driver examinations. DOT medical forms and operator's certificates made reference to both physical exams and drug testing. These two activities have now been separated. Random drug testing has replaced scheduled drug testing within most transportation sectors, and reference to drug tests has been removed from the DOT commercial driver exam card.

Nuclear Regulatory Commission (NRC) drug testing provisions differ from those of other federal agencies in that they represent a fitness for duty rather than a deterrence program. NRC permits on-site screening; if an individual tests positive, he/she is removed from safety-sensitive duties until confirmation results are received (21). Screening cutoff levels may be lower for marijuana and cocaine, testing for other drugs is allowed, and alcohol testing is required.

Department of Defense contractors are required to have a drug-free workplace program, but drug testing is not mandated. While EAPs are mandated for federal agencies, they are not required to be offered to private sector employers or defense contractors covered by drug testing regulations. Instead, the regulations require that individuals be informed about any available counseling, rehabilitation, and EAPs.

TYPES OF WORK-SITE DRUG TESTING

There are six major situations in which drug testing is performed at the work site:

Preemployment/Preplacement/Applicant/at Hire

This is the most prevalent form of drug testing. For federal employees, it is limited to those in safety-sensitive positions and all military personnel. But many private employers require preemployment drug tests of all those entering the workplace. Preplacement testing can include employees who are transferred and/or promoted to covered positions and those who are returning to work after extended absences. Although the Americans with Disabilities Act (ADA) prohibits preoffer employment *medical tests and examinations,* it specifically allows preoffer testing for Schedule I to IV drugs under the Controlled Substances Act.

Postaccident/Postincident

Testing may be required after an accident, incident, and/or safety violation. Each employer must define specific conditions under which postaccident testing is required. The DOT regulations define conditions that trigger postaccident testing, e.g., accidents that lead to personal injury or those resulting in property damage. Postaccident specimens must be collected quickly, often after-hours and away from the usual collection site. In anticipation of this, the employer should explore available collection options. Proper urine and alcohol collection procedures, chain-of-custody forms, and analytic methods must be observed in the emergency department or other clinical setting. A growing trend among states is to reduce or eliminate workers' compensation and/or unemployment benefits among workers having a positive alcohol or drug test at the time of the accident/incident. This presumption of voluntary intoxication is considered to be contributory negligence on the part of the worker (22).

Reasonable Cause/Reasonable Suspicion

This testing is performed when there is reason to believe that the employee's behavior and/or appearance suggest use of drugs in violation of company policy or agency rules. A supervisor must document the behavior and usually obtain the approval of a second supervisor prior to testing. Indications for testing can include unsafe practices, violating operating rules, changes in personality, erratic attendance, or aberrant behavior.

Random

Unannounced random drug testing provides the highest deterrent against drug use. Usually, names of employees in specific safety-sensitive jobs (e.g., pilots, drivers or security personnel) are included in a pool, from which individuals are randomly selected. Tests are conducted on short notice, e.g., within 1 to 3 hours. To maintain the deterrent effect, employees who have already tested negative remain within the pool, subject to retesting at any time. It is crucial that information about the dates of random testing, locations, and employees to be tested be kept confidential.

Random testing also raises the greatest threat among rank-and-file employees and concerns of civil libertarians about the invasion of individual privacy and possible unreasonable search and seizure. Random testing among private companies of *all employees* regardless of job category has led to employee relations concerns and legal challenges. Employers are urged to adopt policies that are reasonable, as well as legally defensible, which recognize that the vast majority of employers are not illicit drug users, and which presume innocence rather than guilt.

A few states prohibit employers from conducting random drug testing unless required by federal regulations; other state laws may restrict random drug testing to positions that are defined as safety-sensitive.

Return to Duty and Follow-up

An employee who has previously failed or refused a drug test is often required to provide drug-free urine before returning to work. Current DOT regulations require employees completing a rehabilitation program to have unannounced follow-up testing for a minimum of six tests over 12 months after returning to duty.

Periodic

Employers may require drug testing as part of fitness-for-duty or other examinations. Because these exams are scheduled in advance, recreational users can abstain from drug use prior to testing and positive rates tend to be low. Periodic drug tests are not included in current DOT regulations, except for maritime employees in conjunction with the U.S. Coast Guard license and document renewal.

The SAMHSA National Household Survey of Drug Abuse has tracked the prevalence of different kinds of drug testing (23). Figure 9.2 shows the percentage of full-time workers age 18 to 49 who reported different kinds of workplace testing. Two trends emerge: at-hire testing is most prevalent, followed by reasonable suspicion, postaccident, and fi-

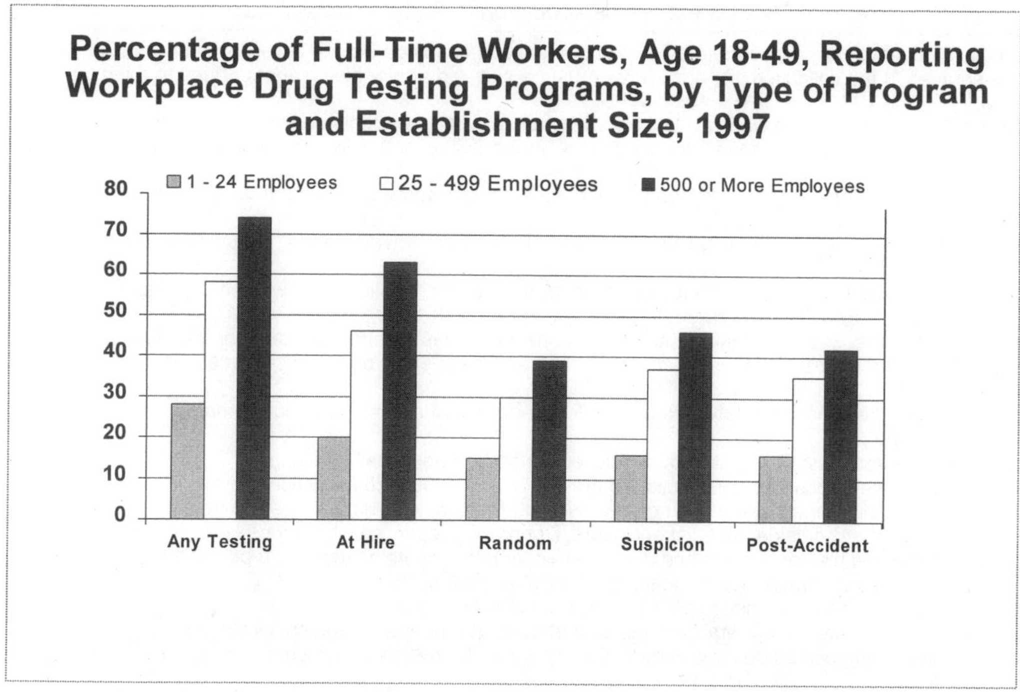

FIG. 9.2. Percentage of full-time workers age 18 to 49 who report different kinds of workplace testing. [From U.S. Department of Health and Human Services, Substance Abuse and Mental Health and Services Administration. *Worker Drug Use and Workplace Policies and Programs: Results from the 1994 and 1997 National Household Survey on Drug Abuse.* DHHS Publication Number (SMA) 99-3252, September 1999.]

nally random testing; and employers with 500 or more employees are at least three times more likely to perform each kind of drug test when compared to employers with 1 to 24 employees.

URINE COLLECTION

Drug testing can be broken down into three steps: (a) collection of the specimen and completion of custody and control forms; (b) laboratory analysis for screening and confirmation of positive tests; and (c) review, verification, and reporting to the employer of test results.

Urine collection is particularly crucial because so many errors occur here. It is important during the urine collection process that each donor be treated with respect and be allowed the maximum reasonable privacy, while minimizing the opportunity to substitute or adulterate urine specimens. Attention to detail in completing the custody and control form is also essential (24). Most positive drug tests that are invalidated are due to improper urine collection or documentation. The DHHS Mandatory Guidelines and DOT rules provide excellent urine collection procedures, summarized in Table 9.2 (25,26). DOT urine specimen collection must be performed by collectors who have completed a qualification training course and demonstrated proficiency by five consecutive error-free “mock” collections. Refresher training is required every 5 years. Additionally, any collector of a DOT specimen who makes an error in collection that results in cancellation of a specimen must undergo error correction training that reviews correct procedures and requires three mock collections related to the error that was committed.

There are three ways to conduct urine collection. In *private* collection, the donor provides a specimen in a carefully prepared separate room with complete privacy. In *monitored* collection, the urine collection is conducted in restroom or other facility that offers partial privacy, e.g., inside a stall with partitions that block direct view. A licensed health professional of either gender may monitor urine collection; a non–medically licensed collector must be the same

TABLE 9.2. *Urine specimen collection procedures*

The collection site must be secure to prevent unauthorized access during the collection process.

Water sources in the collection site enclosures must be secured and/or bluing agent added to toilet tank and bowl.

Employees are required to have individual privacy when providing a specimen except under the following circumstances, when collection under direct observation (witnessed collection) can occur (mandatory or optional):

1. The employee presents a specimen that is outside the accepted temperature range of 90–100°F (mandatory).
2. The collector observes the employee attempting to tamper with, adulterate, or substitute the specimen (mandatory).
3. A previous specimen was canceled by the laboratory as an "invalid result" with no medical explanation for the specimen invalidity (mandatory).
4. A previous test was canceled because a split specimen was not available to reconfirm a positive, adulterated, or substituted test (mandatory). The employee's last provided specimen was determined to be diluted.
5. The employee is having a return-to-duty or follow-up test after previously having had a verified positive test (optional).

Specific procedures must be followed during collection of the specimen, including:

1. Collector reviews positive identification of the donor (e.g., photo identification).
2. Donor removes unnecessary outer garments (e.g., coat, jacket, hat) and leaving hand-carried items (e.g., purse, briefcase) outside the toilet enclosure. Donor may retain wallet or money clip.
3. Donor empties his/her pockets and display the contents. Any items that could be used to adulterate or substitute the specimen must be left outside toilet enclosure.
4. Donor washes and dries hands prior to collection of specimen.
5. Donor receives separately wrapped and sealed collection container and specimen bottle(s).
6. Collector accompanies donor with collection container to the toilet enclosure, where the urine specimen is provided.
7. Donor hands filled collection container to collector; both maintain eye contact with specimen until it has been poured into specimen bottle(s) and labels/seals are placed over the bottle caps, and collector has written date and donor has initialed the tamper-proof labels.
8. Collector checks temperature of the specimen within 4 minutes after receiving specimen from donor.
9. Collector checks specimen volume (at least 45 mL for a split specimen). If donor cannot provide a sufficient volume of urine, partial specimen is discarded, and donor is provided up to 40 ounces of fluids to drink and up to 3 hours to provide the specimen while remaining at collection site.
10. Collector inspects specimen for unusual color, odor, or other physical qualities that may indicate attempt to adulterate specimen.
11. Collector pours at least 30 mL of specimen into a specimen bottle (bottle A) and, if a split collection, the remainder of specimen (at least 15 mL) into second specimen bottle (bottle B).
12. Collector places lid/caps on specimen bottle(s) and then applies tamper-evident label/seals.
13. Collector writes data on label/seals. Donor is asked to initial the label/seals once affixed to bottle(s).
14. Donor reads, completes, and signs donor certification section of custody and control form.
15. Collector completes and signs chain of custody section of custody and control form, recording date and time of collection and name of delivery or courier service.
16. Collector writes any remarks on custody and control form, places copy of custody and control form and sealed specimen bottle(s) in polyurethane bag and bag into hard-sided shipping container if being shipped by express courrier.
17. Collector gives copy of custody and control form to donor, who may leave.
18. Collector distributes other copies of custody and control form to medical review officer (MRO), designated employer representative, and keeps collection site copy.

Adapted from urine collection handbooks and guidelines published by the U.S. Department of Health and Human Services, Substance Abuse and Mental Health and Services Administration, Division of Workplace Programs and the U.S. Department of Transportation, Office of Drug and Alcohol Policy and Compliance. See refs. 24 to 26.

gender as the donor. The third form of collection is under *direct observation* of the urine exiting the urinary meatus—so-called, witnessed collection. When a specimen is collected under direct observation, the observer must be of the same gender as the donor, even if medically licensed.

Following collection, the collector and the donor should keep the sample in constant view until it is properly sealed and labeled. The collector places a tamper-proof seal on the specimen bottle's cap and down the sides of the bottle, together with an identification label showing the date and specimen identification number. The tested individual must initial the label to certify that it is the specimen collected from him or her.

If an employer has requested both a federally mandated drug test for the "DHHS-5" (or "SAMHSA-5") and a test for additional drugs, separate specimens must be collected (separate urine voids into separate containers) for the federally mandated test and for the additional drugs. Separate custody and control forms must be used for each specimen. It is unacceptable to pour any remaining urine from the void for the federally mandated test into another container for additional drug testing. However, if another federally authorized examination is being performed at the same time (e.g., DOT driver exam), it is acceptable to use any remaining urine for a dipstick urine analysis.

Split Samples

An employer may authorize or require a split specimen to be collected. Split specimens are required for all DOT urine collections. A split specimen is obtained from a single void into one collection receptacle; 30 cc are then poured into the first (primary or bottle A) specimen container. The remainder (at least 15 cc) is poured into a second (secondary, split, or bottle B) specimen container. The split specimen is sent along with the primary specimen to the laboratory. The split specimen is tested only if the primary specimen tests positive, substituted, or adulterated, and the employee requests reanalysis of the split. The reanalysis is performed at a second DHHS-certified laboratory by GC/MS only for the analyte that was positive initially at the laboratory's lower limits of detection or for specimen validity testing if the initial specimen tested substituted or adulterated. If the split specimen analysis fails to reconfirm the initial test result, the overall test should be reported to the employer as *canceled* and a report filed with the DOT's Office of Drug and Alcohol Program Compliance.

Custody and Control Forms

All drug tests require the use of a custody and control form, which includes chain-of-custody tracking for the handling of the specimen. The current SAMHSA urine collection form has five slightly different paper copies for the laboratory, MRO, employer, donor, and collection site. The laboratory copy may not contain the name of the donor, only the Social Security or other identification number. SAMHSA forms may not be used in non–federally regulated testing; however, most drug testing laboratories supply custody and control forms for use in nonfederal testing.

The specimen and forms are sealed in transport bags and boxes prior to courier pickup.

LABORATORY ANALYSIS AND SPECIMEN VALIDITY TESTING

Federally regulated urine drug tests must be analyzed in the approximately 60 laboratories certified by SAMHSA under the National Laboratory Certification Program. A list of currently certified laboratories is published regularly in the *Federal Register (27)*. Some laboratories have federal and nonfederal sections, so it is important to specify whether a drug specimen should be analyzed under SAMHSA provisions. Because of rigorous internal open and blind quality control and external blind proficiency testing checks, prices for SAMHSA-certified drug testing are usually higher.

Laboratories use internal chain-of-custody documents to track specimens in-house. From the accessioning area where specimens are logged in and stored, aliquots are removed and sent initially for screening and later, if necessary, for confirmation tests. Screening is first performed using one of several Food and Drug Administration (FDA)-approved immunoassay methods. Screening tests are recorded as positive, negative, or unable to be performed. If the screen is positive, then another aliquot is taken from the specimen for confirmation testing for the drug(s) detected in screening. GC/MS confirmation provides quantitative results, which may be reported routinely to the MRO.

SAMHSA also permits laboratories to perform specimen validity testing under specific guidelines (28). Validity testing determines whether the specimen is consistent with human urine, whether specific adulterants or foreign substances were added, and whether it was substituted or diluted. If the pH is <3 or >11, the specimen is considered adulterated. Other adulterants that can be tested for include nitrite >500 µg/mL, glutaraldehyde, chromate, bleach, peroxide, and ammonia. If urine creatinine is <20 mg/dL, then the specific gravity is also tested. If creatinine is ≤ 5 mg/dL *and* specific gravity is ≤ 1.001 or ≥ 1.020, then the specimen is considered to have been substituted, i.e., inconsistent with human urine. If specific gravity is >1.001 and <1.003, along with creatinine <20 mg/dL, then the specimen is considered to be dilute but still a valid specimen. If the laboratory is unable to test the specimen because some substance appears to be interfering with the screening and/or confirmation tests but adulteration criteria are not met, the laboratory reports the specimen as being *invalid*.

When the laboratory identifies a specimen as negative, it is discarded. Nonnegative specimens (i.e., positives, adulterated, substituted, or invalid) are frozen and retained at the laboratory for at least one full year in case the analysis is questioned and retests must be performed. The laboratory must retain all specimen records for a minimum of 2 years. Laboratories must also send to each employer a semiannual statistical report of all testing conducted, but this does not contain individual results.

Occupational physicians can help employers meet their obligations to submit quality control specimens. DOT requires that larger employers (>2,000 employees) submit one quality control specimen to their laboratory for every 100 employee specimens tested. Because the laboratory should now be able to identify these "external blind proficiency tests," ID numbers, signatures on labels, and other information should appear just as if they were typical specimens. Blind specimens can be known negatives, purchased specimens that are positive at a given cutoff level, adulterated, or diluted. If a laboratory misreports a blind specimen, the laboratory should be notified and an attempt made to investigate the error. Because of its significance, any false-positive test should also be communicated immediately to the DOT or other federal agency for immediate investigation. If verified, a single false-positive test could result in the laboratory's certification being suspended.

A laboratory's certifying scientist must review all drug testing data, quality control, and chain-of-custody documents and certify that the test results are positive, adulterated, substituted, or invalid specimen. MROs may request laboratory reanalysis of specimens, e.g., of the primary specimen, when there is some question as to the validity of findings. If a split specimen was collected, this second bottle is analyzed only at the donor's request (and often the donor's expense) at a difference DHHS-certified laboratory as communicated through the MRO.

DHHS has issued guidance to laboratories regarding "fatal flaws" that constitute grounds for rejecting a specimen, in which case the MRO will report the test as *canceled*. These are outlined in Table 9.3. Nonfatal flaws can be corrected by receiving a signed statement of correction from the appropriate individual, e.g., the collector. Because affidavits permit an otherwise unacceptable sample to be tested, laboratories have been requested to retain specimens not suitable for testing for a minimum of 5 working days to allow for correction in documentation.

The cutoff levels issued by DHHS for both screening and confirmation tests are shown on Table 9.4. The screening level for marijuana of 50 ng/mL represents a variety of metabolites; the confirmation cutoff level of 15 ng/mL represents one specific metabolite: delta-9-tetrahydrocannabinol-9-carboxylic acid. The cocaine screening level of 300 ng/mL is also for various metabolites, whereas the confirmation cutoff level of 150 ng/mL is for benzoylecgonine. For opi-

TABLE 9.3. *Fatal flaws of Department of Transportation (DOT) mandated drug testing programs*

Specimens presented to laboratories should be rejected for testing when any of the following procedural errors occur.

Permanently fatal flaws
- Specimen ID numbers on specimen bottle and custody and control form do not match.
- Specimen ID number is omitted on specimen bottle.
- Donor SSN or ID number is omitted on custody and control form unless "refusal of donor to provide" is stated in remarks section.
- Both collector signature and collector printed name are missing.
- Insufficient specimen volume (less than 30 mL).
- Specimen bottle seal is broken or shows evidence of tampering.
- Specimen shows obvious adulteration (i.e., color, foreign objects, unusual odor).

Correctible flaws (MRO can accept as corrected by getting a signed statement of correction from the person committing the error)
- Collector's signature is omitted from certification statement.
- No donor signature and no remark explaining failure to sign.
- Certifying scientist's signature is omitted on laboratory copy of the drug testing custody and control form for a nonnegative test result.
- Non-DOT form is used in error for a DOT-mandated test.

From U.S. Department of Transportation, Office of Drug and Alcohol Policy and Compliance. Part 40 Procedures for workplace transportation drug and alcohol testing programs. *Federal Register* 2000 (December 19); 65:79462; *Federal Register* 2001 (August 9);65:41944. Summarized from Subpart I—Problems in Drug Tests.

TABLE 9.4. *Department of Health and Human Services (DHHS) cutoff levels for drugs of abuse*

Drugs	Initial (screening) ng/mL	Confirmatory (GC/MS)
Marijuana metabolites	50	15[a]
Cocaine metabolites	300	150[b]
Opiate metabolites	2000	
Morphine		2000
Codeine		2000
Acetylmorphine		10
Phencyclidine	25	25
Amphetamines	1000	
Amphetamine		500
Methamphetamine		500

[a]As delta-9-tetrahydrocannabinol-9-carboxylic acid.
[b]As benzoylecgonine.
GC/MS, gas chromatography/mass spectrometry.
From U.S. Department of Health and Human Services, Alcohol, Drug Abuse, and Mental Health Administration. Mandatory guidelines for Federal Workplace Drug Testing Programs. *Federal Register* 1994 (June 9);59:29908. Section 2.4—Laboratory Analysis Procedures.

ates and phencyclidine (PCP), the screening and confirmation levels are identical. The confirmation test for 6-acetylmorphine (6-AM) is performed whenever the morphine confirmation level exceeds the cutoff; a positive 6-AM is pathognomonic for recent heroin use. Screening levels for amphetamines of 1,000 ng/mL are paralleled by confirmation cutoff levels of 500 ng/mL each for amphetamine and/or methamphetamine.

When repeat analysis is requested or when split samples are tested for positives, only GC/MS confirmation is performed. Under these circumstances, cutoff levels do not apply; the analyte is tested at the laboratory's lowest limit of detection. The cutoff is not used because over time, some analytes can degrade or adhere to the sides of the specimen container. In contrast, the original cutoff levels are still in effect when checking split specimen validity, i.e., for creatinine, specific gravity, nitrite, and other adulterants.

In federally regulated testing, laboratory results must be reported directly to an MRO. In non–federally regulated testing, results may be permitted to go directly to the employer, although a growing number of states now require use of an MRO, especially for positive results. Results may be communicated electronically by facsimile, teleprinter, or modem; a written copy of the custody and control form must also be provided for any specimen that is not negative. Laboratory results may not be communicated to the MRO by telephone.

REVIEW OF TEST RESULTS BY A MEDICAL REVIEW OFFICER

The MRO designation and role emerged from federal regulations, which first referenced a "medical review official." The 1988 DHHS mandatory guidelines governing drug testing under the federal Drug-Free Workplace Program described the MRO as "a licensed physician...who has knowledge of substance abuse disorders and has appropriate medical training to interpret and evaluate an individual's positive test result together with his/her medical history and any other relevant biomedical information." The 2001 DOT regulations require MROs to "be knowledgeable about and have clinical experience in controlled substances abuse disorders, including detailed knowledge of alternative medical explanations for laboratory confirmed drug test results...be knowledgeable about issues relating to adulterated and substituted specimens as well as the possible medical causes of specimens having an invalid result...be knowledgeable about...the DOT MRO guidelines and the DOT regulations applicable to the employers for whom you evaluate drug test results, and...must keep current on any changes to these materials" (29).

Under federally regulated testing, the MRO receives all results from the laboratory, including a certified copy of the custody and control form for all tests that are not negative. By receiving, reviewing, interpreting, verifying, and reporting drug test results, the MRO plays a vital role in protecting individuals from being inappropriately labeled as drug users, with adverse consequences. Approximately 15,000 MROs have received 2-day training offered by the ACOEM, American Society of Addiction Medicine, Federal Aviation Administration, DOT, and other organizations. MRO manuals have been published by SAMHSA (30), DOT (31), and professional societies such as the American College of Occupational and Environmental Medicine (32), and the Medical Review Officer Certification Council (33). DHHS and DOT regulations that enumerate specific duties of MROs are summarized below (6,18).

The MRO must perform an administrative review of the custody and control form for each specimen to assure it was completed in conformance with federal regulations and/or the employer's policy and procedures. Negative laboratory results with a flawed custody and control form must be reported as a *canceled test,* rather than negative, unless a correctable flaw has been repaired by receipt of a signed statement of correction.

The MRO must understand the urine collection procedures, custody-and-control form completion, and analytic procedures. Deviance from procedures may lead the MRO to cancel results, while documentation that prescribed procedures were carefully followed permits the MRO to discount statements from a donor that a collection site person or laboratory adulterated or tampered with the sample.

The most critical MRO function is to interpret and verify each positive, adulterated, substituted, or invalid test result. The MRO must personally attempt to contact each individual whose test was not negative and to provide him/her with an opportunity to provide a legitimate medical explanation. DOT has issued detailed procedures for verifying each of these different types of results. The MRO should follow the steps outlined in the MRO/Donor Interview Guidelines (Table 9.5) and the MRO/Donor Contact Record/Verification Sheet (Fig. 9.3).

However, before reporting verified positives, an MRO must personally speak with individuals with nonnegative results unless (a) an individual refuses to talk with the MRO; (b) the MRO has been unable to reach the individual through at least three attempts in 24 hours, and a designated employer representative can document that a message was delivered for the donor to contact the MRO and 3 days have elapsed; or (c) neither the MRO nor the employer representative has been able to reach the donor within 10 days of receipt of test results.

The MRO may ask the laboratory for the concentration of the detected drug. The MRO may authorize

TABLE 9.5. *MRO/donor interview guidelines*

Identify yourself as a physician serving as the MRO for the specific employer, with the duty of receiving and reviewing drug test results.

Establish the identity of the applicant or employee (i.e., full name, SSN or employee ID number, date of birth).

Inform the employee that medical information discussed during the interview is confidential, and may be disclosed only under special circumstances (e.g., impact on fitness-for-duty) as required by law.

If the employee holds a medical certificate under a DOT agency (e.g., airline pilot or train engineer), advise the employee that information regarding drug test results and information supplied by the employee will be provided to the DOT agency as required.

Tell the employee you are calling about the specific drug test he/she underwent on the specific date and at the specific location. Inform the employee for what drug the specimen tested positive. If applicable, explain the meaning of adulterated, substituted, or invalid test results and provide an opportunity for the donor to explain how such a result might be possible. If you believe the explanation to be plausible, explain how the donor can arrange at his/her own expense a referral evaluation by a medical examiner acceptable to provide confirmatory evidence.

If the employee requests the quantitative levels of the confirmed positive results, provide him/her with it, if available. If quantitative levels are not available, the MRO should request them from the laboratory. However, pending quantitative levels should not delay verification decisions.

Ask for recent medical history, when appropriate, regarding use of prescription medication, over-the-counter (OTC) drugs, dental, ear-nose-throat (ENT), ophthalmologic, or other medical procedures, and food ingestion if pertinent to help explain a positive test result.

Request that the employee provide medical records or documentation of prescription for controlled substance when appropriate. Set a specific deadline for receipt of the medical records.

Request the employee to undergo a medical evaluation, when appropriate (e.g., to provide clinical confirmation of opiate abuse, or to substantiate physiological basis for substituted specimen). Provide assistance with medical evaluation, including explaining to the examiners their role, responsibilities, and limits to what they can do (e.g., must perform additional substance abuse testing at a SAMHSA-certified laboratory). Review written report of referral physician and make your MRO assessment as to its significance.

Notify the employee that he/she may request a retest of the split (or original) specimen at another laboratory and, if appropriate, provide information about payment for retest in accordance with employer's policy. Tell the employee that a retest will not delay verification of the initial test result.

When the verification process is complete, inform the employee that the designated employer representative will be notified.

If the test result was verified positive or as a refusal to test, inform the employee of any substance abuse professional or employee assistance program made available by the employer, as appropriate.

Offer to answer any further questions.

Give your name and telephone number in case the donor has any further questions or wishes to provide further information.

Adapted from MRO guidelines published by the U.S. Department of Health and Human Services and the U.S. Department of Transportation.

MRO – DONOR Contact Record/Verification Sheet

DONOR NAME:________________________________Telephone Number:________________________
Type of Test: [ ] Federal; [ ] Non-Federal; [ ] Other:________________
Donor SS# or ID: ____________-_______-____________ Employer: ____________________________
Donor Phone (Day) ____________________ Donor Phone (Night) ______________________________
Drug Screen Panel: ______________________
Specimen ID Number: ____________________________ State Verification:____________________
Date Collected: _____________ Date Results Rec'd: ___________ Med. Dept. Rec'd:____________
Positive Metabolite:____________________ Quantitation: ________________________
Reason for Interview:[ ]Positive; [ ] Invalid/Unsuitable; [ ] Adulterated; [ ]Substituted
Reason for Test: [ ] Pre-employment; [ ] Random; [ ] Post-accident; [ ] Reasonable Suspicion;
[ ] RTD; [ ] Follow-up; [ ] Periodic; [ ] Other _________

_____ 1) Contact Attempt Record:

Date	Time	Result	Date	Time	Result
a.			c.		
b.			d.		

_____ 2) Company Notification: *If unable to perform interview after 3 contact attempts in 24 hours,* notify (DER) of need to talk with donor. Name of DER contacted:_________________________; Date__________; Time________

_____ DER reports that donor was told to contact MRO: Date________; Time________ - (starts 72 hr clock)

DONOR INTERVIEW

_____ 3) Sample MRO statement:
"Hello, My Name is _____________, the medical review officer for (EMPLOYER) ______________________________ serving to receive and review the results of your company's drug testing program.

_____ 4) Verify Donor Identity
_____Am I talking to (Name of Donor)? [ ] YES [ ] NO
_____Did you have a drug screen on (Date) at (Location) using a _______________sample?
_____Were you satisfied that the sample you gave was collected, labeled and sealed in your presence? [ ] YES [ ] NO
_____Can you tell me the last 4 numbers of your Social Security #?

_____ 5) Points to be made (General for All Interviews)
"The reason I am speaking to you personally is because the results of the drug test have been received and it is a ______ (positive, adulterated, substituted, invalid/unsuitable) test. The purpose of this interview is to provide you an opportunity to voluntarily share information with me that might explain this result, such as anything from your medical history, prescriptions, recent treatment or something in your diet. Based upon this information, I can make the best final determination of the result. There are a few things important for you to know: 1) If any further medical evaluation is needed you must comply with such a request and that failure to do so is the same as refusing to discuss the test result; 2) I am required to report to third parties ***without your consent*** drug test results or medical information affecting performance of safety-sensitive duties, and, 3) Before informing any third party about valid medication you may be taking, I will, if you arrange it, discuss the matter with your prescribing physician to see if a safer medication can be prescribed. You have the option of not discussing the matter with me if you choose. Do you have any questions at this point?"

(For adulterated add:) "The finding of ***specimen adulterated*** means that the laboratory discovered materials in your urine sample not consistent with human urine."

A

FIG. 9.3. MRO–DONOR Contact Record/Verification Sheet. (Adapted from checklist prepared by Ronald D. Springel, MD, MRO, C-SAPA.) *(continued)*

(For substituted add:) "The finding of ***specimen substituted*** means that the laboratory discovered that the specimen you submitted was so watery or dilute that it was not consistent with human urine. This was determined by measuring a substance that do not normally occur or that it contains substances expected to be present but in a concentration so high that it is called creatinine and by measuring the specific gravity of the sample. Specific gravity is a measurement reflecting the amount of dissolved solids in the urine and creatinine is a normal breakdown product found in urine."

"You have the right to present to me legitimate medical information that could explain the laboratory results. If you wish to do this, please be advised that the burden of proof is on you to show:
(For adulterated only:) "...that this substance can normally occur in your urine in the amount found."
(For substituted only:) "...that you can normally produce urine that is as dilute as that found in this test."

Do you have any information of this type? If you wish, you may have up to five days to provide me with this information. Bear in mind that you may need a medical examination to determine whether these things normally occur in your urine and you are responsible for bearing any expense. If you wish, I will attempt to find a physician acceptable to both of us to perform this evaluation." [ ] Donor accepts [ ] Donor declines

_____ 6) Inquire directly about illicit drug usage:
CLAIMS PERSONAL USE: [ ] YES; [ ] NO; Details:______________________________

_____ 7) Inquire directly about any factors that might explain a positive result and record below:

Prescription Drugs [ ] yes [ ] no
a.______________________________ c.______________________________

b.______________________________ d.______________________________

PRESCRIPTION VERIFICATION:
Rx #________________ Date________ Dr.____________________ Quant.________
Drug________________ Pharmacy ____________Phone__________RPh.____________

RECENT MEDICAL Rx: [ ] SUTURES; [ ] NOSEBLEED; [ ] SURG. PROCEDURE

OVER-THE-COUNTER DRUGS:
[ ] Vicks

DIET: Poppy Seeds: [ ] Yes; [ ] No

_____ 8) Request for review of medical records OR examination when appropriate.

_____ 9) SAMPLE REANALYSIS [ ] YES [ ] NO
SPLIT ANALYSIS: [ ] DECLINED [ ] REQUESTED Date funds received:___
LABORATORY CHOSEN FOR SPLIT SAMPLE ANALYSIS:______________________________
Database RECORD #:___________ SPECIMEN ID:_______________

_____ 10) For DOT: Inform donor of consequences of a positive test and where to obtain a list of resources for resolving problems associated with alcohol or drugs. SAP Referral: [ ] Yes [ ] No

B _____ 11) Offer to answer any questions; give name and phone #.

FIG. 9.3. *Continued.*

reanalysis of the original sample. Consultation with the toxicologist or laboratory certifying scientist can also be helpful.

Many prescription and over-the-counter (OTC) drugs can cause positive tests. Verification of legitimate medical explanations for positive tests often requires clinical judgment. For example, tetrahydrocannabinol, the active ingredient of marijuana, is used as an antinausea agent for cancer patients under the prescription name Marinol, a Schedule III substance under the Controlled Substances Act. Although inhalation of sidestream marijuana smoke is often offered as an explanation for a positive test, toxicology studies have not confirmed this as a feasible explanation for a positive test. Cocaine is used in ear, nose, and throat (ENT) ophthalmology and surgical procedures, such as bronchoscopy or injection of TAC (tetracaine, adrenalin, and cocaine) for suturing skin lacerations.

It is important to distinguish between the *d* (dextro) and *l* (levo) stereo isomers of both amphetamine and methamphetamine. The *d*-form is associated with illicit drug use, but many prescription drugs can also

MRO VERIFICATION

DONOR NAME____________________ COMPANY DER CONTACT & PHONE____________________

DATE VERIFICATION COMPLETED AND DONOR NOTIFIED OF RESULTS_______________

DATE EMPLOYER TOLD RESULTS____/____/____(__:__hrs) REPORTED TO:_______________

DATE FEDERAL AIR SURGEON (FAA ONLY) NOTIFIED:______________________________

MRO VERIFICATION WORKSHEET

FINAL VERIFIED RESULT: ____**POSITIVE** ____**NEGATIVE** ____**REFUSAL TO TEST** ____**CANCELED TEST**
____**DRUG(S) FOUND**______________________________
____**SPECIMEN ADULTERATED/SUBSTITUTED** ____**INVALID/UNSUITABLE (RECOLLECT [ ] YES [ ] NO)**
____**SPECIMEN DILUTE**
____**UNABLE TO CONTACT (72 HR RULE/10 DAY RULE)**

COMMENTS: ____

SIGNATURE OF MEDICAL REVIEW OFFICER DATE

C

FIG. 9.3. *Continued.*

test positive for *d*-amphetamine or *d*-methamphetamine. In addition, high doses of OTC drugs such as Vick's inhaler can cause a positive *l*-methamphetamine. It is recommended that the MRO request from the laboratory *d*- and *l*-isomer separation on confirmed methamphetamine specimens. Even with the elevated opiate cutoff levels of 2,000 ng/mL, ingestion of poppy seed paste can cause positive tests. For this reason, DHHS regulations require that verification of an opiate test as positive be accompanied by (a) clinical evidence of opiate misuse, (b) the identification of the heroin metabolite 6-AM, or (c) levels above 15,000 ng/mL (in which case the burden of proof shifts to the donor to demonstrate prescription and authorized use). Clinical signs include admission of use during the medical history, physical findings, or behavior fitting the *Diagnostic and Statistical Manual of Mental Disorders,* fourth edition (DSM-IV) definitions of opiate abuse ascertained by a trained medical professional (34).

Another issue in MRO judgment involves the use of medication prescribed for one's spouse, child, other relative, or acquaintance. DOT guidance has recommended that these be verified as positive, representing unauthorized use of controlled substances. Unless this issue is specifically addressed in company policy, consideration of whether spousal use is legitimate or unauthorized drug use remains an MRO judgment. It is best to resolve such issues in advance through consultation with the employer. Use of a dated prescription issued to the donor could be another judgment call, although the medication was authorized for that individual. It is important for the MRO to obtain written documentation substantiating authorized drug use, i.e., from treating physicians and/or pharmacists. DHHS has issued guidance that use of medically prescribed marijuana, while lawful in some states, does not constitute an acceptable medical explanation for a positive test result. Most MROs similarly do not accept use of prescription medication obtained in a foreign country as an acceptable medical explanation for a positive test.

If the laboratory reports a specimen as substituted or adulterated, the MRO must discuss the result with the donor. If the donor provides a plausible medical explanation for the low creatinine and specific gravity, or the presence of an adulterant, such as a rare metabolic disease, the MRO may give the donor up to 5 days to undergo an independent medical evaluation by a physician acceptable to both the donor and MRO. In this case, the MRO will explain to the examining physician the DOT test process and the consequences of a substituted or adulterated test. Any additional urine tests that are obtained must be conducted in a DHHA-certified laboratory. The MRO will seriously consider and assess the referral physician's written recommendations. If a reasonable medical explanation is presented, which is highly unlikely, the MRO will cancel the test; otherwise, the result is reported as refusal to test.

After full consideration of all the information from the laboratory, the donor, treating physician, or other sources, the MRO must make the final verification determination. Tests can be reported to the employer as (a) positive, (b) negative, (c) canceled (due to administrative errors, failure to reconfirm a split specimen, or an invalid specimen), or (d) refusal to test (tampering with the specimen, adulteration, substitution, or refusal to undergo an examination requested by the MRO, e.g., for an opiate positive). Specific comments must be made to the employer, including the name of the drug for a positive test and the reason for a canceled test or a refusal to test. MRO-verified results may be telephoned to the employer representative, but must be reported in writing within 24 hours of verification following safeguards to protect confidentiality. Verified positives or refusals to test may also be reported to a designated substance abuse professional, EAP contact, or federal management official with the power to recommend or take administrative action. Under federal programs, employers are not routinely entitled to quantitative results, but must be told the specific drug for which the test was positive.

SUBSTANCE ABUSE PROFESSIONALS

An increasingly vital role is played by substance abuse professionals (SAPs), who evaluate employees who have violated DOT drug and alcohol regulations and make recommendations concerning appropriate education, treatment, follow-up testing, and aftercare (35). According to DOT regulations, SAPs must be licensed physicians or psychologists, social workers, certified employee assistance professionals, or drug and alcohol addictions counselors certified by acceptable national organizations. Like MROs, SAPs must undergo qualification training, complete an examination by a nationally recognized professional or training organization, and have a minimum of 12 hours of pertinent continuing education every 3 years.

Unlike the MRO interview, which can be performed by telephone, SAP evaluations must be performed face to face. The initial evaluation is a clinical assessment and evaluation, after which the SAP must refer every individual who has violated DOT drug and alcohol regulations for the most appropriate course of education and/or treatment. Appropriate education may include self-help groups such as Alcoholics Anonymous, community lectures, or drug and alcohol education courses. Appropriate treatment may be inpatient hospitalization, partial inpatient treatment, or outpatient counseling, with or without aftercare. Following education and/or treatment, the SAP must also perform a follow-up clinical evaluation to determine successful compliance and recommend to the employer whether the employee is ready to return to duty. If the employee has not demonstrated successful compliance, then the employee may not return to safety-sensitive duty and the employer may take adverse personnel actions. If the SAP determines that the individual needs ongoing aftercare, the employer may include this in a return-to-work agreement. The SAP also must determine the number, frequency, and duration of follow-up drug and/or alcohol tests, which must include for those in DOT safety-sensitive positions a minimum of six tests during the first 12 months and may last for as long as 5 years. The SAP can terminate the requirement after the first year of testing. These follow-up testing requirements follow the employee from one employer to the next. SAPs must issue written reports after both the initial and follow-up (return-to-duty) evaluation (36).

ALCOHOL TESTING

In 1991, Congress passed the Omnibus Transportation Employee Testing Act, which extended testing for controlled substances to include testing for misuse of alcohol in preemployment, random, reasonable suspicion, postaccident, and posttreatment testing in most transportation sectors (37). It also provided legislative authority for drug and alcohol testing for mass transit vehicle operators, controllers, and maintenance workers. The Act did not apply to the oil and gas or maritime industries, thus comprehensive alcohol testing requirements were not included in the DOT's RSPA or USCG regulations. The 1994 final rules required those subject to urine drug testing to also undergo alcohol breath testing (38). In effect, these regulations broadened the previous deterrent program into a fitness-for-duty program. Prohibited alcohol conduct for individuals in qualified safety-sensitive functions includes (a) having a breath alcohol concentration of 0.04 or greater, (b) consuming alcohol within 4 hours (8 hours for FAA flight crews) of performing duty, (c) consuming any alcohol while on duty, (d) consuming alcohol after an accident before a test has been conducted or within 8 hours (whichever comes first), and (e) refusing to take an alcohol test. Since implementation of the DOT regulations, many private sector employers have also instituted breath alcohol testing using similar standards.

Employment alcohol tests may be conducted anytime between the preplacement exam and first performing safety-sensitive functions. Postaccident tests are required for employees whose performance could have contributed to an accident as soon as possible, preferably within 2 hours. Random tests may be performed just before, during, or just after performing safety-sensitive functions. Reasonable suspicion testing is based on the observations of a supervisor trained in recognizing signs of alcohol misuse. For those returning to duty after evaluation and rehabilitation, at least six tests are required in the first 12 months.

Although screening may use oral swabs for testing saliva, all confirmation tests must use evidential grade breath testing devices approved by the National Highway Traffic Safety Administration (NHTSA). NHTSA publishes a conforming products list (39). Confirmation tests require a permanent record of results and identification of the individual tested (e.g., a printed result of sequentially numbered tests), capability of testing blank air samples, and discrimination between alcohol and acetone, which can be produced by fasting or diabetics in ketosis. A 15-minute wait is required between the initial screening and confirmation test. The confirmation value is the final result. Testing must be conducted by a trained, certified breath alcohol technician (BAT) who has demonstrated proficiency in a NHTSA-approved course (40). Only in the Federal Railway Administration is blood alcohol testing permitted for postaccident testing. The Federal Motor Carrier Safety Administration allows an alcohol test conducted by the police to substitute for the employer-required postaccident test.

The consequences of having a breath alcohol concentration of 0.04 or greater include immediate removal from safety-sensitive duty. Return to work is permitted only after evaluation and rehabilitation, as well as return-to-duty and follow-up testing. The regulations call for temporary removal from safety-sensitive duty if the alcohol concentration is between 0.02 and 0.04 for specific amounts of time (e.g., 8 hours) as specified by DOT agency rules. SAP evaluation and return-to-duty and follow-up testing are not required for return to work following a breath alcohol test result of 0.02–0.039. This two-tier provision underscores the DOT's concern that even low levels of alcohol are inconsistent with safety. Although correlated with blood alcohol levels, the breath alcohol results stand on their own merit and do not require conversion to blood alcohol concentrations.

CURRENT ISSUES

Individual Privacy and Confidentiality vs. Public Health and Safety

Drug testing programs must balance carefully the individual right to privacy and personal freedom versus public health and safety needs. The federal drug testing regulations seek to protect the individual against false accusation of illicit drug use and, in the collection process, to balance the right to privacy against unreasonable search and seizure, a Fourth Amendment constitutional protection. For this reason, directly witnessed specimen collection is permitted only in instances of likely specimen adulteration or substitution. Federally regulated drug testing is also restricted to those in safety-sensitive job positions. Although private sector drug testing is not so restricted, health professionals are urged to be sensitive to privacy issues, to recognize that the vast majority of those tested are not illicit drug users, and to assure each individual confidentiality and respect. Of note is the 2002 U.S. Supreme Court's decision to uphold the constitutionality of random drug testing of all high school students participating in extracurricular activities (41).

DOT regulations effective in 2001 require MROs to release medical information to a third party (the designated employer representative, physician, or health care provider responsible for determining medical qualification; a substance abuse professional; and/or the DOT agency or National Transportation Safety Board) if the information is likely to result in disqualification or if continued performance of the employee's safety-sensitive function is likely to pose a significant safety threat.

Specimen Dilution and Substitution

A quarrelsome issue for MROs has been interpretation of dilute specimens. By water loading, donors can reduce their urine creatinine to <20 mg/dL and the specific gravity of urine to <1.003. A urine specimen that meets these criteria is called "dilute" unless it meets the criteria for being substituted. However, when a laboratory reports a specimen as being both dilute and negative, DOT guidelines require that it be verified as a negative test. DOT regulations now allow an employer that receives a report of a dilute negative test the option of ordering an immediate recollection from that donor (not under direct observation). The employer must accept the result of the second test, even if it again comes back as a negative dilute.

Challenges to substituted tests have been made by employees of the airline industry. In response, DOT now requires the MRO to provide the donor with an opportunity to present a plausible medical explanation. If the MRO believes there might be a reasonable basis for such a finding, an additional medical evaluation may be permitted by the MRO. Because an analysis of more than a decade of all patient records at a major New England teaching hospital was unable to reveal a single instance of a patient with both creatinine <5 mg/dL and a specific gravity <1.001, such an explanation for a substituted specimen is extremely unlikely (42).

Adulterated and Invalid Specimens

A sizable industry has sprung up promoting products that can be added to urine and purport to invalidate urine drug tests. Commercially available products include UrinAid! and Mary Jane's Superclean 13, Klear, Stealth, and Whizzies. In response to urine specimen adulterants containing soap, bleach, glutaraldehyde, chromates, nitrites, peroxides, acids, and other substances, laboratories are developing sophisticated adulteration panels. DHHS has proposed specific procedures for testing for adulterants, so that laboratories performing specimen validity testing will follow consistent procedures (43). If a specimen is reported as being adulterated, the MRO should report this to the employer as a refusal to test.

Specimens that cannot be tested because of some interfering substance, and for which no adulterant can be identified, are reported by the laboratory as invalid. In response to an invalid test, MROs are encouraged to talk with the laboratory forensic toxicologist and must interview the donor. Tolectin (tolmetin—a nonsteroidal antiinflammatory medication), Flagyl (metronidazole—an antifungal and antibacterial agent), and Cipro (ciprofloxacin—an antibacterial agent) are known prescription medications that may interfere with some immunoassay tests. If a suitable explanation is identified, the MRO should report the test as canceled, with no follow-up needed. If there is no suitable explanation, then the MRO should inform the employer that another specimen must be collected immediately under direct observation.

MRO Training and Credentialing

Because of concerns about the quality of MRO services, federal officials urged establishment of voluntary MRO credentialing and certification within the private sector. Physicians seeking to demonstrate their competence in a competitive marketplace and a litigious environment showed strong interest in MRO credentialing. The Medical Review Officer Certification Council (MROCC) was established in 1992 by ACOEM, with partners including the American Medical Association, the College of American Pathologists, the American Academy of Clinical Toxicologists, the American Academy of Medical Toxicology, and other medical specialty societies. MROCC eligibility requires at least 12 hours of approved MRO training, followed by a rigorous written certifying examination (44). Certificates are valid for 6 years. In 2001, the DOT published rules requiring MROs to receive initial qualification training in specified subjects, to receive at least 12 hours of continuing medical education in pertinent subjects every 3 years, and to pass an examination by an approved national certifying body. Such bodies include the American Society for Addiction Medicine (ASAM), the American Association of Medical Review Officers (AAMRO), and MROCC.

Evidence of Drug Testing Effectiveness

Many studies have shown a strong association between illicit drug use and increased absenteeism, accidents, injuries, disciplinary measures, and health care costs (45,46). NIDA surveys indicate that the prevalence of drug use among high school seniors and employees dropped significantly from 1985 to 2000 (47). The former is believed due to health education, and the latter in response to a broad-based deterrent program, which includes education and drug testing. Relatively few studies have looked at the ability of drug testing programs to reduce either the prevalence of drug use or consequent effects (48,49). The Federal Railroad Administration has noted a significant decrease in the number of accidents, accompanied by a steady drop in the rate of positive drug tests in postaccident testing (50). Figure 9.1 shows the steady and dramatic drop in the percent of positive drug tests in workforce testing, from 18.1% in 1987 to 4.7% in 2000. Many successful corporate case studies are reported by the Institute for a Drug-Free Workplace (51).

Americans with Disabilities Act

The ADA specifically defines testing for controlled substances as not constituting a medical test. Thus drug testing is permitted at any time, including prior to an employment offer. Additionally, ADA distinguishes current and former drug users. Those who test positive (i.e., current users) are excluded from protection under ADA; but former drug users are protected. Employers may require periodic, unscheduled testing for a reasonable period of time to assure that former users are successfully rehabilitated. However, a positive test automatically voids ADA protection. In contrast, testing for alcohol is considered a medical test and may not be performed prior to the employer's making a job offer. Users of alcohol and drugs may also be held to the same performance standards in the workplace as all other employees, including attendance, productivity, and conduct.

On-site Testing

In federally regulated testing, the NRC has long permitted on-site drug testing as part of a fitness-for-duty program. On-site testing is not permitted under other deterrence-based federal agency regulations. However, an increasing number of non–federally regulated employers have adopted on-site screening as a valuable way to assure that employees are fit for duty to perform highly safety sensitive jobs. Employees testing positive can immediately be removed from duty pending results of confirmation tests. Unfortunately, several studies of instant on-site testing kits have shown a wide variation in sensitivity and specificity. As might be expected, the most sensitive tests produce many false positives, as determined by confirmation tests; the most specific tests produce many false negatives.

Choice of Drug Panel

Even when testing only for the DHHS-5, considerable MRO dialogue is required with those testing positive. However, employers often seek to reduce the accidents, injuries, absenteeism, and medical costs caused by inappropriate use of other controlled substances and prescription drugs not covered by current federal regulations. Medical review of laboratory results becomes essential when testing for commonly used prescription medications such as barbiturates and benzodiazepines.

Analysis of Hair, Oral Fluid, and Other Matrices

Gradually the quality of laboratory methodology has improved for testing hair, sweat, and saliva for controlled substances. A committee of the DHHS Drug Testing Advisory Board (DTAB) has drafted proposed standards for use of these tests, which are still under scientific investigation and policy review (52). Many toxicologists do not believe that this technology has been sufficiently validated to replace urinalysis. Issues include challenges of standardization, blind specimen quality control, impact of adulterants, and secondary or environmental exposure. However, an increasing number of employers in the non–federally regulated sector are using these tests.

CONCLUSION

This chapter has briefly reviewed the wide-ranging area of drug and alcohol testing, laboratory analyses, and medical review of results. Because drug-testing programs cannot assure a drug-free workplace, the importance of preventive efforts, employee assistance, and rehabilitation programs cannot be overemphasized. Well-trained MROs should be an integral part of any drug-testing program. As drug testing becomes increasingly complex, litigation will increase, placing the collection facility, laboratory, MRO, and SAP at growing risk.

A positive drug test identifies an individual to be at high risk of impaired work performance. However, a positive test means only the presence of a drug above the cutoff level at the time of testing. It does not mean that the individual was under the influence, impaired, or addicted. Furthermore, the quantitative test result cannot distinguish between the recreational user and the drug addict. Occupational health professionals need to help employers understand these limitations.

Alcohol and drug abuse often reflect dissatisfaction with one's life, be it personal or at work. Employers must seek ways to foster healthier work environments, filled with challenge, support, creativity, and human concern—in short, high-level wellness. Addressing these issues will help solve the drug problem our society faces.

REFERENCES

1. Peat M. Personal communication from Clinical Director of Dynacare Laboratories, Houston, TX, June 2002.
2. Peterson K. Employee drug screening: issues to be resolved in implementing a program. *Clin Chem* 1987;33: 54B.
3. ACOEM Committee Report. Drug screening in the workplace—ethical guidelines. *J Occup Med* 1991;33:651.
4. Reagan RF. Drug-free federal workplace executive order 12564. *Federal Register* 1986(September 17);51 (180):32889.
5. U.S. Congress. Public Law 100-71. 101 Stat. 468, July 11, 1987. See *http://www4.law.cornell.eduuscode41ch10.html*.
6. U.S. Department of Health and Human Services, Substance Abuse and Mental Health Services Administration. Mandatory guidelines for Federal Workplace Drug Testing Programs; Final guidelines. *Federal Register* 1988(April 11);53(69):11979. These were revised in the *Federal Register* 1994(June 9);59:29908, and in brief in the *Federal Register* 1998(November 13);63:63483.
7. U.S. Department of Transportation, Office of the Secretary. Procedures for Transportation Workplace Drug Testing Programs, Final Rule. *Federal Register* 1989(December 1);54(230):49854. See also Interim Final Rule. Federal Highway Administration. *Federal Register* 1990(February 1);55(22):3546.

8. U.S. Nuclear Regulatory Commission—Fitness-For-Duty Programs; Final Rule and Statement of Policy. *Federal Register* 1989(June 7);54(108):24468.
9. *Skinner v. Railway Labor Executives Association,* 109th Supreme Court, 1989.
10. U.S. Department of Health and Human Services, Substance Abuse and Mental Health Services Administration, Division of Workplace Programs. Guidance for Selection of Testing Designated Positions (TDPs). *http://workplace.samhsa.govframesframe_fed.htm.*
11. U.S. Department of Labor, Bureau of Labor Statistics. Survey of Employer Anti-drug Programs. Washington, DC, Report 760, 1989.
12. American Management Association. *www.amanet.orgresearchpdfsmedicl2.0.pdf.*
13. U.S. Department of Health and Human Services, Substance Abuse and Mental Health Services Administration. An Analysis of Worker Drug Use and Workplace Policies and Programs. DHHS Publication Number (SMA) 97-31-42, July 1997.
14. U.S. Department of Health and Human Services, Substance Abuse and Mental Health Services Administration. Summary of Findings from the 1999 National Household Survey on Drug Abuse. DHHS Publication Number (SMA) 00-3466, August 2000.
15. U.S. Department of Health and Human Services, Substance Abuse and Mental Health Services Administration. Worker Drug Use and Workplace Policies and Programs: Results from the 1994 and 1997 NHSDA. DHHS Publication Number (SMA) 99-3252, September 1999.
16. U.S. Department of Health and Human Services, Substance Abuse and Mental Health Services Administration. Drug Use Among U.S. Workers Prevalence and Trends by Occupation and Industry Categories, DHHS Publication Number (SMA) 96-3089, May 1996.
17. Zwerling C, Ryan J, Orav EJ. The efficacy of preemployment drug screening for marijuana and cocaine in predicting employment outcome. *JAMA* 1990;264:2639.
18. Sheridan JR, Winkler H. An evaluation of drug testing in the workplace. In: Gust SW, Walsh JM, eds. *Drugs in the workplace: research and evaluation data.* NIDA Research Monograph 91. U.S. Department of Health and Human Services; Alcohol, Drug Abuse, and Mental Health Administration; National Institute on Drug Abuse, 1989:195–216.
19. U.S. Department of Transportation, Office of Drug and Alcohol Policy and Compliance. 49 CFR Part 40: Procedures for transportation workplace drug and alcohol testing programs. *Federal Register* 2000(December 19);65:79462; *Federal Register* 2001(August 9);65:41944.
20. U.S. Department of Transportation, Federal Highway Administration. 49 CFR: Section 391.41-391.49, Subpart E: Physical Qualifications and Examinations and Subpart F: Files and Records.
21. U.S. Nuclear Regulatory Commission. *Federal Register* 1989(June 7);54:24494. Amended at *Federal Register* 1991(August 26);56:41926; *Federal Register* 1993(June 3);58:31469; *Federal Register* 1994(January 5);59:507. See CFR Part 26, Fitness for Duty Programs: *http://www.nrc.govreading-rmdoc-collectionscfrpart026index.html.* Section 26.24 deals with chemical and alcohol testing.
22. Judge WJ. "Outside the Circle": the impact of drug testing on Workers' Compensation. Tort and Insurance Practice Section, American Bar Association, 1991.
23. U.S. Department of Health and Human Services, Substance Abuse and Mental Health Services Administration. Worker Drug Use and Workplace Policies and Programs: Results from the 1994 and 1997 NHSDA. DHHS Publication Number (SMA) 99-3252, September 1999.
24. U.S. Department of Health and Human Services, Substance Abuse and Mental Health Services Administration, Division of Workplace Programs. Urine Specimen Collection Handbook for the New Federal Drug Testing Custody and Control Form. OMB Number 0930-0158, Exp. Date: June 30, 2003.
25. U.S. Department of Transportation, Office of the Secretary. DOT Urine Specimen Collection Guidelines for the U.S. Department of Transportation Workplace Drug Testing Programs. (49 CFR Part 40). Version 1.01. August 2001. Can be downloaded from *http://www.dot.govostdapcprog_guidance.html.*
26. U.S. Department of Health and Human Services, Substance Abuse and Mental Health Services Administration. Center for Substance Abuse Prevention Technical Report 12: Urine Specimen Collection Handbook for Federal Workplace Drug Testing Programs, 1996.
27. U.S. Department of Health and Human Services, Lists of SAMHSA-certified drug testing laboratories can be found at the following Web sites:
http://www.access.gpo.govsu_docsacesaces140.html
http://www.drugfreeWorkplace.gov
http://www.health.orgWorkplace.
28. U.S. Department of Health and Human Services, Substance Abuse and Mental Health Services Administration, Division of Workplace Programs.
29. U.S. Department of Transportation, Office of Drug and Alcohol Policy and Compliance. 49 CFR Part 40: Procedures for transportation workplace drug and alcohol testing programs. *Federal Register* 2000(December 19);65:79462; *Federal Register* 2001(August 9);65:41944. See Section G—Medical Review Officers and the Verification Progress. 40.121—Who is qualified to act as an MRO?
30. Vogl WF, Bush DM. Medical Review Officer Manual for Federal Workplace Drug Testing Programs. CSAP Technical Report 15; DHHS Publication No. (SMA) 97-3164, 1997.
31. U.S. Department of Transportation, Office of the Secretary. Medical Review Officer Guide. October 1990.
32. Peterson KW, ed. *Medical Review OfficerDrug and Alcohol Testing Syllabus and Medical Review OfficerDrug and Alcohol Testing Resource Manual.* Arlington Heights, IL: American College of Occupational and Environmental Medicine, 2002.
33. Swotinsky RB, Smith DR. *The Medical Review Officer's Manual: MROCC's Guide to Drug Testing,* 2nd ed. Beverly, MA: Occupational and Environmental Medicine Press, 2002.
34. *Diagnostic and statistical manual of mental disorders* (DSM-IV), 4th ed. Washington, DC: American Psychiatric Association, 1994.
35. U.S. Department of Transportation, Office of Drug and Alcohol Policy and Compliance. Part 40 Procedures for workplace transportation drug and alcohol testing programs. *Federal Register* 2000(December 19);65:79462; *Federal Register* 2001(August 9);65:41944. See Sub-

part O—Substance Abuse Professionals and the Return-to-Duty Process.
36. U.S. Department of Transportation. Office of Drug and Alcohol Policy and Compliance. The Substance Abuse Professional Guidelines, August 2001.
37. Omnibus Transportation Employee Testing Act of 1991, Public Law No. 103-272.
38. U.S. Department of Transportation. Drug and Alcohol Testing Programs; Final Rules. *Federal Register* 1994 (February 15);59(31):7302.
39. U.S. Department of Transportation, National Highway Traffic Safety Administration. Highway Safety Programs; Model Specifications for Devices to Measure Breath Alcohol. *Federal Register* 2000(July 21);65 (141):45419.
40. U.S. Department of Transportation. Breath Alcohol Technician (BAT) Training and Screening Test Technician (STT) Training, DOT Model Courses. Available through the Transportation Safety Institute, 4400 Will Rogers Parkway, Suite 205, Oklahoma City, OK 73108, Tel. 405-949-0036, ext. 323; Fax (405) 946-4268.
41. U.S. Supreme Court. *Board of Education of Independent School District No. 92 of Pottawatomie County (Oklahoma) et al. v. Early et al.* on Writ of Certiorari to the United States Court of Appeals for the Tenth Circuit. No. 01-332. Decided June 27, 2002.
42. Barbanel CS, Winkelman JW, Fischer GA, et al. Confirmation of the Department of Transportation criteria for a substituted urine specimen. *J Occup Environ Med* 2002;44(5).
43. U.S. Department of Health and Human Services, Substance Abuse and Mental Health Services Administration, Division of Workplace Programs. Notice of Proposed Rulemaking: Mandatory Guidelines for Federal Workplace Drug Testing. *Federal Register* 2001(August 21);66(162):43876.
44. Medical Review Officer Certification Council, 1821 Walden Office Square, Suite 300, Schaumburg, Illinois 60173, Tel. (847) 303-7210; Fax (847) 303-7211; Obtain Application By Fax-On-Demand: (630) 851-9702; e-mail: *mrocc@mrocc.org*; Internet: *http://www.mrocc.org*.
45. Crouch DJ, Webb DO, Butler PF, et al. A critical evaluation of the Utah Power and Light Company's substance abuse management program: absenteeism, accidents and costs. In: Gust SW, Walsh JM, eds. *Drugs in the workplace: research and evaluation data.* NIDA Research Monograph 91, U.S. Department of Health and Human Services; Alcohol, Drug Abuse and Mental Health Administration, 1989:169–193.
46. U.S. Department of Health and Human Services, Substance Abuse and Mental Health Services Administration. Worker Drug Use and Workplace Policies and Programs: Results from the 1994 and 1997 NHSDA. DHHS Publication Number (SMA) 99-3252, September 1999.
47. National Institute on Drug Abuse, National Institutes of Health, Monitoring the Future: National Survey Results on Drug Use, 1975–1999, 2 volumes, NIH Publication Number 00-4802, August 2000, *http://www.MonitoringTheFuture.org*.
48. Zwerling C, Ryan J. Preemployment drug screening: the epidemiologic issues. *J Occup Med* 1992;34(6):595.
49. Upfal M, Peterson KW. Preemployment drug screening: the epidemiological issues. [Letter to the Editor, with response by the authors.] *J Occup Med* 1993;35(1):8.
50. Federal Railroad Administration, Office of Safety. *Reducing substance abuse in the railroad industry—a success story.* [Unpublished.] Presented to the 71st Annual Meeting of the Transportation Research Board, 1992.
51. Current WF. Does drug testing work? Institute for a Drug-Free Workplace, 1301 K. Street, NW, Washington, DC 20005, 1993.
52. U.S. Department of Health and Human Services, Substance Abuse and Mental Health Services Administration, Division of Workplace Programs. Minutes of the Drug Testing Advisory Board (DTAB) are posted on the SAMHSA Web site and at *http://www.workplace.samhsa.gov*. Updates of proposed revisions to the Mandatory Guidelines for Workplace Drug Testing include provisions for testing other matrices, including hair, sweat patch and oral fluids are also posted on this site.

FURTHER INFORMATION

Peterson KW, ed. Medical Review Officer/Drug and Alcohol Testing Syllabus and Medical Review Officer/Drug and Alcohol Testing Resource Manual. Published by the American College of Occupational and Environmental Medicine, 1114 N. Arlington Heights Road, Arlington Heights, IL 6000-47704; *www.acoem.org*.
A compendium of materials for ACOEM's ongoing MRO/Drug and Alcohol Testing training courses. Materials are updated at least annually to contain the latest available information in this rapidly evolving field.

Swotinsky RB, Smith DR. *The Medical Review Officer's Manual: MROCC's Guide to Drug Testing,* 2nd ed. Occupational and Environmental Medicine Press, 2002.
A succinct condensation of the DHHS and DOT drug and alcohol testing regulations, with useful tables and charts. It was completely updated in 2002 and will be revised as needed.

Swotinsky RB, ed. *MRO Update Newsletter*. Published by the American College of Occupational and Environmental Medicine, 1114 N. Arlington Heights Road, Arlington Heights, IL 6000-47704; *www.acoem.org*.
Published 10 times a year, MRO Update contains clear, concise, and practical articles and news about the latest regulations, research, and changes in technology, state laws and the marketplace.

SAMHSA's toll-free Drug Free Workplace Helpline: 1-(800)-843-4971. Provides consultation to health professionals, employers, and labor representatives on developing drug-free workplace policies and programs. It is linked to the National Clearinghouse for Alcohol and Drug Information (1-800-729-6686), which provides model policies, available publications, and literature searches, and lends videotapes on drugs in the workplace.

FMCSA Electronic Bulletin Board Service: 1-(800)-337-3492. After dialing into this service by modem, the user can download drug and alcohol testing regulations. Users also post questions and responses to questions in the "Motor Carrier Safety" conference.

DOT Fax-on-Demand Service: 1-(800)-225-3784. DOT's service offers documents on topics such as alcohol testing, drug testing, forms and lists, DOT news releases, and order forms for regulation reprints. New users will want to request the list of documents first, and then call back for specific items from the list.

Useful Internet sites include the following:

- ***DOT's Office of Drug and Alcohol Policy and Compliance (ODAPC)*** **[http://www.dot.govostdapc]** contains sections on recent news and upcoming events, drug and alcohol testing regulations, program guidance material, operating administrations program managers, and links to other federal and nonfederal sites.
- ***SAMHSA's National Clearinghouse for Drug and Alcohol Information*** **[http://www.health.orgworkplace]** is a rich resource that contains all the regulations, manuals, and guidance materials that SAMHSA publishes, along with information for employers and small businesses.
- ***Government Printing Office Gate*** **[http://www.gpo.ucop.edu]** offers a search engine for finding articles in the *Federal Register* and other government publications. Search "drug test or alcohol test" in the *Federal Register* to find recent drug and alcohol testing rules.
- ***Lawsinhyand*** **[http://lawsinhand.dtstatelaws.com]** is a resource for legal, medical, and scientific information. It is an on-line library of information related to employment drug and alcohol testing, containing more than 3,000 court decisions (complete text and summarized) and federal and state statutes and regulations. Subscribers can ask questions and receive input from medical, legal, and administrative experts and other subscribers.
- ***Join Together*** **[http://www.jointogether.orgsa]**. This address lists recent news related to substance abuse.

MROCC **[http://www.mrocc.org]**. The Medical Review Officer Certification Council (MROCC) home page describes MROCC and the MRO certification exam, provides an application for the exam, and has instructions for the MROCC fax-on-demand service.

APPENDIX: ACOEM DRUG SCREENING IN THE WORKPLACE: ETHICAL GUIDELINES

Drug and alcohol abuse constitute a significant problem in the workplace, contributing to impaired productivity and job performance, increased accidents and injuries, violations of security, theft of company property, and diminished employee morale. The federal government and many companies have adopted policies regarding the use of drugs, as well as instituting a variety of drug screening, control, and rehabilitation programs.

Appropriate constraints must be observed in order to ethically screen employees and prospective employees for the presence in their bodies of drugs, including alcohol, that might affect ability to perform work in a safe manner.

The following guidelines deal only with ethical issues involved in drug screening in the workplace. Other important considerations that must be addressed in the design and implementation of a drug screening program include biologic factors concerning rates of absorption and elimination of drugs, technical factors relating to specificity and accuracy of analyses, legal safeguards, regulatory requirements, and employee relations concerns.

ACOEM recommends strongly that employers obtain expert legal, medical, and employee relations advice before making a decision to require screening of employees or applicants for drugs. Such experts also should be involved in the actual structuring and implementation of any program of screening of employees and applicants for drugs.

These guidelines are pertinent to drug testing done under the following circumstances: preplacement assessment, job transfer evaluation, periodic mandatory medical surveillance, postincident/accident, for-reasonable-cause, and random testing of those in safety and security-sensitive positions, special work fitness examinations, and monitoring of employees who are under treatment for drug abuse, including alcohol, as a condition of continuing employment....

The following features should be included in any program for the screening of employees and prospective employees for drugs:

1. A written company policy and procedure concerning drug use and screening for the presence of drugs should exist and be applied impartially.
2. The reason for any requirement for screening for drugs should be clearly documented. Such reasons might involve safety for the individual and other employees or the public; security needs; or requirements related to job performance.
3. Affected employees and applicants should be informed in advance about the company's policy concerning drug use and screening. They should be made aware of their right to refuse such screening and the consequences of such refusal to their employment.
4. Where special safety or security needs justify testing for drugs on an unannounced and possibly random basis, employees should be made aware in advance that this will be done from time to time. Care should be taken to assure that such tests are done in a uniform and impartial manner for all employees in the affected group(s).
5. Written consent for screening and for communication of results to the employer should be obtained from each individual prior to screening.
6. Collection, transportation, and analysis of the specimens and the reporting of the results should meet stringent legal, technical, and ethical requirements. The process should be under the supervision of a licensed physician.
7. A licensed physician who is qualified as a medical review officer should evaluate positive results prior to a report being made to the employer. This may require the obtaining of supplemental

information from the employee or applicant in order to ensure that a positive test does not represent appropriate use of prescription drugs, over-the-counter medication, or other substances that could cause a positive test.

Training of the medical review officer should include the pharmacology of substance abuse, laboratory testing methodology and quality control, forensic toxicology, pertinent federal regulations, legal and ethical requirements, chemical dependency illness, employee assistance programs, and rehabilitation.

8. The affected employee or applicant should be advised of positive results by the physician and have the opportunity for explanation and discussion prior to the reporting of results to the employer, if feasible. The mechanism for accomplishing this should be clearly defined.
9. The employee or applicant having indication of a drug abuse problem should be advised concerning appropriate treatment resources.
10. Any report to the employer should provide only the information needed for work placement purposes or as required by government regulations. Identification to the employer of the particular drug(s) found and quantitative levels is not necessary, unless required by law. Reports to the employer should be made by a physician sensitive to the various considerations involved.

The use of a drug screen as part of a voluntary periodic examination program can be acceptable ethically if adequate safeguards as to confidentiality can be assured. It seems probable at present that inclusion of a drug screen as part of a voluntary periodic examination program may lead to a significant reduction in participation, with consequent loss to the nonparticipants, of the benefits of the examination. Potential health benefits should be carefully weighed against potential losses to health before a decision is reached on this matter.

If carefully designed and carried out, programs for the screening of employees and applicants for drugs, including alcohol, serve to protect and improve employee health and safety in an ethically acceptable manner.

American College of Occupational and Environmental Medicine
Approved by Board of Directors
February 9, 1991

10

Accreditation of Occupational Health Services

Dennis Schultz

OVERVIEW

Accreditation is a process used to certify that an organization meets certain criteria. The accreditation body must have a defined *set of standards,* which represent value or excellence, and a *defined process* by which the organization's performance is judged against these standards. Usually the organization applying for accreditation begins its preparation with a program of evaluation and improvement. It obtains the standards and performs a comprehensive self-assessment reviewing its policies, procedures, and practices. The organization identifies deficiencies, improves these areas, and repeats its evaluation to assure improvement. Once this process is completed, the organization requests that the accrediting body evaluates its program. Usually the accrediting body conducts an on-site survey with independent auditors.

Medical organizations may pursue accreditation for a variety of reasons. Traditionally, accreditation of ambulatory facilities was voluntary and done to improve quality of care and gain recognition. Under these conditions, the value of accreditation depends on the relevance of the standards to the specific medical organization, the value of the standards in assuring and improving quality of care, the quality of the survey process, and the reputation of the accrediting body.

Hospital accreditation began as a voluntary process, but by the mid-1960s, it had become a financial necessity. Accreditation was required for reimbursement under federal insurance plans. Now, similar regulations have been enacted for certain ambulatory facilities, primarily surgical centers. For these facilities accreditation has become a necessity. If current legislative and insurance trends continue, accreditation will extend into the office setting starting with office-based surgery. However, these changes have not yet affected occupational health settings where accreditation continues to be a voluntary process. Ideally, accreditation meets all of the facility's needs. It improves quality, is of value, and fulfills requirements for certification and billing.

A number of organizations offer accreditation for health care organizations (1). Currently, there are two primary accreditation organizations available to occupational medical clinics or in-plant medical departments. These are the Joint Commission on Accreditation of Healthcare Organizations (JCAHO, also known as the Joint Commission) and the Accreditation Association for Ambulatory Health Care (AAAHC). JCAHO was formed in 1951 as the Joint Commission on Accreditation of Hospitals (JCAH). Its sole focus was hospital accreditation. Starting in the mid-1960s, JCAH began expanded accreditation services to other types of inpatient health care facilities. In 1975 it began ambulatory accreditation with the formation of the Accreditation Council for Ambulatory Health Care. The Council was disbanded in 1979, replaced by a Professional and Technical Advisory Committee. In 1987 JCAH changed its name to JCAHO, reflecting greater involvement in nonhospital health care organizations. It renewed its commitment to ambulatory accreditation with the publication of the *Accreditation Manual for Ambulatory Health Care* in 1996 (2).

AAAHC was formed in 1979, in response to the Joint Commission's disbanding of the Accreditation Council for Ambulatory Health Care. Several organizations that had been involved with the JCAHO's Ambulatory Council withdrew their support and became founding members of AAAHC. These organizations included the American Group Practice Association, the Group Health Association of America, the Medical Group Management Association, the Freestanding Ambulatory Surgical Association, the American College Health Association, and the National Association of Community Health Care Centers.

Currently, AAAHC has grown to 17 member organizations. AAAHC has expanded its accreditation services, but its sole focus continues to be ambulatory settings.

The American College of Occupational and Environmental Medicine (ACOEM) became a member of AAAHC in 1987. In 1991, ACOEM strengthened its commitment to accreditation with a formal endorsement supporting the development of standards of practice, the achievement of these standards through self-evaluation, and the participation in accreditation to demonstrate that the standards have been met (3). The following year, 1992, ACOEM formally recognized AAAHC as the accrediting body for occupational health organizations (4). Working together, ACOEM and AAAHC developed standards for occupational health services, which are reviewed and revised annually. Because of the affiliation between ACOEM and AAAHC and the strength of the occupational health standards, the remainder of this chapter discusses accreditation under AAAHC.

AAAHC is a nonprofit corporation whose goal is to assist ambulatory health care organizations in providing high-quality care in the most efficient and economically sound manner possible. AAAHC achieves its goal through a voluntary, peer-based accreditation program that is focused on education and counseling (5).

During the past 20 years, AAAHC has become the leader in ambulatory accreditation. It has been recognized and accepted by a variety of third-party payers that require accreditation. Examples include commercial carriers, health maintenance organizations (HMOs), and governmental agencies. It has also been recognized as equivalent accreditation for Joint Commission network affiliation.

ACCREDITATION UNDER AAAHC

Criteria used by AAAHC are published in the *Accreditation Handbook for Ambulatory Health Care.* This document represents the efforts of thousand of experts in the delivery of ambulatory health care. Standards are reviewed and revised annually. ACOEM's board of directors is involved in any modifications or revisions of the section addressing occupational health services.

The standards make up about half of this 100-page document. Background information, appendices, and self-directed questionnaires constitute the remainder of the booklet. AAAHC standards are brief, simple, and clearly written. The format, which is the same for each standard, begins with one or two opening sentences defining and setting goals for the service or entity. Next it lists a series of characteristics of accreditable organizations, which delineate objectives. Most of the standards are written in general terms so they can be applied to all ambulatory settings.

There are 24 chapters that are divided into two groups: core and adjunct standards. *Core* standards apply to all organizations and address issues common to ambulatory health care delivery such as patient rights, administration, facilities, and records. *Adjunct* standards address specific services or activities and apply only if the organization offers the services listed. One of the adjunct standards is for occupational and employee health services. This arrangement of core and adjunct standards provides consistency between all ambulatory health care organizations while offering specific guidance for organizations offering specialized services. The standards can be applied to any occupational health program—in-plant, hospital based, or solo or group practice.

Survey Eligibility

AAAHC's goal is to provide quality accreditation services to a wide variety of ambulatory health care organizations. This goal is reflected in the eligibility requirements for accreditation surveys. The organization's primary activity must be provision of health services and it must have been in operation for at least 6 months. Either the organization or its parent organization must be a formally organized, legal entity. If required, the organization must be licensed to provide services and must be in compliance with appropriate regulations. Medical care must be under the direction or supervision of a physician. The health care organization must also share facilities, equipment, and patient care records among its members providing patient care. There is an early option survey for organizations that are licensed in their state but have not been in operation for 6 months.

Survey Process

Preparation for the survey starts with a review of the *Self-Assessment Manual* published by AAAHC. This serves as a blueprint to assess an organization's status and to guide the organization's effort to become accredited. Much of the manual consists of AAAHC standards subdivided into their component parts. The organization completes a checklist, which rates its current level of compliance on a five-point scale for each component. The manual also provides worksheets to guide the organization in assessing and improving performance. AAAHC standards do not require that an organization use the manual to achieve compliance, but the manual provides a reasonable approach for most organizations.

Usually, the first step of the self-assessment process is creation of an accreditation committee or team. Collectively, the members of this team should be knowledgeable about all aspects of the organization's operations, be capable of implementing change, and be committed to the process of self-assessment and accreditation. Once the committee is formed, it names a chairperson and divides primary responsibilities for the standards among its members. These individuals enlist the support of other organization members, begin the process of assessment, and plan for needed changes. One of the goals at this step of the process is to involve as much of the organization as possible. Ultimately, everyone will be affected by the accreditation process. Through regular meetings, the team creates a timetable for the project and monitors progress.

The self-assessment process may take months to years, depending on the status of the organization. Certain AAAHC standards require that programs be in place long enough to demonstrate effectiveness. It may take a year to gather sufficient information to demonstrate that a quality improvement program is effective. Changes in medical records are best made over the course of a year. The same holds true for changes in the way staff or physicians are evaluated or assigned clinical privileges. Once the self-assessment is completed, the organization obtains, completes, and submits the Presurvey Questionnaire, published by AAAHC. Responses to these questions form the basis for AAAHC recommendations about the structure and timing of the on-site survey. AAAHC also offers consulting services to help organizations improve their quality and achieve accreditation.

The survey consists of an extensive on-site evaluation of the organization's policies, procedures, and operations. The process relies heavily on the abilities of AAAHC surveyors, who are volunteers, chosen and trained by AAAHC. Surveyors may be practicing health care providers or health care administrators. AAAHC training focuses on using the surveyors' experience to evaluate the organization and to apply the standards fairly.

AAAHC determines the composition of the survey team and the duration of the survey. If the organization has multiple practice sites, AAAHC will also determine which of the sites will be evaluated. These determinations are based on characteristics of the organization. The initial survey consists of at least one surveyor spending a minimum of one day at the site. If the organization provides services at several sites, then at least 50% of the sites are usually surveyed. AAAHC matches surveyors and organizations, so individuals performing the evaluation are knowledgeable about the practice setting. For example, occupational health professionals are used for occupational health site visits. The organization is consulted prior to the on-site assessment. It may request a surveyor with particular experience or expertise. It may also decline to have a particular surveyor perform the evaluation. The organization may not request a specific surveyor. The organization is also involved in planning the site visit. AAAHC strives to minimize the impact of the survey on the organization's day-to-day operation.

The cost of a site visit varies with the type and size of the health care organization. Currently, the minimum charge is $3,000 for an office-based surgery practice. This assumes the survey can be completed using one surveyor for 1 day. Surveying an office practice with several physicians usually requires one or two surveyors for 1½ to 2 days. A typical charge for this survey is $5,000 to $6,000. Site visits for large ambulatory care organizations, clinics, or HMOs are much more involved. They may require three to four surveyors working 3 to 4 days. Costs will increase with the number of practice sites, number of practitioners, and types of medical services. AAAHC determines the cost after analyzing the Presurvey Questionnaire; however, the association's staff members will provide rough estimates based on preliminary information.

A primary goal of the surveyors is to determine if the organization is in compliance with the intent of the standards. The surveyors use a variety of information to assess the extent of compliance, such as written documentation of policy and procedure manuals, patient information brochures, patient chart reviews, internal audit information, and answers to detailed questions concerning implementation. Surveyors also use information from interviews, observations from the on-site visit, and public comment. The organization must demonstrate that it understands and is in compliance with the standards. AAAHC does not require extensive policies and procedures, though this is a common means for organizations to demonstrate compliance. If the organization does have extensive policies and procedures, these must be understood by the organization's members, must be consistent with AAAHC standards, and must be applied in the organization's day-to-day operations. In these situations, compliance with the standards must be evident in both policy and action.

A second goal of the surveyors is to educate and provide consultation to the organization. The surveyors have a formal meeting with representatives of the organization at the end of the site visit. At the meeting they discuss their findings, answer questions, and make suggestions for improvement. The organization may refute the findings or provide additional information that the surveyor may not have reviewed. The surveyors' written report and conclusions are submitted to the accreditation committee of the board of directors of AAAHC, which will determine whether the organization is accredited.

Accreditation can be granted for either 1 or 3 years. AAAHC can also decide to defer accreditation if there are deficiencies likely to be corrected within 6 months. If it's a new organization being reviewed under the early-option program, the maximum duration of accreditation is 1 year. AAAHC may also deny accreditation. There is a formal policy for appeals and the organization can apply for reevaluation immediately. The organization receives a completed Survey Report Form, which outlines the survey findings. It also receives an evaluation form, which it uses to critique the accreditation process. In addition to scheduled surveys, AAAHC performs unannounced surveys on a random sample of accredited organizations. These surveys are brief, limited, and focused. Their purpose is to identify any significant changes in quality of care or other factors affecting accreditation status. They are also a component of AAAHC's internal quality assurance programs. Unannounced surveys are used by many accreditation programs, including any involved in Joint Commission networks. Surveyors are practicing health professionals, who understand the challenges of an announced survey. They make every effort to minimize the effect of the survey on the daily routine and operation of the facility.

AAAHC STANDARDS

Core Standards

As noted, chapters are divided into core and adjunct standards. Core standards apply to all organizations. The following eight topics constitute AAAHC's core standards.

Patient Rights

The first of the core standards addresses patients' rights, specifically the obligations of the organization to the patient. It requires that the organization protect patients' dignity and confidentiality, provide them with proper information about their medical condition, encourage patient participation in medical decisions, and inform patients of their respective rights and responsibilities. Specific examples of topics included in this chapter are the organization's policy concerning payment, provision of after-hour care, the accuracy of the organization's advertising, and whether the organization informs patients of their right to change physicians or refuse treatment.

Governance

The second standard addresses governance, the relationship between the organization and its governing body. The chapter delineates the basic responsibilities of a governing body, such as setting the mission, goals, and objectives for the organization, assuring adequate facilities and personnel, determining organizational structure, adopting policies and procedures, and providing oversight for quality improvement. Other areas of responsibility are physician appointments and credentialing, risk assessment, and staff improvement. The standard specifically requires compliance with Centers for Disease Control (CDC) guidelines for the prevention of transmission of blood-borne pathogens (6) and compliance with Occupational Safety and Health Administration (OSHA) regulations (7). It also requires involvement with local agencies for facility or community emergencies.

Lastly, the governance chapter requires a comprehensive program for identifying, reporting, analyzing, and preventing adverse incidents. Adverse incidents include unexpected patient deaths, illness, or injury. They also include "near misses," errors in process, procedures, or medical care that have the potential for harming patients or staff. The chapter describes required elements of the program, including a process for identifying the causative factors leading to the adverse outcome or breach in procedures or care, a process for reporting the event to internal and external bodies, and a process for correcting problems or improving the organization's operation through development of an action plan. The plan must address responsibilities for implementation, time lines, strategies, and ongoing monitoring to assure the implementation has been effective.

Administration

The third core standard notes that the organization must be administered in a manner that assures quality health care and is consistent with its mission, goals, and objectives. Many topics in this standard are similar to those in governance; however, the focus is on *executing* the policies and procedures. Issues addressed include the enforcement of policies, the steps taken to comply with applicable laws, and the method of evaluating performance. The standard is broadly divided into personnel policies and procedures and administrative policies and procedures. This standard also requires assessment of patient satisfaction.

Quality of Care

The fourth core standard requires that the organization provide high-quality, cost-conscious health care. Most of the standard addresses medical management issues such as accuracy of diagnosis, appropriateness of treatment and referrals, and duplication of services. Generally, these types of questions are addressed through patient chart audits. The standard also addresses training and credentialing of health care providers, highlights the importance of adverse event reporting, and requires obtaining translators when possible. Community emergency preparedness and disaster planning are also addressed in this chapter.

Quality Management and Improvement

The fifth and most challenging of the core standards addresses how the organization monitors and improves its processes and outcomes. Like the previous standard, it addresses quality of care issues; however, the standard is much more comprehensive. The organization's quality management and improvement program must include (a) peer review for health care providers, (b) quality assessment including outcome measurement and benchmarking, (c) a program to improve quality, and (d) a risk management program. These programs must be integrated. They should be an active part of the day-to-day operation of the organization.

Clinical Records

The sixth core standard addresses all aspects of medical records from legibility to confidentiality and from organization to security. The standard notes the type of information that should be included for any clinical encounter, that telephone contacts be documented, and that records be managed properly. The handbook includes a Clinical Record Worksheet to guide the assessment of clinical care and medical records.

Professional Improvement

The seventh core standard discusses professional improvement. The organization must strive to improve the competence and skills of its members. Issues include continuing education, support for library services, and credentialing.

Facilities and Environment

The last of the core standards addresses the adequacy of the organization's facilities, equipment, and internal safety procedures. In addition to fire safety and emergency preparedness, this standard addresses accommodations for individuals with disabilities, parking issues, smoking policy, appropriate design of patient areas and examination rooms, the organization's hazardous materials program, and facilities maintenance.

Adjunct Standards

AAAHC has 16 adjunct standards, each addressing a different clinical activity or service. The individual standard is only applied if the organization provides the service described in the chapter. Following are summaries of the most pertinent of these standards.

Occupational and Employee Health Services

Chapter 1 addresses occupational and employee health services. It is divided into two subchapters. The standards in this chapter were developed in conjunction with ACOEM. They embody the principles of occupational medicine and are worthy goals for all organizations providing occupational health services. The opening statement sets the primary goals of occupational and employee health services as (a) assuring a safe and healthy workplace for employees and patients through the recognition, evaluation, and control of illness and injury in or from the workplace; and (b) meeting the needs of the individuals served.

The occupational health chapter is divided into two sections. The first, titled "Employee Health in Health Care Settings," applies to health care facilities, such as surgical centers or offices, which provide limited occupational health services to their own employees. This section contains four brief standards. The first addresses protection from biologic hazards. Topics such as hepatitis B vaccination, blood-borne pathogen exposures, and immunization programs are included. The second addresses chemical hazards and hazard communication compliance. The third discusses physical hazards such as violence in the workplace and ergonomics. The last discusses record keeping.

The second section, titled "Occupational Health Services," is more comprehensive and applies to occupational health facilities or departments. This section contains 13 standards listed as A through M. Standards A through E provide general guidelines for occupational medical care. Standards F through M address specific occupational health services. The initial standards usually apply to all occupational health facilities, while the later standards apply only if the organization provides the specific services discussed.

A. This standard extends patient rights to employees. It requires that individuals who agree to laboratory testing or medical examinations at the request of their employer be informed of the purpose and scope of the evaluation, the role of the examiner, confidentiality protections, information that may be conveyed to the employer, and whether medical follow-up is necessary.
B. This standard requires that occupational health services be accurately portrayed. It has the effect of expanding "honesty in advertising" from patients to employees, companies, and other purchasers of occupational health services.
C. This standard requires access to appropriate resources needed to evaluate workplace hazards such as an industrial hygienist, ergonomist, toxicologist, occupational health nurse, and physicians board-certified in occupational medicine. It also requires reference material and continuing medical education in occupational health.
D. This standard lists several characteristics of quality occupational health services. It notes that services should be provided with an understanding of the individual's workplace and work demands, that they include preventive counseling to reduce potential hazards, that they address the relation of work exposures and medical findings or disorders, and that they address whether the individual can perform essential job functions.
E. This standard requires that the elements noted above be reflected in the medical records in addition to relevant communications about the individual to employers, insurance carriers, or others.
F. This standard addresses medical care for individuals with occupational injury or illness. It requires special attention if there is a delay in recovery, if the problem is recurrent, or if there are residual permanent impairments.
G. This standard addresses work placement examinations such as preplacement, transfer, or fitness for duty examinations. It indicates they should address current health and ability to perform the job as well as the extent and duration of recent health changes affecting job performance.
H. This standard addresses medical surveillance evaluations. It requires that health professionals have specific knowledge about the hazardous agent. This includes the agent's effects, permissible and actual exposure levels, biologic monitoring results, and regulatory requirements. It also recommends that surveillance data be analyzed for trends if feasible.
I. This standard addresses examinations mandated by state or federal statutes. Examples are medical examinations for commercial truck drivers and medical evaluations for respirator use. The standard requires that health providers performing these exams be knowledgeable about their role and responsibilities under the law. It also requires that they have access to the regulation and to relevant reference materials.
J. This standard addresses laboratory or medical testing programs. Examples of this type of service include urine testing for drugs of abuse, blood lead determinations, and audiograms. The standard requires that these testing programs be consistent with the law, under specific written protocols, and with appropriate medical oversight.
K. This standard is a general statement about consulting in occupational health. It requires that the consultant's role and responsibilities be clearly defined.
L. If the occupational health services include educational or training programs, these are covered by this standard. Such programs must have written objectives, be tailored to their specific audience, include an evaluation process, and use results to improve program quality.
M. Some occupational health programs are responsible for components of community preparedness or emergency response. These services are addressed in this standard. It requires that the disaster plan address various scenarios, estimate morbidity and mortality, include plans for medical management of those affected, and be done in collaboration with local emergency planning committees. Toxicologic exposure plans address identification and management of those affected and assures sufficient training.

Immediate/Urgent Care Services

Several other adjunct chapters may apply to an organization, depending on the type of services the organization provides. If the organization provides urgent care in addition to occupational services, then

Chapter 14, Immediate/Urgent Care Service, applies. This standard requires that the organization be accurate in describing its services, that it sees only patients who can be appropriately treated in an urgent care setting, and that it has appropriate staff and facilities.

Testing: Diagnostic Imaging and Laboratory Services

AAAHC's *Handbook for Accreditation* has two adjunct chapters addressing diagnostic testing. Chapter 16, Pathology and Medical Laboratory Services, discusses laboratory testing. Chapter 17, Diagnostic Imaging Services, covers radiographs. The basic issues in both standards are the same. They consider staffing, facilities, equipment, safety, record management, and quality improvement.

Other Professional and Technical Services

Services such as occupational therapy, physical therapy, psychologic services, health education, and audiology are covered by an adjunct standard 20, Other Professional and Technical Services. This chapter is general and brief. It notes that services must be appropriate to the needs of the patient. There must be appropriate staffing and facilities. In addition, evaluation of the services must be consistent with other AAAHC standards.

Other Standards

There are 11 other adjunct standards. Some of these may also apply to organizations providing occupational health services. Individual standards cover emergency, pharmaceuticals, teaching and publication activities, research activities, and others.

PROBLEM AREAS IN ACHIEVING ACCREDITATION

If organizations encounter problems in accreditation, it is usually in one of three areas: clinical records, quality management and improvement, or occupational health services.

Clinical Records

Deficiencies in medical records are among the most common problems seen in surveys. The clinical record worksheet in the handbook provides 16 specific areas that are used to judge care and medical records. The standard indicates that records must be legible, accurate, current, accessible, and have a common format. All information, including test reports, dictated notes, and hospitalization records, must be reviewed. In addition, the chart must clearly note allergies. The occupational health standard notes additional elements that should be included in the records, including an appropriate occupational history. Problems can arise in any of these areas, but *a common problem is failing to adequately document the patient encounter*.

The medical record is the primary source of information about patient care. It is used by all accrediting bodies including AAAHC. To evaluate care, the medical records must provide sufficient detail so that an outside reviewer can (a) determine the patient's primary complaint, (b) independently confirm the patient's diagnosis based on reported findings, (c) confirm that the treatment was appropriate and necessary, and (d) confirm that the patient's care was appropriate over time. Records must be complete and legible.

There are many ways organizations generate and manage medical records. These range from handwritten notes stored in folders to computer-generated notes archived as an electronic database. The specific solutions for charting deficiencies vary from one practice setting to the next. But regardless of the practice setting or medical record format, practitioners must be convinced and reminded that documentation is important. Charts and forms can be designed in ways to facilitate documentation and provision of quality services. The same holds true for computer-assisted charting. Fortunately, deficiencies in documentation are easy to identify and can usually be solved with a minimum of effort. Unfortunately, organizations generally have to institute an ongoing program to assure that improvement is maintained. The occupational health chapter has several additional requirements for the content of medical records. This includes documenting work exposures, preventive counsel, restrictions, or accommodations.

Quality Management and Improvement

A second common problem area for accreditation is the quality management and improvement chapter. A variety of factors influence the quality of health services. Many factors are relatively easy to assess, such as the adequacy of personnel, staff credentials and training, and the adequacy and maintenance of equipment and facilities. Managing these elements of quality is addressed in several of the core chapters.

By contrast, the quality improvement chapter focuses on processes, outcomes, and improvement. These are more difficult to define, measure. and manage.

AAAHC's quality improvement chapter requires peer review, outcome measurement, benchmarking, quality improvement, and a risk management program. Of these, peer review is the most established process and the least likely to cause problems in accreditation. Quality improvement initiatives and outcome measurements tend to be the most difficult. As with other standards, AAAHC lists characteristics of acceptable programs, rather than mandating specific programs or program structure. It does require that the organization systematically review its operations and develop comprehensive programs appropriate to its practice setting. Meeting the intent of this chapter requires commitment and dedication. Quality management and improvement are critical for any organization striving for excellence.

Peer Review

The first requirement in the quality management chapter is peer review, the process of having one health care provider review the care provided by a second. Generally, peer review is done through chart audits. Care is commonly judged against medical criteria. AAAHC's standard requires a formal peer review program. At least two physicians or dentists must be involved. Results from peer review must be integrated into other elements of quality management such as granting clinical privileges and quality improvement. This standard also requires that health care providers participate in developing the criteria used to judge their care.

Peer review is one of the older quality improvement techniques. Over the years, it has gained wide acceptance. Now, most organizations have established peer review processes. The most challenging part of peer review programs is gaining the support of the health care providers as the program is being implemented. Providers may mistakenly assume that the goal of peer review is to identify individuals for punitive measures, or that using criteria to judge care substitutes "cookbook" medicine for clinical judgment. Neither assumption is true. The process of developing criteria causes providers to review their own approach to medical management, generates discussion, and ultimately creates consensus. The process, in and of itself, usually improves quality of care. It also allays fear about peer review and forms the foundations of a strong program. Peer review can identify individuals who are practicing poor medicine. But more commonly, peer review validates that the organization is providing quality care. Peer review is also an important source of suggestions for quality improvements, identifying system changes that support delivery of quality care. These suggestions may involve patient forms or records, equipment, test reports, transcription, medical staff responsibilities, or patient flow within the center.

Outcome Measurement and Benchmarking

In the past, quality assurance programs have focused on structural and process measurements. But recent trends are to directly measure outcomes of care. Outcome assessments are measurements of end points that represent improved health, reduced risk, or other health quality improvement parameters. Benchmarking involves comparing these outcome assessments against results from other organizations and against established standards of best practice. AAAHC accreditation requires outcome measurement for both clinical and nonclinical parameters. It also requires benchmarking. The standard notes that the organization must identify *key indicators* or outcomes, collect information on these on an ongoing basis, analyze measurements for trends over time, and then benchmark the data. Benchmarking should compare data to other organizations and to state, local, or national standards. If benchmarking shows deficiencies, the organization is required to demonstrate improvement.

The standard does require a comprehensive program of monitoring, measuring, comparing, and improving outcomes. But it does not mandate the number or type of outcome measurements. Nor does it require comparison to a specific database or norm. Establishing these parameters and determining appropriate comparison data are left to the organization.

Organizations with comprehensive programs usually measure a variety of variables including health care outcomes, financial outcomes, efficiency measurements, safety audits, and patient satisfaction. The most important clinical variables will be measured continually and be benchmarked against best practices. Occupational medicine facilities will commonly include lost or restricted workdays, days until discharge from care, recurrence rates for injury, rates for permanent impairment or restrictions, and cost per case. Commonly these data are stratified by diagnosis, such as low back disorders. Other variables may be monitored episodically, quarterly, semiannually, or annually, for defined periods of time. Patient satisfaction surveys and safety and internal audits are commonly approached in this manner. Data from these audits are usually compared to previous years' data to identify changes or trends. Internal audit data are not usually benchmarked against other organizations. However, they can be if the organization is part of a network or owned by a corporation that has other occupational health facilities. Other outcome measurements may be done only once, to determine whether a problem exists.

The primary issue with clinical benchmarking is finding appropriate comparison data. AAAHC requires comparison with similar organizations and with local, state, or national normative data. If the organization is part of a network, then results may be compared to other affiliated facilities. Journal articles and medical textbooks can provide clinical outcome measurements, but it may be difficult to directly compare these results to those of the clinic. Factors such as age, gender, and type of work may affect outcomes. To make meaningful comparisons, clinic data may need to be adjusted to account for biases. The organization should be comprehensive and resourceful in its search for normative and comparison data. The state's workers' compensation program may be a source of data. Some disability guidebooks provide information for common occupational conditions (8). As benchmarking becomes commonplace, more private organizations will develop normative databases. Acknowledging problems in identifying benchmark data, AAAHC has created the Institute for Quality Improvement (IQI). This not-for-profit subsidiary will gather and analyze clinical outcome data for groups of organizations. The organization, with the help of the research staff at IQI, will set parameters for the study. Each organization collects data from its own patients and submits it to IQI, which analyzes the data and writes the performance measurement report. IQI has produced a number of studies covering a range of ambulatory services from cataract extraction to asthma management (9). Copies of these reports are available through IQI. The advantage of using this approach is that outcome measurements are specific to the organization's setting, and directly comparable from one organization to the next.

Quality Improvement Program

The preceding standards mandate that the organization measures its performance and identify areas for improvement. This section, Quality Improvement Program, mandates that the organization use the data to make sustained, measurable improvements in quality and performance. AAAHC does not require a specific quality improvement program; rather, it provides a list of characteristics for the program and for quality improvement initiatives. The program must be active, integrated, and comprehensive. Each specific initiative must include measuring the problem, implementing an improvement, remeasuring the problem, and reanalyzing the situation to determine if any further action is required. AAAHC provides a template to document and evaluate individual quality improvement initiatives. Organizations commonly modify the template and use it to guide and report their individual quality improvement initiatives. Here are the questions that AAAHC audits ask: (a) Was an important problem or concern identified? (b) Were the frequency, severity, and source of the problem evaluated (measured)? (c) Were corrective measures implemented? (d) Was the problem reevaluated? (e) If the problem persisted, were alternative measures taken? (f) Were the results reported to appropriate personnel and a governing body?

Successful quality improvement programs draw on all sources of information for quality improvement initiatives, including peer reviews, audits, patient surveys, suggestions, outcome measurements, and benchmarking. The program must be comprehensive in scope and continuous in operation. It seeks to include all the organization's members. Successful programs require commitment at all levels of the organization, beginning with the governing body.

The actual structure of the program varies between organizations. Larger organizations may have a several-tier program with a single committee monitoring all activities; topic subcommittees addressing areas such as clinic outcomes, utilization management, facilities, or administrative issues; and study groups addressing specific questions. Small organizations may have several individuals who review all data, manage all concerns, and implement all improvement studies.

Quality improvement initiatives are documented as quality studies. The most difficult quality improvement study is usually the first one. The key to doing a first study is keeping the study simple and focused. The more easily defined the study question and outcome, the easier it is to understand, complete, and document the study. The same principles generally hold true for subsequent studies. Multiple studies implementing small changes are generally more easily understood and effective than a large study with multiple interventions and complex outcomes. The more experienced the organization becomes in performing initiatives, the more intuitive this quality improvement model becomes. Eventually all issues will be approached using the same basic steps: define and measure the problem, implement a change, and remeasure to assure improvement. Once the pattern is well established, the program will sustain itself.

Risk Management

The last requirement of the quality management and improvement standard is a risk management program. A major focus of risk management is preventing accidents, injuries, and other adverse occurrences. A recent Institute of Medicine report addressing medication errors and others that affect patient safety highlights how important these issues have become (10). Effective risk management programs also have the effect of minimizing financial liabilities for the organization. Programs that meet AAAHC standards are designed to protect the life and welfare of the organization's patients and employees. The program has a designated person or committee to serve as director. The program must review clinical records and policies. It must include staff education. The content of the risk management program must be tailored to the organization. AAAHC lists topics that should be considered in designing a program. These cover a wide range of issues from unauthorized prescribing to compliance with antitrust regulations and emergency preparedness. AAAHC surveyors will assure that the organization has considered all major sources of adverse outcomes or liabilities and that it has developed a comprehensive program appropriate for its setting. All risk management programs must include a comprehensive, structured, and effective monitoring system for adverse patient outcomes, as was noted in the governance section.

Practice Guidelines

Practice guidelines are sets of directions or principles used to assist health care practitioners with decisions concerning appropriate medical management. AAAHC standards do not mandate the use of practice guidelines, but most organizations integrate them into their quality improvement program. A major impetus to develop and use guidelines came in the mid-1980s when they were viewed as a mechanism to reduce variation in medical care and improve medical quality (11). Initially, practice guidelines reflected the opinions of medical experts. But guidelines based solely on consensus panels were replaced by evidence-based guidelines that relied on medical literature interpreted by panels of medical experts. Over the past several years there has been an explosion of guidelines produced by private, professional, and governmental agencies. Many of these are accessible through the National Guidelines Clearinghouse (12). This catalogue of evidence-based clinical practice guidelines is sponsored by the Agency for Healthcare Research and Quality (AHRQ), which has also created a number of practice guidelines, including one for acute low back pain (13). The American College of Occupational and Environmental Medicine has published a set of guidelines tailored to occupational health settings (14).

Practice guidelines are commonly used to create peer review criteria. Providers will review relevant practice guidelines, interpret them in light of their patient population, and by consensus create chart audit criteria. Practice guidelines can also be used to analyze outcome measurements or benchmark results. Differences between the organization's practice pattern and those listed in the practice guidelines may explain differences in outcome measurements. This analysis commonly provides suggestions for quality improvement initiatives. Finally, practice guidelines can be used to analyze adverse patient outcomes. The purpose here is to establish if the organization was following accepted standards of care and determine where problems may have arisen. In each of these cases, practice guidelines do not replace clinical judgment. But these documents do provide a consensus guide for care based on scientific evidence and critical review.

Occupational Health Services

Prevention

The third common problem area is the occupational health services standard. The focus of this chapter is prevention. The focus of other standards are treatment. This difference, combined with an emphasis on workplace hazards and compliance with labor regulations, demands a different approach to providing occupational health services. If organizations fail to identify this difference, they will not comply with this standard.

The goal of occupational health services is to assure a safe and healthy workplace, which requires identification, evaluation, and reduction of workplace hazards. The only way of accomplishing this task is through understanding of the workplace and the potential hazards. Thus, the standard requires education in occupational health and knowledge of the patient's specific work environment, which must be applied to all aspects of patient or employee care.

For example, job titles usually don't provide enough information to perform preplacement examinations.

One forklift operator may never lift weights in excess of 10 pounds and work in a dust-free environment, whereas another may routinely lift 50 pounds while working in areas with high lead dust levels. Foundry work can run the spectrum from high physical demands under harsh work conditions for individuals working in melting, pouring, or shake out, to light physical demands under nonhazardous conditions for individuals doing inspection, testing, or sampling. To make meaningful determinations regarding placement, health care providers must understand the worker's job and the workplace environment.

If practitioners perform surveillance examinations, they must be knowledgeable about the type of work performed and the potential exposure. If the surveillance exam is prompted by exposure to lead, the practitioner should understand the significance of blood lead levels, and be able to interpret values in light of the patient and the work. A blood lead level of 25 μg/dL may present a cause for alarm or for celebration, depending on the specifics of the situation. Factors such as the patient's ambient lead exposure, previous lead levels, use of protective equipment, history of past exposure, age, gender, and current medical conditions all play a role. While the standard doesn't require expertise in occupational medicine, it does require that the practitioner be knowledgeable and have access to reference materials including a physician with expertise and credentials in occupational health.

Treatment

Providers must also be knowledgeable about the work environment in delivering care to injured workers, a responsibility that is critical in making recommendations regarding job placement. The primary goal of treatment is to restore function and reduce disability. Encouraging the individual to return to normal home and work activities as soon as feasible is part of the treatment strategy. To make meaningful recommendations for work placement, the practitioner must understand the demands of the various jobs and the effects of the individual's medical condition on performance. Using this information, the practitioner can judge when the patient is able to safely return to work, assist the employer in temporary job placement while the patient is recovering and provide guidance in implementing reasonable accommodations. The occupational health standard also requires special review if patients are not improving as expected, if injuries are recurrent, or if injury results in permanent restrictions or limits.

Regulations

Another difference between occupational health and primary care services are the applicable rules and regulations. Practitioners should be knowledgeable about occupational safety and health standards, workers' compensation statues, Department of Transportation regulations, the Americans with Disabilities Act, and any others that affect the provision of services. Compliance with these regulations should be reflected in the organization's practices, policies, and procedures. There should be copies of applicable regulations as well as appropriate reference materials.

Integration with Other Standards

Finally, the specific goals of the occupational health services standard should be reflected in all other relevant AAAHC standards. Documentation must include the preventive activities, knowledge of the workplace, and compliance with all applicable rules and regulations. The organization must be able to demonstrate that the preventive services are characterized by quality, efficiency, effectiveness, and continuous improvement.

PRACTICAL CONSIDERATIONS

Interpreting the Standards

AAAHC's standards focus on characteristics or attributes common to all organizations providing quality occupational health services. To do this, the standards must be general. General standards, combined with differences in the structure and function of occupational health facilities, mean that organizations must carefully consider what the standards mean for their setting. If they fail to interpret the standards, they will fail in their efforts to comply with the standards. Two examples follow.

The governance chapter requires that the governing body be responsible directly, or by delegation, for the activities and operation of the organization. In most cases, the governing body is the board of directors. For most ambulatory facilities, responsibilities are not delegated, but addressed directly by the board itself. Reports of credentialing, quality improvement, as well as changes in policy and procedures are reviewed and approved by the board. Communication between the board and the facility medical director and administrator is direct. But if the medical department is part of large, nonmedical corporation, such as a printing company, manufacturing firm, or assembly operation, the situation is more complex. The board does not directly interact with the medical department. It operates by delegating governance responsibilities to other persons or entities within the organization. Before facilities in these companies can demonstrate compliance with the governance chapter, they must establish what person or entity is responsible for the medical department. Once this is done, the organization must demonstrate that communication and governance through the responsible party meets the intent of the standard. Commonly there are also two lines of authority for governance and administrative responsibilities. Medical issues, such as approval of standing medical orders, credentialing, and medical quality improvement, are managed by the chief medical officer. Administrative responsibilities, including supervision of nonmedical staff, administrative and personnel policies, and procedures, may be managed by someone else. If this is the case, the organization must show that both areas are properly administered and governed, and that there is effective coordination of activities.

The occupational health standard also requires access to personnel and resources needed to evaluate workplace hazards. It provides examples, such as an industrial hygienist, ergonomist, toxicologist, occupational health nurse, and a physician board-certified in occupational medicine. But the standard doesn't state which resources are required or how they should be provided. Comprehensive occupational health facilities generally have a certified occupational health nurse and a board-certified occupational health physician on staff. They may have an industrial hygienist, toxicologist, and ergonomist available as consultants. But none of these individuals is specifically required. The organization must carefully review the services it provides and the patient population it serves. It must assure that it has the resources required to meet the needs of these individuals.

To comply with any of AAAHC's standards, the organization must first understand the intent of the standard and how the standard applies. It is critical that the organization interpret the standard in light of its structure, its function, and the needs of its patient population. It must be systematic in its approach to the standard, use sound reasoning, and be able to justify its decisions.

Preparing for the Survey

The amount of time required to prepare for a first survey ranges from 3 months to 2 years. Time requirements vary with the types of changes that need to be implemented and the amount of resources the organization is willing to dedicate to the process. More time is required if the organization needs to implement a quality improvement program, make changes in medical records, or make changes affecting the evaluation process of its providers. Completing a quality improvement study takes time. In addition to implementing a change, the process includes two outcome measurements, one before and one after the change is made. Therefore, it is usually best to allow 12 months for the first quality study. It is also reasonable to allow at least a year for any changes in patient charting or chart organization. Usually charts are converted to a new system at the time the patient is seen. Within 12 to 18 months all active patients should have been seen and their charts would have been changed. The same applies to changes in health care provider evaluations. These evaluations are usually done annually. So after 1 year, all providers would have been evaluated under the new protocol. Of course, all these changes can be done more rapidly if the organization wishes to dedicate additional staff to the project. All active patient charts can be converted to a new chart system in several days. Quality initiatives can be completed in 4 months. Provider evaluations can be done over several weeks. Compressing the process into shortened time frames usually requires several staff members working on the project on a full-time basis. It is far easier to start in advance and allow the documentation supporting accreditation to accumulate gradually.

In some cases, an organization may not have anyone experienced in accreditation or knowledgeable about AAAHC standards. Reading the self-assessment guide and calling AAAHC for questions or visiting a recently accredited facility will eventually lead to an understanding of accreditation. However, it is more efficient to send a staff member to an AAAHC accreditation workshop. These 2-day seminars provide all the information needed to prepare for accreditation. When the individual returns, he or she can serve as a trainer for other staff. Occasionally, facilities will choose to hire a consultant. AAAHC has a consulting subsidiary, Healthcare Consultants International (HCI), which provides a variety of services to prepare for accreditation and improve quality. HCI also offers self-assessment manuals and policies and procedures. HCI can be contacted through AAAHC.

A couple of months prior to the survey, most organizations perform a "mock survey," in which accreditation committee members review each of the standards, considering how they are going to document compliance. As part of this process, they should have set aside manuals, minutes, reports, or certificates that they will be using for the survey. About a week before the survey, they should do a comprehensive inspection of their facilities. Areas to review include fire extinguishers, emergency exits and signs, medications for expiration dates, security of unfiled charts, Material Safety Data Sheets (MSDSs) for cleaning agents and chemicals, equipment maintenance, or calibration logs and cleanliness. A brief inspection should be repeated the day before the survey. The surveyors will need a private area to work, stocked with all the written material the organization is offering in support of accreditation. The organization should be prepared to present credentialing and personnel files, to pull patient charts based on criteria provided by the surveyor, and to present their quality management and improvement programs. Ideally, key individuals in the accreditation process should be available for questions.

Demonstrating Compliance

Organizations use a wide variety of approaches in demonstrating compliance with the standards. A patient bill of rights is commonly used to highlight the organization's commitment to its patients. It is posted in patient areas, distributed to patients, and used in staff training. Governance and administration are closely related. Much of the material used to document compliance with one supports compliance with the other. Policy and procedure manuals are not required by AAAHC but are valuable in documenting compliance. If manuals are used, they should be up to date and accurately reflect how the organization operates. AAAHC surveyors use interviews and observations to validate an organization's written documentation.

The chart audit is the primary means by which surveyors evaluate quality of care and clinical records. Patient medical records must be complete, legible, and accessible. In addition to documenting the rationale for treatment, they should demonstrate understanding of the patient's work environment and the individual's job. At a minimum, they should contain a focused occupational history. If problem lists are used, they should be current. Allergies should be displayed prominently and consistently in all records. There should be policies regarding record retention and management, and release of information. Interviews should confirm that the policies are being followed.

Documentation of peer review, outcome measurements, and quality studies is important in demonstrating compliance with the quality management and improvement chapter. Equally important is the organization's approach and rationale to its program's design. It should be able to explain why it has chosen specific elements of its program.

There are several keys to complying with the occupational health standard, but foremost is demonstrating an understanding of the workplace. Documenting a thorough, focused occupational history for each patient is an important first step. This should be supplemented by information from the workplace. MSDSs and monitoring data are important in cases involving chemical exposure. Job descriptions are valuable in making determinations about placement, but there is nothing as valuable as visiting the workplace for developing an understanding of job tasks, demands, and hazards. Job site visits can be done as part of an introductory company tour, as a preliminary step in participating in a surveillance project, or in the context of caring for an individual patient. Documenting that health providers routinely perform job site visits is compelling evidence that an organization is committed to quality occupational health services. In addition to an occupational history, the medical record must document preventive counsel. This may be advice about using a respirator, review of how to use hearing protection, suggestions about proper lifting, or advice about how to modify the job to reduce ergonomic demands. The organization must be able to explain how patients with delayed recovery, recurrent injuries, or permanent impairments are identified and handled. The organization's references should include regulations covering the different types of exams performed. Health care providers performing regulatory exams should be able to discuss their roles under the statutes.

In all of these cases, AAAHC relies on the expertise of its surveyors to determine whether or not the organization is in compliance. The organization must convince the surveyor that it understands the standards and that the standards are embodied in the organization's policies and operations. The surveyor will be knowledgeable and experienced in the area of occupational health services and will understand the issues surrounding care. If there is a question about the adequacy of a provider's knowledge of the workplace for a specific patient, the surveyor can ask the provider to describe the workplace and its hazards. If there are questions about release of information, the surveyor can ask medical records personnel what is required before they release records to an employer. Surveyors will focus on the standards that provide the greatest challenge to organizations. The surveyors will attempt to determine how the organization operates on a day-to-day basis.

RATIONALE FOR ACCREDITATION

There has been a dramatic increase in the number of organizations undergoing accreditation over the past 5 years. Much of the growth has been in surgical centers where accreditation is required for certification or payment. The next area of growth will likely be office-based surgical practices. Accreditation has become common in certain primary care settings such as large multispecialty clinics, community health centers, and college health centers. The impetus for accreditation for these organizations is participation in managed health care plans, participation in Joint Commission networks, or recognition as providing quality health services. Accreditation in smaller primary care offices is less common. Future changes in legislation, however, may increase requirements for accreditation in these settings. The American Academy of Family Physicians and the American College of Obstetrics and Gynecologists have recently joined AAAHC. This demonstrates increased interest of primary care providers in accreditation.

Currently 1,500 organizations have been accredited by AAAHC, a 400% increase over the past 10 years. All types of facilities have been accredited, from single physician offices to large clinic networks. Accreditation of occupational health facilities is not required for state certification, insurance reimbursement, or participation in managed care. As a result, overall rates of accreditation in occupational health facilities are low. However, accreditation may be popular in certain practice settings. For example, the Department of Energy (DOE) strongly encourages AAAHC accreditation for all of its on-site medical departments. As a result, it is likely that medical facilities at national laboratories or other DOE sites are accredited. Multispecialty clinics also have higher rates of accreditation. Occupational medical clinics in these settings are also familiar with accreditation processes.

Most occupational health facilities are not in these settings. Their primary reason to pursue accreditation is to improve the quality of their services. Those that undergo accreditation find it worthwhile. Accreditation focuses the attention of the organization on evaluating and improving its services. It guides staff members through an assessment of all of their internal processes. It challenges them to compare their outcomes to others. It uses surveyors who are knowledgeable and experienced in occupational health. And it provides recognition for a job well done. All occupational health facilities should consider AAAHC accreditation. If they do not pursue accreditation, they should consider using AAAHC's standards as a reference for evaluating and improving their services.

OTHER CERTIFICATION REQUIREMENTS

Organizations providing occupational health services should be aware of other certification programs and requirements. The Clinical Laboratory Improvement Act (CLIA) requires registration and certification of all laboratories, including offices performing basic laboratory tests. OSHA also has certification requirements that vary from standard to standard. Examples of OSHA mandates include equipment and training requirements for individuals performing audiograms and pulmonary function tests, and general accreditation requirements for laboratories performing biologic tests. In certain situations OSHA requires special certification programs, such as CDC certification for laboratories performing blood lead levels and participation in certain quality assurance programs for laboratories performing cadmium tests. There are special laboratory and training requirements for organizations providing drug tests under the Department of Transportation regulations.

AAAHC MEMBER ORGANIZATIONS

AAAHC member organizations include the following: American Academy of Cosmetic Surgery, American Academy of Dental Group Practice, American Academy of Dermatology, American Academy of Facial Plastic and Reconstructive Surgery, American Academy of Family Physicians, American Association of Oral and Maxillofacial Surgeons, American College Health Association, American College of Obstetricians and Gynecologists, American College of Occupational and Environmental Medicine, American Society of Anesthesiologists, American Society for Dermatologic Surgery, Federated Ambulatory Surgery Association, Medical Group Management Association, Outpatient Ophthalmic Surgery Society, Society for Ambulatory Anesthesia, National Association of Community Health Centers.

REFERENCES

1. Viswanathan HN, Salmon JW. Accrediting organizations and quality improvement. *Am J Managed Care* 2000;10(6):1117–1130.
2. Joint Commission on Accreditation of Healthcare Organizations. History of the Joint Commission. Available at *http://jcaho.orgtrkhco_frm.html*.
3. ACOEM. Endorsement of self-evaluation processes leading to accreditation. *American College of Occupa-*

tional and Environmental Medicine Executive Policy Manual. 1991(July);14(D):G-15.
4. ACOM. Endorsement of AAAHC. *American College of Occupational and Environmental Medicine Executive Policy Manual.* 1992(July);14(A):G-15.
5. Accreditation Association of Ambulatory Health Care. Who, what, why. Available at *http://www.aaahc.orgaboutwhowhatwhy.shtml.*
6. CDC. Updated U.S. Public Health Service Guidelines for the Management of Occupational Exposures to HBV, HCV, and HIV and Recommendations for Postexposure Prophylaxis. *MMWR* 2001;50(RR-11):1–54.
7. Occupational Safety and Health Administration, U.S. Department of Labor. OSHA regulations and compliance. Available at *http://www.osha.govcomp-links.html.*
8. Reed P. *The medical disability advisor: workplace guidelines for disability duration.* Beverly Farms, MA: OEM Press, 1998.
9. Institute for Quality Improvement. Studies. Available at *http://www.aaahci.orgstudies.shtml.*
10. Kohn LT, Corrigan JM, Donaldson MS. *To err is human: building a safer health system.* Institute of Medicine. Washington, DC: National Academy Press, 2000.
11. Chassin MR. Practice guidelines: best hope for quality improvement in the 1990s. *J Occup Med* 1990;32(12): 1199–1206.
12. National Guideline Clearinghouse. Available at *http://www.guidelines.govindex.asp.*
13. Bigos SJ, ed. *Acute low back problems in adults.* Rockville, MD: Agency for Health Care Policy and Research, 1994.
14. Harris JS, ed. *Occupational medicine practice guidelines.* American College of Occupational and Environmental Medicine. Beverly, MA: OEM Press, 1997.

FURTHER INFORMATION

AAAHC and Affiliated Organizations

AAAHC and its affiliated organizations, HCI and IQI, provide a variety of information and services for accreditation and quality improvement. IQI focuses on research and publication. A primary activity is performing clinic outcome studies used for benchmarking. HCI was created to provide consulting and education. AAAHC produces two documents used for accreditation. The first is the *Accreditation Handbook for Ambulatory Health Care.* This provides all of AAAHC's accreditation standards. It contains several questionnaire appendices addressing risk management, analysis of quality assurance programs, and clinical chart reviews. It also has the presurvey questionnaire and a survey application. The standards are revised annually. The second document is the *Self-Assessment Manual,* which can be used in conjunction with the handbook. It lists the standards in checklist form and provides work forms that guide an organization through its efforts to achieve accreditation. The third document, *Medical Event Reporting Special Report,* was created by IQI. It discusses issues related to medical event reporting in ambulatory settings. IQI also offers completed clinical performance measurement studies. HCI produces a series of manuals to assist an organization in preparing for accreditation or improving its operations. It also offers consultants who will assist the organization in all aspects of preparing for accreditation. All publications are available through AAAHC in Wilmette, IL, at 1-(847)-853-6060. Information can also be obtained at *http://www.aaahc.org.*

Joint Commission on Accreditation of Healthcare Organizations

Currently the only other national organization accrediting significant numbers of ambulatory facilities, such as occupational health centers, is the Joint Commission. Many hospital-based occupational health centers have undergone JCAHO accreditation in conjunction with accreditation of other hospital clinics. JCAHO has extensive ambulatory accreditation guidelines designed to apply to any ambulatory settings. It does not have any standards specific to occupational health facilities. Its accreditation standards can be obtained through the Joint Commission in Oakbrook Terrace, IL, at 1-(630)-792-5000. Information can also be obtained at *http://www.jcaho.org.* The Joint Commission also offers consulting services. There are consulting organizations, such as Occupational Health Resources (OHR), that provide specific information about how Joint Commission standards apply to occupational health facilities and strategies for successful accreditation. OHR can be reached at 1-(800)-444-8432 or at *http://www.systoc.comdefault.asp.*

Other Accrediting Organizations

The International Organization for Standardization (ISO) is well known for its industrial certification programs. ISO is made up of national standards institutes from countries throughout the world. Historically, ISO has produced technical specification standards that cover everything from the size and shape of sheet metal screws to the dimensions of credit cards. But more recently, it has produced generic standards for managing quality, the ISO 9000 standards. These can be applied to any organization from manufacturing to health care. Unlike Joint Commission or AAAHC standards, they do not provide any guidelines specific to medical care. Some medical organizations have applied ISO 9000 to their management programs. Information about ISO 9000 certification is available at *http://www.iso.orgisoeniso9000-14000index.html.*

The Utilization Review Accreditation Commission (URAC), also known as the American Accreditation Healthcare Commission, began in 1990. Initially, it provided accreditation only to utilization review organizations. With time, URAC expanded its programs. It is not involved in accrediting health facilities, but it does offer accreditation for workers' compensation health care networks and for workers' compensation utilization management programs. Its standards address issues like personnel, procedures, processes, grievances, confidentiality, and quality management. Information about URAC's workers' compensation programs is available at *http://www.urac.orgprogramsworkerscompnet.htm*.

Crossing the quality chasm: a new health system for the 21st century.

Institute of Medicine. Washington, DC: National Academy Press, 2001.

This is a 350-page report from the Institute of Medicine's Committee on Quality of Health Care. The committee was created in 1998 to identify strategies for achieving substantial improvement in quality of health care. The report discusses the current status of the health of our population and of the health care delivery system. It makes a variety of recommendations for change. The report does not specifically address occupational health facilities or accreditation. But it is a valuable resource for those interested in quality, quality improvements, current issues in health care delivery, and future trends.

11
Health and Productivity

Dee W. Edington and Wayne N. Burton

> That men in general should work better when they are ill fed than when they are well fed, when they are disheartened than when they are in good spirits, when they are frequently sick than when they are generally in good health, seems not very probable. Years of dearth, it is to be observed, are generally among the common years of sickness and mortality, which cannot fail to diminish the produce of the industry.
>
> —Adam Smith, *The Wealth of Nations,* 1776

Occupational medicine continues to expand its understanding of the workplace and the role of the occupational health care professional. The emerging field of health and productivity is still developing the tools, metrics, and methodology to measure the impact of health on employee performance. Whereas the prevention and treatment of illnesses and injuries related to work is at the core of occupational medicine, understanding the role of health in facilitating high levels of productivity will continue to uncover emerging roles for occupational medicine. These emerging roles have both direct and indirect outcomes related to the financial success of an organization.

Worker productivity has been measured since the early 1900s, especially in manufacturing type jobs where there is a clear connection to work and an objective measure of output. These measures were related to presenteeism, e.g., the number of widgets produced per unit of time. Productivity of white collar and the emerging knowledge worker has been and continues to be a less exact science. Furthermore, the link between worker health and worker productivity has only recently received increasingly more attention. This chapter describes the relationships between worker health and worker productivity. This link has been made possible by the relatively new measurement and data management techniques and the linking of diverse health care and productivity databases. The diagram in Fig. 11.1 shows the relative contribu-

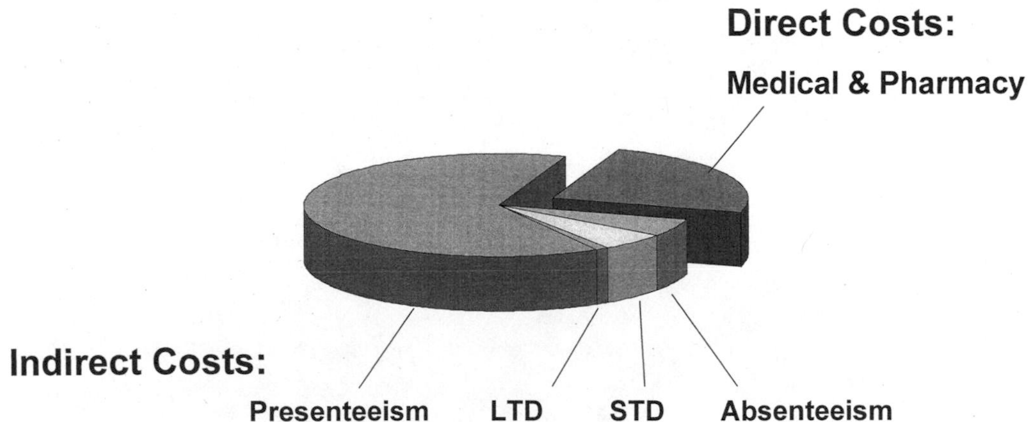

FIG. 11.1. Direct and indirect costs of poor employee health and productivity. (Source: Unpublished data from a large financial services corporation.)

tions of direct and indirect costs of poor employee health and productivity.

COMPONENTS OF WORKER PRODUCTIVITY

The losses in worker productivity due to health-related problems are an indirect cost to corporations and society that are largely unmeasured. Absenteeism and disability costs are significant contributors to an incomplete estimate of the total loss of productivity resulting from impaired health. These time-off-the-job measurements are the most common measurable components of productivity in most work environments. Even in measuring time off the job, one does not always capture the true loss of productivity, since many work tasks, especially with white collar or knowledge workers, remain on someone's desk until the person returns to work. Thus, often the task still gets done but the time frame is delayed, which may or may not cause productivity decreases downstream from the original worker. Nevertheless, time off the job is the most commonly accepted measure of worker productivity.

Absenteeism

Absenteeism refers to time off the job. In most organizations, absenteeism has a wide variety of forms, including scattered absence, sick days, short-term disability, long-term disability, family medical leaves, discretionary leaves, and unpaid leaves. Even more detailed absences are recorded by some organizations to include jury duty, military leave, and public service leave.

Presenteeism

Most of the early work on productivity concentrated on presenteeism, which is the amount of work accomplished while on the job or output per unit of time. While the concept is relatively straightforward, the measurement of presenteeism is a major challenge for any organization. In fact, nearly every job classification has inherent definitions that require a unique solution in order to get a true measure of productivity. The decrease in productivity measured by presenteeism is typically unrelated to absenteeism or disability absences. Presenteeism is the decrement in performance associated with remaining at work while impaired by risk factors or health problems. Presenteeism can be measured in terms of costs associated with decreased or slowed output, failure to maintain a production standard, additional training time, and errors in the work produced.

It is therefore reasonable to assume that workers' health is related to their ability to be maximally productive. For example, workers suffering with low back pain may be limited in the weight they can lift or in the postures that they can be expected to maintain on the job. A worker with carpal tunnel syndrome may be limited in the amount of keyboard work that can be performed. A worker suffering from a depressive disorder may be limited in tasks requiring cognitive speed and interpersonal skills.

To approximate the decrease in productivity for workers who remain at work with health problems, studies have utilized both objective measures of productivity as well as self-reported measures of productivity.

Quality of the Work

Quality of the work is an important contributor to the total value of the output of the work. If quality is low, then waste increases and the work often has to be repeated by the worker, a co-worker or supervisor. An important component of quality can be customer satisfaction, including on-time delivery and the number of errors. An evaluation of on-the-job productivity ideally takes into consideration the quality of the work performed.

Work-related Disability

On-the-job injuries and accidents occur, but it is well documented that when safety is a high priority of an organization the accident rates typically decline dramatically. Effective safety programs can reduce on-the-job accident rates and workers' compensation claims. Furthermore, participation in work-site health promotion programs has been demonstrated to lower workers' compensation claims. For example, among those with workers' compensation claims, health risk appraisal participants at Xerox were found to have an average savings of $1,238 per worker per year compared to non–wellness program participants (1). Health risk status as calculated from a health risk assessment questionnaire (e.g., exercise, blood pressure, body mass index, etc.) is also related to individual costs for workers' compensation. Nearly 85% of the costs of workers' compensation could be related to excess health risks in the population at Xerox. The implication is that an organization could manage workers' compensation costs by providing workers with programs that result in health risk reduction and the avoidance of additional risks.

Worker Recruitment, Retention, and Turnover

Substantial indirect costs to a corporation are associated with recruitment and retention of workers. This is especially important when unemployment is low and there is significant competition for qualified workers. Although a competitive salary and benefits are important in attracting and retaining employees, a variety of other benefits are also important, including the corporate culture and values in regard to employee health and well-being.

Safety and Health

According to the U.S. Bureau of Labor Statistics, in 2000 a total of 1.7 million injuries and illnesses occurred in private industry, which required recuperation away from work beyond the day of the incident (2). In 1999 the National Safety Council estimated the total annual cost of occupational injuries at $125 billion: $62.0 billion for wage and productivity losses, $19.9 billion in medical costs, $25.6 billion in administrative expenses, and $16.7 billion in additional employer costs (3). Healthy People 2010 has established a goal of reducing work-related injuries to 4.6 injuries per 100 full-time workers (4). Occupational Safety and Health Administration (OSHA) recordable injuries and illnesses and lost time cases data are available for most industries. OSHA recordable data can be expressed as cases per 200,000 hours worked, which is the number of events per 100 employees working for 1 year.

One of the most measurable ways to improve worker productivity is by reducing work-related injuries and illnesses. Comprehensive management of workers' compensation losses includes prevention by the identification of potential workplace hazards, early provision of appropriate medical services, and flexible return to work policies and programs. Transitional return to work from a work-related illness or injury can be beneficial to both the worker and the employer (5,6). Safety is an important component of a total corporate health and productivity management program for many companies. These programs may include safety program training, regulatory compliance, and management of workers' compensation benefits.

Productivity Metrics (Presenteeism)

Measurement of on the job productivity is a much more difficult task. Productivity metrics are dependent on distinct job classifications. Specific measurement tools will have to be developed for unique job classifications within a corporation. An organization has the challenge of developing specific job productivity measures for a variety of job classifications or determining if self-administered questionnaires can be applied across several job categories or even the whole company to approximate the work lost due to lower productivity. In general, worker productivity is related to a worker's health and job requirements. A job may be classified as primarily working with people, things (tools), or data. For example, a customer service worker is primarily interacting with people but also may need to enter information into a computer (tool) and review information about the customer (data). A disease such as depression could profoundly impact a customer service worker's presenteeism. In contrast, a mechanic suffering from depression might experience significantly less job productivity impact from depression. However, the mechanic with low back pain might be significantly impaired in the ability to complete tasks that involve the use of tools. Different health disorders and diseases can have a differential impact on the worker's presenteeism.

OBJECTIVE MEASURES OF WORKER PRODUCTIVITY

If a worker's task can be exactly modeled and measured, then that job is a good candidate for the development of an objective measure of worker productivity. A good example of this type of productive measure occurred at a credit card telephone call center (7). A worker's productivity index (WPI) was developed to measure the productivity of customer service call center operators. A major credit card company employed the customer service operators. Employees at this facility answer inquires from customers about their credit card accounts, make customers and potential customers aware of product offerings, and perform several other customer service tasks. These employees' workstations have a telephone connected to a computer system. The computer is programmed to record data elements of each and every telephone call to the workstation, including the time that a customer waits in the queue, the length of time the customer spends on the call with the service representative, the amount of time spent holding, the amount of time between calls when the employee is doing paperwork or researching information, and the amount of time the employee spends logged off the system. This information was analyzed and placed into algorithms to determine the performance goals among the employees with similar telephone call center tasks. The WPI was calculated using the algorithms derived from the employee's presenteeism together with absenteeism and short-term disability absence.

Productivity Measurement Questionnaires

In general, objective measures of productivity in the workplace are rarely available, and when they are available they are specific to the job classifications. There are relatively few jobs that involve tasks that are easily counted and that have such records available. Some jobs where such tracking is done include telephone call centers, package deliveries, and assembly line piecework jobs. However, such objective measures, where available, are important to validate self-reported measures of presenteeism. Such validation of self-reported productivity is being conducted at workplaces involving telephone call centers, claims data entry, and other jobs that have objective measures of productivity.

There are several publicly available self-reported productivity questionnaires. A recent publication reviewed the strengths and weaknesses of the following questionnaires:

Endicott Work Productivity Scale (EWPS)
Health and Labor Questionnaire (HLQ)
MacArthur Health and Performance Questionnaire (MHPQ)
SF 36
Stanford/American Health Association Presenteeism Scale (SAHAPS)
Work Limitations Questionnaire (WLQ)
Work Productivity and Activity Impairment Questionnaire (WPAI) (8).

Worker Replacement Costs

Calculating the cost of replacing workers off the job is critical to understanding the implication of lost productivity. There are several methods available for making this calculation (9). The most straightforward method is called the lost wages method. This is simply the number of hours/days absent times the rate of compensation. Ideally, one would have the exact rate of compensation for the individual workers or, at least, a rate per job classification. Total compensation, to include both direct and indirect benefits would be an even better metric. The authors discuss the valuation of work loss and present a model to more fully incorporate indirect costs attributed to the company and society. The result of the additional costs of on-the-job time substantially increases the costs attributed to work replacement.

WORKER PRODUCTIVITY AND RISK FACTORS

Ideally, organizations would attempt to promote and protect the health of their employees at as early an age as possible. Compliance with and adherence to preventive services is one of the least expensive and most effective strategies to contribute to the good health of employees. Health risks appraisals and health fair screenings for preventive services and risk factors raise the employees' awareness of their current and future health status. Once awareness is raised, the employer has an opportunity to facilitate maintenance of preventive services and a good health status. There is now a wealth of information relating healthy behaviors and risk factors to future disease and to levels of productivity, especially data related to excess absent days and short-term disability related to risk factors and participation in wellness programs (10–15).

The opportunities for proactive health management occur throughout a typical work-site population. The illustration in Fig. 11.2 indicates where disease management, screening and preventive services, and low-risk maintenance and risk reduction programs can be most effective in maintaining and improving health status within the workforce (16). Each employee is somewhere on the continuum, from no risk factors, to recovery from the acute effects of the disease, to learning to live with the chronic nature of the disease. Essentially, there are health management services for everyone. The overall objective is to maintain low-risk status or to facilitate risk reduction in each individual. At the no-risk end of the continuum, preventive services and low-risk maintenance programs can be provided to these individuals to maintain their already good health status. At the disease end of the continuum, case management and disease management programs are appropriate, as well as other programs to help employees maintain and improve their health status. The vast majority of employees are in the middle section of the continuum, and here, preventive services, screening, low-risk maintenance, and risk-reduction programs are appropriate to allow employees the opportunity to improve their health status through a variety of options.

The same risk factors that are precursors for disease have impact on hours of lost productivity. In a study of call center operators, the presence of each of the several individual risk factors was assessed for its impact on hours of lost productivity. As shown in Fig. 11.3 and somewhat surprisingly, the impact of the risk factors on illness days and short-term disability was considerably less than their impact on presenteeism (7).

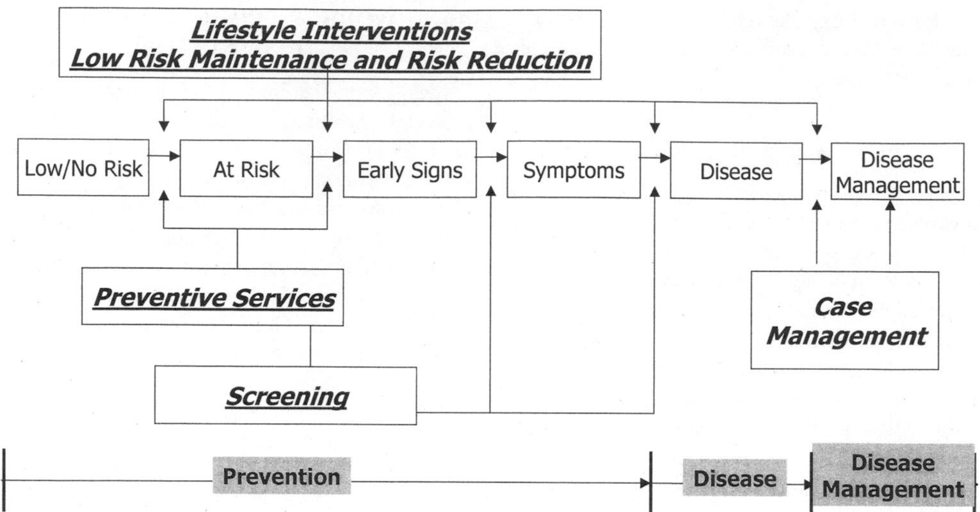

FIG. 11.2. Continuum of health status and opportunities for corporate health management programs. (From Musich SA, Burton WN, Edington DW. Costs and benefits of prevention and disease management. *Dis Manage Health Outcomes* 1999;5[3]:153–166.)

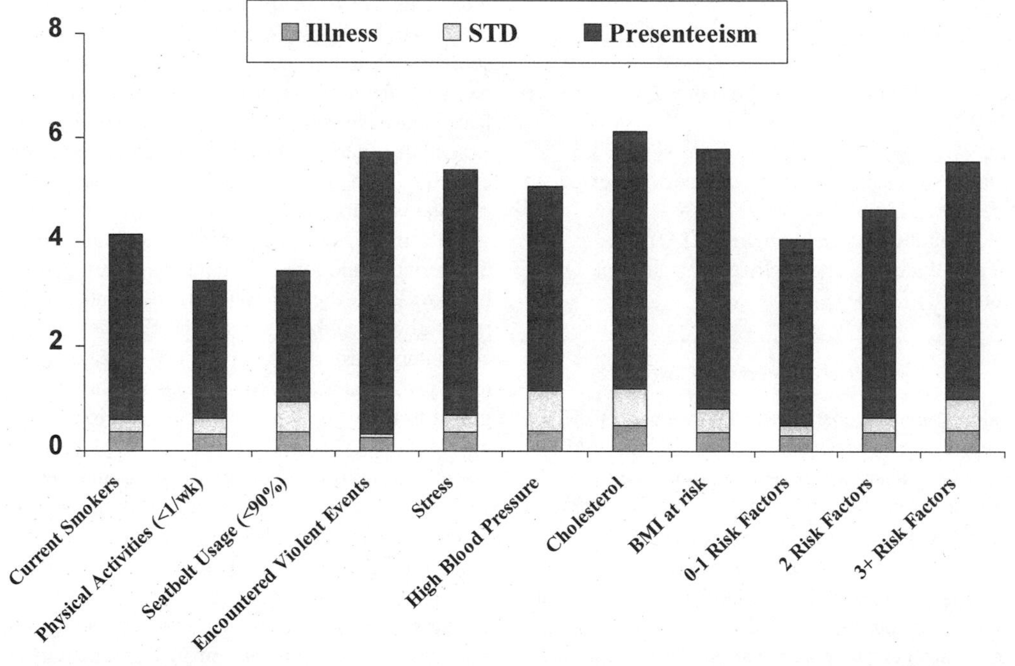

FIG. 11.3. Health risks related to the number of hours of productivity lost per week. (From Burton WN, Conti DJ, Chen C-Y, et al. The role of health risk factors and disease on worker productivity. *J Occup Environ Health* 1999;41[10]:863–877.)

WORKER PRODUCTIVITY AND DISEASE

Chronic medical conditions account for significant medical disability and lost productivity costs for corporations. As the workforce in the United States ages over the next several decades, appropriate management of these conditions will be important to assure a healthy and productive workforce.

There has been a proliferation of new and more expensive therapies for diseases. Evaluation of the value of such therapies should include their impact in reducing worker absenteeism and increasing worker productivity (17,18). One group of investigators examined the number of work-loss days and work-cutback days attributable to the presence of 29 common medical conditions in the U.S. population using data from a nationwide survey of 3,032 individuals aged 25 to 74 years. Participants were questioned regarding how many days out of the past 30 days they were "totally unable to work or carry out your normal household work activities because of your physical health or mental health," and how many additional days in the past 30 they were able to work but had to "cut back on work or how much you got done because of your physical or mental health." Data on absenteeism that included scattered sick days and short-term disability absence were combined with lost productivity data. The average number of work-impaired days for employed individuals was 0.9 workdays per month. The authors noted a dose-response relationship between the number of chronic medical conditions and the probability of any work impairment. At least one illness-related work-loss or work-cutback day was noted by 22.4% of the respondents. Participants with cancer reported the highest prevalence of impairment (66.2%) within the past 30 days and the greatest number of days with impairment in the past 30 days (16.4 days). Additional common causes of impairment included ulcers, major depression, and panic disorder.

Other researchers have demonstrated a dose-response relationship between self-reported health risk factors recorded on a health risk appraisal questionnaire with medical claim costs, short-term disability workdays lost, scattered absence workdays lost, and on-the-job productivity for workers (7). This information can be used to prioritize work-site disease screening and management programs as well as in the selection of appropriate benefit plan design options.

The health of a population has been associated with a higher productivity in a country (19). There is a positive relationship between the health of a country's population and its per capita income. Average life expectancy for a country is directly correlated with the per capita income. As the average income increases in a country, it increases the ability of the population to purchase goods and services that can improve health. Healthier workers have less absenteeism for their own illness and the need to care for ill family members. Investments in international development that lead to healthier populations should lead to greater economic development.

The primary disease drivers of health care costs are heart disease, cancer, diabetes, depression, and stroke, among others. What has recently become clear is that the primary disease drivers of productivity are arthritis, asthma, digestive disorders, headaches, flu, stress, and back pain, among others. This latter set of diseases is relatively low cost in health care but high in productivity loss.

The above relationship is illustrated in Fig. 11.4, which shows the contribution of the presence of several diseases to illness days, short-term disability, and presenteeism in a study of call center operators (7). The set of diseases impacting on hours of lost productivity include those typically associated with high medical costs plus those chronic diseases most often associated with lower long-term medical costs, including allergies, asthma, digestive disorders, and mental health.

There is increasing concern about the rise in pharmaceutical costs among workers, employers, pharmacy benefits managers, managed care companies, and other purchasers of health care. Corporate medical directors are frequently asked by benefit managers about the value of new medications or more expensive medications to treat a variety of diseases. Over $100 billion is now spent in the United States on prescription medications. Costs for older workers and retirees have been skyrocketing for many reasons, such as increased cost, increased utilization of medications, newly identified patients, and new medications to treat previously untreated conditions. The value of pharmaceuticals should take into consideration many factors including the potential impact on worker productivity (20). For example, does a newer medication allow a worker to return to work sooner and be more productive? Two decades ago, acquired immune deficiency syndrome (AIDS) was, in general, not treatable, resulting in a relatively short life span after diagnosis. Today with treatment, AIDS is now considered a chronic disease with a significant life span for most workers. Several examples are presented below of chronic diseases that, when treated appropriately, can be controlled, with significant improvement in worker productivity.

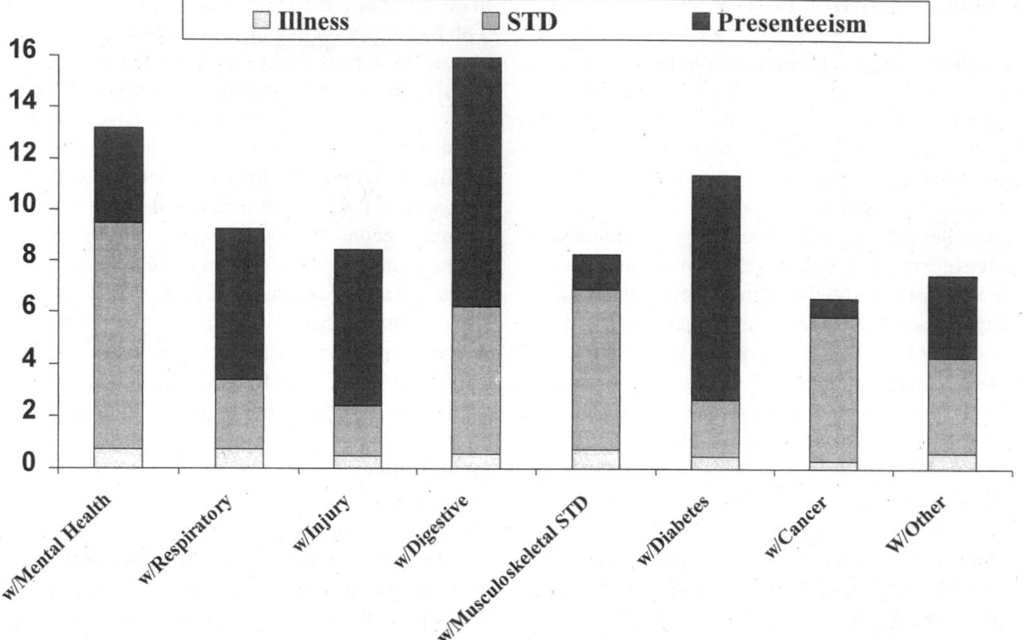

FIG. 11.4. Disease states related to the number of hours of productivity lost per week. (From Burton WN, Conti DJ, Chen C-Y, et al. The role of health risk factors and disease on worker productivity. *J Occup Environ Health* 1999;41[10]:863–877.)

Significant challenges for U.S. corporations have been the control of health care costs and how to increase worker productivity. An evolving new perspective by companies is to view health care as a strategic investment in the health and productivity of the workforce. Some newer treatments and medications have been demonstrated not only to improve the health of workers but also to improve their productivity. The ability of appropriate pharmaceutical solutions to influence worker productivity is critical to high levels of productivity in most workforces.

Allergies

Allergic reactions are common in an estimated 15 to 39 million individuals in the United States. This condition is responsible for approximately 10 million physician office visits annually in the U.S. It is estimated that 12% of American working women and 10% of working men suffer from allergic disorders. The impact of allergic reactions on medical expenses, workplace absence days, and, perhaps more importantly, productivity while on the job is a major expense for employers. The productivity loss associated with allergic disorders is related in general to a decrement in on-the-job productivity rather than to absences from the workplace. Workers with allergies were found to have a decline in on-the-job productivity with increasing pollen counts during allergy season. Computerized worker productivity measurements in a credit card telephone call center were combined with self-reported allergic disorder symptoms and medication use prior to and during allergy season (21). The indirect cost of allergies in telephone customer service representatives was shown to be a 10% reduction in presenteeism during the height of the pollen season. For those customer service representatives on effective medication, the decreased productivity was not observed during the ragweed pollen season.

The effect of allergies on worker productivity is of a continuing interest, including the effects of antihistamine pharmaceuticals to control the allergic reaction. One group of investigators used a retrospective database that linked medical claims including prescription medication claims for workers of a large insurance company who were medical claims processors. They observed that workers prescribed a sedating antihistamine were up to 13% less productive than workers prescribed nonsedating antihistamines (22). First-generation antihistamines, which are generally available without a prescription, may be effective in controlling symptoms but can cause drowsiness and impairment in the performance of various tasks. For example, a randomized, placebo-controlled trial in the Iowa driving simulator compared the effects of diphenhydramine (50 mg), a first-generation antihistamine, fexofenadine (60 mg), a second generation antihistamine, placebo, and alcohol (approximately 0.1% blood alcohol concentration) on driving performance (23). The authors report that participants had significantly better performance after using alcohol or fexofenadine than after taking diphenhydramine. However, self-reported drowsiness ratings were not a good predictor of impairment. An unpublished study (William Bunn, M.D., personal communication) reports increased work-related injuries for employees using first-generation antihistamines. Some authors have recommended that workers should use nonsedating antihistamines to avoid work-related accidents and injuries (24). Seasonal allergic symptoms can be controlled with a variety of medications including allergy desensitization injections, sedating and nonsedating antihistamines, nasal corticosteroids, and other medications. The older antihistamines have been linked to accidents and injuries in the workplace (25). Newer nonsedating antihistamines may increase worker productivity with fewer side effects.

Arthritis

Arthritis includes more than 100 different diseases affecting the joints and other connective tissues of the body. It can result in pain, stiffness, and reduced flexibility of the joints in addition to other symptoms. Arthritis and related conditions affect nearly 43 million Americans, making it one of the most common diseases in adults. By 2020, an estimated 60 million Americans will be affected with arthritis. Arthritis is a leading cause of disability, and cost-effective treatments are now available to reduce the economic burden of arthritis in the workplace (26). Fourteen percent of employed women and 9% of employed men report having arthritis (27).

While osteoarthritis is more prevalent among older workers, affecting 80% of adults over the age of 55, rheumatoid arthritis (RA) affects a younger working population between the ages of 35 and 50. The direct and indirect cost of the disease is approximately three times the cost for those without the disease (28). The estimated direct and indirect costs from a worker disabled with RA to the employer were $17,822 vs. $6,131 for non-RA employees. The annual total employer cost per RA employee for medical, pharmaceutical, and work loss was estimated to be $9,693. Ergonomically designed jobs and, when indicated, prescription medications have now enhanced the quality of life and allow most workers with appropriate treatment to be productive in the workplace.

Asthma

Asthma affects more than 27 million American adults and is one of the leading causes of lost productivity in the workplace (29). It accounts for an estimated 14 million workdays lost annually in the United States. At work productivity loss has been estimated at 8.2 days per year per employee suffering with asthma working at less than 90% of capacity (30). Asthma is a controllable disease for the vast majority of sufferers. The value of work-site–based asthma education and disease management programs has been demonstrated (31,32). These investigators reported on the value of a work-site–based program that improved asthma control and improved worker productivity as measured by a self-reported decrease in worker absenteeism. An individualized asthma care training program for adults with severe or uncontrolled asthma demonstrated statistically significant increases in functional status and productivity and decreases in the number of days absent from work due to asthma (33). Participants reported a decline in absenteeism from 5.7 days per month at baseline due to asthma to 2.4 days. The number of days of reduced productivity declined from 4.3 days per month at baseline to 2.0 days per month at 12-month follow-up. A study in the managed care setting showed that patients treated by physicians with expertise in treating asthma had better control of asthma and were less likely to miss work (34).

The National Institutes of Health has published treatment guidelines for the treatment of asthma (35). These guidelines are the basis for most disease management programs and include the following general recommendations:

1. Initiate a partnership with the patient with asthma.
2. Reduce inflammation, symptoms, and exacerbations.
3. Monitor and manage asthma over time.
4. Promptly treat asthma exacerbations.

Following these treatment guidelines should result in reduced absenteeism and increased worker productivity.

Headache

Common forms of headaches include tension, cluster, and migraines. Migraines are the most debilitating and nearly 60% of the missed workdays due to headaches are related to migraines. Nonmigraine headaches are not as debilitating but are more likely to result in lower productivity when the patient is on the job. Nonmigraine headaches account for over 60% of reduced effectiveness on the job. Thus, although the direct costs of headaches are relatively low, except for the chronic migraine patient, the indirect cost of headaches is relatively substantial (36).

The complexity of the several phases of migraines increases the extent of its impact on worker productivity. The preheadache phase, which could last for 24 hours or more, plus the headache phase and the postheadache phase indicate that a single migraine could impact productivity for as long as 8 days. Although the direct costs related to migraine are relatively small, the costs in terms of lost productivity are high. Up to 40% lost productivity has been reported during the 8 days of the attack. It has also been estimated that the indirect cost of migraines account for approximately 75% of the total costs, with medical costs accounting for the direct costs (37).

In a large U.S. population survey involving over 20,000 respondents to a questionnaire, 17.6% of women and 5.7% of men reported having one or more headaches a year that met the International Headache Society criteria for migraine. Similar results were confirmed in a survey of a major financial services company in the United States (38). This condition peaks during the prime working years, ages 25 to 55 years. The majority of the economic burden to employers is attributable to lost on-the-job productivity. Migraineurs report an average of 3.2 actual lost workdays annually, and an additional 4.9 workdays lost due to reduced effectiveness on the job (36). The cost to U.S. employers is approximately $13 billion annually because of missed workdays and impaired work function.

Migraineurs can prevent some attacks by eliminating triggers for the headaches. Nonprescription and prescription medications are available for the treatment once a migraine headache occurs. For employees with frequent migraines, medications are available that may actually prevent migraines.

Two questionnaires have been developed for specific use in migraineurs. The migraine adaptive cost-effectiveness model combines the costs of time lost both from work and nonwork activities with medical resource and medication use. The Migraine Work and Productivity Loss Questionnaire (MWPLQ) estimates the impact of migraine and migraine treatment and was found useful in comparing the effectiveness of different drugs for the treatment of migraine (39,40).

Diabetes Mellitus

Diabetes mellitus affects approximately 5.9% of Americans and was estimated in 1997 to account for $44 billion in direct and $54 billion in indirect costs (16). The Diabetes Control and Complications Trial (DCCT) demonstrated that good control of diabetes could delay the onset and slow the progression of many diabetic complications and thereby result in avoidance of costs related to complications of diabetes. There are an estimated 8 million Americans diagnosed with diabetes and another 8 million undiagnosed. Of the 8 million diagnosed Americans, up to 800,000 have type 1 diabetes and 7–7.5 million have type 2 diabetes. In 1997, workers with diabetes accounted for approximately 14 million disability days lost as well as an average of 8.3 days off from work annually compared with 1.7 days for people without diabetes or other chronic conditions (41). Corporations are in a unique position to proactively address the potential complications of diabetes through work-site–based educational programs (42).

It has been shown that diabetes can significantly impact worker productivity in a telephone call center employee population (7,43,44). A work-site–based diabetes education program can result in improved control of diabetes in workers and would be expected to result in decreased complications and disability over time.

Influenza

Influenza occurs annually in the United States and the impact of this disease on workplace productivity can be significant (45,46). Although the burden of this disease can be great, the potential for prevention is high, especially with a work-site influenza vaccination program. Influenza causes increased work absenteeism, decreased productivity, and increased health care costs during flu season. Several studies have now demonstrated the effectiveness of work-site–based flu shot programs and some studies have shown a return on investment (ROI). Vaccinating healthy working adults was on average cost saving, with mean savings of $13.66 per person vaccinated (47). Workers with influenza-like illness missed 2.8 days of work per episode of illness and reported reduced effectiveness and inability to resume normal work activities for a mean of 3.5 days after the onset of symptoms (48).

Workers who received an influenza vaccine, through a randomized control trial, reported 25%

fewer episodes of upper respiratory illness than workers given the placebo and 43% fewer days of sick leave from work due to upper respiratory illness. The authors estimated a cost savings of $46.85 per worker vaccinated (49).

The value of a work-site influenza vaccination program was shown to be more effective in employees over the age of 45 (50). Others reported a cost per saved lost workday for an influenza vaccination program of $22.36 and a reduction in sick days (51). Influenza vaccination reduced lost workdays by 32%; however, it was not found to be economically beneficial in most years (52). An intranasal flu vaccine was found to be safe and effective in healthy, working adults in a year when influenza A was the predominate virus. This vaccine resulted in fewer lost days of work, including a 17.9% reduction for severe febrile illness and a 28.4% reduction for febrile upper respiratory tract illnesses (53).

Gastrointestinal Disorders

A variety of gastrointestinal disorders can result in absenteeism and lost worker productivity, such as gastroesophageal reflux disease (GERD), ulcer disease, and irritable bowel syndrome. Approximately 60 million Americans have GERD symptoms that in most cases are mild. One study reported that 45% of a population had GERD symptoms at any point in time and approximately 18% had symptoms on a weekly basis (54). In addition to lifestyle modification, a variety of highly effective medications are now available to treat this disorder. GERD has been reported to affect worker productivity (55,56). Researchers found that 42% of patients with peptic ulcer disease (PUD) and 41% with GERD reported lost work productivity accounting for an estimated $606 and $237, respectively, in wage costs over a 3-month period. Untreated patients reported a 6% productivity loss in patients with PUD and a 3% productivity loss in patients with GERD.

Historically, treatment for GERD included lifestyle changes such as changes in diet and the use of medications such as over-the-counter antacids and/or the use of H2-receptor antagonists such as ranitidine or cimetidine to control stomach acid. In rare situations, surgery was performed. More recently, proton pump inhibitors (PPIs), such as omeprazole, have been used for the treatment of GERD. The role of the bacterium *Helicobacter pylori* in GERD is controversial at this time, as well as the potential eradication in the control of GERD symptoms. PPIs tend to be more expensive than other medications; however, they may be more effective in controlling symptoms in some patients. Various analyses have reported that in some patients PPIs may be more cost-effective (57,58).

Similarly, irritable bowel syndrome (IBS) has been reported to be second only to the common cold as a cause of absenteeism from work and school. Approximately 20% of the general population has reported symptoms of IBS. It is characterized by alterations in bowel habits and abdominal pain or discomfort. Women are affected more commonly, with a female to male ratio of 2:1 or 3:1 (59). A survey of 5,430 U.S. households found that individuals with IBS symptoms reported missed work or school an average of 13 days per year (60). Hahn et al. (61) reported on a random sample of 1,000 patients in the United States and the United Kingdom and found that one third of the IBS patients reported an average of 1 to 2 workdays absence every 4 weeks (61). At the present time there are a limited number of pharmaceutical treatments available.

Mental Health Disorders

Depression is a major health problem in the United States that is often unrecognized and undertreated. Greenberg et al. (62) estimated the annual cost to employers of major depression is $43 billion in terms of work loss and reduced productivity. Depression is readily treatable, with response rates to medication and/or psychotherapy in excess of 80% to 90%. Major depression is associated with both a significant increase in work loss and a decrease in worker productivity. A 1997 report noted that major depression was one of the five most impairing condition in the U.S. with regard to work loss and decreased worker productivity (63,64).

For an individual employer, the financial burden for mental health disorders such as depression, is derived from medical claims data where indirect costs go largely unmeasured. An important study examined the health care resource utilization and at-work productivity for employees with and without anxiety and other mental health disorders (65). The authors studied 2,222 workers at a large U.S. insurance claims processing company at multiple nationwide locations. Inpatient, outpatient, and pharmaceutical medical claims and objective productivity information on these workers were analyzed. The number of medical claims processed by each worker each day measured worker productivity. Over a 30-month period, 14.9% of the workers were diagnosed with a mental disorder, with the most prevalent disorder being depression. Over this period, 7.4% of workers were diagnosed with depression. Although workers with mental health disorders accounted for less than 15% of the population, they accounted for 31% of all worker medical costs. No significant difference was noted in annualized absenteeism for workers with and without a diagnosed mental health disorder, with the exception of workers with depression plus another mental health disorder. At-work productivity also demonstrated no difference for workers with and without a mental health disorder. A study of telephone call center workers did demonstrate a difference in worker productivity for employees who had returned from a short-term disability absence for a mental health disorder, but the difference was not as great as for other medical disorders such as diabetes mellitus (7).

How can the finding that workers with mental health disorders have relatively normal at-work job productivity be explained? The most logical explanation is that workers treated for mental health disorders have effective treatment and the productivity of these workers reflect the improvement of productivity from such therapy. In fact a recent literature review supports such an explanation (66). Four clinical trials in the 1980s documented a significant reduction in the prevalence of a self-reported decrease in at-work productivity with treatment for mental health disorders (67). Such research is important for benefit plan design decisions in regard to parity for mental health benefits (68).

ROLE OF THE CORPORATE MEDICAL DEPARTMENT IN MANAGING WORKER PRODUCTIVITY

The corporate medical director can play a key role in the health and productivity of the workforce and in the direct and indirect success factors of the organization. Clearly, health and safety are important areas of responsibility for occupational health professionals. It is now clear that similar factors that drive success in maintaining the health and safety of the workforce are influential in determining the productivity of the workforce (69).

The corporate medical department can maximize its role by integrating its data management system and including data related to productivity, such as scattered absences, short-term and long-term disability, workers' compensation claims, and other available data sets (70). In the 1980s, corporations implemented several disability management programs. Several such programs have been described in the literature. The goal of such programs was to ensure that employees with job limitations were placed in appropriate jobs and assisted in the control of disability costs. A major automotive manufacturing corporation implemented a variation of the above description. As a result, over the subsequent 3 years total disability leave rates fell approximately 50% (71). A major financial services corporation described the results of an in-house disability management program. The overall short-term disability average duration declined 20%.

The corporate medical department can play an important role in managing the indirect costs of worker health. Work-site health promotion or wellness programs can play an important role in avoiding unnecessary or prolonged disability absences (72). Similarly, the quality of health care may play a role in disability absences. For example, such an absence may be prolonged by delays in a worker's receiving appropriate medical care and or testing (73).

The role of the corporate medical department has truly expanded to include the impact of worker health on corporate productivity and profitability in addition to its more traditional role of enhancing worker health in terms of disease and safety.

REFERENCES

1. Musich SA, Napier D, Edington DW. The association of health risks with Workers' Compensation costs. *J Occup Environ Med* 2001;43(6):534–541.
2. U.S. Bureau of Labor Statistics. Injuries, illnesses, and fatalities. *http://stats.bls.goviifhome.htm*.
3. National Safety Counsel. *Injury facts*. 1999 edition. Itaska, IL: NSC, 1999.
4. U.S. Department of Health and Human Services. *Healthy People 2010*. Washington, DC: DHHS, 2000.
5. McGrail MP, Tsai SP, Bernacki EJ. A comprehensive initiative to manage the incidence and cost of occupational injury and illness. *J Occup Environ Med* 1995;37: 1263–1268.
6. Bunn WB, Pikelny DB, Slavin TJ, et al. Health, safety, and productivity in a manufacturing environment. *J Occup Environ Med* 2001;43:47–55.
7. Burton WN, Conti DJ, Chen C-Y, et al. The role of health risk factors and disease on worker productivity. *J Occup Environ Health* 1999;41(10):863–877.
8. Riedel JE, Lynch W, Baase C, et al. The effect of disease prevention and health promotion on workplace productivity: a literature review. *Am J Health Promotion* 2001; 15(3):167–191.
9. Berger ML, Murray JF, Xu J, et al. Alternative valuations of work loss and productivity. *J Occup Environ Med* 2001;43(1):18–24.
10. Serxner S, Gold D, Anderson D, et al. The impact of a worksite health promotion program on short-term disability usage. *J Occup Environ Med* 2001;43(1):25–29.
11. Serxner SA, Gold DB, Bultman KK. The impact of behavioral health risks on worker absenteeism. *J Occup Environ Med* 2001;43(4):347–354.
12. Yen L, Edington DW, Witting P. Prediction of prospec-

tive medical claims and absenteeism: costs for 1,284 hourly workers from a manufacturing company. *J Occup Med* 1992;34:428–435.

13. Edington DW. Emerging research: a view from one research center. *Am J Health Promotion* 2001;15(5): 341–349.
14. Bertera RL. The effects of behavioral risks on absenteeism and health-care costs in the workplace. *J Occup Med* 1991;22:1119–1124.
15. Halpern MT, Shikiar R, Rentz AM, et al. Impact of smoking status on workplace absenteeism and productivity. *Tobacco Control* 2001;10:233–238.
16. Musich SA, Burton WN, Edington DW. Costs and benefits of prevention and disease management. *Dis Manage Health Outcomes* 1999;5(3):153–166.
17. Kessler RC, Greenberg PE, Mickelson KD, et al. The effects of chronic medical conditions on work loss and work cutback. *J Occup Environ Med* 2001;43:218–225.
18. Greenberg PE, Birnbaum HG, Kessler RC, et al. Impact of illness and its treatment on workplace costs: regulatory and measurements issues. *J Occup Environ Med* 2001;43(1):56–63.
19. Bloom DE, Canning D. The health and wealth of nations. *Science* 2000;287:1207–1209.
20. Goetzel RZ, Ozminkowski RJ, Meneades L, et al. Pharmaceuticals—cost or investment? *J Occup Environ Med* 2000;42:338–351.
21. Burton WN, Conti DJ, Chen C-Y, et al. The impact of allergies and allergy treatment on worker productivity. *J Occup Environ Med* 2001;43(1):64–71.
22. Cockburn IM, et al. Loss of work productivity due to illness and medical treatment. *J Occup Environ Med* 1999;41(11):948–953.
23. Weiler JM, Bloomfield JR, Woodworth GG, et al. Effects of fexofenadine, diphenhydramine, and alcohol on driving performance. *Ann Intern Med* 2000;132:354–363.
24. Hennessys S, Strom BL. Non-sedating antihistamines should be preferred over sedating antihistamines in patients who drive. *Ann Intern Med* 2000;132:405–407.
25. Gilmore T, Alexander BH, Mueller BA, et al. Occupational injuries and medication use. *Am J Ind Med* 1996; 30:234–239.
26. CDC Web site on Chronic Disease Prevention. Prevalence of disability and associated health conditions—United States, 1991–1992. *MMWR* 1994;43(40): 730–731, 737–739.
27. National Health Interview Survey. *Third National Health and Nutrition Survey, 1988–1994,* 1996.
28. Birnbaum HG, Barton M, Greenberg PE, et al. Direct and indirect costs of rheumatoid arthritis to an employer. *J Occup Environ Med* 2000;42(6):588–596.
29. Mannino DM, Homa DM, Akinbami LJ, et al. Surveillance for asthma—United States, 1980–1999. *MMWR* 2002;51(SS-1):1–13.
30. Sullivan SD. The economic cost of asthma. *Med Interface* 1994;7[suppl]:17–18.
31. Burton WN, Schultz AB, Connerty CM, et al. Asthma disease management: a worksite-based asthma education program. *Dis Manage* 2001;4(1):3–13.
32. Burton WN, Connerty CM, Schultz AB, et al. Bank One's worksite-based asthma disease management program. *J Occup Environ Med* 2001;43(2):75–82.
33. Zimmer LO, Almond MJ, Jones D, et al. One-year outcomes from a computer-based disease management program: the Individualized Asthma Care Training Program (IACT). *Dis Manage* 2000;3:65–73.
34. Wu AW, Young Y, Skinner EA, et al. Quality of care and outcomes of adults with asthma treated by specialists and generalists in managed care. *Arch Intern Med* 2001; 1621:2554–2560.
35. U.S. Public Health Service. *National Institutes of Health, National Heart Lung and Blood Institute. Practical guide for the diagnosis and management of asthma.* NIH publ. No. 97-4053, October 1997.
36. Schwartz BS, Stewart WF, Lipton RB. Lost workdays and decreased work effectiveness associated with headache in the workplace. *J Occup Environ Med* 1997; 39(4):320–327.
37. Stang P, Cady R, Batenhorst A, et al. Workplace productivity: a review of the impact of migraine and its treatment. *Pharmacoeconomics* 2001;9(3):231–244.
38. Burton WN, Conti DJ, Chen C-Y, et al. The economic burden of lost productivity due to migraine headache: a specific worksite analysis. *J Occup Environ Med* 2002; 44(6).
39. Davies GM, Santanello N, Gerth W, et al. Validation of a migraine work and productivity questionnaire for use in migraine studies. *Cephalalgia* 1999;19(5):497–502.
40. Warshaw LJ, Burton WN, Schneider WJ. Role of the workplace in migraine disease management. *Dis Manage Health Outcomes* 2001;9(2):99–115.
41. American Diabetes Association. *Economic consequences of diabetes mellitus in the United States in 1997.* Alexandria, VA: American Diabetes Association, 1998.
42. Diabetes and the workplace: how employers can implement change. Employers Managed Health Care Association, 2001.
43. Burton WN, Connerty CM. Worksite-based diabetes disease management program. *Dis Manage* 2002;5(1):1–8.
44. Burton WN, Connerty CM. Evaluation of a worksite-based patient education intervention targeted at employees with diabetes mellitus. *J Occup Environ Med* 1998;40(8):702–706.
45. Couch RB. Influenza: prospects for control. *Ann Intern Med* 2000;133:992–998.
46. Couch RB. Prevention and treatment of influenza. *N Engl J Med* 2000;343(24):1778–1787.
47. Nichol KL. Cost-benefit analysis of a strategy to vaccinate healthy working adults against influenza. *Arch Intern Med* 2001;161:749–759.
48. Keech M, Scott AJ, Ryan PJ. The impact of influenza and influenza-like illness on productivity and healthcare resource utilization in a working population. *Occup Med* 1998;48:85–90.
49. Nichol KL, Lind A, Margolis KL, et al. The effectiveness of vaccination against influenza in healthy, working adults. *N Engl J Med* 1995;333(14):889–893.
50. Musich S, Adams L, Broder J, et al. Preliminary evaluation of a worksite influenza vaccination program: the experience of the progressive corporation. *Worksite Health* 1996;3(4):27–34.
51. Campbell DS, Rumley MH. Cost-effectiveness of the influenza vaccine in a healthy, working-age population. *J Occup Environ Med* 1997;39(5):408–414.
52. Bridges CB, Thompson WW, Meltzer MI. Effectiveness and cost-benefit of influenza vaccination of healthy working adults. *JAMA* 2000;284(13):1655–1663.
53. Nicol KL. Effectiveness of live attenuated intranasal in-

fluenza virus vaccine in healthy, working adults. *JAMA* 1999;282:137–144.
54. Locke GR II, Talley NJ, Fett SL. Prevalence and clinical spectrum of gastro-esophageal reflux: a population-based study in Olmsted County, Minnesota. *Gastroenterology* 1997;112:1448–1456.
55. Oliveria SA, Shristos PJ, Talley NJ, et al. Heartburn risk factors, knowledge, and prevention strategies: a population-based survey of individuals with heartburn. *Arch Intern Med* 1999;159:1592–1598.
56. Henke CJ, Levin TR, Henning JM, et al. Work loss costs due to peptic ulcer disease and gastroesophageal reflux disease in a health maintenance organization. *Am J Gastroenterol* 2000;95:788–792.
57. Skoutakis VA, Joe RH, Hara DS. Comparative role of omeprazole in the treatment of gastroesophageal reflux disease. *Annu Pharmacother* 1995;12:1252–1262.
58. Sridhar S, Huang J, O'Brien BJ, et al. Clinical economics review: cost-effectiveness of treatment alternatives for gastro-esophageal reflux disease. *Aliment Pharmacol Ther* 1996;10:865–873.
59. Longstreth GF. Irritable bowel syndrome: a multibillion-dollar problem. *Gastroenterology* 1995;109:2029–2031.
60. Drossman DA, Li Z, Andruzzi E. U.S. householder survey of functional gastrointestinal disorders: prevalence, sociodemography, and health impact. *Dig Dis* 1993;38: 1569–1580.
61. Hahn BA, Yan S, Strassels S. Impact of irritable bowel syndrome on quality of life and resource use in the United States and United Kingdom. *Digestion* 1999;60:77–81.
62. Greenberg PE, Stiglin LE, Finkelstein SN, et al. The economic burden of depression in 1990. *J Clin Psychiatry* 1993;54:405–418.
63. Conti DJ, Burton WN. Economic impact of depression in a workplace. *J Occup Environ Med* 1994;36(9):983.
64. McCunney RJ. Health and productivity: a role for occupational health professionals. *J Occup Environ Med* 2001;43(1):30–35.
65. Berndt ER, Bailit HL, Keller MB, et al. Health care use and at-work productivity among employees with mental health disorders. *Health Affairs* 2000;19(4):244–258.
66. Simon GE, Barber C, Birnbaum HG, et al. Depression and work productivity: the comparative costs of treatment versus nontreatment. *J Occup Environ Med* 2001; 43:2–9.
67. Mintz J, Mintz LI, Arruda MJ, et al. Treatments of depression and the functional capacity to work. *Arch Gen Psychiatry* 1992;49:761–768.
68. Goetzel RZ, Osminkowski RJ, Sederer LI, et al. The business case for quality mental health services: why employers should care about the mental health and well-being of their employees. *J Occup Environ Med* 2002; 44:320–330.
69. Brady W, Bass J, Moser R, et al. Defining total corporate health and safety costs—significance and impact. *J Occup Environ Med* 1997;39(3):224–231.
70. Burton WN, Conti DJ. Disability management: corporate medical department management of employee health and productivity. *J Occup Environ Med* 2000;42 (10):1006–1012.
71. Mobley EM, Linz DL, Shukla R, et al. Disability case management: an impact assessment in an automotive manufacturing organization. *J Occup Environ Med* 2000; 42(6):597–602.
72. Goetzel RZ, Ozminskwski RJ. Health and productivity management: emerging opportunities for health promotion professionals for the 21st century. *Am J Health Promotion* 2000;14(4):211–214.
73. Warshaw LJ, Burton WN. Cutting the costs of migraine: role of the employee health unit. *J Occup Environ Med* 1998;40(11):943–953.

FURTHER INFORMATION

Riedel JE, Lynch W, Baase C, et al. The effect of disease prevention and health promotion on workplace productivity: a literature review. *Am J Health Promotion* 2001;15(3): 167–191.

Good introduction to the scope of the issue. The authors provide several benchmark case studies and annotated major articles important to this developing field.

Aldana S, Pronk N. Health promotion programs, modifiable health risks, and employee absenteeism. *J Occup Environ Health* 2001;43(1):36–46.

Review of health risks and employee absenteeism and the influence of participation in employee health promotion programs.

Institute for Health and Productivity Management Web site at *www.ihpm.org*.

The goal of the institute is provide a clearinghouse for materials related to helping employers measure and improve the health and productivity of its workforce. One of the resources available is a catalog of existing public-domain questionnaires to measure on-the-job presenteeism.

12

Health Promotion

Molly J. McCauley and Robert J. McCunney

Health promotion, defined as the science and art of helping people change their lifestyle to move to an optimal state of health (1) through a combination of efforts to enhance awareness, encourage behavior change, and create environments that support good health practices, has as its goal individual movement toward a state of optimal health, which is a balance of physical, emotional, social, spiritual, and intellectual health. Yet, in an effort to support individuals' health goals, the scope of health promotion practice today has evolved and strives to change physical, social, and normative environments. To begin, a brief look at definitions will help to put this evolution in perspective.

The dominant view of health promotion that emerged in the mid- to late-1970s was in response to a growing disillusionment with the limits of medicine, pressure to contain health care costs, and a social and political climate that emphasized self-help and individual control over health (2). Later the vision of health promotion that was articulated by the surgeon general in the 1979 Healthy People Report set the stage for programs that not only brought attention to helping individuals modify health behaviors but also punctuated the importance of physical and social environments (2). The notion of going beyond the focus on the individual was enhanced even further by the definition of health promotion as stated by the World Health Organization (WHO) in the mid-1980s: "Health promotion is a process of enabling people to increase control over and improve their health and represents a mediating strategy between people and their environments, synthesizing personal choice and social responsibility in health" (2).

As a result of more than two decades of program proliferation, health promotion is now central to work-site programming and is recognized as an integral part of occupational health practice. Indeed, the work site is viewed as one of the most popular venues for promoting health and preventing disease (3). Several studies provide evidence that health promotion is firmly embedded in the fiber of U.S. business. One study to determine the prevalence of activities at small work sites was conducted by American Business Lists. Over 3,000 companies, all having between 15 and 99 employees, were surveyed. Based on the responses of 78% of those polled, 25% indicated that they were offering at least one health promotion program, specifying occupational safety, cardiopulmonary resuscitation (CPR), and back injury prevention as the most common programs (4). Another survey, the 1994 National Health Interview Survey, used the responses of 5,219 respondents who were employed and completed the section on work-site health promotion (5); 43% of the respondents acknowledged access to smoking cessation programs, 31% to general health education programs, and 31% to screenings; 32% indicated that they were participants in some program at the work site. However important all such studies are as evidence of the growth of work-site health promotion over the years, the preeminent study is and has been the National Health Promotion Survey, conducted by the United States Office of Disease Prevention and Health Promotion in 1985, 1992, and 1999. The 1999 survey concluded that 90% of work sites with 50 or more employees offer at least one health promotion activity compared to 81% of work sites in 1992 and 65% in 1985 (6). Aside from documenting the growth and prevalence of health promotion, the 1999 survey contributes to the understanding of both the content and context of work-site health promotion. Consider a few of the survey highlights as follows:

- 84% of companies want to keep employees healthy.
- 79% have smoking policies.
- 18% offer health risk appraisals (HRAs).
- Blood pressure, cholesterol, and cancer screening are the most available interventions.
- 39% report that senior management ranks employee health near the top of its business priorities.
- 94% report that health care costs are a concern for management.
- 10% offer financial incentives.
- 74% are evaluating their programs.
- The average number of programs offered by an employer is 12 (5).

Given this current understanding of programming nationally, there is another document that provides a template for future direction. This compilation of the nation's health promotion and disease prevention objectives, Healthy People 2010, is published by the U.S. Department of Health and Human Services. One specific challenge for the work site is continued programming growth, setting a target for 75% of work sites with 50 or more employees to offer *comprehensive* health promotion activities with special emphasis placed on comprehensive design versus single program offerings. Another challenge is to significantly increase the number of employees who participate, again with a target of 75%. In conjunction with Healthy People 2010, the federal government will establish tracking mechanisms for ten of the leading health indicators. This will be valuable information for planning health promotion in the future. It has been noted that of particular interest to this tracking effort are the physical activity and overweight/obesity indicators (7).

Most certainly, the national initiatives of the past 20 years have fueled the growth of work-site health promotion and disease prevention in the United States. The work-site drivers have been equally as influential. There has been a desire on the part of employers to manage health care costs, decrease absenteeism, improve productivity, improve employee morale, recruit and retain employees, enhance the corporate image, and contribute to the health and well-being of their human resources. As such, the stated mission of work-site health promotion is to support these interests of senior management (8). The good news is that there is growing empirical evidence that work-site health promotion is contributing to the achievement of management goals. Throughout this chapter, documented evidence of impact and outcomes is highlighted.

Growth in the number of programs as well as new national targets for advancing the health of Americans are not the only distinguishing differences in health promotion over the past 6 years. Implementation models have been tested and challenged; programs have been evaluated and results published; and the literature has been reviewed in order to summarize health impact, cost savings, and implementation effectiveness. As a result, there is an emerging body of knowledge that serves to applaud the progress made in health promotion practice and challenge health professionals to continue these efforts. For those who deliver occupational health services and will be asked to assess, design, develop, implement, and evaluate health promotion programs, this chapter presents the most current view of the following issues:

- The rationale and justification for work-site health promotion
- A systematic process for getting started and starting over
- The scope of comprehensive programs
- Implementation options—what works and what doesn't
- Evaluating the effectiveness of health promotion
- The future: facing the challenges and the opportunities.

RATIONALE AND JUSTIFICATION FOR WORK-SITE HEALTH PROMOTION

Over the years increased attention has been directed to documenting the effect of work-site health promotion programs on health care costs, absenteeism, health outcomes, and employee health and work-related attitudes. There is now a compelling body of evidence that there are positive results, thereby providing substantive rationale to invest in programming. This section presents an overview of findings over the past years.

Health Care Costs

Recognizing that 94% of the 1999 National Health Promotion Survey respondents indicated that a top management concern is health care costs, it would follow that there is great interest in understanding the potential impact of health promotion on these costs. Controlling health care costs paid by employers is complex and part of an ever-growing national dilemma (9–11). Currently, 13 cents out of every dollar spent in the U.S. economy is spent on health care (12). Annual increases in health care spending dropped from 12.2% in 1990 to 4.8% in 1997 due to employers moving to managed care plans, low medical-specific inflation, and price cuts extracted from providers (8). Now, however, the single-digit increases are a thing of the past, and double-digit increases are once again the norm. The average health plan is expected to cost employers $4,853 per employee in 2000, representing an increase of $110 per employee over 1999 (13). Such increases can only affect business profitability, with concomitant impact on employees' benefits, wages, and job security, so it is not unreasonable for management to ask, "What will health promotion programming do to impact health care costs?"

Programs from the 1980s presented early evidence that health promotion and positive health behaviors can reduce heath care costs. Live for Life, Johnson & Johnson's program, documented a mean annual inpatient cost increase for active program participants of $42, as compared to a $76 increase for nonparticipants (14). Control Data's cross-sectional study of insurance data showed that smokers experienced 18% higher medical claims and that people with hypertension are 68% more likely to incur claims in excess of $5,000 per year (15).

More recent studies continue to add to the body of evidence that health promotion does impact on health care costs for employers, understanding that the type of programming and the degree to which health risks can be influenced are critical variables.

The conclusions from one group of studies demonstrated that results are heavily dependent on the type of intervention. The University of Michigan's Health Management Research Center studied U.S. employees who were participating in health promotion programs, and concluded that employees in comprehensive programs experienced moderation in medical costs while employees in awareness/assessment programs had medical costs that continued to rise (16). Citibank NA conducted a quasi-experimental employee study of 11,194 participants and 11,644 nonparticipants. They concluded that their return on investment (ROI) was $4.56 to $1, and attributed these results to the high-risk intervention focus of their program (17). A study by Proctor and Gamble (P&G) of participating vs. nonparticipating employees' total and lifestyle-related medical care costs found that they were significantly different at 3 years as compared to baseline. At baseline, total participant vs. nonparticipant costs were 2% different and at 3 years participant costs were 29% lower. P&G concluded that there was a strong association between the program and the results, and indicated that the key success factor was one-on-one high-risk counseling (18).

The findings from two other studies that address health care costs are specific to health risks. The HERO study is indeed a benchmark study to the extent that it documents, using a large database, that high-risk employees cost employers more money. The study controlled for multiple risk conditions and demographic confounders in order to increase the confidence levels of the estimates. The health care costs of 46,026 employees from six companies were examined, and those costs were tracked for 3 years after completion of a health risk appraisal. Employees at high risk in seven of the ten risk categories had significantly higher expenditures than those at low risk. Specifically, health care costs were higher for employees at high risk for depression by 70%, for stress by 46%, and for high blood glucose by 35%. Individuals with a multiple risk profile for heart disease had costs 228% higher, for psychosocial problems 147% higher, and for stroke 85% higher (19,20). Notably, there were three health risks, when analyzed as independent variables that did not show evidence of increased health care expenditures. They were high cholesterol, excessive alcohol use, and poor nutrition habits (19,20). One other study of 2,898 municipal employees in Birmingham, Alabama, found a significant difference in both health care costs and utilization for those in the cardiovascular disease, psychosocial disease, and multiple risk groups (21).

Aside from the studies and reviews noted above, the work of Ken Pelletier over the last 10 years has afforded health professionals a source of reference in connection with the findings from key health and cost-effectiveness outcome studies. His reviews and analyses have contributed significantly to an aggregate understanding of the studies that have formed the foundation of work-site health promotion's science base. Each of his four summary articles (22–25) succinctly overviews each evaluation and the time period studied. In turn, they highlight the purpose of the evaluation, the study design, study period, and findings. His first review featured 24 studies (22), his second 23 (23), his third 26 (24), and his fourth 11 (25). The one notable difference between the first three reviews and the fourth is that in the fourth the programs had to meet specific criteria to be included. Specifically, those programs had to be comprehensive, ongoing, integrated, and consistent with corporate objectives (25). In summary, all of Pelletier's reviews portray a historical perspective of the evolution of the research design, data analysis, and intervention sophistication that is taking place in work-site health promotion. There were positive results during the 1980s, and while there have been content and context changes during the 1990s, the results continue to be positive. Pelletier contends that the positive findings from these studies cannot be cavalierly dismissed as "no evidence," and he believes that it continues to be increasingly possible to prove both cost-effectiveness and cost-benefit (23).

Absenteeism

Simply stated, employees who are absent from the job are not productive employees. Business not only pays the health care bill for an ill or injured employee, but also incurs the cost of salary continuation when an employee is absent. The impact that health promotion has on absenteeism, therefore, is significant. If healthier employees are absent less, they are certainly more productive. However, the extent to which this variable of interest has been studied is far less than the analyses of health care costs and health outcomes.

Yet, there were early studies that indicated positive results. Johnson & Johnson examined absence in terms of sick hours and found that Live for Life participants report 20 fewer hours of sick time per year than nonparticipants (26). Avoiding payment for 2½ days of absence per employee per year across an entire employee population would dramatically reduce payment of salary dollars that are not associated with productivity. Likewise, a 2-year Dupont study of 41 sites with a health promotion program as compared to 19 control sites without any health promotion documented a 14% decline in sickness, absence, or disability days at the program sites and only a 5.8% decline at control sites (27).

Health Outcomes

One premise upon which health promotion programs are justified is the ability to focus on the preventable aspects of morbidity and mortality in the U.S. The leading causes of death and disease today have been linked to major risk factors. It has been estimated that many years of life are lost to premature death (28), and there is evidence that the prevalence and levels of preventable risk factors in employed populations are high (29). Efforts directed toward reducing these risk factors are the essence of work-site health promotion.

The fact that actual health risks are reduced has been the easiest to document. AT&T's Total Life Concept (TLC) program reported significantly greater improvements among study group participants than control group participants for diastolic blood pressure, serum cholesterol, type A behavior, and body weight after just 1 year (30). After 2 years, the significant improvements were maintained, and resulted in a decrease in health age, as well as reduced population scores for total mortality, heart attack morbidity, and cancer morbidity (31).

The above is just one example of the hundreds of published studies that report the health impact of health promotion programs. While this body of literature is far too extensive to review comprehensively in this chapter, there are two noteworthy review articles that summarize the work in this area over the last 15 to 20 years.

The first article reports a review of 365 articles covering 11 major health areas. Experts from each of the health areas reviewed the published studies and rated them for the rigor of the study design (from two to five stars) and the conclusiveness of the results (from weak to conclusive). Over half of the studies had four- and five-star ratings for design, and as a whole the body of literature was deemed to be indicative to acceptable for positive results (32). The authors note that this compares most favorably to a 1986 review done by Warner et al. (33), who concluded that published findings were weak. They further note that this body of literature is comparable to and even superior to the body of literature supporting the outcomes of medical interventions (32).

The second article was a review of 47 studies and the results from 35 programs. Again the published studies were rated on the rigor of the study design and the conclusiveness of the results. The authors concluded that:

- risk reduction for high-risk employees is the greatest in the context of comprehensive programming;
- work-site health promotion reduces health risks under the conditions of (a) personal and consistent counseling, and (b) sufficient program duration;
- there can be a cautious optimism about work-site health promotion (34).

If risk reduction does eventually translate to actual reduction of morbidity and mortality, companies compound the short-term benefit of a healthier workforce with the long-term savings from reduced health care costs and utilization, as well as from decreased disability absence.

Attitudes Toward Health and the Company

Positive attitudes toward the employer, a necessary ingredient of high morale in the workforce, were a highly valued outcome by key corporate executives in the early 1980s. Companies experiencing change and transition and equally concerned about the well-being of the employees sought to document attitude change.

Did employees have a better attitude toward health and did it make a difference in how they viewed their work and the company? The answer is yes and no.

Johnson & Johnson found a significant attitudinal improvement in employees at participating Live for Life companies. Measures were favorable for organizational commitment, supervision, working conditions, job competence, pay and fringe benefits, and job security (35). AT&T documented attitudinal changes as well. After 1 year of ongoing Total Life Concept programming, participants reported a belief that they could affect their own health and were committed to change health behaviors (30). Additionally, participants perceived that AT&T cared about their welfare, were enthused about their work, and were satisfied with working conditions (30). However, the positive job-related effects attained after 1 year were negated at 2 years, likely due to the organizational and operational changes that occurred during that time. This finding suggests that, while health promotion can positively influence attitudes toward the company, the presence of a program cannot eliminate the consequences of job/work-related transition, ambiguity, and uncertainty.

Since those early studies, there is very little documentation about attitudes and satisfaction. Anecdotally, there is no doubt that programs contribute to levels of satisfaction. What is lacking is the important correlation between satisfaction, health risks and health care costs. Studies that document the correlation of these critical qualitative variables (attitudes and satisfaction) with quantitative results will contribute significantly to the field's understanding of program strengths and weaknesses as well as to an understanding of the context of the program, specifically, the culture and norms of the workplace. It is likely that this is a sensitive area for managers, especially human resources (HR) managers with accountability for health promotion programs, and may explain why there is so little analysis and reporting of attitudes and satisfaction.

A SYSTEMATIC PLANNING PROCESS—GETTING STARTED AND STARTING OVER

Given that 90% of companies with 50 or more employees are offering at least one health promotion activity, it is not likely that there are many companies starting a program for the first time. But companies are always starting over. With every change in the company, every new finding about a health risk or disease, and every new program type that comes into favor, there is an opportunity to recycle the planning process. The possibilities for program scope, the options for delivery, and the potential for targeting not only risks and diseases but also select subsets of the employee population are extremely varied. Appropriate choices depend on the characteristics of the employee population coupled with the goals of both the program and the business. A systematic planning process is the key to immediate and ongoing success. The getting started steps include establishing a vision, mission, and goals, and assessing data. In the practical world these steps are not sequential as one might expect. If management can articulate a vision, mission, and goals, it is likely that data have influenced the direction. And as planning proceeds it is also likely that additional data will influence the vision, mission, and goals. So the process as it unfolds is iterative rather than sequential.

Establishing the Vision, Mission, and Goals

At the outset of planning, a clear description of the expectations of the health promotion program is essential. The stakeholders, key executives, and business managers need to articulate a vision for the future in light of initiation of or change in the health promotion program. How will the program link to the business strategy, how will it contribute to the management of human resources, how will it enhance corporate image/positioning? Based on that input from top management, the mission and goals for the program can be formulated by program staff. The mission statement, at a very high level, explains why the program exists as a function of the business. And finally, the goals are broad statements about the expected results of the program. Save the objective setting for much, much later when the specificity of who will be doing what by when can be added.

Data Collection

Employee assessment, taking the form of surveys and focus groups, is a good place to begin regardless of whether this is a first-time effort or a recycling effort. The goal is to understand the wants and needs of the population, as well as the ethnic, cultural, social, and organizational characteristics. Such assessment activities offer employees an opportunity to comment during the development stage, which may enhance interest and participation. Focus groups identify a myriad of issues (among them the strengths and weaknesses of an existing program if there is one in place) and highlight the barriers and helpers that the program is currently facing or may face in the future.

During focus groups, unofficial leaders who may emerge are invaluable as employee committee members and in soliciting co-workers' participation.

Management interviews gather another perspective, that of the leadership and supervision in the company. It is critical that the needs of the business are understood and that the issues of managers are taken into consideration. The concern of "What's in this for me?" cannot be ignored; anything short of a win-win for both the employee and the manager sets the stage for failure. Interviews give valuable insights into the level of commitment within the organization and the degree to which financial support and personal involvement can be expected.

Health care cost data (inpatient, outpatient, and pharmacy), illness/injury absence data (short-term disability and workers' compensation), and demographic data should be used to determine the major categories of disease that are driving costs, and for which groups of employees. Using company health care cost and absence data to prepare a profile by the major diagnostic categories (MDCs) and the diagnostic related groups (DRGs) could be extremely informative. In some cases the specificity of an International Classification of Diseases ICD-10 code may be helpful. For example, a company may find that there is significant spending for musculoskeletal problems and thus may want to establish targeted interventions for these problems. Summary information about pharmacy claims, highlighting expenses by therapeutic group, may lead a company to address depression or allergies if significant expenditures are in those areas. Additionally, a demographic overview can portray specific employee groups that may benefit from targeted interventions. A young female population with a high rate of complications from pregnancy may benefit from a pregnancy management program, or an older female population may benefit from an osteoporosis program.

Data from HRAs can be used to develop an aggregate view of population risk, information that is essential to program planning. Computerized HRAs use a set of algorithms developed from investigations of large populations as the basis for interpretation. While some authors have suggested that employee populations have risks similar to those of the general population (36), company-specific data are more readily accepted by management, thereby building a case for the administration of the HRA, even if on a periodic basis. Baseline administration of an HRA and interval readministration can help gauge the effect of the program on employee risk factors, health behaviors and readiness to change.

Finally, program participation and employee satisfaction is particularly important when a program is being reassessed. What did employees like or dislike? What did they elect to participate in and why? Consider a 24-hour telephone access program with low participation. If most employees have this service available through their health plan or physician practice group, then the participation will be low. In the case of this example if the data had been established in advance through surveys and interviews, this type of program may never have been initiated.

Once all the data noted above have been collected, it is time to assimilate this information and begin molding a plan that will (a) include content acceptable to both the employees and management, (b) allow for implementation within the scope of the resources available, (c) incorporate strategies and methods that take into consideration employee preferences and the needs of the operation of the business, and (d) consider measures indicative of both short-term and long-term results. Scope of programs, implementation options, and evaluation considerations are delineated in the next three sections of this chapter.

SCOPE OF PROGRAMS FOR HEALTH PROMOTION

Programs can range from health awareness campaigns, to educational seminars, to biologic screenings, to multiple session behavior change courses. The important feature of all approaches is to leverage positive employee health behaviors supported by the workplace environment. Whatever the topic of interest, the goal has been, and continues to be, to support employees in personal achievement and maintenance of positive health behaviors. Yet as the scope of programming has taken on new dimensions through the incorporation of demand and disease management initiatives, complementary goals have emerged. Specifically, those goals focus on providing support for employees and their families to use self-care appropriately, to be an informed consumer of health care, and to effectively manage chronic disease in order to avoid symptom progression and complications.

Whether the approach is to focus on a single health topic, to address multiple health risks or behaviors at the primary prevention level, or to implement across the health continuum through primary, secondary, and tertiary prevention, the best rule of thumb for choosing the specific intervention(s) is to let the data guide decision making. Categories of illness and injury accountable for high medical costs and absenteeism, prevalent health risks, employee interests, and population demographics are factors to be considered.

This section presents highlights of the features and benefits of some of the popular programs offered in the business setting today: preventive screenings/examinations, smoking cessation, exercise/aerobics, eating habits/nutrition/cholesterol, weight management, blood pressure control, stress management, employee assistance, demand management, disease management, environmental and organizational interventions, and other programs of interest. Although each program component is only briefly discussed, more detailed descriptions are available in the references.

Preventive Screenings/Examinations

Biologic screenings and preventive examinations are central to early detection of disease and, thereby, to prevention efforts. The findings can provide actual measurements for a health risk appraisal, raise awareness about a particular disease, motivate the participant to take action, and contribute important variables for program evaluation.

At the work site there are two options for screenings and preventive examinations. One is that they are actually conducted on-site and the other is that educational programs are held to encourage employees to see their personal provider. There are pros and cons for both options. The former option provides convenience and access, but the downside may be that there is no physician consultation about the findings. While the latter option places employees in contact with their personal physician, it is very likely that they will never seek the services.

Cancer screenings and/or related educational programs are popular work-site offerings and for good reason: 500,000 Americans die each year from all types of cancer. That translates to approximately 1,500 deaths a day, and there are 1 million newly diagnosed cancer cases each year. The good news is that taking steps to reduce risk factors can prevent 50% of all cancers. The fact that there are four cancers (breast, prostate, colon, and lung) that represent 50% of the U.S. cancer burden (37) punctuates the importance of screening and education in those areas. In addition, opportunities for screening and education exist in the area of skin cancer to counter the 4% increase in malignant melanoma each year (38). Historically for cancer screenings the value of age-, risk-, and history-specific screening has been documented (39), and at present the latest edition of the U.S. Clinical Preventive Services Guidelines (40) serves as a valuable resource for targeting appropriate populations. While there are many examples of successful programs in the literature that help program managers to determine educational content and implementation methods, just a few are cited here as examples:

- One study of skin cancer helps in the selection of the central messages for a skin cancer screening. This study found that users of sunscreens with sun protection factor (SPF) 30 spent 25% more time in the sun, which alone raises one's risk for skin cancer (38). Based on this finding, it is imperative that urging use of SPF 30 sunscreen be coupled with messages about limiting time in the sun (total number of hours) and avoiding sun exposure completely between 12 noon and 3 p.m.
- Recent computer modeling to determine the impact of mammography on breast cancer detection and diagnosis concluded that the incidence of metastatic breast cancer would be reduced 66% with a mammography every 9 months and 78% with a mammography every 6 months (41). This investigation demonstrates the importance of keeping up to date with the most recent recommendations of the National Cancer Society and the National Cancer Institute so that work-site programs and benefit coverage are compatible with validated science.
- The Next Step Trial, a work-site colorectal screening program, targeted auto industry employees at high risk for colorectal cancer. There were 5,042 workers from 28 work sites, randomized as control or intervention sites. The employees at the control sites had screening only, while the employees at the intervention sites had screening plus nutrition education and phone contact. Over a 2-year period, compliance with recommended screening schedules and proper nutrition was greater for the employees at the intervention sites (42).

Conducting blood pressure measurements as well as the blood values (lipids and glucose) as part of an HRA process adds to the validity of the estimated risk, and therefore enhances the value of the reported results for the participant. Likewise, these screenings are popular as stand-alone interventions due to the emphasis placed on hypertension, hyperlipidemia, and elevated blood sugar as major risk factors for cardiovascular disease and diabetes.

No screening is complete without appropriate follow-up. One study of cholesterol screening follow-up conducted by Blue Cross and Blue Shield of Maryland found that the most successful predictor of referral completion after the screening itself was a cholesterol level equal to or greater than 240 mg/100 mL

(43). Another study of referral compliance after public cholesterol screening found that individuals with prior history were 10% to 15% more likely to initiate follow-up (44). These studies are but a few examples of which participants may take action, leaving us with the challenge of targeting messages to participants least likely to take action.

More recently, osteoporosis screening has received a great deal of attention due to the fact that osteoporosis is now treatable and screening devices are available. This attention is also due to the fact that the prevalence of osteoporosis has been empirically quantified. One in two women and one in eight men over 50 will develop osteoporosis (45). The National Osteoporosis Foundation (NOF) recently launched a multiyear campaign designed to bring attention to the importance of weight-bearing exercises for bone health, making this a key educational message in connection with screening. NOF is looking for partners to disseminate this message. NOF is an excellent source for educational materials and has developed risk-screening questionnaires. It is also noteworthy that the National Institutes of Health recently convened an expert panel to consider guidelines and recommendations for osteoporosis screening. The consensus, as published in the proceedings of the meeting, was that more research is needed to determine who should be screened, the best method for screening, and the frequency of screening. This will be an area to follow closely as companies continue to sponsor such screenings.

Smoking Cessation

Smoking-related issues have taken center stage in recent years. There has been continued research, legal action against the tobacco companies, and smoking bans imposed for public places. By now there is no doubt that smoking is the single lifestyle behavior that has the greatest impact on health. There are 430,000 tobacco-related deaths each year, with associated medical care costs of $50 billion (46). It remains the single most important preventable cause of death in our society (47). Still, one in four U.S. adults smoke (46). While this rate of smoking reflects great progress from the 35% to 40% rate of 20 to 25 years ago, there is still much to be done, especially given current concerns related to secondhand smoke.

Recognizing that the individuals who are still smoking may be the ones who will experience the most difficulty quitting, and recognizing that only one in 20 who try to quit will be successful (47), it is imperative that the interventions with the greatest potential for success are the ones that are implemented. Some findings from recent studies can be helpful as programming decisions are made:

- A study supported by the Robert Wood Johnson Foundation concluded that cognitive-behavioral interventions coupled with pharmacotherapy yield 40% quit rates for the highly motivated, least addicted individuals (48).
- A study conducted at three aerospace industry work sites in California tested for differences between three programmatic approaches: a traditional smoking cessation program, a multicomponent program plus telephone counseling, and a multicomponent program plus team competition and cash incentives. After 12 months, the two multicomponent programs had 37% and 30% quit rates, while the traditional program had an 11% quit rate (49).
- The Working Well Trial surveyed employees at 90 blue-collar work sites, designated as intervention and control sites, about their tobacco use behaviors at baseline and after 2½ years. Interesting gender differences were found. Women quit more than men under the intervention conditions, and women quit more with a specific intervention than without (50).

These few studies suggest that program managers should consider adding pharmacotherapy, delivering multicomponent smoking cessation interventions, and targeting women. Another perspective, broader in scope, is based on a general review of 79 smoking cessation/tobacco policy evaluations (51) that rated program process and impact as follows: (a) group programs are more effective; (b) tobacco policies reduce consumption at work; and (c) minimal interventions, competitions, and medical interventions produce "indicative" results, while incremental efforts produce "suggestive" results. In support of implementation planning, guidelines published by the U.S. Department of Health and Human Services in July 2000 cite proven interventions that can increase an individual's likelihood of success. In addition, many structured programs that address the addictive and behavioral components of smoking are readily available through the American Cancer Society, the American Lung Association, the American Heart Association, and Smoke-Anon. These organizations provide program material and sometimes group facilitators. Hospitals and health maintenance organizations are also resources for smoking cessation.

Keeping in mind that the variables for success, program duration, educational content, and support mechanisms need to be determined. Program duration can range from 5 or 6 consecutive days to once weekly for 8 to 10 weeks. Program content should address the physiologic as well as the psychosocial and addictive characteristics of smoking. The support strategies may include a buddy system, behavioral contracting, use of incentives, telephone counseling, and use of a nicotine supplement. Employees may also respond favorably to self-help, self-paced programs learning methods, and some may choose alternatives such as hypnosis, acupuncture, and biofeedback. Since no single method works for everyone, offering different program options affords smokers the opportunity to find the program that works for them.

As emphasized in "Reducing Tobacco Use," a report by Surgeon General David Satcher that was presented in August 2000 at the 11th World Conference on Tobacco or Health, individually focused interventions cannot stand alone. In this report the surgeon general critically analyzes not only educational and clinical methods but also regulatory, economic, and social methods. Therefore, as work-site practitioners, our work is not done when there is a plan for individual programming. Efforts toward the implementation of work-site smoking policies as well as the organizational institutionalization of programs are imperative (52). A national survey conducted in 1986 found that 27% of work sites limited smoking to a particular area and, upon readministration in 1992, 87% of work sites had either a complete ban or restricted areas (53). It is estimated that smoke-free workplaces in the U.S. have reduced the number of cigarettes smoked each year by 2% (54). A legitimate concern about instituting a workplace smoking policy has always been employee reaction. One study of employees working in medium-sized businesses found that employees who were former smokers or never smoked wanted total bans. Employees who were smokers wanted designated areas. Preferences aside, all employees perceived smoking and environmental smoke as hazardous to health (55). What an excellent foundation to build upon when implementing a workplace smoking policy—the elimination of a documented health hazard.

Fitness/Aerobics

Sixty percent of U.S. adults are inactive or underactive, making the prevalence for inactivity more than twice that of smoking (56). Moreover, American Sports Data, Inc. *(Americansportsdata.com)* estimates that just 20% of the population performs one physical activity 100 times a year. That is down from 23% in 1990. The more this country is faced with a decline in physical activity, the more evidence there is that physical activity has proven health benefits. It has been shown that physical activity markedly reduces risk for endometrial cancer (57), brings about a 20% reduction in risk for breast cancer (58), and reduces one's risk of developing diabetes by 59% (59). Higher levels of physical activity have been associated with reduced incidence of coronary artery disease (CAD) (60), and all-cause mortality is 3.4 times greater for the least fit men and 4.6 times greater for the least fit women (61). There is also the impact on osteoporosis, asthma, depression, and stress. Evidence also exists that exercisers cost less in health care expenditures. A study of all participants in the University of Kentucky Wellness Program found that exercisers had an average health care claim of $207 vs. the average claim of $266 for nonexercisers (62). Yet, in spite of the documented linkages, most Americans are still not active. The workplace can make a significant contribution to this national dilemma by making exercise convenient and accessible for the "already exercising" as well as providing the motivation and support for nonexercisers to engage in a regular program.

The goal of a fitness/aerobics component is to improve cardiovascular fitness, increase strength, and improve flexibility. The psychosocial benefits, as well as improved morale, attitude, and productivity, also cannot be overlooked. To implement a fitness program, it is not necessary to have a fully equipped on-site facility. There can be on-site group exercise classes and walking routes, negotiated rates at quality community facilities, and financial incentive programs as alternatives. When establishing financial incentives, be sure that the criteria are clearly communicated and that simple administrative processes have been established.

Regardless of where employees exercise, individual exercise routines should be tailored to the needs of the person and of sufficient intensity and duration to be beneficial to health (63). Exercise screening (risk factor review, personal health history, heart rate, blood pressure, and cholesterol) is recommended before entry into any program, with additional testing (submaximal or maximal exercise electrocardiography) as indicated by a protocol that quantifies risk factors. Exercise testing can be conducted using a bicycle ergometer with results guiding the development of a safe and beneficial exercise program. For more detailed information about screening and testing, refer to the American College of Sports Medicine (ACSM) Guidelines publication listed in the Further Information section.

Aside from implementing the strategies for exercise itself, there is an important educational component. Employees need to understand the benefits of regular exercise and they need help with self-efficacy, self-regulation, and outcome expectations so that there will be better adherence to a regular exercise program. Individuals attending four 1-hour sessions that enhance those three constructs showed statistically significant improvement pre- to postprogram (64). This suggests that this type of social-cognitive intervention is worth consideration.

Finally, better studies of work-site exercise programs are needed. A 1998 review of 26 studies involving nearly 9,000 subjects concluded that the typical work-site program has yet to demonstrate an increase in physical fitness/physical activity. The studies were viewed as having poor scientific quality based on design and validity of measures (65). As professionals, that is an acceptable empirical conclusion, but as practitioners we need to ask some hard questions. Are the proper techniques being used to reach nonexercisers? Are we encouraging exercise or merely supporting membership? Are we building a culture that supports and rewards exercise?

Although coordinating a fitness program is resource intensive, the well-documented physical, social, and emotional benefits make that resource investment worthwhile.

Eating Habits/Nutrition/Cholesterol

What do Americans think about healthful eating? What should they be eating? A telephone survey of 800 consumers conducted by the American Dietetic Association provides an answer to the first question. The survey found that 40% of Americans believe that a nutritious diet is important but report not following one, 30% report having made significant dietary improvements, and 30% are not concerned about healthful eating (66). The second question is not easily answered but there are certainly many guides and resources. One such resource is "Dietary Guidelines for Americans, 2000" (67), released by the U.S. Department of Agriculture and the Department of Health and Human Services in May 2000, which recommends exercise, includes expanded food pyramids, calls for smaller servings, emphasizes attention to calories, and directs attention to fat consumption no matter what that fat is called.

The messages are strong—there is a great deal to do in this area. People don't recognize the importance of healthy eating; they face many barriers to the adoption of a nutritious diet, and they are confused about the messages. The challenge is clear—educate about the benefits, help with skills building to transcend barriers, and simplify the messages.

Reports from the National Heart, Lung, and Blood Institute (NHLBI), dietary guidelines of the National Cancer Society, and results of several clinical investigations support the role of nutritional programs as a pathway to reducing preventable illness. In addition, specific work-site studies add to the body of knowledge about what to do and why:

- **Go beyond "education only" programming**—502 employees at eight work sites in the Denver area were randomized by site into three groups, each of which was offered a different level of intervention. There were four education-only (printed materials and lunch and learn) sites; there were two group nutrition sites; and there were two self-paced nutrition program sites. Employees at the group nutrition sites and the self-paced program sites modified their behaviors and related risks greater than the employees at the "education only" sites (68).
- **Include learning sessions to examine predisposing factors, enabling factors, and stages of change**—The Next Step Trial studied three psychosocial constructs (predisposing factors, enabling factors, and stages of change) to determine their relationship to the intake of fats, fiber, fruits, and vegetables. The results showed strong, statistically significant relationships between all of the constructs for fat and fiber intake (69).
- **Incorporate environmental interventions**—A 3-year study of nutrition-related environmental interventions at 55 work sites found that employees improved eating practices and reported feeling better as compared to employees at 56 work sites where there were no environmental interventions. The intervention included more fruits and vegetables and meals lower in fat in the cafeteria, as well as labeled snacks in the vending machines (70). In addition to the improved eating practices, the employees at the intervention sites reported more positive perceptions about access to healthy food and information, coworker encouragement, and management concern.

General nutrition and healthy eating habits aside, cholesterol has had a central position in the context of the healthy eating controversy for years. NHLBI initiated a National Cholesterol Education Program in 1985 to increase public awareness of cholesterol as a risk factor. Results of the MRFIT study substantiated that levels of cholesterol above 180 mg/100 mL needlessly increase the risk of coronary heart disease (CHD) among middle-aged American men (71). The Framingham Study confirmed that relationship, noting that when plasma cholesterol levels increase, so does the incidence of CHD (72). Most recently a published review of three studies that had tracked 82,000 males for three decades revealed that the men with high cholesterol (240 and above) were two to three times more likely to die from a heart disease–related death than men with a cholesterol reading of 200 or below (73). Led by decades of research, it is clear that we cannot forget about cholesterol/total fat education. However, recent wisdom suggests that the messages be simplified so that program participants understand more easily how to adopt low fat eating patterns.

Weight Management

Approximately one in two U.S. adults is overweight or obese, representing a 25% increase over the past three decades. The National Health and Nutrition Examination Survey (NHANES III) of 16,884 adults determined that 63% of men and 55% of women had a body mass index (BMI) of 25 or greater. Further, analysis of the survey documented that the prevalence of two or more chronic conditions increased as the severity of obesity increased (74). Increased severity of obesity is specifically associated with high risk for and prevalence of hypertension, type II and gestational diabetes, cardiovascular disease, gallbladder disease, osteoporosis, large birth weight babies, and certain cancers (71,74,75).

Another view of overweight and obesity comes from a study conducted by the Centers for Disease Control and Prevention (CDC). A telephone survey of 100,000 adults was conducted and as a result the CDC concluded that 17% of adult Americans are obese and 50% overweight. Based on these findings, it is estimated that obesity alone increased 50% between 1991 and 1998 (76).

Today obesity is of great concern and is noted to be the second leading preventable cause of death after smoking (77). The strong recommendation that obesity and overweight be treated aggressively is a call to action.

There is no single approach to weight management. Participants tend to lose weight if they first understand their own eating patterns and the influences upon those patterns and then learn how to modify those patterns without getting into a cycle of deprivation. Given behavioral counseling, necessary support, and long-term follow-up, the chances for success are enhanced. External motivation such as wanting to look better is sometimes adequate to initiate weight loss; however, internal motivation is the prime determinant for maintenance of weight loss. The combination of caloric restriction and exercise seems to work best, as long as psychosocial and cultural influences are not ignored (78). Furthermore, in light of the dramatic increase in obesity and the associated burden of the comorbidities, work-site programs should consider incorporating clinical oversight and a pharmacologic agent.

Blood Pressure

Screening for hypertension is not new to occupational health. In fact, work-site treatment and education programs have been shown to be more effective in achieving compliance and reduction of health care costs than treatment by any other type of community-based program. Specifically, studies have found that the workplace is a useful setting for hypertension management and that screening, case identification, and referral, linked to rigorous work-site follow-up, achieves optimal blood pressure control (79). A structured educational component is an essential adjunct to any hypertension detection and treatment program. Hypertension control requires adequate diagnosis and appropriate follow-up. Screening for hypertension often lacks strong educational and follow-up elements, in which case participants do not seek the necessary diagnostic tests and treatment required to achieve control. Provision of follow-up care that includes behavioral contracting and support groups enhances compliance in 70% to 80% of cases (80).

Using reliable criteria and protocols, organizations can easily provide routine treatment for employees with high blood pressure, while continuing to ensure that a relationship with the primary care provider is maintained. A periodic visit to an occupational health professional provides the opportunity for accurate monitoring coupled with counseling about diet, exercise, weight control, and stress management that can complement the care and treatment of the employee's personal physician.

Stress Management

Health risk appraisals (HRAs) and other stress assessment tools are readily available to employers as a way to quantify stress in the population. While the HRA indicates the degree to which stress is a high, moderate, or low risk in the population, other stress assessment tools help to further define employee stress. Do employees experience more stress on the job, at home, or socially? Do employees have and practice appropriate coping skills? Are employees experiencing associated physical and emotional symptoms? Armed with this information, a wide variety of programs can be planned that address stress and stress management.

These programs are integral to any comprehensive health promotion program and are highly sought interventions by employees and managers alike. More importantly it is of value to address stress due to the proven associations with many illnesses and higher health care costs. Stress potentially plays a role in cardiovascular disease, asthma, skin disorders, and peptic ulcer, among others; and individuals at high risk for stress have health care costs 46% higher that those at low risk (19). Effective stress management techniques can improve employees' ability to cope with stress, improve their sense of well-being, and reduce the likelihood of stress-related symptoms. See Chapter 28 for a detailed description of stress and appropriate interventions.

Employee Assistance

The prevalence of alcohol abuse among employee populations has been estimated to be between 5% and 10% (81). In addition, 20% of the adult population suffers from various types of psychiatric disorders that would benefit from treatment (81). Depression costs the economy $44 billion annually, $24 billion of which is due to lost workdays. It is the primary diagnosis in up to 20% of disability claims and is the secondary diagnosis in up to 65% of disability claims (82). Furthermore, it is known that individuals at high risk for depression have health care costs that are 70% higher than those at low risk for depression (19). These significant problems can best be addressed by the incorporation of an employee assistance program (EAP) into the company suite of services. EAPs have emerged as a viable strategy for early detection, short-term counseling, appropriate referral, and follow-up. For alcohol-related issues, most EAPs work closely with self-help groups (e.g., Alcoholics Anonymous and Al-Anon), inpatient psychiatric services, and intensive outpatient programs. Referrals to EAPs can originate from management, peers, family members, or the medical community. Yet, most EAPs report that approximately half of the people are self-referred.

Establishing an EAP needs to begin with a clear policy statement regarding how emotional/behavioral problems will be addressed. Guidelines for participation need to be developed at the same time. Voluntary participation that ensures confidentiality is essential. Case management practices as well as the responsibilities of the employee need to be clearly articulated.

A counselor can be made available in several ways. Small companies can contract with a mental health practitioner or organization to provide service either on- or off-site. Often this service is on a per capita basis; however, a fee-for-service arrangement can also be made. Larger companies may find it more cost-effective to hire their own staff, and indeed this may add value because the internal resource may better understand company and management issues. Unionized companies have found it advantageous to make the EAP a joint labor/management initiative. Not only can a collaborative effort support relations between the union and the company, but also it may foster participation.

Other EAP components can be valuable adjuncts to the existing secondary prevention strategies. Lectures and seminars on aging, child rearing, change, violence, relationships, career conflicts, and communications are excellent primary prevention initiatives. In addition to enhancing psychological and emotional well-being, seminars that address self-esteem, assertiveness, commitment, and self-efficacy also enhance employees' ability to make effective health behavior change.

It is important to keep in mind and to prepare management for the fact that a good EAP will and should increase alcohol-, drug-, and mental health–related claims. The increase is generally noted within the same quarter as the first EAP contact, and there is a probability of increased claims expenditures for the following 11 quarters (83). In the end, that is a small price to pay for the avoidance of more significant claims in the future.

Employee assistance programs, as an integral part of an organization's occupational health services, contribute to the productivity and bottom line of the business, as well as to the well-being of both the employee and the company.

Demand Management

During the last decade, employers, motivated by the desire to improve health care utilization patterns and contain health care costs, have incorporated medical self-care and consumer empowerment activities into the scope of work-site programs. The primary goal of demand management is to control medical care costs by enhancing the participants' sense of responsibility for their own health and health care decisions (78), unlike health promotion, which has as its primary goal the improvement of health. In the context of demand management, health improvement is a secondary benefit.

More specifically, demand management interventions support the needs of employees at the point along the health continuum where they are faced with the symptoms, diagnosis, and treatment of illness and injury. They strive to:

- reduce unnecessary heath care utilization,
- encourage appropriate treatment decisions,
- eliminate delays in seeking appropriate medical care, and
- reduce the severity and discomfort of symptoms.

The most prevalent forms of demand management now included as part of work-site programming are toll-free health advice lines, medical self-care texts, prenatal care, presurgery counseling, case management for select illnesses or injuries known to generate high medical costs, and health consumer education. Each of these interventions, if carefully selected based on known health care costs and utilization, has great potential for short-term savings, a real plus in the mix of programs that generally yield long-term cost savings. Specifically, there have been reports of a 10% to 20% reduction in costs related to physician visits and emergency room (ER) utilization (84).

Employers should exercise great caution when implementing demand management to select a quality vendor and work with their health plans to ensure that there is no duplication of effort. These programs are extremely supportive of the needs of employees and their families when facing symptoms, illness/injury, and care decision making.

Disease Management

Disease management, like demand management, has become popular as a work-site program within the past decade and similarly has the potential to yield short-term savings if appropriately targeted and implemented. These interventions are designed to support the needs of employees at the point along the health continuum where they have been diagnosed with and are living with a chronic disease. Today 70% of medical care spending is caused by preventable illness (85), so it reasonably follows that there is tremendous potential to impact health care costs in the process of helping to manage chronic disease. The goal of disease management is to prevent progression and complications of the disease and to help individuals maintain optimal quality of life.

Back Care programs are a good example and have evolved over the years from educational sessions, to "back schools" (exercise-based), to chronic condition initiatives, and for good reason. Back pain is the second most common reason for work absence in the United States, with *work-related costs* of approximately $11 billion annually (86). It is estimated that the *total cost* of work-related back pain in the United States was $49.2 billion in 1992, representing 34% of all direct and indirect costs for occupational injuries (87). Studies of earlier program strategies have been equivocal as it relates to cost-effectiveness and lasting health behavior change (88); yet, there is evidence that an exercise intervention (eight 1-hour classes) does improve self-reported disability due to back pain (89). Thus, it is not unreasonable to implement a more integrated educational, exercise, pain management, and support strategy to help individuals manage and cope with the chronicity of back problems.

A diabetes intervention is another good example. Diabetes affects 5% to 10% of Americans and is estimated to cost $45 billion in direct and $47 billion in indirect expenditures. Health care costs (1992 dollars) for a person with diabetes averages $11,157 annually compared to $2,600 for a person without diabetes (90). Findings suggest that incorporation of individual counseling, exercise, and weight loss are important:

- **Individual counseling**—First Chicago, National Bank Division, studied employees who met monthly with a health educator. After 3 months, blood glucose, glycohemoglobin and hemoglobin A_{1C} all showed a significant decline as compared to baseline levels (90).
- **Exercise**—1,200 men with type 2 diabetes were followed for 12 years. The findings revealed that the men in the low-fit group were more than twice as likely to die as compared with the men in the high-fit group (91).
- **Weight loss**—618 overweight adults between 30 and 50 years of age were followed for 16 years. At the end of the 16 years, those individuals that had lost between 8 and 15 pounds had a risk for diabetes that was 33% lower than those who had not lost weight, and those who had lost greater than 15 pounds had a risk 51% lower. This study suggests that losing just 1 to 2 pounds a year and keeping it off reduces one's risk of diabetes (92).

Asthma, depression, and CAD are also popular as disease management programs and worth consideration, again if the conditions are prevalent, costly, and driving excessive utilization in the targeted population.

Environmental and Organizational Interventions

The programs that have been highlighted thus far are those with an individual focus, although the importance of environmental interventions has been punctuated for smoking, healthy eating, and exercise interventions.

We now briefly address the controversy about self-responsibility for health versus social responsibility (2). Some maintain that the health promotion landscape today exemplifies the continuing tension between stressing personal responsibility and improving the social and environmental context (3). While there is a tendency to hold individuals responsible for their health because of the role that personal health behaviors play in accidents, illness, and premature death, the social context cannot be ignored. Consider the notable health disparities by socioeconomic status and race as an example. It is maintained by Minkler (2) that encouraging individual change can have only limited impact because (a) maintenance of positive health behaviors is difficult, and (b) the trend curve for disease keeps moving. Therefore, she urges a balanced approach to programming inclusive of broader social and environmental interventions.

In consideration of the importance of both environmental and organizational interventions, work-site health professionals are urged to work diligently with management to incorporate the "culture of health" in the workplace and to investigate workplace practices that have an impact on employee health and well-being.

Management support is key. Indeed it is the foundation for a workplace culture of health. Strong and unwavering management support that does not wane in light of business pressures results in high participation rates and counters program attrition. It contributes to a positive psychosocial work environment that is known to impact employee health behaviors. In this type of work environment, employees feel valued, have a sense of job control, are satisfied with the process of work itself, and perceive that management has a positive view of health (34).

There are three studies worth noting that further help to support consideration of organizational interventions:

- The architects of a study at Pacific Lumber Company considered decreased absenteeism, tardiness, and health care costs/utilization as organizationally valued outcomes. This study concluded that there is an impact on organizational commitment as a result of the employer's demonstrated interest in employee health and well-being. However, absence and tardiness are not impacted. Yet, when there is a positive perception of the job itself, job stress, supervision, job security, and the work environment, organizational commitment as well as absence and tardiness are significantly impacted (3). The study suggests the value of working with management to improve the system of work as part of a work-site health promotion effort.
- Twenty companies in western New York participated in a quasi-experimental study. The companies were divided into experimental and comparison companies, with the experimental companies receiving the intervention. The intervention, targeting HR managers, was a specially designed training seminar, and the goal was to increase organizational support for employee heart health programs. The experimental companies reported a fourfold difference in organizational support over the comparison companies (93).
- There is evidence, based on a study conducted by the Department of Health/Exercise Sciences at the University of Delaware, that health promotion programs do not significantly impact job satisfaction. Job design and the psychosocial aspects of the work environment are noted to be influential (94). As was suggested as a result of the findings from the Pacific Lumber Company's study, it is of value to work with management to improve the system of work, in this case specifically job design and the psychosocial aspects of work.

It is apparent that the organizational domain presents a significant challenge to work-site health promotion professionals. There is a need for more involvement and research in this area that calls for collaboration across health professionals, management experts, and academics. Environmental and organizational interventions are not as easy to integrate, but should not be lost to the myriad of interventions designed for the individual. Let us commit to being diligent in our efforts to balance that landscape of programming mentioned earlier.

Other Programs of Interest

There are several other programs that have proven merit as part of work-site programs. They are viable considerations depending on the interests of employees and management.

Flu Vaccine Program

Many companies now offer flu vaccines to employees on an annual basis. The goal is to impact absence due to flu and flu-related illness. Therefore, the more employees who are immunized the greater the impact. It has been proven that the predictors of acceptance for flu vaccination are perceived effectiveness of the vaccine, the unlikelihood of side effects, and previous vaccination (95). Communicating information about the need for and effectiveness of the vaccine as well as facts about side effects could positively influence participation.

Occupational Health Protection

Integrating occupational health protection as a component of health promotion has many benefits. A study of work sites in California concluded that there is a greater capacity to lower health risks, utilize the skills of an interdisciplinary team, and emphasize both the environmental and personal factors impacting health (96).

Women's Health Program

Some companies with a high percentage of female employees focus on a targeted women's health program. Breast self-care, breast exams, mammography screening, Pap smears, and gynecologic consultations are generally included. When there is a large percentage of the female population in the childbearing years, it is not unusual to find prenatal educational and exercise programs, lactation rooms, and childcare facilities on-site.

IMPLEMENTATION OPTIONS: WHAT WORKS AND WHAT DOESN'T

Having considered the rationale for programming and selected appropriate content, we now turn to implementation choices. It is time to bring the target audience to the center of planning and assure that implementation works for them. It is time to examine available resources and apply them effectively. It is time to detail implementation processes and logistics. The reality is that implementation is never complete. It is an iterative process, just like determining rationale and selecting content. Attending to the day-to-day impact of implementation and monitoring changes in the workforce and the business are essential to successful planning.

The Target Audience

For many years executives, management, and white- and pink-collar workers were the primary target for health promotion programs. Today the literature is replete with information about programs designed for special populations. There are reports of back care programs for offshore petroleum workers (97) and municipal workers (98). There are programs that target casino workers (99), police officers (100), and school personnel (101). A hypertension control program was designed for minority and unskilled employees (102), and a special program was designed to meet the needs of oil refinery employees (103). Needless to say, no two of these programs would have exactly the same implementation planning process. There is no cookie-cutter approach—one size does not fit all. The implementation team must ensure that the specific needs and interests of the population are met.

Unfortunately, it has been documented that only about 25% of programs are implemented in response to the explicit needs and views of employees (104). This fact serves as a driver to investigate the potential for forming employee partnerships and utilizing employees in responsible roles. Three studies emphasize the possibilities that exist for working with employees as program advisors and implementation coordinators:

- The Working Well Trial had an interest in understanding the characteristics of employee groups (employee advisory boards, EABs) that contribute to their success. They found group autonomy, management involvement, and institutionalization of programs to be critical factors (105).
- The Treatwell 5-a-Day study used EABs to implement a nutrition program with great success. The EABs were able to adapt the program to the site and gain management support. The number of events directly correlated to the number of hours spent by the EAB members, and the resulting behavior change within the employee population at the intervention sites as compared to the control sites was favorable. Employees at the intervention sites reported a 19% increase in their consumption of fruits and vegetables as compared to a 7% increase at the control sites (106).
- The Arizona 5-a-Day Peer Health Education Program was designed for public sector labor and trade employees. The program goal was to achieve a lasting change in fruit and vegetable consumption among multicultural employees. Peer health educators, a cadre of informal opinion leaders, were used to influence behavioral norms and disseminate tailored messages. They met with employees one-on-one, in small groups, and in large groups. Knowledge, attitudes, and consumption were impacted; there was a change in the normative environment, and contacts continued even after the program ended (107).

The time and effort that it takes to involve employee groups pay off. It requires training and a system to monitor activities and impact, but there is no doubt that the end result is worth the investment.

Again, depending on the business, planners may need to factor in the needs of employees in remote work locations, shift workers, and telecommuters. Additionally, the employee's family and company retirees should be considered because they contribute significantly to the company's health care expenditures. Families can provide support for employee behavior change, while a focus on retirees can influence their lifestyle, health risks, and in turn the high demand they place on the health care system.

The subject of targeting the population and meeting the needs of the audience also requires discussing motivational readiness/stages of change (108,109). The first attempt at conceptualizing the process of change was in the 1960s when the process was described as a sequence of knowledge change, then attitude, and then practice. Around the same time, diffusion of innovation with its five stages of adoption—innovation development, dissemination, adoption, implementation and maintenance—was conceptualized, followed by the notion of behavioral intention—one intends to engage in a behavior or one intends not to engage in a behavior. In the early 1970s, the health behavior adoption model was a one-stage model that predicted behavioral intentions based on selected beliefs. In the late 1970s and early 1980s that model was adapted and six stages, each with its own counterforces and supporting factors, were delineated: interest, awareness, evaluation, decision, behavioral trial, and establishment of a habit. During that same time frame (late 1970s/early 1980s), Prochaska and Velicer (110) conceptualized the transtheoretical model with five stages of change—precontemplation, contemplation, readiness, action, and maintenance. In the context of these five stages of change, the authors acknowledged the constructs that mediate readiness (self-efficacy, decisional balance, cognitive processes, behavioral processes) and recognized the concepts of counterforces and support factors. Many studies, too numerous to mention here, have examined the application of the stages of change to adoption of a behavior and have clearly documented the associations with risk for heart disease (111), adoption of a moderate-intensity exercise program, stopping smoking, and making a dietary change (109). Given this extensive body of knowledge and research, professionals would be remiss not to assess employee readiness to change and tailor interventions accordingly. We would also be remiss not to have great respect for the process of changing a health behavior. It is difficult, it is longitudinal, and it is lifelong.

Program Resources

How will the program be staffed? How will the program be funded? Should incentives be used? What might be gained from working with the company's managed care plans?

Staffing

Selecting staff may be as easy as turning over programming to existing staff that has the essential skills, or it could be as difficult as hiring a new staff or selecting qualified vendors, or both. Do not assume capability based on credentials and referrals, but screen to specific criteria, assuring that experience and knowledge are substantive and that effective interpersonal, writing, presenting, and management skills exist. Select vendors on the basis of details presented in a Request for Information (RFI) and a Request for Proposal (RFP), and once selected ensure that contracts are carefully negotiated and measurable performance specifications are in place.

Funding

Adequate resources are required if the program is to be a success. A poorly implemented program on a shoestring budget is very different from a cost-effective program. If a budget allocation will compromise the quality of the intervention, it is recommended that the pros and cons of implementation be carefully weighed. A solid business case is generally a must in today's business environment and increases the chance of securing a reasonable budget allocation. Stakeholders may fund ongoing planning and development activities, yet when it comes to implementation there are options:

1. Management pays full costs. Inherent to this approach is the fact that management supports employee health and stands to benefit from both the health care cost savings and the human resource aspects of the program.
2. Employees pay full costs. They too stand to benefit from increased levels of health and well-being.
3. Costs are shared. Under this arrangement all parties who stand to benefit make a financial commitment, setting up a win-win situation.

Incentives

Motivating participation and health behavior change are the stated goals of an incentive offering. What follows is the assumption that the participation and initial behavior change efforts will lead to the adoption of a positive lifestyle on a long-term basis. Everything from shoelaces and water bottles to wellness days and financial incentives has been used as program incentives. And while this strategy has met with short-term success, there is ongoing controversy about the efficacy of incentives. There is research that indicates that external reinforcers are not effective and may even have potential negative consequences (112). This research advances the notion that external prods may undermine internal motivation, which is ultimately the foundation for sustained healthy behaviors. Given the controversy, it is clear that more research is needed in this area. For now, practitioners are at least cautioned to "do no harm" (112). The way to address that concern is to implement incentives with great caution. It is important to (a) establish clear criteria that potentially allows all participants to "win" at some level, (b) communicate openly and directly, and (c) have a simple and efficient tracking process in place. And by far the greatest caution is to avoid anything that can in any way be perceived by the employees as a negative, coercive incentive. Any incentive process viewed as negative will foster mistrust and damage the credibility of the program. While the incentive may drive the achievement of high participation and accomplishment of an immediate goal, it could be at a very high price.

The Role of Managed Care

Managed care health plans, having health as a fundamental plan tenet, have emerged recently as players in work-site health promotion. First some facts about managed care. Three-fourths of Americans are covered by managed care. Managed care spending for prevention is 4% to 5% on the average and in some cases as low as 1%. Managed care spending for health promotion averages from $2 to $6 per member per year with three fourths of the plans doing minimal health promotion (8). Yet, employers increasingly conclude that health promotion is a service of the managed care plans and that internal resource commitment is a duplication of effort. To counter this position, occupational health professionals need to understand the current scope and efficacy of the plan services.

A recent survey of HMOs found that:

- 63% offer classes,
- 77% use newsletters,
- 73% provide brochures,
- there is no targeting of programs to those with greatest need, and
- cardiovascular risks are the most common topics.

The conclusion of the researchers was that the current state of health promotion in managed care is insufficient to meet its promise of prevention. Furthermore, they recommend that employers lobby for inclusion of more health promotion criteria in Health Employer Data and Information Set (HEDIS), and for health insurance discounts for employers offering company-sponsored programs, making the depth of the discounts commensurate with the comprehensiveness of the program (8). Another viable strategy is to have specific annual performance objectives for prevention/health promotion written into the managed care contracts.

Program Logistics

Scheduling

It is often difficult, based on the needs and nature of the business, to select times for lectures, classes, screenings, special events, and counseling sessions. Seeking balance between the needs of the business and convenience and access for the employees is one way to guide decision making. Times for sessions and appointments may range from 6 a.m. when drivers pickup vehicles at a central garage to 10:30 p.m. when third-shift employees arrive at the plant. Scheduling during break time, lunchtime, before work, and after work ensures maximal access. However, the optimal time may be during work hours, primarily because of the strong message of organizational support and commitment that this sends. Finally, nontraditional time frames should be considered, such as Saturday morning at the ballpark or Sunday afternoon at the company picnic.

Location

Location, long recognized as the number one variable in real estate, is equally important in the context of program implementation. If programs target special populations, their churches, clubs, and community centers may afford the greatest appeal. If programs are for telecommuting or virtual office employees, reaching them in the home via print, Web sites, and audiovisual material may work best. These methods would work equally as well for retirees, as would an intervention at their senior citizen clubs. No longer is the work-site classroom or clinic the location of choice. The plant floor, the entrance to the cafeteria, and the break room are locations that enhance opportunities for health-related learning, discussions, and monitoring. When considering location, adhere to the paramount rule: "Meet them where they are."

EVALUATING THE EFFECTIVENESS OF HEALTH PROMOTION

General Characteristics

The scope of the program evaluation and the level of analysis vary depending on the setting and available resources. Nonetheless, the evaluation component should be developed at the beginning of the program when considering the interests of all stakeholders. Carefully weigh the issues of data collection and storage, time intervals, and evaluation partners such as an academic institution, a vendor, or a managed care plan. Without an evaluation plan, the effects of a health promotion program will not be systematically measured and the ability to justify continuing a program may be lost. In addition, the data from evaluation can be used as continuous feedback for quality improvement efforts.

The design of the evaluation should be carefully considered and can range from a pre/post design to a randomized controlled study. The prevailing wisdom today suggests that evaluations require more rigor and that studies at the minimum must employ a quasi-experimental design and at best call for experimental designs with randomized controls (8). Larger scale studies are needed to provide more conclusive evidence of the value of health promotion.

Goals and objectives for both the program and the evaluation must be clearly stated. Management may be interested in lowering costs and rates of absenteeism; occupational health professionals may be most concerned with reducing risk factors and impacting morbidity and mortality. The evaluation plan, therefore, should reflect a consensus, with stated goals that satisfy the interest of all concerned parties. Evaluations can be focused on measures of process, impact, and outcomes (113).

Process evaluation measures the participant's perception of the program. A logical indicator of program success is participation numbers and percentages. Beyond the numbers, process evaluation provides information about what was helpful and what was not, what should be changed and how, and what could be improved. It is important to acknowledge that there is little correlation between positive perceptions and change in health risk. For example, although participants in a high blood pressure program may find the information valuable, attend regularly, and rate the instructor highly, their blood pressure may not be lower at the end of the program. Nevertheless, such measures are useful and may be the earliest source of program feedback that can easily formulate a story for management.

Impact evaluation measures the extent to which an intervention has had an immediate effect on biometric measures and risk factors. These measures are more objective than those obtained in process evaluation, as they can indeed be observed or measured. Impact evaluation is more difficult and expensive to conduct, as it encompasses measures such as blood pressure, cholesterol, weight, body fat, and HRA risk factors. Self-reported behaviors that influence risk analysis as a measure of impact should be used with caution. Although the behaviors are a measure of impact, the more reliable way of assessing impact is through direct observation, which is obviously more labor and resource intensive.

Outcome evaluation determines the effect of interventions on the company or employee population as a whole. It measures subsequent consequences in terms of quality of life and economic benefits from the physiologic and psychological changes (114). Health status improvements as measured by changes in morbidity and mortality, and social benefits as measured by improved quality of life are examples of outcomes. Reduced health care costs, reduced absenteeism, fewer on-the-job accidents, and improved employee morale (based on factor analysis) are essential indicators. A major caution of designing outcome evaluation is that beneficial effects may take years to detect.

In consideration of a template for evaluation, there is a guide recently developed and released by the CDC entitled "A Framework for Program Evaluation" (115). The framework was developed to be a practical resource for public health professionals and serve as a tool with potential to bring some consistency to evaluation efforts. The framework has six steps and four standards as follows:

Steps	Standards
Engage stakeholders	Utility—evaluation users are satisfied
Describe the program	Feasibility—evaluation is practical
Focus the evaluation design	Propriety—evaluation is ethical
Gather credible information	Accuracy—evaluation is correct
Justify conclusions	
Ensure that lessons learned are shared	

The CDC wants to advance this framework with the goal of achieving optimal evaluations, specifically meaning that all steps and standards are included in any evaluation activity.

Remember to be alert for confounding factors that may affect the measures of interest. For example, revisions in the medical benefits plan, a labor strike, changes in the workforce, and fluctuating business demands all have an effect. Changes in the local community and national events can also influence employee health practices and in turn influence both the impact and outcome evaluation. The influence of the media and national educational campaigns needs to be recognized, especially if there is a measurable impact that is unexplained by the scope of the company's interventions.

Specific Program Evaluation Considerations

Preventive Screenings

Evaluating an on-site screening is very straightforward. The particular measure of interest is recorded as well as rates of participation and employees' satisfaction with the process. In the case of abnormal findings, tracking follow-up action taken is valuable, and finally the actual measure of impact is best reflected through another screening after 6 or 12 months. If participation in a screening is representative of the employee population, overall results afford program managers the opportunity to compare their population to known norms for a particular measure and determine a course of action. For example, 55% of the workforce at a site attended a glucose screening, and 14% of the attendees presented with an elevated blood sugar. Assuming an expected 8% to 10% with positive findings, further investigation of this risk and action planning can be initiated.

Smoking Cessation

The impact of smoking cessation interventions is among the easiest to evaluate because there is one essential immediate measure of success: Did the participant stop smoking by the end of the program? However, continued abstinence after 18 to 24 months is the true measure of success. While individuals generally self-report accurately about their smoking habits, biochemical measures can be used to validate self-report. Carboxyhemoglobin, urinary cotinine, and salivary thiocyanate can indicate the presence and degree of smoking. Associated morbidity and mortality, comparing smokers and nonsmokers, can also be monitored as a measure of outcome.

Fitness/Aerobics Exercise

For fitness/aerobics programs, the measures of interest are improved cardiovascular endurance, strength, and flexibility. Cardiovascular fitness is measured by resting blood pressure and heart rate as well as estimation of maximal oxygen uptake. Measures of strength and flexibility are estimated by using simple grip and sit and reach tests. Percentage of body fat, body weight, total serum cholesterol, and high-density lipoprotein (HDL) can also be used as impact indicators. Long-term morbidity and mortality, particularly for cardiovascular disease, are outcomes of interest. Remember to capture participation data as well because it tells a very strong story about the ability of the program to bring in first-time exercisers and to get regular exercisers to increase the time commitment to and the intensity of exercise.

Eating Habits/Nutrition/Cholesterol

Are employees eating healthier? That's the bottom line. The impact of nutrition interventions is reflected best by changes in dietary habits and biometric indicators. Analysis of pre- and post-dietary intake records allow evaluators to determine if actual changes in eating have taken place relative to intake of fruits and vegetables, fat, fiber, salt, sugars, and total calories. Given the major impact of serum cholesterol as a risk factor for CHD, the biometric measurement of interest is the lipid profile. Attention should be given to the variability of lipid measurements and, when comparisons over time are being made, similar analytic devices should be used to ensure comparability of results. Again, analogous to smoking cessation results, success is a program by-product only when changes in eating behavior and positive changes in blood lipids are maintained over time.

Weight Management

Body mass index (BMI) and body fat are more useful indicators of normal weight/overweight/obesity than total weight, since these values consider height, weight, body frame and muscle mass in the equation. Based on the earlier discussion about a more comprehensive approach to weight management, tracking associated clinical measures and understanding the status of any comorbidity, as well as the individual's psychosocial context, are imperative.

Blood Pressure

Blood pressure control programs have a single-impact measure—a reduced level of blood pressure. Maintenance of reduced levels over time, using standard protocols, is the desired state. Improved self-efficacy and increased quality of life are important for the hypertensive individual living with a chronic disease. And the control efforts of individuals are assessed by their medication compliance, exercise practices, eating behaviors, and weight control. Long-term effectiveness of hypertension control is measured by the avoidance of complications such as stroke, heart attack, and renal disease and their attendant medical costs.

Stress Management

The impact of a stress management program is difficult to measure. Unlike cigarettes smoked, body weight, or blood pressure, stress does not lend itself to easy quantification. Thus, stress management programs are generally evaluated by participant self-report. Differences in pre- and post-stress assessment scores, collected using a validated instrument, provide indicators of participants' perception of their stressors; their ability to recognize physical, cognitive, and emotional responses; and their success in implementing coping strategies. Interpretations of impact need to be approached with caution.

Employee Assistance Programs

Employee assistance programs can be evaluated by measuring the functional status of individuals before and after treatment relative to their diagnosis. Further assessment can be made by analyzing absenteeism, use of the health care system, and health care costs for individuals before and after treatment. Certain impact measures, depending on the diagnosis, can be selected, such as liver function tests, urine and blood tests for the presence of substances, and rate of job turnover. Particularly in this arena, improved well-being, job performance, and quality of life are significant markers. The cost-effectiveness of EAPs can be determined by assessing the return on investment for selected outcome variables. Typical cost-benefit ratios for EAP are reported as $2.50 to $4.00 saved for every dollar invested (116) (see Chapter 28).

Demand Management

Office visits and ER utilization are examples of the measures of demand management interventions. Participation should be comparable to expected norms or better, and an assessment about care-seeking decision making is informative. In other words, are the services supporting appropriate decisions to the extent that employees and their family members are seeking care when they may have thought it was not necessary, and are they applying self-care methods when they are appropriate? Finally, perception is a key measure here, especially when employees report that they are better health care consumers and have a level of comfort that they are making good decisions about diagnostic tests, care, and treatment.

Disease Management

Targeted disease management programs for employees with a targeted diagnosis, as well as educational programs about the disease for the population in general, can be evaluated in two ways: first by specifically tracking the impact on the targeted individuals, and second by profiling the prevalence of the disease in the population and the associated inpatient, outpatient, and pharmacy costs. Obtaining information from claims and pharmacy data about related diseases can be equally helpful for selecting other disease management targets.

Environmental and Organizational Interventions

The impact of environmental strategies is reflected by changes in the particular area of interest (i.e., eating habits) and it may be difficult to tease out the relative impact when other offerings are in place. Therefore, environmental activities become part of the whole, and when changes in eating habits are measured, recognize that the environmental segment played a role in those results. For organizational interventions, if the culture is a culture of health, employees will report that the company, the management, and their co-workers support health programs and positive health behaviors. If the program is "institutionalized," employees will reflect that in reporting organizational health norms (e.g., healthy foods in the cafeteria and at meetings, acceptance by management of time taken to go to a lecture or the fitness center, etc.). Do not sell satisfaction surveys short. They can answer many questions about the quality and effectiveness of program components, and are the missing ingredient for strategy planning if overlooked. Knowing what is right for the company may be very different from doing what is right for the employees.

There are other measures, often neglected in program evaluations, that may be essential to advancing successful implementation in the future:

- Imagine that a measure of employees' perceptions of the determinants of their health behaviors is incorporated. Then, armed with that information, several sessions could be held to help employees fully understand those determinants and the impact they have on their health behaviors. Is it possible that clarity would help an employee deal more effectively with the targeted behavior change?

- Imagine that readiness levels are applied at the outset of every topic-specific program and that employees are counseled about their participation based on the results. Is it likely that participants would be more successful because they are ready for the change process?
- Imagine that self-efficacy for a given behavior is always assessed and that strategies for enhancing that construct are as much a part of the program as the behavioral skills. Is it likely that the improving confidence that the behavior can be practiced at certain times under certain conditions will be a factor for success?

THE FUTURE—FACING THE CHALLENGES AND OPPORTUNITIES

To meet the challenges and opportunities of the future, occupational health professionals need to be prepared to offer the best programs, apply the latest technology, participate in large-scale studies, and collaborate across the professional community.

Current best practices, as identified based on a systematic assessment of work-site health promotion programs (117), serve as a succinct guide to judging the strength of programs in occupational health. These practices were identified based on six criteria: (1) impact/evaluation findings, (2) effectiveness of communication, (3) comprehensiveness of programming, (4) positive incentives, (5) relationship to organizational strategy, and (6) unique and appealing program. The six best practices that emerged were as follows:

1. Program plans are linked to organizational business strategy.
2. There are effective communication strategies applied.
3. Effective (positive) incentives are offered.
4. Evaluation is conducted, results shared, and value of results communicated.
5. The environment is health supporting.
6. There is strong executive support.

Web-based technology is the answer to many of the challenges faced in the past. How do we reach families? How do we have the right information available at the right time? How do we appeal to different ages and stages with diverse health needs? The answer is the Web. Health is the largest market segment on the Web, with approximately 20,000 to 25,000 sites offering health content (118). Therefore, along with the opportunity comes the responsibility to select and promote quality services for the employees and their families. To that end, there is good news to support employers' quest for quality information on the Web. During the first quarter of 2000, 20 on-line health site companies formed a coalition and developed a set of 14 principles that when applied will help to protect consumers from false and misleading health information on the Web (119).

Evaluative studies and the findings that emerge from those studies hold the key to the future. For it is results that convince the stakeholders to continue funding, it is results that prove the value of prevention, and it is results that guide the development of new program strategies. Studies are costly but consider it an investment in the future. Look for evaluation partners, join large-scale studies, and turn to the experts for consultation about study design. Collect and analyze data that will answer the prevailing evaluation questions and at the same time use the data and feedback to continually improve programs, products, and services.

The *professional community* shares similar concerns and interests and is equally concerned about the advancement of health promotion, the audience for health promotion, the methods and strategies, and the results. By reaching out and joining together, we can collaborate to answer some key questions: Are the populations that need prevention most being reached? Are the correct concepts and theories being applied to the practice of health promotion? Are new theories evolving as a result of documented results in the workplace? Are the changes in employees' health behaviors maintained over time? Are the products and services of health promotion cost-effective and cost-beneficial? Over time these questions will be answered and in their place will be new questions. It is the collaborative efforts across the professions that will produce the richest answers.

The best of all worlds is a win-win situation for everyone concerned, where occupational health professionals see the rewarding benefits of disease prevention and health promotion, stakeholders see evidence that health promotion is a viable human resource investment, and employees have access to the resources they need to manage their health and health care.

After more than 20 years, health promotion in the work site is poised for the future. Key leaders, able to articulate a vision for the future, are forging an agenda for health promotion that includes legislative and regulatory activities, enhanced funding for research, and theoretically sound program implementation. Researchers, having learned from past studies, are prepared to support quality evaluations to advance the health promotion knowledge base. Companies are more prepared than ever to commit to prevention as the right thing to do to preserve their organization's financial and human capital.

Health promotion will continue to be propelled by the wisdom of becoming and not merely by the sense of being. It will become what we make it by applying best practices, conducting ongoing research, refining paradigms and models, and continually striving for ultimate state-of-the-art programming that emphasizes positive health behaviors, appropriate use of health care services, and vigilance in the management of chronic conditions for all.

REFERENCES

1. O'Donnell MP, Harris JS. *Health promotion in the workplace,* 2nd ed. Albany, NY: Delmar, 1994.
2. Minkler M. Personal responsibility for health? A review of the arguments and the evidence at century's end. *Health Educ Behav* 1999;26(1):121–140.
3. Donaldson SI, et al. Health behavior, quality of work life, and organizational effectiveness in the lumber industry. *Health Educ Behav* 1999;26(4):579–591.
4. Wilson MG, et al. Health promotion programs in small work sites: results of a national survey. *Am J Health Promotion* 1999;13(6):358–365.
5. Grosch JW, et al. Work-site health promotion programs in the U.S.: factors associated with availability and participation. *Am J Health Promotion* 1998;13(1):36–45.
6. Association for Work-site Health Promotion, William M. Mercer, Inc., U.S. Department of Health and Human Services—Office of Disease Prevention and Health Promotion. *1999 National Work-site Health Promotion Survey: A Report of the Findings.* 2000:1–24.
7. U.S. Department of Health and Human Services, Office of Disease Prevention and Health Promotion. *Healthy People 2010: National Health Promotion and Disease Prevention Objectives.* Washington, DC: U.S. Government Printing Office, 2000.
8. Golaszewski T. The limitations and promise of health education in managed care. *Health Educ Behav* 2000;27(4):402–416.
9. Herzlinger RE, Schwartz J. How companies tackle health care costs: Part I. *Harvard Business Rev* 1995 (July/Aug);69–81.
10. Herzlinger RE. How companies tackle health care costs. Part II. *Harvard Business Rev* 1985(Sept/Oct);108–120.
11. Herzlinger RE, Caulkins D. How companies tackle health care costs: Part III. *Harvard Business Rev* 1986 (Jan/Feb);70–80.
12. Levit K, et al. Health spending in 1998: signals of change. *Health Affairs, The Policy Journal of the Health Sphere* 2000;19(1):124–132.
13. Hewitt Associates, LLC. United States Salaried Managed Health/Health Promotion Initiatives Survey. Lincolnshire, IL, 1999.
14. Bly JL, Jones RC, Richardson JE. Impact of work-site health promotion on health care costs and utilization. *JAMA* 1986;256:3235.
15. Control Data. *Health risks and behavior: the impact on medical costs.* Minneapolis: Milliman and Robertson, 1987.
16. Musich SA, Adams L, Edington DW. Effectiveness of health promotion in moderating medical costs in the USA. *Health Promotion Int* 2000;15(1):5–15.
17. Ozminkowski RJ, et al. A return on investment evaluation of the Citibank, N.A. health management program. *Am J Health Promotion* 1999;14(1):31–43.
18. Goetzel RZ, et al. Health care costs of work-site health promotion participants and non-participants. *J Occup Environ Med* 1998;40(4):341–346.
19. Goetzel RZ, et al. The relationship between modifiable health risks and health care expenditures: an analysis of the multi-employer HERO health risk and cost database. *J Occup Environ Med* 1998;(10):843–854.
20. Whitmer RW, Goetzel RZ, Anderson DR. The HERO Study on Risks and Costs: research findings. *Art of Health Promotion* 1999;2(6):1–8.
21. Weaver MT, et al. Health risk influence on medical costs and utilization among 2,898 municipal workers. *Am J Prev Med* 1998;15(3):250–253.
22. Pelletier KR, ed. Data base research and evaluation results—a review and analysis of the health and cost effective outcome studies of comprehensive disease prevention programs. *Am J Health Promotion* 1991;5:311.
23. Pelletier KR. A review and analysis of the health and cost-effective outcome studies of comprehensive health promotion and disease prevention programs at the work-site: 1991–1993 update. *Am J Health Promotion* 1993;8(1):50–62.
24. Pelletier KR. A review and analysis of the health and cost-effective outcome studies of comprehensive health promotion and disease prevention programs at the work-site: 1993–1995 update. *Am J Health Promotion* 1996;10(5):380–388.
25. Pelletier KR. A review and analysis of the health and cost-effective outcome studies of comprehensive health promotion and disease prevention programs at the work-site: 1995–1998 update. *Am J Health Promotion* 1999;13(6):333–345.
26. Jones RC, Bly JS, Richardson JE. A study of a work-site health promotion program and absenteeism. *J Occup Med* 1990;32:95.
27. Bertera RL. The effects of workplace health promotion on absenteeism and employment costs in a large industrial population. *Am J Public Health* 1990;80:1101.
28. Centers for Disease Control. Premature mortality in the United States: public health issues in the use of the years of potential life lost. *MMWR* 1986;35[suppl 25]:1S.
29. Harris JS, Collins B, Majure IL. The prevalence of health risks in an employed population. *J Occup Med* 1986;28(3):217.
30. Spilman MA, et al. Effects of a corporate health promotion program. *J Occup Med* 1986;28:285.

31. Bellingham R, et al. Projected cost savings from AT&T Communications Total Life Concept (TLC) process. In: *Health promotion evaluation.* Stevens Point, WI: National Wellness Association, 1987, Chapter 3.
32. O'Donnell MP. Health impact of workplace health promotion programs and methodological quality of the research literature. *Art of Health Promotion* 1997;1(3):1–9.
33. Warner K, et al. Economic implications of workplace health promotion programs: a review of the literature. *J Occup Med* 1988;30:105–112.
34. Heaney CA, Goetzel RZ. A review of the health-related outcomes of multi-component work-site health promotion programs. *Am J Health Promotion* 1997;11(4):290–307.
35. Holzbach RL, et al. Effect of a comprehensive health promotion program on employee attitude. *J Occup Med* 1990;32:973.
36. Dickerson OB, Mandelbilt C. A new model for employer-provided health education programs. *J Occup Med* 1983;25(6):471.
37. National Cancer Institute. Statistics 2000. Cancer Facts and Figures. *(http://www.cancer.org).*
38. Autier P, et al. Sunscreen use and duration of sun exposure: a double-blind, randomized trial. *J National Cancer Inst* 1999;19(15):1304–1309.
39. American Medical Association Council on Scientific Affairs. Medical evaluations of healthy person. *JAMA* 1983;249:1626.
40. U.S. Clinical Preventive Services Task Force. *Guide to clinical preventive services.* Baltimore: Williams & Wilkins, 1989.
41. Michaelson JS, et al. Breast cancer: computer simulation method for estimating optimal intervals for screening. *Radiology* 1999;212(2):551–560.
42. Tilley BC, et al. The next step trial: impact of a work-site colorectal cancer screening program. *Prev Med* 1999;28(3):276–283.
43. Fitzgerald ST, Gibbons S, Agnew J. Evaluation of referral completion after workplace cholesterol screening. *Am J Prev Med* 1991;7:335.
44. Maiman LA, et al. Improving referral compliance after public cholesterol screening. *Am J Public Health* 1992;82:805.
45. National Osteoporosis Foundation. Initiatives for National Osteoporosis Month, May 2001 *(http://www.nof.orgprevention).*
46. U.S. Public Health Service. *Treating tobacco use and dependence: a clinical practice guideline.* Silver Spring, MD: Publications Clearinghouse, June 2000 *(http:www.surgeongeneral.gov).*
47. Centers for Disease Control. Cigarette smoking attributable mortality and years of potential life lost—United States, 1990. *MMWR* 1993;42:33.
48. Orleans CT, Cummings KM. Population-based tobacco control: progress and prospects. *Am J Health Promotion* 1999;14(2):83–91.
49. Koffman DM, et al. The impact of including incentives and competition in a workplace smoking cessation program on quit rates. *Am J Health Promotion* 1998;13(2):105–111.
50. Gritz ER, et al. Gender differences among smokers and quitters in the working well trial. *Prev Med* 1998;27(4):553–561.
51. Eriksen MP, Gottleib NH. A review of the health impact of smoking control at the workplace. *Am J Health Promotion* 1998;13(2):83–104.
52. Sorenson G, et al. Durability, dissemination, and institutionalization of work-site tobacco control programs: results from the Working Well Trial. *Int J Behav Med* 1998;5(4):335–351.
53. Beiner L, et al. Impact of the working well trial on the work-site smoking and nutrition environment. *Health Educ Behav* 1999;26(4):478–494.
54. Chapman S, et al. The impact of smoke-free workplaces on declining cigarette consumption in Australia and the United States. *Am J Public Health* 1999;89(7):1018–1023.
55. Mikanowicz CK, et al. Medium sized business employees speak out about smoking. *J Community Health* 1999;24(6):439–450.
56. Marcus BH, Forsyth LH. How are we doing with physical activity. *Am J Health Promotion* 1999;14(2):118–124.
57. Terry P, et al. Lifestyle and endometrial cancer risk: a cohort study from the Swedish twin registry. *Int J Cancer* 1999;82:38–42.
58. Rockhill B. A prospective study of recreational physical activity and breast cancer. *Arch Intern Med* 1999;159:2290–2296.
59. Hu FB, et al. Walking compared with vigorous physical activity and risk of type 2 diabetes in women. *JAMA* 1999;282:1433–1439.
60. Paffenberger RS, et al. Physical activity, all cause mortality, and longevity of college alumni. *N Engl J Med* 1989;314:605.
61. Blair SN, et al. Physical fitness and all cause mortality: a prospective study of healthy men and women. *JAMA* 1990;262:2395.
62. Dunnagan T, Haynes G, Noland M. Health care costs and participation in fitness programming. *Am J Health Behav* 1999;23(1):43–51.
63. McCunney RJ. The role of fitness in preventing heart disease. *Cardiovasc Rev Rep* 1985;6:776.
64. Hallam J, Petosa R. A work-site intervention to enhance social cognitive theory constructs to promote exercise adherence. *Am J Health Promotion* 1998;13(1):4–7.
65. Dishman RK, et al. Work-site physical activity interventions. *Am J Prev Med* 1998;15(4):344–361.
66. American Dietetic Association. *Nutrition and you: trends 2000.* January 2000 *(http:www.//eatright.org).*
67. U.S. Department of Agriculture and the U.S. Department of Health and Human Services. *Dietary guidelines for Americans, 2000,*5th ed. Federal Consumer Information Center (1-888-878-3256), 2000:1–40 *(http://www.usda.govcnpp).*
68. Anderson J, Dusenbury L. Work-site cholesterol and nutrition: an intervention project in Colorado. *AAOHN J* 1999;47(3):99–106.
69. Glanz K, et al. Psychosocial correlates of healthful diets among male autoworkers. *Cancer Epidemiol* 1998;7(2):119–126.
70. Campbell MK. Stages of change for increasing fruit and vegetable consumption among adults and young adults participating in the national 5-a-day for better health community studies. *Health Educ Behav* 1999;26(4):513–534.
71. Stamber J, et al. For the MRFIT Research Group. Is

the relationship between serum cholesterol and the risk of premature death from health disease continuous and graded? *JAMA* 1986;256:2823.

72. Gundy SM. Cholesterol and coronary heart disease. *JAMA* 1986;256:2849.
73. Stamler J, et al. Relationship of baseline serum cholesterol levels in 3 large cohorts of younger men to long-term coronary, cardiovascular, and all-cause mortality and to longevity. *JAMA* 2000;284(3):311–318.
74. Must A, et al. The disease burden associated with overweight and obesity. *JAMA* 1999;282(16):1523–1529.
75. American Society of Anesthesiologists. Annual Meeting of the American Society of Anesthesiologists Proceedings, October 12, 1999.
76. Mokdad AH, et al. The spread of the obesity epidemic in the United States, 1991–1998. *JAMA* 1999;282(16): 1519–1522.
77. Allison AD, et al. Annual death rates attributable to obesity in the United States. *JAMA* 1999;282(16): 1530–1538.
78. Brownell KD. Obesity: understanding and treating a serious, prevalent, and refractory disorder. *J Consult Clin Psychol* 1982;50:820.
79. Alderman MH, Lamport B. Treatment of hypertension at the workplace: an opportunity to link service and research. *Health Psychol*1988;7[suppl]:283–295.
80. Alderman M. Hypertension at the workplace. *Corporate Commentary* 1986;2:1.
81. Grant B, Noble J, Malin H. The epidemiologic catchment area program. *Alcohol Health Research World* 1985;10:68.
82. Office of the Surgeon General. *Mental health: a report of the Surgeon General.* Washington, DC: U.S. Government Printing Office, 2000. *(http://www.surgeongeneral.govlibrarymental healthhome.html).*
83. Zarkin GA, Bray JW, Qi J. The effect of Employee Assistance Programs use on healthcare utilization. *Health Serv Res* 2000;35:77–100.
84. Chapman LS. The role of demand management in health promotion. *Art of Health Promotion* 1998;2(4): 1–9.
85. Orleans CT, et al. Rating our progress in population health promotion: report card on six behaviors. *Am J Health Promotion* 1999;14(2):75–82.
86. Mahmud M, et al. Clinical management and the duration of disability for work-related low back pain. *J Occup Environ Med* 2000;42(12)1178–1187.
87. Dasinger LK, et al. Doctor proactive communication, return-to-work recommendation, and duration of disability after a Worker's Compensation low back injury. *J Occup Environ Med* 2001;43(6):515–525.
88. Symonds T. Back school or pamphlet education: which method is best for industry. *Work* 1998;10(1):49–53.
89. Moffett JK, et al. Randomised controlled trial of exercise for low back pain: clinical outcomes, costs, and preferences. *Br Med J* 1999;319:279–283.
90. Burton WN, Connerty CM. Evaluation of work-site-based patient education intervention targeted at employees with diabetes mellitus. *J Occup Environ Med* 1998;40(8):702–706.
91. Wei LW, et al. Low cardiorespiratory fitness and physical activity as predictors of mortality in men with type 2 diabetes. *Ann Intern Med* 2000;132(8):605–611.
92. Moore LL, et al. Can sustained weight loss in overweight individuals reduce the risk of diabetes mellitus. *Epidemiology* 2000;11(3):269–273.
93. Golaszewski T, Barr D, Cochran S. An organization-based intervention to improve support for employee heart health. *Am J Health Promotion* 1998;13(1):26–35.
94. Peterson M, Dunnagan T. Analysis of a work-site health promotion program's impact on job satisfaction. *J Occup Environ Med* 1998;40(11):973–979.
95. Chapman GB, Coups EJ. Predictors of influenza vaccine acceptance among healthy adults. *Prev Med* 1999; 29(4):249–262.
96. Blix A. Integrating occupational health protection and health promotion: theory and program application. *AAOHN J* 1999;47(4):168–171.
97. Maniscalco P, et al. Decreased rate of back injuries through a wellness program for offshore petroleum employees. *J Occup Environ Med* 1999;40(9):813–820.
98. Myers AH, et al. Back injuries in municipal workers: a case-control study. *Am J Public Health* 1999;89(7) 1036–1041.
99. Shaffer HJ, Vanderbilt J, Hall MN. Gambling, drinking, smoking, and other health risk activities among casino workers. *Am J Ind Med* 1999;36(3):365–378.
100. Richmond RL. How healthy are the police: a survey of life-style factors. *Addiction* 1998;93(11):1729–1737.
101. O'Loughlin J, et al. Screening school personnel for cardiovascular risk factors: short term impact on behavior and perceived role as promoters of heart health. *Prev Med*1996;25(6):660–667.
102. Fouad MN, et al. A hypertension control program tailored to unskilled and minority workers. *Ethnicity and Disease* 1997;7(3):191–199.
103. Talvi AI, Jarvisalo JO, Knuts L-R. A health promotion programme for oil refinery employees: changes of health promotion needs observed at three years. *Occup Med* 1999;49(2):93–101.
104. Harden A, et al. A systematic review of the effectiveness of health promotion interventions in the workplace. *Occup Med* 1999;49(8):540–548.
105. Linnan LA, et al. Measuring participatory strategies: instrument development for work-site populations. *Health Educ Res* 1999;14(3):371–386.
106. Hunt MK, et al. Results of employee involvement in planning and implementing the Treatwell 5-a-Day work-site study. *Health Educ Behav* 2000;27(2):223–231.
107. Buller D, et al. Implementing a 5-a-day peer health educator program for public sector labor and trade employees. *Health Educ Behav* 2000;27(2):232–240.
108. Laitakari J. On the practical applicability of stage models to health promotion and health education. *Am J Health Promotion* 1998;22(1):28–38.
109. Bock BC, et al. Motivational readiness for change: diet, exercise, and smoking. *Am J Health Behav* 1998; 22(4):248–258.
110. Prochaska JO, Velicer WF. Introduction: the transtheoretical model. *Am J Health Promotion* 1997;12(1):6–7.
111. Burn GE, Naylor P-J, Page A. Assessment of stages of change for exercise within a work-site lifestyle screening program. *Am J Health Promotion* 1999;13(3): 143–145.
112. Robison JI. To reward?—or not to reward?: questioning the wisdom of using external reinforcement in health promotion programs. *Am J Health Promotion* 1998;13(1):1–3.

113. Green LW, et al. *Health education planning: a diagnostic approach.* Palo Alto, CA: Mayfield, 1980.
114. Green LW, Lewis FM. *Measurement and evaluation in health education and health promotion.* Palo Alto, CA: Mayfield, 1986.
115. Milstein B, Wetterhall S. CDC Evaluation Working Group: a framework featuring steps and standards for program evaluation. *Health Promotion Pract* 2000;1 (3):221–228.
116. Spicer J, Owen R. *Finding the bottom line: the cost impact of employee assistance and chemical dependency programs.* Center City, MN: Hazelden Foundation, 1985.
117. O'Donnell MP, Bishop CA, Kaplan KL. Benchmarking best practices in workplace health promotion. *Art and Science of Health Promotion* 1997;1(1):1–8.
118. Gomez editorial staff. Medical Web sites: Dot-compromised security and information. Gomez Wire, Health News, February 2, 2000 *(http://www.Gomez.com).*
119. Engler N. Medical Web sites take their pulse. Gomez Wire, Health News, May 11, 2000 *(http://www.Gomez.com).*

FURTHER INFORMATION

Balady GJ, Berra KA, Golding LA, et al. *The American College of Sports Medicine (ACSM's) guideline for exercise testing and prescription*, 6th ed. Philadelphia: Lippincott Williams & Wilkins, 2000.

Cataldo MF, Coates TJ, eds. *Health and industry: a behavioral medicine approach.* New York: John Wiley & Sons, 1986.
A comprehensive text that looks at the relationship among workplace health issues, existing health promotion programs, and the application of behavioral principles in the occupational setting.

Fielding JE. *Corporate health management.* Menlo Park, CA: Addison-Wesley, 1984.
A comprehensive overview of medical issues that affect the workplace. An excellent quantification of the human and financial cost of ill health and a presentation of how to develop programs to deal with these costs.

Kezer WM. *The health workplace.* New York: John Wiley & Sons, 1986.
A practical guide written for the business leader who understands the importance of health promotion but does not know where to begin.

DeJoy D, Wilson MG. *Critical issues in work-site health promotion.* Needham Heights, MA: Allyn and Bacon, 1995.

Glanz K, Lewis FM, Rimer BK, eds. *Health behavior and health education: theory, research, and practice,* 2nd ed. San Francisco: Jossey-Bass, 1997.

Gochman D, ed. *Health behavior: emerging research perspectives.* New York: Plenum, 1988.

Green LW, Lewis FM. *Measurement and evaluation in health education and health promotion.* Palo Alto, CA: Mayfield, 1986.

Green LW, et al. *Health education planning: a diagnostic approach.* Palo Alto, CA: Mayfield, 1980.

O'Donnell MP, Harris JS, eds. *Health promotion in the workplace,* 2nd ed. Albany, NY: Delmar, 1993.

Scofield ME, ed. Work-site health promotion. *Occup Med State of the Art Rev* 1990(Oct–Dec).

Shumaker SA, Schrow EB, Ockene JK, eds. *The handbook of health behavior change.* New York: Springer, 1990.

Sloan R, Gruman J, Allegrante JP. Investing in employee health: a guide to effective health promotion in the workplace. San Francisco: Jossey-Bass, 1987.

13

Principles of Travel Medicine

Jeffrey G. Jones, Donald S. Herip, and David O. Freedman

The world is rapidly shrinking, and more people are traveling than ever before. The world tourism organization estimates that in the year 2000 approximately 700 million people traveled internationally (1). The increased numbers of international postings of workers is mirrored by an increasing number of immigrants working within the United States. For occupational medicine physicians, caring for this international workforce presents special challenges: prevention, recognition, diagnosis, and treatment of communicable diseases, but also minimizing the impact of noninfectious travel-related conditions. This chapter discusses measures for preventing both infectious and noninfectious travel-related conditions.

RISK CONSIDERATIONS

Many factors feed into the prevention equation as it relates to international travel. Geography is important, for it may introduce specific environmental hazards and may also act as an indicator of endemicity of various infectious diseases. Many risk considerations go beyond geography, however, including work activities, political climate, and the social climate of the new location. Some travel conditions are related to travel itself, such as problems associated with flying or with jet lag. The individual traveler's health plays a strong role in the individual's chances of surviving in the specific location. Chronic health conditions, immunosuppression, pregnancy, and traveling with young children also present special challenges.

IMPORTANCE OF EDUCATING THE TRAVELER

Frequently, travelers assume that risk is homogeneous worldwide. In reality, assumptions or behaviors that might be prudent at home could expose the traveler to excess risk while abroad. Food and water, which are assumed to be safe in the developed world, are a source of significant risk in the developing world. Travelers who are not aware of these differences are likely to experience health problems as a result of their ignorance. Similarly, causes of accidents vary throughout the world. In the United States, we are fortunate to have an excellent system of highways and automobiles that are generally well maintained. This is frequently not true in the developing world, where poor highways, different driving practices, and even sharing the roads with animals may present special risks. Clearly, education of international travelers is crucial to their understanding of risk differences, a prerequisite for effective prevention.

PROBLEMS ASSOCIATED WITH TRAVEL

For some travelers, travel itself presents problems. The most common problem occurs in trains upon entering a tunnel (2) or while descending during flight: *acute barotitis media.* This condition results from an imbalance of pressure such that there is a negative pressure in the middle ear (3). Approximately 2% to 10% of flyers, because of problems with eustachian tube dysfunction, allergy symptoms, or upper respiratory infections, have trouble equalizing the pressure in the middle ear (4). Symptoms of ear blockage, followed by pain, tinnitus, vertigo, and conductive hearing loss, occur with descent of the aircraft. Resolution of such symptoms may take several weeks. Barotitis may be prevented through maneuvers that increase the pressure in the middle ear. Swallowing, yawning, chewing, Valsalva's maneuver (holding the nose closed and blowing into the nose), and Frenzel maneuver (Valsalva and swallowing simultaneously) may be effective (3,5). These techniques must be done before or just as symptoms begin, for once there is a great differential pressure, it may be difficult or impossible to equalize the two pressures. The use of decongestants prior to flying decreases the incidence of barotitis (4). For patients with severe barotitis symptoms, myringotomy may be necessary (3).

Deep venous thrombosis (DVT) with associated *pulmonary embolism* is another potential risk of travel, and especially long-haul flying, where it is not unusual to fly for 15 to 16 hours at a time (6). Risk factors for DVT may be specific to the individual or to the flying environment. Factors that predispose individuals to DVT include age >40 years, pregnancy, blood disorders, malignant disease, altered blood clotting, personal or family history of DVT, recent surgery, and estrogen therapy (6). Other predisposing factors that can be specific to flying include hypobaric hypoxia, increased fluid retention in the lower extremities, increased erythropoietin levels, relative dehydration, and relative immobilization (7). DVT may be asymptomatic, but can also cause pain and swelling, and is rarely associated with pulmonary embolism. Techniques useful in preventing DVT include frequent moving around the cabin, intermittent exercising of the calf muscles, staying well hydrated, avoidance of diuretics such as alcohol and caffeine, and use of support stockings (8). For travelers at higher risk, pretravel use of aspirin may be useful (9), although there are no specific data of the efficacy of aspirin in preventing the DVT associated with flying. High-risk travelers may wish to consider low molecular weight heparin as a preventive therapy (10).

Motion sickness is the name given to the symptom complex of pallor, cold sweating, nausea, and vomiting that occurs commonly in people exposed to real or simulated unfamiliar motion. In the correct circumstances, almost everyone can be susceptible, but approximately 5% of the general population is highly susceptible (11). Ship travel is the most potent inducer of motion sickness, followed by planes, cars, and trains. For susceptible patients, the prophylactic use of medications is helpful in preventing symptoms. Oral medications that are effective for this purpose include scopolamine, 0.4 mg to 0.8 mg every 8 hours (12); cyclizine, 50 mg every 4 to 6 hours; dimenhydrinate, 50 to 100 mg every 4 to 6 hours (also available as a chewing gum); meclizine 25 to 50 mg every 24 hours; diphenhydramine 50 to 100 mg every 4 to 6 hours; buclizine, 50 mg b.i.d.; and promethazine, 12.5 to 25 mg every 8 to 12 hours (13). Although not available in United States, cinnarizine, 15 to 30 mg by mouth every 8 hours, is very popular in other parts of the world (14). Scopolamine may also be administered via a dermal preparation, with patches replaced every 72 hours. Once motion sickness is established, parenteral medications are usually required to treat symptoms. Promethazine, 12.5 to 25 mg IM every 6 to 8 hours, is often used for this purpose (13).

Nonpharmacologic treatment of motion sickness has also gained popularity. Ginger (500 to 2,000 mg by mouth every 4 hours) can be effective in preventing motion sickness, and should be considered seriously for pregnant travelers and children (15). Acustimulation (electrical stimulation of P6 acupuncture point) via a device worn like a wristwatch (Relief Band) has also shown some promise as an alternative nonpharmacologic method of reducing motion sickness symptoms (16).

Once adapted to motion, which usually takes about 3 to 4 days, the majority of travelers will not be bothered by symptoms. Upon return to preexposure environment, *mal de debarquement* may occur (17), resulting in a sensation of unsteadiness, until readaptation occurs.

Jet lag is the name given to the symptom complex associated with a mismatch between bodily systems and external environment (18). Jet lag is caused by crossing several time zones, and is most often characterized by daytime fatigue, poor sleep at destination, headache, irritability, poor concentration, gastrointestinal disorders, and reduced performance. It may last up to 5 days after arrival, and is usually more severe in the older traveler (19).

Nonpharmacologic methods that are most useful in alleviating jet leg symptoms include light therapy, exercise, and the use of social time cues. Light is the most important *zeitgeber* ("time giver"), and can be used to advantage (18). For the eastbound traveler crossing five to nine time zones, bright light should be avoided in the morning and sought in the afternoon. For travel to the west, for a similar number of time zones, afternoon and evening light should be sought. Increased physical activity during the habitual rest period is helpful in lessening jet leg symptoms, as is quickly adopting the new meal times and routines. Ensuring good rest the night prior to travel is also helpful in preventing sleep deprivation, which worsens jet lag's symptoms.

Pharmacologic options for lessening symptoms of jet lag include melatonin or short-acting hypnotics. Melatonin, which is available as a dietary supplement in the United States, has considerable variation in purity and quality (20). The use of 3 to 5 mg of melatonin for 4 days at bedtime at the new destination helps to synchronize the internal body clock. Short-acting benzodiazepines promote restful sleep at the new destination. Zolpidem, 5 to 10 mg, is often preferred because of its short half-life and decreased effect on short-term memory (21). It is more effective than melatonin in facilitating sleep during night flights (although the advisability of sleeping on night flights vis-à-vis DVT formation is not clearly defined). It is not advisable to use both melatonin and zolpidem because of increased side effects (22).

COMMON TRAVEL MALADIES

Traveler's diarrhea (TD) is experienced by approximately 40% of people traveling to the developing world. Although TD is a rare cause of death, approximately 1% of travelers who develop TD are hospitalized, 20% are confined to bed, and 40% are forced to change their itinerary as a result of this condition (23). Clearly, TD is a common problem with a large economic impact.

TD is more commonly seen in younger travelers, and 90% of cases occur within the first 2 weeks of travel (24). *Escherichia coli,* and especially enterotoxigenic *E. coli* (ETEC), is the most common cause, although *Campylobacter* species, *Salmonella* species, and *Shigella* are also common etiologies. There is geographic variation in the most likely pathogens for TD. For example, *Campylobacter* and *Salmonella* species are commonly isolated from TD patients in Asia. Destinations with the highest TD risk include Africa, Latin America, the Middle East, and most parts of Asia (24).

Specific safety practices with foods, beverages, and general hygiene can decrease the risk of developing TD. Safe food practices include eating piping-hot food, eating only cooked vegetables (as opposed to cold salad), and eating only peeled fruit. For beverages, boiled or bottled water, carbonated drinks, ultrahigh temperature (UHT) pasteurized milk, and hot tea or coffee are generally quite safe. Carrying one's own toilet paper and having either prepackaged moisturized towelettes or alcohol-based antiseptic gel to cleanse one's hands can lessen the risk of contaminating one's own food.

Some travelers desire or need chemoprophylaxis of TD, and bismuth subsalicylate is modestly effective as such (25). Travelers with underlying bowel disease or diseases where diarrhea might represent a threat to health should consider antimicrobial prophylaxis with fluoroquinolones.

Capacity for self-treatment of TD makes good emporiatric sense. Oral rehydration salts may be necessary to treat severe TD in adults, and may be carried by the traveler. For more mild cases, crackers and soft drinks are sufficient. Antimotility agents such as loperamide or diphenoxylate-atropine are helpful in controlling symptoms, but their use is discouraged in cases of dysentery (diarrhea containing blood). Fluoroquinolones and azalides play a central role in the empiric treatment of TD. Ciprofloxacin, norfloxacin, ofloxacin, and enoxacin have been demonstrated to be effective in controlled trials of TD (26). Azithromycin, an azalide antibiotic, is especially useful against *Campylobacter* infections, which show progressive resistance to fluoroquinolones (27). Azithromycin also represents a good choice during pregnancy. Rifaximin, a new semisynthetic, nonabsorbable antibiotic, may represent an effective tool for treatment of TD once it becomes commercially available (28).

Persistent diarrhea, lasting longer than 2 weeks, has a greater likelihood of being caused by protozoa (including *Giardia, Entamoeba, Cryptosporidia,* or *Cyclospora)* or *Clostridium difficile* (29). In such cases, the causative agents should be specifically sought and, if found, treated. Even with appropriate evaluation, the etiology of chronic TD may be elusive. In some cases, an episode of TD appears to unmask a preexisting gastrointestinal disorder (30).

Sexually Transmitted Diseases

Sexually transmitted diseases (STDs) are the second most common travel-related infection, following TD (31). Casual sexual activity, often of a high-risk variety, is common in travelers. There are several potential reasons for this, including increased use of alcohol, increased sense of anonymity, loneliness, or ready availability of commercial sex workers. Thus, the travel medicine practitioner is strongly advised to have a discussion with the traveler regarding potential risk of STDs and methods to prevent these diseases. Specifically, travelers should be encouraged to carry condoms, preferably ones made in the United States, as they are thought to be more durable than those manufactured in other parts the world (32). The potential for STDs also has implications for surveillance in returning travelers, and they should be given the availability of STD testing.

Emergency contraception may urgently present itself as an issue for female travelers. As it may be difficult to obtain in some countries, women should be briefed on the advisability of carrying emergency contraception with them during travel, and the logistics of its use (33).

TRAVEL MEDICAL KIT

Travelers, and especially those traveling to the developing world, should be encouraged to be as self-sufficient as possible in providing self-care. This translates into carrying a medical kit that includes over-the-counter medicines to use against common symptoms, but also prescription medications that are likely to be needed. These would include medicines for TD, altitude illness, and sleep disturbance (34). Patients who wear contact lenses should consider carrying an antibiotic drop for use should they develop an eye infection while traveling in the developing world, as this could rapidly lead to serious infection and resulting scarring (35).

SEEKING LOCAL CARE

There will be times when it is necessary to use the services of local health care providers. In some parts of the world, blood-borne pathogens may present a risk, as some health care systems may give IM/IV medications or suturing with needles that are not sterile. Thus, the traveler must weigh these possibilities and consider carrying sterile needles (along with a letter justifying these materials). Getting the name of a local health care provider prior to travel can be quite useful not only in providing reassurance, but also in directing the traveler to a practitioner who is likely to provide competent and safe care. Some commercially available databases provide information about the medical care in various cities throughout the world (36), and organizations such as the International Association for Medical Assistance to Travelers (IAMAT) (37) can provide lists of English-speaking practitioners who trained in a Western nation and who follow a specified fee schedule.

INSECT ISSUES

Insects are major vectors of disease in many parts of the world, and methods directed at lessening the risk of bites help prevent disease. Travelers are often most vulnerable to insects while sleeping, so a first consideration is the nature of the accommodations. Many travelers, even if staying in the developing world, will be residing in hotels with air conditioning, where insect risk will be minimal. A mosquito net is a reasonable option, however, if the nature of the accommodations is not known. Thus, knowledge of the living conditions of the individual will help answer the question of whether netting is appropriate. Nets should be treated with permethrin (see below). Insects tend to feed at dusk or dawn, and travelers can also lessen their risk of bites by staying indoors during these times.

Other measures that lessen the risk of insect bites include appropriate use of permethrin and *N,N*-diethyl-M-toluamide (DEET). Permethrin, an organic pesticide, can be used to treat clothing and nets, thus lessening the risk of insect exposure (38). Depending on the concentration of permethrin used, this effect lasts several weeks and up to 1 year. Permethrin may be difficult to find in the developing world, and should be obtained and used prior to traveling. DEET is the active ingredient in many insect repellents. It is the most effective, and best studied, insect repellent on the market, and there are many formulations available, ranging from 5% to 100%, and in solutions, lotions, creams, gels, aerosol and pump sprays, and impregnated towelettes (38). DEET, especially in high concentrations, may damage plastics, rayon, spandex, and other synthetic materials and lens coatings, and should be carefully applied. Polymer-based DEET products have been developed and are more slowly released, lessening the frequency of application. The concomitant use of DEET and sunscreen may lessen the effectiveness of the sunscreen. Effective alternatives to DEET are not available in the U.S., but are being developed in Europe.

ENVIRONMENTAL ISSUES

Differences in temperature are the first and most evident environmental factor noted by the traveler. For travelers to the developing world, the most common difficulty is arrival in a tropical climate where the traveler is not acclimatized to the extremes of heat. Travelers need to be warned about potential difficulties of heat, especially problems with heat-related fatigue, electrolyte imbalance, heat syncope, or even heat stroke. Having foreknowledge of the climate at destination is important in preventing heat-related problems. Wearing appropriate clothing, scheduling physically demanding tasks during the cooler parts of the day, and ensuring adequate hydration with safe fluids are also critical safety measures. Travelers may want to carry powdered sports drinks to use for electrolyte replacement and to make water more palatable during the acclimatization process. Proper care of skin and attention to hygiene can help prevent the maceration of skin and/or fungal infections, which commonly occur when the skin is chronically damp. Carrying antifungal medications may be appropriate for travelers to the tropics.

Travelers going to cold environments without appropriate clothing are at risk for cold-related problems. Again, having knowledge of likely temperatures in the destination environment is an important part of prevention. Emergency kits for dealing with unexpected exposure to cold, such as in a stranded car, should be standard for travelers to cold environments.

As one travels closer to the equator, or to higher altitudes, ultraviolet (UV) radiation becomes an increasing problem. Acute UV overexposure causes sunburn and keratitis. Sunburn is especially worrisome because it prevents normal sweating, which may increase the traveler's risk of heat-related illness. The well-prepared traveler wears sunglasses and appropriate clothing, notably a hat to shade the face and neck, to help avoid extremes of ultraviolet light. Attention should be paid to appropriate use of sunscreens, especially in hot, humid environments or at high altitudes (39). Where possible, travelers to areas with high levels of UV should avoid drugs associated with photosensitivity (40).

Extremes of altitude present hazards that are frequently not anticipated by travelers. There is a wide variation in individual susceptibility to altitude illness, and most people have no knowledge of their own susceptibility prior to going to altitudes. Most travelers tolerate altitudes of up to 10,000 feet without much difficulty. However, once one is sleeping above 10,000 feet, the risk for *acute mountain sickness (AMS), high-altitude pulmonary edema (HAPE), and high-altitude cerebral edema (HACE)* increases (41). Symptoms of AMS include headache, anorexia, nausea or vomiting, insomnia, dizziness, lassitude and/or fatigue. Slow ascent, with adequate time for acclimatization, is the most effective preventive technique. For travelers rapidly going to altitudes above 10,000 feet, prophylactic therapy or standby therapy with Diamox (acetazolamide), 125 to 250 mg PO b.i.d., is helpful in preventing AMS (41). Because most travelers are unaware of altitude-related health problems, they frequently assume that their sickness is related to influenza, a hangover, or dietary indiscretion. For those travelers who develop cough, respiratory distress, or ataxia, HAPE or HACE is a real possibility that demands rapid evaluation and intervention. Descent to lower altitude and supplemental oxygen are the most important treatment modalities. Recent studies suggest that subclinical pulmonary edema is very common, even in modest climbs of average effort (42). If a traveler with a history of altitude-related problems plans to return to altitude, he or she should consult with someone knowledgeable in preventing and treating these problems prior to traveling.

Exposure to fresh water may present infectious hazards in the form of *schistosomiasis* and *leptospirosis.* Schistosomiasis, a parasitic worm, can infect the body through freshwater exposure via intact skin. Thus, primary prevention is avoidance of infested freshwater, and travelers must be made aware of whether they will be in a schistosomiasis zone. If a traveler either inadvertently enters infested water or decides to enter the water based on minimization of risk by locals, it is important for the health care provider to consider serologic testing for infection several months after exposure (43). The serologic testing available at the Centers for Disease Control (CDC) (770-480-7775) is sufficiently specific that a negative test effectively excludes a diagnosis of schistosomiasis (44). Praziquantel is the treatment of choice for this infection, and is generally effective (45). Leptospirosis is found in many freshwaters of the world, and is often associated with adventure travel and water sports. If risks are thought to be high, preventive therapy with doxycycline, 200 mg PO once per week of exposure, can be quite effective in preventing the infection (46), or at least the most severe infections (47).

EMERGENCY CARE OF THE INTERNATIONAL TRAVELER

Many travelers are surprised to find that their health insurance does not cover transport to areas that can provide treatment in case of emergencies, or even treatment outside the United States. Thus, formulating a plan for medical evacuation and treatment of the critically ill or injured traveler is essential prior to the need for such treatment. Travelers' insurance is readily available through many providers in the United States.

VACCINATING TRAVELERS

An important part of protecting the international traveler is the use of appropriate vaccination. This involves tailoring a vaccine plan for the specific traveler, and not just vaccinating based on geography. Important factors in choosing vaccines are the traveler's age, general health, medications, country of origin, and vaccination history. Other factors to consider are the traveler's planned activities; disease patterns in the new destination; the type of accommodations and eating patterns; the duration of the trip; and the available budget for preparation. Individual risk tolerance may also play a role, as does the length of time before departure that the traveler seeks advice. The strength of vaccine recommendations may be affected by considering if the client travels repeatedly or only rarely.

Vaccination of travelers can be effectively organized into three categories: routine vaccines, recommended vaccines, and required vaccines. These categories are discussed below. Early identification of people who are likely to be traveling frequently allows the use of standard vaccine schedules instead of accelerated ones, thus saving money. Supplying travelers with a completed International Certificate of Vaccination allows them to have a record of all administered vaccines, and simplifies subsequent consultations.

Routine Vaccines

Because of high levels of effectiveness of routine vaccines, our infrastructure, and the protective effects of herd immunity, vaccine-preventable infections in the U.S. are relatively rare. Travelers are then surprised to learn that they may be susceptible. Travelers need to be specifically asked about their vaccine status.

Tetanus is found worldwide and frequently results from contamination of even minor wounds. *Clostridium tetani* is the causative agent, and it thrives in the warm, moist soils of the tropics (48). Many Americans, and especially the elderly, do not have immunity to the disease (49). For adults who have completed a primary tetanus series as a child, a booster is suggested every 10 years. If an adult patient has never received the primary vaccine, two doses, spaced 1 to 2 months apart, should be given, followed by a third dose, 6 to 12 months later (50).

Diphtheria generally presents as a sore throat with pseudomembrane, and is spread from infected individuals via droplets. This infection is common in sections of the former Soviet Union and in many countries in the developing world (51). A large percentage of the U.S. population has no demonstrable immunity to diphtheria (52). Optimal protection requires a primary series, followed by a booster every 10 years. The vaccine is usually given in conjunction with tetanus. Primary immunization in the previously unvaccinated is the same as with tetanus, using the Td formulation (50).

Pertussis, or whooping cough, continues to be a common infection worldwide. During the prevaccine era (i.e., prior to the mid-1940s), it was a major cause of morbidity and mortality in the U.S. (53). Protection lasts approximate 10 years after the most recent dose of vaccine, so many adults are vulnerable, since the last scheduled dose for children is when they enter school (54). Because the rate of pertussis among adolescents and adults is increasing, studies are underway to evaluate the new acellular pertussis vaccines for older teenagers and adults (55).

Tremendous progress has been made in decreasing the number of cases of *polio,* and the Western Pacific region of the world was recently certified as polio-free (56). This viral disease is spread via the fecal-oral route and the oral-oral route, and children are the most common reservoirs (57). Most adults have had a primary series, but few adults have gotten boosters unless they were traveling to polio endemic areas, which include sub-Saharan Africa, the Middle East, the Indian subcontinent, and the island of Hispaniola (Haiti and the Dominican Republic). Travelers at risk for polio should have one dose of the injectable inactivated polio vaccine as an adult, assuming they had a primary series as child. If they are unvaccinated, they should receive three doses: the first two separated by 1 to 2 months, and a third dose 6 to 12 months after the second (50).

All cases of *measles* in the U.S. are now thought to have originated abroad, brought to the U.S. by travelers (58). Measles continues to represent a significant health threat in the developing world, and is especially common in sub-Saharan Africa and the Indian subcontinent, where it continues to be a common cause of death in children. Measles is highly contagious, and is spread by direct contact with infectious droplets or by airborne transmission (59). Americans born prior to 1957 are presumed to have had the disease, and are likely to have lifelong protection (60). In the late 1950s and early 1960s the measles vaccine was poorly immunogenic, and because of this, protection was not reliably lifelong. Children now receive two doses of measles vaccine, usually combined with mumps and rubella (MMR). Susceptible travelers should receive at least one dose of the measles vaccine, and preferably two, spaced at least 1 month apart (50). It is also possible to verify that a measles antibody is present serologically.

Rubella and *mumps* vaccines are not standard throughout the world. They are not routinely given even in several highly industrialized countries. These diseases, which usually occur during childhood, are spread by direct or droplet contact with nasopharyngeal secretions. Mumps vaccine rarely has serious side effects. In susceptible women, rubella vaccine is associated with a 10% chance of developing arthritis and 25% chance of developing arthralgia. These symptoms usually persist for a few weeks, but can be prolonged (50).

Varicella, or chickenpox, can be a serious illness in adults. Infection during pregnancy can harm the fetus as seriously as rubella does. The infection is common during childhood, and is spread by direct contact with individuals who have either varicella or herpes zoster (61). In the U.S., the live varicella vaccine is now routine, and has been associated with a dramatic decrease in disease (62). In the developing world, varicella is often the disease of adults (58), so travelers may be more likely to be exposed. Varicella is often associated with serious secondary skin infections, especially in the tropics. If the traveler has no history of varicella infection, it is prudent to check a serologic titer, because up to 90% of people without definite history of chickenpox do have protective antibodies (63). If there is no protective antibody, two doses of the vaccine, spaced 1 to 2 months apart, are indicated, provided there is no contraindication to immunization with a live virus vaccine (50).

Influenza occurs worldwide. Outbreaks have occurred on aircraft and onboard ships. Because the influenza virus changes continually, vaccines are reformulated each year to reflect current trends in infection. There are formulations for the Northern and Southern Hemispheres. Influenza spreads from person to person via droplets, or by fomites contaminated with nasopharyngeal secretions (64). Influenza exists year-round in the tropics and in the Southern Hemisphere's winter season (our summer). All travelers should be encouraged to have the influenza vaccine. Travelers at highest risk for influenza may also benefit from carrying antiinfluenza medication, as it has been shown to shorten the duration of the disease and can make symptoms milder (65).

Streptococcus pneumoniae (pneumococcus) is a common cause of infection, including sinusitis, otitis media, pneumonia, and invasive infections, especially in the older population (66). While drug resistance to this bacterium is increasing in the U.S. (67), the level of antibiotic resistance in the rest of the world is high (68,69). Transmission of the pneumococcus is via respiratory droplets. The 23-valent polysaccharide vaccine that is currently available for adults is recommended for the elderly, smokers (70), and for people with chronic illnesses (66). A conjugate vaccine has been developed for children, but is not yet available for adults (71).

Recommended Vaccines

Vaccines that are recommended for travelers vary according to the specific disease patterns in the countries to be visited, anticipated associations with local people, and the traveler's health status, including past illnesses.

Hepatitis A is highly endemic in most developing countries, and is usually contracted via contaminated food or water. Infection is highly prevalent in the developing world, where, after infection, individuals enjoy lifelong protection (72). Since infection is relatively rare in the U.S., most U.S. travelers to the developing world are at risk. The infection has increasing morbidity and mortality with increasing age, so travelers to the developing world are strongly advised to be protected.

Because so many countries are high risk for hepatitis A, it is generally easier to consider which countries do *not* carry a risk greater than that seen in North America. These would include the countries in Western Europe, as well as Australia and New Zealand. But southern Europe is now considered to have an intermediate level of risk for hepatitis A (73). Two formulations of hepatitis A vaccine are available in the U.S., although there are other formulations abroad. The available formulations, Havrix and VAQTA, are considered to be interchangeable (74). High levels of protection are seen after even one dose of either vaccine. A second dose, given 6 to 12 months after the initial dose, provides long-term immunity. Although the CDC recommends that immune serum globulin (ISG) should be given in conjunction with the vaccine if the traveler is vaccinated less than 1 month before travel (72), there are several lines of evidence to strongly suggest that effective protection occurs very rapidly after receiving the vaccine (58).

In the case of travelers who are more likely to have had the disease, such as the elderly or immigrants from high prevalence countries, it is possible to serologically check for the antibody. However, vaccination of those travelers who may already be protected is not harmful (50).

Typhoid fever is caused by infection with *Salmonella typhi,* and is usually contracted from consuming contaminated food or water. The infection is seen throughout the developing world, and especially on the Indian subcontinent (75). Typhoid fever is potentially quite serious, and is becoming more difficult to treat because of antibiotic resistance (76). Two vaccines are available in U.S. The Ty21a form (Vivotif Berna), is a live-attenuated antigen vaccine, and gives 5 years of protection. Attention must be given to storing and taking this vaccine correctly (50). Typhim Vi is a single-dose, injectable, capsular polysaccharide vaccine that generally has fewer side effects that the older whole-cell killed vaccine, which was recently removed from the market. Typhim Vi gives approximately 3 years of protection (77). A new conjugate *Salmonella typhi* Vi vaccine appears promising in field trials (78).

Hepatitis B is prevalent in many areas of the world, but especially in Southeast Asia, sub-Saharan Africa, and the Amazon basin. The infection is associated with blood or body fluid exposure. In travelers, it may be seen as an STD or after exposure to nonsterile needles or instruments. If a person contracts the infection, there is a 10% chance of developing chronic hepatitis B, with its associated complications (79). In the U.S., hepatitis B vaccine has been routine in children since the early 1990s.

There are two formulations of the hepatitis B vaccine available in the United States: Engerix-B and Recombivax HB (50). Both of these are recombinant DNA vaccines, and there is no risk of the disease from the vaccine. In adults, three doses of the vaccine are required to provide immunity. The normal schedule is one dose at point zero, 1 month, and 6 months. Because this amount of lead time is frequently not available, accelerated schedules may also be used. The standard accelerated schedule is three doses of the vaccine, separated by 1 month. With Engerix-B, a superaccelerated schedule can be used, giving one dose on days 0, 7, and 21 (80). In all of the accelerated regimens, a fourth dose must be given 1 year after the first, to ensure long-term protection. Protection from hepatitis B vaccine is thought to be lifelong in immunocompetent individuals who develop antibody after the initial series (81). A combined hepatitis A and B vaccine (82), Twinrix, is now available in the U.S. The schedules are the same as for hepatitis B.

Meningococcal meningitis, an infection caused by *Neisseria meningitidis,* is spread by respiratory droplets. Although the disease occurs worldwide, the infection is especially prevalent in sub-Saharan Africa during the dry season and in Saudi Arabia during the annual hajj (83). Vaccination is mandatory for entry into Saudi Arabia during this pilgrimage period. Recently, the meningitis vaccine has been recommended for college students because of a high relative risk for incoming freshman living in dormitories (84). In the U.S., only one meningitis vaccine is available: Menomune. This polysaccharide vaccine is protective against groups A, C, Y, and W-135. Protection provided by the vaccine lasts for 3 to 4 years. In the United Kingdom, a conjugated vaccine is available for children (85).

Japanese encephalitis is an arboviral infection common in many parts of Asia. Mosquitoes transmit it, and pigs and aquatic birds are the reservoirs. The disease is a risk primarily if the traveler stays in rural areas (86). Because neurologic sequelae of the disease are common, vaccination of children against this infection is standard in many Asian countries. JE-Vax, a purified, formalin inactivated mouse brain–derived vaccine, is available in the U.S. (50). Primary immunization consists of three doses of the vaccine, given on days 0, 7, and 30. Because about 0.3% of vaccinees experience generalized urticaria, the patient should be closely monitored after vaccination. Reactions can occur up to 10 days after the vaccination. Patients should be instructed on what to do if they begin to experience a reaction. The reaction is more frequently seen in people who have any type of allergic disorder (87). The duration of protection of the vaccine is approximately 3 years.

Deaths from *rabies* are not unusual in many parts of the developing world. Thus travelers should be educated about the dangers inherent in animal contact. Indeed, any bite, scratch, or exposure to saliva on nonintact skin from a mammal may represent risk (59). Management of a potential rabies exposure represents a tremendous logistic problem, because preventive treatment of a rabies exposure includes immediate wound cleansing, the urgent use of rabies immune globulin (RIG), and the vaccine on days 0, 3, 7, 14, and 28 (50). RIG is given in a dose of 20 IU/kg, and is infiltrated directly into the wound, if possible (88). RIG may be difficult to locate in the developing world, and because it is a blood product, has potential safety concerns. The greatest advantage of using preexposure rabies vaccine is that it eliminates the need for RIG.

If the traveler will be in a situation where exposure to animals is likely or where access to medical care will be limited, preexposure rabies vaccine should be strongly considered. There are three rabies vaccines available in the U.S. Human diploid cell vaccine (HDCV) can be administered either intradermally or intramuscularly. Purified chick embryo cell (PCEC) and rabies vaccine adsorbed (RVA) may be given intramuscularly (88). All preexposure rabies vaccine schedules involve giving the vaccine at days 0, 7, and either 21 or 28. In the event of an exposure to rabies, two additional doses of the vaccine are needed on days 0 and 3.

Tuberculosis infects one third of the world's population and causes more than two million deaths per year (89). Although not traditionally considered a travel vaccine, there may be circumstances where the use of BCG (Bacilli Calmette-Guérin), should be offered to the traveler. BCG is a live-attenuated *Mycobacterium bovis,* and is used in most countries to limit the seriousness of tuberculosis infection. BCG has been used worldwide more than any other vaccine (90). It is not used in the U.S. because of concerns over its efficacy, its use making purified protein derivative (PPD) interpretation more difficult, and the relatively low prevalence of tuberculosis in the U.S. In children, BCG would only be recommended for young children who are likely to be exposed to a population where tuberculosis is highly prevalent. It should be thought of as lowering the risk for tubercular meningitis or miliary tuberculosis, but not necessarily for preventing infection with tuberculosis. In adults, BCG should be considered where there will be prolonged time spent in areas with high concentration of TB, especially if it is a multidrug-resistant type (58).

For the routine traveler, the risk of TB is relatively low (91). These travelers can have PPD skin testing before and after travel to high-risk populations. Post-travel testing should be done 8 to 12 weeks after return. If positive, preventive therapy for latent infection should be strongly considered. Traveling to, and working in, a country with a high prevalence of tuberculosis significantly increases the risk of contracting this infection (92).

Tick-borne encephalitis (TBE) is a viral infection found in Eastern Europe, the Balkans, Scandinavia, Russia, and parts of China. It is transmitted by the *Ixodes* tick, the same type that transmits Lyme disease. The tick is found in many rural areas, and is most active between April and August. Thus, the disease is most common in the spring and summer, when ticks are most numerous and are feeding (93). Tick precautions should be taken seriously during these seasons for the traveler who plans outdoor activities. If the traveler anticipates staying in an endemic area for a prolonged length of time, consideration should be given to taking the vaccine. The vaccine is not available in the U.S., but may be obtained in Europe (50).

Required Vaccines

Yellow fever is the only vaccine that is required by the World Health Organization (WHO) in specific situations. Meningitis vaccine is required by the government of Saudi Arabia for pilgrims going on the hajj, but is not required by the WHO.

Yellow fever is a mosquito-borne infection found in the Amazon basin of South America and in sub-Saharan Africa. The disease has no known treatment, and carries a high mortality rate (94). The reservoir for yellow fever is in animals, so no human cases are necessary in order to produce a new infection. The vaccine, which has been around for many years, is highly effective. One injection provides immunity for at least 10 years. It is an egg-based vaccine, and patients with a serious egg allergy should avoid it. It must be given at least 10 days prior to entering a country with yellow fever. Although this live-attenuated vaccine has generally been considered very safe, there have been recent cases where deaths have been associated with vaccination. Immunosuppression and advanced age are relative contraindications to receiving the vaccine. The elderly traveler should be cautioned about the risk of serious adverse effects, including encephalitis and death, from the vaccine. The risk for such occurrences for the general population is about 0.3 per 100,000 doses compared to about 9 per 100,000 doses in travelers 75 years of age or older (95). Although a physician may write a letter that states that the vaccine is contraindicated, to meet the entry requirements for countries, real risk of disease may still be present. If travelers do not wish to accept the risk of the vaccine, they should consider altering their itinerary.

Malaria Prevention

Malaria is an extremely common tropical disease that affects about 40% of the world's population in more than 100 countries. The incidence of malaria is estimated to be 300 to 500 million new cases per year. Each year, malaria kills between 1.5 and 2.7 million people (96). African countries are hardest hit by malaria, both in numbers of cases and in deaths. *Plasmodium falciparum* is the species of malaria that results in the most severe cases and the highest mortality rate. Every year, thousands of travelers enter malaria risk areas, and there are over 1,000 cases of malaria diagnosed among travelers returning to the U.S. (97). In these travelers, *Plasmodium falciparum* and *Plasmodium vivax* account for the majority of cases (97).

Malaria is present in tropical areas between latitude 37 degrees north and 31 degrees south, and lower than 2,500 m in altitude (98). For current information regarding specific malaria risk areas, one can refer to the CDC (99) or the WHO (100). The CDC also maintains a telephone malaria risk information service (888-232-3228). There is also commercially available software that frequently updates changes in the locations and resistance patterns of malaria (36).

Preventing malaria in travelers involves both personal protective measures against mosquito bites and chemoprophylaxis. The use of netting, permethrin, and DEET has already been discussed above. Chemoprophylaxis involves the use of a medication that kills the malaria parasite either in the blood or in the liver. Resistance patterns of the specific type of malaria in the region must be known so that the correct medication can be prescribed. Although there are frequent problems with poor compliance of travelers in taking chemoprophylactic agents (101), there have also been deaths in travelers who conscientiously took an inappropriate chemoprophylactic agent (102). It is imperative that physicians who are managing malarial medications be familiar with drug side effects, drug interactions, and resistance patterns of malaria, especially since this may be a relatively rare problem in occupational medicine, and because drugs and resistance may change quickly. Current treatment guidelines should be consulted (103).

Chloroquine phosphate (trade name Aralen) is an older antimalarial that remains effective in areas where *P. falciparum* has not developed resistance: Central America (west of the Panama Canal), Hispaniola, and in parts of the Middle East. Because of its long half-life, it may be taken one time per week, starting 1 week prior to travel, and continuing until 4 weeks after leaving the malarious area. The tablets may be taken with food to minimize the potential side effects of nausea, vomiting, and diarrhea. Chloroquine can also cause blurred vision and worsening of psoriasis. It should be used with caution in anyone with liver disease (including alcoholism) or in patients taking hepatotoxic drugs (104). The usual weekly adult dose is 500 mg of chloroquine phosphate (equal to 300 mg of the chloroquine base).

Mefloquine (trade name Lariam) is effective in most areas that have chloroquine resistance. The usual adult dose is 250 mg per week, starting 1–2 weeks prior to travel. Mefloquine should also be continued for 4 weeks after leaving the malarious area. The primary side effects for mefloquine are neuropsychological, and include sleep disturbances, vivid dreams, fatigue, dizziness, confusion, worsening of depression, and anxiety. Mefloquine does lower seizure threshold and is an arrhythmogenic agent (104). Some patients note gastrointestinal symptoms including nausea or diarrhea. Mefloquine resistance is been documented along the Thailand border with Myanmar and Cambodia (105,106), so alternative agents should be used in travelers to these areas. Mefloquine is considered safe during the second and third trimesters of pregnancy, but there are limited data on first-trimester use (104).

Doxycycline is a chemoprophylactic agent that can be used where *P. falciparum* malaria is chloroquine resistant or mefloquine resistant. Its chief advantage is its price, since it is available as a generic medication, but it also has the advantage of preventing travel-associated leptospirosis and rickettsial infections (107). The usual daily dosage is 100 mg, starting 1 to 2 days prior to entering a malarious area. It should be continued throughout the trip and for 4 weeks after leaving the malarious area. Possible adverse side effects include nausea, vomiting, diarrhea, photosensitivity, and vaginal yeast infections. Travelers should be reminded to take the doxycycline with a full glass of fluids so as to avoid the potentially severe esophageal ulcer that can occur if the capsule lodges in the esophagus. Travelers using doxycycline should also utilize sunscreen that blocks ultraviolet A to prevent photosensitivity (104), and women taking doxycycline should have treatment available for vaginal candidiasis. Doxycycline should not be used in pregnant or lactating women, or in children younger than 8 years.

Atovaquone/proguanil (trade name Malarone) is a fixed combination antimalarial that is especially useful for short-term travelers. The adult formulation, which has 250 mg of atovaquone and 100 mg of proguanil, should be started 1 to 2 days prior to travel, and continued on a daily basis until 7 days after leaving the malarious area. This combination should be taken with food in order to enhance absorption. It is generally free of serious side effects, but is the most expensive antimalarial (108). Because this combination kills liver-stage malaria parasites, it need be taken for only 1 week after malaria exposure. It does not kill the latent hypnozoite forms of *P. vivax,* however, so additional treatment with primaquine may still be appropriate (109). This combination drug is contraindicated during pregnancy.

Primaquine has activity against all stages of the malaria parasite, including the dormant parasites in the liver, the hypnozoite forms (104). Because of its use after exposure to *P. vivax* or *P. ovale* malaria, this treatment is called terminal prophylaxis. Primaquine can cause hemolytic anemia in patients with a glucose-6-phosphate-dehydrogenase (G6PD) deficiency, so this enzyme level should be measured prior to using the medication. The usual dose for terminal prophylaxis is 26.3 mg per day of primaquine phosphate (15 mg of the base) for 14 days. Primaquine can also be used as a chemoprophylactic agent, although this usage is not Food and Drug Administration (FDA) approved. The dose is 30 mg of the base (two of the 26.3-mg primaquine phosphate tablets) per day starting 1 day before travel and continuing for 7 days after leaving the malarious area (104). Primaquine should not be used in pregnant patients. Drug-related side effects include anorexia, nausea, vomiting, and abdominal pain, and may be reduced by taking the primaquine with food.

Because side effects with any chemoprophylactic antimalarial agent are common, travelers need to be briefed on what to expect and how to minimize any side effects. They also need to have a realistic understanding of the risks of malaria so they will be less tempted to discontinue the medication at the first sign of side effects. There are no international standards on antimalarial medication usage, and travelers may want to try medications that may not even be available in the U.S. These medications may offer a lower side effect profile, but also less protection. Native inhabitants of malaria endemic areas may minimize the severity of malaria because they are semi-immune, thus discouraging the malaria-naive traveler from taking any medication.

Emergency standby treatment of malaria is a concept that has gained popularity, especially for travelers in relatively low-risk areas, but it also poses several difficulties. The concept is that travelers who have already been educated about malaria have medications available to treat themselves should they develop the disease. Self-test kits for malaria are available, but have been shown not to be highly reliable in untrained testers (110,111). Potentially useful medications for standby treatment include pyrimethamine/sulfadoxine (trade name Fansidar), Malarone, and mefloquine. The same medication that has been used, even intermittently, for chemoprophylaxis, should not be used for treatment. Because many foreign health care workers who routinely treat malaria rely more on clinical rather than laboratory findings, malaria smears may not be done. Since an accurate diagnosis has important implications, i.e., whether terminal prophylaxis should be done, the traveler would be encouraged to have a blood smear made at the time of illness that may be read later, upon returning home. Because of shortages of medications needed to treat malaria in the developing world, and the troubling presence of counterfeit malaria medication (112,113), it may be prudent for travelers to carry a treatment dose even if they are on chemoprophylaxis.

SCREENING THE RETURNING TRAVELER

In some situations, it may be prudent to screen the returning traveler for conditions that would not otherwise be evident. This is especially true in the long-term traveler. The screening process should be based on risks specific to the individual, and not just based on geography. A careful history and review of systems is a useful starting place. The traveler who has been sexually active is likely to benefit from screening for HIV and STDs. Because tuberculosis is extremely common in the developing world, the TB skin test may also be prudent, 8 to 12 weeks after returning. Screening returning travelers for parasites is especially troublesome, since it is relatively rare to find serious problems in the asymptomatic traveler. An exception to this is the traveler who has had freshwater exposure, because schistosomiasis may not cause symptoms, or at least the initial symptoms may be mild. For travelers who have had freshwater exposure in a schistosomiasis area, *Schistosoma* serology may be warranted (see above). For other invasive parasites, a blood count with differential, using the eosinophil count as a screen, may be useful. In patients with high-grade eosinophilia returning from the tropics, there is a high likelihood of travel-related infection, especially with helminths (114).

Specific Problems in the Returning Traveler

Recently returned travelers most commonly present with one of the following four types of problems: fever, gastrointestinal symptoms, dermatologic problems, or psychological issues. Although the occupational medicine physician might not provide treatment for the diseases that cause these symptoms, he should have a good understanding of the urgency needed for diagnostic testing, treating, or referring these patients.

Fever in the traveler who has recently returned from the tropics is due to malaria until proven otherwise. Malaria may have many presentations, but the most common feature is fever. Thus, fever, either by itself or with almost any other symptom, should warrant thick and thin blood smears to search for malaria parasites. If four sets of smears, done 12 hours apart by a competent microscopist, are all negative for parasites, it is probably safe to assume malaria is not the cause of the fever (115). However, in the event of a compelling clinical presentation, one is well advised to start treatment for malaria even without a positive smear. Many other conditions cause fever, and in any recently returned traveler, one must also consider meningitis, typhoid fever, dengue fever, leptospirosis, the hemorrhagic fevers, schistosomiasis, rickettsial infection, and others. Appropriate laboratory studies should be undertaken early in the evaluation (116). Expert consultation should be strongly considered.

Gastrointestinal problems in the returning traveler are common. The most common manifestation is diarrhea, although malabsorption syndrome is also frequently seen. Depending on the timing of the symptoms, empiric treatment with antibiotics may be appropriate. In the traveler with acute diarrhea, a quinolone antibiotics or azithromycin would be a reasonable choice. In the traveler who has already been treated for acute traveler's diarrhea, testing for *C. difficile* or parasites, and especially the protozoal parasites, would be a logical step. In this setting, empiric treatment with metronidazole may be useful. At this point, a syndromic approach can help guide further evaluation. Syndromes include malabsorption (either acute or chronic), chronic diarrhea with associated gastrointestinal (GI) symptoms, chronic diarrhea associated with weight loss, and hematochezia (29). It is not unusual to see acute malabsorption as a temporary postinfection phenomenon, due to intestinal disaccharidase deficiency. In this case, specific foods would be expected to trigger symptoms, and the condition usually subsides in several weeks. Chronic malabsorption may result from parasitic causes (three stools for ova and parasites are indicated) or sprue syndromes (quantification of malabsorption and/or small bowel biopsy needed for diagnosis). Chronic diarrhea with chronic GI symptoms, also known as postinfective irritable bowel syndrome (117), is very common, and may represent the unmasking of irritable bowel syndrome. In patients with chronic diarrhea and weight loss who do not have malabsorption, one should consider HIV or noninfectious etiologies, especially colon cancer and inflammatory bowel disease (118). The presence of rectal bleeding, or hematochezia, suggests either infectious processes (such as *C. difficile, Entamoeba histolytica,* or *Campylobacter* sp.) or inflammatory bowel disease. Care must be taken to rule out amebic dysentery prior to using steroids for inflammatory bowel disease. Tuberculosis may cause chronic diarrhea, and can be varied in its presentation (119). In spite of a complete evaluation, no etiology may be found in some cases of chronic diarrhea. Fortunately, idiopathic chronic diarrhea is usually self-limited (120).

Dermatologic problems are a common presenting complaint in the recently returned traveler (121). The most frequently encountered skin lesions are cutaneous larva migrans (or other parasitic infections), residuals of insect bites, pyoderma, or dermatitis as part of a systemic process (122). Cutaneous larva migrans produces a characteristic linear and migratory lesion of the skin that is generally seen at the site of exposure to earth or the beach. It is caused from exposure to hookworm larvae that are found in soil contaminated with cat or dog feces. Leishmaniasis, myiasis, and tungiasis all have a characteristic appearance. Scabies is a common cause of generalized pruritus in returned travelers (123). The most common insect bites in travelers include those of bedbugs, chiggers, midges, mosquitoes, sand flies, and scabies. These bites may cause symptoms in their own right, but may also be vectors for other diseases. Superficial infection of the skin is extremely common in the tropics, as is superficial fungal infection. Swimming-related skin problems include cercarial dermatitis, which is generally found on uncovered skin of bathers in fresh water (124), and seabather's eruption, found on skin under the swimming suit (125). Because the potential for UV exposure is great in the tropics, various photosensitivity and phytophotodermatitides are not unusual in travelers returning from these areas (126).

Psychological problems are common both during travel and upon return. Travel-related problems often manifest as an adjustment disorder (culture shock), and may be lessened through pretravel counseling (127). Psychiatric problems such as substance use disorder, affective disorders, adjustment disorder, and personality disorder are relatively common reasons for needing to medically evacuate workers in foreign countries (128). In returned travelers, psychological problems are strongly related to illicit drug use (129). Interestingly, the homeward move, for many travelers, is associated with just as many adjustment problems (reentry shock) as the outbound move (130).

REFERENCES

1. World Tourism Organization. *http://www.world-tourism.orgnewsroomreleasesmore_releasesjanua... numbers_2001.htm*.
2. Proops DW. Sound advice for tunnel travellers. *Br Med J* 1994;309:426.
3. Brown TP. Middle ear symptoms while flying: ways to prevent a severe outcome. *Postgrad Med* 1994;96: 135–142.
4. Csortan E, Jones J, Haan M, et al. Efficacy of pseudoephedrine for the prevention of barotrauma during air travel. *Ann Emerg Med* 1994;23:1324–1327.
5. Strangerup SE, Tjernstrom O, Harcourt J, et al. Barotitis in children after aviation: prevalence and treatment with Otovent. *J Laryngol Otol* 1996;110:625–626.
6. Lapostolle F, Surget V, Borron SW, et al. Severe pulmonary embolism associated with air travel. *N Engl J Med* 2001;345:779–783.
7. Ansell JE. Air travel and venous thromboembolism—is the evidence in? *N Engl J Med* 2001;345:828–829.
8. Scurr JH, Machin SJ, Bailey-King S, et al. Frequency and prevention of symptomless deep-vein thrombosis in long-haul flights: a randomised trial. *Lancet* 2001; 357:1485–1489.
9. Pulmonary embolism prevention trial collaborative group. Prevention of pulmonary embolism and deep vein thrombosis with low dose aspirin: Pulmonary Embolism Prevention (PEP) trial. *Lancet* 2000;355: 1295–1302.
10. Bendz B, Sevre K, Anderson TO, et al. Low molecular weight heparin prevents activation of coagulation in a hypobaric environment. *Blood Coagulation Fibrinolysis* 2001;12:371–374.
11. Oosterveld WJ, Landolt JP. Motion sickness. In: DuPont HL, Steffen RS, eds. *Textbook of travel medicine and health,* 2nd ed. Hamilton: BC Decker, 2001: 396–403.
12. Wood MJ, Wood CD, Stewart JJ, et al. Comparison of dosage routes for antimotion sickness drugs. *Aviat Space Environ Med* 1987;65:504.
13. Gahlinger PM. Motion sickness—how to help your patients avoid travel travail. *Postgrad Med* 1999;106: 177–184.

14. Shupak A, Doweck I, Gordon CR, et al. Cinnarizine in the prophylaxis of seasickness: laboratory vestibular evaluation and sea study. *Clin Pharmacol Ther* 1994;55:670–680.
15. Schmid R, Schick T, Steffen R. Comparison of seven commonly used agents for prophylaxis of seasickness. *J Trav Med* 1994;1:203–206.
16. Bertolucci LE, Didario B. Efficacy of a portable acustimulation device in controlling seasickness. *Aviat Space Environ Med* 1995;66:1155–1158.
17. Gordon CR, Spitzer O, Doweck I, et al. Clinical features of mal de debarquement: adaption and habituation to sea conditions. *J Vestibular Res* 1995;5:363–369.
18. Suhner A, Petriek J. Jet lag. In: DuPont HL, Steffen RS, eds. *Textbook of travel medicine and health,* 2nd ed. Hamilton: BC Decker, 2001:403–408.
19. Waterhouse J, Reilly T, Atkinson G. Jet-lag. *Lancet* 1997;350:1611–1616.
20. Williamson BL, Tomlinson AJ, Naylor S, et al. Contamination in commercial preparations of melatonin. *Mayo Clin Proc* 1997;72:1994–1995.
21. Darcourt G, Pringuey D, Sallieve D, et al. The safety and tolerability of zolpidem—an update. *J Psychopharmacol* 1999;13:81–93.
22. Suhner A, Schlagenhauf P, Hofer I, et al. Efficacy and tolerability of melatonin and zolpidem for the alleviation of jet-lag. In: Suhner A, ed. *Melatonin and jet-lag.* Dissertation No. 12823. Zurick: Swiss Federal University of Technology, 1998:85–103.
23. Ericsson CD. Travelers' diarrhea. *Infect Dis Clin North Am* 1998;12:285–303.
24. Castelli F, Pezzoli C, Tomasoni L. Epidemiology of travelers' diarrhea. *J Trav Med* 2001;8[suppl 2]: s26–s30.
25. DuPont HL, Ericsson CD, Johnson PC, et al. Prevention of travelers' diarrhea by the tablet formulation of bismuth subsalicylate. *JAMA* 1987;257:1347–1350.
26. Murphy GS, Petruccelli BP, Kollaritsch H, et al. Treatment of travelers' diarrhea. In: DuPont HL, Steffen RS, eds. *Textbook of travel medicine and health,* 2nd ed. Hamilton: BC Decker, 2001:165–176.
27. Kuschner R, Trofa AF, Thomas RJ, et al. Use of azithromycin for the treatment of Campylobacter enteritis in travelers to Thailand, an area where ciprofloxacin resistance is prevalent. *Clin Infect Dis* 1995;21:536–541.
28. DuPont HL. Treatment of travelers' diarrhea. *J Trav Med* 2001;8[suppl 2]:s31–s33.
29. Connor BA. Persistent travelers' diarrhea. In: DuPont HL, Steffen RS, eds. *Textbook of travel medicine and health,* 2nd ed. Hamilton: BC Decker, 2001:177–183.
30. Schumacker G, Kollberg B, Ljungh A. Inflammatory bowel disease presenting as travellers' diarrhoea. *Lancet* 1993;341:241–242.
31. Hawkes S, Hart G. The sexual health of travelers. *Infect Dis Clin North Am* 1998;12:413–430.
32. Mardh PA, Hira SK. Sexually transmitted infections. In: DuPont HL, Steffen RS, eds. *Textbook of travel medicine and health,* 2nd ed. Hamilton: BC Decker, 2001:280–289.
33. Pennachio DL. New approaches to emergency contraception. *Patient Care* 2001;35(5):19–37.
34. Marcus LC. Preparation for travel. In: Wolfe MS, ed. *Health hints for the tropics,* 12th ed. Northbrook, IL: ASTMH, 1998:2–6.
35. Donzis PB. Corneal ulcers from contact lenses during travel to remote areas. *N Engl J Med* 1998;338: 1629–1630.
36. Travax from Shoreland, Inc. P.P. Box 13795, Milwaukee, WI 53213-0795. *www.Shoreland.com.*
37. International Association for Medical Assistance to Travelers (IAMAT). 417 Center Street, Lewiston, NY 14092, *www.iamat.org.*
38. Fradin MS. Mosquitoes and mosquito repellents: a clinician's guide. *Ann Intern Med* 1998;128:931–940.
39. Anonymous. Sunscreens: are they safe and effective? *Med Lett* 1999;41:43–44.
40. Anonymous. Drugs that cause photosensitivity. *Med Lett* 1995;37:35–36.
41. Hackett PH, Roach RC. High-altitude illness. *N Engl J Med* 2001;345:107–114.
42. Cremona G, Asnaghi R, Baderna P, et al. Pulmonary extravascular fluid accumulation in recreational climbers: a prospective study. *Lancet* 2002;359:303–309.
43. Cetron MS, Chitsulo L, Sullivan JJ. Schistosomiasis in Lake Malawi. *Lancet* 1996;348:1274–1278.
44. Tsang V, Wilkins P. Immunodiagnosis of schistosomiasis: screen with FAST-ELISA and confirm with immunoblot. *Clin Lab Med* 1991;11:1029—1039.
45. Shekhar K. Schistosomiasis drug therapy and treatment considerations. *Drugs* 1991;42:379.
46. Takafuji ET, Kirkpatrick JW, Miller RN, et al. An efficacy trial of doxycycline chemoprophylaxis against leptospirosis. *N Engl J Med* 1984;310:497–500.
47. Sehgal SC, Sugunan AP, Murhekar MV, et al. Randomized controlled trial of doxycycline prophylaxis against leptospirosis in an endemic area. *Int J Antimicrob Agents* 2000;13:249–255.
48. Nathan BR, Bleck TP. Tetanus. In: Guerrant RL, Walker DH, Weller PF, eds. *Tropical infectious diseases—principles, pathogens, and practice.* Philadelphia: Churchill Livingstone, 1999:517–526.
49. Gergen PJ, McQuillan GM, Kiely M, et al. A population-based serologic survey of immunity to tetanus in the United States. *N Engl J Med* 1995;332:761–766.
50. Thombson RF. *Travel and routine immunizations—a practical guide for the medical office.* Milwaukee: Shoreland, 2001.
51. Wharton M. Diphtheria. In: Guerrant, RL, Walker DH, Weller PF, eds. *Tropical infectious diseases—principles, pathogens, and practice.* Philadelphia: Churchill Livingstone, 1999:438–442.
52. Chin J, ed. *Control of communicable diseases manual,* 17th ed. Washington, DC: APHA, 2000:165–170.
53. Anonymous. Pertussis—United States, 1997–2000. *MMWR* 2002;51:73–76.
54. Anonymous. Recommended childhood immunization schedule—United States. *MMWR* 2002;51:31–33.
55. Edwards KM, Decker MD, Mortimer EA. Pertussis vaccine. In: Plotkin SA, Orenstein WA, eds. *Vaccines,* 3rd ed. Philadelphia: WB Saunders, 1999:293–344.
56. Anonymous. Certification of poliomyelitis eradication—Western Pacific Region, October 2000. *MMWR* 2001;50:1–3.
57. Chin J, ed. *Control of communicable diseases manual,* 17th ed. Washington, DC: APHA, 2000:398–405.
58. Wilson ME. Travel-related vaccines. *Infect Dis Clin North Am* 2001;15:231–251.
59. Hatz CFR, Thisyakorn USA, Thisyakern C, et al. Other important viral infections. In: DuPont HL, Stef-

fen RS, eds. *Textbook of travel medicine and health,* 2nd ed. Hamilton: BC Decker, 2001:312–324.

60. Anonymous. Measles, mumps, and rubella—vaccine use and strategies for elimination of measles, rubella, and congential rubella syndrome and control of mumps: recommendations of the advisory committee on immunization practices (ACIP). *MMWR* 1998;47 (RR-8):1–57.
61. Gershan AA, Takahashi M, White CJ. Varicella vaccine. In: Plotkin SA, Orenstein WA, eds. *Vaccines,* 3rd ed. Philadelphia: WB Saunders, 1999:475–507.
62. Steward JF, Watson BM, Peterson CL, et al. Varicella disease after introduction of varicella vaccine in the United States, 1995–2000. *JAMA* 2002;287:606–611.
63. Anonymous. Prevention of varicella. *MMWR* 1996;45 [suppl]:1–27.
64. Couch RB. Prevention and treatment of influenza. *N Engl J Med* 2000;343:1778–1787.
65. Gross PA. Vaccines for pneumonia and new antiviral therapies. *Med Clin North Am* 2001;85:1531–1544.
66. Anonymous. Prevention of pneumococcal disease. *MMWR* 1997;46(RR-8):1–25.
67. Whitney CG, Farley MM, Hadler J, et al. Increasing prevalence of multidrug-resistant streptococcus pneumonia in the United States. *N Engl J Med* 2000;343: 1917–1924.
68. Song JH, Lee NY, Ichiyama S, et al. Spread of drug resistant streptococcus pneumonia in Asian countries: Asian network for surveillance of resistant pathogens (ANSORP) study. *Clin Infect Dis* 1999;28:1206–1211.
69. Lalitha MK, Pai R, Manoharan A, et al. Multidrug-resistant streptococcus pneumoniae from India. *Lancet* 2002;359:445.
70. Nuorti JP, Butler JC, Farley MM, et al. Cigarette smoking and invasive pneumococcal disease. *N Engl J Med* 2000;342:681–689.
71. Eskola J, Kilpi T, Palmu A, et al. Efficacy of a pneumococcal conjugate vaccine against acute otitis media. *N Engl J Med* 2001;344:403–409.
72. Anonymous. Prevention of hepatitis A through active or passive immunization. *MMWR* 1999;48(RR-12):1–37.
73. Barnett ED, Reg M, Chen RT. Principles and practices of immunoprophylaxis. In: DuPont HL, Steffen RS, eds. *Textbook of travel medicine and health,* 2nd ed. Hamilton: BC Decker, 2001:232–251.
74. Connor BA, Phair J, Sack D, et al. Randomized, double-blind study in healthy adults to assess the boosting effect of Vaqta or Havrix after a single dose of Havrix. *Clin Infect Dis* 2001;32:396–401.
75. Lee TP, Hoffman SL. Typhoid fever. In: Strickland GT, ed. *Hunter's tropical medicine and emerging infectious diseases,* 8th ed. Philadelphia: WB Saunders, 2000: 471–484.
76. Mermin JH, Townes JM, Gerber M, et al. Typhoid fever in the United States, 1985–1994: changing risks of international travel and increasing antimicrobial resistance. *Arch Intern Med* 1998;158:633–638.
77. Hellel L, Debois H, Fletcher M, et al. Experience with *Salmonella typhi* Vi capsular polysaccharide vaccine. *Eur J Clin Microbiol Infect Dis* 1999;18:609–620.
78. Lin FYC, Ho VA, Khiem HB, et al. The efficacy of a *Salmonella typhi* conjugate vaccine in two- to five-year-old children. *N Engl J Med* 2001;344:1263–1269.
79. Thomas D, Strickland GT. Hepatitis B virus and hepatitis D virus infections. In: Strickland GT, ed. *Hunter's tropical medicine and emerging infectious diseases,* 8th ed. Philadelphia: WB Saunders, 2000:231–235.
80. Block HL, Loscher T, Scheiermann N, et al. Accelerated schedule for hepatitis B immunization. *J Trav Med* 1995;2:213–217.
81. Banatvala J, VanDamme P, Oehen S. Lifelong protection against hepatitis B: the role of vaccine immunogenicity in immune memory. *Vaccine* 2001;19:877–885.
82. Thoelen S, VanDamme P, Leentraar-Kuypers A, et al. The first combined vaccine against hepatitis A and B: an overview. *Vaccine* 1999;17:1657–1662.
83. Scheld WM, Wenger JD, Sousa AQ. Meningococcal infections. In: DuPont HL, Steffen RS, eds. *Textbook of travel medicine and health,* 2nd ed. Hamilton: BC Decker, 2001:365–380.
84. American College Health Association. *http://www.acha.orgresource-infomeningitis-faq.htm.*
85. Maclennan JM, Shackley F, Heath PT, et al. Safety, immunogenicity, and induction of immunologic memory by a serogroup C meningococcal conjugate vaccine in infants—a randomized controlled trial. *JAMA* 2000; 283:2795–2801.
86. Tsai TF, Chang GJJ, Yu YX. Japanese encephalitis vaccine. In: Plotkin SA, Orenstein WA, eds. *Vaccines,* 3rd ed. Philadelphia: WB Saunders, 1999:672–710.
87. Berg SW, Mitchell BS, Hanson RK, et al. Systemic reactions in United States Marine Corps personnel who received Japanese encephalitis vaccine. *J Infect Dis* 1997;24:265–266.
88. Anonymous. Human rabies prevention—United States, 1999. *MMWR* 1999;48(RR-1):1–21.
89. Dye C, Scheele S, Dolin P, et al. Consensus statement. Global burden of tuberculosis: estimated incidence, prevalence, and mortality by country: WHO Global Surveillance and monitoring project. *JAMA* 1999;282: 677–686.
90. Behr MD. BCG—different strains, different vaccines? *Lancet Infect Dis* 2002;2:86–92.
91. Health information for international travel 2001–2002. Atlanta: Centers for Disease Control and Prevention, 2001.
92. Cobelens FG, Van Deutekom H, Draayer-Jansen IW, et al. Risk of infection with Mycobacterium tuberculosis in travellers to areas of high tuberculosis endemicity. *Lancet* 2000;356:461–465.
93. Steffen R, DuPont HL. *Manual of travel medicine and health.* Hamilton: BC Decker, 1999:325–330.
94. Tsai T. Yellow fever. In: Strickland GT, ed. *Hunter's tropical medicine and emerging infectious diseases,* 8th ed. Philadelphia: WB Saunders, 2000:272–275.
95. Martin M, Weld LH, Tsai TF, et al. Advanced age as a risk factor for illness temporally associated with yellow fever vaccination. *Emerg Infect Dis* 2001;7:945–951.
96. World Health Organization. World malaria situation in 1994. *Wkly Epidemiol Rec* 1997;72:269–274.
97. Anonymous. Malaria surveillance—United States, 1997. *MMWR* 2001;50(SS-1);25–44.
98. Sturchler D. Global epidemiology of malaria. In: Schlagenhauf-Lawlor P, ed. *Travelers' malaria.* Hamilton: BC Decker, 2001:14–55.
99. CDC Web site: *http:cdc.gov.govncidoddpdparasites-malariahcp_malaria_drugs.htm.*
100. World Health Organization Web site: *http:who.intith englishgeneral2.htm.*
101. Dorsey G, Gandhi M, Oyugi JH, et al. Difficulties in

the prevention, diagnosis, and treatment of imported malaria. *Arch Intern Med* 2000;160:2505–2510.
102. Anonymous. Malaria deaths following inappropriate malaria chemoprophylaxis—United States, 2001. *MMWR* 2001;50:597–599.
103. Anonymous. Drugs for parasitic infections. The Medical Letter Handbook of Antimicrobial Therapy. New Rochelle: Medical Letter, 2000:104–126.
104. Jong EC, Nothdurft HD. Current drugs for antimalarial chemoprophylaxis: a review of efficacy and safety. *J Trav Med* 2001;8[suppl 3]:S48–S56.
105. Barat LM, Bloland PB. Drug resistance among malaria and other parasites. *Infect Dis Clin North Am* 1997; 11:4.
106. Nosten F, Kuile FT, Chongsuphajaisiddhi T, et al. Mefloquine-resistant falciparum malaria on the Thai-Burmese border. *Lancet* 1991;337:1140–1143.
107. Beallor C, Kain, KC. Doxycycline. In: Schlagenhauf-Lawlor P. *Travelers' malaria.* Hamilton: BC Decker, 2001:210–218.
108. The Medical Letter. Atovaquone/Proguanil (Malarone) for Malaria. *Med Lett* 2000;42:109–110.
109. Looareesuwan S, Chulay JD, Canfield CJ, et al. Malarone (atovaquone and proguanil hydrochloride): a review of its clinical development for treatment of malaria. *Am J Trop Med Hyg* 1999;60:533–541.
110. Trachsler M, Schlagenhauf P, Steffen R. Feasibility of a rapid dipstick antigen-capture assay for the self-testing of travellers' malaria. *Trop Med Int Health* 1999; 4:442–447.
111. Jelink T, Amsler L, Grobusch MP, et al. Self-use of rapid tests for malaria diagnosis by tourists. *Lancet* 1999;354:1609.
112. Sowunmi A, Salako LA, Ogunbona FA. Bioavailability of sulphate and dihydrochloride salts of quinine. *Afr J Med Med Sci* 1994;23:275–278.
113. Newton P, Proux S, Green M, et al. Fake artesunate in Southeast Asia. *Lancet* 2001;357:1904.
114. Schulte C, Krebs B, Jelinek T, et al. Diagnostic significance of blood eosinophilia in returning travelers. *Clin Infect Dis* 2002;34:407–411.
115. White NJ. The treatment of malaria. *N Engl J Med* 1996;335:800–806.
116. Magill AJ. Fever in the returned traveler. *Infect Dis Clin North Am* 1998;12:445–469.
117. McKendrick MW, Read NW. Irritable bowel syndrome—post salmonella infection. *J Infect* 1994;29:1–3.
118. Harries AD, Myers B, Cook GC. Inflammatory bowel disease: a common cause of bloody diarrhoea in visitors to the tropics. *Br Med J* 1985;291:1686–1687.
119. Harries AD, Beeching NJ. Chronic diarrhoea in adults in the tropics: a practical approach to management. *Trop Doct* 1991;21:56–60.
120. Theilman NM, Guerrant RL. Persistent diarrhea in the returned traveler. *Infect Dis Clin North Am* 1998;12: 489–501.
121. Steffen R, Rickenbach M, Wilhelm U, et al. Health problems after travel to developing countries. *J Infect Dis* 1987;156:84–91.
122. Caumes E, Carriere J, Guermonprez G, et al. Dermatoses associated with travel to tropical countries: a prospective study of the diagnosis and management of 269 patients presenting to a tropical disease unit. *Clin Infect Dis* 1995;20:542–548.
123. Caumes E, Lucchina LC. Dermatologic problems abroad and on returning. In: DuPont HL, Steffen RS, eds. *Textbook of travel medicine and health,* 2nd ed. Hamilton: BC Decker, 2001:510–518.
124. Gonzales E. Schistosomiasis, cercarial dermatitis, and marine dermatitis. *Dermatol Clin* 1989;7:291–300.
125. Freudenthal AR, Joseph PR. Seabather's eruption. *N Engl J Med* 1993;329:542–544.
126. Kain KC. Skin lesions in returned travelers. *Med Clin North Am* 1999;83:1077–1102.
127. Stewart L, Deggat PA. Culture shock and travelers. *J Trav Med* 1998;5:84–88.
128. Valk TH. Psychiatric medical evacuations within the Foreign Service. *Foreign Service Med Bull* 1987;268: 9–11.
129. Paz BA, Paz A, Potasman I. Psychiatric problems in returning travelers: features and associations. *J Trav Med* 2001;8:243–246.
130. Dupont RL, Valk TH, Heltberg J. Psychiatric illness and stress. In: DuPont HL, Steffen RS, eds. *Textbook of travel medicine and health,* 2nd ed. Hamilton: BC Decker, 2001:365–370.

14

Economics of Occupational Medicine

Jeffrey S. Harris

Occupational health programs (OHPs) can play an important role in support of the organizations they serve by preserving and enhancing the health and productivity of the workforce. If those managing occupational health services can express the benefits of their services in economic terms, they can demonstrate the effectiveness of their efforts, compete effectively for resources, and accomplish their goals. If not, they may be marginalized or provided inadequate resources. In the latter case, they will have missed a significant opportunity to make key contributions to organizations' success and to the health and well-being of their employees and their dependents.

Using business analysis and presentation is important to this effort. Businesses and government organizations typically have a mission, strategy, and tactics to produce goods and services to satisfy and even delight their customers. The organizations' managers have goals framed in terms of output, market share, profit margin, customer service, and human resource management, among others. In well-run organizations, measurable objectives are set to meet these goals. The mission, goals, and objectives of the OHP should be congruent with and support the mission, goals, and objectives of the organization. It is important to quantify the benefits provided to the organization, its employees, and their dependents to match resource needs with benefits provided, and to focus the operations of the OHP. In this context, the OHP can include medical liaison as well as treatment, consultation, and health management leadership. (See Chapter 19 for the definition of these terms.)

Occupational physicians and other occupational health professionals can contribute to these efforts in a variety of ways. In the face of medical care costs that are increasing faster than the Consumer Price Index, and significant questions about the value received for these large outlays, some occupational physicians have become involved in benefits redesign and in medical management of employee and dependent general health care (see Chapter 19). Occupational health professionals can also act as liaisons with the private medical community to refer employees and dependents to high-quality, lower-cost providers (the two are usually synonymous) (1–3). They may also act as internal consultants in evaluating medical care provided to employees and dependents, including operational management of vendors who provide services ranging from employee assistance, health promotion, and primary care to utilization management and managed care. Occupational health professionals, with training in organizational behavior, management, epidemiology, practice parameters, technology assessment, and the research related to the effectiveness and appropriateness of various diagnostic and therapeutic modalities, are in a unique position to understand the organization's culture and the decision-making process, and to effectively provide an informed point of view, to the benefit of both management and employees (4).

Adverse health effects from the workplace should be prevented by medical surveillance and control of hazardous exposures (see Chapter 41). Strategic health management activities can also reduce morbidity, mortality, and disability caused by a number of diseases through informed co-management by the patient and health professionals (see Chapter 19).

The economic benefits of any of these activities can be evaluated along a number of dimensions, including direct, indirect, and intangible costs. The information presented in this chapter should help occupational health programs plan, manage, and monitor their programs of service. A number of the variables can be used to support continuous quality improvement efforts, which should increase the value of both the consultative and direct-service components of OHPs over a period of time.

Employers are often initially most interested in activities with an immediate economic benefit. Such activities include occupationally related medical treatment services, some aspects of health promotion, and the primary care of nonoccupational illnesses and injuries, which employers would otherwise pay for through their benefits plan. Management of the care purchased with medical benefits, for optimal efficiency and effectiveness of care, can also have a relatively quick payback, depending on the willingness of the provider organizations to work with health management specialists employed by the organization.

"TRADITIONAL" OCCUPATIONAL MEDICAL SERVICES

Many employers, particularly small and mid-sized ones, are most familiar with the prevention, treatment, and management of occupationally related illness and injury. This section reviews the approach to calculating the economic benefits of those activities, and briefly discusses the other traditional role of occupational physicians and other health professionals—that of the medical liaison. In this role, occupational physicians and nurses works with the private medical community and may refer employees to "preferred providers," who are high quality and cost-effective. Occupational health professionals can interact with work-site human resource professionals and community providers about issues such as limited duty, return to work policies, assistance that might be provided with rehabilitation after injury or illness, and perhaps reinforcement of instructions from a private treating physician. The key to these activities has been negotiating and assisting with job accommodation for those who have some degree of medical impairment, and assurance of quality care for those who have a variety of illnesses, injuries, and medically related impairments.

PREPLACEMENT, SURVEILLANCE, AND RETURN TO WORK EXAMINATIONS

The traditional cornerstone of clinical OHPs is the determination of the ability of an applicant or employee to safely perform the essential functions of a job. Preemployment examinations are an attempt to screen employees to prevent placing them in a job that they are physically incapable of performing or in which they would become a threat to the health and safety of other employees with no change in the job. The economic benefits include avoidance of safety problems and injury, and increased productivity. Generally accepted criteria for not placing a person in a specific job are that the person:

- is unable to perform the work for medical reasons, such as impairment (for example, an inability to perform a specific required motion) or because of a history or potential for development of an adverse reaction to substances in the workplace;
- poses a danger to their own health or safety or that of their co-workers;
- has a reasonable and high probability of aggravation or recurrence of a preexisting condition; or
- is unable to attend work on a reasonable basis.

The Americans with Disabilities Act (ADA) has changed the approach to these examinations to some extent, since they now must be performed *preplacement,* that is, after a conditional offer of employment, rather than preemployment. Employers are prohibited from asking a variety of medical questions that are not directly related to the functional requirements of the job. However, the examining physician may obtain complete medical histories on a voluntary basis.

Under the ADA, a thorough attempt must be made to reasonably accommodate the applicant or employee if the person can perform the *essential,* or key, job functions with accommodation before that person is excluded from the position. A careful analysis of the essential functions of the job must be performed before a statement can be made that a documented, measurable impairment prevents the applicant from performing the job without undue hazard to his or her health or safety or that of others. Further, economically viable attempts at reasonable accommodation, which might include splitting of job duties between this employee and others, reasonable assistance with minor aspects of the job, the use of assistive devices, or redesign of the job, must be made before disqualification.

A number of the actions taken under the impetus of reasonable accommodation actually have made jobs safer for all employees. For example, changing the way in which weight is transferred or chemicals are handled should benefit anyone in that position by preventing cumulative trauma disorders (CTDs) or reducing chemical exposures. As an example, suppose that an applicant with a previous history of back pain is denied employment for a position that involves lifting a 30- to 40-lb box or kit to a table, after which the components in the box are assembled. There are a number of fairly obvious challenges to this assessment. First, if this task was relatively infrequent, other employees could be asked to help. A somewhat more expensive but probably more beneficial solution would be to install a device to raise the weight to the work surface, which can be done relatively inexpensively and therefore constitutes "reasonable accommodation." Another solution might be to break the components into smaller lots. In either of the latter situations, the frequency and severity of back strain or regional low back pain in the entire population of employees performing this task would likely drop. These health complaints are often difficult to manage and account for a large proportion of expensive and extended workers' compensation claims (see Chapters 12 and 18).

Here is another example that illustrates the potential pitfalls of lack of preplacement screening: Joe Jones, a 46-year-old white man, has marginally compensated congestive heart failure. He applies for and obtains a higher-paying job forming packing molds using isocyanate resins. No preplacement examination is performed. Joe's congestive heart failure decompensates when he wears the respirator required for protection from isocyanate fumes. At first, he seems merely to be shirking work, but in fact he is severely hypoxic. He is disciplined for failing to do his job up to standards. After his private physician detects his condition, Joe files a grievance for harassment. He applies for and receives workers' compensation and, on the advice of his union, sues the company for gross negligence as well as pain and suffering. His medical expenses are paid in part by the company's benefits plan. His replacement must be trained and brought up to speed.

This situation (which has cost upward of $50,000 in similar real cases) would have been avoided had a preplacement examination, including certification for respirator use, been performed. Cases like this exist in many companies. These costs can be derived from company data or similar cases to calculate the total benefit of a medical placement program.

Anecdotal examples such as this are often cited to provide the economic justification for preplacement evaluation programs. One must take care in using anecdotes to justify OHPs, since they may later prove not to be cost-beneficial. There are in fact few well-done studies of the economic benefits of preplacement screening or medical surveillance programs. Several such studies (reviewed in ref. 5) demonstrated that the yield was highest from the medical history, and that most of the yield was in the area of personal health risk behaviors. This suggests that justifying such programs, while they are intuitively sound, requires a careful, fact-based analysis.

In evaluating the economic effects of medical screening and placement programs, therefore, one would balance the cost of the program against decreases in real or projected cost of work-related illness or injuries. All direct and indirect costs, including medical treatment, time lost from work, supervisory time, and other attributable costs, should be included to obtain a proper analysis. Failure to place employees appropriately using essential job function comparison and cost-benefit analysis may result in preventable costs for replacement and retraining, inefficiency, medical treatment, workers' compensation payments, fines under the ADA, actions under the Vocational Rehabilitation Act of 1974 or various state laws, as well as lost wages.

In contrast, failure to perform careful preplacement examinations and to place workers only in positions for which they are physically and mentally suited may place the employer in a legally precarious position. In addition to lost time and productivity, grievance procedures may be filed. There could be medical and wage replacement costs under workers' compensation. In the context of the ADA, consideration should also be given to savings from agency fines and litigation if accommodations were not provided for impairments. Employers may also be liable under tort law for pain and suffering as well as damages if willful negligence or recklessness can be demonstrated, thus invalidating the protection provided by workers' compensation statutes.

The best demonstration of the effectiveness of a medical screening program would be to show decreases in illness and injury rates and their associated costs following the point at which the program was either installed or upgraded. The value of this type of program depends on levels of hiring, placement needs, economic conditions (which can influence workers' compensation claims), and simple chance in smaller populations. The ultimate value of preplacement evaluations should be considered in the context of a larger, comprehensive program.

MEDICAL SURVEILLANCE

A key duty of the occupational health professional is to monitor health-related data on members of the workforce exposed to chemical, radiation, and other physical hazards and to compare the values for exposed and unexposed groups periodically. If an increased prevalence of abnormal laboratory values or symptoms is detected in an exposed group, the exposure should be quantified and controlled through engineering measures, administrative efforts (e.g., rotating employees), or personal protective equipment, in that order. The economic value of this type of service depends on the cost of the disease avoided, which can be computed for a population of workers if the probability of illness is known for various levels of exposure. The probability at a given exposure is similar conceptually to the attack rate of an infectious disease (probability × number of exposed individuals = expected number of cases). The expected number is then multiplied by the average cost of treating such a case over the worker's lifetime to arrive at a total cost. Subtracting the cost of the surveillance program yields the net cost. (Although these measures may be beyond the capabilities of the average practitioner, such an economic analysis can be conducted by consulting firms or universities.)

For example, if 70% of a group of 4,000 workers exposed to 50 fibers/cc asbestos for 10 years developed asbestosis, and 10% developed mesothelioma, the logic above could be followed to determine cost-effectiveness of the control program. There may be several levels of exposure that could be computed separately. The National Institute for Occupational Safety and Health (NIOSH) criteria documents recommend threshold limit values, and the Nuclear Regulatory Commission (NRC) exposure studies contain extrapolated or actual dose-response curves. Mortality costs may have been avoided also.

There are many examples of preventable occupationally related complaints or diseases that ultimately have caused great expense. Alert practitioners can intervene in cases of back, upper extremity, and other muscle/tendon pain with education, job design change, and conditioning exercises before such cases become disabling or chronic. While the most publicized complaints that come to mind in this area are carpal or ulnar tunnel syndromes, the majority of cases diagnosed under workers' compensation as carpal tunnel and other CTDs are in fact tendonitis or regional pain syndromes, rather than disorders that meet the diagnostic criteria for carpal tunnel or other nerve compression syndromes. Alert practitioners in regular contact with workers in repetitive motion jobs can screen for the discomfort that is an unnecessary effect of poorly designed jobs, improper postures, or deconditioning. In some cases, these complaints may precede disabling tendonitis, rotator cuff syndrome, carpal tunnel, and other CTDs. The practitioner may then recommend job redesign or other preventive interventions. Consistent monitoring and changes in job structure are important modes to prevent the occurrence or worsening of these health complaints and disorders.

Some employees with these health problems find it difficult to return to the same job because of associated emotional trauma. Workers with intermittent back discomfort, for example, may fear a return to the position associated with the cause of their discomfort, even in the absence of serious illness. This fear-avoidance behavior is a risk for delayed recovery. It should be actively managed through counseling by the primary treating physician and graded return to work.

A comprehensive or specific examination may need to be repeated periodically, especially in hazardous occupations and when an employee is considered for transfer to another job. The information then forms the database for a medical surveillance program (see Chapter 41).

Specific total costs avoided from these types of early detection and medical management programs can be determined from workers' compensation records. Direct costs include medical treatment and compensation payments to the employee. Indirect costs include reduced productivity of the impaired employee before definitive treatment, and replacement and retraining costs as well as probable retraining of the affected worker, since such injuries and illnesses may recur if the worker is placed back in the same job.

In many occupations, such as health care and food service, transmission of infections is a hazard to the business as well as to the individuals involved. Detection and control of infections through medical surveillance programs is a vital service, especially at medical centers. The benefits include reduced medical costs and lost time; business interruption is also avoided.

IMMUNIZATION

Immunization is an example of primary prevention resulting from a surveillance program. Workers in health care facilities, prisons, and waste disposal and sanitation are at high risk of hepatitis, influenza, and other blood-, body fluid–, or aerosol-borne diseases. The economic benefit of immunization of workers in these critical community services against influenza (6) and hepatitis B (7) has been demonstrated. Health care workers are also at risk of acquiring and transmitting rubella (8). On-site or community occupational health services are more aware of the specific biologic hazards and able to ensure coverage and monitoring of the employed population (9).

Immunization of workers against tetanus will prevent many visits to medical facilities for prophylaxis of minor wounds. Diphtheria, influenza, and other routine immunizations will prevent considerable lost work time (Table 14.1).

Immunization and malaria prophylaxis for overseas travel is often more accurately and comprehen-

TABLE 14.1. *Recommendations for adult immunizations*

Vaccine	Target population	Dose	Frequency	Comments
Live rubella virus vaccine	Susceptible young adults, females of child-bearing age, health care workers, homeless; HIV-positive patients	0.5 mL SC	Once or as part of MMR	Immunity = at least one dose, positive antibody titer, or physician-documented infection; contraindicated in pregnant women, immunocompromised
Live measles virus dose, vaccine	Susceptible persons born before 1957, overseas travelers born after 1957 to endemic areas, health care workers; inmates; homeless; HIV positive patients	0.5 mL SC	Two doses 1 month apart	Immunity = at least 1 positive antibody titer, or physician-documentedinfection; contraindicated in pregnant women, immunocompromised; MMR preferred if deficient immunity in more than one disease
Live mumps virus dose, vaccine	Susceptible persons born before 1957, overseas travelers born after 1957 to endemic areas, health care workers; inmates; homeless; HIV-positive patients	0.5 mL SC	Two doses 1 month apart	Immunity = at least one positive antibody titer, or physician-documented infection; contraindicated in pregnant women, immunocompromised; MMR preferred if deficient immunity in more than one disease
Varicella zoster vaccine	Adults living in households with children; teachers; day-care employees; institutional staff members; immunocompromised individuals, and corrections staff; college students; military personnel; nonpregnant women of childbearing age; international travelers; household contacts of immunocompromised persons	0.5 mL	Two doses 4 to 8 weeks apart	Varicella vaccination is contraindicated in persons with an anaphylactic reaction to neomycin; avoid use of salicylates for 6 weeks postvaccination
Varicella immune globulin (ZVIG)	Immunocompromised persons; susceptible pregnant women; hospital personnel	125 U/10 kg	Postexposure	Obtain history of exposure; contact = 1 hour indoors in close contact
Tetanus and diphtheria toxoids	Adults with unknown or unclear immunization history	0.5 mL IM	Two doses 4 weeks apart; booster in 6–12 months	
	All adults; travelers; IV drug users; homeless; pregnant women	0.5 mL IM	Every 10 years	Contraindicated in persons with previous severe hypersensitivity to Td
Polio virus vaccine	Health care workers with inadequate immunization history; travelers to endemic areas	eIPV IM or oral	Two doses 4–8 weeks apart Two doses 1 month apart then in 6–12 months	Booster can be OPV Booster for high exposure
Inactivated influenza virus vaccine	Health care workers; essential community services; heart disease, pulmonary disease; diabetes; renal disease; pregnancy is not contraindication; hemo-globinopathies; immunocompromised; inmates and staff; group home residents and staff; homeless; persons over 65 years of age; workers	0.5 mL IM	Annually	Contraindicated with egg allergy

continued

TABLE 14.1. *continued*

Vaccine	Target population	Dose	Frequency	Comments
Pneumococcal polysaccharide vaccine	Health care workers; smokers; alcohol abusers; splenic dysfunction or absence; transplant patients; congestive heart failure; COPD; diabetes; chronic renal disease; persons over 65 years of age; homeless	0.5 mL SC or IM	Once	Booster in 6 years for transplants, CRF; can be given with influenza at a different site
Hepatitis A vaccine	Persons traveling to or working in countries with high or intermediate endemicity of infection; homosexual men; drug users; lab workers working with HAV or infected primates; clotting factor disorders; chronic liver disease	1.0 IM	Initial, 6 months	
Hepatitis A immune globulin	Postexposure: close personal contacts, day-care center staff, food handlers, common source infections; travelers to endemic areas (see above)	0.02 mL/kg	Immediate	Screen for immunity prior to use. Dose depends on body weight
Hepatitis B vaccine	Health care workers; lab workers; morticians; sewer and sanitation workers; emergency services workers; prostitutes; inmates and staff of correctional and mental institutions; persons with multiple sexual contacts or other STDs; transplant patients; dialysis patients; household or sexual contacts of HBV infected persons; factor VIII and IX recipients; pregnant women	Varies by product	Varies by product	There are 2,3, and 4 dose series depending on the product used
Human diploid cell rabies vaccine	Veterinarians and assistants; animal handlers; field workers; travelers to endemic areas	1 mL HDCV	3 doses at days 0,7, and 21 or 28 for the primary series, then one booster if less than 1:5 serum dilution	There are 3 forms of the vaccine. Serologic testing for immunity by rapid focus fluorescent inhibition test every 6 months for continuous exosure, and every 2 years for frequent exposure
Meningococcal vaccine	Asplenia; HIV infected patients; travelers	0.5 ml SC	Every 3 years	Quadrivalent vaccine
Anthrax vaccine	Workers with imported animal products; lab workers exposed to *B. anthracis*			
Plague vaccine	Veterinarians and assistants in western U.S.; field workers exposed to rodents or fleas	0.1 mL IM, then 0.2 mL	Initial at 1 month and 5 months	Vaccine no longer available. Antibiotic prophylaxis may be used in endemic areas or occupations
Smallpox	Exposed laboratory workers; health care workers In recombinant vaccine trials			

COPD, chronic obstructive pulmonary disease; CRF, chronic renal failure; HAV, hepatitis A virus; HDCV, human diploid cell vaccine; HRIG, human rabies immunoglobulin; MMR, measles-mumps-rubella vaccine; STD, sexually transmitted disease.

sively done at the workplace because of the volume of cases and the need to avoid business interruption. Recommendations for immunization and prophylaxis for overseas travelers change frequently because disease distribution patterns often shift. The occupational physician should consult the Centers for Disease Control (CDC) or International Association for Medical Assistance to Travelers for the latest recommendation by country. The CDC's *Health Information for International Travelers* (10) is a valuable guide, as is *Control of Communicable Diseases in Man* (11). This material is available on the World Wide Web as well (12).

In general, travelers should have their primary immunizations for childhood diseases completed and updated. These illnesses are still quite common in developing countries. Generally, the manifestation of these illnesses is more severe in adults. In addition, travelers should be actively immunized against typhoid, cholera, yellow fever, influenza, hepatitis B, plague, and rabies, depending on their destination, occupation, and potential for contact with the respective pathogens. Prophylaxis against malaria and immunization against hepatitis A and B are also important to avoid unnecessary illness, business interruption, and emergency repatriation. Recommendations are listed in Table 14.2. (See Chapter 17 for a detailed discussion.)

Many employees can be reached at the work site who would not otherwise have their immunizations up to date. Cost savings per case of infectious disease prevented include avoidance of the cost of business interruption, repatriation expenses, and treatment, as well as replacement and retraining costs that would have resulted had workers not been immunized (13).

TREATMENT OF JOB-RELATED INJURIES AND ILLNESSES

Treatment of injuries and illnesses on site can be cost effective for a variety of reasons (see Chapter 18) Time lost to travel to a health facility and wait for treat-

TABLE 14.2. *Recommended immunizations for travelers*

Vaccine	Dose/type	Comments
Tetanus and diphtheria	Booster; primary series if unimmunized	Both common in underdeveloped countries
Measles, mumps, rubella	Live vaccine; if unimmunized	MMR if more than one deficient; endemic in the Third World, may be imported by unimmunized individuals
Poliovirus	Remaining doses of eIPV if not fully primarily immunized	Exposure exists in Asia and Africa; may use OPV for boosters or to complete the series Booster for partially immunized
Rabies	Preexposure series, then booster every 2 years or with low titer	For travel to areas with high incidence, particularly children
Hepatitis B	Preexposure series	For travel to or residence in endemic areas, particularly arctic, East Asia, and sub-Saharan Africa
Hepatitis A	Primary immunization >4 weeks prior prophylaxis with immune globulin	Travel to or work in endemic areas: Mexico, Central and South America, Greenland, Africa, Middle East, China, Southeast Asia
Meningococcus	Tetravalent polysaccharide	Travel to endemic areas
Plague	Primary series; booster at 6 months Booster every 1–2 years	Vaccine no longer commercially available
Typhoid	Four oral or IM doses; reimmunize every 5 years	Recommended for travel in areas such as rural Africa, Asia, Central and South America
Yellow fever	One dose primary immunization, booster every 10 years	Reported cases in Africa and South America. Available from a federally designated vaccination center
Japanese B encephalitis	Primary series 3 doses	Rural or prolonged exposures in areas of risk
Cholera	No longer recommended	
Smallpox	No longer recommended	

Contact the U.S. Centers for Disease Control Information Services Office in Atlanta at 888-232-3228 for current recommendations by country.

OPV, oral poliovaccine.

ment is avoided. The actual cost of treatment is usually less because the plant health center is not a for-profit operation. This is largely dependent upon the size of the employee population and the sophistication of the on-site medical service. Finally, physicians and nurses who are familiar with the work environment usually have a better understanding of the toxicity of substances used, individual workers' backgrounds, attitudes and risks, and factors involved in injuries that may complicate the recovery process. The costs saved include differential prices between facilities, avoided time lost for workers and supervisors, reduced length of absence postincident, and the differential costs of more accurate treatment compared to cases managed elsewhere. In particular, it has been demonstrated that the quality and appropriateness of care delivered to many patients receiving workers' compensation can be much more variable than that for general medical care (14,15). On-site care may be of greater consistency.

Workers' compensation case rates may also be reduced because the employee is absent less than a half day [i.e., not a lost workday by Occupational Safety and Health Administration (OSHA) criteria], which can affect workers' compensation insurance premium rates, depending on the carrier's definitions and state workers' compensation regulations. Where on-site treatment is not feasible, community-based occupational health services can also save time by prompt treatment and effective management of work-related injuries.

There are a number of examples of very cost-effective on-site care, both for general medical care and for comprehensive care. A comprehensive health management program at Northern Telecom, Inc., demonstrated significant decreases in cost for both work-related injuries and non–work-related illnesses (16). Gillette Company calculated substantial savings based solely on decreases in absenteeism (17). There are a number of other examples as well (18).

REHABILITATION AND RETURN TO WORK

Knowledge of the job is critical for appropriate placement of workers returning to work following an illness or injury. The occupational physician can prescribe modified duties in light of availability of proper assignment and medical limitations.

There are physical, mental, and financial advantages for the worker in an early return to work. First, return to work benefits the injured worker, who becomes a part of the work milieu again. Improvements in perception of self-worth that result can aid in the recovery process. Second, many musculoskeletal problems such as regional low back pain become worse with inactivity. Inactivity is one of the risks for significant delays in functional recovery. Further, the rate of return to work declines substantially after several months' absence and is very low after 6 months to a year. Many of these employees could work in some capacity if graduated accommodation were made (see Chapter 18). From a financial standpoint, many employees, after a certain period of time, receive only partial wage replacement when absent for illness or injury of any sort. Therefore, there is benefit from return to work for both the employer and the employee. With modified work of value, an employee who can work at 70% capacity costs only 30% in replacement, as opposed to 100% if absent. Savings in these cases derive from disability costs avoided (by comparison to similar unmanaged cases) and other intangible benefits. Successfully rehabilitated workers and their friends often have increased loyalty to the organization.

An example of the benefit of a traditional occupational health program that includes on-site services and modified duty should illustrate the cumulative effect of these measures. The key measure used is the absence rate, or proportion of total available work hours lost to absence. A major Canadian firm with three plants in Ontario and one in Quebec retained the services of an occupational health physician. The rate of absence for all illness and injury had been 9.5%, not uncommon for heavy industry. After 1 year of occupational medicine service in one plant, the absence rate was 8%, while it remained at 9.5% in the others. By year 4, the rate had fallen to 6.5%. The health service was then extended to a second plant; its absence rate fell to 7.0% by year 2. This meant that 1,000 workers were required where 1,025 were needed before. The health program cost $50,000 per 1,000 employees; the savings were $650,000 for a net of $600,000, plus uncalculated savings for retraining, inefficient function of replacement workers, and business interruption.

CONSULTING ACTIVITIES

Beyond the clinically based activities of placement, surveillance, treatment, medical management, and rehabilitation, occupational health professionals often serve as internal consultants to an organization in areas of industrial hygiene, job modification, employee assistance, and other special problems. These activities can prevent health problems, both primarily and secondarily. The cost-effectiveness of consulting activities can be measured by savings resulting from the program recommendations. For example, if consultation results in prevention of exposure to a toxic substance, savings are the net of disease costs minus the cost of engineering controls. Or, if cases of alcoholism are treated early through an effective employee assistance program (EAP) that the physician recommended, part of the savings are due to the consultation activities.

Industrial Hygiene Consultation

Occupational health practitioners have the opportunity to prevent illnesses and injuries caused by chemical and physical hazards at the work site in several ways. They can advise managers about the presence, nature, and magnitude of hazards. They can also evaluate the adequacy of barriers and procedures intended to protect employees from exposure, both by inspection and by epidemiologic surveillance of the workforce. The occupational physician should work closely with the industrial hygienist if one is available. The hygienist will usually measure air levels of toxins and evaluate barriers, while the physician can predict and monitor health effects based on analogous structures of chemicals, the literature, and surveillance examinations. The physician must be aware of industrial hygiene measures in his or her areas of responsibility and correlate them with observed health effects, if any. The object is to ensure that the workplace is safe (see Chapter 1).

Reductions in injury and disease rates attributable to improvements in industrial hygiene and safety can be calculated by measuring reductions in workers' compensation insurance costs, and the value of enhanced productivity resulting from reduction of restricted and lost workdays. This latter figure can be derived by comparing restricted and lost workdays before and after the intervention on the OSHA 200 Log, or the net of workers' compensation costs on Workers' Compensation Board reports. The value of lost time should be multiplied by a factor of 3 to 10 to reflect the cost of business interruption, retraining, and associated costs (19). These savings should be offset against the cost of industrial hygiene controls (amortized over their expected useful life) and placement and biologic monitoring programs.

Because workers' compensation insurance provides benefits for health problems until the person is considered functionally "permanent and stationary." Not uncommonly, payments may be made for 10 or more years. Results can be seen much more rapidly in self-insured programs. In addition, if time-based case management is used in these cases, and employees can be returned to work much more quickly, savings can be realized that much faster (20).

Intangible effects of control measures include avoidance of liability for delayed or negligently caused health problems, and enhanced public image. These figures are difficult to pinpoint; however, they can be valued within broad limits.

Workers' compensation costs increased from $25 billion in 1980 to $60 billion in 1991. With greater awareness of issues such as chemically caused disease, regional pain complaints, and repetitive use injuries, as well as high inflation in medical care costs, this escalation is expected to continue. Prevention efforts may well modify this steeply rising curve.

NEWER OCCUPATIONAL SERVICES

Employee Assistance Programs

A small number of employees at most work sites use significantly more medical services than other employees and are absent a great deal because of somatization of psychological conflicts. Resolution of these somatization disorders by providing cognitive services has resulted in benefit-cost ratios of up to 10:1 (21,22).

One good example is a comprehensive program that is an extension of an EAP program. At First Chicago National Bank, the EAP acts as a gatekeeper for a comprehensive mental health effort that includes concurrent psychiatric hospital utilization review, consulting psychiatrists, and some other features of case management. Mental health care costs have decreased as a proportion of total outlays, and the cost per covered employee was kept constant during a 5-year period while other benefits were inflating dramatically. The cost of inpatient mental health care dropped significantly during that time period (23). Similar effects have been noted in other settings as well (24).

EAPs also provide savings by early intervention in mental health problems, which can prevent hospitalization and long-term illness. Nonproductive conflicts between employees and supervisors can be resolved early, as can performance problems due to stress or substance abuse (see Chapter 28) (25). It should be noted that performance problems not related to an illness or injury are the province of the supervisor and not occupational health professionals, who should be careful to separate the two issues.

Transitional Work

Injury and reinjury in taxing jobs can be prevented by gradually increasing workload or time at the job. This is termed "transitional work." Protocols are available for acclimation schedules according to total workload over time. Medical personnel must work with supervisors to ensure that appropriate modified work is available. Reductions in injury rates and associated expenses can be costed in a manner similar to that described above. The value obtained from reconditioning workers appears to significantly outweigh the cost of professional time and lost production. It is clear that on-site transitional duty is much less expensive and more supportive of reintegration than extensive simulated work conditioning and work hardening performed by clinics off-site (26,27).

ON-SITE MANAGEMENT OF NONOCCUPATIONAL ILLNESS AND INJURIES

Many employers, especially those who are self-insured, have noted the advantages of providing comprehensive health care for both occupational and nonoccupational illnesses and injuries at the work site. Advantages include earlier treatment with reduced morbidity, better health supervision, ready access to practitioners who understand the work environment, and lower unit cost. Access and quality can be improved in several ways. The employee, in turn, does not need to take half a day or longer off from work to travel to a medical facility and wait in the waiting room; this scenario involves lost wages, and also interferes with production and work duties. Easier access to medical care frequently results in earlier treatment and reduction in severity of illness and resultant lost time. Physicians familiar with the work environment can be expected to recommend modified work duties that will be of benefit to the organization and the employee, and not aggravate or prolong the condition (28).

Physicians, as well as nurses, nurse practitioners, and physician assistants under appropriate supervision, can perform on-site treatment. Allied health professionals such as nurse practitioners and physician assistants can provide many clinical and nonclinical services at significantly lower cost. The quality of care has repeatedly been demonstrated to be comparable to traditional services and often with evidence of better patient empathy on the part of the allied providers (29). In the majority of cases treated by mid-level providers, the physician becomes a team leader rather than a direct provider of care.

According to the United States Chamber of Commerce, fewer than 40% of employed people have a primary care physician. Some patients may have trouble selecting an appropriate physician or gaining timely access to treatment. For these employees, on-site facilities improve access and may improve the quality of care. As an alternative to on-site treatment or for chronic or complex cases, the occupational physician can play a valuable role in facilitating referral to high-quality specialists and reduce anxiety and morbidity. Referred cases can also be tracked against a control group to assess the effects of the occupational health programs on total cost per case, including indirect costs.

Political difficulties can surface when an organization provides services on site or when an occupational health clinic for small business is established. Local physicians in particular may feel threatened with a loss of patient volume. Since fewer than half of employed people have a primary care physician, however, this fear is not justified. In fact, referral patterns from a well-run occupational health program greatly benefit the local medical community (see Chapter 1).

Occupational health programs designed to serve smaller companies in the immediate geographic area can have similar benefits to an organization. These programs focus on the work environment; thus, they are apt to be aware of special occupational medical concerns, in a manner similar to on-site programs.

Direct economic benefits of on-site treatment of both occupational and nonoccupational health problems include lost time saved and lower unit cost because of use of allied health professionals or contract arrangements with physicians at a community occupational health program. Indirect savings include decreased morbidity for specific cases, with imputed savings in absence and medical care costs. Whether on-site programs are appropriate or cost-effective for any organization depends in large part on the number of employees, the type of business operation, and the resultant need for occupational medical services. At the Morgan Guarantee Trust, for example, the on-site medical program provides primary care services and has been able to negotiate significant discounts for laboratory, x-ray, and consultative services from local medical providers, resulting in a significant savings to the company (30). The Goodyear Tire and Rubber Company and Nestle's provide primary care to employees and dependents on site, apparently at significant savings (31). Southern California Edison has integrated its on-site primary care clinics into its preferred provider organization. Apparently, by reducing overhead and medically unnecessary treatment, a savings also resulted (32). At General Electric, on-site physical therapy decreased lost workdays by 32%, and overall cost by 37% for workers' compensation low back pain claims (33). A similar savings was demonstrated at several plants at Northern Telecom, Inc. (34).

CHRONIC DISEASE MANAGEMENT

Management or co-management of certain conditions such as hypercholesterolemia, diabetes, asthma, coronary artery disease, and hypertension may be more effective at the work site, primarily because of ease of access to medical care, close follow-up, and coordination with managing physicians (35). Routine contact with allied health personnel and referral back to the primary care physician for medications have resulted in improved control of hypertension at lower cost (36,37). Peer pressure also contributes to these success rates. Lost time for follow-up visits is also decreased when the services are provided on site. Further, work accommodations for disabilities in such patients can be made more efficiently.

Economic benefits of on-site chronic disease monitoring include reduced absence for treatment and increased compliance with treatment regimen, which reduces morbidity and mortality from the disorder. Over a period of several years, these benefits can be documented (38). In the shorter run, they can be determined from data available from federal and voluntary agencies applied to the demographics of the employee population (39).

SELF-CARE AND WISE USE OF COUNSELING AND EDUCATION

Education of patients in self-care for minor illnesses and injuries has reduced health care costs. Benefit costs declined 17% to 35% in one study for those who participated in self-care education (40). There are many other examples (41). A variety of allied health care practitioners can effectively provide and coordinate this counseling and education. One interesting way of increasing awareness of the medical system, as well as saving a significant amount of money, is to have workers audit their hospital bills for accuracy. A reward can be given for errors discovered.

Educating employees in the best way to use the medical care system has resulted in increases in the quality of care and substantial decreases in inappropriate utilization. This training may take the form of printed material or discussions with a health care professional (42–44).

CASE AND DISEASE MANAGEMENT

Case management of both chronic diseases and catastrophic and complex cases can have a significant effect on total costs. Close management of seriously ill, injured, or chronically ill employees or those undergoing treatment is valuable to avoid unnecessary procedures, ensure appropriate therapy, and aid in proper discharge planning as well as early return to work. Often this consists of ensuring physician compliance with evidence-based practice guidelines (45). Careful case-control–type comparisons are needed to ensure reasonably accurate estimates for care that was avoided.

HEALTH PROMOTION AT THE WORK SITE

Impact of Lifestyle on Health and Costs

Since the economic impact of lifestyle-related disease on health care costs has been more clearly recognized, health promotion programs have become increasingly common at the work site. The trend has continued to accelerate since the last edition of this book. The primary yield from preplacement and screening exams, as noted above, is information on unmanaged lifestyle health risks. Costs for lifestyle-related problems have been estimated at 10 to 15 times as much as work-related illness and injuries. Interactions between lifestyle and certain occupational exposures (e.g., smoking and asbestos) further compound the problem.

The leading causes of death as well as morbidity in the United States today are heart disease, cancer, stroke, chronic obstructive pulmonary disease, injuries, pneumonia, diabetes, suicide, chronic liver disease, and human immunodeficiency virus (HIV) (46). This appears to represent the continued aging of the population and ongoing lifestyle risks despite medical advances. In the last edition of this chapter, injuries ranked fourth and influenza ranked fifth (47). It appears that influenza immunization, child restraints and seatbelt requirements and programs, airbags, and other safety programs have had a significant effect, so that other causes have eclipsed accidents and influenza. Heart disease accounts for 31.4% of all deaths, down from 37.5% at the time of the last edition, and cancer another 23.3%, up from 22.2%. Both of these disorders are lifestyle related. In terms of years of life lost before age 65, the leading lifestyle-related causes are unintentional injuries, cancer, heart disease, suicide and homicide, and HIV infection (48). The leading causes for these problems were tobacco use, diet and activity patterns, alcohol misuse, microbial agents, toxic agents, motor vehicles, firearms, sexual behavior, and illicit use of drugs, in that order (49). Harris and Fries (50) provide a full listing of the linkages between lifestyle risk factors and mortality, morbidity, disability, and productivity.

The effects of lifestyle on premature mortality are shown in Table 14.3 (51). The prevalence of these risk factors in employed populations has changed rather dramatically in recent years, and should be determined

TABLE 14.3. *Relative risk of death for a 35-year-old with designated risk factors*

	Heart disease		Cancer		Stroke		Injury		Chronic obstructive pulmonary disease		Influenza/ pneumonia	
Risk factor	M	F	M	F	M	F	M	F	M	F	M	F
Sedentary lifestyle	2.5	1.4	—	—	—	—	—	—	—	—	—	—
Cigarette smoking	2.0	2.0	10.0	10.0	1.2	1.5	7.0	7.0[a]	4.0	4.0	3.2	1.2
Hypertension	2.0	2.2	—	—	2.0	2.2	—	—	—	—	—	—
Obesity	1.3	1.3	—	[b]	—	—	[c]	[c]	—	—	—	—
Diabetes	3.0	4.0	—	—	[d]	—	—	—	—	—	—	—
Elevated cholesterol	2.0	2.0	—	—	2.0	2.0	—	—	—	—	—	—
Positive stool occult blood	—	—	2.0	2.0	—	—	—	—	—	—	—	—
Failure to self-examine breast	—	—	—	2.0	—	—	—	—	—	—	—	—
Failure to obtain Pap smears	—	—	—	7.0	—	—	—	—	—	—	—	—
Irregular use of seat belts	—	—	—	—	—	—	1.5	1.6	—	—	—	—
Heavy alcohol use	[d]	—	[e]	[e]	4.0	4.0	—	—	—	—	3.0	3.0

[a]Automobile injury.
[b]Elevated risk for some cancer, such as ovarian cancer.
[c]Elevated but unquantified risk in morbid obesity.
[d]Elevated risk; estimates vary.
[e]Elevated risk for cancer of pharynx, esophagus; synergistic with tobacco use.
Adapted from Hall J, Zwemmer JD. *Prospective medicine.* Indianapolis: Methodist Hospital, 1979.

for each group by obtaining health risk appraisals and pooling the results. The self-reported prevalence for some risks, such as uncontrolled hypertension, sedentary lifestyle, and nonuse of seat belts, has declined sharply in recent years. Cigarette smoking has dropped somewhat in some demographic groups and increased in others. Other risk factors, such as obesity, have not changed significantly. The proportion of premature mortality due to risk factors in a typical employed group can be calculated by multiplying the prevalence of the risk factor by the relative risk. Thus, a factor with a moderate risk but a high prevalence, such as a sedentary lifestyle (upward of 60% in many groups of older workers) would cause many more deaths than smoking (with a prevalence of less than 15%) in this age group (persons 60 to 69 years of age). Some diseases caused by smoking, such as cancer, cause the majority of attributable deaths in younger age groups, in which heart disease is not so prevalent. Excess mortality and morbidity in those with risk factors increase sharply after age 30 (Fig. 14.1).

Each case of heart disease that requires coronary bypass can cost over $50,000 (depending on the part of the country in which it is performed and the managed care arrangements involved) in direct costs, and as much as triple that amount in wage replacement and other indirect costs. The treatment for lifestyle-related cancers such as lung cancer can cost more than $50,000 per patient. There are one million new cases of cancer per year, of which over half are lifestyle related (52). Life insurance costs should be added to these costs, significantly increasing the total outlay. There are additional indirect costs for retraining and replacement.

Medical care costs per nonfatal case for typical employee groups with lifestyle-related diseases can be determined for each employed group. Costs vary substantially depending on risks, health plan design, and employee demographics. The data on the proportion of this morbidity that is preventable are not as well studied, but one review of medical records noted that the 13% of patients with one or more serious risk factors incurred the same medical care costs as the other 87% and had five times the number of major complications (53).

Effects of Health Promotion Efforts

There is evidence from both epidemiologic studies and clinical trials that morbidity and mortality are reduced if risk factors are decreased (54). Studies on the net cost-effectiveness of health promotion programs demonstrate a significant positive benefit-to-cost ratio (55). A framework for the analysis of the cost-effectiveness of health promotion programs has been provided in a recent publication (56).

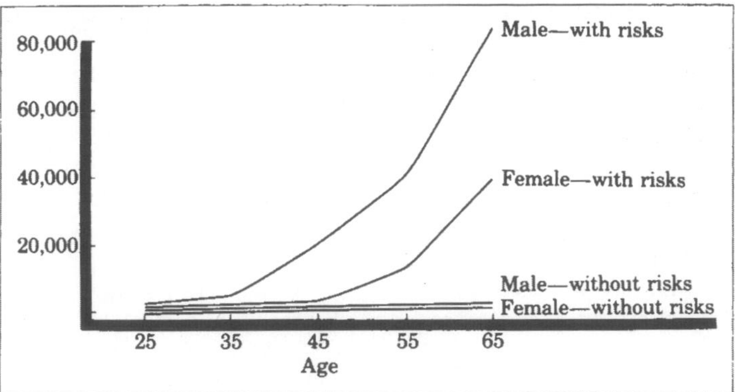

FIG. 14.1. Cumulative heart disease deaths (per 100,000) in the United States, 1980 estimate. Risks include blood pressure, 160/100; weight, 50% over the ideal; cholesterol, 300 mg/100 mL; sedentary lifestyle; and one pack of cigarettes per day. (Data from Hall J, Zwemmer JD. *Prospective medicine.* Indianapolis: Methodist Hospital, 1979.)

Screening to Promote Health

While much of the risk screening done today is nonproductive, early detection of hypertension, hypercholesterolemia, and cervical and breast cancer has a significant benefit-cost ratio. In asymptomatic individuals, other tests, such as chest and back films, multichannel chemistries, and resting and stress electrocardiograms, are of minimal value and may result in unnecessary costs involved in ruling out false positives (57).

Cost savings for illnesses such as upper- and lower-respiratory infections, adverse reproductive outcomes, and some gastrointestinal diseases that could be affected by health promotion have been demonstrated (58). Other studies demonstrating a positive benefit-to-cost ratio include Johnson & Johnson's Live for Life Program (59) and Travelers' Taking Care Center (60). It is frequently necessary to follow participants for up to 10 years to document long-term benefits (61). Nonetheless, reductions in health risks can result in significant savings in benefits, retraining and replacement costs, business interruption, and improvements in performance and employee morale.

MEDICAL BENEFITS QUALITY AND COST MANAGEMENT

Benefit Design Consultation

Astute occupational medicine physicians can be of great value to a company's benefits organization by recommending appropriate medical services to be covered (including preventive services) and reimbursement schemes that discourage the use of medically unnecessary services. Conversely, the physician can recommend and/or arrange for more appropriate services and audit fees. They can also assist employees in auditing their hospital bills.

Utilization Management: The Gatekeeper Concept

Medical practice patterns vary significantly in different areas of the country, often with little discernible difference in treatment outcome. To curtail medically unnecessary services, almost all insurers and some self-insured companies require employees to clear hospitalizations and diagnostic procedures or use defined practitioners; otherwise, benefits and coverage may be reduced. Other companies have authorized third-party services to review the need for hospitalization or surgery and to determine whether alternative measures, such as outpatient surgery, can be used.

Precertification and concurrent reviews of hospitalizations have led to steep drops in inpatient service use as criteria are tightened. In one of the few controlled studies, private review of hospitalization decreased inpatient days by 11%, total hospital expenditures by 7%, and total expenditures by 6%. Admissions in this study dropped by about 13% (62). Savings may have been offset to some extent by increased spending on outpatient care and the cost of administration of the program. An Institute of Medicine (IOM) study concluded that the evidence was not researched well enough to provide a definitive answer (63). One study, published after the IOM report, of employers in the Houston area found that utilization review significantly reduced total monthly inpatient charges but increased total monthly outpatient charges, with a resulting net gain in cost (64). It should be noted that the shift across from inpatient to outpatient settings can be controlled by using both inpatient and outpatient utilization management. It has also been noted that the program's impact is greatest at the onset (65), because of a "sentinel" effect. If criteria and guidelines can be progressively tightened over a period of time, utilization will decrease.

Second opinions regarding certain surgical procedures have resulted in nonconfirmation rates of 17% to 50%. Later reviews, however, show that the actual rate of avoided surgery was less than 1% in the Medicare program, prompting the Healthcare Financing Administration to focus on a few selected procedures (see Chapter 19). Level of care monitoring has resulted in savings of up to $500,000 per identified provider. These providers were outliers, identified by state peer review organizations, who changed their practice patterns after education. As the foregoing implies, a few providers often generate a tremendous amount of excess cost for little if any benefit to patients (66,67). Savings in these areas can be calculated from company insurance payment rates compared to data for optimal case management for age, gender, and disease category.

Changes in Economic Incentives

Incentives in benefits plans that contribute to inappropriate utilization include full payment for services. Introduction of substantial deductibles and copayments can reduce costs by one third (68). Full reimbursement for inpatient or emergency department treatment but partial or capped reimbursement for outpatient therapy or surgery also contributes to inappropriate care. Incentives for healthy lifestyles, such as reduced premiums or copayments for nonsmokers, have the potential to improve employee health.

Putting Providers at Risk

Capitated payment systems, whereby the provider of health care is at some risk for ordering testing and treatment of questionable benefit and in turn responsible for keeping patients healthy, have proved to be effective in managing health care costs (69). Comparing the capitation payment to the cost of the parallel conventional insurance plan can follow the benefit of this change. Another purchasing method of payment, which has price but not volume controls, is payment on the basis of diagnostic related groups (DRGs) (70). Government programs have adopted both approaches in many areas.

As described in Chapter 19, in the most comprehensive situation, occupational physicians can administer managed health care programs, which have been shown to provide significant decreases in costs or cost increase rates, and to improve the quality of care (71).

ACKNOWLEDGMENT

The author would like to acknowledge Jack Richman, M.D., for his contributions to the first edition of this chapter.

REFERENCES

1. Donabedian A. Quality and cost: choices and responsibilities. In: Harris JS, Belk HD, Wood LW, eds. *Managing employee health care costs: assuring quality and value.* Beverly Farms, MA: OEM Press, 1992:13–18.
2. Peterson KP, Loeppke RR. Population health management in managed care. In: Harris JS, Loeppke RR, eds. *Integrated health management: the key role of occupational medicine in managed care, disability management, and integrated delivery systems*. Beverly Farms, MA: OEM Press, 1998.
3. Harris JS. Managed occupational health. In: Harris JS, ed. *Managed Care: Occupational Medicine State of the Art Reviews* 1998;13(4):625–643.
4. Moser R Jr. *Effective management of occupational and environmental health and safety programs,* 2nd ed. Beverly Farms, MA: OEM Press, 1999.
5. Harris JS, Collins B, Majure IL. Prevalence of health risks in an employed population. *J Occup Med* 1986;28:217.
6. Immunization Practice Advisory Committee. Prevention and control of influenza. *MMWR* 1985;34:261.
7. Recommendations for protection against viral hepatitis. *MMWR* 1985;34:23.
8. Advisory Committee on Immunization Practices and Hospital Infection Control Practices Committee. Immunization of Health Care Workers. *MMWR Recommendations and Reports* 1997;46:1–42.
9. Harris JS. Blood borne diseases. In: DiBenedetto DD, Harris JS, McCunney RJ, eds. *The OEM manual of occupational health and safety,* 2nd ed. Beverly Farms, MA: OEM Health Information Press, 2000.
10. Division of Global Migration and Quarantine (DQ), National Center for Infectious Diseases (NCID), Centers for Disease Control and Prevention (CDC). *Health Information for International Travel, 2001–2002.* Atlanta: CDC, 2001. Available from the National Technical Information Service, (PB 2002103854) at 888-232-3228, or the Public Health foundation at 877-252-1200.
11. Benenson AS, ed. *Control of communicable diseases in man, 17 ed.* Washington, DC: American Public Health Assoc., 1999.
12. *www.CDC.gov/mmwr.*
13. Koplan JP. Benefits, risks, and costs of immunization programmes. In: CIBA Foundation. *The value of preventive medicine.* London: Pitman, 1985.

14. Harris JS, et al. Business as usual may mean going out of business. *National Council on Compensation Insurance Digest* 1989;4:25.
15. Harris JS, Bengle AL III, Makens PK, et al. *Striking the balance: an analysis of the cost and quality of medical care in the Texas Workers' Compensation system.* Austin: Texas Research and Oversight Council on Workers Compensation, 2001.
16. Dalton BA, Harris JS. A comprehensive approach to corporate health management. In: Harris JS, Belk HD, Wood LW, eds. *Managing employee health care costs: assuring quality and value.* Beverly Farms, MA: OEM Press, 1992:181–191.
17. Greer WT. Presentation to New England Medical Association, Boston, 1992.
18. Fass PH, Carr RW, Larkin GN, et al. The corporate medical department and managed care. In: Harris JS, Loeppke RR, eds. *Integrated health management: the key role of occupational medicine in managed care, disability management and integrated delivery systems.* Beverly Farms, MA: OEM Press, 1998:85–89.
19. Brady W, Bass J, Moser R Jr., et al. Defining total corporate health and safety costs—significance and impact. *J Occup Environ Med* 1997;39:224–231.
20. Harris JS. Wise up to workers' compensation. *Financial Executive* November/December 1992.
21. Harris JS. Managing health: what employers can do about health care costs. In: Meyer J, McLennon K, eds. *Care and cost: current issues in health policy.* Boulder: Westview Press, 1989:167–202.
22. Harris JS. Working paper for the Institute on Health and Productivity. Dallas: Institute on Health and Productivity, 1999.
23. Burton WN, Conti DJ. Value of managed mental health benefits. In: Harris JS, Belk HD, Wood LW, eds. *Managing employee health care costs: assuring quality and value.* Beverly Farms, MA: OEM Press, 1992:151–153.
24. Burgess AG, et al. *Investing in workplace productivity—innovations in managing indirect mental health costs.* Washington, DC: National Institute of Mental Health, 1999.
25. Lippman H. This is not your father's EAP. *Bus Health* 1999;17(12):42. MacAlister E. Does an employee assistance programme benefit employers and employees alike? *Occup Med (Lond)* 1999;49(7):465–466. Rotarius T, Liberman A, Liberman JS. Employee assistance programs: a prevention and treatment prescription for problems in health care organizations. *Health Care Manag (Frederick)* 2000;19(1):24–31.
26. Harris JS, Bengle AL III, Makens PK, et al. *Returning to work: an examination of existing disability duration guidelines and their application to the Texas Workers' Compensation System.* Austin: Texas Research and Oversight Council on Workers Compensation, 2001.
27. Harris JS, Bengle AL III, Makens PK et al. *Striking the balance: an analysis of the cost and quality of medical care in the Texas Workers' Compensation System.* Austin: Texas Research and Oversight Council on Workers Compensation, 2001.
28. Walsh DC. *Corporate physicians: between medicine and management.* New Haven: Yale University Press, 1987.
29. Scharon GM, Bernacki EJ. Corporate nurse practitioners. *Business and Health* 1984;1:26.
30. Schneider WJ. A corporate medical department's role in medical benefits. In: Harris JS, Belk HD, Wood LW, eds. *Managing employee health care costs: assuring quality and value.* Beverly Farms, MA: OEM Press, 1992:171–174.
31. Bryant M. Comeback for the company doc? *Business and Health* 1991;9(2):44–45, 48–50.
32. Geisel J. Company-run clinics cutting health care costs: an interview with Jacques Sokolov. *Business Insurance* March 5, 1990.
33. Galvin RS. Personal communication.
34. Dalton BA, Harris JS. A comprehensive approach to corporate health management. In: Harris JS, Belk HD, Wood LW, eds. *Managing employee health care costs: assuring quality and value.* Beverly Farms, MA: OEM Press, 1992:181–191.
35. Harris JS, Fries JF. The health effect of health promotion. In: O'Donnell MP, ed. *Health promotion at the workplace,* 3rd ed. Albany, NY: Delmar, 2001.
36. Aldana SG. Financial impact of health promotion programs: a comprehensive review of the literature. *Am J Health Promotion* 2001;15:296–320.
37. Erfurt JC, Foote A, Heirich MA. The cost-effectiveness of work-site wellness programs for hypertension control, weight loss, and smoking cessation. *J Occup Med* 1991;33(9):962–970.
38. Musich SA, Burton WN, Eddington DW. Costs and benefits of prevention and disease management. *Dis Manage Health Outcomes* 1999;5:153–166.
39. Harris JS, Fries JF. The health effect of health promotion. In: O'Donnell MP, ed. *Health promotion at the workplace,* 3rd ed. Albany, NY: Delmar, 2001:1–21.
40. Vickery DM, et al. Effect of self-care education program on medical visits. *JAMA* 1983;250:2952.
41. Fries JF, Koop CE, Sokolov J, et al. Beyond health promotion: reducing health care costs by reducing need and demand for medical care. *Health Affairs* 1998;17:70–84.
42. Lorig K. *Patient education: a practical approach.* Thousand Oaks, CA: SAGE, 1996.
43. Harris JS, Goldstein JR, Tager MJ. *Wise moves.* Chicago: Great Performance, 1986.
44. MacStravic S, Montrose G. *Managing health care demand.* Gaithersburg, MD: Aspen, 1998.
45. Couch JB, ed. *The physician's guide to disease management.* Gaithersburg, MD: Aspen, 1997.
46. National Center for Health Statistics. *Advance report of final mortality statistics, 1998.* Washington, DC: National Center for Health Statistics, 2000.
47. U.S. Department of Health and Human Services. *Healthy People 2000 Review, 1998–1999.* Washington, DC: U.S. Department of Health and Human Services, Public Health Service, 1999.
48. Fielding JE. Occupational health physicians and prevention. In: Harris JS, Belk HD, Wood LW, eds. *Managing employee health care costs: assuring quality and value.* Beverly Farms, MA: OEM Press, 1992:154–166.
49. McGinnis JM, Foege W. Actual causes of death in the United States. *JAMA* 1993;270:2207–2212.
50. Harris JS, Fries JF. The health effect of health promotion. In: O'Donnell MP, ed. *Health promotion at the workplace,* 3rd ed. Albany, NY: Delmar, 2001:1–21.
51. Hall J, Zwemmer JD. *Prospective medicine.* Indianapolis: Methodist Hospital, 1979.
52. National Center for Health Statistics. *Advance report of final mortality statistics, 1998.* Washington, DC: National Center for Health Statistics, 2000.

53. Zook CJ, Moore FD. High cost users of medical care. *N Engl J Med* 1980;302(18):996–1002.
54. O'Donnell MP. The financial benefits of health promotion. In: O'Donnell MP, ed. *Health promotion in the workplace,* 3rd ed. Albany, NY: Delmar, 2001.
55. Aldana SG. Financial impact of health promotion programs: a comprehensive review of the literature. *Am J Health Promotion* 2001;15:296–320.
56. Anderson DR, Serxner SA, Gold DB. Conceptual framework, critical questions, and practical challenges in conducting research on the financial impact of worksite health promotion. *Am J Health Promotion* 2001;15: 281–288.
57. U.S. Preventive Services Task Force. *Guide to clinical preventive services,* 2nd ed. Baltimore: Williams & Wilkins, 1996.
58. Dalton BA, Harris JS. A comprehensive approach to corporate health management. In: Harris JS, Belk HD, Wood LW, eds. *Managing employee health care costs: assuring quality and value.* Beverly Farms, MA: OEM Press, 1992:181–191.
59. Bly JL, Jones RC, Richardson JE. Impact of worksite health promotion on healthcare cost and utilization: an evaluation of Johnson & Johnson's Live for Life program. *JAMA* 1986;256:3235.
60. Lynch WD, et al. Impact of a facility-based fitness program on the number of absences from work due to illness. *J Occup Med* 1990;32:9.
61. The Multiple Risk Factor Intervention Trial Research Group. Mortality rates after 10.5 years for participants in Multiple Risk Factor Intervention Trial: findings related to a priori hypotheses of the trial. *JAMA* 1990;263: 1795–1801.
62. Gray BH, Field MJ. *Controlling cost in changing patient care? The role of utilization management.* Washington, DC: National Academy Press, 1989.
63. Appel FA. Testimony before the National Academy of Sciences Institute of Medicine. Committee on utilization management by third parties. *J Qual Assur* 1988;10 (3):6–7.
64. Custer WS. *Employer healthcare design, plan costs, and health care delivery.* Washington, DC: Employee Benefits Research Institute, 1989.
65. Khandker RK, Manning WG, Ahmed T. Utilization review savings at the micro level. *Med Care* 1992;30:1043.
66. Harris JS. *Cost effective health care.* Nashville: Northern Telecom, 1988.
67. Harris JS, Bengle AL III, Makens PK, et al. *Striking the balance: an analysis of the cost and quality of medical care in the Texas Workers' Compensation system.* Austin: Texas Research and Oversight Council on Workers Compensation, 2001.
68. Brook RH, et al. Does free care improve adult health? Results from a randomized clinical trial. *N Engl J Med* 1983;309:1426.
69. Harris JS. Does managed care manage healthcare costs effectively?—It depends. In: Harris JS, Belk HD, Wood LW, eds. *Managing employee health care costs: assuring quality and value.* Beverly Farms, MA: OEM Press, 1992:131–135.
70. Gold M. Health maintenance organizations: structure, performance, and current issues for employee health benefits design. In: Harris JS, Belk HD, Wood LW, eds. *Managing employee health care costs: assuring quality and value.* Beverly Farms, MA: OEM Press, 1992:117–125.
71. Gold M. Health maintenance organizations: structure, performance, and current issues for employee health benefits design. In: Harris JS, Belk HD, Wood LW, eds. *Managing employee health care costs: assuring quality and value.* Beverly Farms, MA: OEM Press, 1992:117–125.

SOURCES

Advisory Committee on Immunization Practices. Vaccinia (smallpox) vaccine recommendations of the Advisory Committee on Immunization Practices. *MMWR* 2001;50 (RR-10):1–25.

Advisory Committee on Immunization Practices. Prevention and control of influenza: recommendations of the Advisory Committee on Immunization Practices. *MMWR* 2001;48(RR-4):1–44.

Advisory Committee on Immunization Practices. Prevention and control of influenza: recommendations of the Advisory Committee on Immunization Practices. *MMWR* 1999;48(RR-4):1–28.

Advisory Committee on Immunization Practices. Prevention of hepatitis A through active or passive immunization: recommendations of the Advisory Committee on Immunization Practices. *MMWR* 1999;48(RR-12):1–37.

Advisory Committee on Immunization Practices. Prevention of varicella: updated recommendations of the Advisory Committee on Immunization Practices. *MMWR* 1999;48(RR-06):1–4.

Advisory Committee on Immunization Practices, and Hospital Infection Control Practices Advisory Committee. Immunization of health care workers. *MMWR* 1997;46 (RR-18):1–43.

Advisory Committee on Immunization Practices. Prevention of plague: recommendations of the Advisory Committee on Immunization Practices (ACIP). *MMWR* 1996 (RR-14):1–15.

Advisory Committee on Immunization Practices. Prevention of varicella: recommendations of the Advisory Committee on Immunization Practices (ACIP). *MMWR* 1996; 45(RR-11):1–25.

Advisory Committee on Immunization Practices. General recommendations on immunization: recommendations of the Advisory Committee on Immunization Practices. *MMWR* 1994;43(RR-1):1–55.

Advisory Committee on Immunization Practices. Update on adult immunization recommendations of the Immunization Practices Advisory Committee. *MMWR* 1991;40 (RR12):1–52.

Gardner P, Eickhoff T, Polland GA, et al. Adult immunizations. *Ann Intern Med* 1996;124:35–40.

Gardner P, Schaffner W. Immunization of adults. *N Engl J Med* 1993;328:1252.

Updated U.S. Public Health Service Guidelines for the management of occupational exposures to HBV, HCV, and HIV and recommendations for postexposure prophylaxis. *MMWR* 2001;50(RR11):1–42. www.cdc.gov/mmwr/.

15

Educational Opportunities

David J. Tollerud and Edward A. Emmett

This chapter discusses educational options and sources of information for practicing physicians interested in expanding their knowledge and skills in the delivery of occupational and environmental medicine (OEM) consultative and clinical services. The bulk of the chapter deals with training in the specialty of OEM, but the education of physicians-in-training and continuing medical education (CME) are also briefly addressed. Resources are listed where information on OEM training and education can be obtained. Particular attention is given to the training opportunities for physicians wishing to make a midcareer shift into the field, since, among recognized medical specialties, OEM has arguably the most developed educational structure to support a career transition.

OEM AND THE PHYSICIAN-IN-TRAINING

Almost all physicians in clinical practice see patients who are or were working. In delivering quality medical care, physicians are aided by knowing what kind of work their patients do and how it may affect their health. Every week hundreds of thousands of workers visit their physicians for advice on work with reference to certain illnesses or injuries. Clinicians must decide when their patients have recovered sufficiently to return to work, whether their illness could have been caused or aggravated by work, and whether work site modifications are necessary. To make these assessments, an understanding of the work environment is essential.

Despite this, in the United States OEM remains a field in which most practitioners do not have formal training. The Institute of Medicine's Subcommittee on Physician Shortage in 1991 recommended a series of measures to alleviate the shortage of practitioners in OEM, most of which focused on increased education and training opportunities at all levels of medical education (1,2). The Institute of Medicine has also recommended that "all primary care physicians be able to identify possible occupationally or environmentally induced conditions and make appropriate referrals for follow-up" (3). The fund of knowledge required to meet such a standard of care includes familiarity with principles of preventive medicine as well as OEM, clinical skills in occupational history taking, a basic knowledge of common occupational and environmental diseases, and an understanding of the United States regulatory system and workers' compensation system. Unfortunately, most medical school curricula do not adequately expose students to the field at an early stage in their medical education. A survey of medical schools in 1996 found that, of 116 of 126 schools responding, 24% had no curricula content in environmental medicine (EM). Those who did include EM gave an average of 7 hours of instruction. Only 68% of schools reported having faculty with OEM expertise (4). Case formats for medical student education (5) and for use in structured examinations in OEM have been published (6). Most medical schools associated with hospitals that offer residency training programs in OEM (see *www.acgme.org* for list) will arrange elective rotations in OEM for medical students or residents training in other fields.

The Accreditation Council for Graduate Medical Education (ACGME) now requires some element of occupational medicine training in accredited family medicine training programs (7). Other boards and specialty areas such as internal medicine are likely to follow.

NEED FOR PHYSICIANS IN OEM

In a study published in 1991 entitled *Addressing the Physician Shortage in Occupational and Environmental Medicine,* the Institute of Medicine estimated a current shortage of 3,100 to 5,600 physicians with special competence in OEM (1). This includes primary care physicians and other specialists who have undertaken some form of training or have acquired significant practical experience in OEM. The estimated shortage of fully trained specialists in OEM was 1,600 to 3,500.

Increasingly, U.S. corporations are using external sources of medical care for their employees. Although large companies may have well-staffed occupational medical programs at many of their plants and laboratories, the bulk of Americans work in small plants, in service organizations, or for themselves, and do not have easy access to competent occupational medical advice. The result is that a growing number of primary care physicians and specialists are caring for employees with potentially work-related illnesses and injuries. For the clinician interested in providing OEM services, an understanding of the basic principles of the specialty is crucial. An increased supply of physicians in the United States, coupled with a change in funding of health care, has also motivated many physicians to seek alternative means to broaden their practices. The need for OEM services has stimulated the development of occupational and environmental health programs at hospitals, emergency rooms, and group practices.

What Is an OEM Physician?

To understand educational needs, one must address the question: What is *different* about OEM? The most fundamental distinction is that OEM is a specialty that focuses on the *prevention* of illness and injury.

Thus one goal of OEM practitioners is to deliver consultative and clinical services designed to prevent illness and injury. Often a sentinel illness or injury will provide the lead for identifying a problem workplace. What sets the OEM practitioner apart is the desire and expertise to go to the workplace and help formulate measures that will prevent recurrence of the condition among other workers. In instances where illness is identified, the physician must have enough knowledge about the workplace and specific job activities of the patient to render a judgment as to the relative contribution of the workplace. To competently deliver OEM services, one must be more than just a good clinician.

In most private practices, the clinician waits for the patient to come to the clinic with certain symptoms, makes a diagnosis, and prescribes a course of treatment. The OEM physician deals primarily with a healthy workforce and often focuses on medical surveillance of workers to identify potentially hazardous exposures at a stage when disease can be prevented (see Chapter 38). A large proportion of OEM clinical practice also focuses on the treatment of acute injuries and their follow-up as well as treatment of extended soft tissue pain. In this context, the physician needs to be aware of how work may have led to the illness or injury and the consequences or prevention. Other factors come to bear as well, including determination of a person's ability to work with a physical impairment (disability). The practitioner needs to think in terms of *populations of workers* and have an understanding of epidemiology and biostatistics to interpret trends in illness or presence of certain sentinel abnormalities in disease or laboratory surveillance measures (7). The effective physician interacts comfortably with people from business, labor, and regulatory organizations in the day-to-day practice of the specialty. He or she may be called upon to develop policies regarding occupational and environmental health and safety issues. The ability to conceive and implement new programs requires a unique type of involvement on the part of the physician. Clinical skills, communication, and teamwork skills and a broad understanding of public health, business, and law are essential to effectively carry out these complex tasks.

Beyond the treatment and prevention of occupational injury and disease, OEM physicians may be involved in assisting corporations or public sector organizations, governments, or unions with such areas as disability management and reducing the work and productivity impact of nonoccupational injury and disease, increasing the safety of products and processes, optimizing human relations practices, the reduction of global health care costs, and regulatory compliance (8).

OEM is devoted to the prevention and management of occupational and environmental injury, illness, and disability, and the promotion of the health and the productivity of workers, their families, and communities. Through training and experience, the OEM physician should bring specific competencies to achieve this mission. A reference set of competencies for OEM has been defined and published by a panel of the American College of Occupational and Environmental Medicine (ACOEM) (7). This list indicates the rather broad range of skills necessary to practice good OEM.

SPECIALIZATION AND RESIDENCY TRAINING PROGRAMS

Board Certification and Accredited Training in Occupational Medicine

Board certification in occupational medicine is administered through the American Board of Preventive

Medicine (ABPM). Eligibility to sit for the annual certifying examination is determined by a thorough review of each applicant's credentials and experience (9).

Pathways to eligibility include completion of an accredited residency in occupational medicine followed by a period of relevant practice experience. Requirements for board certification are periodically revised. Potential applicants are urged to obtain current information from the ABPM *(www.abprevmed.org)*. Currently the requirements include at least satisfactory completion of an ACGME-approved year of clinical internship, an academic year [master of public health (MPH) or equivalent], and a supervised practicum year in occupational medicine. An alternative pathway to certification by the ABPM is available to individuals who graduated from medical school before January 1, 1984. Applicants for the alternative pathway must successfully complete graduate-level courses in biostatistics, epidemiology, health services administration, and environmental health, but do not need to have completed the supervised practicum year training requirement. There are recertification requirements for those who were certified by ABPM after 1997.

Oversight and accreditation for occupational medicine residencies are provided by the ACGME through its residency review committee (RRC) for preventive medicine. The RRC develops special requirements for approved residency training programs and reviews their progress on an annual basis (Table 15.1).

A description of the special requirements for occupational medicine residency training can be found in the *Directory of Graduate Medical Education Programs* (10), which is updated annually. Information on accredited programs can be obtained from the ACGME *(www.acgme.org)*.

TABLE 15.1. *Accredited residencies in occupational medicine—October 2000*

University of Alabama Medical Center
University of California (Irvine)
University of California (Los Angeles)
University of California (San Francisco)
Loma Linda University
University of Colorado
University of Connecticut
Yale–New Haven Medical Center
George Washington University
University of South Florida
Emory University
University of Illinois College of Medicine at Chicago
Cook County Hospital/Cook County Board of Commissioners
University of Iowa Hospitals and Clinics
University of Kentucky Medical Center
Johns Hopkins School of Hygiene and Public Health
Uniformed Services University of the Health Sciences
Harvard School of Public Health
University of Massachusetts
University of Michigan School of Public Health
HealthPartners Institute for Medical Education, St. Paul, Minnesota
St. Louis University School of Medicine
UMDNJ–Robert Wood Johnson School of Medicine
Mount Sinai School of Medicine
Duke University
University Hospitals/University of Cincinnati College of Medicine
University of Pittsburgh Graduate School of Public Health
University of Pennsylvania Medical Center
Meharry Medical College
United States Air Force (USAF) School of Aerospace Medicine
University of Texas School of Public Health
University of Texas Health Center at Tyler
University of Texas Medical Branch, Galverston
University of Utah
University of Washington School of Public Health and Community Medicine
West Virginia University
Medical College of Wisconsin

Two Pathways to Specialty Certification in OEM

Since at least the mid-1960s, entry into the advanced practice of OEM has been characterized by two different career paths: traditional residency and mid-career shift. For physicians graduating from medical school prior to 1984, the ease of a midcareer shift has been aided by the availability of the alternate pathway to obtaining board certification in occupational medicine. More recently other options have become available to physicians making a midcareer shift to OEM.

Those going into the specialty through traditional residency training have generally become interested in OEM in medical school, undergraduate college, or during another residency (typically internal medicine, an internal medicine subspecialty or family practice). Either after an initial transitional clinical residency year or in combination with internal medicine or family practice, the resident completes the academic and practicum years required by the ABPM, typically both years at the same institution.

This traditional residency career path has been almost obligatory for those going into academic research positions and for many government agency posts, and has been desirable for some corporate positions, especially for those dealing heavily with toxicology or policy. A number of individuals with this type of training have risen to the most senior positions in the profession and in multinational corporations.

The strengths of those taking this career path included their formal training in the academic, preventive, research, and regulatory aspects of OEM. A potential weakness is the lack of extensive clinical experience to develop a maturity of clinical judgment around complex medical and social issues, especially where the resident has not also completed training in a primary care specialty.

Those going into the specialty midcareer typically have had a number of years of medical experience (often in internal medicine, family practice, or emergency medicine), began to work part-time in occupational medicine, and found they enjoyed and had a penchant for the practice of occupational medicine. Many of these physicians pursued no formal training other than entry-level CME courses (such as ACOEM's basic curriculum). Those who took corporate jobs (which were plentiful in the 1970s and 1980s) were trained on the job or through mini-residencies that offered more extensive training. Because of the limited scope of activities in many corporations, on-the-job training could be quite narrow in scope. Traditional residency training was seldom an attractive option for the midcareer shift physician for reasons of cost and logistics, but also because the style and content of the training was not always appropriate to the trainee's level of medical maturity.

Many residents who graduated from medical school before 1984 were able to sit for the ABPM certification examination through the alternative pathway option described below, and, although their pass rate was lower than that for residency trained physicians, many passed and became certified. The strength of these physicians lay in their clinical judgment, broad medical experience, and medical maturity, and they are attractive to many corporate employers, to freestanding occupational health clinics, and to some hospital-based clinics particularly outside the academic medical centers. Their relative weaknesses lay in the academic, preventive, research/scientific, and regulatory aspects of occupational medicine, and in environmental medicine. Just as with the traditional residency training career path, a number of individuals making a midcareer shift to occupational medicine rose to the most senior positions in the professions and in multinational corporations.

A recent trend has been the application of a competency paradigm for training, allowing the training and professional development needs for both traditional residency trained and midcareer-shift physicians to be evaluated against the same set of outcome requirements, even though their initial skill base may be very different. Training is then directed at achieving a common set of competencies by the end of the training experience. Appropriate sets of professional competencies for those practicing OEM have been published under the auspices of ACOEM and have been developed by a number of training programs for their own use. It is generally acknowledged that the application of competency-based learning in occupational medicine residency training has been very successful.

The last several years have seen two developments in education, which offer substantial new possibilities to enhance the training and skill development of those wishing to enter OEM through either path (11). Distance learning techniques made possible by advances in information and communication technology allow academic and didactic material to be learned off-campus at a time and place chosen by the student. The trainee can be freed from the constraints of time and location, which previously limited academic education. "Executive type" (or "on-job, on-campus") master's degrees programs have also been developed that require a series of 2- to 5-day periods of attendance on campus, distributed over 2 years or longer.

Most recently, innovative practicum year training experiences have been developed to help a midcareer shift into occupational medicine. This type of program works through a combination of supervised clinical experiences and projects in a number of specified areas of OEM. The resident works at an approved work site under local competent professional supervision. There are periodic, strongly interactive, didactic sessions at the home institution, and the full-time program faculty visit the resident's work site to monitor and guide both the resident's performance and the resident supervisor relationships. Some months of training rotation may be required at the mother institution.

Traditional Residency Training Programs for OEM

In 2000, 38 residency training programs in occupational medicine were accredited by the ACGME in the United States, an increase from 25 in 1966 (10). Occupational medicine residencies vary widely in size (ranging from 1 to over 10 residents). Nationwide, approximately 75 to 100 physicians graduate each year. The academic and clinical focus varies from program to program, but all provide trainees with the fundamental academic and practical knowledge to practice occupational medicine in a variety of settings.

Occupational medicine residency training includes three distinct components. The first year consists of an ACGME-accredited clinical internship (PG1). Many programs do not offer this clinical year, but require applicants to have completed at least 1 year of internship or residency before beginning the occupational medicine residency.

The second year of the residency consists of a broad curriculum of study, generally leading to an MPH or equivalent degree. Required courses include biostatistics, epidemiology, health services organization and administration, environmental and occupational health, and social and behavioral influences on heath. An additional didactic component, often included in the third-year practicum phase, addresses environmental physiology, occupational disease, toxicology, industrial hygiene and safety, ergonomics, and topics in worker evaluation and clinical program administration. Many programs have added a focus in environmental medicine to address the increasing public concerns over the potential health impact of environmental chemicals and pollutants. The Agency for Toxic Substances Disease Registry (ATSDR), for example, publishes clinical case series in environmental medicine that some residency programs have incorporated into their curriculum (see Appendix B).

The third year of the typical residency program consists of a series of rotations provided at a variety of occupational medicine settings to gain practical experience. Termed the *practicum,* this phase of training usually includes supervised training at industrial sites, occupational medicine clinics, labor organizations, and government agencies such a the Occupational Safety and Health Administration (OSHA), National Institute for Occupational Safety and Health (NIOSH), and ATSDR. Some residencies require additional training in certain specialties of importance to the practice of occupational medicine, such as dermatology, pulmonary medicine, and neurology.

Residency training has been supported by NIOSH grants, the military, by scholarships from the Occupational Physicians Scholarship Fund (OPSF), and, to a quite limited extent, by hospital or university funds. NIOSH provides some degree of funding to most training programs through the education and research centers (ERCs) and training program grants. However, such grants generally cover only a fraction of training costs. Residency programs also rely on scholarships, corporate grants, income from consultative and clinical services, and a variety of innovative funding mechanisms. A significant source of scholarship support is OPSF established with donations from corporations, individuals, and the ACOEM. Unlike most graduate medical education, which receives significant support from hospitals in exchange for clinical services, occupational medicine residency programs are only rarely sponsored by hospitals, although there is in fact no barrier to using hospital funds for this purpose.

NONTRADITIONAL RESIDENCY TRAINING FOR MIDCAREER PHYSICIANS

Brief descriptions of training programs are given in this section. The respective program directors should be consulted for up-to-date information.

Nontraditional Academic Year Training

Several types of academic training programs are now available that allow the practicing physician, over time, to complete the academic year training requirement without having to leave his or her employment. These include distance-learning MPH degree programs (e.g., Medical College of Wisconsin), on-job on-campus MPH programs (e.g., University of Michigan), and executive type MPH programs (e.g., Columbia School of Public Health). All have been successfully developed and are available to physicians wishing to enter the specialty practice of occupational medicine. These academic-year programs can be taken by residents in traditional residency training in OEM, but may have their greatest application to physicians making midcareer shifts.

The Medical College of Wisconsin offers an MPH degree through its academic program in occupational medicine. After a 1-day orientation session at the Medical College of Wisconsin in Milwaukee, students complete the program on a self-study basis, with curricular materials sent to the participants' homes. Interim examination and review are accomplished by computer linkage (via modem) between the students' home computers and computers at the Medical College of Wisconsin. Course work is completed at the student's own pace, with computer quizzes taken (at home) after each segment. Final examinations are conducted at the Medical College of Wisconsin or at other cooperating institutions by special arrangement. Most students take several years to complete the degree program. Information can be obtained from the Medical College of Wisconsin, MPH degree programs *(www.mcw.edu).*

The University of Michigan offers the On Job/On Campus Program, which affords practicing physicians in the region an opportunity to complete an accredited residency program on a part-time basis. The program includes a didactic component leading to an MPH degree in occupational health and a practicum component that may be taken independently. During the didactic component, students attend classes for a 4-day period (Thursday through Sunday) each month for 24 months. Information can be obtained from the University of Michigan School of Public Health *(www.sph.umich.edu)*.

Columbia University in New York City offers an executive MPH in health services management, which should allow a physician to complete a satisfactory curriculum to meet academic year curriculum requirements for occupational medicine. This weekend program for working professionals is offered through the Division of Health Policy and Management. The executive MPH is a structured program in which the school's core curriculum and concentration courses are prescheduled and taught on one weekend a month, Thursday through Sunday, over a set period of 2 years. Further information can be obtained from Mailman School of Public Health, Department of Health Services Management, through *www.columbia.edu*.

Nontraditional Practicum Year Training

At the time of this writing there are three accredited practicum-year training programs that allow a physician to obtain part or all of the supervised practicum training from a site where he or she is employed full-time in the practice of OEM. All are tuition-based.

The external track of the OEM residency at the University of Pennsylvania Medical Center is available to physicians employed full-time in occupational medicine at a facility that has a suitable breadth of activities and an appropriate local supervisor. The program is competency-based, emphasizes skill acquisition, and is arranged around both general competencies and seven modules: the worker; the workplace; hazard recognition and control; disability and work fitness; environmental health, risk assessment, and risk communication; population-based occupational medicine; and organization management. Each resident completes a project from his or her workplace in each competency module. There is a structured, highly interactive program for 3 days a month (a Thursday, Friday, and Saturday) in Philadelphia. A faculty supervisor visits the work site four times a year. The program is heavily interactive with approximately 300 hours of face-to-face contact with a resident. Limited assistance with tuition and/or travel may be available to selected trainees based on need criteria, through a grant from NIOSH.

The practicum program at the Medical College of Wisconsin is available to physicians who are employed full time at a suitable field site, generally a light or heavy industrial facility, where the resident has a supervisor with suitable certification and experience in occupational medicine. The resident must make visits to Milwaukee at least quarterly to interact with departmental faculty and to visit industrial sites in the Milwaukee area. There are regularly scheduled teleconferences. Residents complete a didactic curriculum with required readings and assigned activities corresponding to the programs educational objectives.

During the on-job, on-campus supervised practicum year training at the University of Michigan, students integrate practical experience on the job with residency training requirements during a 2-year work-study period. Students attend eight quarterly advanced workshops and also complete a minimum of 4 months of field rotations at the University of Michigan in major industries with a comprehensive program in occupational medicine and industrial hygiene. Field rotations are arranged and supervised by the University of Michigan faculty.

CME AND RELATED EDUCATIONAL RESOURCES

A number of CME and alternative educational opportunities are available through professional societies, books, and periodicals for physicians who desire to acquire additional competence in selected areas of OEM and who do not wish to take sufficient periods of time away from professional commitments to attend a residency training program.

Professional Societies

The ACOEM sponsors seminars and courses related to the specialty. In addition to postgraduate seminars and courses offered at the national meetings in the spring and fall of each year, the college periodically sponsors 1- or 2-day courses of particular interest to practitioners. Examples include medical review officer (MRO) courses and seminars on the Americans with Disabilities Act (ADA). The ACOEM also offers the basic curriculum, a structured series of three 2-day segments designed to provide the non–occupational medicine specialist with useful information and an introduction to OEM. An outline of the basic curriculum presented at recent ACOEM meetings is presented in Table 15.2. Further information and registration forms for the basic curriculum can be obtained from the ACOEM education office, and membership information is available through the ACOEM membership office (1114 North Arlington Heights Road, Arlington Heights, IL 60004-4770) *(www.acoem.org)*.

TABLE 15.2. *Basic curriculum in occupational medicine*

SEGMENT 1: Foundations, epidemiology, and lung disorders
Learning objectives: Upon completion of this educational activity, learners should be able to:
- List objectives of occupational and environmental health and safety programs
- Obtain medical histories to define the relationship of health problems to occupational or environmental exposures and activities
- Locate and use sources of professional assistance for managing occupational and environmental health problems
- Apply management and administration techniques and principles in planning, consulting, organizing, team building, directing, facilitating, and evaluating occupational and environmental health and safety programs
- Utilize biostatistics and epidemiology principles to analyze data and evaluate scientific studies related to occupational and environmental medicine (OEM)
- Discuss the principles used to design, implement, and evaluate occupational and environmental medical surveillance and monitoring programs
- Discuss legal and ethical implications of occupational and environmental health and safety programs
- Administer and evaluate occupational histories of patients with lung problems due to occupational and environmental exposures

SEGMENT 2: Toxicology and psychology
Learning objectives: Upon completion of this educational activity, learners should be able to:
- Describe the fundamentals of toxicology
- Identify the scope of workplace psychological issues including workplace stress, shiftwork stress, jet lag, and substance abuse
- Describe workplace drug testing and the role of the medical review officer (MRO)
- Identify, diagnose, and treat occupational dermatoses
- Consider reproductive health issues in the workplace
- Apply case management principles and return to work evaluation
- Identify the role of the occupational physician in emergency preparedness
- Define the fundamental concepts in risk analysis
- Discuss the basics of workplace noise-induced hearing loss
- Investigate low back problems efficiently

SEGMENT 3: Industrial hygiene and specific workplace health concerns
Learning objectives: Upon completion of this educational activity, learners should be able to:
- Describe work-site evaluations
- Review fundamentals of industrial hygiene
- Discuss essentials of upper extremity evaluations
- Consider fitness to work in relation to cardiac problems
- Define an approach to the evaluation of occupational or environmental disorders of the neurologic system
- Apply a plan for preventing infectious disease hazards in the workplace, including needlestick injuries and tuberculosis
- Recognize common physical hazards in the workplace including radiation, heat, cold, vibration, and light
- Develop an approach to ergonomic assessment of the workplace

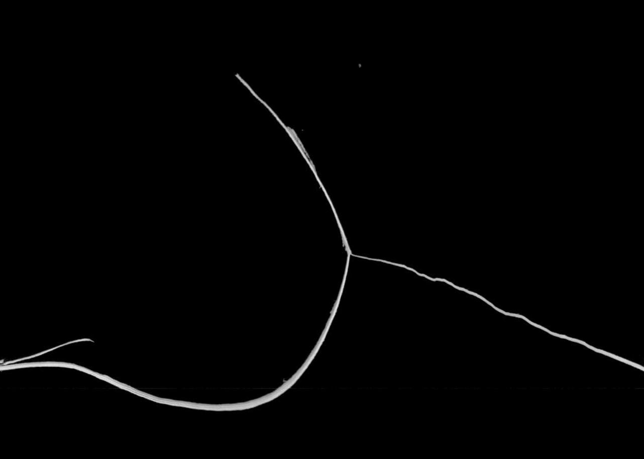

In addition to the national organization, regional groups have formed component societies of ACOEM. These components hold regular meetings and support CME activities at the local and regional level. Membership is coordinated through the ACOEM national office.

A number of other professional and medical specialty organizations provide some educational programs related to occupational medicine. Many of these organizations include segments on occupational medicine in their national meeting programs with varying points of emphasis. Universities and medical schools also offer programs related to OEM, including some extensive courses spanning 2 weeks or more. Interested practitioners are encouraged to contact the medical school or university in their area.

Education and Research Centers

ERCs were established by NIOSH to provide multidisciplinary educational resources in occupational health. Each center was required to maintain at least three of the four educational components of occupational health as determined by NIOSH: occupational medicine, occupational health nursing, safety, and industrial hygiene. These centers continue to provide an important educational resource for physicians and other health professionals seeking additional information and expertise in occupational medicine. In addition to their full-fledged training programs, ERCs provide CME opportunities, ranging from 1-day conferences and short courses to extended educational programs of several weeks' duration. A catalogue of educational programs and courses can be obtained from individual ERCs or from NIOSH *(www.cdc.gov/NIOSH)*.

Schools of Public Health

Schools of public health, of which 26 are accredited in the U.S., provide another important educational resource in areas such as epidemiology, biostatistics, toxicology, health services administration, environmental health, and behavioral sciences. Most schools offer curricula leading to the MPH degree, and many accept students on a part-time basis. In addition, some occupational medicine residency programs and ERCs are affiliated with schools of public health.

Information on entrance requirements and admission procedures can be obtained by contacting the registrar at the school of interest or the Association of Schools of Public Health (ASPH) *(www.ashp.org)*.

Federal and State Agencies

Educational programs are also offered by federal, state, and local governmental agencies. NIOSH has created a comprehensive curriculum for use by primary care residency training programs to teach the fundamentals of OEM to nonspecialists. NIOSH and other programs in the Centers for Disease Control (CDC) offer internships and fellowships, many of which are relevant to the practice of occupational and environment medicine.

NIOSH and other federal agencies, including OSHA, the Environmental Protection Agency (EPA), and ATSDR also provide educational materials and sponsor seminars that may be useful to the practitioner seeking additional information on selected aspects of occupational and environmental medicine (see Appendix B). Two particularly useful series are the NIOSH Current Intelligence Bulletins, which relate recent information on workplace hazards, and the Current Environmental Health issues. NIOSH also publishes a yearly update of current permissible exposure limits (PELs), available from the agency. A nongovernmental organization, the American Conference of Governmental Industrial Hygienists (ACGIH) publishes a pocket-sized booklet of threshold limit values (TLVs), and biological exposure indices (BEIs). The ACGIH also publishes documentation of the TLVs and BEIs, a useful reference for the theoretical basis for these standards and an extensive bibliography.

Journals and Computer Databases

Prominent journals with significant content in OEM and related topics are listed in Table 15.3. The *Journal of Occupational and Environmental Medicine,* founded in 1959, is the official publication of the American College of Occupational and Environmental Medicine.

In addition, many specialty journals frequently contain articles relevant to the occupational medicine practitioner, particularly in the areas of pulmonary medicine, dermatology, allergy, and rehabilitation medicine.

TABLE 15.3. *Journals with significant occupational medicine content*

American Association of Occupational Health Nurses Journal
American Industrial Hygiene Association Journal
American Journal of Industrial Medicine
American Journal of Preventive Medicine
American Journal of Public Health
American Journal of Respiratory and Critical Care Medicine
Applied Occupational and Environmental Hygiene
Archives of Environmental Contamination and Toxicology
Archives of Environmental Health
Chest
Clinical Toxicology
Environmental Health Perspectives
Health Physics
International Archives of Occupational and Environmental Health
Journal of the American Medical Association
Journal of Occupational and Environmental Medicine
Journal of Risk Analysis
Journal of Toxicology
Journal of Toxicology and Environmental Health
Occupational and Environmental Medicine (formerly *British Journal of Industrial Medicine*)
Occupational Health and Safety
Occupational Medicine (published by the Society of Occupational Medicine)
Preventive Medicine
Scandinavian Journal of Work Environment and Health

A useful review of selected occupational medicine literature can be found in the monthly publication *Occupational and Environmental Medicine Report.* The report contains reviews and comments on articles of general interest to occupational and environmental medicine practitioners (see Further Information, below).

Computerized databases such as the National Library of Medicine's MEDLARS on-line network provide a rapid, efficient mechanism for literature searches and data retrieval for specific topics. MEDLARS is an on-line network of approximately 20 bibliographic databases. (See Chapter 16 for a guide to retrieving medical literature.) This service is available directly from the National Library of Medicine or via subscription to commercial on-line services. Many medical libraries offer literature search services or assistance in preparing a search. For medical literature, MEDLINE provides an excellent resource within the MEDLARS system. Other databases of potential interest for more specialized searches include CANCERLIT (cancer literature), CHEMLINE (chemical dictionary on-line) for information on specific chemical substances, and TOXLINE (toxicology information on-line) for information related to published human and animal toxicity studies.

Information on computer programs and databases can also be obtained from the ACOEM Computers in Occupational Medicine Section, which publishes the *Directory of Occupational Safety and Health Software.* For information or a copy of the catalogue, write to the ACOEM Office (1114 North Arlington Heights Road, Arlington Heights, IL 60004) *(www.acoem.org).*

Books and Other Reference Materials

A recommended library for occupational physicians, developed by the publications committee of the ACOEM Council on Education, is included in Appendix F. A useful series of quarterly monographs entitled *Occupational Medicine: State of the Art Review* provides current information on selected topics. Each issue consists of an in-depth review of a specific subject, with contributions by experts in the field (see Further Information, below).

CONCLUSION

The actual educational training needed for the practice of OEM varies depending on factors such as previous experiences, current responsibilities, and access to training opportunities. Residency training is ideal, although other forms of education, including the ACOEM core curriculum, provide an introduction to the discipline. Keeping abreast of journals and attending local and national professional society meetings can be an invaluable means to stay current and meet colleagues who face similar challenges.

REFERENCES

1. Institute of Medicine. *Safe work in the 21st century: education and training needs for the next decade's occupational safety and health personnel.* Washington, DC: National Academy Press, 2000.
2. Rosenstock L, et al. Occupational and environmental medicine: meeting the growing need for clinical services. *N Engl J Med* 1991;325:924.
3. Institute of Medicine. *Role of the primary care physician in occupational and environmental medicine.* Washington, DC: National Academy Press, 1988.
4. Schenk M, Popp SM, Neale AV, et al. Environmental medicine content in medical school curricula. *Acad Med* 1996;71:499–501.
5. Pope AM, Rall DP, eds. *Environmental medicine: integrating a missing element into medical education.* Washington, DC: National Academy Press, 1995.
6. Schenk M, Popp S, Bridge P, et al. Effectiveness of an occupational and environmental medicine curriculum as indicated by evaluation of medical student performance on an objective structured clinical examination. *J Occup Environ Med* 1999;41:954–959.
7. Committee Report. Occupational and environmental medicine competencies—v1.0. *J Occup Environ Med* 1998;40:427–440.
8. Emmett EA. What is the strategic value of occupational and environmental medicine? *J Occup Environ Med* 1996;38:1124–1134.
9. DeHart RL. Establishing eligibility for examination in the specialty of occupational medicine. *J Occup Med* 1986;28:303.
10. American Medical Association. *Directory of graduate medical education programs.* Chicago: AMA, 1999.
11. Emmett EA, Green-McKenzie J. External practicum-year training in occupational and environmental medicine—the University of Pennsylvania Medical Center program. *J Occup Environ Med* 2001;43(5):501–511.

FURTHER INFORMATION

Occupational and Environmental Medicine Report. Published by OEM Health Information, 8 West Street, Beverly Farms, MA 01915-2226, 1-978-921-7300, 1-800-533-8046.

Published since 1987, this monthly periodical critiques occupational medicine-related articles that appear in a wide range of professional journals. Each issue includes a special report focused on a practical aspect of occupational medicine.

Occupational Medicine: State of the Art Reviews. Published by Hanley & Belfus, 210 South 13th Street, Philadelphia, PA 19107, 1-800-962-1892.

This quarterly publication addresses occupational and environmental medical topics in considerable depth. Each issue includes at least six to ten scholarly and academic articles on the particular topic as medical surveillance or occupational lung disease.

16

Computers and Informatics in Occupational Medicine Practice

Kent W. Peterson, Todd D. Kissam, and Barry A. Cooper

Computers, automated data, the Internet, telecommunications, and other aspects of health informatics offer an ever-expanding set of opportunities to improve the quality and cost-effectiveness of occupational health (OH) services. Yet the task of deciding when and how to use these resources can be daunting for experienced computer users and computer-neophytes alike.

There are three basic uses of informatics in occupational medical practice. The first is office automation involving the use of software programs for word processing, spreadsheet analysis, project planning, communication graphics, client contact, Web browsers and e-mail programs, personal assistants, computer utilities, and similar functions. These programs, which can be linked together through local and wide-area networks and synchronized with hand-held devices, serve as the basic building blocks of an information system and can prove extremely useful to the OH practitioner.

Occupational and environmental health applications are the second use, with applications of database management systems being tailored to the occupational health user. Some are focused on a single purpose, for example, generating random numbers for drug testing or preparing the Occupational Safety and Health Administration (OSHA) report of first injury. Others handle multiple purposes and are usually described as occupational practice management systems or occupational health information systems (OHISs). The latter are designed for occupational health clinics operated by hospitals, freestanding clinics and chains, or solo practitioners who serve many clients, or run in-house by employers. Some large employers have developed integrated health data management systems (IHDMS), linking data from many different corporate functions (e.g., personnel, benefits, risk management, medical and nursing, environmental health and safety).

The third set of informatics tools is large text libraries and powerful information databases that are available via CDs, hand-held computers, or electronic Internet links to a server. These can include regulations, regulatory guidelines or interpretations, chemical inventories, toxicology databases, health information sources, and many more kinds of information.

This chapter discusses the benefits of automation; the establishment of an occupational health information system based on a clear understanding of user processes and specifications; currently available occupational health and safety software; practical guidelines for evaluating, selecting, or developing a system; and the future direction of occupational health information management technology.

BENEFITS OF COMPUTERIZATION AND APPLICATIONS

Advantages of Automation

A growing number of hospitals, clinics, corporate employers, and consultants rely on occupational health practice management software. The following list provides insight into some of the advantages they are experiencing:

Clerical costs at one clinic were reduced by 30% when they switched to a computerized clinic management system.

At many clinics, data entered once are now automatically incorporated into dozens of documents at multiple sites, without error.

OH providers gain a greater understanding of individual practice profiles by analyzing data from thousands of medical records.

An OH clinic gains new business due, in part, to its reputation for providing quick, follow-up reports in a clear, highly customized format.

A corporate medical director is able to target specific disease management interventions and demonstrate cost-effectiveness through an IHDMS.

Computers are quickly becoming essential management tools with valued applications in all aspects of OH. The use of a successful OHIS can significantly improve an organization's ability to achieve its goals through (a) improved efficiency, accuracy, and productivity; (b) enhanced quality, decision making, and documentation; (c) regulatory compliance and litigation assistance; and (d) the ability to inexpensively create supplemental and new services, such as Web sites customized to meet highly specific client and employee needs. Advantages of computer automation include the following:

Improved Efficiency, Accuracy, and Productivity

Tasks are accomplished faster and cheaper, with significant staffing economies possible. The consequent improvements in efficiency and accuracy result in greater productivity than that obtained using manual methods.

Computers provide users with instant access to vast amounts of data organized in standardized and customized formats. Using relational databases, information can be entered once and automatically duplicated in designated data fields on command. Standard forms and reports can be regularly generated to meet highly specific requirements. Greater efficiency can also be achieved through direct electronic interface of test equipment and calculation programs that help reduce errors while enhancing speed.

Warning: Many companies justify the implementation of an OHIS based on projected cost savings from potential staffing cuts due to increased efficiency. A successful OHIS does increase efficiency, but staffing is generally not reduced. They are, instead, reassigned to other tasks that could not be accomplished previously.

Enhanced Quality, Decision Making, and Documentation

An OHIS can prove a valuable tool that results in higher levels of quality assurance, documentation, and professional decision making than manual methods. This is a very tangible benefit that most companies undervalue when generating their OHIS requirements.

For example, the quality of decision making can improve by allowing more time and more immediate access to relevant information. Through the computer's powerful ability to organize and present data, managers and clinicians can analyze information from a variety of perspectives. The more quickly and easily data are transformed into information, the more effectively it can be used in analysis and in the development of more thoughtful decisions. The growth of automated decision-support tools, e.g., disability duration guidelines or Web-based information, means that clinical guidance can be made concurrently with care, rather than retrospectively.

Regulatory Compliance and Litigation Assistance

With sophisticated computer-assisted information retrieval, analytical and reporting capabilities, regulatory compliance programs are more likely to remain effective, avoiding costly fines, penalties, and investigations. Litigation costs may also be reduced due to improved reporting and documentation, although some legal challenges continue regarding the admissibility of electronic medical records.

Provision of Supplemental Services

The use of an OHIS allows organizations to provide supplemental services with little additional costs. Virtually all OHIS components have a database kernel. This means that once a service is provided to an individual, the results of that service (the data) are stored in the computer within a database (an easily accessible file). Relational databases allow supplemental services to be provided to groups for almost no additional cost.

For example, a hearing conservation program prints customized follow-up letters to participants based on a computer analysis that identifies individuals who require medical follow-up and/or education on hearing protection. If the needed data are available, a financial analysis of potential fiscal liability is generated based on hearing test results and other analyses.

OCCUPATIONAL HEALTH INFORMATION SYSTEMS

Evolution of OHIS

The development of OHISs has paralleled the evolution of general computer-based information systems.

First Generation: Mainframe Systems

The first generation of OHIS came on-line in the 1970s. Because these systems were mainframe computer–based, only the largest companies could afford the millions of dollars for the hardware and the even more millions for the software development. Some of these companies tried to recoup their investment by selling the software to other companies. This was met with limited success due to the lack of flexibility in meeting other companies' needs.

Most of these systems were large data storehouses. Huge amounts of data (and money) were poured into these systems, but very limited provisions were made for getting the data out in usable form. This fatal flaw caused most systems to fail. Even extensive modifications of these systems could not fully meet the users' needs. These systems had to be scrapped. Surviving mainframe systems used database software.

All mainframes (and their systems) have a closed architecture, which is proprietary to a single company and not accessible for outside vendors to use or enhance. The specifications are protected by patents. In an open architecture system, the plans and specifications for the computer hardware are in the public domain, so any vendor can reproduce or improve the hardware. As a result of competitive pressure involved with open systems, they are cheaper and will continue to become even more so.

It was during this period that medical departments began to become prisoners of their data processing (DP) departments. When DP departments implemented the OHIS, they applied the same methodology of back-charges used for other departments (e.g., accounting or engineering). This charge-back method turned DP into an internal profit center, allowing DP to build an empire by showing how much money it was making instead of answering to the criticism of how much money it was costing. The result was that most medical departments were charged for every page printed and for every medical record stored or accessed. One large chemical company's DP department charged $1.65 each time a medical record was looked at. Instead of having a system that encouraged use and thereby increased the efficiency of the department, the system discouraged use by punishing the user.

Second Generation: Minicomputer Systems

The second generation of OHIS came on-line in the late 1970s through the 1980s. These systems, recognizing the limitations of proprietary, single-purpose mainframe systems, were based on minicomputers, which are cheaper than mainframes and easier to use but not as powerful. Hospitals, midsize companies, and the largest clinics and consultants all could afford minicomputer hardware, but few could afford the investment in generating the software to create an OHIS.

Some minicomputer OHIS used early database technology, acquiring flexibility to meet different client needs. Unfortunately, the price of customization was prohibitive and minicomputers did not allow a migration path that took advantage of new developments in database and personal computer (PC) technology.

Although minis have a closed architecture, by using a UNIX operating system they can allow the software to be independent of the hardware (see Future Directions for Occupational Health Information Management Technology, below).

Third Generation: Microcomputers

Although microcomputers first appeared in the 1970s, the IBM PC and compatibles and Macintoshes appeared in the 1980s.

PCs were the first systems with inexpensive connections to modems, scanners, medical testing equipment, compact disc read-only memory (CD-ROMs), etc. This fact has greatly enhanced the usability of these systems. The IBM-compatible PC represents an open architecture.

In the past decade, PCs and Macs have gained power at a rate never seen before in the computer industry. This increase of power and ever lowering of price has resulted in the sale of hundreds of millions of PCs. The marketplace is so large that over 500,000 software packages are in existence.

OHIS have been implemented on both stand-alone and networked PCs. Most of these systems now use databases with fourth-generation languages. This results in more flexibility as well as cheaper systems.

Fourth Generation: Internet Connected or Web Based

Many companies continue to use mainframes or minicomputers to maintain their large databases. The connections to this database from internal departments, field employees, vendors, and partners have become complex. The Internet represents a technology that can both reduce the complexity and enhance the value of OHIS (1). The Internet provides both low- and high-speed connections among most computers in the world. Internet access software programs (browsers) provide an easy-to-use tool for linking computers and data to a desktop PC. Privacy is a major issue. Two technologies using the Internet address privacy issues: (a) An Intranet is a company-based network that appears as a limited private Internet to a user. (b) A virtual private network (VPN) is a private subset or portal of the Internet. Only users who have special software (and who are allowed membership) are part of the VPN (this could include various departments within a company, employees, patients, clients, vendors, consultants, etc.).

As the hardware has evolved from mainframe to mini to micro to "net based," the politics of OHIS has also evolved. Systems have migrated from being data processing–controlled to user-controlled. This shift has caused turf wars between the medical and other departments and the central data-processing structure within companies. This requires the OHIS user to become not only more technically competent but also more politically savvy.

USING THE INTERNET AND DATABASES TO DELIVER HIGHLY CUSTOMIZED OCCUPATIONAL HEALTH SERVICES

Most OH clinic administrators understand the importance of customer loyalty as they periodically fight price wars with their competition. Clients can often be seen jumping back and forth among providers to gain a few dollars here, a concession there. Increasingly, technology-rich customer relationship management (CRM) strategies allow loyalty to be earned on an enterprise level in much the same way it has been earned on a smaller scale for centuries—one customer at a time (2). Providing customers with highly customized services that they grow to rely on can enhance important personal relationships. With each communication (e.g., each touch point) viewed as an opportunity to learn about customer needs and preferences, information can be stored on electronic databases and shared throughout the organization in real time, creating continuously improving service. Harnessing computer and Internet technologies makes it easier to shift clients away from price-sensitivity by gaining a competitive advantage based on delivering highly individualized services developed with the help of these continually updated knowledge bases. By gaining a more comprehensive understanding of their most valued clients, organizations can become better able to attract similar, more profitable new customers with the help of sales force automation tools included in these CRM programs.

Perhaps most rewarding are the employee health and productivity gains possible when OH organizations work in tandem with their clients and partners to harness these powerful technologies in the delivery of employee health services on a one-to-one basis.

The early to mid-1990s saw the introduction, with varying levels of success, of back-office corporate efficiencies such as integrated health-data management systems (see below) and larger enterprise resource planning (ERP) initiatives. Sales force automation (SFA) also got its legs at this time and has provided the technologic underpinnings for today's sophisticated CRM solutions. CRM programs help companies focus on one customer at a time by linking front-office data silos and communication lines in marketing, sales, and customer service. This customer-centric way of doing business becomes even more powerful when applied to the Web, becoming a global initiative often referred to as e-CRM (electronic CRM). Rapid CRM sector growth includes development of vertical industry CRM "flavors" (e.g., in the financial industry), with robust health care delivery applications, sometimes referred to as health care relationship management (HRM), yet to be fully realized.

Much of this revolution in the way we do business is made possible because of the startling and continuing growth of the Internet and the World Wide Web in our daily lives and business affairs. Highly sophisticated, integrated database programs are enabling organizations to establish individualized interfaces with customers and their employees. As these developments evolve, OH marketing and delivery innovations will follow. Just as the Web makes on-line shopping a personalized experience, even in what has been referred to as the Internet's "Kitty Hawk era," OH professionals working with their technology colleagues can fashion a new standard for delivering highly personalized, useful and cost-effective services. OH (or, perhaps, e-OH) organizations can embrace this movement to fit the specialized needs of their customers and patients. Along the way, many mistakes and missteps will be made, but net progress should result.

To achieve optimal results, top management must support a thorough review and reengineering of the business processes that will be assisted by these emerging technologies. The technologies never lead the way, but follow thoughtful planning and reorganization. Early initiatives should target relationships with a subset of most valued clients (or for the corporate medical director, most valued internal customers such as divisions, plants, or high-risk employee groups). This calls for learning how to assess customer value and communicating these findings throughout your organization. Recruiting key employees to work across departmental lines to deliver one-to-one service to VIP client groups can help ensure future success and greater acceptance of the

CRM approach within the corporate culture, where turf will be closely guarded.

Applying one-to-one principles when providing employee health services is likely to be more technology intensive given the pure numbers involved. One exciting approach can provide the homebound injured worker with a highly customized 24-hour-a-day, 7-day-a-week Web portal providing easily accessible resources to help speed recovery and return to work (RTW). Case management tracking can be facilitated through self-reporting and wireless monitoring of vital signs and biometrics related to medication reactions and other critical issues. These customized Web sites can provide audiovisual, perhaps animated, patient-education messages targeted to the injured worker's diagnosis and RTW plan. Motivational reviews of rehabilitation exercises, for example, can be offered on a scheduled basis. Hyperlinks can speed the patient to needed community services and support groups, and provide relevant uplifting entertainment. Knowledgeable, supportive health professionals can host on-line self-help groups. E-mail communications with caregivers and case managers are also possible. Optional communication links to the employee's company might help homebound individuals stay in touch with and motivated about work-site developments.

The challenge for OH professionals is to use emerging technologies and other e-business tools to create innovations that could not have been imagined just a few short years ago. In explaining why becoming Internet-compliant is mission critical, industry consultant Jim Dickie puts it well: "It's not easy, it's not cheap, and it's not optional. That is a sobering lesson, but an exciting one. If you're ready to take it to heart—welcome aboard" (3).

MANAGED CARE AND THE GROWTH OF PRACTICE GUIDELINES

Nowhere has the role of computers in OH been more dramatic than in the managed care arena. As technology has become more sophisticated, elaborate expert systems now can be applied to individual practice decisions. Expert systems are rule-based computer programs that can make sophisticated decisions while incorporating feedback to continually improve their performance based on the rules or principles programmed into them. If properly managed, these systems can contribute to quality-improvement and cost-containment initiatives. If poorly managed, they can prove counterproductive and limit the individual provider's ability to practice appropriate, high-quality medicine.

Sophisticated systems are now used by case management companies to improve acute care, short- and long-term disability management, and workers' compensation outcomes. By applying utilization review and case management techniques previously used exclusively for major illnesses and injuries, computers are now being applied to more common clinical occupational-medical cases, such as cumulative trauma disorders.

As the gatekeepers of a disability management system judged out of control (workers' compensation costs alone topped \$100 billion in 2002), OH providers can be central players in a growing cost-containment movement that recognizes that wage-related benefit expenses are inexorably linked to medical decisions and costs. Large self-insured companies, major insurers, third-party administrators, workers' compensation preferred provider organizations (PPOs), state workers' compensation systems, and other vendors and service companies have come to rely on computer-assisted solutions to assure quality and stem the perceived cost crisis.

The technology of OH managed care is taking shape. It features utilization review and case management programs supported by medical guidelines, protocols, and databases. The medical community's charge is to use these sophisticated tools to help ensure the cost-effective delivery of care, carefully monitoring both resource use and quality.

The guidelines, protocols, and systems are usually based on International Classification of Diseases, ninth or tenth edition (ICD-9 and ICD-10) codes and Current Procedural Terminology, fourth edition (CPT-4) codes. Some are keyed to job demands and capabilities measures. Computerized case management systems can feature disability duration guidelines, clinical practice guidelines, and sophisticated scheduling and follow-up programs. They are increasingly available through administrative services contracts, licensure, or as part of insurer and third-party–administered (TPA) services. As these tools evolve, they are beginning to include coded elements of the patient's medical history, physical examination, laboratory tests, imaged x-rays, electrocardiograms (ECGs), and other digitized documents.

The full impact of these developments on OH practice remains to be seen. Totally automated electronic medical record systems are still not in widespread use, but are gaining acceptance. Current decision-support systems do not provide sufficient information to establish the correct diagnosis and procedure. Forward-looking organizations recognize the variability of each case, and the importance of individual patient reactions to psychosocial factors and treatment interventions. However, there have also been disturbing examples of high technology being inappropriately applied in a field that defies simple solutions. Examples are overzealous case managers insisting that employees return to work based solely on absence duration guidelines, and utilization review systems at times overly stridently creating the need to obtain preapproval before rendering care (sometimes referred to as "1-800-may-I").

The caveats are clear. The technology available through computer programs should be used to assist knowledgeable professionals to do their jobs more efficiently and accurately. Guidelines should be used as reference points, not to make complex, subjective decisions. A hierarchical decision-making process can help to ensure that the most appropriate professionals are involved in authorizing exceptions to expert system-generated recommendations. In a typical model, a nurse case manager with access to medical guidelines and treatment protocols is responsible for determining when additional input is needed from a physician, vocational rehabilitation, or other specialist.

Most commercial clinical protocols are based on proprietary criteria, often not subject to public scrutiny or peer review. Yet, collectively, they may ultimately establish a new paradigm. Fortunately, the American College of Occupational and Environmental Medicine (ACOEM) practice guidelines have set a high standard for evidence-based protocols in the occupational arena. As this technology evolves, the medical profession has a stake in ensuring that valid guidelines are developed and that they are applied with proper professional oversight.

INTEGRATED HEALTH DATA MANAGEMENT SYSTEMS (IHDMS)

Some corporations are using IHDMSs for help in making complex decisions. Implementation of an IHDMS can help to prevent unnecessary duplication of effort, foster coordination among units, and provide a clearer picture of the company's health expenditures and priorities. These systems may include disability and general health benefits; occupational health services, wellness, and safety programs; and related databases (e.g., personnel) that cut across departmental lines for employees, dependents, and retirees. They may also be linked to larger enterprise resource planning systems.

The corporate medical department can play a central role in developing IHDMS. Optimally, the director of OH services should provide leadership in the description of processes and user specifications (see below) to be supported by the system, ensuring that high-priority programs are included. Opportunities to better target and evaluate OH programs should be developed, periodically reengineering critical processes to ensure that they contribute optimally to the organization's mission. Team-building processes are inherent in establishing and maintaining IHDMSs that cut across multiple corporate functions. Minimally, the medical department should work with other departments and key vendors to help ensure that their computer systems evolve compatibly.

In the absence of an IHDMS, corporate health professionals should consider the need for establishing one. If a full system is not feasible, partial integration may be realistic. A subgroup should set out to review company and vendor databases with an eye to optimizing their utility.

OH clinic managers should be aware of opportunities to assist client corporations as they work toward health-data system integration. For some clients, this will mean providing systems design assistance, while others may benefit from more active clinic participation in day-to-day data management and exchange. Clinics providing ongoing services to corporations have a vested interest in ensuring that the net effectiveness of their services is not masked by cost-shifting or tracking errors.

Establishing an OHIS/IHDMS

Developing an OHIS requires a clear understanding of the processes to be supported. Well-conceived user specifications help ensure that the system will perform the necessary functions required. This is true for either off-the-shelf software programs or for those written in-house. If the system is to be custom-built, either by an in-house department or by consultants, system developers should create preliminary system specifications documents based on detailed user specifications. This will help ensure that the software optimally assists essential OH processes.

The following steps should be carefully considered (also see Practical Guidelines for Evaluating, Selecting, and/or Developing Software, below):

Identify the needs of each system user and follow through with precise requirements. The overall requirements for a system are generated from these needs. Example: The system is needed to support a hearing conservation program by generating letters to employees who have had a temporary hearing threshold shift (TTS). A requirement is to generate up to 50 letters per day within 20 working days of the audio testing. Additional precise requirements would add the following qualifier: The system needs to generate up to 50 letters per day and be received by the employee (at home) within 20 working days of the audio testing for a cost (including data entry, processing, and quality control) not to exceed $2.00 per employee tested.

Employ a multidisciplinary approach in generating user specifications and system requirements. Requirements need to be generated by a task force with representatives of all affected departments in order to help ensure that systems will support commonly agreed upon processes and specifications.

Evaluate the implemented system against the goals/requirements. What if requirements are not met? What is the schedule for their implementation? The requirements need to be concise and complete enough so that the successes and the failures of the system are easily recognized.

Budget sufficient funds for ongoing system modifications. Unfortunately, most systems are never finished. Finishing the last 10% of a system can represent 50% of the entire systems cost, yet this last 10% frequently separates success from failure.

Build in flexibility to adjust to changes over time. (Here's where relational databases prove valuable.) If the system cannot adapt to a changing organization, then the system has failed. Restructuring, downsizing, acquisitions, new product development, and new business directions need to be part of the requirement discussions. A section addressing contingencies (e.g., "How the system will perform if the following happens...") needs to be part of the finished requirements. This is another reason for a multidisciplinary approach.

Develop systems using open architecture to help ensure OHIS hardware and software flexibility. Closed systems can restrict flexibility and increase the ultimate cost of the system.

Components of an OHIS

Below, we discuss possible components of a comprehensive OHIS/integrated health-data management system. Many components can be integrated within a single, structured relational database. Alternatively, several relational databases can share properly coded data elements.

General Office Automation

One of the most important components of an OHIS—indeed, perhaps the most important component—is support of the office staff in the pursuit of everyday tasks. Word processing, spreadsheets, contact and time managers, project timelines, electronic mail, and Web access are all important parts of general office automation support. Without integration of these functions, the OHIS might not be used. Most users already have these support programs on their desktop computers and they do not want to (a) learn new systems, (b) have two computers on their desk, or (c) leave their desk in order to do their job. Fortunately, Windows-based systems allow shared use of commercial software and specialized OH applications.

Personnel Data

Almost every OHIS requires information about the company (e.g., sites) and employees (e.g., name, mailing address, date of birth, gender, Social Security number, and other demographic information). Because of employee turnover or relocation, this information needs to be easily updated, indicating the last date the information was changed. The most sophisticated systems now use data from company personnel databases, either through periodic extracts or from real-time linkages, where the actual data are stored in the personnel database.

Benefits Information

In an era of medical cost containment, linkage with benefits information can be valuable. Such information may include medically related absence and use of sick leave, health care utilization, workers' compensation, general health claims and costs, and detection of occult occupational diseases that are being treated by the general medical community.

Work History and Job Tracking

Current job titles, classifications, and prior job histories can become especially important in medical surveillance studies where test results or health outcomes are monitored for all workers in particular jobs, or those with selected exposures. Job histories can be particularly important when employees at the same locations are used as a control group to compare against workers exposed to hazardous substances.

Functional Job Requirements

Compliance with the Americans with Disabilities Act (ADA) requires OH professionals to have more information than just a current job title. Understanding functional job requirements—including physical, psychological, social, and environmental demands—becomes critical in medical assessment. Such descriptions should distinguish between essential and marginal job functions. This area can be managed with a relatively simple computer application. Specialized software is available to help develop functional job requirements.

Job Capabilities and Work Restrictions

Traditionally, OH professionals have identified employee work restrictions (e.g., unable to lift more than 50 pounds, blind, sensitized to TDI, or may not operate hazardous equipment requiring use of upper extremities). Job restrictions have often been systematized for use in medical or personnel information systems. The ADA challenged OH professionals to state an individual's capabilities rather than limitations (e.g., able to lift up to 50 pounds, can be exposed to dust if uses a respirator, can stand for 2 hours before requiring a 15-minute rest). Contemporary systems will also list reasonable job accommodations recommended or made.

Appointment Scheduling

In busy OH clinics, computerized appointment scheduling is a valuable asset, and can issue reminder and follow-up notices to employees and facilitate tracking those who miss scheduled appointments. Such a system can also schedule future appointment dates for people requiring periodic medical evaluations.

Regulatory Requirements

Through simple automated text-retrieval systems, computers can help track current company policies and state or federal medical requirements, including the periodicity of required examination procedures.

Medical Record Keeping and Retrieval

Computerized systems can summarize dates of past exams and appointments, leaving actual medical information in hardcopy or electronically imaged records. OH clinics are automating critically important information. A number of employers and health care providers have adopted paperless medical records (4). Coding of health history (see below) and physical findings can significantly increase the value of these systems, but clinicians who insist on using free text notes may resist development. It is now well established that the electronic medical record is admissible as evidence in legal proceedings, and the Health Insurance Portability and Accountability Act (HIPAA) discussed below provides may safeguards to electronic medical information (5). Procedures such as storing backup paper medical records signed by the health professional should be considered.

Health History

Most medical histories are completed on paper; however, key historical information is often entered into computers for archiving and comparison over time. Many employers have developed optically scannable health histories; some medical departments use interactive health histories. Interactive histories allow hundreds of questions to be included in a branching tree format, designed so that each employee sees only a fraction of the total available items. This requires use of key branch points (e.g., gender, use of tobacco, or key symptoms for each organ system). Automating health history information can help assure appropriate medical follow-up of positive symptoms and can even direct the physical examiner to do the most beneficial, cost-effective physical exam procedures. It can also allow tailoring of periodic examinations to individual risk.

Medical Examination Results

Occupationally relevant test results are often automated, e.g., audiometry, spirometry, vision, respiratory fit, ECG, x-ray, specialized occupational tests and the hands-on physical examination. The Health Level Seven (HL7) standards (see Linkage to Other Systems and Databases, below) have helped ensure data transmission and compatibility. Immunizations and medical treatment can be included as well. Automation allows comparison of results over time, and calculations, such as TTSs for hearing, can be automatic. The computerization of medical examination results and related surveillance activities can be optimized by ensuring that they meet user specifications. Health screening technology is moving toward direct computer interface of screening equipment, allowing greater efficiencies, immediate quality control, and even comparison with prior results at the time of testing.

Medical Problems and Treatments: Procedure and Disease Coding

As clinical care has moved toward the problem-oriented health record (POHR), master problem lists are increasingly sought. A problem-oriented occupational health record can include important medical diagnoses, required job-related examinations, medical surveillance, respirator clearance, risk factors, and other key information. These can be correlated to encounter notes (SOAP notes—subjective history, objective findings, assessment, and plan). Computers can be used to support this function through the use of coded problem lists. And software is available to help code medical diagnosis by ICD-9, ICD-10, or CPT-4 codes.

Injury Monitoring and Management

Many computer systems record the federal and state OSHA reports of first injury or illness, generating forms to assure regulatory compliance. Tracking injuries by location and job can identify high-risk situations in need of followup and monitor patterns of injury and illness.

Case Management, Disability Management, Tracking, and Follow-up

As disability costs skyrocket, computers are used to monitor absence and to compare absence against anticipated duration codes, flagging individuals whose absence has exceeded a threshold (i.e., outliers) (5,6); increasingly, these systems help to manage cases proactively in cooperation with clinical providers. Case managers seek computer support to help contact workers and supervisors, monitor clinical care, record anticipated return to work dates, schedule independent medical evaluations, and record free text notes.

Health Promotion, Health Risk Appraisal, Risk Reduction, and Demand Management

Automating risk factor information such as blood pressure, cholesterol, weight, fitness, and smoking status can assist health promotion programs. For example, individuals at high risk can be identified for targeted follow-up, health education mailings, and scheduled revisits. Computerized health-risk appraisals range from inexpensive public-domain software to highly sophisticated, commercially available systems (7). Aggregate reports profile the health status of a population and can even project health benefit expenses related to modified risk factors. Specialized programs include diet and nutrition analysis, fitness evaluation, and body composition and stress profiles. Systems can track those at high risk and monitor participation in risk reduction, medical self-care, and informed consumer programs.

Drug and Alcohol Testing

Random drug testing requires use of random-number generators to select individuals for testing on short notice. Specialized programs track individuals in a pool eligible for testing, urine collection procedures, laboratory test results, review by a medical review officer (MRO) of positive findings, and reporting of verified results to the employer. The very important need for data security demands a high level of care in automating such information. U.S. Department of Transportation regulations make it clear that drug-testing records should be maintained separately from other general medical records (8).

Employee Assistance Programs (EAP)

EAP counselors often keep separate medical records. Automated EAP systems or EAP components of an OHIS with restricted access allow generation of activity reports, tracking, and follow-up of individual cases, and group reporting for evaluation purposes.

Medical Surveillance

A medical surveillance module tracks required examinations and assures that every employee has been tested. This module can link to appointment scheduling systems and record pertinent test results.

Chemical Inventory

Manufacturers and users of chemicals must track chemicals used to comply with the OSHA hazard communication standard (HazCom). More than 50,000 different chemicals are used in the U.S. Tracking the ingredients of mixtures is especially challenging, especially when formulations are proprietary. This information is often linked to OHIS.

Exposure Monitoring

Because industrial hygiene (IH) measurements generate a high volume of data, they have become increasingly automated. Potentially hazardous substances, appropriate measurement techniques, required periodicity of sampling, and actual measured exposures are included. Eight-hour time-weighted average exposures can be easily calculated. By linking IH data with job and personnel information, individuals requiring medical surveillance can be identified. Flags can be set to identify any area exceeding allowable exposures, either by company action levels or external standards. Workplace exposures can be tracked by location or by groups of individuals.

Toxicology Information

Under the OSHA HazCom, employers must compile and make available to employees copies of Material Safety Data Sheets (MSDSs). Many companies have automated this information for substances that they manufacture. A number of vendors have compiled large numbers of MSDSs. CD-ROMs or telecommunication links to large databases allow rapid access to MSDSs and other toxicology information. These databases include CHEMINFO, Regulatory Information on Pesticides Products (RIPP), Transport of Dangerous Goods (TDG)/hazardous materials (49 CFR), Chemical Evaluations Search and Retrieval System (CESARS), the National Institute for Occupational Safety and Health (NIOSH) Registry of Toxic Effects of Chemical Substances (RTECS), the Combined Health Information Database (CHID) of the National Institutes of Health, and the Superfund Amendments and Reauthorization Act (SARA) Title III.

Safety and Training

Information frequently tracked by computer includes personnel protective equipment, employee training (e.g., hazard communication), audits and inspections, fire, and other safety information. Systems are being designed to include centralized incident reporting and tracking.

Financial and Administrative Information

OH clinics require information on clients, services rendered, invoicing, accounts payable and receivable, direct and indirect revenues, and other financial reports. They also may want to reconcile revenues for referrals to other clinic or hospital departments. Corporate OH departments as well must accurately account for services charged back to operating organizations. Billing can be complicated when employers want a single consolidated invoice for multiple services provided by different elements of a hospital or clinic. Many features of a general ledger may be needed.

Quality Monitoring and Improvement

Tracking of quality and performance indicators has grown from reengineering and continuous quality improvement movements within companies. In health care, outcome measures are being identified to monitor quality of care. We are moving into an era of using practice guidelines and parameters to provide real-time decision support at the time care is given, rather than retrospectively. Feedback and documentation are increasingly being required by certification groups such as the Joint Commission on Accreditation of Healthcare Organizations (JCAHO) and the Accreditation Association for Ambulatory Health Care (AAAHC).

Analytic and Reporting Capabilities

While most OHISs still function largely as passive electronic storage cabinets, they must be able to report data in a variety of flexible formats. Increasingly, computer systems add features such as error checking, determining if values are beyond acceptable ranges, and flagging situations requiring follow-up. As total quality management becomes woven throughout OH, software systems are beginning to track variation in provider performance, e.g., variation in absence duration for selected conditions by provider. Systems are beginning to incorporate decision support technology that prompts the provider to make appropriate decisions. Examples include medical practice guidelines and protocols, such as those for diagnosing, treating, monitoring, and managing low back pain and soft tissue injuries. Most OHIS products come with formatted standard reports. Customized reports generated by the user using ad hoc queries must be easily generated.

Epidemiologic and Statistical Analysis

The most demanding reporting capabilities are those of epidemiologic analysis. Epidemiologic studies require correlation of many data elements (e.g., numerator as well as denominator information on employee populations). Often test results or health outcomes are compared to workplace exposures or jobs. Standard and proportional mortality ratios require tracking of appropriate disease coding for all deaths. Cancer registries have often been maintained by selected industries that manufacture or use toxic substances.

Linkage to Other Systems and Databases

Increasingly, clinics and employers are moving toward the integration of health data within OHIS or IHDMS. Users must consider whether data from inexpensive, single-purpose software programs can be imported into larger integrated systems (including broader ERP systems). Similarly, occupational health clinic users may need to obtain selected data from, and share it with, other corporate databases for purposes of industrial hygiene monitoring, chemical inventories, safety, and personnel data management.

Health Level Seven (HL7) is one of several ANSI-accredited standards developing organizations (SDOs) operating in the health care arena producing standards (sometimes called specifications or protocols) for clinical and administrative data. HL7's mission is "to provide standards for the exchange, management and integration of data that support clinical patient care and the management, delivery and evaluation of healthcare services. Specifically, to create flexible, cost effective approaches, standards, guidelines, methodologies, and related services for interoperability between healthcare information systems" (9). These standards address the definition of the data to be exchanged, the timing of the interchange, and the communication of certain errors to the application. They also support security checks, participant identification, availability checks, exchange mechanism negotiations, and, most importantly, data exchange structuring.

OHISs must support HL7 standards if they are to efficiently link to external systems such as insurance carriers, TPAs, hospitals, etc.

CURRENTLY AVAILABLE SOFTWARE

Most occupational health and safety software products currently available fall into several general categories.

Occupational Health Clinic Management and Tracking

The most prevalent category of commercial software addresses the focused needs of OH clinics. Almost two dozen commercial software programs are available on PC platforms. Most include demographic and administrative information, appointment scheduling, injury/illness care and absence tracking, reporting capabilities, clinical results, and accounting and financial management. Some include alcohol and drug testing, hazard exposure and other environmental information, and ergonomics capabilities. Most vendors have fewer than 100 installed clients, so no software is dominant. Of interest is the continual entry of new software products into this competitive arena. Clinic management systems licensing fees are usually in the $5,000 to $25,000 range, with smaller annual maintenance/renewal fees.

Injury, Absence, Disability, and Case Management

Many proprietary managed care software products focus on injury reporting and disability case management. These range from simple programs that complete OSHA 200 logs or provide absence duration guidelines, to full-scale disability case management systems that support case managers.

Ergonomics and Health Promotion

At least a dozen software programs perform health risk appraisal; most use algorithms developed by the Emory University Carter Center Update of the Centers for Disease Control and Prevention public domain program. A few have a more sophisticated risk computation science base and provide communication designed to motivate health behavior change. Other health promotion software programs perform dietary nutrition analysis, fitness evaluation, and ergonomics assessment, focused on the spine and upper extremities (9).

Chemical and Environmental Monitoring and Regulations

Many programs have been developed for safety, industrial hygiene, toxicology, emergency response, and environmental medicine needs. Some provide rapid access to large chemical databases by use of CD-ROM or telecommunication linkages. Others enable employers to comply with federal regulations, including OSHA, SARA II, and TOSCA. Some are PC-based, and others link with mainframe computers.

Epidemiology and Statistics

Many low-cost epidemiologic analysis software packages exist. Most of these build upon standard statistical analysis capabilities, but are tailored to the needs of epidemiologists.

INTEGRATED HEALTH DATA MANAGEMENT SYSTEMS (IHDMS)

Only a few large-scale systems are available that track personnel, medical, industrial hygiene, safety, toxicology/MSDS, and, occasionally, benefits information. During the past decade, a number of expensive integrated systems have dropped out of the marketplace, mostly because they could not operate in a Microsoft Windows environment. Available systems now operate on a PC platform, with workstations linked by PC networks or the Internet. Full-scale IHDMSs can cost many millions of dollars to develop.

PRACTICAL GUIDELINES FOR EVALUATING, SELECTING, AND/OR DEVELOPING SOFTWARE

The following recommendations are based on the authors' many years of experience working with OHISs.

Evaluating and Selecting Software

Define Clearly Your Needs and Intended Use

As is so often true in life, "knowing yourself" can make the critical difference in selecting one product over another. The great American philosopher Moon Mullins once said, "If you don't know where you're going, any road will do." It is here that a clear understanding of user processes and specifications should begin. Interdisciplinary task forces can be invaluable if they involve users and internal customers as well as local information-system people. These groups can not only help obtain a buy-in from key players, but also help avoid making a technically elegant decision that won't meet user needs. It is helpful to define goals and identify priorities in decreasing order. The entire group should sign off before proceeding.

Areas to address include the following:

Program objectives and processes, e.g., regulatory compliance, patient scheduling, tracking and billing, information storage and ready access, employee education, behavior change.

Users, e.g., degree of computer sophistication at all levels—end users, operators, systems managers.

Use, e.g., stand-alone task or part of integrated department or company-wide IHDMS.

Feedback—what specific information will be needed; what reports?

Resources available—personnel, computers, software, other users.

Size of operation and volume of data processing.

Speed and turn-around time—How quickly do you need data entry and reports? Could data entry/processing be done off-site?

Group data needs—management reports, measures of success.

Clear identification of needs can save a lot of time by helping to eliminate many products. Consider the analogy of house hunting: What would happen if a realtor had to show a buyer every property on the market? An internal or external consultant can help enormously. Successful systems are usually simple, user friendly (or at least tolerable), and flexible enough to adapt to changing needs. In short, first define needs; then look at software; finally, select hardware.

Explore the Various Available Software Packages and Make the "Buy/Build" Decision

Evaluate your options in terms of how they meet your needs. Most vendors are product oriented (i.e., they will try to sell you what they have to offer, convincing you that they have just what you need). Look around thoroughly and be aware of the range of choices. None may suit your needs exactly, hence the potential need for customization. Even if one product meets your purposes today, your needs are likely to evolve, and the software must follow suit or be discarded. But developing even the simplest program from scratch is fraught with hazard (e.g., time, money, and the frustration of re-creating the wheel). There is no magic bullet.

If you elect to build your own software program, check the literature and contact organizations that have done it. Always become familiar with commercially available alternatives and conduct a cost-benefit analysis before embarking on a major program development effort. Enlist the participation of other departments and establish an integrated program as appropriate. Beware of the many pitfalls of developing a system, described in the next section.

Try Out the Software Thoroughly and Contact Current Users

Do this once you are in the ballpark. No amount of talking or reading of marketing materials will substitute for making arrangements with a vendor to have a few hours of actual hands-on work at the keyboard. Having a demonstration at an existing user site can be instructive. Run a number of sample employees, patients, exams, or industrial hygiene measurements through the system; put it through the paces. Every vendor uses examples that put its best foot forward. What about the typical person in your intended audience? Try to discover the limitations of the system you are considering. Talk with several experienced users of the product.

Look Carefully at the Organization and the Key People with Whom You Will Be Dealing

How long has the organization been in existence and what is its history? Is it stable? What is its financial condition? Will it be able to provide continued support after the next recession? How many clients does it have? How large is its programming staff? Are the annual renewal fees and number of current customers sufficient to support a programming staff? How long have the actual programmers worked with the vendor? What is their continuous quality improvement (CQI) process, if any? How does it work? How do they involve their customers in CQI?

What are the backgrounds and qualifications of the principals and of those with whom you will be dealing on a day-to-day basis? This is important because although many purchasers believe they are buying a product, in reality they are buying a service and a relationship. Like most relationships, the true test comes after the purchase when the sky is dark, the winds are blowing, and hailstones are falling. Talk to other clients who will have similar uses to yours. Does the organization come through and deliver as promised?

Review the Sample Contract or Agreement

Do the vendor offer field tests, trial use of software, and a money-back guarantee if it doesn't work or if you are not satisfied? Look at users' manuals and documentation; find out what kind of training, customer support, and software support is available. Is remote support provided, e.g., linking your computer directly to the vendor's modem? Will you have access to the source code, possibly in an escrow account held by a third party, in case the company goes out of business?

Make Sure There Is Enough Flexibility to Meet Your Needs

Perhaps an off-the-shelf product is all you need, but you may well want to customize things later on. This may be simple or complex, costing tens of thousands of dollars. For example, how easy is it to add variables (e.g., new questions to a questionnaire), to telecommunicate, or to export data for external storage or processing? What is the organization's track record in customizing its product for other clients? How close to budget and time did it come? What about data analysis, storage, transfer, software limitations, import/export capabilities, compatibility?

Look Closely at Group Data as a Valuable Resource

What group reports are available, and do they report what you need, e.g., can they report employees by location, payroll code, job class, or other variables? Will they give you what you need to present to management, e.g., on the health or illness of a defined population, or the potential cost savings or degree of improvement over time? What data summarization and query capability exists, and how complex is the query language? Many million-dollar systems have been developed or purchased without adequate consideration being given to analysis and reporting. How easy is report generation? Can you design your own reports without needing software customization?

Regulatory Compliance

Does software meet current OSHA, HIPAA, and other regulatory requirements? Does the vendor keep abreast of regulations?

Connectivity

How does the software connect to other systems? This includes both internal company specific applications (human resources) and external systems (insurance claim databases). Are external devices connected using the HL7 standard? Connectivity can occur at different levels. The lowest level concerns documentation of file interchange formats. The highest level could be a VPN, allowing seamless connections to your users using a browser on their desktop PC. One example of the value of connectivity is in quantifying in a hospital- or group practice–based OH clinic the "downstream" revenues of referrals to other departments or specialists.

Working with a Software Vendor

Once you have decided to purchase or develop a software system, the next challenge is how to work more effectively with a vendor or developer.

Know Your Needs Well: Plan the Program Completely

Again, the most important single thing you can do is to think through your needs as clearly as possible at the beginning. Then plan carefully. Failure to plan is planning to fail. Planning the whole program not only helps you to select the correct software package in the first place, but aids enormously along the way. As health care professionals, we tend to be crisis oriented. Yet it often comes as a surprise to hear we help create crises around us. Careful planning—doing it right the first time—usually prevents turmoil and wasted effort, netting a large saving of time and money. For example, if you are asked to cost-justify a program or show its effectiveness in the workplace, you are more likely to succeed if the right data are collected from the beginning.

Make Your Needs Clear to Internal Developers and Information System Specialists

Information system specialists can often help you think through program options and make good choices at the beginning (e.g., data needed for later program evaluation). However, manage their consultation. Beware of DP departments that are motivated to extend or consolidate their empire.

Clarify What You Are Buying

What comes with the package and what will cost extra? What other services can the vendor provide? The price may never be lower than when you are negotiating the first dollar spent. What will cost extra? Get clarification in writing on such features as assistance in program design and evaluation, data analysis, graphics, and reporting.

Develop Measured Indicators and Benchmarks

Working with a vendor to develop, customize, enhance, or maintain a system is challenging. Having agreed-upon criteria for success (or failure) and benchmarks for measuring how the effort is progressing (or not) helps to objectify the process.

Cross-train Two People to Be Liaisons with the Vendor

If you have multiple sites using software, it is useful to have all go through one coordinator. Developing in-house competence will become an asset. But have more than one person trained, so there is backup support in case of illness, absence, early retirement, or job transfer.

Clarify Customer Support, Periodic Updates, and Annual Fees

Be clear about what services are covered under the basic licensing/purchase fee and what costs extra. Be willing to pay annual maintenance fees. Make certain that the vendor has a sufficient ongoing revenue stream to maintain the software and continually improve it. You want to make sure that your vendor is in business in the future.

Get to Know the People: Build a Positive Relationship

Offer your questions, comments, and suggestions freely. The squeaky wheel gets the oil. More importantly, an interested customer can bring out the best in a software team.

Train Your Users

The best computer system in the world will sit idle unless the users are trained and motivated. New computer systems change the way people work, which can be quite threatening. Ask the vendor or a skilled training group for help. Training should address the transition from traditional ways of working. Doing double duty of front-end data entry while maintaining an old system leads to decreased productivity and disillusionment.

FUTURE DIRECTIONS FOR OCCUPATIONAL HEALTH INFORMATION MANAGEMENT TECHNOLOGY

In this Information Age, data have become an important form of currency. Occupational health is just coming into the forefront of this powerful new technology.

Quick access to the right information is the goal of all information systems. Currently, there are no standardized building blocks for assembling OHIS. The technologies described below represent the foundation stones of these building blocks. It will be years before the foundation is complete and OHIS/IHDMSs begin to reach their full potential.

Legal Climate and Regulation

Food and Drug Administration Regulation of Medical Software

The Food and Drug Administration (FDA) has regulated the software used on some medical devices since 1987. In 1997, the FDA submitted an updated policy for public comment.

The previous policy did not affect OHIS as long as a gatekeeper (defined by FDA as "competent human intervention") was involved. Example: Consider a system for hearing conservation that automatically interfaces the audiometer to the computer system that generates the follow-up letters. If the audio results are entered into the system without being flashed on the screen for technician acceptance or rejection (without a human seeing them first), the system would be subject to FDA's policy.

The proposed policy extends what software is covered and requires certification and auditing of software depending on risk. The future impact on OHIS will be determined by the FDA's final definition of "diagnosis of disease and other condition, or...treatment, or prevention of disease..." as it relates to medical device software.

The continued use of a gatekeeper on ECG diagnostic machines, audiometers, and any other device that makes diagnosis of findings is recommended until the FDA policy is clarified.

Reasonable Accommodation Under the ADA

The ADA requires employers to provide accessible telephone and computer systems to employees, if needed, and to provide reasonable job accommodations. Potential enhancements for an OHIS might include image intensification of forms and video display terminals (VDTs), and speech recognition for the visually impaired. The Job Accommodation Network (JAN) at 800-526-7234 is an excellent resource on available technology.

The Health Insurance Portability and Accountability Act of 1996 (HIPAA)

HIPAA, also known as the Kassebaum-Kennedy law, contains five principles:

1. Consumer control: The standards provide consumers with important new rights, including the right to see a copy of their medical records, the right to request a correction to their medical records, and the right to obtain documentation of disclosures of their health information.
2. Accountability: The statute includes new penalties for violations of a patient's right to privacy. These penalties include, for violations of the privacy standards by the persons subject to them, civil monetary penalties of up to $25,000 per person, per year, per standard. There are also substantial criminal penalties applicable to certain types of violations of the statute that are done knowingly: up to $50,000 and 1 year in prison for obtaining or disclosing protected health information; up to $100,000 and up to 5 years in prison for obtaining protected health information under false pretenses; and up to $250,000 and up to 10 years in prison for obtaining protected health information with the intent to sell, transfer, or use it for commercial advantage, personal gain, or malicious harm.
3. Public responsibility: Privacy protections must be balanced with the public right to support such national priorities as protecting public health, conducting medical research, improving the quality of care, and fighting health care fraud and abuse. For example, public health agencies routinely use health records in their efforts to protect the public from outbreaks of infectious diseases. The new standards clarify how such information should be released.
4. Boundaries: With few exceptions, an individual's health care information should be used for health purposes only, including treatment and payment. For example, a hospital could use personal health information to provide care, teach, train, and conduct research and ensure quality. However, employers who also function as health care providers or health plans would be barred from using information for nonhealth purposes like hiring, firing, or determining promotions. Similarly, insurers could not use such information to underwrite other products, such as life insurance.
5. Security: Organizations that are entrusted with health information must protect it against deliberate or inadvertent misuse or disclosure. The standards require each covered organization to establish clear procedures to protect patients' privacy, designate an official to monitor that system, and notify its patients about their privacy protection practices. In addition, those who get information and misuse it would be subject to the penalties outlined in the proposal.

These comprehensive national medical record privacy standards are complex and subject to continuing legislative review. OH programs appear to be affected in the following areas:

Basic Rights for Individuals

Individuals will be able to obtain access to protected health information about themselves, which would include a right to inspect and obtain a copy of such information. The right of access would extend to an accounting of disclosures of the protected health information for purposes other than treatment, payment, and health care operations. (Health information is any information, whether oral or recorded in any form or medium, that is created or received by a health care provider, health plan, public health authority, employer, life insurer, school or university, or health care clearinghouse; and that relates to the past, present, or future physical or mental health or condition of an individual, the provision of health care to an individual, or the past, present, or future payment for the provision of health care to an individual.)

Individuals would have a right to receive a written notice of information practices. The primary purpose of this notice would be to inform individuals about the uses and disclosures that a covered entity (see below) would intend to make with the information, the notice also would serve to limit the activities of the covered entity—an otherwise lawful use or disclosure that does not appear in the entity's notice would not be permitted.

Some uses of data would require an individual's authorization. These uses would include, but would not be limited to, the use of protected health information for marketing of health and nonhealth items and services; the disclosure of protected health information for sale, rent, or barter; the use of protected health information by a non–health-related division of the same corporation, e.g., for use in marketing or underwriting life or casualty insurance, or in banking services; the disclosure, by sale or otherwise, of protected health information to a plan or provider for making eligibility or enrollment determinations, or for underwriting or risk rating determinations, prior to the individual's enrollment in the plan; the disclosure of information to an employer for use in employment determinations; and the use or disclosure of information for fund-raising purposes.

Individuals would have the right to request amendment or correction of protected health information that is inaccurate or incomplete.

Covered Entities

Covered entities include health plans, health care clearinghouses, and health care providers who transmit any health information in electronic form in connection with a transaction. Health care means the provision of care, services, or supplies to a patient and includes any preventive, diagnostic, therapeutic, rehabilitative, maintenance, or palliative care, counseling, service, or procedure with respect to the physical or mental condition, or functional status, of a patient or affecting the structure or function of the body.

Covered entities would be required to establish policies and procedures to limit the amount of protected health care information used or disclosed to the minimum amount necessary to meet the purpose of the use or disclosure, and to limit access to protected health information only to those people who need access to the information to accomplish the use or disclosure.

Covered entities would also be required to satisfy the requirements of the security standards, by establishing policies and procedures to provide access to health information systems only to persons who require access, and implement procedures to eliminate all other access. Thus, the privacy and security requirements would work together to minimize the amount of information shared, thereby lessening the possibility of misuse or inadvertent release.

The impact of these regulations on components of OHIS can be minimized by the removal of individually identifiable health information (health information created or received by a health care provider, health plan, employer, or health care clearinghouse that could be used directly or indirectly to identify the individual who is the subject of the information).

Information would be presumed not to be "identifiable" if:

1. All of the following data elements have been removed or otherwise concealed: name; address, including street address, city, county, zip code, or equivalent geocodes; names of relatives and employers; birth date; telephone and fax numbers; e-mail addresses; Social Security number; medical record number; health plan beneficiary number; account number; certificate/license number; any vehicle or other device serial number; Web URL; Internet protocol (IP) address; finger or voice prints; photographic images; and any other unique identifying number, characteristic, or code (whether generally available in the public realm or not) that the covered entity has reason to believe may be available to an anticipated recipient of the information.
2. The covered entity has no reason to believe that any reasonably anticipated recipient of such information could use the information alone, or in combination with other information, to identify an individual. Thus, to create de-identified information, entities that had removed the listed identifiers would still have to remove additional data elements if they had reason to believe that a recipient could use the remaining information, alone or in combination with other information, to identify an individual. For example, if the occupation field is left intact and the entity knows that a person's occupation is sufficiently unique to allow identification, that field would have to be removed from the relevant record.

Electronic signatures, electronic data interchange, coding standards, are other areas in which the regulations can impact OHIS.

COMPUTER HARDWARE

Growing Capacity and Shrinking Size

To appreciate the benefits of computer technology, consider that if the car had evolved like the computer chip, today's Rolls Royce would cost $100 and allow you to drive 10,000 years on one tank of gas.

Computer processors are doubling to tripling in performance every 3 years. To increase speed (electricity travels only 11.8 inches in a billionth of a second), everything must also get smaller.

Hard disk drives are also getting smaller, faster, and increasing in capacity (a 100 to 1 improvement in 10 years). Technologies under development ensure the continuing of this trend for at least the remainder of this decade.

Pricing Trends

In 1982, a basic office PC cost $7,500 for the hardware and $750 for the software (software was 9.1% of total system cost). By 1993 a basic office system had dropped in price to $1,800, while the software cost had risen to $1,200 (software increased to 40% of the total system cost). *The good news:* The price of hardware has decreased by 80%. *The bad news:* Not only did the cost of software increase by 60%, but the percentage that software represents as a part of the entire system increased from 10% to 40%.

Overall, the combined price of software and hardware will continue to decrease. However, software will continue to take more and more of the pie. Currently, hardware costs are but a fraction of those for software.

Decentralizing from Mainframe to Mini to Micro

Virtually all Fortune 500 companies are involved with downsizing (the movement of systems from mainframe to minicomputer or microcomputer). The cost and performance advantages of PC-based systems make the movement from mainframes to PCs inevitable.

High-speed Internet/VPN Connectivity

The ability to move large amounts of information (including images) from one user to another (either within the company or to an external user) will make high-speed data connections mandatory.

Imaging

Computers do a cost-effective job of storing numbers and characters; however, the ability to store images (photographs, graphs, x-rays etc.) is still expensive. A full-featured x-ray computerization system can cost $500,000. As economies of scale occur, the price of imaging systems will become a fraction of their current cost. This will result in new applications of imaging; within 5 years, imaging will be a common feature of OHISs. Imaging is a good idea when rapid access of multiple concurrent users is needed, or when many copies of selected portions of medical records are needed.

The technology of scanning in pages of medical records and storing them as images is being successfully implemented by a number of corporate medical departments. These images are easily retrieved in digitized format that can take the place of hardcopy medical records. Notes can be attached that do not print out with the record. When signed, these paperless medical records are legally acceptable documents. Although imaged records can be indexed by type, they are not relational database files. Therefore, imaged information cannot be sorted or compared for analysis purposes.

Pen Computers

Pen computers are like clipboards with a computer underneath that can recognize your handwriting. They are useful for field data acquisition and for computerization (of the data entry) of forms (checking off boxes). Although current high prices prohibit widespread use, economies of scale will lower their price enough so that pen computers will replace scanners or keyed data entry in certain components of an OHIS. Physical exam and personal medical history are two examples (10).

Personal Data Assistants

Personal data assistants (PDAs) have witnessed explosive growth in the general market. These devices have been likened to an "external cerebral cortex," being able to store thousands of names and addresses, years of daily schedules, extensive notes and to-do lists, and, with wireless linkage to the Internet, serve as pagers and download e-mail from anywhere. Current devices readily synchronize to a desktop or laptop computer and have color screens, removable memory chips for backup, and can plug in extensive information libraries. For OHIS they can be viewed as smaller versions of pen computers. Because they are targeted to the general public (vs. the workplace for pen computers), the price is substantially lower. The lower price will have a trade-off with size and performance, but the PDAs will find a role in OHISs where pen computers remain too cumbersome and expensive (11–13).

COMPUTER SOFTWARE

Growing Storage and Memory Requirements

As the functions and features of an OHIS become more complicated and numerous and as users demand that systems be easier to use and work on different types of computer hardware, the software grows bigger and slower.

The bad news: Future software will continue this trend, doubling in size every few years. This means faster systems with more memory [random-access memory (RAM)] and larger disk systems will be required. *The good news:* The evolution of the hardware will more than make up for the above, still at prices lower than today's.

Fourth-generation and Higher Level Languages

It costs an estimated $100,000 per year to maintain live-ware (salary, benefits, office space, computer software/hardware for a programmer). To generate more complex OHISs, the productivity of the programming staff must increase. With each generation of language, there is a five- to tenfold increase in productivity. Fourth-generation languages write much of the code based on simpler instructions. Many of the PC-based database languages are fourth generation. A fifth generation is being developed (it may become the Holy Grail of programming), but will not be available in the next few years.

OPERATING SYSTEMS

There are two main alternatives for an operating system on a PC: Microsoft or not Microsoft.

Unix/Linux

Unix/Linux was originally a minicomputer operating system predominantly used in research. It is powerful (good for multiple CPUs), and good software is available but complicated. It is used by many of the computer systems accessed via the Internet, and is recommended for scientists and for large-scale database servers. Linux has become a real option for developers and Internet applications.

Windows

Windows has been issued in the following recent editions: Windows 98, Windows XP, and Windows 2000 (successor to Windows NT). Upgrading an operating system can be very expensive. Sometimes hardware needs to be upgraded and all applications will need to be reloaded. Most businesses have recently upgraded their systems to Windows 2000. In general, Windows 2000 is targeted to business (desktops, servers, and laptops) and Windows 98/XP is for the home.

Networks

Increasingly, office systems also have a network operating system (NOS). There are two types:

Peer-to-Peer

Each computer can share data with every other computer but there is no central server. This works well for simple file and printer sharing among 20 or fewer systems. (Windows 98/NT/2000/XP are good choices.) Most small-office or home-based networks are peer-to-peer. (A small-office or home network is an efficient way to obtain high-speed Internet access by sharing a cable or xDSL modem.)

Server-based

Each computer is connected to one or more servers (centralized systems dedicated to making the connections among the desktop (or users) computers. Use of dedicated servers (both file and application) allows the connection of more systems to the network without degradation of performance. Server-based networks can have thousands of connected desktops. Novell and Windows 2000 are the current state-of-the-art server-based NOSs.

Client Servers

Computer networks often connect to large databases. These databases may be present on a different computer called a client server. Most new OHISs are likely to be developed using a client server approach. Information and data are requested from a server and then made available on the local PC in the user's choice of database software (e.g., Access, Visual FoxPro). The server may be another PC, a PC with multiple processors, a minicomputer, or even a mainframe. In most cases, the local PC will request the data needed in SQL (a standard relational database dialect). Client-server system architecture allows greater performance and flexibility.

Information Access

Telecommunications

High-speed nationwide data networks are a reality. We can expect the cost of remote data access to continue to decrease as these fiber-optic networks come on-line. The Internet, a worldwide network of networks, is accessible through commercial on-line services and local access providers. The accompanying chapter in this volume provides more information.

Dropping modem prices and faster transmission speed are dramatically increasing telecommunications availability, especially as higher-speed telephone connections are becoming available, e.g., DSL, ADSL.

Storage Devices (CD-ROM, CDR, DVD)

Certain components of an OHIS, such as MSDSs and x-rays, require vast amounts of data. The following storage devices are durable and can handle large amounts of data:

CD-ROM drives are capable of storing 650 MB (like audio CDs), and are mostly read-only. Writing on a CD requires a CDR system. DVD drives can store almost 3 gigabytes of data and 20- "gig" drives are coming. Recordable DVD drives are just becoming available and may replace CDR drives in the next few years.

Connectivity

Medical Testing Equipment

As new models of medical testing equipment (e.g., audiometers, tonometers, spirometers) are introduced, they have added the necessary hardware and software to allow connection to an OHIS. Although most of these current interfaces are crude and require technical competence to be able to program, in 2 to 3 years these initial growing pains will fade. These are governed by an HL7 standard (see Linkage to Other Systems and Databases, above).

Other Systems

Because much of the information needed by an OHIS is available on other computer systems within the company, OHISs tend to store duplicated data. Yet current systems can also be expensive to connect to other company systems so that data can be shared. Many of the above technologies (e.g., client server, object-oriented database) will remove the difficulty and cost of these data connections.

Future state-of-the-art systems that use fax boards, modems, electronic mail, cellular telephones, and other technology will be heavily interconnected and may not require wire/cabling (wireless) to make these connections.

Centralized DP vs. User Control

The turf wars over who controls and supports OHIS within organizations will increase in intensity over the next 3 to 5 years. The resolution of conflict in most companies will be the narrowing of focus and breakup of the DP empire that currently exists. The user will have increased options and responsibilities for systems, with DP providing support on request.

SUMMARY

The OHIS of the future will be PC-based utilizing a multiprocessor client server. Each of the nodes (connected desktop systems) will use a fourth-generation language and an object-oriented database as the underlying software. Much of the system software will be shared with other OHIS users, and system changes will be both inexpensive and quick to perform. Connections to other local company applications (other departments), vendors, and to key information sources will be transparent using Internet, Intranet, and VPNs. The system will store images of forms and x-rays using DVDs. All equipment, whether testing or pen-based, will be directly connected to the system. Employees and clients with disabilities will gain improved access to the system. The performance of the hardware will far exceed anything available today, but will be cheaper than current systems. The software will be isolated from the hardware, allowing physical pieces of the system to be replaced, transparent to the user, as better technologies become available. All of the above will result in a system that is more productive and flexible.

REFERENCES

1. Eder LB, ed. *Managing healthcare information systems with Web-enabled technologies*. Hershey, PA: Idea Group Publishing, 2000.
2. Baldwin FD. Customer relationship management (serving stakeholders catches on enterprise-wide). *Healthcare informatics.* February, 2002 (also see *www.healthcare-informatics.com).*
3. Siebel TM, House P. *Cyber rules—strategies for excelling in E-business*. New York: Currency Doubleday, 1999:268.
4. Kadas RM. The computer-based patient record is on its way (HMOs, the economy and HIPAA will drive adop-

tion). *Healthcare Informatics* February, 2002 (also see *www.healthcare-informatics.com)*.

5. Reed P. *The medical disability advisor: workplace guidelines for disability durations,* 4th ed. Boulder, CO: Reed Group, 2001.
6. Work Loss Data Institute. *Official disability guidelines: top 200 conditions,* 7th ed. Corpus Christi, TX: Work Loss Data Institute, 2001.
7. Hyner GC, Peterson KW, Travis JW, et al. *SPM handbook of health assessment tools.* Pittsburgh: Society of Prospective Medicine and the Institute for Health and Productivity Management, 1999.
8. U.S. Department of Transportation, 49 CFR Part 40, Section 40.321-40.333, August 2001.
9. Health Level Seven (HL7). *www.hl7.org*.
10. Morrison M. *The unauthorized guide to pocket PC.* Indianapolis: Que, 2001.
11. Carlson J. *Palm organizers,* 2nd ed. Berkeley, CA: Peachpit Press, 2002.
12. Johnson D, Broida R. *How to do everything with your palm handheld,* 2nd ed. New York: Osbourne/McGraw-Hill, 2001.
13. Monahan T. Hot and cold on PDAs (competition among manufacturers is heated, but doctors are still lukewarm about handhelds). *Healthcare Informatics* May, 2002 (also see *www.healthcare-informatics.com)*.

FURTHER INFORMATION

The most in-depth source of OHIS software information is the *Directory of Occupational Health Informatics* published by the Medical Informatics Section of the American College of Occupational and Environmental Medicine (ACOEM). Now in its 11th edition, the 190-page directory is available from ACOEM (cost: $95; $75 to ACOEM/AAOHN members) at *www.acoem.orgpubspubs.htm*.

Briefer listings of occupational health and safety software are published in the annual software edition of the journal *Occupational Health and Safety and Software Packages in Occupational Health and Safety,* published by the Canadian Centre for Occupational Health and Safety.

Useful and active occupational health internet sites include the Occupational Safety and Health Administration at *www.osha.gov*; the Duke University OEM Forum at *dmi-www.mc.duke.eduoem*; the Agency for Toxic Substances Disease Registry at *www.atsdr.cdc.govscience*; and the National Institute of Occupational Safety and Health at *www.cdc.govniosh*, both parts of the Centers for Disease Control and Prevention at *www.cdc.gov*; and the American College of Occupational and Environmental Medicine at *www.acoem.org*.

USEFUL GENERAL REFERENCE TEXTS

Berkowitz LL. Clinical informatics tools in physician practice. *Healthcare Informatics* April, 2002 (also see *www.healthcare-informatics.com)*.

Dick RS, Steen EB, Detmer DE, eds. *The computer-based patient record: an essential technology for health care (revised edition).* Committee on Improving the Patient Record, Institute of Medicine. Washington, DC: National Academy Press, 1997 (also see *www.nap.edu* to read this book on-line at no charge).

Networking health: prescriptions for the Internet. Committee on Enhancing the Internet for Health Applications: Technical Requirements and Implementation Strategies, Computer Science and Telecommunications Board, National Research Council. Washington, DC: National Academy Press, 2000 (also see *www.nap.edu* to read this book on-line at no charge).

Rice RE, Katz JE, eds. *The Internet and health communication: experiences and expectations.* Thousand Oaks: Sage Publications, 2001.

Shortliffe EH, Perreault LE, Wiederhold G, eds. *Medical informatics: computer applications in health care and biomedicine,* 2nd ed. Stanford: Stanford Medical Informatics, 2000.

17

International Occupational Medicine

William B. Bunn and Sadhna Paralkar

International occupational medicine is distinct from traditional occupational medicine as practiced in the United States. Rather than having responsibility only for injuries or illnesses due to workplace risks, as in the U.S., international practice also includes the health care of employees and families for all diseases. Therefore, the occupational physician must understand the national health system of the host country, and then provide appropriate support for national workers, national managers, and expatriates. This chapter discusses traditional health risks of the workplace, and the health care of workers and families not related to occupational exposures.

HEALTH RISKS RELATED TO OCCUPATION

The health risks internationally related to occupation are similar to the risks experienced in developed countries; however, exposures may be quantitatively greater. The use of chemicals, minerals, and other substances that have significant economic value despite health risks are a major global issue. For example, asbestos, pesticides, leaded gasoline, lignite coal, chlorinated hydrocarbons, and many other substances that are banned or are highly regulated in the U.S. are still widely used globally. In developing countries, lignite coal provides necessary home and commercial heat, pesticides protect crops and kill mosquitoes that transmit malaria, asbestos serves as a high temperature insulator, and chlorination purifies water that prevents millions of deaths from infantile diarrhea. These factors make health care in developing countries vastly more variable and complicated than in developed countries. In each international setting, it is important to understand the risk-to-benefit ratio. An excellent example of risk reduction is asbestos. Asbestos was used for centuries, but achieved significant industrial use only in the 20th century. Asbestos has significant advantages over materials for fire protection and in certain high-temperature insulation uses; it is used in many developing countries. The advantages of asbestos are related not only to industrial use, but also to its fire protective qualities (e.g., on ships). The noncancer risk of lung disease was recognized early in the industrial history of asbestos, but the cancer risk was clearly defined only in the 1960s. Given the use of this potentially injurious fiber globally, the need for protective practices that reduce friability and the need for respiratory protection becomes an issue not commonly faced in the U.S.

Similarly, there are chemical agents widely used internationally that are not found in the U.S. or most developed countries. Pesticides are the most obvious example but vinyl chloride, dioxins, PCBs, and other chlorinated compounds are not regulated, or are regulated less vigorously than in the U.S.

In addition to chemical risks, biologic risks are a much more serious concern. Although bacterial and viral diseases have been the traditional focus, the global impact of emerging infectious diseases such as prions/mad cow disease has been significant. Malaria is the second largest cause of lost life-years (with infantile diarrhea being the most dangerous infectious disease). Although generally not occupational, the care of workers demands knowledge of the risk of malaria and malaria prevention. Blood-borne diseases are much more prevalent globally. Hepatitis B and C and HIV pose much greater risks in certain parts of the world (e.g., hepatitis B and C in Asia, HIV in Africa), and have major impact on workers' productivity. Rare occupational diseases in the U.S., such as anthrax, are seen globally.

Physical hazards are also global risks. Heat, cold, radiation, and other physical hazards may be much greater risks globally. Although heat is an issue for certain areas in developed countries, tropical countries have unique risks caused by heat and humidity. Conversely, working in high and low latitudes (e.g., oil fields) can produce significant risk from cold. Radiation is a physical hazard in certain situations (high altitude) and certain geographic locations. For example, exposure from ingestion of food and water are significant issues in atomic-bomb test areas of the former Soviet Union. Ergonomic risks are also increased in many countries. Lasers are not commonly regulated outside of developed countries, nor are many other nonionizing radiation sources. Noise and hearing loss are rarely considered significant occupational issue in developing countries.

OCCUPATIONAL RISK OF WASTE HANDLERS

There are also unique job-related occupational risks outside developed countries, for example, there are significant risks to waste disposal workers. The disposal of waste is a unique occupational risk in developing countries. Wastes if centrally disposed contain a mixture of solid waste, biologic waste (biohazards), toxic wastes, and chemicals. The waste streams are not separated.

The waste collection system in developing countries is primitive and requires lifting and unprotected waste handling. Exposure to infectious agents is constant, and significant increases in diarrhea and respiratory diseases including tuberculosis are reported globally. Blood-borne diseases such as hepatitis and HIV are also increased.

Bioaerosols are generated through waste handling in all countries. When lifting is required, the risks are exacerbated by increased respiratory rate and by mouth breathing. Allergens are dispersed when waste is not in closed containers and allergic risks are elevated. Endotoxin and mold-exposure levels are elevated in waste disposal workers. Particulate matter exposure is increased from both the waste disposal and the consistent exposure to vehicle exhaust. Waste dumps usually have elevated particulate levels, particularly during the dry season. Burning of wastes also increases particle exposures. Volatile organic compounds are commonly emitted as gas from wastes, especially when solid and chemical/toxic wastes are disposed together. Heavy metals, including high lead levels, have been reported in waste disposal workers.

SUSCEPTIBILITY

Workers' susceptibility is also an issue of major significance. Child labor is a common practice in many countries. Children are uniquely susceptible to many types of occupational risks (e.g., lead), and are also subjected to greater risk of significant injury in certain situations. In addition, women may need to take special precautions during pregnancy or while nursing.

War and extreme poverty increase occupational and nonoccupational risks. The risks to the professional or volunteer soldier are significant, as are the civilian workers' risks during periods of violence. Migrant workers, who are a major portion of the workforce in developed and developing countries (e.g., in the Middle East), are at much greater risk of injury or illness. These workers have both occupational (e.g., lack of protective equipment such as hearing protection) and nonoccupational (e.g., infectious disease) risks. The housing and lifestyle of migrant workers are also significant risk factors.

A special issue is the susceptibility of workers who immigrate to areas with different patterns of infectious disease (e.g., malaria). Although they are immune to most childhood diseases in their original country of habitation, the disease patterns in other countries produce increased risk. The issue is significant in developed countries where workers (e.g., domestic workers exposed to childhood illnesses such as chicken pox) may not be immune by a previous infection or vaccination.

OCCUPATIONAL HYGIENE/INDUSTRIAL HYGIENE IN THE INTERNATIONAL SETTING

The demand for occupational hygiene services and its impact on safety and health vary widely. In African countries where agriculture dominates, there is little demand for occupational hygiene. Therefore, the equipment needed for accurate analytic testing and the laboratories required may not be available. In developed countries, air monitoring is usually conducted on a regular basis. Even if quantitative exposure levels are not obtained, hazard recognition is important in occupational health. Many occupational hazards can be recognized and quantitatively assessed without special equipment (noise, temperatures, and volatile solvents).

GLOBAL OCCUPATIONAL ISSUES

Standardization of medical surveillance and care, exposure limits, measurement systems, audit programs, policies, and procedures/regulations is a major international challenge. Although the International Standards Organization's (ISO) 14000 environmental management systems have helped create a common approach, standard diagnosis and treatment of occupational diseases also will pose a challenge in the coming years. No occupational standard has been developed on a global scale.

Additionally, the reconciliation of the use and abuse of workers with special risks such as child labor and migrant workers, and the use of toxic chemicals, will continue to pose significant challenges.

INTERNATIONAL HEALTH PROGRAMS

The support and oversight of international occupational and environmental medicine (OEM) programs extend considerably beyond the traditional hazard-based programs previously described. In many countries, OEM programs provide nonoccupational health care that is not provided by governmental programs for expatriates, short-term assignees and visitors, managers, workers and their families, and in some cases extended families.

The first challenge is the care of expatriates, short-term assignees, and visitors. For most expatriates and short-term assignees in major corporations, the legally required level of care is defined as "Western-style" health care. The provision of this level of care is a major challenge in countries where private health care is not available, and the quality of access to national health care may not meet this standard.

Domestic managers also expect health care benefits beyond the provisions of care of the national government. However, health care benefit plans have not developed for the workforce due to nationalized health care, the lack of private providers, and cost. The provision of care for domestic managers can be an insurance plan covering private care or care by private providers, and special hospital care similar to the care provided to expatriates.

The workforce is generally provided health care that is considered to be at the high end of the general population's care. For countries with well-developed national health-care systems, additional support may be provided. If adequate care is not available to assure a healthy, productive workforce, significant supplemental care may be needed. For example, outpatient care may be provided on-site or in the residential area of the workers. Special hospital rooms may be purchased and specifically equipped. Occasionally hospitals are built and staffed.

To build and maintain these health care programs requires significant planning, on-site evaluation and negotiation, and regular follow-up visits. The initial site visit to establish a program includes visits to local clinics and hospitals to determine which facilities provide the quality of care necessary for each group. These visits normally assess outpatient clinics, inpatient care, emergent care, intensive care, laboratories and blood banks, and radiology and other diagnostic procedures. The outpatient clinics utilized by the employees' families receive a similarly detailed review.

In addition to the evaluation of clinical services, access to care must be assured and a mechanism of payment must be established. For example, access may be difficult for expatriates who will be categorized as immigrant in status. Hospitals often require large cash deposits for treatment and care.

The evaluation must always include an examination of the health risks of the country. Special screening before expatriation may be necessary for expatriates or travelers with high risk (e.g., respiratory disease if there is significant air pollution). There may also be unique risks for infectious disease (e.g., malaria, tuberculosis, AIDS). The combination of special risks and the availability of medical care must be combined to generate a risk assessment and action plan for individuals or groups of individuals.

The visit also includes an evaluation of occupational hazards and assurance that programs comply with health, safety, and environmental regulations. Meeting with local regulators is recommended.

Finally, emergency transportation and evacuation plans must be developed. In most developing countries the first consideration is transportation to the local medical facility for the victim of an injury or illness. Effective community based ambulances are not commonly available, particularly for accidents. In addition, transfers to specialty hospitals must be assessed as well as the transfer vehicles. If evacuation is needed, the method of transfer for illnesses or injuries of each severity must be established (ground, commercial air, private jet) and the regional, continental, and global medical care destinations must be identified. In each case access and method of payment must be established.

Expatriate Health

Expatriate families provide a unique occupational challenge. The cost of unplanned or emergency repatriation varies from $500,000 to $1,000,000 per employee; thus, careful screening and special preparation of expatriates is necessary. The most common cause of repatriation is the physical or mental health of the spouse. Mental health is especially important because the risk of psychological instability and drug usage is much higher for expatriates. In addition,

Western-style psychiatric support is rarely available even in many developed countries.

Procurement of quality pharmaceuticals locally or importation of pharmaceuticals is difficult. International transportation of drugs prescriptions by mail is generally not legal, and hand-carrying medications for workers and family members by other workers is often necessary. Some drugs that are legal in the United States, like Ritalin (methylphenodate hydrochloride), are illegal in many other countries. Analytical labs may not be available to test drug levels or to conduct special studies like clotting times.

Special infectious disease risks also apply to family members. Maintaining malaria prophylaxis is challenging, especially in children because their medication choice is limited. Supporting individuals with underlying diseases is difficult.

Constant and consistent communication with expatriates and expatriated families is of paramount importance. In addition to health risks, special safety concerns like the increased risk of traffic accidents and death, or of criminal activity, must be communicated clearly.

It is necessary to control anticipated occupational exposures, especially if direct measurement of exposures is not possible. If testing is conducted, the maximum occupational-exposure limits may vary between or within countries. Commonly, the recommended exposure levels by the World Health Organization (WHO) and threshold limit values by the American Conference of Governmental Industrial Hygienist (ACGIH) are utilized; however, each country may have not only unique exposure limits, but also unique units of measurement. In addition, testing for toxic substances not utilized or not used in certain applications may be necessary, as well as an assessment of potential cost-effective substitutes.

18

Workers' Compensation

Jeffrey S. Harris

Occupational health professionals (OHPs) can play a pivotal role in providing and improving the care for ill or injured workers financed by workers' compensation insurance programs. In addition to providing direct care, OHPs can and should provide clear and factual information as input for decisions made by nonmedical insurance claims personnel; coordinate communications among employers, injured workers, and payers; manage care and absence from work; and support the dispute process to ensure fair and effective resolution of work-related health concerns.

Underlying all these roles is complete and accurate information acquisition, analysis, and decision making, which in turn require that OHPs know and apply complete and careful history taking; review of medical records and reports; physical examination; consideration of treatment alternatives, risks, and benefits; and explanation of their analytic and decision-making processes to nonmedical personnel making payment and service authorization decisions. Providers are often irritated with the workers' compensation system and with payers or case managers. A focus on functional recovery, prompt and complete communication, complete information and analysis, and a reasoned and neutral approach will improve the current, somewhat dysfunctional system to the benefit of injured workers and their families as well as employers and society in general.

This chapter discusses the history, provisions, organization, clinical best practices, and management of workers' compensation.

WORKERS' COMPENSATION SYSTEM

Workers' compensation systems typically consist of legislation, regulations, a governmental oversight and administrative body, insurance or other financing mechanisms, medical care services, disability management, and rehabilitation services. State and federal workers' compensation laws, rules, and regulations define and govern benefits eligibility and coverage, selection of providers, the dispute resolution process, and often care management and safety and preventive services. Most systems include a prevention component and financial incentives that are designed to encourage safer work conditions. The legal and regulatory framework is governmental; either government entities or private employers, insurers, health care organizations, and other vendors may finance and administer the insurance, medical, and disability management functions, depending on the jurisdiction involved.

State, federal, and private workers' compensation funds and insurers finance services to cure and relieve adverse health effects of work. They also provide wage replacement to mitigate the economic consequences of ill health. In some cases rehabilitation, transportation, and legal expenses are also covered. All state and provincial laws, and systems for federal workers in North America provide for these benefits regardless of fault for the industrial illness or injury. Some other systems, such as those for railroad workers (the Federal Employers Liability Act) and merchant seamen (the Jones Act), require that liability be proven (see below).

Evolution of Modern Workers' Compensation Laws

Knowledge of the development of workers' compensation laws is important to understand the continuing debates about the intent of the legislation and programs, coverage, benefits, the "rules of engagement," litigation of cases, and the roles of employers, employees, payers, and health care providers. History can provide some perspective to those engaged in a confusing system that can appear inequitable or insensitive to the well-being of workers, on the one hand, and costly and of sometimes dubious benefit, on the other. There is no perfect system; governments and interest groups are constantly trying to institute what they perceive to be improvements.

Workers had been injured or killed in the course of employment for centuries without compensation. The problem of loss of wage-earning capacity gained greater public attention during the Industrial Revolution as machinery caused proportionally more injuries and deaths, and extended families that could care for workers and replace their economic contributions were less available. As modern production techniques were adopted, the amount of mechanical force and chemical energy used to produce products increased and the rate of injury increased as well (1).

As attitudes about the rights of workers and employers changed, common law in Europe and the United States evolved to enable workers to recover damages if a person was injured at work. By the turn of the 20th century in the U.S., workers could bring successful lawsuits against employers for injuries suffered on the job. Common law held that a "master" or employer was responsible for injury or death of employees "resulting from a negligent act by him." However, injured workers had to prove that their injuries were due to employer negligence, which resulted in a slow, costly, and uncertain legal process. As a result, workers often did not receive needed medical care or wage replacement in a timely manner.

In addition, there were a number of accepted common-law defenses when an employee sued an employer. The employer could claim that the employee contributed to the injury (contributory negligence), that he or she had assumed risk by taking the job (assumption of risk), or that negligent acts of fellow workers were responsible for the injury (co-employee doctrine). By the end of the 19th century it was generally accepted that these defenses and the employer's greater legal resources placed the employee at a significant disadvantage.

The situation changed between 1870 and 1910. First, there was an increased public awareness that placing the burden of industrial illness and injury on workers might be unfair. This attitude resulted in political pressure by reformers to make recovery of lost wages and lost earning capacity easier and faster. A countervailing trend between 1900 and 1920 involved the adoption of employers' liability laws in many states. These laws were intended to modify common-law defenses and limit employers' liability.

Neither of these initiatives led to equitable and timely compensation for injured workers. As a result, a series of "no-fault" workers' compensation laws were passed on a state-by-state basis. Workers' compensation laws represented a compromise or "lesser peril" for both employers and employees. These laws were supposed to ensure rapid payment to injured workers for lost wages and medical costs regardless of fault. In exchange, employers' liability for occupational injuries, illness, and death was limited if they participated in a compensation system. Under this system, employers generally were exempt from damage suits, unless gross negligence could be proved (see Chapter 2). The benefits from workers' compensation being the only means of compensation for illnesses or injuries is termed "exclusive remedy." This concept of "exclusive remedy" meant that workers exchanged the uncertain right to sue for damages for prompt and certain medical care and wage replacement under workers' compensation insurance.

The initial workers' compensation law enacted in the U.S. was the Federal Employers Liability Act (FELA) enacted in 1906 and revised in 1908 in response to public demand for protection of railway workers. At that time one railway worker in 300 (2) was killed and one in 30 injured annually, with little ability to bring suit for recompense. The first state workers' compensation laws were passed by nine states in 1911. The first comprehensive Canadian laws were enacted in 1915. Mississippi was the last state to pass a workers' compensation law, in 1949. Today there are workers' compensation statutes in all 50 states, American Samoa, Puerto Rico, the U.S. Virgin Islands, and all provinces in Canada. The Federal Employees' Compensation Act of 1916, as amended, administered by the Office of Workers' Compensation Programs (OWCP) of the Department of Labor covers federal employees. The Federal Employees Liability Act covers railroad workers. The Jones Act of 1920 covers merchant seamen. The Longshoremen's and Harbor Workers' Compensation Act (LSA) of 1927 covers workers other than seamen performing duties on or adjacent to the navigable waters of the U.S., which are under Federal jurisdiction. The LSA provides workers' compensation for both public and private employees engaged in maritime work. It has been extended to cover employees on U.S. defense bases outside the U.S. and workers on U.S.-funded contracts outside the U.S. It is also administered by the OWCP (3).

Occupational disease laws were not passed until 1917, starting in Massachusetts and California; all states' laws did not cover occupational diseases until 1976. Part of the reason for the slow adoption of occupational disease compensation laws was a fear of liability because of the long latencies of disease and the lack of a definite onset of many occupational diseases. In addition, the sudden trauma of an occupational injury, which was generally used to define compensability, was missing, so that expansion of coverage required a change in thinking.

Goals and Objectives of Workers' Compensation

Workers' compensation systems are not simply mechanisms for financing patient care. Workers' compensation laws were instituted to "make workers whole" in a timely manner, to remediate physical damage and prevent economic hardship, and to provide incentives to prevent occupational health problems. Much of the research on workers' compensation is in fact in the economic and legal literature. OHPs should keep the goals and objectives of workers' compensation in mind when dealing with workers, employers, payers, utilization review personnel, and case managers. This broad perspective will ensure that the immediate and longer-range objectives are achieved to benefit the worker presenting for care, his or her dependents, and the larger working population.

The goals of workers' compensation systems are the following:

- Prevent work-related illness and injury.
- Make injured workers whole physically, mentally, and/or economically.
- Return workers to productive work in their original, or, if necessary, some alternative capacity.

The first goal may be implied rather than stated overtly. The safety function may be located in another area of government, but it is usually present. The second goal may be stated in economic terms, but it uses medical care to effect restoration of functional ability. The third goal embodies the underlying intent of workers' compensation. While the original goal was economic protection, the more modern approach aims for return to preinjury wage-earning capacity.

The objectives of workers' compensation, more specifically stated are to:

1. Provide sure, prompt, and reasonable income and medical benefits to work-accident victims, or income benefits to their dependents, regardless of fault.
2. Provide a single remedy and reduce court delays, costs, and workloads arising out of personal injury litigation.
3. Relieve public and private charities of financial drains related to uncompensated industrial accidents.
4. Eliminate fees paid to lawyers and witnesses as well as time-consuming trials and appeals.
5. Encourage maximum employer interest in safety and rehabilitation through appropriate experience-rating mechanisms.
6. Promote frank study of causes of accidents (rather than concealment of fault), reducing preventable accidents and human suffering (4).

Types of Workers' Compensation Systems

Workers' compensation systems may be no-fault or adversarial. State and provincial systems in the U.S., Canada, Australia, and other countries were originally designed as no-fault systems to hasten and regularize the delivery of benefits in exchange for limited liability of employers. National combined health systems, which include work-related illnesses and injuries, in New Zealand, Scandinavia, the United Kingdom, and elsewhere provide medical benefits regardless of cause, and deal with income replacement separately. Other systems, such as FELA for railroad workers and the Jones Act, are tort systems in which the worker must prove employer fault, and which do not have caps on compensation. The type of system may or may not influence the pattern of medical care provided.

Compensation laws are elective or compulsory. Under an elective law, the employer may accept or reject the compensation act. If employers reject it, they lose the common-law defenses of assumption of risk, negligence of fellow employees, and contributory negligence. While this approach used to mean that the laws were in effect compulsory, many employers in Texas and New Jersey are opting out of the compensation system to better manage medical and disability costs. Currently, workers' compensation laws are elective only in New Jersey, South Carolina, and Texas. Opting out is under consideration in Louisiana.

Coverage

There were 126.6 million workers covered by workers' compensation insurance in 2000, an increase of 2.8 million from 1999 (5). The covered payroll, or wages paid to covered workers, was $4.4 trillion, an increase of 8.3% from 1999.

Workers' compensation statutes cover all industrial and most service employment; however, very small businesses, business owners, farm labor, domestic service, and casual employees may be exempted from the laws. As a result, workers' compensation laws cover an estimated 97% of the American workforce covered by unemployment insurance, which in turn is estimated at 97% to 98%. All federal workers are covered as well. Many jurisdictions provide workers' compensation for all or certain classes of public employees. Minors, defined as those under the legal age of majority, are covered by workers' compensation; as an incentive to protect underage workers, some jurisdictions provide double coverage or penalties if minors are injured or killed at work.

Merchant marine and railroad workers are generally not covered by state workers' compensation acts, but may seek damages under FELA. The Federal Black Lung Act (Title Four of the Federal Coal Mine Safety and Health Act of 1969 as amended in 1972, 1978, and 1981) provides benefits for total disability or death caused by black lung disease. The Division of Coal Mine Workers, the Department of Labor's workers' compensation programs, and the Social Security Administration administer this act. Armed forces personnel injured in the line of duty are covered by the military health care system while on active duty, and by the Veterans Administration after discharge.

The Federal Social Security Disability Program pays benefits to disabled workers under the age of 66 when disability is expected to last 12 months or longer or results in death. The federal Social Security tax finances benefits. Combined Social Security, disability, and workers' compensation benefits may not exceed 80% of average current earnings before disability.

Benefits

Benefits are provided for wage replacement, medical and legal expenses, and permanent impairment. Lump-sum compensation is paid for certain scheduled physical damage or loss of function such as the loss of a body part, whereas medical and wage replacement payments are made whenever there is a wage loss related to work. A growing number of states are also requiring rehabilitation benefits. Impairment is defined as a loss of or damage to a body part or function due to illness or injury, whereas disability is defined as the inability to perform a specific task based on the functional requirements of the job, education, social factors, and other issues in addition to the medical impairment (6). In fact, one can be impaired but not disabled. Generally, physicians determine impairment and personnel administrators or supervisors determine disability.

Medical benefits are generally provided without dollar or time limits and are typically paid directly to providers in state workers' compensation systems. Many states have fee schedules for payments of medical costs. Some managed care organizations have negotiated discounts from these fee schedules. Providers are prohibited from billing patients for the difference between the amount paid by the payer and their usual charges (a practice called "balance billing"). Most of these schedules apply to physician or chiropractic outpatient care only; inpatient care and facility fees have been compensated at 100% of charges, although there is a trend toward payment by diagnosis-related group (DRG), per diem, or fee schedule. There is also a trend toward managing reimbursement for pharmaceuticals.

Many workers' compensation claims, called "medical only," require medical treatment, but do not result in lost time or impairment. When there is lost time, income replacement payments are made on a weekly basis according to a formula expressed as a percentage of wages. Most states have maximum and minimum limits; some states limit the total number of weeks payable. The highest weekly state payments are $1,031 in Iowa, $956 in Illinois, $949 in the District of Columbia, $923 in New Hampshire, $838 in Connecticut, and $831 in Washington and Massachusetts. In Canada, the highest maxima are $898 in the Yukon Territory, and about $850 in British Columbia, the Northwest Territories, and Ontario. Maximum benefits under the Federal Employees' Compensation Act are $1,495 per week, and $934 under the LSA (7). The lowest weekly maxima are $65 in Puerto Rico, $250 in Guam, $311 in the Virgin Islands, $316 in Mississippi, and $375 in Arizona and Georgia. Maxima are also relatively low in the most populous states of New York and California. The maxima are increased periodically by either cost-of-living adjustments or legislative action.

Disability, as used in workers' compensation, is defined as "temporary and total" (i.e., the employee must be absent from work for a period of time), "permanent and total," "temporary and partial" (i.e., restricted work if possible), or "permanent partial." Lump-sum awards are made for the permanent partial disability. Permanent partial is divided into nonscheduled and scheduled impairments. Most workers' compensation other than "medical only" involves temporary total disability or the need to be absent from work for more than one-half day [the Occupational Safety and Health Administration (OSHA) definition]. Temporary total disability definitions vary by state.

Most states limit compensation to two thirds of previous wages and cover all medical costs. Several states have more generous benefits. Self-insured employers must offer benefits at least equivalent to those required by state statutes. For a variety of reasons, some employers have elected to offer benefits equivalent to or coordinated with their short-term disability programs, which typically fully replace wages. Because these payments are tax exempt, they actually exceed the value of the average weekly wage. FELA, the Jones Act, veterans' benefits, and the Federal Black Lung Act have separate benefits schemes.

The penalties for failure to provide workers' compensation insurance tend to be minimal. For example, in Delaware the fine is $1 per employee, per day with a $25 minimum. In general, most fines are in the range of $500 to $10,000. In some states there are criminal penalties and jail terms. In Alaska, failure to insure is considered a class B or C felony. In New Mexico, the employer may be enjoined from doing business in the state if compensation insurance is not provided (8).

Adequacy of Coverage and Reimbursement

There is considerable dispute about the adequacy of workers' compensation coverage. In 1972, the National Commission on State Workers' Compensation Laws recommended 84 revisions in state systems to improve compensation, make the state laws more consistent, and remove certain inequities. However, most states have not made the revisions, 19 of which were considered essential. There have been recommendations for federal workers' compensation coverage to ensure equity and uniformity; however, these proposals have repeatedly been defeated. Differences in benefits have created effective wage differentials between states based on workers' compensation premiums or payments, similar to cross-border differentials in labor costs.

Some authorities believe that only a fraction of cases of work-related disease are covered by workers' compensation. The remainder of compensation for workers with these diseases comes from Social Security, welfare, pensions, veterans' benefits, and private insurance (9). Provisions of occupational disease coverage require that death or disability result within 1 to 5 years after exposure. The latency period may be significantly longer than 5 years in many cases for illnesses such as asbestosis or pneumoconiosis. Further, several states pay benefits only if exposure lasts longer than a specified period. There are time limits on filing, which typically are 2 years after last exposure or onset of disability. These restrictions generally place the employee at a disadvantage since it is not always clear what the causal agent was, with the exception of certain unusual diseases such as mesothelioma (10).

Financial Aspects of Workers' Compensation

Total benefits paid for medical care and cash benefits for impairment and wage replacement rose dramatically during the 1980s, and then declined sharply during most of the 1990s (11). Wage replacement costs had increased at almost twice the rate of the general wage index. As the economy improved and changes were made to workers' compensation statutes in the early 1990s, these costs stabilized.

Benefits payments were $43.4 billion in 1999. This was a 2.5% increase from 1998. The total payout for benefits has been in the $40 billion range, with some fluctuation, for the entire decade of the 1990s. Relative to the total payroll of covered workers, benefits payments declined from 1.09% to 1.05% of payroll. This is an average, and varies widely by business type and occupation. It was the seventh consecutive year of such a decline.

Employer costs for workers' compensation were $53.3 billion, an increase of 0.9%. Again, as a proportion of wages, employers' direct costs for workers' compensation insurance premiums declined from 1.37% of covered payroll in 1998 to 1.29% in 1999, the sixth consecutive year of decline. The cost per covered worker in 1999 was $430. Estimates of indirect costs for income loss in excess of benefits, lost productivity, and business interruption are generally thought to be about three times that amount (12).

Medical care costs as a proportion of benefits paid have been about 40% for the 1990s, rising to 42.4% in 1999. In general, these costs have risen two to three times faster than the medical consumer price index.

These costs have affected where companies locate, have driven a number of insurance companies to leave certain state markets, and have brought attention to the often fragmented management of real or allegedly occupationally related illness and injury, and the quality and quantity of medical care provided under workers' compensation statutes.

Insurance Markets

Employers can purchase insurance from state funds in 27 states, from commercial insurers, or they may self-insure. Self-insurance is permitted in all states and territories except Guam, Puerto Rico, the Virgin Islands, and Wyoming. In Texas, the insurance commission must approve self-insurance. The largest firms, which include about 1% of employers in the U.S. and employ 10% to 15% of the workforce, are self-insured. These employers are able to spread risk within their own workforce because of their size. Twenty-eight states and the LSA authorize group self-insurance for smaller employers, who pool their risks and liabilities.

Midsized firms (14% of employers, 70% of employees) generally purchase workers' compensation insurance on the commercial market. This insurance is risk rated according to the firm's own experience. The smallest firms (85% of employers, 15% of employees) are class rated, which is essentially a payroll tax based on industry-wide illness and injury history.

The administrative and legal frameworks of all workers' compensation programs are under state control. There are three fundamental provisions of all workers' compensation programs when claims are contested. First, the insurer or self-insured company is entitled to contest permanent disability claims and in most cases all claims. Second, state compensation boards or court systems adjudicate all contested claims. Third, the burden of proof is on the worker in any contested case.

Financial Condition of the Insurance Industry

In the last decade, the "loss ratios," the ratios of payout to premiums collected, have averaged 110% to 120%. In other words, insurers were losing between 10% and 20% more than they were collecting. Many insurers therefore withdrew from the workers' compensation insurance market. In most states, a "residual market" enables uninsurable companies to obtain insurance. A surtax, known as a residual market load, is imposed on purchasers of commercial insurance. This surtax provides an incentive to self-insure, insure through an association or risk pool, or seek other methods of financing to avoid this tax.

It is widely believed that there is cost shifting from Medicare, Medicaid, and other government programs, as well as from private insurance, because cost containment programs have succeeded in those areas, but have not been widely used in workers' compensation (13). This shifting is due in part to a confounding by administrative requirements and long time frames involved in workers' compensation. There is also a belief that all medical bills must be paid, although, in fact, few statutes or regulations make that statement. The correct statement is that medically necessary care must be reimbursed.

Incentives and Disincentives

Workers' compensation insurance grew up as part of the property and casualty insurance sector. At the time the laws were enacted, there was little medicine could do for acute traumatic injuries, and health and life insurers were reluctant to write this coverage because of a perception that there might be "moral hazard," which means that the employee could seek unnecessary care for gain. The chief emphasis at the time the laws were passed was on loss.

Immediate Versus Delayed Investment and Rating

One reason why workers' compensation costs have not led to an increased investment in loss control technology or prevention is that it is generally less expensive to buy insurance now than to install costly engineering controls. Due to the time value of money, paying insurance premiums over a 10-year period is less expensive in current dollars than paying a lump sum to install control technologies today. This is particularly true in the case of occupational diseases, which may take many years to appear.

Risk Spreading and Payment Lags

For those who are fully insured, compensation insurance premium calculations are a disincentive to improve loss control. Most premiums are calculated on a 3-year average of losses. There is also a significant retention of funds to cover the payout or "tail," which typically runs off in a long curve, peaking in the first or second year and tailing off over up to a 10-year period. The tail is apparently increasing. It is difficult, therefore, to see an immediate effect on cash outflow with a reduction in accident frequency.

By spreading risk through insurance, insurance pools, or large employee populations, financial incentives to avoid a catastrophe or other major losses have been diluted. Incentives to improve one's loss record in order to reduce costs have also been blunted. The situation has changed somewhat for self-insurers and experience rated employers as workers' compensation costs have escalated rapidly. However, the attitude for diffusing or delaying costs remains and is subject to change (14).

Perverse Incentives Within Organizations

In many companies or nonprofit organizations, losses are not allocated back to the department in which they were incurred. This policy is an intracompany version of risk spreading that provides a disincentive to improvement and safety records.

Further, many managers have productivity incentives. They therefore prefer not to return employees to work on limited duty. This disincentive clearly prevents rapid return to work, which is associated with shorter recovery times and reduced payments. The availability of light work or modified duties is key to reducing accident severity rates. Several studies show that absenteeism and disability with low back pain are significantly reduced when light duty is available (15,16).

Provider and Patient Incentives

With reductions in group-health benefits, there has been a tendency to ascribe injuries to the work site, since workers' compensation will pay 100% of the medical bills and provide wage replacement (17). As group health benefits continue to be reduced or are eliminated by smaller employers, this incentive to use the workers' compensation system is expected to increase. Because workers' compensation pays 100% of charges, there has been an apparent increase in hospitalization rates as well as cost shifting. Managed care organizations seem to be very careful about assuring that compensable injuries are classified as such to ensure payment outside the prepayment system.

There is also an economic incentive to undertake workers' compensation claims as benefits payments increase. The National Council on Compensation Insurance (NCCI) demonstrated that a 10% increase in indemnity benefits leads to a 4% increase in the frequency of claims (18).

Dissatisfaction with one's job, monotonous and repetitive tasks, and the feeling of fatigue at the end of the workday are associated with greater absenteeism and disability leave (19,20). A study at the Boeing Corporation revealed that a major predictor of absence from work was poor performance evaluation, and another was conflict with supervisors (21). These studies also noted that workers who do not enjoy their jobs or communicate well with peers are more likely to file and maintain compensation claims.

Rehabilitation programs, which are mandated in many workers' compensation insurance programs, are based on a social service model that is in direct conflict with the compensation model. The goal of rehabilitation programs is to restore function, whereas one goal of workers' compensation, although probably an unintended one, is compensation for disability. In workers' compensation the law is construed as a right to benefits. Rehabilitation takes a clinical point of view, whereas workers' compensation may seem like a reward system to some. The incentives for rehabilitation are increased social rewards and self-esteem, whereas in workers' compensation the more disabled a person becomes, the higher the award (22,23). Rehabilitation programs work best when they make as few changes in the client's premorbid life as possible, including return to the same job and the same occupation.

Legal Factors

Attorney involvement was the strongest predictor of disability in one extensive study (24). In New York State an analysis of almost 3,000 cases demonstrated that with attorney involvement much of the diagnostic testing conducted was frequently repetitious and unnecessary. The quality of medical records was poor (25). In general, the probability of surgery was higher with attorney involvement, and when indications were less than clear, the outcome was poor (26,27). When comparing settlements for the same impairment, settlements were significantly greater with attorneys involved, but the claimants received less than half the settlements (28). Because the amount of a settlement relates to the perception of disability, there is a financial incentive to portray the claimant as significantly disabled, which probably explains the increased use of tests and surgery. The proportion of litigated cases is increasing rapidly. It is now estimated that over 50% of the cases in California and Texas are represented by attorneys and in this supposedly "no-fault" system.

EPIDEMIOLOGY OF OCCUPATIONAL DEATH, ILLNESS, AND INJURY

Mortality

There were 6,023 work-related fatalities in the U.S. in 1999, down from 6,055 in 1998 despite an increase in employment (29); 43% were due to transportation incidents, 17% to objects and equipment, 15% to assaults and violent acts, 12% to falls, and 9% to harmful substances or environments. Motor vehicle accidents accounted for over half the transport fatalities. The number of homicides at work has declined almost 40% from 1994 to 1999. Homicide dropped from second to third among leading causes. Accidental work deaths per 100,000 population have dropped more than 83% from 1912 to 1999.

The occupations with the highest relative risk are construction, which accounts for 20% of fatalities but only 6% of the workforce. The leading cause was falls. Other occupations with high relative risk include agriculture (tractor-related), forestry and fishing (falling trees), transportation and public utilities (vehicle crashes), and mining. Men, the self-employed, and older workers suffered more fatal injuries than their employment shares would suggest.

These data were derived from the Census of Fatal Occupational Injuries. This Bureau of Labor Statistics (BLS) program uses diverse state and federal data sources and cross-references source documents such as death certificates, workers' compensation records, and government-mandated reports.

TABLE 18.1. *Bureau of Labor Statistics (BLS) estimates of occupational injury and illness incidence rates for selected industries, 1989*

Industry	SIC code	Incidence rates: Total cases	Lost workday cases	Nonfatal cases without lost workdays	Lost workdays
Private sector		8.6	4.0	4.6	78.7
Agriculture, forestry, and fishing		10.9	5.7	5.2	100.9
Agricultural production	01–02	12.2	6.2	6.0	101.9
Agricultural services	07	9.7	5.3	4.5	99.8
Forestry	08	11.4	5.6	5.7	132.4
Mining		8.5	4.8	3.7	137.2
Metal mining	10	8.5	4.7	3.8	133.0
Coal mining	12	11.6	8.3	3.2	254.8
Oil and gas extraction	13	7.6	3.8	3.9	111.7
Crude petroleum and natural gas	131	3.3	1.6	1.8	41.6
Natural gas liquids	132	4.1	1.1	3.0	28.8
Oil and gas field services	138	12.1	6.0	6.0	184.7
Nonmetallic minerals, except fuels	14	7.9	4.4	3.5	90.2
Construction		14.3	6.8	7.5	143.3
General building contractors	15	13.9	6.5	7.4	137.3
Residential building construction	152	11.4	6.1	5.3	131.7
Nonresidential building construction	154	16.9	7.2	9.7	148.1
Heavy construction, except building	16	13.8	6.5	7.3	147.1
Highway and street construction	161	14.1	6.5	7.6	139.0
Heavy construction, except highway	162	13.7	6.5	7.1	150.6
Special trade contractors	17	14.6	6.9	7.7	144.9
Plumbing, heating, air conditioning	171	15.7	6.3	9.4	116.0
Painting and paper hanging	172	9.4	5.0	4.4	137.2
Electrical work	173	13.1	5.3	7.8	105.6
Masonry, stonework, and plastering	174	16.0	8.3	7.7	179.3
Carpentry and floor work	175	13.0	7.1	5.9	134.8
Roofing, siding, and sheet metal work	176	18.3	10.0	8.3	247.1
Manufacturing		13.1	5.8	7.3	113.0
Durable goods		14.1	6.0	8.1	116.5
Lumber and wood products	24	18.4	9.4	9.1	177.5
Logging	241	19.5	11.7	7.7	307.8
Sawmills and planing mills	242	18.6	9.6	9.0	187.3
Millwork, plywood, and structural members	243	17.7	8.8	8.9	151.2
Wood containers	244	16.2	9.0	7.2	180.9
Wood buildings and mobile homes	245	25.2	11.0	14.2	164.9
Furniture and fixtures	25	16.1	7.2	8.9	124.9
Household furniture	251	15.5	6.9	8.5	113.1
Office furniture	252	17.5	7.5	9.9	162.7
Public building and related furniture	253	19.6	8.5	11.0	163.5
Stone, clay, and glass products	32	15.5	7.4	8.1	149.8
Flat glass	321	21.9	7.3	14.5	116.6
Glass and glassware, pressed or blown	322	14.2	6.5	7.6	139.7
Products of purchased glass	323	16.9	6.7	10.1	120.8
Structural clay products	325	17.1	7.9	9.2	179.0
Pottery and related products	326	15.8	9.2	6.6	186.7
Concrete, gypsum, and plaster products	327	15.8	8.2	7.6	167.1
Miscellaneous nonmetallic mineral products	329	13.7	6.7	7.0	132.4
Primary metal industries	33	18.7	8.1	10.5	168.3
Blast furnace and basic steel products	331	16.7	6.8	9.8	166.8
Iron and steel foundries	332	25.4	10.8	14.7	183.6
Primary nonferrous metals	333	19.9	7.6	12.2	159.9
Nonferrous rolling and drawing	335	15.3	7.1	8.2	149.2
Nonferrous foundries (castings)	336	20.9	10.0	10.9	193.7
Fabricated metal products	34	18.5	7.9	10.7	147.6
Metal cans and shipping containers	341	16.2	6.5	9.7	128.1
Cutlery, hand tools, and hardware	342	14.8	6.2	8.5	131.7

TABLE 18.1. *Continued*

		Incidence rates			
Industry	SIC code	Total cases	Nonfatal Lost workday cases	cases without lost workdays	Lost workdays
Plumbing and heating, except electric	343	20.3	7.8	12.5	128.7
Fabricated structural metal products	344	21.3	9.6	11.7	167.9
Screw machine products, bolts, etc.	345	14.7	5.9	8.8	89.5
Metal forgings and stampings	346	23.1	8.7	14.4	186.8
Metal services	347	15.9	7.4	8.5	132.9
Ordnance and accessories	348	10.2	4.5	5.7	96.7
Miscellaneous fabricated metal products	349	16.7	7.5	9.2	138.3
Industrial machinery and equipment	35	12.1	4.8	7.3	86.8
Engines and turbines	351	13.9	5.2	8.6	112.3
Farm and garden machinery	352	18.7	6.8	11.8	102.7
Construction and related machinery	353	16.3	6.7	9.7	116.5
Metalworking machinery	354	12.7	4.6	8.1	78.4
Special industry machinery	355	13.9	5.3	8.6	89.5
General industrial machinery	356	13.7	5.4	8.3	98.0
Computer and office equipment	357	3.8	1.9	1.9	41.7
Refrigeration and service machinery	358	16.8	7.0	9.8	125.6
Industrial machinery, n.e.c.	359	12.9	5.1	7.9	94.8
Electronic and other electric equipment	36	9.1	3.9	5.1	77.5
Electric distribution equipment	361	12.0	4.8	7.2	92.0
Electrical industrial apparatus	362	11.1	4.6	6.4	98.4
Household appliances	363	18.0	7.1	10.9	127.3
Electric lighting and wiring equipment	364	10.8	4.8	6.0	100.8
Household audio and video equipment	365	10.0	4.6	5.4	96.3
Communications equipment	366	4.7	2.1	2.6	43.6
Electronic components and accessories	367	6.6	2.9	3.7	55.2
Transportation equipment	37	17.7	6.8	10.9	138.6
Motor vehicles and equipment	371	22.6	8.5	14.1	173.9
Aircraft and parts	372	10.1	3.7	6.4	70.2
Ship and boat building and repairing	373	38.0	15.6	22.4	343.9
Railroad equipment	374	20.9	9.7	11.2	181.0
Guided missiles, space vehicles, parts	376	4.8	2.2	2.6	39.7
Instruments and related products	38	5.6	2.5	3.1	55.4
Search and navigation equipment	381	3.6	1.6	2.1	35.6
Measuring and controlling devices	382	6.4	2.9	3.4	62.7
Medical instruments and supplies	384	7.4	3.4	4.0	74.3
Photographic equipment and supplies	386	5.2	2.2	3.1	49.3
Miscellaneous manufacturing industries	39	11.1	5.1	6.0	97.6
Musical instruments	393	10.7	4.6	6.1	78.5
Toys and sporting goods	394	13.3	6.2	7.1	112.2
Pens, pencils, office, and art supplies	395	10.1	4.6	5.5	94.4
Costume jewelry and notions	396	7.2	3.4	3.8	82.7
Nondurable goods		11.6	5.5	6.1	107.8
Food and kindred products	20	18.5	9.3	9.2	174.7
Meat products	201	27.1	13.5	13.7	250.9
Dairy products	202	15.2	7.9	7.3	156.5
Preserved fruits and vegetables	203	17.5	8.3	9.2	148.8
Grain mill products	204	13.1	6.7	6.4	139.8
Bakery products	205	13.5	6.9	6.6	153.9
Sugar and confectionery products	206	14.2	6.9	7.3	118.8
Fats and oils	207	15.3	7.7	7.5	164.8
Beverages	208	17.7	9.1	8.6	165.1
Miscellaneous foods and kindred products	209	16.3	8.4	7.9	139.3
Tobacco products	21	8.7	3.4	5.3	64.2
Textile mill products	22	10.3	4.2	6.1	81.4
Broadwoven fabric mills, cotton	221	8.5	2.7	5.8	57.1
Broadwoven fabric mills, man-made	222	8.0	3.4	4.6	72.1

TABLE 18.1. *Continued*

Industry	SIC code	Total cases	Nonfatal Lost workday cases	cases without lost workdays	Lost workdays
		Incidence rates			
Broadwoven fabric mills, wool	223	9.7	5.2	4.5	118.8
Narrow fabric mills	224	11.5	5.4	6.0	96.7
Knitting mills	225	9.0	4.2	4.8	73.4
Textile finishing, except wool	226	11.6	5.1	6.5	89.2
Carpets and rugs	227	13.8	4.9	8.9	94.3
Yarn and thread mills	228	11.7	4.1	7.6	83.5
Apparel and other textile products	23	8.6	3.8	4.8	80.5
Men's and boys' suits and coats	231	8.9	4.3	4.6	98.8
Men's and boys' furnishings	232	11.3	5.5	5.8	126.9
Women's and misses' outerwear	233	4.9	1.8	3.0	45.1
Women's and children's undergarments	234	7.2	2.8	4.4	53.1
Hats, caps, and millinery	235	10.7	4.7	6.0	108.3
Girls'and children's outerwear	236	8.0	3.5	4.5	72.3
Miscellaneous apparel and accessories	238	6.9	3.3	3.6	60.9
Miscellaneous fabricated textile products	239	11.6	5.1	6.5	84.6
Paper and allied products	26	12.7	5.8	6.9	132.9
Paper mills	262	11.9	4.7	7.2	137.5
Paperboard mills	263	12.1	4.9	7.3	126.5
Paperboard containers and boxes	265	13.2	6.3	6.9	133.7
Printing and publishing	27	6.9	3.3	3.6	63.8
Newspapers	271	7.2	3.4	3.8	72.3
Periodicals	272	3.2	1.7	1.4	39.4
Books	273	6.5	3.1	3.4	55.5
Commercial printing	275	7.9	3.7	4.2	68.7
Manifold business forms	276	9.8	4.2	5.6	73.6
Blank books and bookbinding	278	9.6	5.0	4.7	88.9
Chemicals and allied products	28	7.0	3.2	3.7	63.4
Industrial inorganic chemicals	281	5.9	2.6	3.2	54.8
Plastics materials and synthetics	282	6.3	2.9	3.4	62.2
Drugs	283	5.8	2.9	2.9	55.0
Soap, cleaners, and toilet goods	284	8.5	4.0	4.5	72.4
Paints and allied products	285	10.4	5.0	5.4	85.3
Industrial organic chemicals	286	6.1	2.5	3.6	55.1
Agricultural chemicals	287	7.8	3.5	4.3	63.3
Miscellaneous chemical products	289	8.7	4.1	4.5	82.8
Petroleum and coal products	29	6.6	3.3	3.3	68.1
Petroleum refining	291	5.3	2.6	2.7	56.6
Asphalt paving and roofing materials	295	10.2	5.1	5.1	108.7
Rubber and miscellaneous plastics products	30	16.2	8.0	8.2	147.2
Tires and inner tubes	301	15.4	9.2	6.2	170.4
Rubber and plastic footwear	302	16.8	8.2	8.7	157.4
Hose and belting and gaskets and packing	305	13.8	6.4	7.4	110.1
Fabricated rubber products, n.e.c.	306	17.1	8.6	8.5	150.4
Miscellaneous plastics products, n.e.c.	308	16.4	7.9	8.5	146.8
Leather and leather products	31	13.6	6.5	7.1	130.4
Leather tanning and finishing	311	25.0	13.9	11.0	290.0
Footwear, except rubber	314	13.3	6.0	7.3	117.4
Transportation and public utilities		9.2	5.3	3.9	121.5
Railroad transportation	40	7.7	5.8	1.9	153.3
Local and interurban passenger transit	41	9.6	5.5	4.1	125.3
Local and suburban transportation	411	12.0	7.2	4.8	143.2
Taxicabs	412	4.9	3.0	1.9	77.9
School buses	415	9.0	4.3	4.7	88.9
Trucking and warehousing	42	13.5	7.9	5.6	205.0
Trucking and courier services, except air	421	13.4	7.9	5.5	210.0

TABLE 18.1. *Continued*

Industry	SIC code	Incidence rates: Total cases	Nonfatal: Lost workday cases	cases without lost workdays	Lost workdays
Water transportation	44	12.1	7.3	4.8	263.1
Water transportation of freight, n.e.c.	444	10.0	6.4	3.6	167.1
Transportation by air	45	14.2	8.2	5.9	138.2
Air transportation, scheduled	451	14.5	8.5	6.0	142.3
Transportation services	47	4.3	2.4	1.9	47.9
Communications	48	3.1	1.7	1.4	33.2
Electric, gas, and sanitary services	49	8.0	4.0	3.9	73.0
Electric services	491	6.0	2.6	3.4	51.0
Gas production and distribution	492	7.2	3.5	3.7	53.8
Combination utility services	493	6.7	3.8	2.9	71.0
Water supply	494	10.6	5.9	4.7	81.3
Sanitary services	495	18.7	10.6	8.1	192.6
Wholesale and retail trade		8.0	3.6	4.4	63.5
Wholesale trade		7.7	4.0	3.8	71.9
Wholesale trade—durable goods	50	6.7	3.3	3.4	55.8
Lumber and construction materials	503	11.5	6.1	5.4	114.1
Electrical goods	506	4.3	2.2	2.1	37.1
Machinery, equipment, and supplies	508	7.7	3.6	4.1	55.3
Wholesale trade—nondurable goods	51	9.3	5.0	4.3	96.3
Groceries and related products	514	13.3	7.5	5.8	140.1
Petroleum and petroleum products	517	5.1	2.6	2.6	53.4
Retail trade		8.1	3.4	4.6	60.0
Building materials and garden supplies	52	9.8	4.8	5.0	78.1
General merchandise stores	53	10.7	5.0	5.7	82.6
Food stores	54	11.6	4.9	6.7	102.5
Automotive dealers and service stations	55	6.9	2.7	4.1	50.8
Apparel and accessory stores	56	3.0	1.3	1.7	21.7
Furniture and home furnishing stores	57	4.7	2.4	2.3	40.3
Eating and drinking places	58	8.5	3.2	5.3	49.4
Miscellaneous retail	59	4.2	1.9	2.3	37.5
Finance, insurance, and real estate		2.0	0.9	1.1	17.6
Depository institutions	60	1.4	0.6	0.9	12.2
Insurance carriers	63	1.7	0.7	1.0	14.0
Real estate	65	4.8	2.5	2.3	45.2
Services		5.5	2.7	2.8	51.2
Hotels and other lodging places	70	10.8	4.7	6.1	80.3
Personal services	72	3.6	1.9	1.7	42.9
Business services	73	4.7	2.4	2.3	48.3
Service to buildings	734	8.0	4.2	3.8	83.6
Auto repair, services, and parking	75	6.7	3.0	3.6	61.1
Miscellaneous repair services	76	8.6	4.4	4.2	73.8
Health services	80	7.3	3.8	3.5	76.7
Nursing and personal care facilities	805	15.5	8.8	6.6	181.8
Hospitals	806	8.5	4.2	4.2	78.7
Legal services	81	0.5	0.2	0.3	5.9
Educational services	82	3.5	1.5	2.0	26.8
Social services	83	5.7	2.8	2.9	46.5
Residential care	836	9.3	4.3	4.9	79.7
Museums, botanical, zoologic gardens	84	6.2	3.0	3.3	51.2
Engineering and management services	87	1.9	0.9	1.0	13.2

SIC, Standard Industry Code; n.e.c., not elsewhere classified.
Adapted from Bureau of Labor Statistics Supplementary Data System, 1989.

Morbidity

A total of 5.7 million injuries and illnesses were reported in private industry workplaces in 1999, resulting in a rate of 6.3 cases per 100 equivalent full-time workers (30). This represents a 4% drop in the number of cases and a 2% increase in the number of hours worked. This is the lowest rate since the BLS began reporting this information in the early 1970s.

The most marked drop was in the goods-producing sector, with a drop from 11.9 per 100 full-time equivalents (FTEs) in 1994 to 8.9 per 100 FTEs in 1999. Among goods-producing industries, manufacturing had the highest incidence rate (9.2 per 100 FTEs). Within the service-producing sector, transportation and public utilities reported the highest rate at 7.3 per 100 FTEs.

While there has been great improvement in the rate of work-related health problems, there is still considerable room for improvement compared to benchmarks. For example, in 1989, the OSHA recordable lost workday incident rate was 78.7 per 100 workers. During that same year, DuPont's lost workday rate was 0.05, and Johnson & Johnson, which had announced a goal of displacing DuPont as the corporate leader in safety, had a lost workday incidence of 0.14 lost workdays per 100 workers. In other words, the national lost workday incidence per 100 workers was approximately 1500 times worse than DuPont's, and 500 times worse than Johnson & Johnson's. One of the most effective approaches to managing workers' compensation is significant improvement in workplace safety.

Of the 5.7 million total injuries, 2.7 million, or 47.4%, were lost workday cases. In the OSHA reporting system, lost workday cases include days in which the employee was at work but with restrictions. The lost workday rate of 1.9 per 100 workers was the lowest ever reported. Days with restrictions appear to be replacing lost workday cases (Fig. 18.1). The manufacturing rate for restricted activity days (2.4) was higher than the rate of cases with days away from work (DAW) (2.2). In all other types of occupation, the DAW rate was higher than the restricted day rate. Overall, 1.7 million cases with DAW were reported in 1999.

Ninety-three percent of the nonfatal occupational illness and injury cases were reported as injuries. Truck drivers had the highest rate in 1999 (141.1 per 200,000 hours worked, usually equivalent to 100 FTEs), only a slight decline from 1993. The rates for nonconstruction laborers and nursing aides and orderlies, the next two most prevalent occupations, declined 33% and 26%, respectively, during that time period.

The remaining 7% of cases were reported as occupational illnesses. Manufacturing accounted for 60% of these cases. Two thirds of the cases of occupational illness were attributed to repeated trauma; of these, 70% were in manufacturing.

The longest median durations away from work were carpal tunnel syndrome (CTS) (27 days), fractures (20 days), and amputations (18 days). Grouped by mechanism, repetitive motion cases had the longest median absence (17 days).

Men accounted for 66% of lost workday cases, while comprising 59% of the workforce by hours

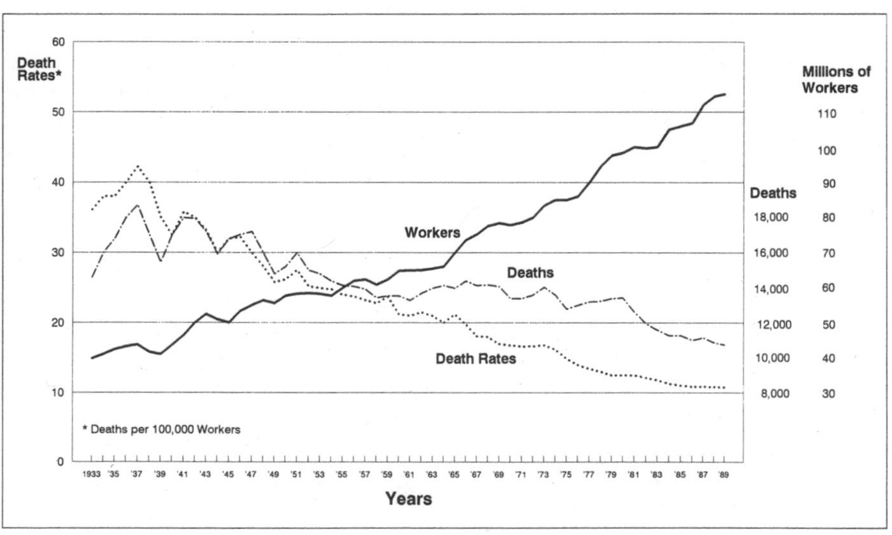

FIG. 18.1. Workers, deaths, and death rates. Source: National Safety Council, 1991.

worked. Operators, fabricators, and laborers led all occupational groups, accounting for 42% of the total DAW cases. The most common causes of lost workday cases were overexertion, primarily in lifting; being struck by an object; and falls on the same level.

Parts of Body and Nature of Injuries

In an analysis of 12 states' workers' compensation data for 1998 by International Classification of Diseases ICD-9 code, soft tissue complaints accounted for many of the top ten diagnostic groups for all workers' compensation cases. The top ten in Texas, for example, included low back soft tissue complaints (17%), shoulder soft tissue complaints (7%), neck soft tissue complaints (6%), hand and wrist superficial trauma (4%), knee internal derangements (3.8%), hand and wrist soft tissue complaints (3.4%), multiple body parts soft tissue complaints (3.2%), low back nerve compression (2.4%), ankle and foot soft tissue complaints (2.4%), and hand and wrist nerve compression (2.4%) (31).

According to OSHA statistics, the back was the body part most commonly affected by disabling work incidents, accounting for about a quarter, or 424,300 cases of the 1.7 million total. Finger injuries were next (149,500 cases), then knees (128,000) and shoulder injuries (93,800).

The most common types of disabling injuries and illnesses were sprains and strains (739,700), bruises and contusions (156,000), cuts and lacerations (132,400), and fractures (113,700). A total of 27,900 cases of CTS requiring DAW were reported in 1999, ranking 6th overall. There were 16,600 tendonitis cases with DAW reported as well.

Reporting of Injuries and Illnesses

A number of authors have documented significant underreporting of work-related disorders for various reasons (32–35). Reasons for underreporting include fear of reprisal, a belief that pain is a normal consequence of aging or work, lack of management responsiveness to previous complaints, and a desire not to be moved to another job. Corporate safety objectives may have an indirect effect on reporting, as managers attempt to reduce injury rates to meet goals (36).

OPERATIONAL OVERVIEW OF THE WORKERS' COMPENSATION SYSTEM

It is important for all participants in the workers' compensation system to understand one another's roles and responsibilities, in order to have this conflict-prone system function more smoothly. Employers, employees, payers, regulators, and health care providers all have important roles to play.

Reporting of Claims

When a work-related health concern occurs, it is important to engage the workers' compensation system as soon as possible to ensure that appropriate benefits are paid promptly and to begin to manage care and time off work. When a serious injury occurs at work, the first medical priority is typically to obtain medical care. In those cases, the urgent or emergent care provider is the first point of contact and should report the case as soon as possible. However, many health concerns now are not acute. In these cases, the worker may report the problem to the employer, or may seek discretionary medical care directly. In most states, employers, employees, and providers all have the obligation to report some information about the problem to the payer and to the state regulatory body. In a few states, such as Washington, the employer is not part of the reporting cycle. A number of studies, most of them internal to insurers, have shown that the sooner the claim is reported, the more rapid the return to work and the lower the total cost.

Claim and Case Management

Ideally, the payer or third-party claims administrator, the provider, and the employer would work as a closely coordinated team to ensure prompt determination of benefits eligibility, payment, proactive management of care and disability, and prevention of exacerbation, recurrences, and additional health problems. This typically requires advance planning and discussion. It also requires education of employees about their rights and responsibilities under the workers' compensation system, and their involvement in prevention of health problems at the work site. While some employers and payers are reluctant to inform workers about workers' compensation for fear of inducing fraudulent claims, this has not proven to be a problem. Workers in fact appreciate the consideration. The discussion can be included in safety initiatives, to emphasize the preventive aspect.

The Payer Role

Payers, whether insurers, third-party administrators managing claims for employers, or self-administered employers, must comply with legal requirements for fair and timely benefits administration. The best practice is to assume active management of all aspects of the case, including management of care, management of absence from work, and prevention of recurrences as well as benefits eligibility. Alternatively, occupational health professionals can act as case coordinators, ensuring timely information exchange, appropriate and efficient medical care, and management of disability through modified or transitional work.

Determining Benefits Eligibility

Once a health problem is reported to the payer or claims administrator, insurance claims personnel known as adjusters, examiners, or claims managers must decide whether the problem is indeed related to work to determine entitlement to benefits. In the terms used in claims management, is there an injury related to work? The classic paradigm for workers' compensation has been that of acute injury. Most statutes, discussions, information, and lay literature in the field refer to "injuries" and "injured workers" even though the issue may be an occupational illness, cumulative trauma, or concern about exposure rather than a discrete health effect.

Claims professionals generally do not have medical backgrounds; they are typically recent college graduates from a variety of fields. Their job training typically focuses on legal requirements for benefits coverage and payment. Medical training is usually minimal, and generally does not include evidence- or consensus-based criteria for causation, medical necessity, therapeutic effectiveness, or disability management. Consequently, the basis for causation decisions may be based on the circumstances surrounding the complaint, often using the injury paradigm, or the claims adjudicator may seek medical input. The typical method of property/casualty adjudication, which references the coverage and benefits limits in the insurance policy, is not relevant here, since these limits are set by statute and regulation. The governing issue is whether the complaint was reasonably causally related to work duties and exposures.

The two traditional criteria for eligibility for workers' compensation benefits are termed arising out of employment (AOE) and in the course of employment (COE). The second issue, whether the worker was in fact engaged in job duties at the time the health problem occurred, is generally an administrative one. The first, whether the health problem arose out of employment, follows from the source of exposure to the agent of illness or injury. In the case of direct trauma, these decisions are relatively obvious. However, the exposure for occupational diseases and some other problems such as work-related musculoskeletal disorders (WMDs) can occur over time. Further, there may be exposure to potential agents such as lifting, keyboard work, noise, fumes, and so on at home as well as at work. In these cases, the entitlement to benefits hinges on a thorough history of all sources and amounts of exposure, and plausible experimental or epidemiologic evidence linking the exposure to a specific health problem. An occupational medicine professional should most appropriately do this information gathering and analysis, either as part of the patient encounter or in collaboration with the claim adjuster.

Claims are approved for accepted injuries or accepted body parts. Typically this means that an adjuster will agree to pay for care for an arm, leg, or low back, or some combination of parts of the body, or for damage to a system such as the respiratory system. Subsequent care is then questioned only if it is directed at a different area or system. Claims are not typically accepted for a specific diagnosis. The NCCI and other associations in this field have perpetuated this somewhat arcane system by creating coding schemes that are based on injured body part and rather broadly defined injuries, rather than on diagnoses. The consequence is that care will be paid for aging changes and unrelated diagnoses as well as the original complaint. For example, if a worker with a strain or tendonitis of the forearm later develops CTS, the connection is not usually questioned, even though these entities are not etiologically related. Responsible occupational physicians would not treat such "migrating diagnoses" without reconsidering work-relatedness and reevaluating specific etiologic factors and potential workstation and work practice changes. However, many practitioners have done so, with questionable results.

In addition, some insurers have accepted responsibility for age- or lifestyle-related changes after an initial health problem. In one example, the heart was accepted in the 1970s when a worker had chest pain for unexplained reasons. Thirty years later, after many years of high cholesterol, high blood pressure, and smoking, the worker developed overt coronary artery disease. His physician claimed that the problem was work related, and the insurer paid for the treatment, until an astute case manager questioned the work-relatedness of the problem. Behaviors of this sort drive up costs and contribute to the general attitude among insurers that health care providers may not be entirely neutral or altruistic in their care of workers. The result is increased conflict and delay, often to the detriment of the worker in this supposedly no-fault system.

Care Management

There is a clear need for proactive external medical management of workers' compensation cases because of the wide variations in the quality and quantity of medical care, and the absence of medical expertise under the present property and casualty insurance framework. As noted, workers' compensation claims examiners or adjusters are primarily concerned with complying with legal requirements of the workers' compensation system, including prompt payment, although they often sincerely believe that they are managing medical care by reviewing bills for appropriateness, by arranging care, or even by becoming involved in preauthorization.

Standards, criteria, and protocols have not been widely applied to those cases paid for by workers' compensation. The need for standards and criteria is made more urgent by the fact that many of the current major categories of occupational illness or injury are nonspecific, subjective complaints such as back and wrist pain that can only be effectively managed with carefully constructed criteria and constant reference to physical signs. As mentioned above, in many cases, imaging studies only confuse the issue unless they are applied judiciously; otherwise, the chances of a false-positive result and subsequent misdiagnosis and unnecessary surgery are extremely high (37,38).

Time-based disability management of workers' compensation cases is also critical. For example, it has been demonstrated repeatedly that the average recovery time for uncomplicated low back pain is 2 days of bed rest and 8 days of partial disability before complete return to function (39). However, comparison of recommendations of the American College of Occupational and Environmental Medicine and several other consensus panels (40) of population studies revealed that while the average length of time absent from work for both back pain and wrist pain is in the range of 4 to 15 weeks (41,42), the expert consensus was 1 to 3 weeks.

Payers and employers may employ nurse or medical social work case managers to coordinate complex medical care, to identify issues that might delay functional recovery, or to act as a patient advocate to ensure appropriate and timely care (43). Some more forward-thinking organizations have occupational health nurses manage cases from the date of injury or the date of report, to ensure timely, appropriate care and to coordinate return to work on modified duty if necessary. In the best cases, these medical personnel work in teams with claims adjusters, with each team member using his or her expertise effectively. In many cases, unfortunately, case managers are often consulted only after months of care or absence from work, when expectations and patterns have already been established.

Many payers and employers have also engaged physicians as medical directors, to advise claims and human resource personnel, to coordinate care, or to work with community or network physicians on treatment options and job modification. This coordination and management has streamlined care, prevented drug interactions and unnecessary procedures, improved patient education, and improved disability management in the best cases.

Claims Review and Intervention

It is not infrequent for workers' compensation claims to be left open for long periods, up to years, without medical reevaluation or assessment of the employee's status. Many anecdotal studies have demonstrated that significant backlogs of cases have been left open without reexamination of liabilities amounting to millions of dollars for many mid- to large-sized employers. Periodic medical reviews of these cases can be quite revealing. Additional medical evidence or reevaluation of the claimant may be in order. It is not infrequent for many disorders to resolve spontaneously, as this is the natural history of many nonspecific complaints, dermatitis, and other work-related complaints. Cases that do not meet criteria should be reevaluated immediately, and attempts made to settle or close the cases as quickly as possible. Disability management can be based on either medical treatment or recovery guidelines or disability management guidelines, which are time based.

Another critical role for the occupational physician is to examine the record of the injury to determine if it is, in fact, causally related. This is not the "causality" used by claims examiners, but a question of whether an injury is mechanically or epidemiologically plausible based on exposure to the work site during the time course of the injury. Some estimates are that over half of the occupationally related claims that are paid may not, in fact, be related to the work site. Use of careful clinical judgment as well as standards and criteria should allow the occupational physician to state an informed opinion about the relationship of the inciting event to the alleged resultant injury.

We should note here that the role of care manager can and perhaps should be assumed by the occupational physician treating the patient. In some states, the primary treating provider is specifically responsible for coordinating care. Unfortunately, in many cases, both the payer and the provider default on this responsibility, allowing conflicting or less than efficacious care from several sources to occur.

Provider Networks

Another aspect of care management is the development and management of networks of physicians to treat workers' compensation cases. Networks are often formed to secure discounted fees from physicians and facilities. With careful selection criteria, advance agreement on regular communication with employers and payers, agreement to manage absence from work, and regular feedback on adherence to evidence-based practices, networks can provide better quality care and disability management. At the present time, many payers "rent" networks from specialty companies rather than form and manage their own. They therefore have less control of the quality of care. In addition, many have mistaken large networks for value. Very large, inclusive networks are difficult to manage and typically have as wide a variation on quality of care as the general medical community. Smaller, more selective networks with monitoring and feedback mechanisms incorporated into their daily operation produce a higher quality of care at lower net cost (in the author's experience with a major workers' compensation insurer).

Assisting with creation of exclusive or preferred provider panels is an important area for physician involvement. Because of the highly variable patterns of diagnosis and treatment, which typically vary markedly from group health patterns of treatment (25), it is imperative that occupational physicians carefully screen and agree with specific providers in the evaluation and management of workers' compensation cases. It would be preferable if treating physicians and chiropractors would agree to protocols before treating a company's employees. Even in states with employee choice of physician, most employees do not have physicians and will use providers suggested by the employer, at least initially. It should be noted that the treating physicians should be very skilled at patient interaction so that they do not antagonize employees, who then choose other, probably less skilled and more variable, physicians or seek legal representation.

The Employer Role

Employer involvement in the management of work-related illnesses and injuries ranges from virtually none other than paying the required insurance premium to integrated management of injury prevention, reporting, initial care, return to work, and continuous improvement of the workers' compensation system. The employer role at a minimum includes immediate reporting of work injuries or illnesses. Another minimum recommendation should be returning the injured worker to work quickly in a modified or transitional position.

OSHA and its designated state agencies mandate prevention of recurrences and injury to others in similar jobs. Given the current complex, laborious, and expensive state of workers' compensation management, prevention and avoidance of the system are key. Attention to job design, job placement, education, and reduction of personal risk factors will result in significant reduction of injury rates. Preplacement evaluations directly related to the bona fide occupational qualifications of the job should be conducted, particularly in light of the Americans with Disabilities Act. One of the better ways of constructing functionally based accurate job descriptions that reflect the physical demands of the jobs is to use panels of workers who actually do that job (44). It is not clear what the role of strength testing is at this point (45). It is clear that physically fit individuals seem to have a lower rate of injury and recover more quickly (46).

Strategic Management

Occupational health professionals working with employers can provide leadership in the strategic and tactical management of workers' compensation at the work site. This involves a series of steps: assessing the present situation, envisioning the desired future, providing gap analysis between the two, developing a strategic plan, and providing tactical implementation.

Analysis of the present situation would involve bringing together disparate sources of data to obtain an accurate profile of the costs, sources, and treatment patterns for compensable injuries. One would also want to estimate indirect costs such as supervisory time, retraining, and business interruption.

It is also important to assess the employee perceptions of treatment and compensation of injuries, general attitude toward management, perceived management attitudes toward safety, perceived safety of the workplace, and other issues. There is now a substantial literature documenting the role of the employment climate in creating health concerns and in the filing of workers' compensation claims (47,48). Employers would do well to remediate these circumstances to reduce costs and improve productivity, if not for humanitarian reasons (49,50).

Other data that should be examined are the organizational location of workers' compensation management and flow of the process of injury management, including the management of the injured worker, information, and regulatory and administrative issues. The organizational fragmentation of the typical workers' compensation system within a company often presents a challenge to the management of compensable injuries and illnesses. It is frequently not clear who is in charge of the entire system. It may also be unclear who is in charge of the direct relationship with the injured worker. These processes therefore tend to move rather slowly, and workers can "fall through the cracks."

Once these data have been analyzed and presented to management, targets can be set and a vision of the organization of the program in the future can be established. Gap analysis is simply a comparison of the future vision with the current reality. It is entirely likely that a relatively major reorganization of the function would be appropriate if the typical degree of fragmentation and lack of medical management are discovered. However, it is also important to note that significant regulatory and administrative issues are involved with workers' compensation, so that all viewpoints must be taken into account in designing a maximally effective system. Both preloss and postloss issues should be dealt with. System design would include the design of a more effective data management capability, which captures desired data elements and provides feedback to supervisors and providers.

Disability management should be assessed and improved. This system might include policies for disability management, institution of modified duty, and a feedback system to constantly assess how well disability is managed. Length of disability by diagnosis is a good initial statistic to track.

If the use of vendors is contemplated, proposals can be requested using a structured form based on the analysis of the current situation. Benchmarks can be established for performance, either from the current situation or from comparison with best procedure companies. It is important to assure that data management is adequately addressed. Once answers to very clear proposals are received, they can be assessed against predetermined evaluation criteria.

Using a strategic approach and process quality improvement techniques, management of workers' compensation can be significantly improved. Mapping the flow of the workers' compensation management process can provide the starting point for constant improvement using total quality management procedures. Employers and employees will benefit in many ways, including increased job satisfaction, better financial performance, and decreased mortality and morbidity.

Information Requirements

A lack of complete and timely information is one reason that there is delay in treatment authorization, variance in treatment, and a general failure to improve the quality of care and administration in workers' compensation. There is a great need for information systems that tie the various participants in the system together. These systems should collect and manage data that go beyond the current mandated state reports to include clinical, employment, and other relevant data. They should also apply business and clinical rules to aid both medical and nonmedical decision makers. Finally, they should store data in such a way that reports on relative performance and comparison to best practices and benchmarks are available as management and quality improvement tools.

Without these information systems, it will be difficult to improve workers' compensation system performance.

OCCUPATIONAL PHYSICIAN'S CLINICAL ROLE IN WORKERS' COMPENSATION

At a minimum, physicians caring for workers with health concerns should provide excellent care and foster functional recovery. Doing so requires a broader and arguably more neutral approach than nonoccupational health care. In addition to diagnosing the problem and providing treatment, physicians should take a complete occupational history to determine causation, understand the hazards that caused the problem to prevent further adverse effects, facilitate functional recovery using modified work and other proven effective methods, and dispassionately evaluate impairment at maximal medical improvement. Excellent management of workers' compensation provides a challenge to the administrative and clinical skills of the occupational physician. The effort, however, can benefit both the injured worker, by providing more effective medical care, and the employer, by increasing availability for work and decreasing unnecessary costs.

Prevention

Properly focused preplacement and periodic examinations can prevent later health problems, if a mismatch between job demands and capabilities can be detected and accommodated. Examples range from allergies to lifting capacity (see Chapter 41). Once an injury has occurred, the occupational physician can again prescribe work activities that are compatible with the worker's current capabilities and that will support functional recovery (51).

Clinical Care

The physician or other health professional can play a pivotal role as diagnostician, medical expert on causation and evidence-based medicine, and care and disability manager. To do so, one must obtain a detailed health and work history; perform a careful and complete, yet focused, physical examination; and use analytic skills to make and explain the most effective recommendations at each stage of the care of the ill or injured worker. An explicit analysis is particularly important to guide the lay reader such as an adjuster or judge through the logic leading to conclusions and treatment plans. The description of the clinical process below follows the format recommended by the American College of Occupational and Environmental Medicine's *Occupational Medicine Practice Guidelines* (52).

Initial Presentation

Both a detailed history and a careful, focused physical examination are important to the accurate evaluation of the patient with a work-related illness or injury. The diagnosis and a carefully reasoned opinion about the role of work in the etiology of the problem are pivotal in determining eligibility for medical benefits. Insurance claims personnel are not usually medically trained, so the explanation of diagnosis and causality in lay language is important to the fair determination of benefits. For potential cumulative exposure problems, such as low back pain, neck pain, impingement syndrome, rotator cuff tears, epicondylitis, tendonitis, CTS, and so on, carefully documenting the total exposure, and very specific symptoms that result, including onset and impairment of nonwork activities, allows a reasonable determination to be made. The physician should not assume that the claims adjuster is familiar with the epidemiologic evidence of association between specific exposures and diagnoses. The literature, or meta-analyses such as practice guidelines (53), should be cited to support or question these associations.

History

For patients with an occupational injury, clarifying the mechanism of injury provides direction to focus the physical examination. In direct trauma, the physician should inquire about the amount of force involved, the direction and impact of the force, and the specific symptoms that followed. The precise location of any discomfort, and specific restrictions of motion are important, as well as an exact description of any deformity. This information provides clues to the potential damage present and directs diagnostic testing. A number of studies and protocols, such as the Ottawa ankle rules, for example, outline the minority of cases likely to require radiographs.

In exertional complaints, such as back or shoulder pain following lifting or moving objects, or even with no history of specific trauma, the physician should determine the load, number of repetitions, and resulting specific symptoms, including gradual or acute onset, radiation of pain, and associated symptoms. The total duration of exposure to these forces is important as well (54). Many such complaints are the result of repeated subclinical overload. In these cases, it is important to understand what other activities the patient does or can do outside of work. Often activities of daily living provide a description of what impairment and residual abilities are present.

With occupational illnesses such as CTS or ulnar nerve compression, it is again necessary to determine and record the specific type and location of symptoms the patient is experiencing. These complaints are frequently misdiagnosed, leading to inappropriate treatment. Further, if they are present, they have a number of nonoccupational etiologies as well. Occupational illnesses such as respiratory disease require a complete cumulative exposure history as well. Controversial diagnoses such as multiple chemical sensitivity, chronic fatigue syndrome, or myofascial pain syndrome require both a careful history and examination of the literature to verify that there is any evidence linking the diagnosis, if correct, to work (see Chapter 29).

Physical Examination

The physical examination for many occupational illnesses and injuries should be focused but include areas in which lesions might cause similar complaints. For example, with hand pain or paresthesias, one should examine the hands but also the neck in case the symptoms are those of a cervical radiculopathy (55). In both cases, a careful neurologic examination, including the specific distribution of any sensory deficits, reflex strength, motor strength, and provocative maneuvers, should be specifically documented. Findings should include inspection, palpation, auscultation, range of motion, and limb circumferences as appropriate (see Chapters 22 and 30). Normal or negative findings should be documented as well. Both historical and physical findings, or their absence, are critical for later analysis.

Role of Testing

The role of imaging and electrophysiologic and laboratory tests depends on the nature of the complaint and the time from the onset of the problem. In work-related cases in many states, imaging and electrophysiologic tests are used at rates two- to tenfold higher than in similar cases that are not thought to be work related (56). These tests are not generally useful in the soft tissue complaints that dominate workers' compensation claims. They have very low yield as screening tests. They should be reserved for confirmation of clinical findings prior to invasive procedures, or for attempts at clarifying the minority of symptoms that remain after the expected healing period (57,58).

Red Flags

Researchers in evidence-based medicine have identified a group of mechanisms of injury, symptoms, and signs that could indicate potentially serious conditions (59). These should be ruled out or treated. Most physicians are rightly concerned that these problems, such as occult fractures, infections, and cauda equina syndrome, not be missed. In contrast, conditions like cord compression should not be mistakenly diagnosed. After red flags are ruled out, the health professional can apply practice guidelines to effectively and efficiently treat and rehabilitate common health complaints in workers (60).

Diagnosis

If there is a specific injury or disease clearly present, the clinician should arrive at the diagnosis based on unique and specific symptoms and signs, as well as the force and direction of injury, or dose and duration of exposure for occupational diseases. Precision is important for several reasons. First, decisions about causation are predicated on correlation of the diagnostic entity with known associated factors (see below). Second, treatment, activity modification, and disability duration are keyed to diagnosis in available descriptive studies, protocols, pathways, and practice guidelines. Perhaps most important in the longer term, all available literature analyses and practice guidelines have concluded that procedures for entities such as spinal fusions, nerve compression in the back, neck, and extremities, and internal derangements of the knee and shoulder should only be undertaken to correct lesions that are known to benefit from the procedure balancing risks and benefits. The fivefold variance in procedure rates among states and communities observed in workers' compensation suggests that either diagnostic inaccuracy or inappropriate procedure use are at play. The many studies documenting the adverse effects of inappropriate surgery suggest that more precise case selection would reduce this individual and societal burden.

When a clear, specific lesion is not present, more general diagnoses or even use of diagnostic groups of synonymous diagnoses (e.g., "low back pain" for lumbago, nonspecific low back pain, psychogenic back pain, and similar diagnoses) is appropriate to deal with the diagnostic ambiguity. Even larger groupings, for example including low back strain, commonly diagnosed to conform to the injury paradigm required in workers' compensation statutes, in this group, are appropriate because the treatments recommended for all these entities are similar. The expected recovery time is also similar. There may actually be a benefit in using somewhat nonspecific terms in these very common cases, in that the clinician avoids labeling and "medicalizing" entities that are not fully understood and whose natural history is spontaneous recovery in days to weeks in the absence of iatrogenesis or adoption of the sick role. The patient can be reassured that a more serious problem is not present, and to gradually resume activity per an agreed-upon plan (61,62).

Work-relatedness

Properly determining a relationship between work and a health concern requires precise diagnosis and careful consideration of the available high-grade evidence linking the complaint and work site factors. One must consider temporal sequence, dose or force, biologic plausibility, and other factors to make a logical judgment (63–65).

The legal definition of causality in workers' compensation is that it is "more likely than not" due to work, or a 51% probability in the physician's opinion. The best practice is to form that opinion quantitatively, based on available scientific evidence about the causation of the diagnostic entity rather than conjecture.

Several legal concepts are important in this context. "Exacerbation" is used to mean an increase in symptoms from any disorder caused by work. It is sometimes referred to as "a lighting up or flare-up" of a pre-existing disorder. "Aggravation" is used to mean a change in a pre-existing condition which causes a temporary or permanent increase in disability, or creates a need for additional or different medical treatment. This term typically is used to describe increase in disability from a previous work-related complaint.

"Apportionment" is the process of determining if a portion of a worker's *permanent* disability is due to a cause other than the current injury. The other cause can be non-occupational or a different occupational condition or claim (see Chapter 7).

Initial Care

Since the majority of work-related health complaints come to the physician's attention because of complaints of pain, one of the practitioner's concerns should be pain relief. Treating pain appropriately is helpful to the patient, and also allows mobilization and rehabilitation to occur promptly (67).

Activity, both practitioner-aided and self-directed, is very important to the resolution of many soft tissue complaints, within appropriate increasing limits. Inactivity clearly results in worsening symptoms and may lead to chronic pain in many cases (68–70).

Immobilization of the injured or painful area may clearly be needed in problems such as fractures, dislocations, or complete ligament tears, but it should be used judiciously in strains or pain syndromes such as low back pain. The problems with more than a short duration of bed rest have been noted above. There are similar issues with neck immobilization. Newer approaches to orthopedic and physical medicine emphasize resumption of motion as soon as practical to avoid loss of function and painful inflexibility. Hinged braces or periodic range of motion exercises are helpful in this regard.

Both passive and active physical medicine are widely used in musculoskeletal complaints. Passive modalities such as heat, cold, ultrasound, and electrical stimulation are intended for pain relief. In addition, the latter two are believed to reduce inflammation or hasten healing, as are ionto- and phonopheresis. However, there is no high-grade evidence to affirm these beliefs (71). Passive modalities appear to be useful primarily to facilitate active therapy and self-directed exercise programs. Most state practice guidelines now recommend passive modalities alone only briefly, and then only to enable resumption of activity (72).

Chiropractic and osteopathic manipulation appear to offer relief in the first month of low back pain (73,74). Physical therapists use somewhat similar techniques, but these are just beginning to be researched in a structured way, and appear to vary a good deal by practitioner. Evidence of effectiveness of any of these methods in longer-term therapy is lacking.

There is a great deal of physical therapy used in workers' compensation cases. Aside from widespread use of passive modalities, manipulation, and deep tissue massage, therapists develop and guide structured incremental activity programs to improve range of motion, balance, motor strength, and other areas of musculoskeletal function that may be impaired or painful. The objective is restoration of function. A second objective should be independence, so that patients can and will exercise regularly on their own. These programs should have measurable objectives and be agreed upon between the therapist and the treating physician. In the absence of careful management, therapy can continue far past the point where any reasonable gains in function have been made. This is not efficacious, and does not foster functional recovery.

Follow-up

Many commonly used guidelines recommend frequent follow-up visits to ensure that patients understand care instructions, have their questions answered, and in the case of nonspecific musculoskeletal complaints, are assured that recovery can be expected in days to weeks. Occupational health nurses or nurse practitioners can do some follow-up and counseling.

If patients with complaints of musculoskeletal discomfort have not recovered in 4 to 6 weeks, further investigation may be called for to be sure that an unusual problem has not been missed. At that point, carefully reasoned use of imaging or electrophysiologic tests may be indicated to clarify ambiguous findings. Algorithms are available that summarize a clear approach to ambiguous problems. These are the consensus of conservative, thoughtful physicians about the most efficient way to identify treatable problems without engaging in counterproductive or ineffective testing and treatment that would foster a disability mentality.

If the initial history did not yield risk factors for delayed functional recovery (75), such as family or work dysfunction, litigation, economic issues, and so on, these should be sought when the patient's recovery trajectory does not meet the expected milestones (76). At this point also, illness behaviors may have developed, or the patient may perceive interpersonal or economic incentives to maintain the sick role (77,78). If risks or behaviors that would delay recovery are found, then the OHP should develop a plan, perhaps in concert with behavioral specialists, to manage the factors and behaviors toward resumption of a productive role (79).

A referral to a conservative specialist in the body area in question can be quite helpful in ruling out remediable pathology. In a few cases of complex pain disorders, referral to a multidisciplinary team for evaluation may be useful to establish a psychosocial as well as medical treatment plan.

Surgery may be indicated after failure of a trial of conservative therapy for surgically amenable problems such as meniscus, ligament, or rotator cuff tears. One must be sure that there is an entity that has a positive benefit to the risks involved. Low back surgery for anything other than nerve root compression that fails conservative therapy, for example, has a high failure rate and often-questionable anatomic logic, accounting for the many cases of failed back surgery.

Disability Management

Disability should be managed proactively to ensure functional recovery (80,81). Progressive activity modification is the foundation of functional recovery from many common musculoskeletal problems. The word *functional* warrants some explanation. The strong consensus among occupational health, physical medicine, internal and family medicine, orthopedic, and neurology practitioners is that the objective of care for musculoskeletal disorders and other health problems that present primarily with complaints of pain is to resume function, rather than to ensure complete absence of pain. Such complaints can involve somatization, family or work conflict, depression, and other issues as well as organic dysfunction. Restoring function removes the focus from somatic sensations and places it on resuming a meaningful role at home and at work.

The practitioners' role in functional recovery is a pivotal one. In workers' compensation, they are asked to opine about or determine the residual abilities of an injured worker as he or she recovers. These abilities are usually framed in terms of functions such as lifting, repetitive hand motion, overhead work, standing, sitting, kneeling, and so on. The practitioner is usually asked how long the worker can perform the functions, and how much weight can be lifted. Most often the answers are an informed guess. Formal functional capacity evaluation makes sense intuitively, but has not been proven effective, and is often costly. While the worker is recovering, statements about functional ability can be estimates or based on consensus with the worker. More accurate permanent restrictions may require a formal, task-based functional capacity evaluation.

Insurers usually do not ask these structured questions for several months after the patient's initial presentation. Proactive physicians, however, will submit a list of work abilities, or their inverse, restrictions, with the report of each patient visit. These reports typically are sent to the payer with a bill for services. To ensure appropriate placement in a safe modified position, therefore, the treating physician should also send a copy to the employer.

As a best practice, the practitioner should lay out a plan for increasing activity in whatever areas are temporarily impaired. Alternatively, activity can be increased based on the clinical condition at each visit. At the same time that work activities are defined, practitioners can prescribe or agree on an activity program that will strengthen injured areas, restore flexibility, increase aerobic capacity, and reduce pain. This program can start with the physical therapist's use of modalities, if needed, progress to monitored activity, and finally to a self-directed program. Activities should be described in specific terms of repetitions, load, distance, or duration. Aerobic activity is an important part of any functional recovery program, with flexibility, dexterity, and strength components added as indicated.

Guidelines for functional recovery based on BLS levels of job effort (ranging from sedentary to very heavy, based on lifting amounts) are available as a source of comparison and benchmarks to alert one to delayed recovery. These are either descriptive of current return to work patterns (82–84) or on a consensus of experienced practitioners (85), or a combination of the two.

Recent research has documented the assumption that the content and quality of the doctor–patient interaction as well as employer behaviors and offers of modified duty have a significant effect on the rate and timing of return to work after an occupational illness or injury. Discussing treatment options and pain management, as well as activities the worker can do safely, was significantly correlated with more rapid return to work and lower claims costs in a recent large multistate survey of injured workers. Agreeing on a return to work date had a similar effect, as did offers of modified work and employer attempts to understand the worker's capabilities upon return (86).

Coordination and Communication

Occupational health programs have marketed case coordination successfully to employers who wish to ensure rapid case resolution. It makes sense as an analogy to management of cases in family practice, although there are more parties involved in occupational health cases, and some medical information should not be disclosed to the employer. The added time and expense involved, lack of interest, or lack of skill may militate against practitioners' or their organizations' performing this role. But it is an essential role to assure rapid functional recovery and reintegration into the workforce.

As noted above, the best practice in the insurance industry is for the claim adjuster or case manager to maintain immediate and frequent information exchange among the worker, the health care provider, and the employer. However, this best practice is not common practice. If no one assumes the role, delayed recovery or inappropriate treatment often results.

Closing the Case

When the injured worker has recovered to the extent possible, the attending physician is typically asked to certify that maximal medical improvement (MMI) has been reached. This is usually the point at which further medical care would not have further substantial benefit. It does not mean that the worker might not require palliative care or care for an exacerbation of a problem in the future. The physician may also be asked to forecast the future medical needs of the patient. This opinion should be as quantitative as possible.

At MMI, the attending physician may also be asked to rate any residual impairment (87). California asks the attending physician to describe the patient's impairment; the rater at the state disability evaluation unit then assigns a rating based on the language that the physician used. Words such as "mild" and "occasionally" are on the scales that are used in these rating assignments. In other states, such as Washington, the treating physician may be asked to assign actual values. This is a somewhat specialized skill that many physicians are not comfortable with. There is also the potential that the patient will not agree with the rating, although the practitioner might show the patient the rating formulas to demonstrate that there is an objective basis for the value assigned.

In most states, impairment is based on loss of motion, amputation, loss of strength, or other objective findings. Rating systems in use include several state-specific systems and the various editions of the American Medical Association's (AMA) *Guides to the Evaluation of Permanent Impairment* (88). California allows impairment for subjective findings such as pain and paresthesias. One area that is frequently misused is assigning impairment for imaging findings or past surgery, even if there are no clinical correlates. This is allowed in the AMA system, although it is controversial, but not in a number of state systems.

Independent Medical Examinations

Occupational health providers may be asked to perform independent medical examinations or evaluations (IMEs), which are performed by a disinterested party with no medical or treatment affiliation between the provider and the injured party in the case. IMEs may be requested at any point in the case, most often when a claims adjuster believes that the claimant is at MMI. In general, the number and frequency of the evaluations and who can perform them is not regulated. Oregon limits IMEs to three per case, and Texas allows only one every 6 months. California, Washington, Colorado, and Texas require certification as an independent examiner. Colorado requires training, and Texas will as of 2003. California and Washington require chiropractors to be trained (89).

There are recommended formats for these evaluations (90,91). The specific information to be acquired and analyzed depends on the questions posed by the requester of the evaluation.

The best IMEs are those that answer the questions posed in an objective manner based on a careful and explicit analysis of prior testing and treatment if required, and on a focused yet complete history (complaint, work, social, and personal) and careful physical examination (92,93). The descriptions of recommended histories and physical examinations above apply to IMEs as well as direct care. The logic and evidence leading to all conclusions would be explained understandably to the lay reader (94,95).

IMEs may be used to analyze causality, determine whether the claimant has achieved MMI, analyze and opine about the appropriateness of prior or proposed treatment, determine whether further tests or treatment are needed, or calculate an impairment rating, among other reasons. Most IMEs are obtained to analyze causation or to quantify impairment.

SUMMARY

The workers' compensation system was intended to provide medical care and disability benefits promptly, regardless of fault. While it does provide care and benefits to many workers with health concerns, conflict, political self-interest, and poor quality medical care and disability management have plagued the system. Occupational health professionals can provide excellent clinical care, dispassionate and informed analysis of causation of work-related complaints, and leadership in the strategic management of workers' compensation by employers and payers. If the OHP performs these services effectively, there can be great benefit to workers, their families, and society as a whole.

REFERENCES

1. Ashford NA, Andrews RA. Workers' compensation. In: Rom W, ed. *Environmental and occupational medicine,* 2nd ed. Boston: Little, Brown, 1996.
2. Elisburg D. Workers' compensation. In: Demeter SL, Andersson GBJ, Smith GM, eds. *Disability evaluation.* St. Louis: Mosby and the American Medical Association, 1996:36–44.
3. McLellan JD Jr. Overview of various disability systems in the United States. In: Demeter SL, Andersson GBJ, Smith GM, eds. *Disability evaluation.* St. Louis: Mosby and the American Medical Association, 1996:20–30.
4. U.S. Chamber of Commerce, Statistics and Research Center. *2001 Analysis of workers' compensation laws.* Washington, DC: U.S. Chamber of Commerce, 2001.
5. Mont D, Burton JF Jr, Reno V, et al. *Workers' compensation: benefits, coverage, and costs.* 2000 new estimates. Washington, DC: National Academy of Social Insurance, 2002.
6. Cocchiarella L, Andersson GBJ, eds. *Guides to the evaluation of permanent impairment,* 5th ed. Chicago: American Medical Association, 2001.
7. U.S. Chamber of Commerce, Statistics and Research Center. *2001 analysis of workers' compensation laws.* Washington, DC: U.S. Chamber of Commerce, 2001.
8. U.S. Chamber of Commerce, Statistics and Research Center. *2001 analysis of workers' compensation laws.* Washington, DC: U.S. Chamber of Commerce, 2001.
9. Ashford NA. *Crisis in the work place: occupational disease and injury.* Cambridge, MA: MIT Press, 1976.
10. Ashford NA. *Crisis in the work place: occupational disease and injury.* Cambridge, MA: MIT Press, 1976.
11. Mont D, Burton JF Jr, Reno V, et al. *Workers' compensation: benefits, coverage, and costs.* 2000 new estimates. Washington, DC: National Academy of Social Insurance, 2002.
12. Brady W, Bass J, Moser R Jr, et al. Defining total corporate health and safety costs—significance and impact. *J Occup Environ Med* 1997;39:224–231.
13. Ducatman AM. Workers' compensation cost shifting: unique concern of providers and purchasers of pre-paid health care. *J Occup Med* 1988;28:1174.
14. Butler RJ. Wage and injury rate response to shifting levels of workers' compensation. In: Worrall GD, ed. *Safety in the work place: incentives and disincentives in workers' compensation.* Ithaca, NY: ILR Press, 1983:61–86.
15. Wiesel SW, Feffer HL, Rothman RH. Industrial low back pain: a prospective evaluation of a standardized diagnostic and treatment protocol. *Spine* 1984;9:199–203.
16. Harris JS, Bengle AL III, Makens PK. *Striking the balance: an analysis of the cost and quality of medical care in the Texas workers' compensation system.* Austin: Research and Oversight Council on Workers' Compensation and Med-Fx, LLC, 2001.
17. Ducatman AM. Workers' compensation cost shifting: unique concern of providers and purchasers of pre-paid health care. *J Occup Med* 1988;28:1174.
18. National Council on Compensation Insurance. Annual Statistical Bulletin, 2000 ed. Boca Raton, FL: NCCI, 2002.
19. Vallfors B. Acute, sub-acute, and chronic low back pain: clinical symptoms and absenteeism in the work environment. *Scand J Rehab Med* 1985;[suppl II]:11:1–98.
20. Bigos SJ, et al. Back injuries in industry: a retrospective study. III. Employee-related factors. *Spine* 1986; 11:252.
21. Bigos SJ, et al. The prospective study of work perceptions and psycho-social factors affecting the report of back injury. *Spine* 1991;16:1–6.
22. Berkowitz M. Rehabilitation and workers' compensation: incompatible or inseparable? In: Borba P, Appel D. *Benefits, costs, cycles in workers' compensation.* Boston: Kluwer Academic Publishers, 1990.
23. Haddad GH. Analysis of 2,932 workers' compensation back injury cases: the impact on cost of the system. *Spine* 1987;12:765–769.
24. Worrall GD, et al. Age and incentive response: low back pain workers' compensation claims. Presented at the Fourth Annual NCCI Seminar on Economic Issues in Workers' Compensation, 1985.
25. Haddad GH. Analysis of 2,932 workers' compensation back injury cases: the impact on cost of the system. *Spine* 1987;12:765.
26. Fager CA, Friedbert SR. Analysis of failure and poor results of lumbar spine surgery. *Spine* 1980;5:87–94.
27. Long DM, et al. Clinical features of the failed back syndrome. *J Neurosurg* 1988;69:61–71.
28. Derebery VJ, Tuttle RH. Delayed recovery in the patient with a work compensable injury. *J Occup Med* 1981;24: 829–35.
29. Bureau of Labor Statistics. U.S. Department of Labor News, Release USDL 00-236. Washington, DC: U.S. DOL, 2000.
30. Bureau of Labor Statistics. U.S. Department of Labor News, Release USDL 00-357. Washington, DC: U.S. DOL, 2000.
31. Harris JS, Bengle AL III, Makens PK. *Striking the balance: an analysis of the cost and quality of medical care in the Texas workers' compensation system.* Austin: Research and Oversight Council on Workers' Compensation and Med-Fx, LLC, 2001.
32. Pransky G, Synder T, Dembe A, et al. Under-reporting of work-related disorders in the workplace: a case study and review of the literature. *Ergonomic* 1999;42:171–182.
33. Morse T, Dillon C, Warren N, et al. Capture-recapture estimation of unreported work-related musculoskeletal disorders in Connecticut. *Am J Ind Med* 2001;39: 636–642.
34. Dembe A. Access to medical care for occupational disorders: difficulties and disparities. *J Health Soc Policy* 2001;12:19–33.
35. Glazner JE, Borgerding J, Lowery JT, et al. Construction injury rates may exceed national estimates: evidence from the construction of Denver International Airport. *Am J Ind Med* 1998;34:105–112.
36. Rosenman KD, Gardiner JC, Wang J, et al. Why most workers with occupational repetitive trauma do not file for workers' compensation. *J Occup Environ Med* 2000; 42:25–34.
37. Borenstein DG, Wiesel SW. *Low back pain: medical diagnosis and comprehensive management,* 2nd ed. Philadelphia: WB Saunders, 1997.
38. Brigham CR, Harris JS. Low back pain part II: administrative disability and workers' compensation issues. *Occup Environ Med Rep* 1990;4:92.
39. Deyo RA, Diehl AK, Rosenthal M. How many days of bed rest for acute low back pain? A randomized clinical trial. *N Engl J Med* 1986;315:1064.
40. Bruckman RZ, Rasmusson HL. *Workers' compensation*

healthcare management guidelines. Seattle: Milliman & Robertson, 1998.

41. Harris JS, Bengle AL III, Makens PK, et al. *Returning to work: an examination of existing disability duration guidelines and their application to the Texas workers' compensation system*. Austin: Texas Research and Oversight Council on Workers' compensation, 2001.
42. Reed PR. *The medical disability advisor,* 3rd ed. New York: LRP Publishers, 1997.
43. Harris JS, Hall JC, Ossler C. Case management: prevention and management of delayed functional recovery. In: Harris JS, et al., eds. *Evaluation and management of common health problems and functional recovery in workers: the ACOEM Occupational Medicine Practice Guidelines*. Beverly Farms, MA: OEM Health Information, 1997:6-1–6-12.
44. Nylander SW, Carmean G. *Medical standards project final report,* 3rd ed. San Bernardino, CA: San Bernardino County, 1984.
45. Himmelstein JS, Andersson GBJ. Low back pain: risk evaluation and pre-placement screening. In: Himmelstein JS, Pransky GS, eds. Worker fitness and risk evaluations. *Occup Med* 1988;3:255–269.
46. Brigham CR, Harris JS. Low back pain part II: administrative disability and workers' compensation issues. *Occup Environ Med Rep* 1990;4:92–96.
47. Bigos SJ, et al. Back injuries in industry: a retrospective study. III. Employee-related factors. *Spine* 1986;11: 252–256.
48. Bigos SJ, et al. The prospective study of work perceptions and psychosocial factors affecting the report of back injury. *Spine* 1991;16:1–6.
49. Moon SD, Sauter SL. *Beyond biomechanics: psychosocial aspects of musculoskeletal disorders in office work.* Bristol, PA: Taylor & Francis, 1996.
50. Sullivan T, ed. *Injury and the new world of work.* Vancouver: UBC Press, 2000.
51. Harris JS. Prevention. Pre-placement and periodic examinations; secondary prevention; tertiary prevention, surveillance. In: Harris JS, et al., eds. *Evaluation and management of common health problems and functional recovery in workers: the ACOEM Occupational Medicine Practice Guidelines.* Beverly Farms, MA: OEM Health Information, 1997:1-13–1-17.
52. Harris JS, et al., eds. *Evaluation and management of common health problems and functional recovery in workers: the American College of Occupational Medicine Practice Guidelines.* Beverly Farms, MA: OEM Health Information, 1997.
53. Harris JS, et al., eds. *Evaluation and management of common health problems and functional recovery in workers: the American College of Occupational Medicine Practice Guidelines.* Beverly Farms, MA: OEM Health Information, 1997.
54. Harris JS. General approach to initial assessment: medical history. In: Harris JS, et al., eds. *Evaluation and management of common health problems and functional recovery in workers: the ACOEM Occupational Medicine Practice Guidelines.* Beverly Farms, MA: OEM Health Information, 1997:2-1–2-4.
55. Harris JS. Neck and upper back complaints: forearm, hand, and wrist complaints. In: Harris JS, et al., eds. *Evaluation and management of common health problems and functional recovery in workers: the ACOEM Occupational Medicine Practice Guidelines.* Beverly Farms, MA: OEM Health Information, 1997:10-1–10-28, 13-1–13-27.
56. Harris JS, Bengle AL III, Makens PK. *Striking the balance: an analysis of the cost and quality of medical care in the Texas workers' compensation system.* Austin: Research and Oversight Council on Workers' Compensation and Med-Fx, LLC, 2001.
57. Harris JS, et al., eds. *Evaluation and management of common health problems and functional recovery in workers: the American College of Occupational Medicine Practice Guidelines.* Beverly Farms, MA: OEM Health Information, 1997.
58. Bruckman RZ, Harris JS. Occupational medicine practice guidelines. In: Harris JS, ed. Managed care in occupational medicine. *Occup Med State of the Art Rev* 1998;13(4):679–691.
59. Bigos SJ, Bowyer O, Braen G, et.al. *Acute low back problems in adults, Clinical practice guideline No. 14.* Rockville, MD: U.S. Department of Health and Human Services, Public Health Service, Agency for Health Care Policy and Research. AHCPR Pub. No. 95-0642, 1994.
60. Bruckman RZ, Harris JS. Occupational medicine practice guidelines. In: Harris JS, ed. Managed care in occupational medicine. *Occup Med State of the Art Rev* 1998;13(4):679–691.
61. Harris JS. Low back complaints. In: Harris JS, et al., eds. *Evaluation and management of common health problems and functional recovery in workers: the ACOEM Occupational Medicine Practice Guidelines.* Beverly Farms, MA: OEM Health Information, 1997:14-1–14-30.
62. Bigos SJ, Bowyer O, Braen G, et al. *Acute low back problems in adults, Clinical practice guideline No. 14.* Rockville, MD: U.S. Department of Health and Human Services, Public Health Service, Agency for Health Care Policy and Research. AHCPR Pub. No. 95-0642, 1994.
63. Guidotti TL. Applying epidemiology to adjudication. *Occup Med* 1998;13:303–314.
64. Harber P, Harris JS. Work-relatedness. In: Harris JS, et al., eds. *Evaluation and management of common health problems and functional recovery in workers: the ACOEM Occupational Medicine Practice Guidelines.* Beverly Farms, MA: OEM Health Information, 1997:4-1–4-9.
65. Bunn WB, Johnson CL. Causation in workers' compensation. *Occup Med* 1996;11:113–120.
66. Harris JS. Prevention. In: Harris JS, et al., eds. *Evaluation and management of common health problems and functional recovery in workers: the ACOEM Occupational Medicine Practice Guidelines.* Beverly Farms, MA: OEM Health Information, 1997:1-1–1-11.
67. Harris JS. Initial approached to treatment. In: Harris JS, et al., eds. *Evaluation and management of common health problems and functional recovery in workers: the ACOEM Occupational Medicine Practice Guidelines.* Beverly Farms, MA: OEM Health Information, 1997:3-1–3-9.
68. Deyo RA, Diehl AK, Rosenthal M. How many days of bed rest for acute low back pain? a randomized clinical trial. *N Engl J Med* 1986;315:1064.
69. Mayer TG, Gatchel RJ, Polatin PB. *Occupational musculoskeletal disorders: function, outcome, and evidence.* Philadelphia: Lippincott Williams & Wilkins, 2000.
70. Nordin M, Andersson GBH, Pope M. *Musculoskeletal*

disorders in the workplace: principles and practice. St. Louis: Mosby, 1997.

71. Harris JS, et al., eds. *Evaluation and management of common health problems and functional recovery in workers: the American College of Occupational Medicine Practice Guidelines.* Beverly Farms, MA: OEM Health Information, 1997.
72. Harris JS, Bengle AL III, Makens PK. *Striking the balance: an analysis of the cost and quality of medical care in the Texas workers' compensation system.* Austin: Research and Oversight Council on Workers' Compensation and Med-Fx, LLC, 2001.
73. Shekelle PG, Adams AH, Chassin MR, et al. *The appropriateness of spinal manipulation for low back pain.* Santa Monica, CA: Rand Corporation, 1991.
74. Andersson GB, Lucente T, Davis AM, et al. A comparison of osteopathic spinal manipulation with standard care for patients with low back pain. *N Engl J Med* 1999;341(19):1426–1431.
75. Harris JS, Ossler C, Hall JC. Case canagement: prevention and management of delayed functional recovery. In: Harris JS, et al., eds. *Evaluation and management of common health problems and functional recovery in workers: the ACOEM Occupational Medicine Practice Guidelines.* Beverly Farms, MA: OEM Health Information, 1997:6-1–6-12.
76. Harris JS, Wolens D. Pain behavior, inconsistent findings, and motivation for self-care and recovery. In: Harris JS, et al., eds. *Evaluation and management of common health problems and functional recovery in workers: the ACOEM Occupational Medicine Practice Guidelines.* Beverly Farms, MA: OEM Health Information, 1997:7-1–7-13.
77. Proctor T, Gatchel RJ, Robinson RC. Psychosocial factors and risk of pain and disability. *Occup Med* 2000;15:803–812.
78. Ensalada LH. The importance of illness behavior in disability management. *Occup Med* 2000;15:739–754.
79. Aranoff GM, Feldman JB, Campion TS. Management of chronic pain and control of long-term disability. *Occup Med* 2000;15:755–770.
80. Canadian Medical Association. *The physician's role in helping patients return to work after an illness or injury (www.cma.cainsidepolicybase19973-1.htm).* Ottawa: Canadian Medical Association, 1997.
81. Harris JS, Ossler C, Hall JC. Cornerstones of disability management. In: Harris JS, et al., eds. *Evaluation and management of common health problems and functional recovery in workers: the ACOEM Occupational Medicine Practice Guidelines.* Beverly Farms, MA: OEM Health Information, 1997:5-1–5-5.
82. Bruckman RZ, Rasmusson HL. *Workers' compensation healthcare management guidelines.* Seattle: Milliman & Robertson, 1998.
83. Reed PR. *The medical disability advisor,* 3rd ed. New York: Lippincott-Raven, 1997.
84. Work Loss Data Institute. *Official disability guidelines.* Corpus Christi: Work Loss Data Institute, 2000.
85. Harris JS, et al., eds. *Evaluation and management of common health problems and functional recovery in workers: the ACOEM Occupational Medicine Practice Guidelines.* Beverly Farms, MA: OEM Health Information, 1997.
86. Harris JS, Bengle AL III, Makens PK, et al. *Returning to work: an examination of existing disability duration guidelines and their application to the Texas workers' compensation system.* Austin: Texas Research and Oversight Council on Workers' compensation, 2001.
87. Cox RAF, Edwards FC, McCallum RI. *Fitness for work: the medical aspects.* Oxford: Oxford University Press, 1995.
88. Cocchiarella L, Andersson GBJ, eds. *Guides to the evaluation of permanent impairment,* 5th ed. Chicago: American Medical Association, 2001.
89. Harris JS, Christian JH, Brigham CR, et al. *Improving independent medical examinations.* Olympia, WA: Washington Dept. of Labor and Industries, 2002.
90. Brigham CR, Babitsky S, Mangraviti JJ. *The independent medical examination report: a step-by-step guide with models.* Falmouth, MA: SEAK, 1996.
91. Kraus J. The independent medical examination and the functional capacity evaluation. *Occup Med* 1997;12: 525–556.
92. Harris JS, Brigham CR. Independent medical examinations. In: Harris JS, et al., eds. *Management of common health problems and functional recovery in workers: the ACOEM Occupational Medicine Practice Guidelines.* Beverly Farms, MA: OEM Health Information, 1997.
93. Talmadge JB. Assessment and management of upper and lower extremity impairment and disability. *Occup Med* 2000;15:771–788.
94. Demeter SL. Disability evaluation. *Occup Med* 1998; 13:315–324.
95. Guidotti TL. Evidence-based medical dispute resolution in workers' compensation. *Occup Med* 1998;13:289–302.

19

Health Care Management

Melissa D. Tonn

Employers and the federal government are the two largest purchasers of health insurance in the United States. Occupational medicine is the field in medicine that focuses on the health issues impacting employers, employees, and the workplace. It would then seem natural for occupational physicians to be integrally involved with both employers and health insurance carriers in addressing corporate health care expenditures and the substantial threat to U.S. business competitiveness resulting from the staggering increases in the cost of providing health benefits to employees. However, this has not historically been the case. Corporate medical directors and consulting occupational physicians have not consistently positioned themselves as the resident health benefit experts, or even part of the team that determines how and where employer health care dollars are expended or in choosing among the available health plans or disease management options. As employers scramble to keep health care costs from putting them into financial intensive care, occupational physicians have an opportunity to break out of the customary boundaries and to play an integral role as experts in health care for business and industry.

This chapter defines the specific issues for employers in addressing the rising cost of health care and areas where the occupational physician could have an impact. Issue number one is the recent focus shift from a pure cost containment model to more innovative purchasing methodologies based on informed consumer choice, disease management, outcomes and quality, and cost-sharing arrangements between employers and employees. This shift provides an opportunity for the expansion of the roles of both the corporate medical director and the occupational physician consultant. Such potential can best be realized through the acquisition of knowledge regarding employer-based health benefit programs and the recent developments in program design and health insurance coverage and by thinking strategically about the most appropriate opportunities for health care cost reduction initiatives for a specific employer or for a specific industry. This is not a new strategic approach; occupational physicians have been tangentially involved in the move to integrate health benefits with disability management and workers' compensation. Benefit integration, though, has not been met with overwhelming interest or success. To date, neither the projected cost reductions nor the medical management goals have been fully realized by those employers who have made the shift to an integrated model.

While benefit integration may not have proven as effective in managing cost as projected, many employers are finding that investing in employee health and safety can improve productivity and reduce absenteeism, and that by focusing on quality of care and outcomes they can reduce their total health care expenditures.

EMPLOYER-BASED HEALTH BENEFIT PROGRAMS

Most people with health insurance in the U.S. have received it through their employer. In 1990, 73% of all U.S. citizens with health insurance had coverage through their jobs (1). In 1999, 77% of those with jobs had some health care coverage through their employer, leaving 23% uninsured. The prediction is that by 2009 the number of uninsured working Americans could reach 30% of the labor force. The Health Care Financing Administration (HCFA) has estimated that business spent approximately $250 billion on health care in 1992 (2), and according to recent government projections, health care spending in the U.S. is expected to double over the next decade to $2.6 trillion, with U.S. businesses bearing a significant portion of the tab (Fig. 19.1) (3).

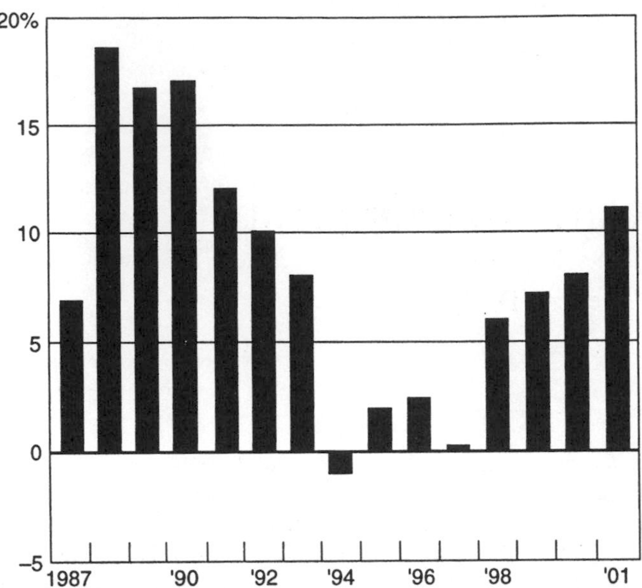

FIG. 19.1. Annual change in average total health benefit costs. Note: Results for 1987–1998 are based on costs for active and retired employees combined. The change in costs from 1998–2001 is based on costs for active employees only. Source: William M. Mercer.

Health insurance in the U.S. has been linked to employment since the 1940s (4). It is sometimes overlooked that medical insurance of any sort in the U.S. is a phenomenon of only the past 60 years. The founding of Blue Cross in 1929 and Blue Shield in 1939 was in part brought about by the Great Depression, as concerns over insolvency led hospitals and doctors to form third-party organizations to finance their operations. The linking of medical insurance to employment was a product of the statutory wage freezes of the World War II era, as both management and labor turned to health benefits as a popular alternative to increase compensation to employees. Health benefits have been tax exempt since their inception, creating a financial incentive for companies to keep offering them.

Providing medical benefits did not become a problem for American business until the 1970s. In 1976, health costs per employee rose 17%, and by the early 1980s, increases in per capita benefits were in the 20% to 24% per year range. The problem began to reach more serious proportions as medical inflation began to outstrip the general inflation rate. The picture just keeps getting uglier—for employers and consumers alike. In 2002, employers expect their health care costs to rise nearly 13%, with some companies expecting increases of 20% or more, according to a survey conducted by the human resources consulting firm William M. Mercer, Inc.

The Mercer survey—of more than 2,800 employers—estimated that the average cost per employee for health care benefits rose 11.2% to $4,924 in 2001. This is the largest increase in 9 years, and reflects a growth rate several times faster than inflation (3). Annual costs for family coverage could reach $10,000 by 2004, up from $7,000 in 2001, according to data compiled by the Washington Business Group on Health. By some estimates, the cost per employee will exceed the average wage by 2030. These double-digit health care cost increases come as a weakened economy is eroding corporate profits, putting businesses in a financial squeeze.

The current thinking among insurance brokers and consultants is that corporate health costs will continue to grow until employers focus their attention on creating value, increasing the cost-sharing with the consumers of the health benefits—the employee and their dependents—and by moving toward a defined contribution approach. In response to rising costs, according to the Mercer survey, 40% of large employers will require employees to pay a higher percentage of total costs in 2002 by raising deductibles and copayments.

That is a particularly troubling trend for a company like General Motors, which spent $4 billion on health care in 2000. Because of agreements with its unions, GM cannot easily make health benefit plan changes. Instead, the company is focusing on ways to better educate employees about costs (3).

Rising Health Care Costs and the Federal Government

The problems associated with rising health costs are not unique to business or private industry. Costs have been increasing throughout the health care system at comparable rates, creating major challenges for the federal government. The government entered the health market with the establishment of Medicare and Medicaid in 1965. The Centers for Medicare and Medicaid Services (CMS), formerly the HCFA, is the federal agency that is the single largest purchaser of health care in the world, with an estimated $476 billion paid for health care services in 2001 on behalf of 70 million disabled, elderly, and poor beneficiaries (5).

In 1965, Congress created Medicare and Medicaid for elderly and poor persons, respectively. Congress vested responsibility for managing Medicare in the Social Security Administration. Medicaid is also subject to federal oversight, but state governments actually operate the programs. In 1977, HCFA was created to manage Medicare and Medicaid.

Since 1996, the agency has been responsible for implementing some 700 provisions of five major laws: the Reconciliation Act of 1996, the Health Insurance Portability and Accountability Act of 1996, the Balanced Budget Act of 1997, the Balanced Budget Refinement Act of 1999, and the Benefits Improvement and Protection Act of 2000 (5). Some of the most expansive provisions contained in these laws called for the agency to regulate private health insurance and to establish electronic-data standards for the entire health care industry. Perhaps the most controversial of all these measures was the Balanced Budget Act of 1997, which reduced Medicare payments to virtually every clinical laboratory, hospital, skilled nursing facility, and home health agency in the U.S., with an estimated total reduction of $112 billion for the period from 1998 through 2002 (6).

Cost Shifting

As the federal government moves to control its health expenditures, the providers of care have historically shifted the burden of payment to the private employers. A consulting firm, Hewitt Associates, estimated that almost 30% of the increases in employer-based premiums of the past decade have been due to this cost shifting (3). Figure 19.2 compares the relative growth of total health expenditures for the U.S. with those for business, clearly showing that employers have experienced a proportionally increased burden.

Small businesses have faced a second cost shift, as large employers often have been able to leverage their size to get discounts from providers and insurers. With the total size of the health care budget growing,

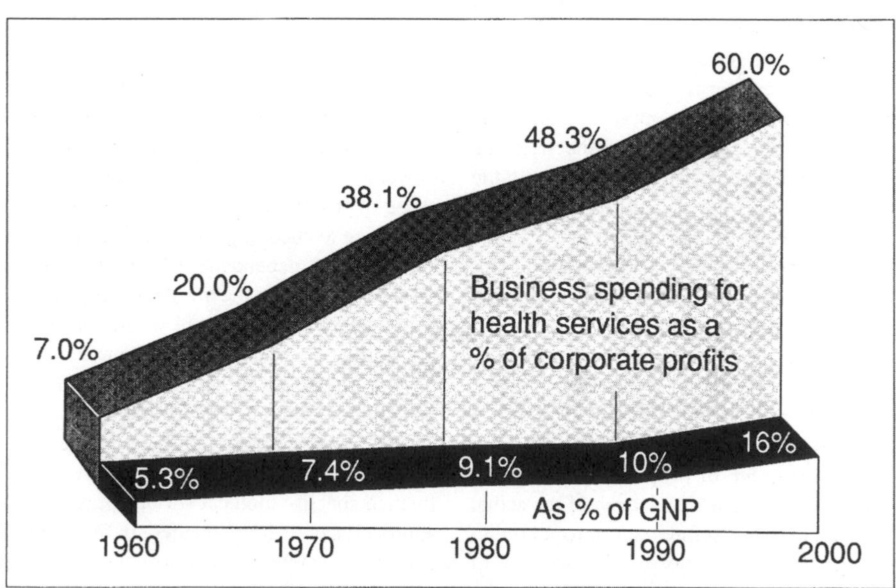

FIG. 19.2. Impact of cost shifting on business health care costs. Source: Agency for Health Care Administration.

the burden has fallen increasingly on small and midsized businesses. When annual health costs increases for business as a whole are stratified by business size, smaller companies may face increases two to three times those of the larger firms.

The Evolution from Managed Care

Since the 1980s, employers have been a prime force in reshaping the delivery of health care in the U.S., and their involvement resulted in what we refer to today as managed care. But, in 2002, it is now official that the massive migration to managed care did not deliver on the promise of long-term price control nor did it result in overwhelming patient satisfaction or improved outcomes (7).

In a pure sense of the term, *managed care* can be defined as a system of medical care designed to control some aspects of that care. It implies some measure of standardization or agreed-upon performance. It also includes a contractual relationship between health care providers and buyers that does not exist in indemnity plans. Contracts allow buyers to specify performance requirements of the supplier (8).

As the term evolved, managed care has been applied to discount pricing as in preferred provider organizations (PPOs), prepayment for care, and to utilization management.

The management arrangement typically is a contract between the providers of health care and a health care financing entity such as a large self-funded employer, an insurance company, a government program, or an independent entity. There is also a separate contract between each employee and the financing organization. Each contract specifies the rights and responsibilities of the parties, but, with the exception of the contract for prepaid care, does not fix the total price of the service. Price and volume management features can occur separately or together, and they can apply to physicians, hospitals, pharmaceuticals, and/or other providers.

The basis for the development of health maintenance organizations (HMOs) was "capitation," which refers only to a payment mechanism—paying a provider a specific sum of money for the ongoing care of a person or group of people for a particular period of time. The sum is set in advance of the actual period of service, and it therefore represents a prediction, or an agreed-on estimate, of the amount of money that will be required to provide that care.

Technically, a contract based on capitation can include or exclude almost any medical service. One can provide payment on a capitated basis, for example, for only primary care visits, for primary care visits and associated laboratory tests, or for only referrals to specialists. Mental health care can be covered or excluded. So can specialty services or surgery, whether or not primary care is included.

Most commonly, however, the person or organization that promises to arrange care under a system of capitation tries not just to buy care, but also to manage it. For a staff-model HMO where the physicians are generally employed by the entity, this is the core business: to accept the risk entailed by prepayment and to configure care so the costs fall within that prepaid amount. In looser aggregations, like physician networks or independent practice associations (IPAs), contracts based on capitation may involve only a small fraction of a specific physician's patients, and managed care may primarily take the form of rules about referrals, requirements for precertification, and selective contracting for ancillary services such as imaging or physical therapy or with hospitals and specialists.

A capitated contract creates some degree of risk. The payment amount is set in advance of the service, and on a population basis it may turn out afterward to have been the wrong amount. Someone has to make up the difference if the capitated fee is too low, and someone stands to gain if it is too high. But nothing about the idea of capitation, as such, specifies who assumes that risk (9).

Insurance Plan Design

A number of insurance plan design changes have been used to alter economic incentives to use medical services. The most common are employee cost-sharing devices meant to spread the cost between the employer and the employee. Some are applied to the purchase of insurance and some are applied at the point of service to encourage responsible purchasing by the employee or dependent. More recently, employers have been debating the merits of defined-contribution plans where the employees would be responsible for managing their own health care purchasing decisions.

The primary design feature intended to impact the demand for insurance or the amount of insurance purchased by the employee is the employee contribution rate. Deductibles and copayments are intended to influence specific medical service purchases. A hybrid approach can be implemented, in the form of flexible benefits or cafeteria plans, which give the employee a budget to purchase various types of insurance and other benefits.

Contribution rates are paid, usually on a monthly basis, by the employee. There are typically two contributions—one rate for the employee and one for dependents. The contribution rate affects only the demand for health insurance. It does not affect the utilization of health care services. Increasing the contribution rate shifts the cost of health insurance from the employer directly to the employees.

Deductibles are a fixed amount that must be paid by the employee before expenses are covered by insurance. Deductibles may be applied to the individual or the family, and may be income linked. Deductibles may provide an incentive for comparison shopping, but once satisfied, the price of the service reduces to a percentage of the cost of the care, usually a percentage in the form of a copayment or 20% of the services provided. Coinsurance is the proportion of the reimbursement that is to be paid by the employee. It can vary by service covered and family income. The effectiveness of coinsurance, or copayments, depends on the employee's responsiveness to price. Most insurance policies have limits called "stop losses," after which copayments no longer apply (8).

Exclusions are generally established in insurance contracts by design. Almost universally, preexisting conditions are not covered for some period. Some plans, especially managed care plans, have a schedule of specific exclusions. Generally these are procedures deemed to be discretionary, experimental, or not medically necessary, such as elective aesthetic procedures, therapeutic abortions, or certain tests and procedures not proven to be effective.

In recent years, more employers are offering their employees defined-contribution plans, in which employees manage their own health care dollars. Under a defined contribution plan, each employee gets a set medical budget, for example, $2,000 per year, which can be spent on virtually any health service. Once that initial money is used up, employees pay for medical costs up to a certain amount out of their own pocket, like a deductible. Beyond that level, the employer begins paying again. If the money is not used, it can be rolled into the following year.

These accounts offer incentives for members to choose generic drugs over brand-name drugs and encourage them to shop around for doctors and medical services.

MANAGING THE DELIVERY OF HEALTH CARE

Utilization Review

Employers began using utilization review as a way of counteracting the incentives toward doing more in the health care system. Utilization review refers to the process in which services are reviewed by third parties to determine if they are medically appropriate and necessary. Payment for services is tied to this review, and only those services deemed necessary by the reviewer are authorized for payment. The most popular forms of utilization review are preadmission or preprocedure certification and concurrent review of inpatient and programmatic services.

Employers have used other forms of utilization review to monitor the delivery of their benefits. Case management is a form of review that attempts to manage the high cost cases early in their course. It is predicated on the fact that 10% of cases in a population can generate greater than 50% of the total costs. Mandatory second surgical opinion programs became popular in the 1980s, based on certain studies that indicated that unnecessary surgeries were a cause of rising health care costs (10).

The newest form of utilization review involves an intensified look at a specific area of high cost benefits, which are "carved out" from the health benefits package as a whole. This has been most commonly done with mental health and pharmacy services.

Quality and Employee Satisfaction

The quality of medical care provided by managed care plans is an increasingly complicated and controversial topic. Traditionally, the quality of care has been measured by professional judgment, often rendered subjectively in individual cases. More recently, as health care delivery and financing are being reordered by the rapid growth of managed care, physicians and the health plans with which they contract are being called to greater account for the quality of service they provide. The scrutiny is coming largely from corporations and the federal government, which are concerned that as health plans compete, they may skimp on services to reduce prices (11). In addition, the managers of many health plans believe that a stamp of approval of the quality of their care from a recognized, independent review agency will help increase their share of the insurance market.

The interests of employers and the plans themselves have catapulted the National Committee for Quality Assurance (NCQA)—a private, not-for-profit organization into the role of the leading accreditor of managed care plans. In a survey of Fortune 500 firms, more than half of the firms surveyed require their plans to have NCQA accreditation, and considerably more use quality criteria in carrier selection. Customer service is the most widely used "quality" requirement in Fortune 500 contracts and more than 60% included requirements for provider access (3).

An employer's willingness to pay more for quality largely depends on how they understand the connection between overall health and productivity. Preserving productivity and controlling medical costs are both good reasons to implement work-site programs and design health benefits that encourage control and prevention of certain diseases.

As one example, diabetes and its complications cost about $32 billion worth of productivity each year. Some 28% of people with diabetes report that the disease limits their activity at work, and those with diabetic complications were 12% less likely to be in the workforce. Another study found that adults with diabetes are absent from work an average of 8.3 days a year, compared to 1.7 days for people without diabetes (12).

A variety of approaches have been introduced within the past decade to address the quality of health care. Approaches such as evidence-based medicine (EBM), total quality management (TQM), accreditation, professional development, patient empowerment, and others have gained popularity. The EBM movement is aimed at helping physicians, patients, policy makers, and payers make health care decisions based on the best evidence available. The inclusion of scientific evidence within clinical practice guidelines has now become more of the standard. Practical, evidence-based recommendations on how to manage health problems are seen as potentially powerful tools for the achievement of effective and efficient care (13).

There is also consensus that assessment and monitoring of clinical performance for both professional development and quality improvement will result in the provision of better quality of care. Such thought processes were the basis for the development by the NCQA of the Health Plan Employer Data and Information Set (HEDIS) indicators for managed care plans. In a review of 48 MEDLINE articles, Schuster and colleagues (13) demonstrated that it is possible to clearly describe many aspects of the quality of care. They suggested that 50% to 70% of the patients in the U.S. receive the recommended care.

Employers, payers, and other authorities expect that systematic data collection, feedback, and the publication of data will improve the quality of care and also reduce health care costs. The assumption is that when health care practitioners are confronted with negative information regarding their performance relative to that of their peers, their behavior will change. Others have found targeted feedback provided by a well-respected peer or opinion leader using clearly credible (e.g., evidence-based) guidelines may be most effective. A multimillion-dollar industry has been created around the publications of performance data in the form of physician report cards or physician profiles as a tool for external accountability (13).

Total quality management (TQM) and continuous quality improvement (CQI) have their roots in the management perspective on quality improvement. The emphasis is not on the performance of the individual clinician, but on the ongoing efforts to improve the whole health care organization with efficient organization of the care process, teamwork, providing a stable infrastructure, and building a culture of quality within the delivery organization. Widespread implementation of TQM has not been achieved in the U.S., in part because physician have not been actively involved in organizational leadership roles within the health care entities such as hospitals and with insurance carriers, and because quality improvement activities have not been focused on the needs of the practitioners or directed at patient-related problems (13).

An innovative approach to the purchasers of health care influencing the quality of care is the Leapfrog Group, a coalition of 60 corporate members that provide health benefits for more than 20 million Americans. Leapfrog members and their employees spend more than $40 billion on health care each year. Armed with data from the Institute of Medicine's 1999 report on errors in medicine, the Leapfrogs have focused on promoting change at the hospital level. The three criteria of measurement chosen by the group are computer physician order entry, evidence-based hospital referral, and staffing hospital ICUs with physicians credentialed in critical care medicine as part of their contract with HMOs. In the case of "founding frog" GM, the company has gone as far as to send teams into the hospitals with experts in manufacturing processes to develop recommendations for improving efficiency. It is expected that improvements in quality will reduce waste and result in cost reductions (14).

Many of the large employers provide quality report cards to their employees at the time of enrollment. Some, like GM, tie a financial incentive to higher quality plans. GM's "benchmark" plans require an employee contribution of only $35 per month for family coverage when the most poorly rated plan would cost the employee $190 a month (14).

OPPORTUNITIES FOR OCCUPATIONAL PHYSICIANS

As health care managers have begun their transition from frustrated payers to educated purchasers, and have sought to understand the process of health delivery, they have found that physicians are crucial participants in this process. As stated by Charles Buck, Staff Executive for Health Care Management at General Electric over 10 years ago (15):

> Speaking as a non-physician with responsibility for corporate-wide "value purchasing" activities, it is obvious that aggressive action on the part of the corporation and its employees, based on quality and value, requires substantial physician input. Are our insurance carriers using appropriate criteria to certify the necessity of procedures? Which of the many and various standards should be used? In selecting preferred networks, are we using the right criteria? What level of quality of care are we justified in claiming? More directly, which hospitals and physicians in a local area have the reputation for, and hopefully are, the highest in quality? Which physicians and hospitals pose problems? What should we do if our employees and their families are currently using "problem" providers? All of these issues arise in any aggressive pursuit of high value medical care on a day-to-day basis. Physician input is critical.

So why has little really changed? Why is it still the case that so few occupational physicians and corporate medical directors are not integrally involved in health care purchasing decisions or actively part of the teams that make the decisions on which health plan and which benefit package to offer in any given year?

While some corporate medical directors have moved to fill the role, many have not. Is it a lack of training or a lack of initiative or is it a narrowed focus on the scope of practice that has been limiting?

The American College of Physician Executives (ACPE), an organization of doctors involved in health care management, has experienced explosive membership growth within the past 10 years and boasts some 12,000 physician members, but only a small percentage of the members are occupational physicians or are physicians employed with non–health care employers. During this same time period, to address the perceived educational requirements of its membership, the American College of Occupational and Environmental Medicine (ACOEM) has developed programs and course offerings focused on a variety of medical management topics. But while the ACPE has been growing and adapting programs to the needs of physicians who are taking the higher level positions within insurance companies, health care systems, and managed care organizations, the business and management courses offered by ACOEM generally have not been well attended.

The traditional scope of occupational medicine practice and the educational offerings have focused on prevention and treatment of work-related illnesses and injuries. Occupational physicians have customarily been hired to staff clinics or to provide consultation under the environmental, health, and safety division of the company, or they are hired to provide expertise in workers' compensation under the risk management department. It has been less common for the occupational physician to have a direct relationship with either human resources or the benefits manager within the organization.

A further explanation for the failure of occupational physicians to take a lead role in health care management is the perceived potential for ethical conflicts. Occupational medicine has long struggled with the ethical dilemma of being between medicine and management. Walsh (16) has developed a model that describes the various functions and ethical conflicts of the occupational physician, which is shown in Fig. 19.3 and Table 19.1. According to this model, there are four distinct areas of occupational medical responsibility. In three of these areas—medical adjudication, environmental health, and health care services—ethical dilemmas abound. For example, in the medical adjudication role, a physician may be responsible for a determination as to the eligibility of an employee for medical disability, where a negative determination could adversely impact that individual's financial status and future employability. Such a determination is typically contrary to the patient advocacy relationship generally expected of a physician. In the environmental health sector and the health care service area, the physician may be faced with employees who have a medical condition that may be worsened by a work activity or exposure, but the employees desire to work at that job for financial reasons, even with the knowledge that they may be jeopardizing their health.

Although these conflicts are real and unavoidable, Walsh argues that occupational medicine has unnecessarily limited its scope by not expanding into a fourth area, that of strategy formulation. Particularly as health care management has evolved from a pure cost-containment model to one of value management, decisions on quality of care may allow the occupational physician to serve the interests of employees and employers simultaneously. Health promotion is one clear activity that achieves this. Involvement in issues such as benefits design and data analysis, how-

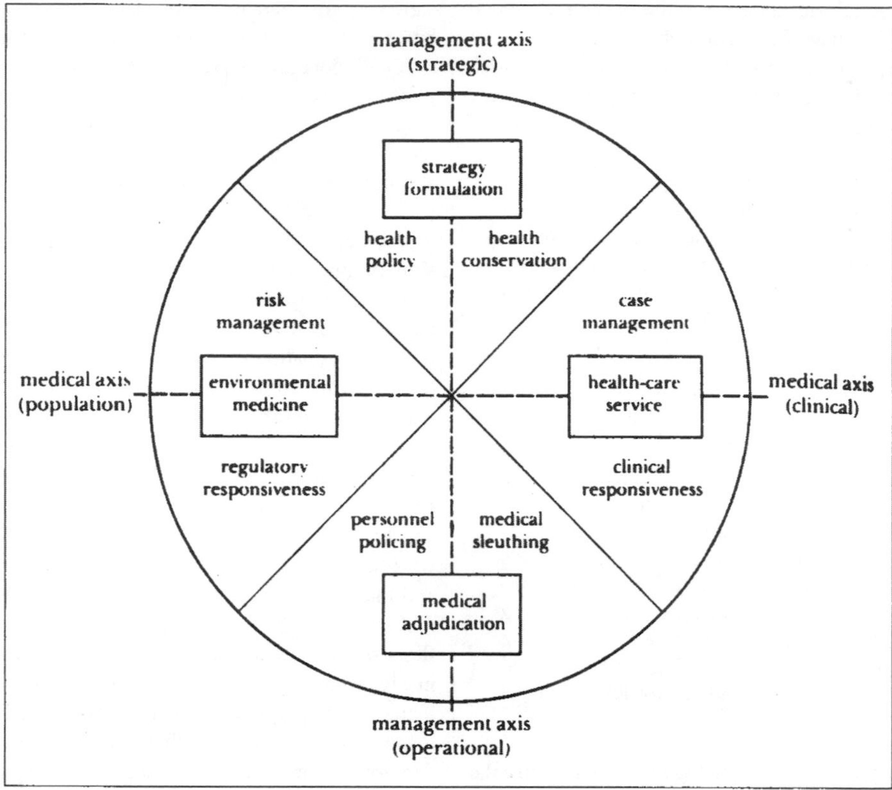

FIG. 19.3. Sectors of corporate physician's role. (From Walsh DC. Employee assistance programs. *Milbank Q* 1982;60:492.)

ever, can serve this purpose as well, as stated by Wood (17).

The corporate physician, in his or her role as protector of the health of workers as individuals and as a productive population, has the inherent interest and the expertise to make judgments about the clinical value of health care purchased for employees, and about the clinical validity of cost control measures, such as utilization review, that assess the appropriateness of the clinical process.

TABLE 19.1. *Three major role sectors for corporate medicine*

	Health care services	Medical adjudication	Environmental health
Historical roots	Emergency treatment, remote locations	Verification of eligibility and claims processing (workers' compensation and benefits associations)	Accident prevention and public health reforms
Functions	Early detection of illness, health conservation, case management	Medical interpretations for industrial relations applications	Risk assessment and management, organizational intelligence
Technique/ expertise	Clinical medicine	Medical administration	Epidemiology, biostatistics, toxicology
Conflicts	Organized medicine, regulators, employees, and public health sector vs. occupational medicine	Costs vs. health mission, line vs. staff	Worker vs. supervisor, in-house vs. outside physicians

Adapted from Walsh DC. *Corporate physicians.* New Haven: Yale University Press, 1987.

For these reasons corporate physicians have a responsibility to assert and insert themselves in the corporate health resource management process. One of the fundamental elements of this responsibility is that the physician be knowledgeable about the needs, the sources, the quality, the analysis, and the meaningful uses for data and the information and knowledge derived therefrom.

HEALTH AND PRODUCTIVITY

Some large employers like Union Pacific Railroad, Bank One, and General Mills have found that by investing in employee health and safety they can boost employee productivity and decrease absenteeism, and in doing so improve their bottom line results. Occupational physicians and corporate medical directors have played integral roles in these organizations in developing and implementing programs and monitoring the outcomes (18).

Union Pacific Railroad identified employee alertness as being a critical factor in both productivity and safety and a decade ago began exploring employee fatigue issues. A study of employees found causes of fatigue were 60% the result of employee behavior and 40% work related (18). "The study taught us dealing with fatigue had to be comprehensive," says Dennis E. Richling, M.D., assistant vice president of health services at the Omaha-based 50,000-employee company. In response, in 1997, the company implemented a comprehensive Alertness Management Program, using education materials, counseling and scheduling changes, Richling reports (18).

General Mills has been able to keep employees at work and save health care dollars by making it convenient for employees to obtain medical services by providing many routine medical services and health-related programs on site. According to Tim Crimmins, M.D., vice president of health and human services for the Minneapolis-based consumer foods company, the on-site clinic has reduced employee time away from work by approximately 30,000 hours annually and has resulted in overall savings of $1.13 million annually (18). Employees can see a gynecologist for Pap smears and mammograms, and they have access to a dermatologist. Dental cleanings are offered, and employees can receive medications on site. The company also invested in an on-site fitness center, which provides yoga, aerobics, and strength-training classes (18).

Allergy problems were identified as contributing to high absenteeism among the 80,000 employees of Bank One, a Chicago-based bank holding company. Of the 20,000 workers who voluntarily took the company's health risk assessment, 40% reported a history of allergies (18). To tackle the problem of absenteeism increasing as the pollen counts increased, Wayne N. Burton, M.D., the medical director, held hour-long lunchtime sessions on self-treatment. Topics ranged from effective housekeeping to the appropriate use of medications (18). According to Burton, productivity "dramatically improved" for allergic employees who took medication. In fact, employees who took medication had the same productivity levels as those who did not suffer from allergies (18).

Learning about health and productivity will be essential for corporate success over the next decade. To address this situation and the lack of research data and expertise, a group of employers decided to become proactive in creating and operating an organized process to advance the science of health enhancement and productivity research. Their commitment launched the Health Enhancement Research Organization (HERO) in 1996. HERO is a national, not-for-profit coalition of employers with concern about and interest in health-related productivity, disease management, and health promotion research. Its members include health care providers, consulting firms, and pharmaceutical manufacturers. Occupational physicians such as David McKenas, medical director of American Airlines, have been actively involved with HERO (19).

The HERO partners realized that no single employer was likely to assume the challenge of creating comprehensive health and productivity research. They postulated that united employers could create a system of synergy for research objectives, expertise, resources, and results. As a facilitator of employer-oriented research, HERO has since conducted and published research on the association between modifiable health risks and individual medical expenditures (19).

HERO has devoted several years to addressing the need for and benefits of health and productivity research. This has been accomplished through regular meetings of senior corporate medical directors and human resources, financial, and benefits executives from Fortune 500 and smaller companies along with individuals from government research agencies, health and productivity scientists, and private practice physicians (19).

Interest in health, productivity, and profit is substantial and growing. Organizations such as the Institute for Health and Productivity Management and HERO are making good progress. In the private sector, William M. Mercer Inc. and the MEDSTAT Group are among the organizations devoting major resources to health and productivity research. In the federal government, not only the National Institute for Occupational Safety and Health (NIOSH) but also the National Institute on Aging and the Agency for Healthcare Research and Quality have interest in the field (19).

PREVENTION AND HEALTH PROMOTION

The prevention of disease has long been within the scope of occupational medicine. Periodic health examinations of individuals are offered by most occupational health clinics, although the actual cost-effectiveness of these examinations is unproven (20). Over the past decade, full-scale health promotion programs have been developed to address the major risk factors and contribution from personal habits of smoking, poor nutrition and lack of exercise. There is emerging evidence that specific types of programs, and specific interventions within these programs, are saving health care dollars (21).

Employee assistance programs (EAPs) have served as initial points of contact for employees with mental health or personal problems and challenges. In most situations, nonphysician counselors provide a triage function to appropriate outside providers. Given that mental health benefits have been the most rapidly rising area of health care benefits, the potential for cost savings by referral to cost-effective providers is substantial. More recently, EAP counselors are performing short-term treatment themselves. Certain programs have been found to have favorable cost-benefit ratios (22).

A third type of prevention activity is educating employees to be informed health care consumers. Some corporate medical centers have been involved in this exercise, for which the data suggest a positive cost-benefit ratio (23).

Helping employees become better consumers is going to be the next big step in cost management, says Rich Ostuw, global director of Group and Health Care Consulting at Watson Wyatt. And that, he says, involves "improving employee benefits communication, helping employees navigate through the system, and giving them the information to make smart choices among alternatives." More that 80% of employers in the Watson Wyatt report intend to use the Internet as a medium to convey information to employees on health plan choices, enrollment, navigating the system, and health and wellness programs.

Demonstrating the value of health outcomes and improving employee education are integral to the future of consumer-driven health care.

In 1994, after serving as the corporate medical director, Pamela Hymel, an occupational physician, was named director of benefits and medical services for Hughes Electronics. Her task was to design and implement a company-wide health management program at Hughes to reduce costs and improve employee well being (24).

According to Hymel, by focusing on case management for a workers' compensation project, her team members had found that they could make a positive impact on overall costs and as a result she believed that they could translate some of the lessons learned in workers' compensation into an integrated disability management program and better health for the workforce. The focus was on reducing the number of disability days for employees, changing behaviors to reduce the instances of disability cases and ultimately reducing costs. WorkWell was Hymel's answer to containing health care costs in a changing environment. WorkWell is an integrated wellness program geared toward those areas where employees can modify lifestyle behavior and impact their overall health and related costs. The program was designed to address modifiable risk behavior for employees in Hughes' self-funded medical plan—it focused on health care costs before they occurred (24).

Hymel compared medical claims to a reference database of preventable conditions. The analysis specifically identified coronary heart disease, low back pain, congestive heart failure, asthma, and diabetes as hot spots (24). In the first 2 years of the program, health care expenses for conditions that had an avoidable component were reduced 7.3%. In particular, cardiovascular disease costs went from 12% of total costs to just 5%. Hymel estimates that Hughes has reduced its disability compensation costs by 35%. In key areas like hypertension, back problems, and breast cancer, expenses have gone down nearly 50% (24).

After completing the health claims review, Hughes subcontracted with Johnson & Johnson to conduct onsite health screenings, or health risk appraisals, focused on the target areas. To encourage participation and create broad employee interest, Hughes offered $200 reduction in health insurance premiums to all participants who completed the program as well as a $50 gift certificate for completing the health risk appraisal (24).

In its third year, the WorkWell health screenings identified 32% of the population as high risk—and 90% of those employees participated in risk reduction programs (24).

SUMMARY

As employers seek alternatives to address rapidly rising health care costs, occupational physicians have an opportunity to expand beyond the traditional scope of practice within the specialty and offer the best available expertise. With a new focus on health and productivity, informed consumer choice, and prevention and health promotion, occupational physicians, as both corporate medical directors and consultants, need to accept the challenge and become experts in the field of health care management.

While opportunities are abundant, it is expertise that the employers are looking for and are willing to pay for. To gain expertise, the occupational physician needs to focus on educational offerings in medical management, become familiar with business and insurance industry publications, and learn to network with employer representatives by attending local business group health-related functions.

Within organizations, corporate physicians need to learn from insurance brokers and health benefits professionals. By using some of what is learned and implementing programs to reduce total health and safety costs, the corporate physician and the medical department can become integral players in health care cost reduction initiatives and not just be viewed as another cost center.

REFERENCES

1. Inglehart JK. The American Health Care system—private insurance. *N Engl J Med* 1991;326:1715.
2. Averbach R. *What business needs to know about health care.* Massachusetts Business Roundtable, 1991.
3. Martinez B. Employers expect health-care costs to rise 13% in 2002. *Wall Street Journal,* December 10, 2001, p. B8.
4. Starr P. *The social transformation of American medicine.* New York: Basic Books, 1982.
5. Inglehart JK. The centers for Medicare and Medicaid services. *N Engl J Med* 2001;345:1920.
6. Crippen DL. *Impact of the Balanced Budget Act on Medicare.* Testimony before the House Energy and Commerce Committee. Washington, DC, September 15, 1999.
7. Lippman H. How the Fortune 500 pick health plans: frustrated by managed care's inability to continue reducing costs, Fortune 500's step up the pressure. *Business and Health Fortune* 2001(June), p. 31–36.
8. Harris J. Does managed care manage health care costs effectively? It depends. Managing employee health care costs—assuring quality and value. Boston: OEM Press, 1992:131–135.
9. Berwick DM. Quality of healthcare. *N Engl J Med* 1996;335:1227.
10. Ruchlin HS, et al. The efficiency of second opinion consultation programs: a cost benefit perspective. *Me Care* 1982;20:3.
11. Epstein A. Performance report on quality-prototypes, problems, and prospects. *N Engl J Med* 1995;333: 57–61.
12. Business and Health Special Report. Keys to workplace productivity. *Mapping Diabetes Management* 2001(December).
13. Grol R. Improving the quality of medical care. *JAMA* 2001;286:2578–2584.
14. Walker L. The state of health care in America 2001. *Business and Health* 2001:44–47.
15. Buck CR. Assessing value in medical care for employees and dependents: an opportunity for occupational physicians. *J Occup Med* 1990;32:1165.
16. Walsh DC. Is there a doctor in-house? *Harvard Business Review* 1984;84:84.
17. Wood LW. A user's view of health care data management. *J Occup Med* 1991;32:264.
18. Lipold AG. Six ideas to boost employee productivity: six different companies benefit from programs addressing employees' special health needs. *Business and Health* 2001(October).
19. Whitmer RW, McKenas DK, O'Donnell MP. *From business and health.* Montvale, NJ:Medical Economics. November/December 2000 edition.
20. Beck HD, et al. Assuring value in medical care for employees and dependents. *J Occup Med* 1990;32:1161.
21. Harris JS. The cost effectiveness of health promotion programs. *J Occup Med* 1991;33:327.
22. Harris JS. Managing health: what employers can do about health care costs. In: Meyer J, McLennon K, eds. *Background papers on health care cost.* Washington, DC: Committee for Economic Development, 1988.
23. Vickery DM, et al. Effect of self-care education program on medical visits. *JAMA* 1983;250:2592.
24. Arapoff J. Staying at Work 2001/2001: the dollars and sense of effective disability management from Watson Wyatt strategy at work: a doctor in the house. www.watsonwyatt.com.

APPENDIX: GETTING INVOLVED

How does the physician get more involved in health care management? Increased involvement in health care management requires two conditions: opportunity and expertise. The opportunities in this area are abundant. As employers struggle with the increasingly sophisticated field of health care, their benefits departments have either contracted with health benefit consultants or added health care managers to their payroll. Few of these benefits professionals are physicians, and they are usually relieved to have a physician help them with issues of utilization review and medical management. The complaint heard among purchasers is not that there are too many occupational doctors involved but that there are too few.

Expertise in health care management requires knowledge of health services research and the economics of health care. The two physician organizations involved in health care management are the American College of Occupational and Environmental Medicine (ACOEM; 55 West Seegers Road, Arlington Heights, IL 60005-3922) and the American

College of Physician Executives (ACPE; 4890 West Kennedy Boulevard, Suite 200, Tampa, FL 33609-2575). ACOEM has a Health Care Cost and Quality Management Committee that sponsors seminars at the semiannual ACOEM meetings. The area of focus in the past decade has been on the value of group health and workers' compensation benefits. ACPE has a committee on corporate medical services, although the organization as a whole has historically been mostly focused on physicians working in the hospital and managed care industries. ACPE offers a three-part physician management series, which presents a thorough introduction to health care management. However, although seminars and courses are useful, a master's-level program in health services administration, business, or public health is necessary to gain true expertise in the field.

Two publications focus on issues of health care management. *Business and Health* is a non–peer-reviewed journal that includes articles on the spectrum of health management issues. It is affiliated with the Washington Business Group on Health and is published monthly through Medical Economics Publishing (5 Paragon Drive, Montvale, NJ 07645-1742).

Health Affairs, an academic journal of health policy published quarterly, is peer reviewed and often referred to as the *New England Journal of Medicine* of the health policy field (2 Wisconsin Circle, Suite 500, Chevy Chase, MD 20815).

A third journal, *Physician Executive,* is peer reviewed and published monthly by ACPE, and has as its focus the issues of physicians as managers. Each issue usually includes one or two articles on health care management.

20

Suspecting Occupational Disease: The Clinician's Role

Rose H. Goldman

Persons suffering from work-related illness enter clinicians' offices every day. Yet consideration of work-related etiologies rarely enters the practitioner's differential diagnosis. As a result, clinicians may miss the chance to make diagnoses that might influence the course of a disease in some and might prevent disease in others (by stopping exposure). The following two cases illustrate the consequences of attention to (or lack of attention to) environmental exposures:

The first case is a man who experienced retrosternal chest pain after applying a paint remover in his basement workshop (1). On admission to the hospital, he showed the paint-remover container to his attending physician. The label cautioned that the product contained 80% methylene chloride and was to be used only with adequate ventilation. The physician made the diagnosis of anterior wall myocardial infarction but apparently did not look further into the health effects of methylene chloride. After discharge, the patient reused the solvent in a similar manner and suffered a fatal myocardial infarction. This tragic ending might have been averted if the history of solvent exposure had stimulated inquiry into the toxic properties of methylene chloride. If the practitioner had known that this substance is rapidly metabolized to carbon monoxide, which can stress the cardiovascular system (2,3), then he could have advised the patient not to use the solvent, particularly in an unventilated area.

In the second case, in contrast, a young man reported fatigue, headache, and skin rash to his physician. He inquired if his problems could be related to his job, in which he machined metal parts and cleaned them with methylene chloride. The physician knew little about this solvent but was suspicious that it might be a contributing factor. He consulted with an occupational physician and learned that overexposure could cause dizziness, headache, excessive fatigue, and skin irritation. The physician then learned that the patient worked in a small, unventilated basement workshop over an open container of solvent. The patient's job was to dip metal parts into the container of solvent, wetting his arms to the elbow, and then hold the dripping parts up to his eye for close inspection. The occupational physician discussed the dangers of these conditions with the patient and recommended methods for decreasing exposure. The employee persuaded the company to install a safer degreasing operation and also changed his own work practices. When those changes were made, his symptoms resolved.

These two cases demonstrate how a physician's level of attention to potential environmental and occupational hazards can lead to strikingly different outcomes.

It is difficult to estimate the full extent of occupational illness in the United States because of the lack of accurate information. The Bureau of Labor Statistics (BLS) in the U.S. Department of Labor reports statistics based on surveys of private companies with greater than 11 employees, excluding the self-employed, farmers, and government employees. BLS reported 5.7 million nonfatal injuries and illnesses, or 6.1 per 100 full-time workers in 2000 (4). Of the 362,500 new illness cases reported, 67% were disorders related to repeated trauma, such as carpal tunnel syndrome and noise-induced hearing loss. Yet even these Department of Labor statistics are underestimates because of underreporting, lack of identification of cases, the tendency to report predominately acute rather than chronic cases, and failure to include all types of employers. Another study used several collected data sets (including the BLS) to produce the following estimates of annual total occupational injury and illness in the U.S.: 6,500 job-related deaths from injury; 13.2 million nonfatal injuries; 60,300 deaths from job-related disease; and 862,200 work-related illnesses (5). Total costs were estimated to be $171 billion. In a study of health maintenance organization (HMO) members with adult-onset asthma, 21% were found to meet criteria for asthma attributable to occupational exposures (6). The general environment also contributes to illness. Air pollution, for example, has been linked to increased rates of mortality, in particular from cardiovascular and respiratory illnesses (7–9). Home exposures to dust mites and cockroaches (10) as well as work exposures (6,11) are thought to have contributed to the increased incidence and mortality of asthma in both adults and children (12).

Clinicians have an important role to play in identifying potential workplace risks and possible work-related health problems in their patients. One obstacle to physicians' recognition of job-related health problems is insufficient education. A survey in 1983 showed that 50% of medical schools taught courses in occupational health, but the average curriculum time was only 4 hours (13). The Institute of Medicine has recommended how to foster the role and education of the primary care physician in environmental and occupational medicine (14). Now practitioners have many resources available to help them learn more about recognizing and preventing occupational diseases and illnesses, including useful review articles on occupational medicine topics (15–19), paperback textbooks (20,21), comprehensive reference textbooks (22), and Web sites that provide educational materials *(www.aoec.org)* and/or lists of other informative Web sites and resources *(www.acoem.org; http://occ-env-med.mc.duke.eduoemindex2.htrm)*.

Another impediment to the recognition of work-related illness is a lack of uniqueness in the clinical manifestations of many occupational illnesses. Wheezing caused by platinum salts, for example, is similar to wheezing due to animal dander or pollen. Oat-cell carcinoma caused by exposure to bis-

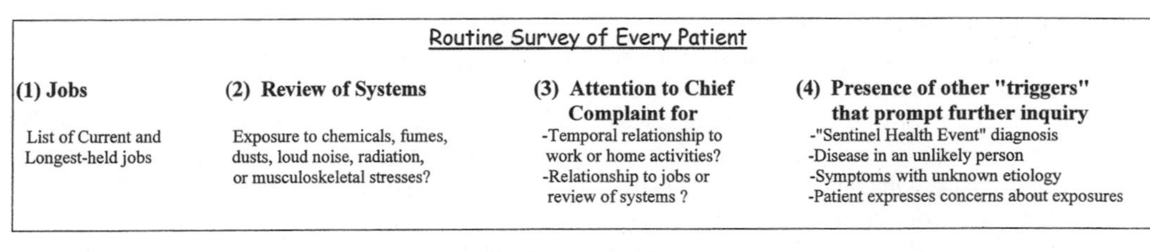

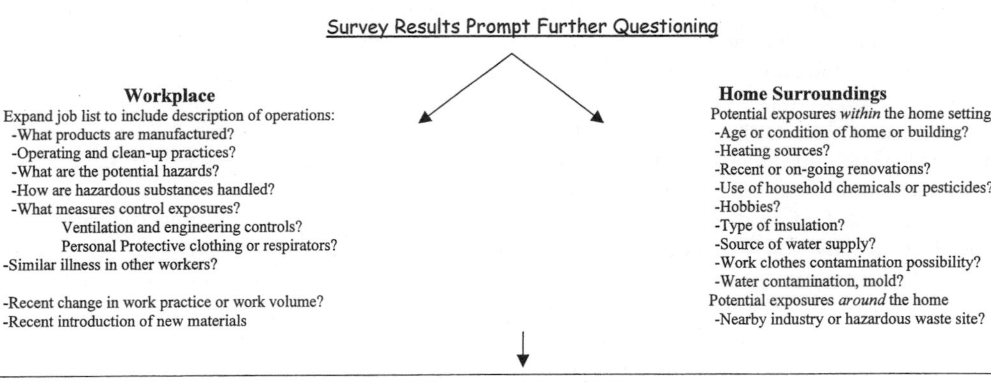

Follow-up and Consultation

May include work or environmental site evaluation, biological monitoring and medical screening, worker compensation claim and appropriate preventive interventions

FIG. 20.1. Systematic approach to history taking and diagnosis of occupational or environmental illness. (From Goldman RH, Peters JM. The occupational and environmental health history. *JAMA* 1981;246:2831, © 1981, American Medical Association.)

chloromethyl ether behaves similarly to that due to cigarette smoking. Hepatitis secondary to hepatitis B virus contracted from contact with blood at work presents in the same way as community-acquired hepatitis; median nerve entrapment related to repetitive motions has the same constellation of symptoms and signs as carpal tunnel syndrome due to pregnancy.

Some exposures cause immediate or subacute symptoms (such as allergic reactions and asthma), while others lead to more delayed effects (such as cancer or pneumoconiosis). A long latency, or the period from initial exposure to presentation of disease, is another factor that leads to underrecognition of some occupational diseases. Asbestosis, for example, can appear 15 to 20 years after first working with the material. Occupational cancer such as mesothelioma can occur 40 years after exposure.

Despite these obstacles, physicians can enhance their recognition of occupational disease by taking a good occupational and environmental (OE) history using an organized approach (Fig. 20.1) (23,24).

OCCUPATIONAL AND ENVIRONMENTAL HEALTH SURVEY OF ALL PATIENTS

Patients with symptoms related to hazardous exposures can present with complaints involving any body system and mimicking ordinary medical diseases (Table 20.1) (23,24). To detect cases of occupational disease, an OE history, even if brief, should be taken on every patient. With this in mind, the first step in the OE history is a brief survey of all patients that could include the following:

1. A list of current and longest held jobs, and a current job description.
2. Attention to the chief complaint (or diagnosis) for clues suggesting a relationship to activities at work or at home.
3. A review-of-systems question about exposures to fumes, dusts, chemicals, loud noise, radiation, or musculoskeletal stresses.
4. Observance of the presence of other triggers that prompt further inquiry, such as a sentinel health event diagnosis, disease in an unlikely person, symptoms with unknown etiology, and/or patient with concerns about exposures.

The importance of a screening survey on all patients is illustrated by a case report of a young man who presented to an emergency room with abdominal pain and vomiting (25). He underwent an appendectomy before it was learned that his job entailed removing lead paint from houses and that the actual cause of his symptoms was lead poisoning. Even a brief occupational history at the time of his presentation could have provided clues to the correct diagnosis and might have avoided an unnecessary operation. His diagnosis of lead poisoning led to the screening of other workers, and to modifications that would prevent lead exposure in other employees.

In looking for a temporal relationship to work, it is preferable to start with nonsuggestive questions, such as "Are your symptoms better or worse at home or at work? Weekends or workdays?" rather than using more leading questions such as "Does work make you sick?" In some cases the screening OE survey suggests a temporal relationship that points to the role of work or environmental factors: the painter who has been scraping old paint and has abdominal pain (lead poisoning); a car painter with a dry, hacking cough that occurs at work or late in the day or evening [delayed bronchospasm due to exposure to toluene diisocyante (TDI), a component in the car paint lacquer]; the mother and other family members who develop headaches in the fall that are worse in the morning and when at home (carbon monoxide poisoning possibly due to a faulty furnace). Finding a temporal relationship between symptoms and exposure is useful, but it is also important to realize that in some cases current exposures do not always lead to immediate symptoms. For example, a lab technician may have been at work for several months before developing itching, hand rash, and wheezing when putting on latex gloves. He might have developed an allergy to latex. In the case of allergic reactions, it may take months of exposure before sensitization and clinical allergy develops. Once the allergic reaction (skin rash and/or asthma) occurs, symptoms can sometimes extend beyond the work period, and then be triggered by exposure to irritants as well.

Symptoms related to current exposures may initially improve on nonworkdays or vacations, but prolonged exposure can lead to the persistence of symptoms beyond the workday. As an example, aching in the wrist and hand of a computer programmer using a mouse might initially resolve with rest in the evenings, on weekends, or vacations. Once chronic tendonitis or nerve entrapment (carpal tunnel or cubital tunnel syndromes) develops, the symptoms can persist into nonwork time and be aggravated by other activities such as biking or gardening.

TABLE 20.1. *Examples of environmental causes of medical problems*

Problem	Agent	Potential exposures
Immediate or short-term effects		
Dermatoses (allergic or irritant)	Metals (chromium, nickel), fibrous glass, epoxy resins, cutting oils, solvents, caustic alkali, soaps	Electroplating, metal cleaning, plastics, machining, leather tanning, housekeeping
Headache	Carbon monoxide, solvents	Firefighting, automobile exhaust, foundry, wood finishing, dry cleaning
Acute psychoses	Lead (especially organic) mercury, carbon disulfide	Handling gasoline, seed handling, fungicide, wood preserving, viscose rayon industry
Asthma or dry cough	Formaldehyde, toluene diisocyanate, animal dander	Textiles, plastics, polyurethane kits, lacquer use, animal handling, latex glove use
Pulmonary edema, pneumonitis	Nitrogen oxides, phosgene, halogen gases, cadmium	Welding, farming ("silo-filler's disease") chemical operations, smelting
Cardiac arrhythmias	Solvents, fluorocarbons	Metal cleaning, solvents use, refrigerator maintenance, auto exhaust
Angina	Carbon monoxide	Car repair, traffic exhaust, foundry, wood finishing
Abdominal pain	Lead	Battery making, enameling, smelting, painting, welding, ceramics, plumbing, radiator repair
Hepatitis (may become a long-term effect)	Halogentated hydrocarbons, e.g., carbon tetrachloride,viral infection	Solvent use, lacquer use, hospital work
Tendinitis, Carpal Tunnel Syndrome, "repetitive strain disorder" (may become a long-term effect)	Repetitive motions, awkward postures, pinching motions, wrist flexion	Assembly work, keyboarding, data entry
Latent or long-term effects		
Chronic dyspnea		
Pulmonary fibrosis	Asbestos, silica, beryllium, coal, aluminum	Mining insulation, pipefitting, sandblasting, quarrying, metal alloy work, aircraft or electrical parts, nylon flocking
Chronic bronchitis emphysema	Cotton dust, cadmium coal dust, organic solvents, cigarettes	Textile industry, battery production, soldering, mining, solvent use
Lung cancer	Asbestos, arsenic, uranium, coke oven emissions	Insulation, pipefitting, smelting, coke ovens, shipyard workers, nickel refining, uranium mining
Bladder cancer	β-Naphthylamine, benzidine dyes	Dye industry, leather, rubber-working chemists
Peripheral neuropathy	Lead, arsenic *n*-hexane, methyl butylketone, acrylamide	Battery production, plumbing, smelting, painting, shoemaking, solvent use, insecticides
Behavioral changes	Lead, carbon disulfide, solvents, mercury, manganese	Battery makers, smelting, viscose rayon industry, degreasing, mfg/repair of scientific instruments, dental amalgam workers
Extrapyramidal syndrome	Carbon disulfide, manganese	Viscose rayon industry, steel production, battery production, foundry, mining
Aplastic anemia, leukemia	Benzene, ionizing radiation	Chemists, furniture refinishing, cleaning, degreasing, radiation workers

From Goldman RH, Peters JM. The occupational and environmental health history. *JAMA* 1981;246:2831. © 1981, American Medical Association.

Exposure to occupational or environmental substances can also aggravate underlying medical conditions. For example, carbon monoxide inhalation, even at the relatively modest levels of exposure encountered during commuter driving in heavy traffic, may precipitate anginal symptoms or decreased exercise tolerance in patients with coronary artery disease (2,3,26). The expression of toxic symptoms is also influenced by the presence of other diseases, genetic traits, medications, and exposure to other hazardous substances. For example, the metabolism of certain poisons may be affected by liver disease, certain medications, concurrent alcohol use, chemicals (such as DDT), and/or any condition that affects liver function.

Other triggers may prompt the need for further inquiry: The presence of a "sentinel health event (occupational)" diagnosis is a disease, disability, or untimely death that is occupationally related and whose occurrence may provide the impetus for evaluations (such as epidemiologic studies or industrial hygiene evaluations) and interventions to prevent future cases (27,28). Table 20.2 is an abbreviated list of these characteristic diagnoses (16).

TABLE 20.2. *Occupationally related unnecessary disease, disability, and untimely death*[a]

ICD-9	Condition	A	B	C	Industry/process/occupation	Agent
011	Pulmonary tuberculosis (O)	P	P,T	P,T	Physicians, medical personnel, medical lab workers	*Mycobacterium tuberculosis*
011, 502	Silicotuberculosis	P	P,T	P,T	Quarrymen, sandblasters, silica processors, mining, metal foundries, ceramic industry	Silica + *Mycobacterium tuberculosis*
020	Plague (O)	P	—	—	Shepherds, farmers, ranchers, hunters, field geologists	*Yersinia pestis*
021	Tularemia (O)	P	—	P,T	Hunters, fur handlers, sheep industry workers, cooks, vets, ranchers, vet pathologists, lab workers, soldiers	*Francisella tularensis, Pasteurella tularensis*
022	Anthrax (O)	P	—	P,T	Shepherds, farmers, butchers, handlers of imported hides or fibers, vets, vet pathologists, weavers, farmers	*Bacillus anthracis*
023	Brucellosis (O)	P	P	P	Farmers, shepherds, veterinarians, lab workers, slaughterhouse workers, field officers	*Brucella abortus, suis*
031.1[b]	Fish-fancier's finger (O)	P	P	P	Aquarium workers/cleaners, breeders/owners	*Mycobacterium marinum*
					Longshoremen	*Mycobacterium marinum*
054.6	Herpetic whitlow (O)	P	P	P	Surgical residents, student nurses, nurses, dental assistants, physicians, orthopedic scrub nurses, psychiatric nurses	Herpes simplex virus
037	Tetanus(O)	P	P	P	Farmers, ranchers	*Clostridium tetani*
042[c]	Human immunodeficiency virus (O)	P	P	P	Health care workers	Human immunodeficiency virus
056	Rubella (O)	P	P	P	Medical personnel, intensive care personnel	Rubella virus
070.0.1	Hepatitis A (O)	P	P	P	Day-care center staff, orphanage staff, mental retardation institution staff, medical personnel	Hepatitis A virus
070.2.3	Hepatitis B (O)	P	P	P	Nurses and aides, anesthesiologists, orphanage and mental institution staff, medical lab personnel, general dentists, oral surgeons, physicians	Hepatitis B virus
070.4	Non-A, non-B hepatitis (O)	P	P	P	As above for hepatitis A and B	Unknown
071	Rabies (O)	P	—	P	Veterinarians, animal and game wardens, lab researchers, farmers, ranchers, trappers	Rabies virus
073	Ornithosis (O)	P	—	P,T	Psittacine bird breeders, pet shop staff, poultry producers, vets, zoo employees, duck processing and rearing	*Chlamydia psittaci*
082.0	Rocky Mountain spotted fever (O)	P	P	P,T	Laboratory technicians, tick breeders, virologists, microbiologists, physicians	*Rickettsia rickettsii*
100.8	Leptospirosis (O)	P	P	P,T	Farmers/laborers	*Leptospira*
115	Histoplasmosis (O)	P	P	P,T	Bridge maintenance workers	*Histoplasma capsulatum*
117.1	Sporotrichosis (O)	P	P	P	Nurserymen, foresters, florists, equipment operators	*Sporothrix schenckii*
147	Malignant neoplasm of nasopharynx (O)	P	P	P	Carpenters, cabinet makers, sawmill workers, lumberjacks, electricians, fitters	Chlorophenols
155M[d,e]	Hemangiosarcoma of the liver	P	P	P	Vinyl chloride polymerization industry	Vinyl chloride monomer
					Vintners	Arsenical pesticides
158, 163	Mesothelioma (MN of peritoneum and pleura)	P	—	P	Asbestos industries and utilizers	Asbestos

continued on next page

TABLE 20.2. *Continued*

ICD-9	Condition	A	B	C	Industry/process/occupation	Agent
160.0	Malignant neoplasm of nasal cavities (O)	P	P,T	P,T	Woodworkers, cabinet and furniture makers	Hardwood dusts
					Boot and shoe industry	Unknown
					Radium chemists and processors, dial painters	Radium
					Chromium producers, processors, users	Chromates
					Nickel smelting and refining	Nickel
					Sawmill workers, carpenters	Chlorophenols
161	Malignant neoplasm of larynx (O)	P	P,T	P,T	Asbestos industry and utilizers	Asbestos
162	Malignant neoplasm of trachea, bronchus, and lung (O)	P	P	P	Asbestos industry and utilizers	Asbestos
					Topside coke oven workers	Coke oven emissions
					Uranium and fluorspar miners	Radon daughters
					Chromium producers, processors, users	Chromates
					Nickel smelters, processors, users	Nickel
					Smelters	Arsenic, arsenic trioxide
					Mustard gas formulators	Mustard gas
					Ion exchange resin makers, chemists	Bis(chloromethyl) ether, chloromethyl methyl ether
					Iron ore (underground) miners	Radon daughters
					Plant protection workers/agronomists	Pesticides, herbicides, fungicides, insecticides
					Welders	Unknown
					Copper smelter and roaster workers	Inorganic arsenic sulfur dioxide, copper, lead, sulfuric acid, arsenic trioxide
					Welders, gas cutters	Asbestos, hexavalent chromium
					Foundry-floor molders and casters	Polyaromatic hydrocarbons
					Dichromate production-floor molders/casters	Unknown
					Chromate production	Chromium dust
					Chromate pigment production workers	Lead chromate, zinc chromate
					Pigment production	Zinc chromate dust
					Steel industry-furnace/foundry workers	Unknown
					Rubber reclaim operations	Unknown
170	Malignant neoplasm of bone (O)	P	—	P	Radium chemists and processors, dial painters	Radium
187.7	Malignant neoplasm of scrotum	P	—	P,T	Automatic lathe operators, metal workers	Mineral/cutting oils
					Coke oven workers, petroleum refiners, tar distillers	Soots/tars/tar distillates
					Tool setters, fitters, cotton spinners, chimney sweeps, machine operators	Mineral oil, pitch, tar
188	Malignant neoplasm of bladder (O)	P	—	P	Rubber and dye workers	Benzidine, α- and β-naphthylamine, magenta, auramine, 4-aminobiphenyl, 4-nitrophenyl

189	Malignant neoplasm of kidney, other, and unspecified urinary organs (O)	P	P	P	Coke oven workers	Coke oven emissions
204.0	Lymphoid leukemia, acute (O)	P	—	P	Rubber industry	Unknown
					Radiologists	Ionizing radiation
205.0	Myeloid leukemia, acute (O)	P	—	P	Occupations with exposure to benzene	Benzene
					Radiologists	Ionizing radiation
207.0	Erythroleukemia (O)	P	—	P	Occupations with exposure to benzene	Benzene
283.1	Hemolytic anemia, nonautoimmune (O)	P	—	P	Whitewashing and leather industry	Copper sulfate
					Electrolytic processes, arsenical ore smelting	Arsine
					Plastics industry	Trimellitic anhydride
					Dye, celluloid, resin industry	Naphthalene
284.8	Aplastic anemia (O)	P	—	P	Explosives manufacture	Trinitrotoluene
					Occupations with exposure to benzene	Benzene
					Radiologists, radium chemists, and dial painters	Ionizing radiation
288.0	Agranulocytosis or neutropenia (O)	P	—	P	Occupations with exposure to benzene	Benzene
					Explosives and pesticide industries	Phosphorus
					Pesticides, pigments, pharmaceuticals	Inorganic arsenic
289.7	Methemoglobinemia (O)	P	—	P,T	Explosives and dye industries	Aromatic amino and nitro compounds (e.g., aniline, trinitrotoluene, nitroglycerin)
					Rubber workers	Aniline, o-toluidine, nitrobenzene
323.7	Toxic encephalitis (O)	P	P	P	Battery, smelter, and foundry workers	Lead
					Electrolytic chlorine production, battery makers, fungicide formulators	Inorganic and organic mercury
332.1	Parkinson's disease (secondary) (O)	P	P	—	Manganese processing, battery makers, welders	Manganese
					Internal combustion engine industries	Carbon monoxide
334.3	Cerebellar ataxia (O)	P	P	—	Chemical industry using toluene	Toluene
					Electrolytic chlorine production, battery makers, fungicide formulators	Organic mercury
354M[f]	Carpal tunnel syndrome (O)	P	P	—	Meat packers deboners	Cumulative trauma
354.0.2.3	Mononeuritis of upper limb and mononeuritis multiplex (O)	P	P	—	Dental technicians	Methyl methacrylate monomer
					Poultry processing—turkey	Cumulative trauma
					Meatpackers, deboners	Cumulative trauma
357.7	Inflammatory and toxic neuropathy (O)	P	P,T	P,T	Pesticide industry, pigments, pharmaceuticals formulators	Arsenic/arsenic compounds
					Furniture refinishers, degreasing operations	Hexane
					Plastic-coated fabric workers	Methyl *n*-butyl ketone
					Explosives industry	Trinitrotoluene
					Rayon manufacturing	Carbon disulfide
					Plastics, hydraulics, coke industries	Tri-o-cresyl phosphate
					Battery, smelter, and foundry workers	Inorganic lead
					Dentists, chloralkali workers	Inorganic mercury
					Chloralkali plants, fungicide makers, battery makers	Organic mercury

continued on next page

TABLE 20.2. *Continued*

ICD-9	Condition	A	B	C	Industry/process/occupation	Agent
					Plastics industry, paper manufacturing	Acrylamide
					Ethylene oxide sterilizer operator	Ethylene oxide
366.4	Cataract (O)	P	P,T	—	Microwave and radar technicians	Microwaves
					Explosives industries, trinitrotoluene workers	Trinitrotoluene
					Radiologists	Ionizing radiation
					Blacksmiths, glass blowers, bakers	Infrared radiation
					Moth repellant formulators, fumigators	Naphthalene
					Explosives, dye, herbicide and pesticide industries	Dinitrophenol, dinitro-o-cresol
					Ethylene oxide sterilizer operator, microbiology supervisors, inspectors	Ethylene oxide
388.1	Noise effects on inner ear (O)	P	P	—	Occupations with exposure to excessive noise	Excessive noise
443.0	Raynaud's phenomenon (secondary) (O)	P	—	—	Lumberjacks, chain sawyers, grinders, chippers, rock drillers, stone cutters, jackhammer operators, riveters	Whole body or segmental vibration
					Vinyl chloride polymerization industry	Vinyl chloride
493.0 507.8	Extrinsic as- T ham (O)	P	P,T	P,T	Jewelry, alloy, and catalyst makers	Platinum
					Polyurethane, adhesive, paint workers	Isocyanates
					Alloy, catalyst, refinery workers	Chromium, cobalt
					Solderers	Aluminum soldering flux
					Plastic, dye, insecticide makers	Phthalic anhydride
					Foam workers, latex makers, biologists	Formaldehyde
					Printing industry	Gum arabic
					Nickel platers	Nickel sulfate
					Bakers	Flour
					Plastics industry, organic chemicals manufacture	Trimellitic anhydride
					Woodworkers, furniture makers	Red cedar (plicatic acid) and other wood dusts
					Detergent formulators	Bacillus-derived exoenzymes
					Crab processing workers	Unknown
					Hospital and geriatric department nurses	Psyllium dust
					Laxative manufacture and packing	Psyllium dust
					Prawn processing workers	Unknown
					Snow crab processing workers	Unknown
495.4	Maltworker's lung	P	P	—	Maltworkers	*Aspergillus clavatus*
495.5	Mushroom worker's lung	P	P	—	Mushroom farm/spawning shed, farmers	Pasteurized compost
495.8	Grain handler's lung	P	P	—	Grain handlers	Erwinia herbicola *(Enterobacter agglomerans)*
	Sequoiosis	P	P	—	Red cedar mill workers, woodworkers, sawmill, joinery	Redwood sawdust, *Thuja plicata*
495.9	Unspecified allergic alveolitis	P	P	—	Cinnamon processing workers	Cinnamon dust, cinnamaldehyde
					Distillery, vegetable compost plant workers	*Aspergillus fumigatus*
					Sawmill workers	Unknown

					Paper manufacture/wood room	*Alternaria,* wood dust
					Snow crab processing workers	Unknown
500	Coalworker's pneumoconiosis	P	P	P	Coal miners	Coal dust
501	Asbestosis	P	P	P	Asbestos industries and utilizers	Asbestos
502M[g]	Silicosis	P	P	P	Quarrymen, sandblasters, silica processors, mining, metal, and ceramic industries	Silica
					Cryolite refining	Cryolite (Na_3AlF_6), quartz dust
	Talcosis	P	P	P	Talc processors, soap stone mining/milling, polishing, cosmetics industry	Talc
503M[h]	Chronic beryllium disease of the lung	P	P	P	Beryllium alloy workers, ceramic and cathode ray tube makers, nuclear reactor workers	Beryllium
504	Byssinosis	P	P	P	Cotton industry workers	Cotton, flax, hemp, and cotton-synthetic dusts
506.0.1	Acute bronchitis, pneumonitis, and pulmonary edema due to fumes and vapors (O)	P,T	P,T	P,T	Refrigeration, fertilizer, oil refining industries	Ammonia
					Alkali and bleach industries	Chlorine
					Silo fillers, arc welders, nitric acid industry	Nitrogen oxides
					Paper and refrigeration industries, oil refining	Sulfur dioxide
					Cadmium smelters, processors	Cadmium
					Plastics industry	Trimellitic anhydride
					Boilermakers	Vanadium pentoxide
					Organic chemicals manufacture	Trimellitic anhydride
570, 573.3	Toxic hepatitis (O)	P	P	P	Solvent utilizers, dry cleaners, plastics industry	Carbon tetrachloride, chloroform, tetrachloroethane, trichloroethylene, tetrachloroethylene
					Explosives and dye industries	Phosphorus, trinitrotoluene
					Fire and waterproofing additive formulators	Chloronaphthalenes
					Plastics formulators	Methylenedianiline
					Fumigators, gasoline and fire extinguisher formulators	Methyl bromide, ethylene dibromide
					Disinfectant, fumigant, synthetic resin formulators	Cresol
584, 585	Acute or chronic renal failure (O)	P	P,T	P,T	Battery makers, plumbers, solderers	Inorganic lead
					Electrolytic processes, arsenical ore smelting	Arsine
					Battery makers, jewelers, dentists	Inorganic mercury
					Fluorocarbon formulators, fire extinguisher makers	Carbon tetrachloride
					Antifreeze manufacture	Ethylene glycol
					Chromate pigment production workers	Inorganic lead
606	Infertility, male (O)	P	P	—	Kepone formulators	Kepone
					Dibromochloropropane (DBCP) producers, formulators, and applicators	DBCP
692	Contact and allergic dermatitis (O)	P,T	P,T	—	Leather tanning, poultry dressing plants, fish packing, adhesives and sealants industry, boat building and repair	Irritants (e.g., cutting oils, phenol, solvents, acids, alkalis, detergents); allergens (e.g., nickel, chromates, formaldehyde, dyes, rubber products)

continued on next page

TABLE 20.2. *Continued*

ICD-9	Condition	A	B	C	Industry/process/occupation	Agent
733.9M[i]	Skeletal fluorosis (O)	P	P	—	Cryolite workers (grinding room) Cryolite refining workers	Cryolite (Na_3AlF_6) Cryolite (Na_3AlF_6)

Key: A = unnecessary disease; B = unnecessary disability; C = unnecessary untimely death; P = prevention; T = treatment.

[a]External causes of injury and poisoning (occupational), including accidents, are classified in the *International Classification of Diseases,* 9th revision, under the E codes.

[b]Original ICD rubric = cutaneous diseases due to other mycobacteria.

[c]From the *International Classification Diseases,* 9th revision, clinical modification (ICD-9-CM).

[d]M, modified ICD rubric.

[e]Original ICD rubric = malignant neoplasm of liver and intrahepatic bile ducts.

[f]Original ICD rubric = mononeuritis of upper limb and mononeuritis multiplex.

[g]Original ICD rubric = pneumoconiosis due to other silica or silicates.

[h]Original ICD rubric = pneumoconiosis due to other inorganic dust.

[i]Original ICD rubric = other disorders of bone and cartilage.

From Mullan RJ, Murthy LI. Occupational sentinel health events: an updated list for physician recognition and public health surveillance. *Am J Ind Med* 1991;19:775.

The occurrence of an illness in an unexpected person (e.g., lung cancer in a nonsmoker) may also stimulate the clinician to delve further into potential contributing environmental or occupational exposures. Sometimes the clinician observes an unusual disease in several patients. Searching for a connection among the cases may reveal that a work exposure is the common link. In fact, an occupational disease may be discovered that has not been previously described. Examples include the first description of occupational cancer, credited to Percival Potts, a surgeon who noted an increased frequency of scrotal cancer among chimney sweeps, which he attributed to the soot collected on their clothes and skin (29); the observation of several cases of angiosarcoma of the liver in employees of a rubber company, which led to the discovery of the causative agent vinyl chloride monomer (30); the detection of a bladder neurotoxin when a group of workers presented with urinary problems, which traced to the toxic effects of a newly introduced catalyst (31); and a high prevalence of sarcoidosis in Salem, Massachusetts ("Salem sarcoid"), linked to employees working in companies making light bulbs and eventually attributed to beryllium exposure (32). In these cases, identification of the causative agents led to better control over exposures and reduction in associated diseases.

Something elicited in the occupational/environmental history survey questions may raise the practitioner's suspicions that the patient's condition is related to an environmental or work exposure, thus prompting further questioning and gathering of information about work and home exposures.

DEFINING AND DESCRIBING THE SOURCES OF EXPOSURE

Workplace

1. List *all* significant jobs.
2. Note places of employment and products manufactured.
3. Obtain a thorough description of the operations performed by the worker on the relevant jobs, including hazardous agents, and protective measures.
4. Inquire about illnesses in other workers on the relevant jobs.

Although a brief list of job titles may be adequate as a part of the screening or initial medical examination, the practitioner evaluating potential occupational illness must take a more detailed history. In the case of latent diseases, an exposure occurring many years before the onset of symptoms may be responsible for the disorder. This point is illustrated by a 47-year-old worker with dyspnea whose roentgenogram showed bilateral pleural thickening and linear reticular parenchymal infiltrates consistent with asbestosis (33). Sixteen years earlier he worked for 9 months in a factory making cigarette filters that contained asbestos.

A worker's description of job duties may reveal potential hazards not suggested by the job title. The worker should describe the tasks he/she performs, the agents handled, and the working conditions. The characterization of hazardous exposure(s) includes the following:

1. Determining the generic name, if a chemical; describing the physical form, if a dust; or determining what form, if radiation.
2. Describing how a substance is handled: What are the operating or cleanup practices? What protective measures are used? Is a respirator worn and properly maintained? Is it the proper respirator given the type and quantity of exposure. Is protective clothing used? Is ventilation adequate? Are there engineering controls?
3. Considering the mode of entry: Is it ingested by eating at the workplace? Inhaled through generation of fumes or vapors? Chance of skin contact and skin absorption?

To characterize the health effects of a chemical substance, it is helpful to know its generic ingredients. To obtain this information, the practitioner can ask the worker or manufacturer for the Material Safety Data Sheet (MSDS) that usually lists the product's ingredients, physical properties, and some environmental protection information. The federal Chemical Hazard Communication Standard (29 CFO 1910.1200) and various state "right to know" laws (34) require that the employer provide employees with detailed information about hazardous chemicals used in the workplace. In general, the worker should be taught about the hazards of certain materials and properly trained in safe work practices. The standard stipulates that the employer must respond to an employee's request for an MSDS within 72 hours. Poison control centers are reliable resources for toxicologic information on many toxins and often can identify the generic name of many trade substances. Once the generic name is known, more information can be found from toxin-oriented texts (35), and by searching the Web and performing literature searches.

The clinician can also obtain more information about the type of hazardous exposures associated with certain jobs or work processes, by consulting references that describe hazards associated with industrial processes (36–39). Sometimes the worker may not have all the specific information concerning the exposures. The practitioner can also ask the patient about contacting the plant physician, manager, or union official to obtain more information, and/or requesting an evaluation by a governmental or private agency. It is frequently very useful to obtain and review any industrial hygiene or air quality evaluations that may have already been performed.

Home Surroundings

The routine survey questions may suggest that the symptoms relate to hazardous materials or conditions in the home. Possible internal sources of hazards in the home environment include household chemicals and pesticides, performance of certain hobbies (40), presence of biologic contamination (41,42), faulty heating system, water and food contamination, and transport of toxic dust or chemicals into the home on work clothes. Due to inadequate labeling, home residents may be inadvertently exposed to hazardous chemicals in aerosol sprays, cleaning fluids, disinfectants, or insecticides (Table 20.3). Methylene chloride, for example, is a frequent component of many household products, such as paint strippers. Rust removers may contain hydrofluoric acid, which can produce deep penetrating burns on skin contact. Without proper handling instructions, people may unsuspectingly develop a variety of symptoms and health problems from the use of these materials. Even mild exposure to certain materials causes allergic reactions in susceptible persons. Dangerous situations may arise when two substances are mixed to produce a more potent cleaning agent. Mixing ammonia and sodium hypochlorite (bleach), for example, can lead to the generation of chloramine gas (43), which in some cases can cause toxic pneumonitis and/or asthma.

The growth and diversification of hobbies may involve the use of various hazardous substances (40), which are then introduced into the household (Table 20.4). If a home studio is poorly ventilated and unkempt, all family members may be exposed to toxic substances.

Concerns over indoor air quality in the home have grown, particularly in reaction to the increasing use of energy-saving insulation, frequently installed without adequate ventilation, and sometimes leading to poor air circulation and the accumulation of potentially toxic agents [e.g., carbon monoxide, volatile organic compounds (VOCs), biologic aerosols] in the air (41,42,44,45).

Dust or chemicals carried into the home on work clothes have led to excessive lead exposure in children (46) and mesothelioma in family members of asbestos workers (47).

External sources of exposures include industrial effluents emitted into the air, water, or grounds of homes. Community contamination from toxic waste sites has been a growing public health concern. Some

TABLE 20.3. *Examples of common dangerous household products*

Product	Potentially hazardous agents
Disinfectants	Cresol; phenol; hexachlorophene
Cleaning agents and solvents	
Bleaches	Sodium hypochlorite (Clorox)
Window cleaner	Ammonia
Carpet cleaner	Ammonia, turpentine, naphthalene: 1.1.1-trichloroethane
Oven and drain cleaners	Potassium hydroxide, sodium hydroxide
Dry cleaning fluids, spot removers	1.1.1-Trichloroethane, perchlorethylene, petroleum distillates
Paint and varnish solvents	Turpentine, xylene, toluene, methanol, methylene, chloride, acetone
Pesticides	Malathion, dichlorvos, carbaryl, methoxychlor
Emissions from heating and cooling devices	
Gas stove pilot light	Nitrogen oxides
Indoor use of charcoal grill	Carbon monoxide
Leaks from refrigerator or air conditioning cooling systems	Freon
Microwave ovens	Microwave radiation
Sun lamps	Ultraviolet radiation

From Goldman RH, Peters JM. The occupational and environmental health history. *JAMA* 1981;246:2831. © 1981, American Medical Association.

TABLE 20.4. *Examples of hazards in hobbies*

Activity	Potential hazard
Painting	Toxic pigments, e.g., arsenic (emerald green), cadmium, chromium, lead, mercury; acrylic emulsions, solvents
Ceramics	
Raw materials	Colors and glazes containing barium carbonate; lead, chromium, uranium, cadmium
Gas-fired kilns	Carbon monoxide
Sculpture and casting	
Grinding silica-containing stone	Silica (silicon dioxide)
Serpentine rock with asbestos	Asbestos
Woodworking	Wood dust
Metal casting	Metal fume, sand (silica) from molding, binders, or phenol formaldehyde or urea formaldehyde
Welding	Metal fume, ultraviolet light exposure, welding fumes, carbon dioxide, carbon monoxide, nitrogen dioxide, ozone, or phosgene (if solvents nearby)
Plastics	Monomers released during heating (polyvinyl chloride), methyl methacrylate, acrylic glues, polyurethane (toluene 2,4-diisocyanate), polystyrene (methyl chloride release), fiber glass, polyester, or epoxy resins
Woodworking	Solvents, especially methylene chloride
Photography	
Developer	Hydroquinone, metal
Stop bath	Weak acetic acid
Stop hardener	Potassium chrome alum (chromium)
Fixer	Sodium sulfite, acetic acid, sulfuric acid
Hardeners and stabilizers	Formaldehyde

From Goldman RH, Peters JM. The occupational and environmental health history. *JAMA* 1981;246:2831. © 1981, American Medical Association.

prominent examples of environmental contamination that have aroused concern include polybrominated biphenyls in Michigan, toxic wastes at Love Canal, and arsenic in Bangladesh. Affected persons usually present to their local physician with their health complaints. When concerned about exposures from external sources, the clinician might inquire whether similar symptoms have occurred in neighbors, the location of the home (near a factory, construction area, or hazardous waste site?), sources of water supply and possibilities for contamination, or any noticeable changes in the neighborhood air or water quality. On rare occasions, sudden environmental disaster occurs, such as railroad or truck collisions, factory fires, or explosions that release toxic materials into the community. Both immediate health problems and delayed effects may develop.

Even when evaluating a presumed occupational health problem, a good history concerning home exposures is essential. For example, in the investigation of elevated blood lead level in a foundry worker, one might learn that a home renovation project involved removal of lead paint, which could be another source of lead exposure.

QUANTIFYING EXPOSURES

Once potential exposures have been identified, the next question is whether or not exposure has actually occurred, and if so to what degree. Documenting and quantifying exposures can involve performing biologic monitoring tests of the affected person as well as evaluating the work or environmental site. Within the office setting the patient can be tested for evidence of exposure in body fluids (biologic monitoring) or of adverse health effects upon target organs. The practitioner must know what agent to look for, the desirable test medium (urine, blood, hair, tissue), appropriate timing, and influences upon test results (48). For example, blood carboxyhemoglobin, a measure of exposure to carbon monoxide, should be performed as soon as possible after exposure since the half-life of carbon monoxide in the body is approximately 4 hours when breathing room air. Urine arsenic is a good marker for recent (but not past) exposure since arsenic is excreted rapidly in the urine within a few days. But recent consumption of seafood can lead to increases in total urine arsenic due to the contribution of nontoxic forms of organified arsenic, thereby leading to mistaken interpretations of elevated arsenic levels. Some chemicals are detected by measurement of metabolites, as in the case of the solvent toluene, which can be assessed with urine metabolites hippuric acid, benzoic acid, and o-cresol. Hair analysis performed by commercial laboratories for multiple toxins and elements have been found to be of poor reliability and accuracy, and have little applicability in most clinical settings (49,50).

Laboratory tests may be performed to look for toxic effects or end-organ damage. As an example, a blood lead concentration could be ordered to assess exposure, and blood urea nitrogen (BUN) and creatinine to look for effects upon the kidneys. Pulmonary function tests and a chest radiograph could assess the effects of past asbestos exposure on the lungs.

It is also important to consider whether the exposed person is particularly vulnerable to the particular exposure. A person with renal disease, for example, might accumulate higher levels of lead than expected secondary to decreased capacity for renal excretion. Children are generally more vulnerable than adults to the effects of toxicants (51).

It is usually important to get exposure information from the environmental location as well, which may involve air sampling, surface samples, water and soil analyses, etc. Sometimes these evaluations can be done privately by certified industrial hygienists and consultants, and in other circumstances through the relevant governmental agencies. These environmental assessments are not only important for diagnosis, but also for planning interventions and prevention of further problems.

FURTHER FOLLOW-UP AND CONSULTATIONS

With exposure data in hand, the clinician can go on to determine if the symptoms and medical findings in the particular patient are consistent with the health effects and time course of toxicity associated with a particular hazardous exposure. In some cases, the correlation between exposure levels (in the environment or the body) and health effects is good, and in other cases poor. Lead, for example, can be measured in air (micrograms per cubic meter) with a reasonable correlation between air levels and blood leads measured in exposed individuals. Although there is considerable individual variation, there is a general correlation between lead exposure and response: in adults, there are usually little or no clinical effects with blood leads below 40 μ/dL; gastrointestinal and cognitive symptoms can appear with levels of 50 μ/dL and above; and anemia seen with levels above 80 μ/dL. In contrast, manganese [of potential importance since an organic form of manganese, methylcyclopentadienyl manganese tricarbonyl (MMT), has recently been approved as a gasoline additive] levels measured in the air are poorly correlated with measurement in the blood. In addition, blood levels of manganese do not correlate well with the appearance of the adverse side effects of manic-depressive symptoms and parkinsonism.

To whom can the practitioner turn for additional consultation and potential intervention? At the local level, state public health or labor departments often have the ability to evaluate work sites. The Occupational Safety and Health Administration (OSHA) performs work-site inspections routinely on a priority basis or at the request of a current worker or management. In some cases, fines may be levied if OSHA standards are violated. Other consultative sources include academically affiliated occupational health clinics *(www.aoec.org)* and worker education groups such as the Coalition for Occupational Safety and Health (COSH) groups. The National Institute for Occupational Safety and Health (NIOSH) in Cincinnati, Ohio, can perform health hazard evaluations (HHEs) of workers and work sites in order to detect work-related health problems. Various government agencies such as NIOSH, the Agency for Toxic Substance Disease Registry (ATSDR), the Environmental Protection Agency (EPA), and their respective Web sites can also provide the practitioner with toxicologic and therapeutic information, published materials on various hazards, and recommendations for further medical care. Experts from any of these sources can investigate the problem further and suggest measures to prevent further exposure or illness in workers at the job site. Industrial hygienists from private consulting groups or from workers' compensation carriers can conduct work-site air monitoring and provide plans for remediating the problems.

For job-related injuries, the practitioner can also help an affected worker obtain workers' compensation when justified (see Chapter 18). The definition of "job related" may vary by state, but usually implies that work responsibilities precipitated, hastened, aggravated, or contributed to the injury or illness. Workers' compensation provides benefits for work time lost, permanent disability, medical care expenses, and rehabilitation. The practitioner should become familiar with the state regulations related to workers' compensation through the medical society or department of health or labor.

SUMMARY

The identification of work- or environmentally related disease is an important task for all practitioners. Thousands of chemical substances are commonly used in industry, and several hundred new substances are introduced to industrial processes each year. Unpredicted health hazards from new processes continue to emerge, and well-known toxins such as lead and certain solvents still escape surveillance and control. Equipped with an awareness and the approach outlined in this chapter, the practitioner can play an important role in the detection and prevention of occupational and environmental diseases.

REFERENCES

1. Steward RD, Hake CL. Paint-remover hazard. *JAMA* 1976;235:398.
2. Allred EN, Bleecker ER, Chaitman BR, et al. Short term effects of carbon monoxide exposure on the exercise performance of subjects with coronary artery disease. *N Engl J Med* 1989;321:1426–1432.
3. Sheps DS, Herbst MC, Hinderliter AL, et al. Production of arrhythmias by elevated carboxyhemoglobin in patients with coronary artery disease. *Ann Intern Med* 1990;113:343–351.
4. Bureau of Labor Statistics. *Summary: workplace injuries and illnesses in 2000.* U.S. Department of Labor, news release, 2001.
5. Leigh JP, Markowitz SB, Fahs M, et al. Occupational injury and illness in the United States: estimates of costs, morbidity, and mortality. *Arch Intern Med* 1997;157: 1557–1568.
6. Milton DK, Solomon GM, Rosiello RA, et al. Risk and incidence of asthma attributable to occupational exposure among HMO members. *Am J Ind Med* 1998;33: 1–10.
7. Dockery DW, III CAP, Xu X, et al. An association between air pollution and mortality in six U.S. cities. *N Engl J Med* 1993;329:1753–1759.
8. Samet JM, Dominici F, Curriero FC, et al. Fine particulate air pollution and mortality in 20 U.S. cities. *N Engl J Med* 2000;343:1742–1750.
9. McConnell R, Berhane K, Gilliand F, et al. Asthma in exercising children exposed to ozone: a cohort study. *Lancet* 2002;359:386–391.
10. Rosenstreich DL, Eggleston P, Kattan M, et al. The role of cockroach allergy and exposure to cockroach allergen in causing morbidity among inner-city children with asthma. *N Engl J Med* 1997;336:1356–1363.
11. Chan-Yeung M, Malo J-L. Occupational asthma. *N Engl J Med* 1995;333:107–112.
12. Anonymous. Asthma—United States, 1982–1992. *MMWR* 1995;43:952–955.
13. Levy BS. The teaching of occupational health in United States medical schools: five-year follow-up of an initial survey. *Am J Public Health* 1985;1985:79–81.
14. Institute of Medicine. *Role of the primary care physician in occupational and environmental medicine.* Washington, DC: National Academy Press, 1988.
15. Menzies D, Bourbeau J. Building-related illnesses. *N Engl J Med* 1997;337:1524–1531.
16. Landrigan PJ, Baker DB. The recognition and control of occupational disease. *JAMA* 1991;266:676–680.
17. Cullen MR, Cherniack MG, Rosenstock L. Occupational medicine. *N Engl J Med* 1990;332:594.
18. Cullen MR, Cherniack MG, Rosenstock L. Occupational medicine II. *N Engl J Med* 1990;332:675.
19. Beckett WS. Occupational respiratory diseases. *N Engl J Med* 2000;342:406.
20. LaDou J. *Occupational and environmental medicine.* Stamford: Appleton and Lange, 1997:845.
21. Levy BS, Wegman DH. *Occupational health: recognizing and preventing work-related illnesses.* Philadelphia: Lippincott Williams & Wilkins, 2000:842.
22. Rom W. *Environmental and occupational medicine.* Philadelphia: Lippincott–Raven, 1998.
23. Goldman RH, Peters JM. The occupational and environmental health history. *JAMA* 1981;246:2831–2836.
24. ATSDR. *Case studies in environmental medicine: taking an exposure history.* Atlanta: Agency for Toxic Substances and Disease Registry, U.S. Department of Health and Human Services, 2000:63.
25. Feldman RG. Urban lead mining: lead intoxication among deleaders. *N Engl J Med* 1978;298:1143.
26. Aronow WS, et al. Effect of freeway travel in angina pectoris. *Ann Intern Med* 1972;77:669.
27. Rutstein DD, Mullan RJ, Frazier TM, et al. Sentinel health events (occupational): a basis for physician recognition and public health surveillance. *Am J Public Health* 1983;73:1054–1062.
28. Mullan RJ, Murphy LI. Occupational sentinel health events: an updated list for physician recognition and public health surveillance. *Am J Ind Med* 1991;19:775–799.
29. Potts P. Chirurgical observations relative to the cataract, polypus of the nose, the cancer of the scrotum, the different kinds of ruptures and the mortification of the toes and feet. *Natl Cancer Inst Monogr* 1963;10:7.
30. Creech JL, Johnson MN. Angiosarcoma of liver in the manufacture of polyvinyl chloride. *J Occup Med* 1974; 16:150–151.
31. Kreiss K, et al. Neurological dysfunction of the bladder in workers exposed to dimethylamino propionitrile. *JAMA* 1980;243:741.
32. Hardy H. Beryllium poisoning: lessons in man-made disease. *N Engl J Med* 1965;273:1188.
33. Goff AM, Gaensler EA. Asbestosis following brief exposure in cigarette filter manufacture. *Respiration* 1972;29:83.
34. Himmelstein JS, Frumkin H. The right to know about toxic exposures. *N Engl J Med* 1985;1985:687.
35. Hathaway GJ, Proctor NH, Hughes JP. *Chemical hazard of the workplace.* New York: Van Nostrand Reinhold, 1996:704.
36. Burgess W. *Recognition of health hazards in industry: a review of materials and processes.* New York: John Wiley & Sons, 1995.
37. Stellman MM. *Encyclopedia of occupational health and safety, vol 2: hazards.* Geneva: International Labor Office/Boyd Printing, 1997.
38. Stellman MM. *Encyclopedia of occupational health and safety, vol 3: industries and occupations.* Geneva: International Labor Office/Boyd Printing, 1997.
39. Sullivan JB, Krieger GR. *Clinical environmental health*

and toxic exposures. Philadelphia: Lippincott Williams & Wilkins, 2001:1323.
40. Duvall K, Hinkamp D. Health hazards in the arts. *Occup Med State of the Art Rev* 2001;16(4):535–702.
41. Seltzer JM. Biologic contaminants. *Occup Med State of the Art Rev* 1995;10:1–25.
42. Burge HA. Aerobiology of the indoor environment. *Occup Med State of the Art Rev* 1995;10:27–40.
43. Reisz GR, Gammon RS. Toxic pneumonitis from mixing household cleaners. *Chest* 1986;89:49.
44. Samet JM, Warbury MC, Spengler JD. State of the art: health effects and sources of indoor air pollution. Part I. *Am Rev Respir Dis* 1987;136:1486–1508.
45. Samet JM, Warbury MC, Spengler JD. State of the art: health effects and sources of indoor air pollution. Part II. *Am Rev Respir Dis* 1988;137:221–242.
46. Anonymous. Occupational and take-home lead poisoning associated with restoring chemically stripped furniture—California, 1998. *MMWR* 2001;50:246–248.
47. Anderson H, et al. Household contact asbestos neoplastic risk. *Ann NY Acad Sci* 1976;271:311.
48. Lauwerys RR, Hoet P. Industrial chemical exposure—guidelines for biological monitoring. Boca Raton: Lewis, 2001:638.
49. Steindel SJ, Howanitz PJ. The uncertainty of hair analysis for trace metals. *JAMA* 2001;285:83–85.
50. Kales SN, Goldman RH. Mercury exposure: current concepts, controversies, and a clinic's experience. *J Occup Environ Med* 2002;44:143–154.
51. Quang LS, Woolf AD. Addressing specific populations: children's unique vulnerabilities to environmental exposures. *Environ Epidemiol Toxicol* 2000;2:79–90.

21

Occupational Pulmonary Disease

Ian A. Greaves

Occupational lung disorders have been recognized for nearly three millennia. Silicosis, for example, was known by ancient Egyptians as a disease of stone cutters and quarry workers, and there was an attempt to prevent the disease by using crude masks to reduce dust exposures. Hippocrates (c. 400 B.C.), in his treatise *Air, Water, and Places,* touched on a number of work-related respiratory disorders. Galen (150 A.D.) alluded to the poisonous atmosphere of sulfur mines. Agricola published a text, *De Re Metallica* (1556), on the hazards of mining. The pioneering Italian physician, Bernadino Ramazzini, in the early 18th century documented a long list of occupations that were associated with adverse respiratory effects, many of which were included in his classic monograph *De Morbis Artificum Diatriba* (1713). The British physician Thackray (1831) was the first to study the dusty trades in modern times, and he clearly described silicosis in sandstone workers, noting that many died before they reached the age of 40.

Awareness of these problems for many centuries has not eliminated them, however. Today, work-related pulmonary disorders still rank among the top ten causes of occupational disability and death in industrialized countries, and are even more severe in many developing nations.

WHAT IS AN OCCUPATIONAL LUNG DISORDER?

An occupational lung disorder can be defined as an acute or chronic lung condition that arises, at least partly, from the inhalation of an airborne agent in the workplace. This definition includes lung diseases that are caused exclusively by workplace exposures, as well as conditions such as asthma that may predate workplace exposures but are exacerbated by them. Broadly speaking, occupational lung disorders fall into five major categories:

1. The pneumoconioses or "dust-related" diseases
2. Irritant reactions
3. Asthmatic responses
4. Hypersensitivity disorders
5. Malignancies

The rates of occurrence of these occupational lung disorders are poorly documented. Data based on workers' compensation claims underestimate the true incidence of many of these disorders; often fewer than 5% of chronic occupational lung diseases are identified as work related, while occupational asthma is probably recognized even less frequently. Occupational lung cancers and mesothelioma are considered only briefly in this chapter, and are considered in more detail in Chapter 23.

DIAGNOSIS OF OCCUPATIONAL LUNG DISEASES

The accurate diagnosis of an occupational cause for lung disease is important for three main reasons.

First, reduction in an individual's exposure to a particular agent may lead to clinical improvement or to arrest of the disease process. Cessation of exposure is most likely to benefit patients with potentially reversible diseases (such as those due to irritant agents, asthma, or other hypersensitivity reactions); reduction or elimination of exposures may not help individuals with one of the pneumoconioses because these disorders are chronic, irreversible, and can progress after cessation of exposure. Second, an accurate diagnosis of the work-relatedness of disease is important for the just and fair financial compensation to the patients for their disability (see Chapter 18).

Finally, an accurate diagnosis may lead to the recognition and prevention of disease among other workers exposed to the same agent.

Patient Evaluation

A physician of first contact is the most likely person to make the diagnosis of many occupational lung diseases, but such a diagnosis can only be made if a physician is in the habit of asking patients about their work. The most important reason for not diagnosing a work-related illness is failing to consider the patient's occupation.

History

Taking an occupational history is described in Chapter 20. Of particular relevance to establishing a work-related cause for lung disease is the *temporal relationship of symptoms to work.* For diseases that cause chronic progressive disability (such as advanced silicosis, asbestosis, or coal worker's pneumoconiosis) generally there is a history of at least 10 years of exposure to the relevant dust; even with 10 years of exposure, however, it may be 20 or more years from first exposure before evidence of a pneumoconiosis appears.

Whenever an occupational lung disease is suspected, the patient should be questioned carefully about *all* jobs (even those as far back as high school) and any relevant hobbies that may be associated with hazardous exposures (for example, arts and crafts that have exposure to toxic pigments; or pigeon-raising and exposure to avian proteins). *Parental occupation* may be relevant also; the families of asbestos workers, for example, have developed asbestos-related diseases from the asbestos dust brought home on work clothes.

More acute disorders, such as irritant responses or acute immune-mediated reactions, are more likely to be related to workplace exposures at the time symptoms first appear. With these conditions it is important to note whether symptoms are better away from work, whether symptoms are worse on any particular day of the week (such as occurs in byssinosis), and whether symptoms are associated with certain jobs or assignments. Sometimes the temporal relationships may be misleading, particularly in some patients with occupational asthma whose symptoms of cough and wheezing may actually be most marked at home during the night or in the early hours of the morning.

Another type of delayed reaction, and one that is very important to consider in the emergency room, is the inflammatory response that occurs in the airways and alveoli following acute inhalation of highly irritant agents such as chlorine, phosgene, and other potent lung irritants. Up to 48 hours after such an acute inhalation, patients may experience *toxic lung edema* with breathlessness, chest tightness, and wheezing. The clinical picture may resemble acute asthma or pulmonary edema from left heart failure.

Irritant reactions to airborne agents are generally dose-dependent and often affect a relatively large proportion of exposed people. Symptoms usually occur within minutes of first exposure. Depending on the water-solubility of the agent, lower respiratory symptoms will be accompanied by eye, nose, and throat irritation; agents having low water-solubility have a greater tendency to affect the deeper lung architecture. Upper respiratory symptoms (allergic rhinitis) may be prominent in patients with occupational asthma.

Information that other workers in the same area or doing similar jobs have been affected similarly is supportive of a work-related etiology. Other workers are more likely to be affected when the condition is dose-dependent (such as an irritant effect or one of the pneumoconioses) than when a degree of hypersensitivity is required (such as for asthma, hypersensitivity pneumonitis, or chronic beryllium disease).

Physical Examination

The findings on physical examination of occupational lung diseases are similar to corresponding nonoccupational disorders. Several of the pneumoconioses, notably simple silicosis or coal worker's pneumoconiosis, may have no abnormal features on examination of the respiratory system. In contrast, the earliest, and sometimes only, clinical finding in mild asbestosis may be fine inspiratory rales at the lung bases. Also, inspiratory rales or rhonchi may be the only abnormal finding following an acute toxic inhalation, and these findings should alert the physician to the possibility of acute lung edema.

No examination of the respiratory system is complete without inspection of the upper airways. Mucosal inflammation is frequently present in the nose, throat, and conjunctivae of workers exposed to irritant gases and fumes, and similar responses can be seen in some hypersensitivity reactions. There are no features of these responses, however, to point exclusively to an occupational etiology.

Laboratory Evaluation

A chest radiograph and simple spirometry are essential to any assessment of occupational lung disease, and both tests should be obtained by the physician of first contact.

Chest Radiography

The chest film is the cornerstone for diagnosis and evaluation of the pneumoconioses (asbestosis, silicosis, coal worker's pneumoconiosis) and beryllium disease, and has been widely used to screen workers exposed to asbestos, silica, coal dust, and beryllium for evidence of lung disease. The chest radiograph is also useful in the diagnosis of hypersensitivity pneumonitides (such as farmer's lung, bird fancier's lung), but of relatively little value in the assessment of occupational asthma.

A standard, clinical interpretation of chest films by a qualified radiologist is adequate for most clinical purposes. When any of the pneumoconioses, asbestos-related pleural disease, or beryllium disease is suspected, however, the chest films should be read according to the classification that has been developed by the International Labor Office (ILO) of the World Health Organization (1). Only radiologists and physicians who have completed special training and passed an examination supervised by the National Institute for Occupational Safety and Health (NIOSH) and by the American College of Radiology are certified to read films according to the ILO classification. These specialists are called *B-readers*.

The standard technique that B-readers use to evaluate chest films is a semiquantitative method for determining the nature, size, and extent of radiographic opacities observed in the lung fields. Additions to the ILO criteria allow grading of pleural shadows also. An important feature of the ILO system is the provision of a standard series of graded radiographs against which a B-reader judges the degree of abnormality present. This approach can be used to classify radiographic changes at a single point in time, or to quantify changes that occur over time. One of the major applications of the ILO system has been in epidemiologic studies of the pneumoconioses.

The intra- and interobserver variability of B-readers in reading chest films has been established (2,3). When presented with the same films on separate occasions, most B-readers show high agreement in their readings at different times; the greatest intraobserver variability is seen with mild abnormalities, particularly with respect to pleural changes and small, irregular parenchymal densities. When the same chest radiographs are read by different B-readers, it is apparent that the experts can disagree substantially. As might be expected, interobserver variability is also greatest for films showing minimal parenchymal or mild pleural changes.

Although chest radiographs can demonstrate radiodense opacities in the lungs, such opacities may not indicate appreciable impairment of lung function or disability of the patient. Uncomplicated forms of silicosis or coal worker's pneumoconiosis typically have scattered, small, rounded opacities visible on the chest radiograph, but lung function is usually well preserved. Also, some inhaled agents (such as particles of iron oxide or barium salts) can produce striking radiographic opacities in the lung fields, but these are simply depositional changes caused by the retention of radiodense particles and do not reflect lung fibrosis or impairment of function.

Lung Function Tests

All patients suspected of having an occupational lung disease should, as a minimum investigation, have ventilatory function tests. Spirometers are now readily available in physician's offices and hospital clinics, while any well-equipped company medical clinic should have a high-quality machine that at least meets the performance standards proposed by NIOSH that have been incorporated into several workplace standards of the U.S. Occupational Safety and Health Administration (OSHA). All spirometers should provide an adequate written record of forced expiratory volumes.

A pneumotachograph is an alternative instrument to the conventional, volume-measuring, bell or bellows spirometer. The pneumotachograph measures flow by recording a pressure drop across a fine metal screen as air passes through; by electronically integrating airflow over time, this instrument creates a volume-time curve similar to the output of a conventional spirometer. Another way of graphing spirometry is the flow-volume curve, in which flow is plotted against lung volume and flows are reported at 25%, 50%, and 75% of the forced vital capacity (Fig. 21.1).

Measurements of the forced expiratory volume in 1 second (FEV_1) and of the forced vital capacity (FVC) are within the capabilities of any physician, nurse practitioner, or nurse. Care is required, however, in obtaining technically satisfactory efforts from the subject. A procedures manual (4) for performing spirometry has been prepared by NIOSH to meet the requirements of the OSHA Cotton Dust Standard, and many laboratories offer spirometry training that has been approved by NIOSH. Another excellent account of spirometry requirements appears in the American

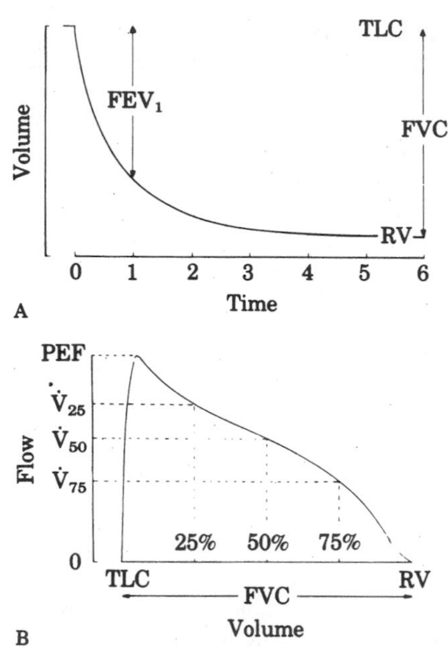

FIG. 21.1. Volume-time (upper tracing) and flow-volume (lower tracing) curves depicting a maximum forced expiratory maneuver. Total lung capacity (TLC) and residual volume (RV) are the beginning and end points, respectively, of a forced vital capacity (FVC). The forced expiratory volume of gas exhaled in 1 second (FEV_1) can be expressed as a ratio (percentage) of the FVC to yield the forced expiratory ratio (FEV_1/FVC%). Peak expiratory flow (PEF) and flows (V) at 25%, 50%, and 75% of the FVC are often derived to describe the relationship of flow to lung volume. Units: volume (liters), time (seconds), flow (liters per second).

Thoracic Society's (ATS) Epidemiology Standardization Project (5).

An important feature of spirometry is *repeatability* of the test in a given individual. In more than 95% of people without lung disease, the two largest values for FEV_1 agree within 200 mL or 5% of the maximum value, and the two largest values for FVC agree similarly. A volume of 200 mL or 5% of the maximum value (whichever is the larger volume) has been used as a test criterion for the validity of the data; tests falling outside this range might represent submaximal efforts and are considered of doubtful value. Patients with respiratory impairment, however, can have difficulty repeating their tests satisfactorily and some judgment is required to assess whether the results in such cases are valid. The opinion of a pulmonary specialist and additional lung function tests that are less effort-dependent may resolve whether the spirometry data are accurate and whether significant respiratory impairment is present.

Respiratory impairment is assigned primarily in terms of abnormal spirometry. By convention, ventilatory abnormalities are described either as being *obstructive* (defined as an abnormally decreased FEV_1 and a decreased FEV_1/FVC ratio) or *restrictive* (an abnormally decreased FVC, with a well preserved FEV_1/FVC ratio). These are purely descriptive terms to imply, respectively, abnormal limitation of airflow from the lungs or a decrease in the number of functioning lung units. Confusion arises, however, when the FEV_1 and FVC are both decreased in a particular patient. In severe asthma, for example, the FEV_1 and FVC are each decreased and the FEV_1/FVC ratio may be mildly decreased. The tendency to describe this as a "combined obstructive-restrictive disorder" should be discouraged; the decrease in FVC in this case is due primarily to premature airway closure during a forced expiration, and is thus part of the overall obstructive disorder. In some diseases, such as conglomerate silicosis, there may indeed be extensive lung fibrosis and airway disease that results in a true, mixed obstructive-restrictive disorder and the term has a sensible meaning in such cases. The term *restrictive disorder* should be reserved for conditions in which there is an acute or chronic loss of functioning alveoli resulting from a parenchymal lung disease (such as pneumonitis, alveolar edema, or lung fibrosis).

Important features of evaluating spirometry are appropriate prediction equations for normal values. An excellent account of normal ventilatory function, and the selection of appropriate normal values for assessing an individual's tests has been published by the ATS (6). Typically, predicted values for FEV_1 and FVC are obtained from a reference group (usually nonsmoking healthy subjects from the general population) and are based on sex, age, and height. There have been several excellent studies of healthy subjects in the United States (5). Perhaps the most representative of these studies involved 8,432 adults from six major cities in the U.S. (7); findings from this group are very similar to the earlier equations published by Knudson and his colleagues (8) that have been used widely for many years. The American Medical Association (9) has recommended the prediction equations of Crapo and co-workers (10), but these equations yield predicted values that are systematically higher than values obtained from other

U.S. population studies, perhaps because Crapo's measurements were obtained at an altitude of 1,400 m (6). The prediction equations of Crapo thus overestimate the abnormality of lung function in many patients and are not recommended.

Most prediction equations for lung function are derived for white Caucasians. Studies among African-Americans have been few and have suffered from small numbers. In practice, predicted values for African-Americans are obtained by multiplying the respective predicted value for white Caucasians by a value between 0.85 and 0.88. For workers, a racial correction factor of 0.87 has been satisfactory for most purposes (6,7). Correction factors are not applied routinely for Hispanics or Asians, whose predicted lung function is generally similar to white Caucasians. The different prediction equations for African-Americans seems to relate to differences in the ratio of upper to lower body size. Upper (symphysis pubis to crown) and lower (symphysis pubis to heel) body segments are approximately equal in most races, but for several African races the lower body segment is longer, on average, than the upper body segment. Thus, for a given standing height, African-Americans often have a smaller upper body segment and therefore a smaller chest cavity, resulting in smaller lungs for a given height and the need to decrease their predicted lung volumes by about 13%.

Evaluation of individuals' lung function has been reviewed critically by the ATS (6). The most common method for expressing lung function relative to the predicted value is as a percentage. Convention dictates that a value of 80% predicted is the cutoff for an abnormal result. Population studies confirm that the standard deviations around the mean predicted values for FEV_1 and FVC are each about 9% to 10% of predicted, so that 80% of predicted is approximately the lower 95% confidence limit for the percent-predicted values. Other lung function tests—including flows at specific lung volumes and the diffusing capacity for carbon monoxide—generally have larger standard deviations, and therefore the use of 80% predicted as their lower 95% confidence limit is not justified. For example, measurements of the carbon monoxide diffusing capacity (gas transfer factor) have a standard deviation of about 20% predicted, and therefore the lower 95% confidence limit is approximately 60% of the mean predicted value.

The practice of using percent-predicted values to assess impairment is so entrenched clinically that it is unlikely to change quickly. This approach, however, can be shown to overestimate lung function abnormality in older and short people, and to underestimate abnormality in younger and tall people. Stated another way, the percent-predicted approach to assessing pulmonary impairment is biased with respect to age and height (5,6). There are sound statistical reasons for using instead the absolute difference between observed and predicted values (6), or the number of standard deviations (z-score) an individual lies from his or her respective mean predicted value (5); recent guidelines published by the American Medical Association have recommended the use of absolute changes or z-scores instead of percent predicted.

Airway Challenge Testing

Bronchial provocation tests are particularly useful when assessing patients with possible occupational asthma. *Nonspecific airway challenge tests* determine whether an individual's airways are unusually "reactive" to a nonspecific bronchoconstrictor stimulus. The most frequently used nonspecific stimuli are either pharmacologic agents (for example, methacholine, histamine) administered by nebulized aerosol; eucapneic hyperventilation of subfreezing dry air (cold air challenge); or submaximal exercise for 6 to 8 minutes. There is fairly close agreement between these various tests of airway reactivity within a given subject.

In occupational settings, a dose-response curve to inhaled methacholine has been used most commonly to assess nonspecific airway reactivity. The results of methacholine challenge are expressed as the inhaled concentration that provokes a 20% decrease in FEV_1 from the baseline level (PC_{20}). The other tests of airway reactivity are less well standardized but have been used in clinical and epidemiologic studies.

Specific airway provocation tests involve exposure of the subject to the agent(s) thought to cause asthma. These tests can be performed in the laboratory or at the work site. The relative merits of where the tests are performed are discussed below (see Occupational Asthma). Specific provocation tests are time-consuming and expensive to perform, and should be undertaken by experienced personnel who have adequate resuscitation equipment immediately on hand. Many industrial agents have "late" asthmatic effects, usually occurring 5 to 8 hours (and up to 24 hours) after exposure, and so it is important to observe the subject's lung function over at least a 24-hour period.

The value of nonspecific tests of airway reactivity lies in the detection of airway hyperreactivity in someone who has normal lung function, or who has mildly abnormal function with little response to a bronchodilator. The demonstration of airway hyperreactivity in such a person suggests an underlying asthmatic disorder, which aids in diagnosing asthma when considered in conjunction with a history of episodic cough, wheezing, chest tightness, or progressive breathlessness, especially in relation to exposure to a known allergen. Specific airway challenge tests are used to determine the etiologic agent(s) for occupational asthma, and to confirm the diagnosis for medicolegal purposes.

Bronchoscopy and Bronchoalveolar Lavage

Fiberoptic bronchoscopy and brushings are established tools for diagnosing malignancy and suspected infections (11). In occupational settings, diseases classified as "extrinsic allergic alveolitis" have been investigated similarly in an effort to recover fungi or spores and to confirm an etiologic diagnosis.

Transbronchial biopsy, another procedure applicable to fiberoptic bronchoscopy, obtains a small fragment of lung tissue for microscopy (11). While diagnosis of malignant lung disease is reasonable using such fiberoptic biopsy methods, a transbronchial biopsy specimen is sometimes too small to make a confident diagnosis of nonmalignant disease, and is subject to substantial sampling error. Occasionally a transbronchial biopsy will include a granuloma, thus confirming a type of interstitial lung disease.

In recent years, video-assisted thoracotomy (VAT) has been used increasingly in place of transbronchial biopsies to obtain lung tissue samples to aid in the diagnosis of patients with diffuse parenchymal disease. Larger samples can be obtained using VAT, with the result that less sampling error and improved diagnostic accuracy might be expected with this method.

Bronchoalveolar lavage (BAL), with recovery of cells from the airways and alveoli, is an investigative tool that has gained increasing popularity over the last 25 years. Although there are some problems when using this approach for diagnostic purposes, the technique is now well standardized and has general acceptance (11). One problem with BAL is the nonspecific nature of many findings in terms of cell counts, protein levels, and enzymes present in lavage fluid. Nevertheless, two occupational settings do seem to have relatively specific BAL findings: chronic beryllium disease and extrinsic allergic alveolitis. In chronic beryllium disease, lymphocytes obtained by BAL can be stimulated in vitro by beryllium salts; lymphocyte transformation in response to beryllium stimulation is an indicator of sensitization to beryllium. In extrinsic allergic alveolitis, BAL characteristically shows a high proportion of suppresser T-lymphocytes.

Immunologic Tests

Immune-mediated occupational lung disorders fall into two main categories: those that cause asthma, and those causing extrinsic allergic alveolitis. The presence of specific immunoglobulin E (IgE) has been demonstrated for several causes of occupational asthma. The sensitivity and specificity of circulating antibodies are highly variable for predicting the allergic reactions occurring in the lung. Not surprisingly, there are patients who have circulating IgE to a particular allergen and who experience no asthma, and there are others who clearly have clinical asthma attributable to a particular agent but have no detectable IgE antibodies to the agent itself or to haptens formed from it.

Similarly, the measurement of circulating IgG precipitins in patients exposed to agents that cause extrinsic allergic alveolitis suffers from low sensitivity and specificity in predicting who has disease. The absence of precipitins does not exclude the diagnosis of allergic alveolitis. Recent evidence suggests that T cells have a substantial role in the pathogenesis of several forms of extrinsic allergic alveolitis. As a result, the conventional notion of these disorders being caused by circulating immune complexes may need to be modified. If a substantial component of the extrinsic allergic alveolitides were mediated by T cells, this could explain why circulating antibodies are poor indicators and predictors of disease.

The condition in which immune testing seems to have the greatest predictive value, and aids in establishing a diagnosis, is chronic beryllium disease. Lymphocytes in the peripheral blood, or obtained by BAL, from sensitized individuals undergo blastic transformation when exposed in vitro to salts of beryllium.

Finally, a rare complication of several pneumoconioses (chiefly silicosis and coal worker's pneumoconiosis, and perhaps asbestosis) occurs in association with rheumatoid arthritis or in the presence of high titers of circulating rheumatoid factor. Large necrobiotic nodules develop in the lungs and frequently cavitate to form abscesses. This disorder is termed Caplan syndrome. There is no convincing evidence that rheumatoid factor, antinuclear factor, or other autoantibodies play a role in the pathogenesis of other occupational lung diseases.

Formulating a Diagnosis

The diagnosis of a work-related lung disease depends first and foremost on the physician considering the possibility and asking patients about their work. Important clues in the history will come from temporal relationships between work and symptoms. Physical examination may contribute some signs of lung disease but will not be specific for an occupational etiology; evidence of other respiratory or skin involvement may be important in determining an environmental cause for the lung disease. Laboratory examination is necessary for an objective determination of respiratory impairment, and laboratory tests are often needed to establish an etiologic diagnosis (for example, challenge testing, immunologic changes, BAL).

Putting all this information together and arriving at a probable work-related cause for lung disease is often straightforward for clinical purposes. The medicolegal consequences of such a diagnosis are more problematic, particularly when compensation or tort liability is involved. The attending physician should not be intimidated, however, by the possible legal outcomes of a work-related diagnosis. Without an accurate diagnosis, some patients with occupational lung diseases may continue to be exposed to toxic agents and progress to severe respiratory impairment. Furthermore, without an accurate diagnosis the unsafe workplace from which a patient comes may continue to expose others to the same hazards.

COMMON OCCUPATIONAL PULMONARY DISORDERS

The Pneumoconioses

The term *pneumoconiosis* (from the Greek *pneumos,* the lung; *konios,* dust; *osis,* a state of—that is, a condition of the lungs resulting from inhaling dusts) was coined by the German pathologist Zenker in the 19th century. A more recent definition has been provided by Parkes (12): "Pneumoconiosis is defined as the non-neoplastic reaction of the lungs to inhaled mineral or organic dusts and the resultant alteration in their structure excluding asthma, bronchitis, and emphysema."

The dust diseases of the lungs are among the oldest occupational diseases known. The chief dusts causing lung problems today are silica, coal, and asbestos. In general, a pneumoconiosis resulting from exposure to one of these agents requires at least 10 to 20 years of exposure. For each of these dusts, the likelihood of developing a pneumoconiosis is proportional to both the intensity and the duration of exposure. Thus, the exposure-response curves for these agents show an effect of cumulative exposure as well as a latent period before effects appear.

The clearance of silica, coal, and asbestos from the lungs occurs very slowly (over months to years) after these agents are deposited in the lung parenchyma. Autopsy studies have shown large amounts of these dusts retained in the lungs of workers who ceased being exposed many years before their death. Thus, it is not surprising that the major dust-related diseases frequently progress in severity after cessation of exposure because a substantial dose of dust remains in the lungs to cause further pathologic changes. Another group of agents, termed *inert dusts,* deposit in the lungs and give rise to mild cellular responses. These deposits sometimes cause striking radiographic changes but are accompanied by little impairment of lung function or disability.

A brief clinical review of the classical pneumoconioses follows. The reader is encouraged to consult more comprehensive accounts in the specific texts and review articles listed below (see Further Information).

Silicosis

Silicosis is the most common pneumoconiosis worldwide and is caused by inhaling one of several forms of crystalline silica (most commonly quartz, tridymite, or cristobalite).

Silica exposures occur in a wide variety of jobs. Granite and sandstone are two important geologic sources of quartz, and people who work in mines or are involved in blasting and drilling operations are at risk of exposure to silica. Other high-risk groups include sandblasters, and foundry workers who grind the surface of iron moldings to remove sand that has been used to make the molds and as a parting agent during the molding process. Cristobalite and tridymite are produced when quartz is heated to high temperatures, and cristobalite is also produced when diatomaceous earth (a form of amorphous or non-crystalline silica) is heated.

Deposition of crystalline silica (silicon dioxide, SiO_2) in the lung parenchyma and airways causes an intense cellular reaction, with infiltration of macrophages, neutrophils, and lymphocytes. Free silica is toxic to macrophages and is cleared relatively slowly from the lungs. Nevertheless, over time, substantial amounts of silica can be found in the hilar lymph nodes of exposed workers as well as in the lung parenchyma.

The characteristic histologic lesion in the lungs and regional lymph nodes is a *granuloma* that has a central, amorphous, hyaline area surrounded by a zone of fibrosis and inflammatory cells. This lesion is termed a *silicotic nodule* and varies in size from less than a millimeter to a centimeter or more in diameter. Silicotic nodules gradually grow in size over time and as cumulative exposure increases.

Nodules 1 to 2 mm in diameter are usually sufficiently radiodense to appear on a chest x-ray. Typically, these small round opacities are more prominent in the upper and middle zones of the lungs, but over time the distribution of nodules becomes more generalized throughout the lungs. Nodules may increase rapidly in size or progress very slowly. Presumably the size and number of nodules in the lung reflect the accumulation of silica at particular sites, and this in turn depends on the rates of deposition and clearance of silica particles. Undefined host factors are probably important also in determining the cellular and fibrotic responses to a given dose.

When silicotic nodules are discrete, the condition has been termed "simple silicosis" or more precisely *chronic uncomplicated silicosis* (13). This condition can be diagnosed readily from the chest x-ray and typically occurs after at least 10 years of exposure to silica dust. Of more concern is progression of the disease to a stage of *conglomerate silicosis* (previously called progressive massive fibrosis). The latter stage results from aggregation of individual silicotic nodules into increasingly larger fibrotic masses. These masses are usually bilateral, occur mainly in the upper and middle zones of the lungs, and are several centimeters in diameter. Advanced conglomerate silicosis produces a butterfly-shaped opacity in the upper lung zones.

In circumstances of unusually high levels of silica dust exposure, acute lung disease can occur with a diffuse inflammatory response throughout the lungs and rapid progression to fibrosis. Silica flower, a very fine silica dust of high purity, has been the most frequent cause of this disorder (14). Acute silicosis resembles alveolar proteinosis, but is more fulminant than the latter and can be rapidly fatal.

Lung function is typically well preserved in workers with chronic uncomplicated silicosis. Mild abnormalities in forced expiratory flows have been reported, but these have been insufficient to cause disability. Once conglomeration occurs, however, lung function is frequently impaired, and functional deterioration may be rapid. A severe restrictive and obstructive disorder can result from the conglomerate lesions, and respiratory failure with cor pulmonale is seen in severely affected workers.

Other pulmonary effects attributable to silica exposure include inflammation and thickening of the pleura (particularly over the lung apices), an increase in risk of pulmonary tuberculosis, and an increased risk of lung cancer. Before the development of effective treatment for tuberculosis, many silica-exposed workers developed tuberculosis and died from this disease. The physician today must still be aware of the possibility of tuberculosis in silicotic workers, particularly when the chest x-ray shows a recent change at one of the apices or the abrupt appearance of an opacity elsewhere.

Chronic cough and phlegm (chronic bronchitis) are common symptoms among workers with heavy silica exposure and those who have silicosis. Phlegm production generally increases in advanced stages of silicosis; recurrent bacterial infections are common. Cavitation and chronic infection occurs occasionally in conglomerate lesions, and these infections may be tuberculous or due to anaerobic bacteria. A rare variant of silicosis occurs in patients who have rheumatoid arthritis or circulating rheumatoid factor; these patients can develop necrobiotic nodules several centimeters in diameter that frequently cavitate and become infected (Caplan syndrome).

In the last two decades there has been increasing evidence that silicosis is associated with an increased risk of lung cancer. The International Agency for Research on Cancer (15) has reviewed the evidence and concluded that silica is a type I (confirmed) human carcinogen. It is unclear, however, whether the increase in cancer risk is confined to subjects with evidence of silicosis or can occur in the absence of lung fibrosis. At this time it appears that any worker with evidence of silicotic nodules in the lungs is at increased risk of lung cancer. Presumably that risk is greater among smokers than nonsmokers, although data are not available concerning possible interactions between smoking and silica.

Because silica exposures are common and lung cancer is a serious, life-threatening condition, prudent public health policy requires that silicosis should be prevented in all its forms, even when it is confined to discrete lung nodules and lung function is well preserved. This implies reducing silica exposures substantially below the current levels occurring in many industries. Dust control methods are available to achieve very low levels of exposure, but economic costs may preclude the widespread use of such improvements, especially in some mining and ore processing operations.

Coal Worker's Pneumoconiosis (CWP)

Coal dust, which is chiefly carbon, produces a relatively mild pulmonary cellular reaction compared with silica. Unlike silica, the characteristic lesion of coal is a pinhead-sized collection of macrophages laden with black coal dust. Typically, these collections are in the vicinity of alveolar ducts and contain increased amounts of reticulin fibers. Such characteristic lesions *(macules)* are initially 1 to 2 mm in diameter, but they too may grow in size and number.

Conglomerate lesions also occur with exposure to coal dust with an outcome similar to that seen with conglomerate silicosis. Advanced CWP with conglomerate lesions is accompanied in most cases by major impairment of lung function and disability attributable to the pneumoconiosis. The factors that promote the sudden development of conglomerate CWP in some coal workers are unknown. Unlike silicosis, which usually shows an orderly progression from uncomplicated silicosis to conglomerate lesions, CWP may progress rapidly from a relatively minor degree of simple pneumoconiosis to the advanced form. The aggressive nature of CWP in some coal workers is surprising because coal is generally less fibrogenic than silica or asbestos. Immune-mediated changes have been proposed to explain the unusual susceptibility of some coal workers to conglomerate CWP, but studies have failed to confirm specific immune features in such workers.

Epidemiologic studies of autopsy data have shown an increased risk of centrilobular emphysema associated with increasing grades of CWP (16). For many years an increased risk of emphysema among coal workers was attributed to cigarette smoking. It is now apparent that coal, alone or in combination with smoking, can cause emphysema in workers with moderate to severe CWP. Because emphysema leads to airflow obstruction, an obstructive abnormality on lung function testing would be expected in workers with CWP. It is unclear, however, whether mild or minimal CWP is associated with emphysema. The presence of an obstructive pattern of lung function tests in a worker with mild CWP will therefore present some difficulty for the physician who wishes to determine the work-relatedness of that individual's condition.

Coal workers frequently have a cough and phlegm that are often accompanied by mild reductions in forced expiratory flows; these features are sometimes referred to as an "industrial bronchitis." The reductions in expiratory flow are thought to reflect either involvement of the alveolar ducts and other small airways in the lungs, or the development of centrilobular emphysema. Not all coal workers with cough and phlegm show these mild impairments of lung function, and not all who have some impairment of ventilatory function have cough and phlegm. Cough and phlegm have no causal role in the production of airflow obstruction, but the symptoms of bronchitis and the function changes may be distinct features associated with cumulative exposure to coal dust. For this reason, it is probably wise to avoid the misleading term "industrial bronchitis" when referring to respiratory impairment in coal workers.

As with silicosis, the presence of rheumatoid arthritis or circulating rheumatoid factor in association with CWP can result in large necrobiotic nodules (Caplan syndrome). Low titers of autoantibodies may be found in many patients with CWP; the significance of these titers is unknown.

Asbestosis

Asbestosis is a form of lung fibrosis of the usual interstitial type that results from inhalation of asbestos fibers. The term *asbestosis* refers only to this type of parenchymal lung disease and excludes pleural thickening or fibrosis that may accompany the parenchymal lesions. An isolated finding of pleural thickening or fibrosis does not justify the diagnosis of *pleural asbestosis,* a term that has no pathologic meaning and has caused confusion.

The interstitial fibrosis accompanying asbestos exposure is indistinguishable histologically from other forms of diffuse lung fibrosis such as idiopathic pulmonary fibrosis. The only feature that is unique to asbestosis is the presence of *asbestos bodies* in the lung tissue. Asbestos bodies comprise an asbestos fiber that has been attacked by alveolar macrophages, with the resulting deposition of proteinaceous materials and iron (derived from digestion of hemoglobin by the macrophage) on the surface of the fiber. Asbestos bodies thus stain positively with Prussian blue and other iron stains, and are often referred to as *ferruginous bodies.* Finding an asbestos body in histologic sections can be difficult, but the diagnosis is established if one can be found.

To produce interstitial fibrosis, there needs to have been exposure to substantial air concentrations (of the order of 2 fibers per milliliter or higher) for at least 10 years, and usually for more than 20 years. Asbestosis is a dose-related disease with a long latency period. Asbestos exposures have occurred in workers in many occupations, including asbestos miners and millers, pipe coverers, asbestos textile workers, various construction trades, and shipyard workers. Some relatives of these workers have developed asbestosis and other asbestos-related diseases from dust brought home on the worker's clothing.

Diagnosis of asbestosis is not as simple as silicosis or CWP. Unlike the other two disorders, mild asbestosis is more difficult to detect with a chest x-ray. The first changes are usually irregular linear densities that are seen initially at the lung bases, and increase in number, coarseness, and extent as the disease progresses. Lung function changes may precede the radiographic changes, with the most prominent early effects being a decrease in FVC and a decrease in the diffusing capacity for carbon monoxide. When other findings are normal, an important clue to possible interstitial disease is the presence of inspiratory rales at the lung bases. Although the presence of inspiratory rales is not pathognomonic of interstitial fibrosis, rales in an asbestos-exposed worker should alert the physician to the possibility of asbestosis, and to the need to monitor this individual's lung function and to obtain a chest x-ray periodically.

Other Pneumoconioses

A large number of other dusts can cause pulmonary abnormalities, including various minerals that contain different forms of silicates, as well as certain metals and their salts. Examples of silicates are kaolin and talc, each of which can cause nodular fibrosis in the lungs of exposed workers and conglomerate lesions similar to those found in advanced silicosis. Several forms of amorphous silica, such as diatomaceous earth and fibrous glass, can also cause respiratory disorders.

Diatomaceous earth is a relatively nontoxic material. The principal health concerns relate to its transformation (by heating to high temperatures, "calcining") into crystalline silica, which causes silicosis in exposed workers. Apart from being a cheap source of silica that can be used as a filler in paints and plastics, diatomaceous earth has been used as a filtering material for wine and beer.

Fibrous glass or, more generally, *man-made vitreous fibers* (MMVFs) have been used for many purposes, chiefly as insulation materials and as substitutes for asbestos. Human exposures to large fibers (such as glass wool) have been associated mainly with irritation of the skin and mucous membranes of the respiratory tract. Animal data suggest that several of the MMVFs can cause lung and pleural fibrosis, and some are carcinogenic in experimental animal models. Epidemiologic studies have indicated a relationship between exposures to certain MMVFs, mainly the group termed "refractory ceramic fibers," and radiographic abnormalities, including pleural thickening and fibrosis. Some MMVFs may also be associated with an increased risk of lung cancer, but a clear relationship has yet to be demonstrated. Data are conflicting regarding the human effects of many MMVFs, but a disturbing trend in industry has been to manufacture synthetic fibers of fine dimensions, similar in size to asbestos fibers. The refractory ceramic fibers are among the finest MMVFs, and most closely resemble asbestos. These fibers have not been in use for very long, but it appears that they have similar properties, and present similar health risks, as asbestos; exposures to these fibers need to be minimized.

Various metals and some of their salts have been shown to cause abnormalities on the chest x-ray. Tin, barium, antimony, and titanium all cause radiodense nodules that are collections of dust-filled macrophages with no fibrotic reaction. These dusts are among a group of agents that have been termed "inert dusts" because they deposit in the lungs but elicit little fibrous reaction.

Irritant Lung Reactions

Many gases, fumes, and aerosols are directly toxic to the respiratory tract, causing dose-related, acute inflammatory responses in the respiratory mucosa or lung parenchyma. The principal sites in the respiratory tract where irritant agents have the greatest effect are determined by their water solubility and particle size. Highly soluble agents dissolve readily in the secretions of the eyes, upper respiratory tract (nose, pharynx), and airways; less soluble agents exert their main effects in the peripheral, small airways and in the lung parenchyma. Particles greater than 10 μm tend to settle out in the upper respiratory tract, those 3 μm to 10 μm settle mainly in the airways, and those less than 3 μm deposit mainly in the lung parenchyma and small airways. It is important to note, however, that the "scrubbing" of inspired air by the upper respiratory tract to remove water-soluble agents and larger particles can be overwhelmed at high air concentrations.

When lung ventilation increases (as during exercise or heavy work), relatively greater deposition is likely to occur in the lower respiratory tract. This reflects less efficient scrubbing of contaminants in the upper respiratory tract, as well as a shift from predominantly nose-breathing to mouth-breathing as the ventilatory rate increases. Mouth-breathing bypasses the nose and reduces further the "scrubbing" action in the upper airways.

Examples of agents causing nonspecific irritant effects are shown in Table 21.1. Highly water-soluble gases or aerosols, such as sulfur dioxide or hydrogen chloride, characteristically produce irritant effects in

TABLE 21.1. *Characteristics of some common irritant gases and fumes*

Agent	Industrial sources and uses	Solubility in water
Ammonia	Production of fertilizers, explosives, various chemicals	High
Cadmium oxide	Jewelry making, silver soldering and brazing, smelting, art pigments	High
Hydrogen chloride	Pickling operations, chemical manufacturing, electroplating	High
Hydrogen fluoride	Etching and polishing glass, plastics manufacture, insecticide	High
Sulfur dioxide	Paper and pulp manufacture, smelting operations, chemical production, combustion of coal	High
Chlorine	Wide use in chemical industry, water purification, bleaching	Moderate
Vanadium pentoxide	Boiler scaling, chemical industry	Moderate
Mercury vapor	Gold extraction, mercury lamps	Low
Oxides of nitrogen	Chemical and fertilizer manufacture, metal processing, silage, welding, manufacture of explosives	Low
Ozone	Disinfectant, bleaching, oxidizing agent	Low
Phosgene	Production of plastics, pesticides, combustion product of chlorinated hydrocarbons	Low

the eyes, nasopharynx, and large airways. Predictably, individuals exposed to these agents may develop sore and watering eyes, sneezing, nasal discharge, coughing, phlegm, and perhaps wheezing. Airflow obstruction can occur as a result of reflex bronchoconstriction. The neural reflex pathways involve afferent nerve fibers in the vagal and glossopharyngeal nerves, and cholinergic efferent fibers in the vagal nerve. Bronchoconstriction from exposure to airway irritants is seen most commonly in asthmatics, who respond at lower air concentrations than do nonasthmatics. The effects of upper respiratory and airway irritants are usually transient and related to the period of exposure; the irritant effects usually resolve promptly on removal from exposure. Among workers, these symptoms tend to improve over weekends or during vacation periods.

Chronic exposure to an agent such as sulfur dioxide can lead to persistent symptoms of cough and phlegm that may take many weeks to resolve after cessation of exposure. Such persistent symptoms probably reflect adaptive responses, including hypertrophy and hyperplasia of mucous glands and goblet cells, that follow chronic inflammation of the airway mucosa. Another important effect of airway irritants is an increased permeability of the airway mucosa to other inhaled agents, such as fine particles, and airway irritants also cause a transient increase in nonspecific airway reactivity even in workers who are not asthmatic. The importance of increases in airway permeability and airway reactivity is unknown, but these appear to be mechanisms whereby exposure to irritant agents and exposure to other agents toxic to the lungs may result in effects greater than the sum of each agent separately; in other words these may be mechanisms by which synergy could occur between irritant agents and other toxic exposures.

Exposures to high air concentrations of water-soluble agents cause extensive inflammatory changes throughout the respiratory tract. In severe cases, this amounts to a chemical burn of the respiratory mucosa from the nasopharynx to the alveoli, and is a medical emergency. The two principal problems encountered from acute irritant toxicity are laryngeal edema (with the possibility of airway obstruction that may require a tracheotomy), and severe lung edema that may require assisted ventilation and oxygen. These serious sequelae of toxic irritants are not always apparent at the time of exposure. Indeed, it is well recognized that these potentially life-threatening outcomes of exposure may be delayed up to 24 to 48 hours after exposure. Quite commonly, individuals will present to an emergency room shortly after exposure to high levels of an irritant and be discharged reasonably well, only to return within 24 hours severely breathless and in need of urgent treatment.

Emergency room management of overexposure to irritant agents is shown in Table 21.2. It is stressed that a careful and prudent policy is to admit to the hospital for 24 to 48 hours of observation those people who appear to be healthy but have been exposed to high levels of an irritant gas, fume, or aerosol, and either have evidence of mucosal inflammation in the upper respiratory tract and conjunctivae, or have rales or rhonchi on auscultation of the chest (regardless of whether there appears to be another plausible explanation for these signs). These comments apply equally to smoke inhalation, which combines expo-

TABLE 21.2. *Principles for the management of acute pulmonary effects from inhaling irritant gases, fumes, and aerosols*

Immediately obtain arterial blood gas measurements and commence oxygen therapy if the patient has any evidence of respiratory impairment.

Take a history of likely toxic exposures from the patient or another informed person from the site of exposure. Pay particular attention to whether carbon monoxide, hydrogen sulfide, or hydrogen cyanide exposures could have occurred. Measure the blood carboxyhemoglobin level if any suspicion of CO exposure. (Commence treatment for hydrogen sulfide or hydrogen cyanide poisoning if there is any suspicion of exposure.)

Examine the eyes, nose, and pharynx for evidence of chemical or thermal burns.

Carefully auscultate the lungs for the presence of rhonchi or rales. Listen over the larynx and trachea for an inspiratory stridor, which is best heard when the subject makes a rapid inspiratory effort.

Measure baseline spirometry if the subject is capable of performing the test.

Obtain an electrocardiograph if the carboxyhemoglobin level exceeds 10% and in anyone who is over the age of 40 years or who has a history of cardiovascular disease.

Obtain a baseline chest x-ray in anybody who may have been exposed to possibly toxic levels. Although frequently normal, the chest x-ray is invaluable if the patient's condition deteriorates and early lung edema is suspected.

Admit to hospital (if only for 24–48 hours of observation) anyone who has evidence of an acute toxic effect from inhalation of an irritant agent. This includes patients with overt abnormalities on testing and those with positive signs on clinical examination of the upper or lower respiratory tract. If in any doubt about discharging patients, hold them for further observation. Those who are discharged after initial evaluation should be advised carefully to return if they feel unwell, and particularly if they develop a cough, wheeze, or breathlessness.

sures to toxic gases, fumes, and particles with the additional problem of thermal burns to the respiratory tract.

Irritant agents that are relatively insoluble in water, such as ozone, phosgene, or the oxides of nitrogen, cause slightly different effects. These agents produce few upper respiratory or airway symptoms, and manifest themselves more insidiously. Following acute severe exposures, the first symptoms are usually a headache and a cough that is triggered by taking a deep breath. A sensation of chest tightness may also be present. The major symptom from these agents, however, is progressive breathlessness attributable to toxic pneumonitis with lung edema. The fulminant condition resembles adult respiratory distress syndrome and carries a similar high mortality risk. Treatment is supportive and recovery occurs slowly. Long-term sequelae of toxic edema include lung fibrosis and occasionally bronchiolitis obliterans. The latter causes chronic irreversible airway obstruction.

Another important sequel of acute exposures to lung irritants is a condition termed "reactive airways dysfunction syndrome" (RADS) (17). Following an acute exposure to agents such as toluene diisocyanate, welding fumes, or other potent respiratory irritants, individuals may experience the onset of asthma attacks or the return of asthma after many years. Airway reactivity is increased in these patients, presumably as a result of the acute toxic insult. Persistent asthma may occur and it appears that RADS is a variant of occupational asthma. A report of 56 people exposed to a formaldehyde spill showed that 3 of 14 (21%) with high exposure developed RADS (18). This high rate of developing RADS suggests that the condition is not rare and needs to be considered whenever someone is exposed to high air levels of a respiratory irritant.

Chronic exposures to low levels of poorly soluble irritants like ozone have also been associated with adverse respiratory effects, notably chronic airflow obstruction and exacerbation of underlying chronic lung conditions. Both ozone and oxides of nitrogen are prominent components of urban air pollution, and exposures also occur in specific work settings. Epidemiologic studies suggest that the workplace hazards of intermittent exposures to high air concentrations of these agents may be more relevant to the production of respiratory impairment than chronic low-level exposures.

Occupational Asthma

Occupational asthma has been defined as "variable airway narrowing causally related to exposure in the working environment to airborne dusts, gases, vapors or fumes" (19). Considerable differences of opinion exist, however, in the interpretation of this apparently straightforward definition. A restrictive definition has been developed in Great Britain by the Industrial Injuries Advisory Council, which defines occupational asthma as a condition that "occurs after a variable period of symptomless exposure to a sensitizing agent at work" (19). Other definitions have included agents that produce bronchoconstriction by mechanisms other than immune sensitization, as well as exacerbation of preexisting asthma by workplace exposures (20).

Some occupational exposures that are known to cause asthma are shown in Table 21.3, which also provides findings for skin testing and circulating IgE antibodies for these various exposures. Van Kampen and colleagues (21) published a more recent literature review up to 1997 of occupational airway sensitizers. As noted by Banks and Wang (22), some forms of occupational asthma share characteristics with atopic or extrinsic asthma (IgE-mediated), but other forms resemble nonatopic or intrinsic asthma (independent of

TABLE 21.3. *Agents causing occupational asthma*

Agent	Industries and occupations	Skin test	Specific IgE antibodies
Vegetable dusts and woods			
Grain	Grain handlers	+	–
Flour (wheat/rye)	Millers, bakers	+	+
Coffee beans	Planters, processors	+	+
Castor beans	Oil producers		+
Tea dust	Tea workers	+	
Tobacco	Tobacco workers	+	+
Western red cedar	Saw millers, carpenters, cabinet makers, other wood workers, construction workers	+	+
California redwood		–	
Oak			–
Mahogany		–	
Colophony (pine resin)	Electronics workers		+
Gum acacia	Printers	+	
Animals, birds, shellfish			
Rats	Animal handlers, laboratory workers, veterinarians	+	
Mice		+	
Guinea pigs		+	+
Rabbits		+	
Pigeons	Pigeon breeders	+	
Chickens	Poultry workers	+	+
Turkeys	Poultry workers	+	+
Crabs	Crab processors	+	
Prawns	Prawn processors	+	+
Oysters	Oyster farmers	+	+
Enzymes			
Subtilisins	Detergent manufacture	+	+
Papain	Meat packaging	+	+
Trypsin	Pharmaceutical workers	+	+
Pepsin	Pharmaceutical workers	+	+
Metals			
Platinum and salts	Pt refining and plating	+	
Chromium salts	Tanning of leather	+/–	+
Nickel	Metal plating	+	+/–
Cobalt	Manufacture of hard metals	+	
Vanadium	Manufacture of hard metals		
Miscellaneous chemicals			
Toluene diisocyanate (TDI)	Manufacture of polyurethane foam, painters, plastics manufacture	+/–	+/–
Diphenylmethane diisocyanate (MDI)	Core makers in foundries, painters	–	+
Phthallic anhydride	Epoxy resins, plastics	+	+
Trimellitic anhydride	Epoxy resins, plastics	+	+
Formaldehyde	Hospital workers, laboratory technicians, chemical workers	–	–
Azodicarbonamide	Plastics and rubber workers	–	
Ethanolamines	Solderers, spray painters, metal machining	–	

+, positive skin test or specific IgE has been reported in affected workers, but not necessarily in all of those affected; –, no reports of a positive skin test or specific IgE antibodies among those who were tested; for many of these agents, however, only small numbers of affected individuals have been examined; +/–, conflicting data: some researchers have found a positive skin test or specific IgE, but other investigators did not.

Data derived from Chan-Yeung and Lam (20).

an IgE-mediated immune mechanism). The latter is mediated by activated T lymphocytes and is accompanied by increased numbers of eosinophils and metachromatic cells in the bronchial mucosa (22). In general, asthma associated with high molecular weight compounds often have an IgE-mediated response, but this is less common with low molecular weight compounds where T-cell–mediated responses may be more important. Atopic persons may be at special risk of asthma caused by some high molecular weight compounds, but many people without atopy can become sensitized and develop asthma in response to occupational exposures. Many times it makes little sense to exclude atopic individuals from workplaces where known sensitizing agents occur because atopy does not appear to be a major predictor for occupational asthma in many cases.

Regardless of the pathogenic mechanisms, occupational asthma is an important clinical condition, and this has become the most common work-related lung disease among workers in economically advanced countries. Estimates of the prevalence of asthma resulting from exposures in the workplace vary from about 5% to 50% of exposed individuals, depending on the particular agent. A large proportion of patients who develop asthma as adults, and many workers who experience worsening of longstanding asthma, actually have an occupational cause for their symptoms.

Several clinical features of occupational asthma need to be stressed. First, although many patients experience typical recurrent episodes of wheezing and breathlessness, in some the onset of symptoms may develop more insidiously and may not show typical acute attacks. Individuals can present with steadily increasing exertional breathlessness with evidence of an obstructive defect on spirometry that often responds incompletely (at least initially) to a bronchodilator. Second, symptoms may not be obviously work related: a sizable fraction of workers with occupational asthma experience their symptoms mainly in the evenings or at night. Also, following exposures to some occupational causes of asthma (e.g., western red cedar, toluene diisocyanate), the recovery period may take several days or weeks. As a result, improvement away from work may be seen only over weekends or during vacation. Unless the physician is aware of these diverse patterns, an occupational cause of asthma will be overlooked.

Once occupational asthma is suspected, the diagnosis involves two steps. First, it is necessary to show that the individual has asthma. The diagnosis can be confirmed either by measuring variations in lung spirometry that occur spontaneously or with treatment, or, if baseline lung function is normal, by showing that the individual has nonspecific airway hyperreactivity (see above). Second, a causal link needs to be established between workplace exposures and alterations in lung function. Sometimes there is only the patient's history to support the work-related nature of the symptoms. Whenever possible, however, direct confirmation should be obtained. Skin tests to the suspected agent(s) and the demonstration of circulating specific IgE antibodies provide evidence of sensitization to the agent(s) being tested, but the sensitivity and specificity of these tests for detecting respiratory sensitization vary greatly for different agents (20,22). Furthermore, not all agents causing occupational asthma seem to exert their effects through IgE-mediated mechanisms.

More direct methods for showing causal relationships involve bronchial challenge with the agent(s) of interest. These challenges can be conducted in the laboratory (where the level and nature of the exposures can be better controlled) or in the workplace (where the offending exposures actually occur). Lung spirometry is obtained before and after a period of exposure, and these tests should be repeated periodically over the next 24 hours to determine whether a late asthmatic response is induced (generally maximal at 5 to 8 hours after exposure). Customarily, a decrease in FEV_1 by 15% or greater of the baseline (prechallenge) value is considered a positive result. Specific bronchial provocation tests are best performed by experienced personnel in a laboratory where the nature of the exposure can be controlled and where urgent treatment can be administered promptly for an acute severe reaction.

Careful thought needs to be given to testing an individual's response to the suspected agent(s) in the workplace. The investigator must be sure that the patient is being exposed to the agent(s) of interest, and that the testing protocol is suitable. One approach has been to perform measurements of ventilatory function before and after a work shift. This is an appropriate method when the timing of exposures and responses during the work period are unknown, and it is useful for screening large groups of workers to identify possible responders, but it is inappropriate for monitoring closely an individual patient with suspected hypersensitivity. Serious reactions to industrial agents have been reported, and some agents (e.g., toluene diisocyanate) can produce severe asthma attacks in sensitized individuals at air concentrations as low as 1 part per billion. If a diagnostic challenge is performed at the work site, measurements of airway function should be obtained frequently within the first 60 minutes of exposure, and thereafter at regular intervals for at least 24 hours, or as determined by the patient's response.

A mini-Wright peak flow meter or similar portable instrument is most convenient for measuring a worker's lung function on the job. Maximum expiratory flow can be obtained at frequent intervals without taking a worker off the job. Self-testing and self-recording of the peak flow measurements can be continued at home to take into account possible late reactions that may occur away from work. Although convenient to use, such peak flow measurements may be inaccurate and should only be used to consider relative changes in lung function over short time periods; they should not be used as a substitute for regular spirometry in assessing whether an individual's ventilatory function is normal. In general, a decrease in peak flow of 20%, or a decrease in FEV_1 of 5% or greater (see OSHA's cotton dust standard, 29 CFR 1910.1000), over a working period is considered an abnormal finding and suggests work-related airflow obstruction.

Whether in the laboratory or at the work site, provocative challenge testing must be aborted and bronchodilator therapy given if the subject becomes acutely distressed, or if the peak flow or FEV_1 drops by 30% or more of the baseline value.

Once a diagnosis of occupational asthma is established, prompt job transfer to an area of no exposure is necessary. Because asthma may be precipitated in some cases by minute levels of the responsible agent(s), the sensitized worker must not work near or even pass through an area where exposure may occur. Sometimes the presence of a substance on a co-workers shoes or clothing can be sufficient to trigger an asthmatic episode. To keep a sensitized individual in an exposed job by using either intensive medication or a respirator cannot be justified on medical grounds; continued exposure could subject that individual to the risk of chronic, irreversible airway obstruction or a potential life-threatening episode of acute asthma.

Some workers with occupational asthma do not recover completely after removal from exposure. These individuals continue to experience episodes of asthma and have persistently hyperreactive airways. Individuals who become sensitized initially to an occupational exposure may go on to develop sensitivities to nonoccupational agents, or they may experience persistent airway narrowing similar to patients with intrinsic asthma.

The probability of recovery from occupational asthma appears to be greatest for those who had the least duration and intensity of exposure, and who subsequently have no further exposure to the agent (19,23). In general, if a patient with occupational asthma has ongoing or recurrent asthma after removal from the workplace, and the asthma can be attributed to initial airway sensitization by a workplace exposure (that is, to the "occupational phase" of the disease), then the current asthma can be regarded as work related for workers' compensation purposes even though that person is no longer exposed to the original sensitizing agent. In other words, if a physician believes that a person's continuing asthma (regardless of the present triggering agent) can be traced to the initial sensitizing event in the workplace, then the present condition should be considered work related.

Another disorder that resembles occupational asthma in many aspects is *byssinosis,* a disease of cotton textile workers and others who inhale cotton dust, flax, or soft hemp. Byssinosis has a characteristic clinical picture of cough and chest tightness occurring on the first day of a working week, but not on other days of the week. As the disease progresses, symptoms may extend into the week further, until eventually the worker has a chronic cough and breathlessness. Occasionally, the condition develops more insidiously; the typical "Monday cough and tightness" are absent and the patient presents with exertional breathlessness. Accompanying the acute Monday symptoms are impairment of ventilatory function that shows an obstructive defect.

The etiologic agent in cotton dust is unknown. An allergic reaction is not responsible, and the most likely causes are either a pharmacologic reaction to a compound in cotton bracts, or a reaction to endotoxin that originates from bacterial and fungal contaminants of the cotton. Whichever agent is primarily responsible for the acute symptoms and lung function changes, it is established that the agent is water-soluble and heat-labile because exposure of byssinotic workers to steamed raw cotton eliminates their respiratory responses.

Hypersensitivity Pneumonitis (Extrinsic Allergic Alveolitis)

The prototype of this group of disorders is *farmer's lung,* a condition that resembles recurrent pneumonia. Fungi that grow in wet hay cause this disorder. Exposures occur when farmers come to use the moldy hay and in the process generate enormous air concentrations of the major fungi *Micropolyspora faeni* and various *Thermophilic actinomyces* species. Patients typically present with recurring episodes of fever, cough, headache, breathlessness, and general malaise that mimic acute infectious disease. Examination reveals an acutely ill patient with few physical signs in the chest (occasional, scattered inspiratory rales may be present). The chest x-ray may be normal, but more commonly shows focal or diffuse infiltrates that may occur anywhere in the lung fields, although the upper zones appear to be affected most often. During the acute illness, the white cell count is elevated and generally shows a left shift; the sedimentation rate and serum immunoglobulins are also increased.

Episodic attacks usually resolve spontaneously within several days after removal of the patient from exposure to the offending agents. With repeated acute episodes, however, there may be progression to lung fibrosis, with a restrictive ventilatory defect and a decreased diffusing capacity for carbon monoxide. When fibrosis is present these changes are irreversible, but progression does not usually occur unless there are further acute episodes. Respiratory failure and cor pulmonale can result from severe lung fibrosis.

Although acute episodes of pneumonic illness are common in this disorder, some patients present with a subacute picture that manifests as slowly progressive shortness of breath. A clinical diagnosis of interstitial fibrosis of undetermined cause has often been made in such patients. The correct diagnosis of an allergic alveolitis can be made by taking a careful history of possible exposures to agents capable of inducing the condition.

Since the initial description of farmer's lung, many other sources (Table 21.4) have been identified as capable of causing the same acute and chronic clinical picture. In rare cases of indoor air pollution, hypersensitivity pneumonitis has also occurred among susceptible people, presumably as a result of fungal spores contaminating air-handling equipment. Culturing air-handling systems, however, can be problematic. Thus, careful clinical assessments in these situations are essential (see Chapter 53 for further discussion).

The pathogenesis of this group of disorders was traditionally thought to involve a type III (immune complex) response to inhaled antigens. It is now believed that the pathogenesis relates more to the high preponderance of T lymphocytes (mainly suppresser cells) found in lung tissue as well as epithelioid granulomas, probably reflecting a type IV (cell-mediated) immune response. Experimental studies in a mouse model have shown that farmer's lung can be transferred to naive mice by T cells from sensitized animals, but cannot be transferred by immunoglobulins from sensitized animals. This certainly suggests a central role for sensitized T cells in the pathogenesis of the disease.

Serum precipitins (IgG) to fungal and other suspected causal agents have been demonstrated in individuals with allergic alveolitis, but similar precipitins can also be found in exposed individuals with no evidence of lung disease; thus serum precipitins are simply thought to reflect exposures to these agents. Bronchoalveolar lavage has a place in the diagnosis and management of extrinsic allergic alveolitis, because a prominent lymphocytosis (chiefly suppresser T cells) is a characteristic finding in the active phase of the disease. A provocative challenge with the suspected allergen should not be used routinely; these agents will make a sensitized individual acutely ill and may precipitate a severe, acute pneumonitis. Moreover, the long-term sequelae of repeated expo-

TABLE 21.4. *Some causes of extrinsic allergic alveolitis*

Condition	Responsible agent(s)	Nature of antigen
Farmer's lung	Moldy hay, grain, straw	*Micropolyspora faeni, Thermoactinomyces vulgaris*
Bird-fancier's lung	Feathers and droppings	Avian proteins
Humidifier fever (air-conditioner disease)	Humidifier aerosols	*Thermophilic actinomyces,* amebae *(Acanthameba, Naegleria gruberi)*
Sauna-taker's disease	Contaminated steam	*Aureobasidium pullulans*
Bagassosis	Moldy sugar cane	*Thermoactinomyces sacchari*
Mushroom worker's lung	Compost dust	Mushroom spores, *Thermophilic actinomyces*
Malt worker's lung	Moldy barley	*Aspergillus clavatus*
Animal handler's lung	Dusts, dander, dried urine, rats, gerbils	Urine and serum animal proteins
Diisocyanate alveolitis	Polyurethane foam production, paints, adhesives	Toluene diisocyanate
Pyrethrin alveolitis	Insecticide aerosols	Pyrethrins

sures is unclear, and a provocative challenge may conceivably initiate or exacerbate lung fibrosis.

The outlook for most patients with one of these forms of extrinsic allergic alveolitis is good if they present before lung fibrosis is extensive and if they cease being exposed to the offending agent(s). Corticosteroid therapy may help ameliorate symptoms and perhaps accelerate recovery during the acute episodes, but corticosteroids have no obvious therapeutic effect once fibrosis has developed. The prophylactic use of steroids to prevent attacks is not recommended. Steroids have reduced the frequency and severity of acute symptoms, but probably do not protect against lung fibrosis.

PREVENTION OF OCCUPATIONAL PULMONARY DISEASES

The prevention of diseases caused by airborne agents falls into three broad approaches:

1. The use of engineering controls, ventilation systems, enclosure of hazardous operations, substitution of highly toxic agents with less toxic agents, and other measures to reduce toxic air levels.
2. The use of personal protective devices (respirators) to reduce the inhaled dose to the lungs of air contaminants.
3. The use of administrative measures to remove from areas of exposure those individuals who are affected or at increased risk.

Of these three measures, the most satisfactory is the first because it focuses on the source of the problem. Many industries have employed engineering controls to reduce exposures. Notable examples include coal mining and cotton textile mills. Substitution of highly toxic with less toxic materials has also been effective in reducing risks to workers, and an example of substitution is the extensive use of fibrous glass to replace asbestos for many insulation purposes.

As preventive measures, personal respiratory protection (respirators) are less satisfactory than reductions in air concentrations because the performance and use of respirators is not always optimal and individuals may receive substantial exposures to toxic agents even while wearing them. A wide range of respirators exist, from simple disposable dust masks to supplied air, full-face respirators. One of the chief reasons respirators fail is that the respirator is inappropriate for the type of exposure. A list of respirators suitable for a wide range of workplace exposures is published and updated regularly in the NIOSH Certified Equipment List, which is available from NIOSH or the U.S. National Technical Information Service (NTIS). Even when respirators appropriate for the particular exposure are used, problems still arise from poor fitting of the respirator on the worker, from incorrect use by the worker, and most importantly from the fact that respirators are often extremely uncomfortable to wear for prolonged periods—some people simply cannot wear certain respirators because they feel claustrophobic.

Merely giving a respirator to a worker does not constitute adequate respiratory protection. Employers are obligated to conduct a respirator program that includes the provision of a respirator appropriate for the exposures encountered, individual fit testing of the respirator on the worker, a training program, and frequent checking and repair of respirators.

Before employees are issued a respirator or assigned to a task that may require a respirator, they must have a medical examination to determine whether they are capable of performing the work and using the respirator (29 CFR 1910.134). Unfortunately, much of the information needed to establish medical guidelines for physicians making these decisions is lacking. While decisions about whether someone can wear a respirator can be based on an interview and assessment of symptoms, it is wise to include an objective measurement of lung function (at a minimum, lung spirometry). As a general rule, anyone with documented respiratory impairment of moderate to severe degree (FEV_1 or FVC <70% of predicted) should not be required to wear a respirator. Asthmatics with normal or mildly impaired lung function should be evaluated based on the job requirements, but should probably be excluded if they require regular medications for asthma or have had an acute asthmatic episode recently. Similarly, individuals who experience claustrophobic symptoms may be incapable of wearing a respirator.

Medical decisions and reasonable accommodations regarding respirator use need to heed the Americans with Disabilities Act, especially if wearing a respirator is considered an essential job function.

If a respirator program is to succeed, there should be a means of assessing its effectiveness among exposed workers. A medical monitoring program may be needed to detect adverse respiratory effects from exposures and to assess whether protection is inadequate in light of the respirator program.

Administrative controls are generally the least effective methods to reduce adverse health effects from airborne toxic hazards. Medical monitoring of ex-

TABLE 21.5. *Occupational Safety and Health Administration (OSHA) standards for occupational respiratory hazards*

Agent	Frequency of examinations	Industrial hygiene	Chest x-ray	Spirometry tests	Other	Reference
Asbestos	Preplacement Annual Termination of employment	Yes	Yes	Yes		29 CFR 1910.1001 29 CFR 1926.58 40 CFR 763
Coke oven emissions	Preplacement	Yes	Yes	Yes	Sputum cytology	29 CFR 1910.1029
	Annual or semiannual[a]					
Cotton dust	Initial	Yes	No	Yes	Standard questionnaire	29 CFR 1910.1043
	Annual or semiannual[a,b,c]					29 CFR 1910.1000

All examinations include a history and physical examination.
[a]Semiannual examinations are required when the worker is 45 years of age or older.
[b]Semiannual examinations are also required if forced expiratory volume in 1 second (FEV_1) decreases by 5% or 200 mL between Monday morning and afternoon; *or* if the FEV_1 is <80% of the predicted value; *or* if there is any significant change in questionnaire findings, pulmonary function, or other diagnostic tests.
[c]If FEV_1 is <60% of the predicted value, the worker must be referred to an expert physician for an opinion.

posed workers and removal of those with early effects is obviously unsatisfactory as a preventive measure because, by definition, the individual is affected by the exposure and there is no guarantee that an early effect will always be reversible or will not progress to more serious disease. Another form of administrative control that is practiced frequently is exclusion of a worker from entering an area of exposure because that individual may be at increased risk. Examples of such policies are to exclude workers with a history of asthma (whether or not it is present currently) or simply atopy alone from being exposed to potent sensitizing agents such as toluene diisocyanate (TDI), a sensible approach because people with asthma usually respond more severely to potent irritants.

All of these approaches to preventing occupational pulmonary diseases have been incorporated in various standards promulgated by OSHA. Exposures to coke oven emissions (which produce lung cancer), asbestos, and cotton dust are the most completely regulated in terms of prevention (Table 21.5). These standards mandate an upper permissible air concentration (permissible exposure level, PEL) for each of these agents, provide details of the minimum requirements for medical monitoring and industrial hygiene measurements, require respirator programs, and in some cases provide recommendations for administrative measures to be taken for affected workers.

One of the consequences of these standards has been the application by industry of new technologies for controlling air levels of toxic agents. Other industries have not needed the impetus of federal regulations to undertake similar retrofitting of old plants and incorporating engineering controls into new plants. If prevention of disease is to succeed, however, it requires the cooperation of workers and management at all levels. Potential toxic exposures are inevitable in some industries, and although many of these hazards can be avoided, others cannot. Many industries are using novel materials and processes that present unknown hazards. A well-informed workforce and an attentive physician can go a long way to anticipating potential airborne hazards and recognizing any early respiratory effects.

REFERENCES

1. International Labor Office. *International classification of radiology of pneumoconioses (revised).* Occupational Safety and Health Science, No. 22 (rev. 1980). Geneva: ILO, 1980.
2. Borbeau J, Ernst P. Between- and within-reader variability in the assessment of pleural abnormality using the ILO 1980 international classification of pneumoconioses. *Am J Ind Med* 1988;14:537–543.
3. Ducatman AM. Variability in interpretations of radiographs for asbestosis abnormalities: problems and solutions. *Ann NY Acad Sci* 1991;643:108–120.
4. Horvath EP, ed. *Manual of spirometry in occupational medicine.* Washington, DC: U.S. Department of Health and Human Services, November 1981.
5. Ferris BG (principal investigator). Epidemiology standardization project. *Am Rev Respir Dis* 1978;118(6, part 2).
6. American Thoracic Society. Lung function testing: se-

lection of reference values and interpretative strategies. *Am Rev Respir Dis* 1991;144:1202–1218.
7. Dockery DW, Ware JH, Ferris BG, et al. Distribution of forced expiratory volume in one second and forced vital capacity in healthy, white, adult never-smokers in six U.S. cities. *Am Rev Respir Dis* 1985;131:511–520.
8. Knudson RJ, Slatin RC, Lebowitz MD, et al. The maximal expiratory flowvolume curve. *Am Rev Respir Dis* 1976;113:587–600.
9. American Medical Association. The respiratory system. In: *Guides to the evaluation of permanent impairment,* 3rd ed. Illinois: AMA, 1990:115–126.
10. Crapo RO, Morris AH, Gardner RM. Reference spirometric values using techniques and equipment that meet the ATS recommendations. *Am Rev Respir Dis* 1981; 123:659–664.
11. Zavala DC. Diagnostic procedures in pulmonary diseases. In: Baum GL, Wolinsky E, eds. *Textbook of pulmonary diseases*, 4th ed. Boston: Little, Brown, 1989:330–331.
12. Parkes WR. *Occupational lung disorders,* 3rd ed. London: Butterworth, 1994.
13. Greaves IA. Not-so-simple silicosis: a case for public health action. *Am J Ind Med* 2000;37:245–251.
14. Banks DE, Morring KL, Boehlecke BA, et al. Silicosis in silica flour workers. *Am Rev Respir Dis* 1981;124: 445–450.
15. International Agency for Research on Cancer (IARC). Silica, some silicates, coal dust and paraaramid fibrils. *IARC monographs on the evaluation of carcinogenic risk of chemicals to humans*, vol 68, 1997.
16. Soutar CA. Update on lung disease in coal miners (editorial). *Br J Ind Med* 1987;44:145–148.
17. Brooks SM, Weiss MA, Bernstein RL. Reactive airways dysfunction syndrome (RADS). *Chest* 1985;88:376–384.
18. Kern DG. Outbreak of the reactive airways dysfunction syndrome after a spill of glacial acetic acid. *Am Rev Respir Dis* 1991;144:1058–1064.
19. Newman Taylor AJ. Occupational asthma. *Thorax* 1980; 35:241–245.
20. Wagner GR, Wegman D. Occupational asthma: prevention by definition. *Am J Ind Med* 1998;33:347–349.
21. Van Kampen. V, Merget R, Baur X. Occupational airway sensitizers: an overview of the respective literature. *Am J Ind Med* 2000;38:164–218.
22. Banks DE, Wang M-L. Occupational asthma: "the big picture." *Occup Med State of the Art Rev* 2000;15: 335–357.
23. Chan-Yeung M, Lam S. Occupational asthma (state of art). *Am Rev Respir Dis* 1986;133:686–703.

FURTHER INFORMATION

Parkes WR. *Occupational lung disorders,* 3rd ed. London: Butterworth, 1994.

The premier text on occupational lung diseases. An excellent and detailed account of the major and uncommon occupational lung disorders. Clear descriptions of the clinical presentations and pathology of the lung.

Ferris BG (principal investigator). Epidemiology standardization project. *Am Rev Respir Dis* 1978;118(vol 6, part 2).

A classic work: a concerted effort by senior respiratory epidemiologists and clinicians to standardize methods for the collection of respiratory health effects data. Includes details for respiratory questionnaires, spirometry and other lung function tests, and radiology of the lung.

Chan-Yeung M, Lam S. Occupational asthma. *Am Rev Respir Dis* 1986;133:686–703.

Yeung M, Grzybowski S. Prognosis in occupational asthma (editorial). *Thorax* 1985;40:241–243.

The above two are older publications but still excellent reviews of occupational asthma.

Banks DE, Wang M-L. Occupational asthma: "the big picture." *Occup Med State of the Art Rev* 2000;15: 335–357.

An excellent and recent review of occupational asthma. Good guidance for the practicing physician.

Becklake MR. Asbestos-related diseases of the lung and other organs (state of art). *Am Rev Respir Dis* 1976;114: 187–227.

Becklake MR. Asbestos-related diseases of the lung and pleura (editorial). *Am Rev Respir Dis* 1982;126:187–194.

The above two are classic summaries of the malignant and nonmalignant effects of asbestos.

Harber P, Schenker MB, Balmes JR. *Occupational and environmental respiratory disease.* St. Louis: Mosby, 1996.

Another excellent overall text on occupational and environmental lung diseases.

22

Musculoskeletal Disorders

Reid T. Boswell and Robert J. McCunney

The diagnosis, treatment, and rehabilitation of musculoskeletal disorders constitute a large portion of clinical occupational medical practice. The physician who provides occupational medical services is likely to encounter patients with sprains, especially to the neck, back, and shoulder; repetitive motion injuries, such as tendonitis and carpal tunnel syndrome; and soft tissue injuries, such as lacerations and contusions. Although some occupational settings are associated with particular types of musculoskeletal disorders, such as decreased urate clearance in lead nephropathy (saturnine gout), fluorosis associated with exposure to fluorine compounds, and autoimmune dysfunction secondary to silicosis, this chapter does not discuss these rare conditions. Rather, it reviews common musculoskeletal disorders, and discusses the diagnosis, treatment, and indications for referral by the primary care physician to an appropriate consultant. Because of space limitations, the full gamut of musculoskeletal disorders that can be caused or aggravated by work cannot be covered.

RATES OF OCCUPATIONAL INJURIES

Musculoskeletal injuries constitute the vast majority of all occupational injuries and illnesses. The Bureau of Labor Statistics (BLS) conducts annual surveys of occupational injuries and illnesses based on a sample of various industries' Occupational Safety and Health Administration (OSHA) 200 Log. In addition, the Supplementary Data System (SDS), established under the 1970 Occupational Health and Safety Act, provides information on compensation claims in the 29 states that participate in the SDS. In 1999, 34% of all recordable injuries and illnesses involved the musculoskeletal system (582,340 out of a total of 1,702,420 recordable cases). Of these musculoskeletal cases, 52% involved the back (302,744 of 582,340) (1).

TABLE 22.1. *Rates per 10,000 workers of Occupational Safety and Health Administration (OSHA) recordable musculoskeletal injuries and illnesses by industry*

Industry	Rate
Nursing and personal care facilities	173.5
Home health services	105.1
Hospitals	93.6
Transportation and public utilities	80.5
Construction	70.1
Manufacturing	48.2
Agriculture	46.0
Finance, insurance, real estate	12.4
All private industry	46.9

Table 22.1 lists the incidence of musculoskeletal recordable cases among select industries in 1999 (1). Because of the enormous importance of back disorders that limit occupational functioning, this chapter pays particular attention to these conditions.

BACK DISORDERS

Acute Back Injuries

Low back problems constitute the most expensive work-related health care problem for people in the 30 to 50 age group (2). Total direct costs for low back disorders, excluding wage replacement, were estimated to be approximately $24 billion in 1990 (3). Indirect costs, such as lost productivity and replacement training costs, are difficult to calculate accurately. In an evaluation of over 900 back injuries, 10% accounted for nearly 80% of total costs for all back injuries and for over 30% of all musculoskeletal injuries (2). Thus, control of costs related to occupational back disorders depends in large part on managing the small percentage of serious disabling conditions.

Risk factors for low back injuries that result in disability include heavy repetitive lifting and pushing and pulling, as well as exposure to industrial and vehicular vibration (3). In addition, other psychosocial characteristics have been identified as significant risk factors for disabling back injury. These include previous back injury claims; job dissatisfaction; poor ratings from supervisors; repetitive, boring tasks; younger age and shorter duration of employment; smoking; and a history of *non*-back injury claims (3,4).

Prolapsed intervertebral discs are most common among persons aged 25 to 45. Major risk factors for prolapsed disc include frequent lifting of objects weighing more than 25 lb, exposure to whole-body vibration, cigarette smoking, and narrow lumbar vertebral canals (5). Possible associations with prolapsed disc include lifting and twisting, sedentary occupations, jobs that require prolonged static positions, lack of flexibility or physical fitness, and pregnancy (5).

Diagnosis of Low Back Pain

Most low back problems related to work are diagnosed and treated by primary care physicians. The clinical approach to evaluating such disorders includes an appropriate history and physical examination, with diagnostic imaging or laboratory testing only when necessary (6).

The causes of low back pain include (a) musculoligamentous injuries; (b) vertebral fractures, including compression fractures; (c) degenerative changes; (d) spinal stenosis; (e) anatomic anomalies, such as spondylolisthesis; (f) herniated intervertebral discs with nerve root compression; (g) systemic diseases, such as cancer, spinal infections, and ankylosing spondylitis; and (h) visceral diseases unrelated to the spine (7). It should be noted, however, that a definitive diagnosis cannot be reached in up to 85% of patients with low back pain (7). Table 22.2 lists the differential diagnosis of low back pain.

TABLE 22.2. *Differential diagnosis of low back pain*

Mechanical low back or leg pain	97%
Lumbar strain/sprain (nonspecific)	70%
Degenerative disease	10%
Herniated intervertebral disc	4%
Spinal stenosis	3%
Compression fracture	4%
Spondylolisthesis	2%
Traumatic fracture	<1%
Congenital disease	<1%
Nonmechanical spinal conditions	1%
Neoplasia	0.7%
Infection	0.01%
Inflammatory arthritis	0.3%
Visceral disease	2%
Pelvic disease (prostatitis, endometriosis, PID)	
Renal disease	
Aortic aneurysm	
Gastrointestinal disease (pancreatitis, cholangeitis, penetrating ulcer)	

PID, pelvic inflammatory disease.
Adapted from Deye, Weinstein. Low back pain. *N Engl J Med* 2001;344:5.

History

Usually, a worker who experiences back pain is likely to describe a precipitating event associated with the discomfort. It is not uncommon, however, for a patient to be unable to relate the onset of back discomfort to a particular incident. Because of certain requirements of the workers' compensation system that encourage the reporting of an *injurious event,* patients tend to relate the discomfort to some specific workplace activity. In the absence thereof, workers' compensation benefits may be denied. In the nonoccupational setting, however, only about one third of back problems are associated with a specific event (8).

Elements of a good clinical history are of value in evaluating back pain. An inquiry should be directed to the onset of pain, its character, duration, radiation, and measures that relieve the discomfort. Questions regarding neurologic symptoms such as pain radiation, especially down the posterior aspect of the leg; numbness or paresthesias in the feet; or weakness can help determine whether nerve route irritation secondary to a herniated disc is present.

Although pain radiation from the back down the posterior aspect of either leg is strongly associated with nerve irritation secondary to an injured disc, such radicular symptoms are not uncommon in acute non–disc-related back disorders. Pain radiation in the "non-disc" back disorder commonly extends to the buttocks and posterior aspect of the upper leg. This is referred pain based on the common embryologic origin of structures that eventually form the low back and muscles, tendon, and ligaments in the posterior thigh. Pain radiation *beyond the knee* is a more ominous finding and is rare in acute back injuries without associated disc herniation.

Patients will often point to the low back region in a circular manner in the vicinity of the sacroiliac joints as the source of their discomfort. Rarely, one particular "trigger point" or local area of tenderness can be elicited. The pain is usually relieved by rest and heat applied to the lower back.

In the course of the medical history, it is helpful to inquire about the nature of the work that the person performs including the availability of mechanical lifting devices and the weight of the material that is expected to be lifted. The National Institute for Occupational Safety and Health (NIOSH) has issued guidelines on safe lifting practices (9), which have been updated (see Chapter 43). Many organizations also restrict the amount of material that can be lifted by the unaided worker.

It is also wise to review whether the patient has had a previous back injury, since back injuries have a high rate of recurrence. In fact, most clinical evaluations suggest that subsequent back injuries usually are more uncomfortable for the patient and require a longer period of time for resolution of the symptoms.

Although nearly all back injuries respond to conservative measures, it is critically important during the history for the physician to evaluate the possibility of an emergency surgical disorder, the cauda equina syndrome. This disorder, secondary to a *centrally herniated* disc, usually results in pain radiation down both legs, saddle anesthesia bowel incontinence, or urinary retention. The predictive value of a negative history of urinary retention is estimated to be 0.9999 (7). Anal sphincter tone is reduced in 60% to 80% of cases (7). Immediate diagnosis and treatment for this condition are imperative. Otherwise, even in the presence of a herniated disc, initial treatment consists of conservative measures.

Physical Examination

The physical examination of the patient with low back pain is comprehensive and aimed at identifying specific pathology. The history and detailed physical

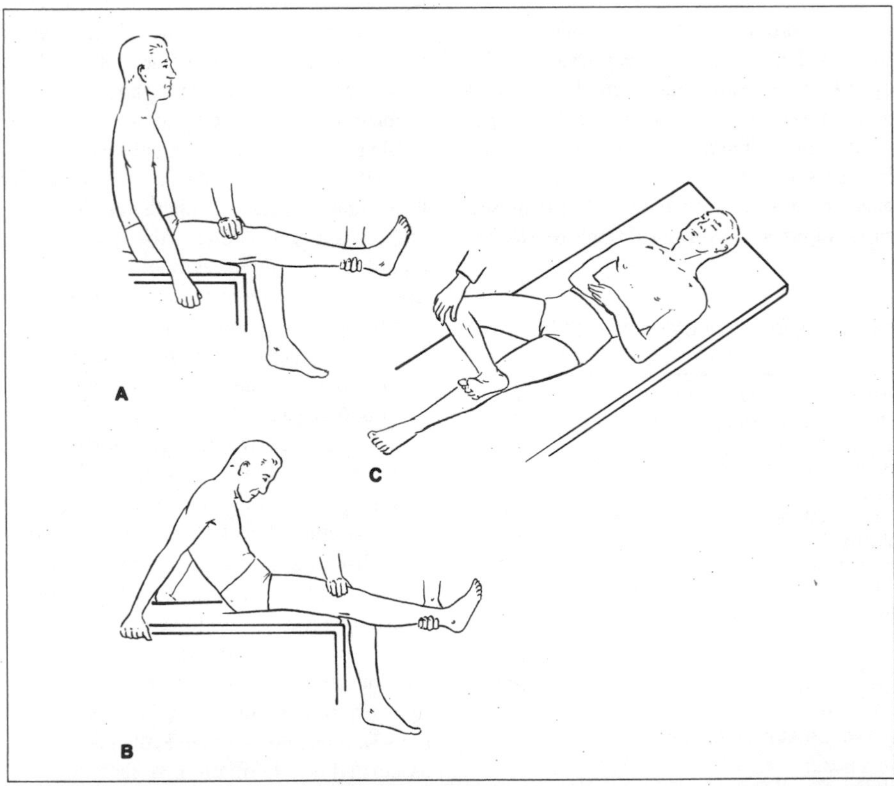

FIG. 22.1. A, B: Straight-leg raising test. In **A** there is no evidence of sciatic irritation. In **B** the test is positive for sciatic or nerve root irritation. Results should be identical in the sitting and supine positions. A positive test elicits pain radiation down the posterior aspect of the leg at 0 to 70 degrees. The production of back pain only is not considered a positive sign. **C:** Patrick's test. Positive when pain is elicited in the hip joint or in the sacroiliac joint region as the heel is placed on the opposite knee and leg and the flexed knee is forced to the table.

examination will rule out disorders that require further testing 85% to 90% of the time. Initially, the patient is observed walking. The gait should be symmetric, and the extent of ankle dorsiflexion and plantar flexion should be noted. This helps verify motor strength. Overall alignment of the spine is then assessed. Patients with spinal stenosis frequently maintain a flexed posture to increase the area of the spinal canal. Similarly, facet joint disease is usually made more comfortable by mild flexion. Conversely, patients with a herniated disc frequently maintain a position of extension. Next, the range of motion of the lumbar spine should be recorded. Paraspinal muscle spasm should be noted, as should any change in spasm with position.

Testing should always then be performed for pain elicited by the straight-leg raising (SLR) test and Patrick's test (Fig. 22.1). The SLR maneuver produces stretch on the sciatic nerve and in the presence of nerve compression should exacerbate pain. The examination is first done with the patient sitting and then in the supine position. *Results should be identical.* A positive test is noted when SLR causes leg discomfort from 0 to 70 degrees. If only back pain is produced, the examination is negative. Dorsiflexing the foot usually exaggerates the leg pain caused by SLR in the presence of a herniated disc. In contrast, plantar flexion should not lead to an increase in pain; when it does a nonorganic etiology of pain is suggested. Many observers find the contralateral SLR test to be very helpful in the diagnosis of a herniated disc; elevation of the nonsymptomatic leg causes sciatic-type pain in the symptomatic leg, which is kept still.

A detailed neurologic examination is then performed. Sensation to light touch, pressure, and vibration is tested in dermatomal distributions L1-S4. The muscle strength of the hip flexors (L1-L3), knee flexors (L2-L4), ankle dorsiflexors (L4), long toe extensors (L5), ankle evertors (L5, S1), and ankle plantar flexors (S1, S2), is sequentially examined and graded. Reflexes are tested for intensity and duration of response. The knee jerk is supplied by L4, while the ankle jerk is supplied by S1. Attempts are then made to elicit ankle clonus and the Babinski reflex.

Finally, a general physical examination should be done, checking for abdominal disorders associated with back discomfort. This approach includes a rectal and, when necessary, a pelvic examination.

Although not exhaustive, the preceding examination aids the physician in determining the etiology of low back pain.

Diagnostic Imaging

Plain films of the lumbosacral spine are of limited value in the diagnosis of acute back pain, unless there is clinical suspicion of vertebral fracture, primary or metastatic cancer, or infection (osteomyelitis). Magnetic resonance imaging (MRI) is the procedure of choice in the diagnosis of herniated intervertebral disc and spinal stenosis (10). Indications for obtaining an MRI of the lumbosacral spine include persistent pain or numbness in a dermatomal distribution; presence of neurologic abnormalities, such as loss of ankle jerk or muscle strength; and presence of neurogenic claudication (pain or neurologic deficits after walking or prolonged standing) (6).

It is important to keep in mind that anatomic evidence of a herniated disc may be found in 22% to 40% of asymptomatic persons. Bulging discs may be seen in up to 81% of asymptomatic persons (11). Therefore, results of MRI or other imaging techniques must be interpreted in light of clinical findings.

Acute Management of Low Back Pain

Most workers with acute low back injuries recover quickly. One study found that 90% of patients with low back pain seen within 3 days of the injury or onset of pain completely recover within 2 weeks (12). The cornerstones of treatment for low back pain arising from a work-related episode are rest and symptomatic relief of the discomfort with rapid return to normal activities as tolerated. If bed rest is advised, it should be for no more than 2 days, after which the patient should be encouraged to ambulate, regardless of whether the pain has improved (13,14). A study found no difference in outcome between groups of patients with nondiscogenic low back pain who were prescribed bed rest, exercises, or return to normal activities (15).

Within the first 24 hours of acute pain, ice applied to the area of discomfort can be helpful. An example of an effective technique is an *ice lollie,* a small paper cup filled with water and then frozen. The patient then peels the top of the paper off the cup, and the frozen cup can be used as a handle by another person to massage the painful area. Alternatively, a bag of frozen peas can be used. Deep muscle spasms and associated pain are often relieved by this simple measure. After the acute phase of the injury, however, locally applied heat through the use of heating pads, whirlpool, or hot baths is usually effective in providing immediate but temporary relief.

The use of nonsteroidal antiinflammatory drugs (NSAIDs) can also aid in symptomatic relief (16). NSAIDs have been consistently shown to be effective for short-term symptomatic relief in patients with acute low back pain, though no specific drug has been demonstrated to be superior (17). The use of muscle relaxants should be reserved for those whose pain interferes with sleep.

The early treatment of those with suspected herniated discs is essentially no different from the treatment of those with nondiscogenic back pain (18). Only about 10% of patients with herniated disc require surgical intervention (11). MRI studies have demonstrated that the herniated disc regrows with time, resulting in partial or total resolution in two thirds of cases after 6 months (19).

Following treatment, the physician must file an appropriate report in accordance with the state's workers' compensation statutes. Prompt filing of reports assists the patient in obtaining income replacement benefits guaranteed by workers' compensation.

Medical Follow-up of Low Back Injury

Because fear and anxiety are often associated with low back pain, it is important for the physician to counsel such patients appropriately. Advising patients that low back injuries do not generally heal in a few days can help them respond better to the treatment process. Failing to advise patients accordingly may lead to frustration in otherwise healthy younger patients (usually between 20 and 50 years old) who are not accustomed to the limitations in activity that are often associated with back pain. In turn, patients may seek other opinions by practitioners, such as acupuncturists chiropractors, and others whose diagnostic acumen may be limited. Unfortunately, so much medical uncertainty is associated with back disorders (in terms of cause, source of pain, and treatment) that these differences of opinions may lead patients to be more confused than helped. Consequently, frequent follow-up evaluations, especially in the early phase of an injury, are advisable. In this period patients often voice their greatest concerns.

During these follow-up evaluations, the physician can inquire about (a) the presence of symptoms noted during the initial evaluation, especially those related to nerve route irritation; (b) the response to treatment; and (c) how the discomfort has affected activities of daily living. After the initial phase of treatment (3–5 days), it is frequently helpful to refer the patient to a physical therapist who is experienced in treating occupational injuries. The therapist can institute passive treatment, such as thermal modalities and ultrasound, and begin range of motion exercises and patient education.

When the patient's condition begins to improve, one should institute gentle exercises, preceded by a hot pack. For stretching, Williams' exercises are appropriate for the patient recovering from the acute phase of a low back injury. The exercises are not intended to produce muscle strength but rather to stretch the large paravertebral muscles and the smaller muscles beneath them. The more these muscles receive gentle stretching, the quicker the resolution of deep muscle spasm. Flexion and extension exercises, however, should not be done to the point of pain, but gradually, so that the individual regains full use of the previously injured area (Fig. 22.2).

Since the recovery process from an acute back injury can be prolonged, physicians will find it of value to be diligent and attentive to detail in note taking during follow-up evaluations. Because of the protracted nature of recovery from many back injuries, subtle improvements may not be easily recognized by the patient. Thus, with proper documentation, the physician can demonstrate that improvements have occurred and in turn encourage the patient toward recovery. The frequency of follow-up evaluations varies considerably and depends on the nature of the disorder, age of the patient, history of previous back disorders, underlying medical conditions, and the type of job to which the patient will be returning. Ideally, patients should be evaluated at least weekly.

During the follow-up period, the physician is advised to take an active role in facilitating a return to work in either a full or a modified-duty capacity. Early return to work (if sufficient improvement has occurred) can be therapeutic from a number of perspectives. Although modified-duty policies may exist at some places of employment, specific recommendations are essential. General terms such as "light duty" should be discouraged in favor of more specific guidelines. For example, the use of long-handled objects such as brooms and rakes can aggravate low back discomfort in many patients. A supervisor unaware of this potential problem may inadvertently assign an injured worker to such a task with the assumption that such work is light duty, especially in contrast to a material-handling position. Any back discomfort that develops as a result of these activities is likely not only to frustrate the worker but also to interfere with the treatment process and affect the patient's trust in the physician and the physician's credibility. Consequently, specific instructions, such as no lifting greater than 20

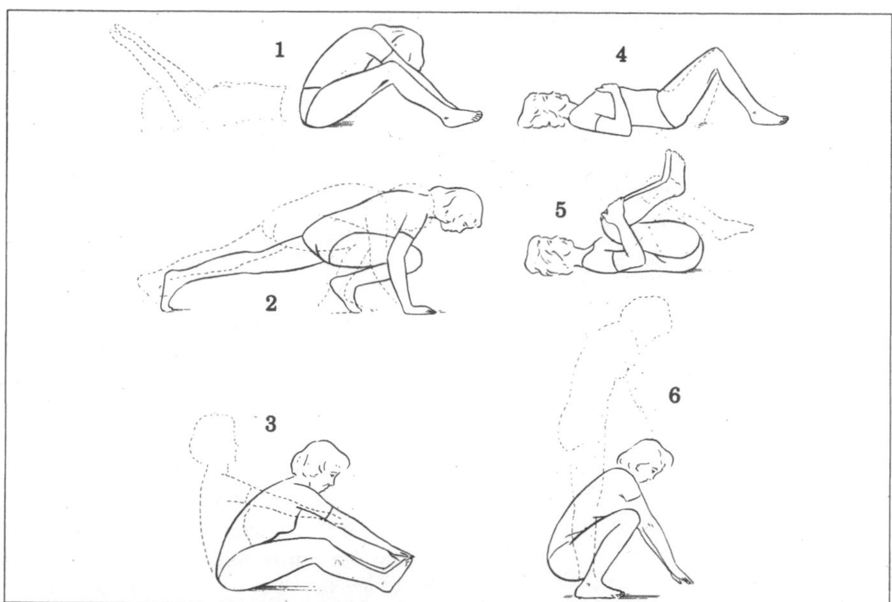

FIG. 22.2. Therapeutic exercises helpful in promoting recovery from a back injury. *Exercise 1* is aimed at developing the abdominal muscles. By varying the distance of the heels from the buttocks, it can usually be accomplished without foot anchorage.

Exercise 2 is aimed primarily at stretching the fascia Was and the iliofemoral ligament, as well as hip flexor muscles. This exercise is frequently not indicated in those individuals who present loose joints and a relaxed attitude. The foot of the extended extremity should be dorsiflexed so that the weight is borne on the ball of the foot and rotated internally so that tension is applied principally to the anterolateral aspect of the thigh. The knee of the extended extremity should remain rigidly fixed in the extended position during the exercise.

Exercise 3 is aimed at restoring lumbosacral flexion and stretching shortened hamstring muscles. It should not be used in those experiencing acute radiating pain into the extremities until these symptoms have been relieved.

Exercise 4 is aimed at developing the gluteus maximus. The pelvis is rotated forward by actively contracting these muscles. The buttocks are lifted off the floor, but the abdomen should remain down and the spine should not be lifted from the floor above the waistline.

Exercise 5 is aimed at stretching the contractures of the erector spinae and all structures posterior to the upright center of gravity at this level. The knees should be pulled to the axillae rather than over the shoulders.

Exercise 6 is directed at restoring flexion of the lumbosacral spine and actively developing the gluteus maximus and the femoral quadriceps. The success of a postural program depends to a large extent on the strength of these two muscles, since the lumbosacral spine can be controlled only by those who have the ability to squat up or down with ease, thus avoiding raising the trunk with the erector spinae muscles. The principle involved in this one exercise would avoid most low back disability if rigidly employed in one's daily activities. The weight should be borne on the heels, and the entire spine should remain flexed at all times during the course of the exercise.

lb or no frequent bending, lifting, or twisting, are preferable. Frequent changes in position to avoid prolonged standing or sitting are also advisable. Fortunately, well over 90% of acute back injuries respond to conservative therapy, and patients are able to return to their original line of work (20).

Useful definitions of levels of work are as follows (21):

Very heavy work involves lifting objects weighing more than 100 lb at a time, with frequent lifting or carrying of objects weighing 50 lb or more.

Heavy work involves lifting no more than 100 lb at a time, with frequent lifting or carrying of objects weighing up to 50 lb.

Medium work involves lifting no more than 50 lb at a time, with frequent lifting or carrying of objects weighing up to 25 lb. Workers with 5% or less back-related permanent partial physical impairment can qualify in this category, but those with higher rates cannot.

Light work involves lifting no more than 20 lb at a time, with frequent lifting or carrying of objects weighing up to 10 lb. Applicants with between 10% and 15% permanent partial physical impairment because of a low back problem should be able to do this type of work.

Sedentary work involves lifting no more than 10 lb at a time and occasional lifting or carrying of articles such as docket files, ledgers, or small tools. Applicants with 20% or 25% permanent partial physical impairment should be capable of this type of work.

Chronic Back Disorders

Chronic back disorders usually refer to back pain that has been present for over 6 weeks and that has not responded to conservative measures. The physician is likely to be asked to evaluate the persistence of a back disorder that has interfered with work capabilities. In this setting, a detailed history and additional laboratory and ancillary procedures are usually necessary to evaluate the possibility of other causes of back pain (Table 22.2).

History

Questions should be directed to the character of the pain. For example, morning stiffness can be associated with underlying inflammatory disorders such as ankylosing spondylitis. Pain in the legs precipitated by walking (pseudoclaudication) relieved by rest, especially by flexion of the hip, may be associated with spinal stenosis. Pain that is steady and aggravated by palpation can be due to tumors or multiple myeloma.

A review of medical records, including results of diagnostic tests and treatment measures, is necessary. In some cases, people have been advised merely to rest for upward of 3 to 4 weeks. But in these settings, the cause of the discomfort may be muscle stiffness and tightness, which can be readily relieved with therapeutic exercises. The physician may also encounter a patient who demonstrates a psychological disturbance or fear and anxiety that interfere with the recovery process and ability to return to work. In the assessment of a chronic back disorder, it is wise to consider these interfering psychological and emotional factors. In one study of 111 patients with chronic low back disorders, nearly half were considered disabled primarily on a psychiatric basis (22). In another report, about 20% of patients admitted to a chronic pain rehabilitation program were "overtly or covertly fraudulent, i.e., seeking by their own volition to maximize monetary gain..." (23).

Although true malingering (factitious symptoms) is rare, emotional issues often interfere with recovery and return to work. Table 22.3 displays some of the nonorganic physical signs in low back pain (24). Figure 22.3 describes aspects of the physical examination that suggest embellishment of symptoms.

TABLE 22.3. *Nonorganic physical signs in low back pain*

Category	Test	Comments
Tenderness	Superficial palpation	Inordinate, widespread sensitivity to light touch over lumbar spine suggests amplified symptoms
Simulation (to assess patient cooperation and reliability)	Axial loading	Light pressure to skull should not significantly increase symptoms
	Rotation	Physician should rotate patient's shoulders, which does not move lumbar spine and should not increase pain
Distraction	Straight-leg raising	Physician asks seated patient to straighten knee; patients with true sciatic tension will arch backward and complain; these results should match those of the traditional, recumbent straight-leg test
Regional		Diffuse motor weakness or bizarre sensory deficits suggest functional disturbances if they involve multiple muscle groups and cannot be explained by neuroanatomic principles
Overreaction		Excessive and inappropriate grimacing

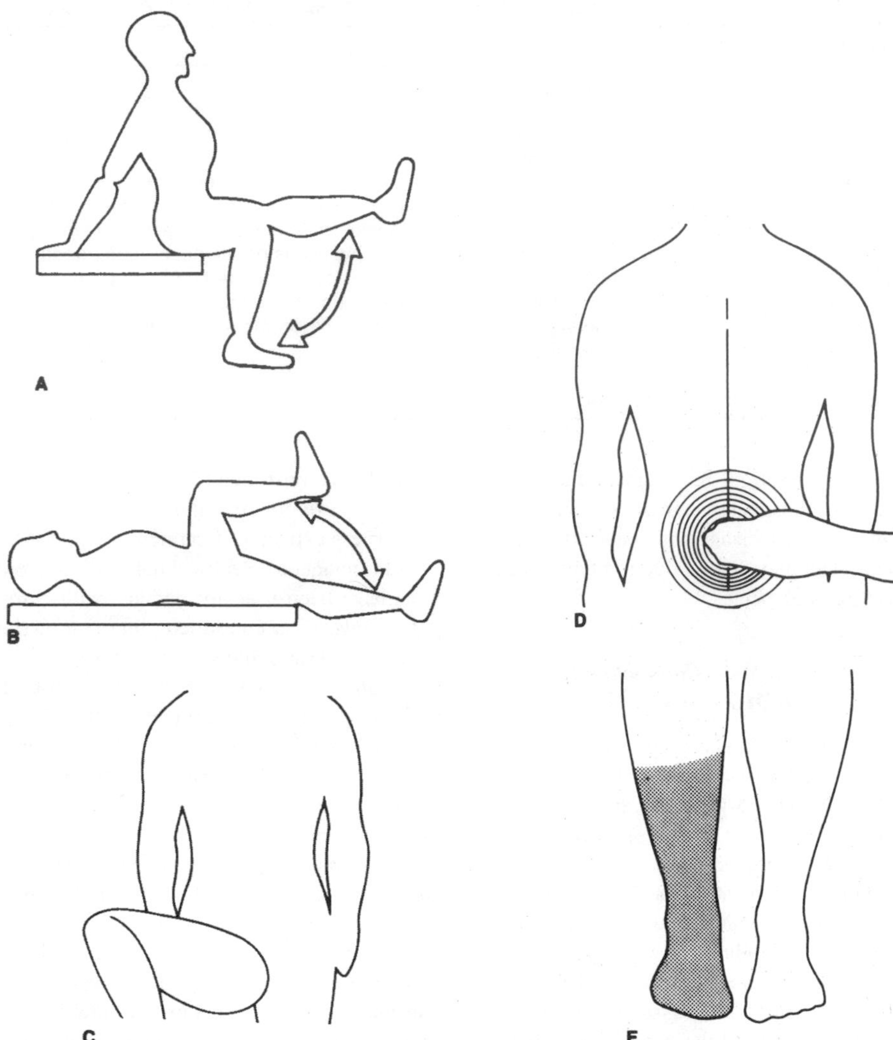

FIG. 22.3. Confusion tests in evaluating chronic back pain and determining validity of physical complaints. **A:** Confusion test 1: knee extension while sitting. If the supine patient has limitation of straight-leg raising, the limitation should be reproducible while the patient is in the sitting position. **B:** Confusion test 2: hip flexion. Patients with lumbar complaints should not experience increased pain when the hip is passively flexed (knee kept in flexion). **C:** Confusion test 3: Faber's test. Patients with lumbar complaints should not experience increased pain when the hip is flexed, abducted, and externally rotated (knee kept in flexion). **D:** Confusion test 4: skin hypersensitivity to touch in the lumbar area. Patients with lumbar complaints should not experience increased pain when the overlying skin is lightly touched. **E:** Confusion test 5: stocking-type numbness in the lower extremities. Patients with lumbar complaints should not have hypesthesia in a stocking-type distribution. (Adapted from William F. Kennedy, M.D., Neenah, Wisconsin.)

Laboratory Testing

Depending on the history and physical examination, appropriate blood testing, especially an erythrocyte sedimentation rate (ESR), may be of value. This nonspecific parameter, if highly elevated, can prompt a search for other disorders such as ankylosing spondylitis, tumors, or infections. Further testing might include human leukocyte antigen HLA-B27 for ankylosing spondylitis or an alkaline phosphatase for

TABLE 22.4. *Laboratory tests of potential value in assessing chronic back pain*

Test	Result
Complete blood count	Elevated in systemic disease
Erythrocyte sedimentation rate	Elevated in infection, tumor, ankylosing spondylitis
Calcium	Elevated in hyperparathyroidism, metastatic tumor; low in advanced osteomalacia
Alkaline phosphatase	Elevated in infiltrative bone disease (tumor), infection (osteomyelitis, diskitis); may be mildly elevated with recent fracture or Paget's disease; a normal glutamyl transpeptidase or 5′-nucleotidase will confirm bone origin
Phosphorus	Increased in renal osteodystrophy, occasionally decreased in osteomalacia
Acid phosphatase	Increased in most cases of metastatic prostate carcinoma
Urinalysis	Abnormal with genitourinary infection of neoplasm
HLA-B27 antigen	Occasionally useful in suspected ankylosing spondylitis with negative or equivocal radiographic changes
Uric acid	Gout
Urine—Bence-Jones protein	Myeloma

Paget's disease. Alterations in serum calcium, phosphorus, and acid phosphatase can also occur in other disorders that are associated with back pain (Table 22.4). A bone scan may be of value if a tumor, infection, or fracture is suspected.

Electromyography/Nerve Conduction Velocity (EMG/NCV)

Electrodiagnostic techniques can help in the diagnosis of nerve route irritation secondary to a herniated disc. A negative EMG, however, does not exclude neural involvement, because early changes secondary to nerve compression from a herniated disc may not be detected within the first few weeks of the disorder. Properly conducted and analyzed studies can confirm clinical findings of abnormal motor or sensory function. In conjunction with other studies, such as MRI (10), EMG/NCV assessment can aid in determining the severity of the disorder. In addition, if conducted at periodic intervals, EMG/NVC studies can indicate areas of improvement.

Treatment

The essential element in treating chronic back disorders without a primary cause is patient education. Patients should be thoroughly instructed in activities of daily living that may relieve or aggravate back discomfort. If a referral to a physical therapy unit has not already been initiated, patients with chronic back pain should be evaluated by an experienced physiotherapist. Physiotherapy has been shown to decrease the severity of pain complaints compared to continued medical treatment alone (25). While chiropractic manipulation may also reduce back pain, the long-term efficacy of manipulation therapy has not been conclusively demonstrated (26). Furthermore, chiropractic is no more effective than physical therapy, which is a far less expensive treatment option (25).

Transcutaneous electrical nerve stimulator (TENS) units have been used for patients with chronic back pain. However, a controlled clinical trial showed no benefit of TENS units versus placebo for chronic back pain (27). The use of steroid injections has been another option in the treatment of chronic back pain. In a double-blind, randomized trial of steroid injections versus placebo in patients with chronic mechanical low back pain, no significant difference was seen in reported improvement in pain over 6 months (28). A recent meta-analysis concluded that there is no convincing evidence that injection therapy is useful for chronic low back pain (29).

Referrals to a neurosurgeon or an orthopedic surgeon should only be considered when surgery is a reasonable option for treatment of low back pain. Present indications for surgical referral are listed in Table

TABLE 22.5. *Indications for surgical referral among patients with low back pain*

- Sciatica and probable herniated discs
  - Cauda equina syndrome (emergency)
  - Progressive or severe neurologic deficit
  - Persistent neuromotor deficit after 4–6 weeks conservative treatment
  - Persistent sciatica (with or without low back pain) with consistent clinical and neurologic findings
- Spinal stenosis
  - Progressive or severe neurologic deficit
  - Persistent and disabling back and leg pain
- Spondylolisthesis
  - Progressive or severe neurologic deficit
  - Associated with spinal stenosis
  - Severe back and leg pain with severe functional impairment for >1 year

22.5 (11). There is evidence that antidepressants (especially serotonergic-nonadrenergic antidepressants) can relieve chronic pain independent of their antidepressant properties (30).

Rehabilitation and Return to Work Status

Determining a patient's ability to return to a job after a back injury can be problematic. In most cases, patients with back injuries are able to return to their original type of work without any restrictions. In other cases, however, especially in those rare disorders that require surgery, considerable alterations may be necessary. Where repeated episodes of back injury have occurred, it may be worthwhile to refer the patient to a physical therapy unit for a work-hardening program. These types of programs are designed to educate patients in proper lifting techniques and gradually to build up their endurance to handle physically demanding jobs. Particular attention to body mechanics, posture, and physical exercise can be instrumental in reducing the risk of future injury.

Prevention of Back Injuries

Because of the prevalence of back problems in the occupational setting, numerous measures have been attempted to prevent, control, and reduce the rate of these disabling ailments. No one preventive approach has proved effective in all situations, and no one specific intervention has been sufficient to reduce the impact of back disorders (31). Back belts and education regarding lifting techniques have not been shown to be effective in preventing back injuries (32,33). An effective preventive program depends on the coordination of a number of efforts, including proper selection and placement, appropriate job design, and maintenance of health through education and physical fitness. Aerobic exercise combined with back and leg strengthening can reduce the frequency of recurrent low back pain (34). Coupled with early recognition and prompt and efficient treatment of back injuries, these preventive measures can reduce the rate of back disorders, which result in the second leading cause of absences from work. (Upper-respiratory infections, such as colds and influenza, lead the list.)

Proper Selection and Placement

Ideally, people at risk of suffering from back injuries could be identified based on a review of individual characteristics and job requirements. Unfortunately, no specific set of criteria applies to all situations. During the preplacement evaluation, attention can be directed toward previous job responsibilities and episodes of back injuries, since the best predictor of future back injuries is past history of a back injury (35). Once a history regarding previous injuries has been obtained, physical examination is unlikely to add any useful information regarding a prospective employee's risk for future back injury (36).

A review of proposed job duties during the examination is essential. The physician should inquire as to the frequency that materials might be lifted, their respective weight, and the availability of lifting devices. It can be complicated to properly place a patient with a history of back injuries, but no current symptoms and a normal examination, in a material-handling position. Many factors affect whether another back injury will occur, including level of motivation, physical fitness, and circumstances beyond the patient's control.

An abnormality that may be noted during a physical examination is leg length inequality. Population studies, however, have demonstrated that leg length discrepancies of up to 4 cm are not associated with an increased incidence of low back pain. For patients with greater than a 2.5-cm congenital shortening, the use of a small lift in the shoe may increase physical comfort.

It has been suggested that certain personality types may be at greater risk of back injuries; however, evidence supporting such claims is lacking. But psychological testing has been shown to predict an individual's response to treatment (37). In fact, one study of 200 workers' compensation cases suggested that psychological factors play a major role in back injuries that occur in workers' compensation settings. The study employed the Minnesota Multiphasic Personality Inventory (MMPI) to measure psychological function (38) and showed that one third of the workers' compensation cases referred for psychological evaluation were back disorders. The authors suggested that psychological disability may profoundly affect an existing physical impairment. The results indicate that a referral to an appropriate therapist may be of value in assessing the many factors involved in long-term disability.

Lumbosacral Spine Films

Lumbosacral spine films have been used since the 1920s to identify conditions of the lower back that might predispose one to future injury (39). Such efforts, however, have failed to meet their promise and are strongly discouraged for routine use (40,41). One particular abnormality, however, of the sacrohorizontal angle (i.e., the relationship between the superior border or S1 and a horizontal plane) has been associated with an increased incidence of low back pain only if the angle exceeds 70 degrees. Another abnormality, spondylolisthesis, however, occurs in 2% to 10% of the population (24) and does not appear to increase the risk of back injuries.

Another common condition, narrow disc space, for example, is not associated with an increased rate of low back pain. The rate of disc degeneration varies, and a strong genetic component to its development appears to exist. In rare cases, severe disc generation that occurs at an early age may contribute to low back pain in some people.

Strength Testing

Isometric strength testing conducted in relation to the requirements of the job has been suggested as a means of predicting those at an increased risk of back injury (42–44). Measurements of physical capacity have also been recommended as a means of predicting those susceptible to injuries. Although both strength and fitness testing have been advocated for their preventive value, the true impact of these interventions on occupational back disorders has yet to be determined.

Maintenance of a Healthy Back

Once a worker begins a job with a higher risk of back injuries, efforts should be directed to controlling the development of these disabling conditions. The foremost consideration in preventing back injuries is appropriate job design. Proper design of material-handling positions has been estimated to reduce up to one third of compensable low back injuries (8). Ergonomics, the science of fitting the job to the person, is an essential component of efficient job design.

Other techniques that can be used at work to control back injuries include guidelines for weights that one can lift without overexertion. For example, some transportation industries as well as the U.S. Postal Service limit the amount of weight that can be lifted without mechanical support to 70 lb or less. If the physician learns that a job requires lifting objects more than 100 lb, efforts should be directed to the use of mechanical lifting devices. NIOSH has established guidelines for safe lifting (9); however, the appropriateness of the biomechanical criteria proposed has recently been challenged (45).

Most training programs include basic measures that emphasize the following aspects of lifting (8): (a) keep the object close to the body; (b) lift slowly, smoothly, and without a jerking, erratic motion; (c) lift without twisting; (d) maintain good physical fitness; and (e) lift with the knees bent.

Physical fitness programs have also been promoted as effective in preventing back injuries (46). A study of the Los Angeles Fire Department showed a decrease in injuries between 1971 and 1978 that was attributed, in part, to better fitness levels. The rate of injuries dropped from 2,134 in 1971 to 1,814 in 1977 without an accompanying change in the size of the workforce or job duties (47). These findings were contradicted, however, in a study of aircraft workers, which showed no correlation between levels of cardiovascular fitness and back injuries (48). Persons with previous back injuries who participate in formal "back school" prevention programs have shown a reduction in the incidence of new injuries (49) and a reduction in mean absenteeism for back pain complaints (50).

The physician who is asked to recommend a preventive back program for a local organization is advised to consider a number of issues, including (a) medical data related to back injuries, (b) investigations (job review, in particular) related to the accidents at work, (c) job requirements, and (d) an individual's work capacity.

Coordinating the above measures and implementing prompt and efficient treatment that includes therapeutic exercises can control the incidence of back pain and its related sequelae. Employers must be informed about the need for frequent education of both supervisors and workers on proper back care and lifting techniques. Vigilant review of active back injury cases and appropriate reevaluation prior to return to work are essential.

SHOULDER DISORDERS

A variety of shoulder injuries are common in the occupational setting. *Impingement syndrome,* also referred to as rotator cuff tendonitis or subacromial bursitis, develops when the tendons of the rotator cuff are compressed when the shoulder is flexed and elevated. Repeated impingement can lead to inflammation of the tendons, which can extend to the subacromial bursa. Symptoms of pain may be acute or chronic and the patient may have a history of specific overuse, particularly above shoulder level. Strength and range of motion are often normal, but there will be pain on resisted forward shoulder flexion at 90 degrees while the arm is held extended and internally rotated ("impingement sign"). Treatment consists of antiinflammatory medications, ice, and rest, with subsequent physical therapy referral for range of motion and stretching exercises. Steroid injection should be considered if the patient shows no initial improvement.

Bicipital tendonitis is similar to impingement syndrome in that the proximal bicipital tendon becomes inflamed from repetitive motion. The patient usually has pain in the bicipital groove and on resisted forearm flexion. Treatment is similar to that for impingement syndrome.

Rotator cuff tears usually result from acute injury, but may be chronic. Examination reveals weakness on arm abduction through 60 degrees. MRI is usually required to confirm the diagnosis. Partial or chronic tears can be treated conservatively with strengthening and range of motion exercises. Complete tears should be evaluated by an orthopedic surgeon for consideration of surgical repair.

Recurrent glenohumeral subluxation can occur following acute shoulder dislocation resulting from a torn glenoid labrum (Bankart lesion) or a fracture of the humeral neck ("fracture dislocation"). Anterior instability is diagnosed by the "apprehension sign," wherein the patient becomes apprehensive when the shoulder is abducted and externally rotated. The patient may also give a history of a painful feeling of the joint being "out of place." Posterior instability is diagnosed when the patient is apprehensive when the arm is placed in forward flexion to 90 degrees in full internal rotation and some adduction and the arm is directed posteriorly. Conservative treatment, consisting of strengthening exercises, should be undertaken initially. If unsuccessful, or if posterior instability is present, orthopedic referral should be considered.

Acromioclavicular (AC) separation results from direct trauma to the AC joint. There is tenderness over the AC joint and pain on any shoulder motion. X-rays of the affected shoulder, with and without weights, reveal displacement of the AC joint. First-degree separation is an incomplete AC ligament tear without joint subluxation, second degree is some joint subluxation, and third degree is full tear of the AC ligament and coracoclavicular ligament with obvious subluxation. First- and second-degree separation can be treated with an arm sling, ice, and antiinflammatory medications, followed by strengthening exercises 1 to 3 weeks after the injury. Third-degree tears should be referred to an orthopedic surgeon for possible surgical correction.

Other diagnoses to consider when a patient presents with a shoulder injury or pain are glenoid labrum tears, pericapsulitis, osteoarthritis, and SLAP (superior labrum, anterior, and posterior) tears. SLAP tears require diagnosis by arthroscopy when conservative treatment is unsuccessful.

KNEE INJURIES

Traumatic injuries to the knee may result from direct external trauma, hyperextension, or varus or valgus twisting injuries.

Tears of the medial or lateral meniscus occur as a result of twisting with the foot planted. Pain is usually immediate followed by swelling, and there may be a history of "giving way," "locking," or "clicking" on ambulation. McMurray's test is performed with the hip flexed to 90 degrees and knee flexed to 90 degrees. The knee is then rotated either internally (lateral tears) or externally (medial tears), and the hip and the knee are gradually extended. If pain is elicited, the test is positive, but there is a high rate of false negatives. There is often localized joint line tenderness, which may be the only finding on examination. Definitive diagnosis requires MRI or arthroscopy. Initial treatment consists of immobilization for 1 to 3 weeks with ice and antiinflammatory medications, followed by a quadriceps strengthening program. If pain persists, or if the patient has a history of locking or concurrent ligament tears, referral to an orthopedist should be initiated.

Injuries to the medial and lateral collateral ligaments occur with a twisting injury or externally applied trauma. The ligament may be stretched or partially torn (sprain) or completely torn. Medial collateral ligament injuries are more common. One should check for collateral ligament instability by stabilizing the femur with the knee held at 0 degrees and then flexed to 20 degrees with slight external rotation. Varus and valgus stress should be applied, making sure that there is good muscular relaxation; comparison should always be made with the unaffected knee. For acute injuries, x-rays should be performed to rule out an associated fracture. Coexistent meniscal or cruciate ligament tears may be present. Sprains can be treated with immobilization and ice for 24 hours; then progressive weight bearing can be allowed. Orthopedic referral should be made if instability is present or if an associated meniscus tear cannot be ruled out.

Anterior cruciate ligament (ACL) injuries occur when force is applied to a slightly flexed knee or in twisting injuries. Often, a "pop" with immediate swelling may be noted at the time of the injury. The anterior drawer test is performed by applying anterior force to the fibia with the knee flexed at 90 degrees. This test can be performed in the supine position with the foot at 0 degrees, 30 degrees internal rotation, and 30 degrees external rotation with immobilization by sitting on the foot. The test can also be performed in the sitting position without foot immobilization. Muscular relaxation (especially of the hamstrings) is essential. Results should always be compared with the unaffected side. Lachman's test is performed by stabilizing the femur with one hand and applying anterior force to the tibia with the knee flexed at 30 degrees. The pivot-shift test is performed by applying valgus stress to the knee in extension with the tibia internally rotated, and slowly flexing the knee to about 30 degrees. A "pop" with pain suggests ACL laxity. Diagnosis often requires MRI for confirmation. If there is evidence of ligament instability, one should immobilize the knee and refer the patient to an orthopedic surgeon.

Posterior cruciate ligament (PCL) tears are usually associated with a severe injury involving other structures. Isolated PCL tears are uncommon, but can occur with externally applied trauma to the anterior tibia with the knee flexed. The posterior drawer test is performed by applying posterior force to the tibia with the knee flexed at 90 degrees. Frequently the tibia is in a posterior sagging position ("spontaneous posterior drawer") and it may appear that the anterior drawer is positive, when in fact the examiner is simply pulling the tibia into the anatomically correct position. One should always check the initial position of the tibia and evaluate if there is a firm anterior end point when performing the anterior drawer test. Treatment for isolated PCL tears consists of quadriceps strengthening and gradual return to normal activities. When other structures are involved, referral to an orthopedist is advised.

Diagnoses to consider if the patient has no specific history of trauma include patellofemoral pain syndrome (chondromalacia patellae), anserine tendonitis, osteoarthritis, and prepatellar or infrapatellar bursitis.

CUMULATIVE TRAUMA DISORDERS

Cumulative trauma disorders, also referred to as repetitive motion injuries, are conditions that are thought to be due to the repetitive performance of a similar task, rather than an injury that results from a single traumatic event (51). Cumulative trauma disorders (CTDs) primarily affect the upper extremities, especially the wrist, and include such disorders as carpal tunnel syndrome, wrist tendonitis, ulnar nerve entrapment, epicondylitis, shoulder tendonitis, and hand–arm vibration syndrome (51).

While the understanding of the pathophysiologic mechanism for these disorders has remained controversial (52), the reported incidence of CTDs has risen steadily since 1982 (50). This apparent increase may be attributable, in part, to improved awareness, diagnosis, and reporting of CTDs. Table 22.6 displays the rates of repetitive trauma cases recorded on OSHA 200 logs, and Table 22.7 lists the rates of these types of disorders, which peaked in the early 1990s and have been declining over the past 5 to 6 years. Under the new OSHA reporting requirements, specific cases of repetitive trauma are not separately reported on the OSHA 300 log.

TABLE 22.6. *Rate of illness cases per 10,000 workers (recordable repetitive trauma)*

1992	36.8
1993	38.3
1994	41.1
1995	37.8
1996	33.5
1997	32.0
1998	28.5
1999	27.3

From Bureau of Labor Statistics, U.S. Department of Labor, March 2001.

TABLE 22.7. *Rates of repeated trauma disorders (per 10,000 full-time workers) by selected industry: 2000*

Meat products	484.6
Transportation equipment	259.6
Food products	180.6
Apparel and other textile products	104.3
Medical instruments and supplies	103.1
Manufacturing	89.2
Instruments and related products	87.8
Electronic and other electrical equipment	72.9
Pharmaceuticals	54.1
Industrial machinery and equipment	45.1
Chemical and allied products	38.2
Printing and publishing	34.8
Health services	16.9
Transportation and public utilities	14.5
Wholesale and retail trade	8.5
Construction	3.7
All private industry	26.3

Carpal Tunnel Syndrome

Carpal tunnel syndrome refers to compression of the median nerve as it traverses the carpal tunnel in the wrist. The tightly bound carpal bones form the dorsal, medial, and lateral walls on the carpal tunnel. Anterior and superior to these bones is the transverse carpal ligament, a dense, nonresilient structure. The carpal tunnel, which is beneath this ligament, contains the median nerve, nine flexor tendons, and their tendon sheaths. At this point, the median nerve has motor fibers to a number of muscles in the hand including the opponens pollicis, abductor pollicis brevis, and the first and second interosseous muscles. The nerve also gives rise to the sensory branches of the midpalm, the palmar aspect of the first 3½ digits, and the dorsal tips of the fingers.

In a study of 652 workers in jobs with specific hand force and repetitive characteristics, the prevalence of carpal tunnel syndrome ranged from 0.6% among workers in low-force, low-repetitive jobs to 5.6% among workers in high-force, high-repetitive jobs. When the authors controlled for potential confounders, the odds ratio for the high-force repetitive jobs was more than 15 ($p < .001$) compared to the low-force repetitive jobs (53). A study among women showed that risk factors for developing carpal tunnel syndrome include history of previous musculoskeletal complaint, obesity, and older age (especially among past users of oral contraceptives). There was no association with psychologic problems or non-musculoskeletal pain complaints (12).

NIOSH proposed a case definition for work-related carpal tunnel syndrome in 1989 (54). The NIOSH criteria are (a) symptoms suggestive of carpal tunnel syndrome (paresthesia, hypoesthesia, or pain in distribution of the median nerve; (b) objective findings, which can include either a positive Tinel's or Phalen's sign, decreased sensation in the distribution of the median nerve, or abnormal electrodiagnostic findings of the median nerve across the carpal tunnel; and (c) evidence of work-relatedness (frequent, repetitive, or forceful hand work on affected side; sustained awkward hand position; use of vibrating tools; prolonged pressure over wrist or palm; or temporal relationship to work). A study examining the validity of this case definition concluded that reliance on physical examination alone for objective evidence resulted in a significant number of false-positive and false-negative results (55).

Controversy over the diagnostic criteria for this disorder has probably led to a significant amount of overdiagnosis of this condition (51).

History

The patient with carpal tunnel syndrome may experience numbness, burning, and tingling in the first 3½ digits. A frequent complaint also noted is coldness and clumsiness of the hand accompanied by weakness and dropping of objects. Some patients awaken from sleep with numbness and tingling in the hand, which they shake to relieve the discomfort.

Virtually any condition that increases the contents of or decreases the size of the carpal tunnel and in turn compresses the median nerve can lead to the problem. Nonoccupational disorders associated with carpal tunnel syndrome include rheumatoid arthritis, diabetes, degenerative arthritis, gout, hypothyroidism, congenital defects such as anomalous muscles, and acute trauma to the wrist. Any condition that results in edema of the hand or wrist, such as trauma, reflex sympathetic dystrophy, or pregnancy, can also cause carpal tunnel syndrome.

Clinical evaluation usually reveals that the little finger (fifth) is not involved and that numbness may be precipitated by gripping a steering wheel; holding tools such as pliers, power screwdrivers, and torque wrenches; or using a broom or kitchen utensil. If a person experiences these symptoms, careful attention should be directed to the possibility of carpal tunnel syndrome.

Physical Examination

The physical examination should focus on assessing the wrist for range of motion in flexion, extension, and lateral and medial mobility. Tapping the dorsum of the wrist anterior to the median nerve (Tinel's sign) can induce numbness in affected persons. Phalen's sign is performed by asking the patient to volar flex the wrist and maintain the position for 60 seconds. If tingling develops in the distribution of the median nerve, that is, the thumb, index, middle, and radial aspect of the ring finger, the test is positive. A study examining the validity of various history taking and physical examination tools for evaluating carpal tunnel syndrome concluded that traditional findings, including nocturnal paresthesias, Phalen's and Tinel's signs, thenar atrophy, and two-point vibratory and monofilament sensory testing are of little diagnostic value. Hand symptom diagrams, hypalgesia, and thumb abduction strength testing are helpful in the diagnosis of carpal tunnel syndrome (56).

Proper evaluation of carpal tunnel syndrome includes a review of other conditions that can cause pain and numbness in the wrist such as thoracic outlet syndrome, brachial plexus lesions, peripheral neuropathy, and herniated cervical discs with nerve root compression.

Electromyography/Nerve Conduction Velocity

The most useful tool in the diagnosis of carpal tunnel syndrome is measurement of EMG/NCV. EMG/NCV studies can confirm clinical findings and aid in the determination of the location and degree of nerve entrapment, if present. These studies are strongly suggested before formulating a diagnosis and initiating a referral to an orthopedic or hand surgeon for surgical correction. New portable nerve conduction testing devices have been shown to have a high level of agreement with traditional EMG/NCV (57).

Treatment

Initial treatment of carpal tunnel syndrome can be conducted by the primary care physician. A volar splint with the wrist held in mild dorsiflexion applied prior to sleep can often be effective; the same splint can be used in settings associated with discomfort. If the patient has an illness that contributes to carpal tunnel syndrome, it should be treated initially. NSAIDs can also be effective. Traditionally, patients are instructed to wear splints at night only. However, full-time splint wearing may result in better outcomes (58).

Once carpal tunnel syndrome develops, the condition usually progresses or at best stabilizes. Eventually, clinical management focuses on the need for and value of surgical correction. Ideally, these decisions are best coordinated by the primary care physician and a consultant in orthopedic or hand surgery. Issues such as the presence of motor weakness, the type of job and availability of reassignment, and the needs and interests of the patient should be considered.

Injections with corticosteroids in the carpal tunnel can relieve symptoms, but it is not clear whether the effects are long lasting (59,60).

Surgical decompression of the carpal tunnel usually relieves a significant amount of pain, although numbness might persist. Whether numbness is a permanent sequela depends in part on the duration and severity of the nerve entrapment. Elderly patients and those with long-standing symptoms, especially muscle weakness and thenar atrophy, may continue to experience numbness and weakness, although pain and discomfort are usually relieved by surgery. A recent study concluded that disability outcomes were better among those with work-related carpal tunnel syndrome treated surgically versus those treated nonsurgically (61).

Preventive interventions are essential to avoid progression or recurrence of carpal tunnel syndrome. A workstation analysis should be performed, and the risk factors should be identified. Workstations should be redesigned to reduce tasks that require prolonged extension or repetitive motion of the wrist.

Wrist Tendonitis

Although traumatic disorders of the tendons of the hand are serious occupationally related injuries, they tend to be relatively uncommon. But irritation of the tendon, referred to as tendonitis, is common in jobs that require frequent and repetitive motions, usually of the upper extremity, especially the hand and elbow but also the shoulder. Sites that may contribute to problems include the muscle, tendon, synovium, tendon sheath, and tendon insertion. Irritation of these structures can occur from repetitive motion activities as well as unaccustomed or severe use of the hand.

A common problem is that associated with excessive or forced repetitive motion that results in irritation of the tendon or its sheath. Ultimately, motion of the affected fingers causes pain and crepitations noted on palpation. The disorder is more accurately described as tenosynovitis, which can progress to the point that the tendon sheath thickens. Restricted motion of the joints of the hand can then result.

One particular type of tenosynovitis is de Quervain's syndrome. The sheaths of the extensor pollicis longus (short thumb extensor) and abductor pollicis longus (long thumb abductor) become thickened. This condition may be traumatic in origin, especially with repeated abduction and extension of the thumb. Diagnosis is made by noting tenderness to palpation of the tendons in the first dorsal compartment of the radial aspect of the wrist. Finklestein's sign is another diagnostic sign that may be helpful. In this maneuver, the patient adducts the thumb into the hand, resting on the palm. The physician then applies an ulnar deviation force to the wrist. The test is positive if this maneuver elicits pain in the first dorsal compartment. In de Quervain's syndrome and in other causes of tendonitis not due to systemic or local infectious disease, the hand should be placed at rest by splinting with a thumb spica splint or with an appropriate support. Systemic NSAIDs and application of local heat can relieve discomfort. In some cases, careful injection of corticosteroids into the first dorsal compartment provides dramatic and long-lasting relief.

Hand–Arm Vibration Syndrome

Hand–arm vibration syndrome, formerly known as vibration white finger, is a condition seen in workers who use handheld vibrating tools. Common presenting symptoms are numbness, tingling, or pain in the fingertips and hands that may progress to weakness and loss of fine motor coordination (62). The pathophysiology of vibration finger probably involves three types of vascular disorders: digital organic microangiopathy, a digital vasospastic phenomenon, and arterial thrombosis in the upper extremities. In addition, vibration can directly affect sensory nerves, causing numbness (63). NIOSH has published diagnostic criteria for hand–arm vibration syndrome (64). The diagnosis is based primarily on the occupational history, and other disorders that can cause hand paresthesias (Raynaud's phenomenon, collagen vascular disorders, or carpal tunnel syndrome) should be ruled out with appropriate laboratory testing (62).

Treatment is aimed at preventing progression of the disease. Careful review of the use of the vibrating tool is essential and consideration of job modification should be made. In some cases, the worker may be unable to use any vibrating equipment. NSAIDs may be helpful in reducing pain. Vasodilators or calcium channel blockers hold some promise in treating the underlying vasospastic episodes (62). If carpal tunnel syndrome is coexistent, wrist splints may be of some benefit.

Epicondylitis

Two relatively common musculoskeletal conditions that occur at work are lateral and medial epicondylitis of the elbow. These disorders result from excessive stress on the muscle groups around the elbow and forearm. In lateral epicondylitis the extensor supinator group of muscles is involved, whereas in medial epicondylitis the flexor pronator muscles are affected. Although these conditions, especially lateral epicondylitis, are frequently associated with sporting activities ("tennis elbow"), use of a hammer, screwdriver, or masonry tools can also precipitate the disorder. Generally, no loss of elbow function occurs; however, pain develops in the affected area of the elbow. Distal radiation of the pain is often associated with a firm grip.

Examination usually reveals tenderness on palpation over the lateral epicondyle, the site of the insertion of the extensor and supinator muscles supplying the wrist. Symptoms are usually reproduced by asking the patient to extend the wrist against resistance. Medial epicondylitis follows a similar course to that of lateral epicondylitis; however, symptoms are usually reproduced by wrist flexion against resistance or by firm palpation of the medial humeral epicondyle.

Primary treatment of both of these disorders requires that the patient refrain from aggravating activities. The administration of systemic NSAIDs, limitation of motion of the elbow through splints and supports, and local heat are advisable initially. Prolonged and marked restriction of activities is ill advised because of the potential for developing stiffness and tightness and ultimately a "frozen" joint. Local infiltration of the affected areas, especially over the trigger site, with 1% lidocaine mixed with a solution of corticosteroids may produce immediate resolution of the symptoms. Repeat injections should be avoided. In general, however, these conditions are apt to recur, especially if the person returns to the same job without changes in job design or work practices.

Other Nerve Entrapment Syndromes

Repetitive motion of the upper extremities can also result in entrapment of the median, ulnar, and radial nerves in other locations (51). *Pronator teres syndrome* involves entrapment of the median nerve in the forearm, while *radial tunnel syndrome* refers to entrapment of the radial nerve by repetitive motion of the extensor muscles of the forearm. *Cubital tunnel syndrome* is when the ulnar nerve becomes entrapped from external pressure over the cubital tunnel at the elbow.

NECK INJURIES

Neck injuries involving muscular strain and spasm are common in the occupational setting (65). For neck injuries in which there is any suspicion of subluxation of the cervical vertebra, immediate immobilization and prompt emergency evaluation are essential. Most acute neck strains result in some degree of overstretching of the paracervical musculature and trapezius muscles. *Cervical strain* usually refers to forced flexion and extension of the neck ("whiplash"), resulting in pain that is often delayed by 12 to 24 hours. *Trapezius strains* are caused by sudden twisting of the neck, often associated with shoulder extension or arm abduction. These types of strains are extremely common and usually respond to conservative treatment with ice or moist heat, NSAIDs, and muscle relaxants (66). Initial treatment is similar to that for low back strains. In cases in which the patient has persistent pain, referral to a physical therapist may be helpful.

Herniations of cervical intervertebral discs are not as common as herniated lumbar discs. However, if the patient has persistent pain or numbness radiating to the shoulder or arm and persistent or progressive abnormal neurologic findings on examination, MRI is indicated to rule out impingement of a cervical nerve root. Nerve conduction studies can be a helpful adjunct in assessing cervical radiculopathies due to a variety of causes. Neurosurgical referral is appropriate if a cervical nerve root is compromised or if spinal stenosis is present.

Occupational cervicobrachial disorder (or "fibromyalgia") refers to neck and shoulder pain associated with repetitive extension of the arms above shoulder height either in static postures or with low external loads (41). This disorder is difficult to treat and frequently requires complete workstation redesign or job transfer. Physical therapy, antiinflammatory medications, and muscle relaxants may be of some benefit in initial treatment of this disorder. If trigger points are identified, an injection with a combination of anesthetic (such as lidocaine) and corticosteroids may provide some relief.

REFERENCES

1. Bureau of Labor Statistics, U.S. Department of Labor, March 2001.
2. Spengler DM, et al. Back injuries in industry: a retrospective study. I. Overview and cost analysis. *Spine* 1986;11:241.
3. Frymoyer JW, Cats-Bavil WL. An overview of the costs and incidence of low back pain. *Orthop Clin North Am* 1991;22:263.
4. Daltroy LH, et al. A case-control study of risk factors for industrial low back injury: implications for primary and secondary prevention programs. *Am J Ind Med* 1991;20:505.
5. Kelsey JL, Golden AL, Mundt DJ. Low back pain/prolapsed intervertebral disc. *Rheum Dis Clin North Am* 1990;16:699.
6. Quinet RJ, Hadler NM. Diagnosis and treatment of back ache. *Semin Arthritis Rheum* 1979;9:261.
7. Deyo RA, Rainville J, Kent DL. What can the history and physical examination tell us about low back pain? *JAMA* 1992;268:760.
8. Snook SH. The design of manual handling tasks. *Ergonomics* 1978;21:963.
9. NIOSH Technical Report. *Work practices guide for manual lifting.* DHHS (NIOSH) publication No. 81-122. Washington, DC: U.S. Government Printing Office, March 1981.
10. Modic MT, Ross JS. Magnetic resonance imaging in the evaluation of low back pain. *Orthop Clin North Am* 1991;22:283.
11. Deyo, Weinstein. Low back pain. *N Engl J Med* 2001; 344:5.
12. Coste J, et al. Clinical course and prognostic factors in acute low back pain in an inception cohort study in primary care practice. *Br Med J* 1994;308:577–580.
13. Deyo RA. Bed rest for low back pain: how much is enough? *N Engl J Med* 1986;315:1064.
14. Naddell, Feder, Lewis. Systematic reviews of bed rest and advice to stay active for acute low back pain. *Br J Gen Pract* 1997;47:647–662.
15. Malmivaara, et al. The treatment of low back pain-bed rest, exercises, or ordinary activity? *N Engl J Med* 1995;332:351–355.
16. Muckle DS. Comparative study of ibuprofen and aspirin in soft tissue injuries. *Rehabilitation (Bonn)* 1974; 13:141.
17. Van Tulder, et al. Non steroidal anti-inflammatory drugs for low back pain: a systematic review within the framework of the Cochrane Collaboration Back Review Group. *Spine* 2000;25(19):2501–2513.
18. Saal JA, Saa JS. Nonoperative treatment of herniated lumbar intervertebral disc with radiculopathy: an outcome study. *Spine* 1989;14:431.
19. Bozzao, et al. Lumbar disc herniation: MR imaging assessment of natural history in patients treated without surgery. *Radiology* 1992;185:135–141.
20. Brown JR. Factors contributing to the development of low back pain in industrial workers. *Am Ind Hyg Assoc J* 1975;26–31.
21. Wiesel SW, Ferrer HL, Rothman RH. *Industrial low back pain.* Charlottesville, VA: Michie, 1985.
22. Aaronoff GM. Pain treatment: is it a right or a privilege? *Clin J Pain* 1986;1:187.
23. Florence DW. The chronic pain syndrome. *Postgrad Med* 1981;70:217.
24. Waddell G, et al. Nonorganic physical signs in low-back pain. *Spine* 1980;5:117.
25. Koes BW, et al. The effectiveness of manual therapy, physiotherapy, and treatment by the general practitioner for nonspecific back and neck complaints: a randomized clinical trial. *Spine* 1992;17:28.
26. Koes BW, et al. Spinal manipulation and mobilization for back and neck pain: a blinded review. *Br Med J* 303:1298.
27. Deyo RA, et al. A controlled trial of transcutaneous electrical nerve stimulation (TENS) and exercise for chronic low back pain. *N Engl J Med* 1990;322:1627.
28. Cavette S, et al. A controlled trial of corticosteroid injections into facet joints for chronic low back pain. *N Engl J Med* 1991;325:1002.
29. Nelemaus, et al. Injection therapy for subacute and chronic benign low back pain. *Spine* 2001;26(5): 501–515.
30. Fishbain, et al. Evidence-based data on pain relief with antidepressants. *Ann Med* 2000;32(5):305–316.
31. Troup JDG. Causes, prediction, and prevention of back pain at work. *Scand J Work Environ Health* 1984;10: 419.
32. van Poppel, et al. Lumbar supports and education for the prevention of low back pain in industry: a randomized controlled trial. *JAMA* 1998;279:1789–1794.
33. Daltroy, et al. A controlled trial of an educational program to prevent low back pain injuries. *N Engl J Med* 1997;337:322–328.
34. Lahad, et al. The effectiveness of four interventions for the prevention of low back pain. *JAMA* 1994;272: 1296–1291.
35. Snook SH. Low back pain in industry. In: *American Academy of Orthopedic Surgeons Symposium on Idiopathic Low Back Pain.* St. Louis: Mosby, 1982.
36. Bigos SJ, et al. A prospective evaluation of pre-employ-

ment screening methods for acute industrial back pain. *Spine* 1992;17:922.
37. Bigos SJ, et al. Back injuries in industry: a retrospective study. III. Employee-related factors. *Spine* 1986;11:252.
38. Repko GR, Cooper R. A study of the average workers compensation case. *J Clin Psychol* 1983;39:287.
39. Bohart WH. Anatomic variations and anomalies of the spine: relation to prognosis and length of disability. *JAMA* 1928;92:698.
40. Present AJ. Radiography of the lower back in pre-employment physical examinations. Presented at the ACR/NIOSH Conference, January 11–14, 1973. *Radiology* 1979;8:261.
41. Rowe ML. Are routine spine films on workers in industry cost or risk benefit effective? *J Occup Med* 1982;24:41.
42. Biering-Sorensen F. Physical measurements as risk indicators for low back trouble during a one year period. *Spine* 1984;9:106.
43. Keyserling WM, Herrin GD, Chaffin DB. Isometric strength testing as a means of controlling medical incidents on strenuous jobs. *J Occup Med* 1980;22:332.
44. Chaffin DB, Herrin GD, Keyserling WM. Pre-employment strength testing: an updated position. *J Occup Med* 1978;20:403.
45. Gracovetsky S. Determination of load. *Br J Ind Med* 1986;43:120.
46. Litchfield MM, Freedson PS. Physical training programs for public safety personnel. *Clin Sports Med* 1986;5:571.
47. Mealey M. New fitness for police and firefighters. *Phys Sport Med* 1979;7:96.
48. Battie MC, et al. A prospective study of the role for cardiovascular risk factors and fitness in industrial back complaints. *Spine* 1989;14:141.
49. Brown KC, et al. Cost effectiveness of a back school intervention for municipal employees. *Spine* 1992;17:1224.
50. Versloot JM, et al. The cost effectiveness of a back school program in industry: a longitudinal controlled field study. *Spine* 1992;17:22–27.
51. Rempel DM, Harrison RJ, Barnhart S. Work-related cumulative trauma disorders of the upper extremity. *JAMA* 1992;167:838.
52. Hadler NM. Cumulative trauma disorders: an intragenic concept. *J Occup Med* 1990;32:38.
53. Silverstein BA, Fine LJ, Armstrong TJ. Occupational factors in carpal tunnel syndrome. *Am J Ind Med* 1987; 11:343.
54. Matte TD, Baker EL, Honchar PA. The selection and definition of target work-related conditions for surveillance under SENSOR. *Am J Public Health* 1989;79 [suppl]:21.
55. Katz JN, et al. Validation of a surveillance case definition of carpal tunnel syndrome. *Am J Public Health* 1991;81:189.
56. D'Aray, McGee. The rational clinical examination: does this patient have carpal tunnel syndrome? *JAMA* 2000; 283(23):3110–3117.
57. Median nerve latency measurement agreement between portable and conventional methods. *J Hand Surg* 2000; 25(1):73–77.
58. Walker, et al. Neutral wrist splinting in carpal tunnel syndrome: a comparison of night-only versus full-time wear instructions. *Arch Phys Med Rehabil* 2000;81(4): 424–429.
59. Gonzalez, Bylak. Steroid injection and splinting in the treatment of carpal tunnel syndrome. *Orthopaedics* 2001;24(5):479–481.
60. Dammers, Veeving, Vermeuleu. Injection with methylprednisone proximal to the carpal tunnel: randomized double blind trial. *Br Med J* 1999;319(7214):884–886.
61. Shin, et al. Disability outcomes in a worker's compensation population: surgical versus nonsurgical treatment of carpal tunnel syndrome. *Am J Orthop* 2000;29(3): 179–184.
62. Pyykko I. Clinical aspects of hand-arm vibration syndrome: a review. *Scand J Work Environ Health* 1986;12: 439.
63. Noel. Pathophysiology and classification of the vibration whole finger. *Int Arch Occup Environ Health* 2000; 73(3):150–155.
64. *Criteria for a recommended standard: occupational exposure to hand-arm vibration.* National Institute for Occupational Safety (NIOSH), Department of Health and Human Services publication No. 89-106, September 1986.
65. Brisson PM, Nordin M, Zettenberg C. Neck and upper extremity impairment. In: Rom WN, ed. *Environmental and occupational medicine,* 2nd ed. Boston: Little, Brown, 1992:719–720.
66. Birnbaum JS. *The musculoskeletal manual,* 2nd ed. Philadelphia: WB Saunders, 1986:31–38.

FURTHER INFORMATION

Birnbaum JS. *The musculoskeletal manual,* 2nd ed. Philadelphia: WB Saunders, 1986.

A basic guide to diagnosis and management of musculoskeletal problems for the non-orthopedist.

Bureau of Labor Statistics. *What every employer needs to know about OSHA recordkeeping.* Report No. 412-413, 1978.

Guidelines to maintenance of records under the Occupational Safety and Health Act of 1970.

Isernhagen SJ. Principles of prevention for cumulative trauma. *Occup Med State of the Art Rev* 1992;7:147.

A comprehensive review of occupational cumulative trauma problems and methods of prevention.

Keim H, ed. Low back pain. *Ciba Clin Symp* 1988;39:1.

Primer on the treatment of low back injuries.

O'Donoghue DH. *Treatment of injuries to athletes.* Philadelphia: WB Saunders, 1984.

Pariapour M, et al. Environmentally induced disorders of the musculoskeletal system. *Med Clin North Am* 1990;74:347.

A review of the pathophysiology, epidemiology, diagnosis, and treatment of musculoskeletal injuries, including psychosocial and organizational factors.

Rowe ML. *Orthopaedic problems at work.* Fairport, NY: Perinton, 1985.

A practical guide to the diagnosis, treatment, and rehabilitation of common work-related musculoskeletal disorders. Written by an orthopedic surgeon with over 20 years' experience in evaluating occupational musculoskeletal problems.

Seeger LL. MRI of the musculoskeletal system. *Orthopedics* 1992;15:437; Bassett LW, Gold RH. Magnetic resonance imaging of the musculoskeletal system. *Clin Orthop Rel Res* 1989;244:17.

Both articles are good reviews of the principles, indications, and limitations of this diagnostic modality.

23
Occupational Cancers

Arthur Frank

In 1775, while recuperating from a broken leg suffered after being hit by a horse-drawn carriage, Sir Percival Pott had time to put pen to paper and wrote about his experience with cancers of the scrotum seen among young chimney sweeps. This became the first written documentation of an occupational cancer (1), even though it took until well into the 20th century for it to be understood that the polycyclic aromatics in soot were the cause of these skin cancers. Cancer continues to be one of the diseases people fear most, and workplace and environmental exposures play a significant role in the development of the many manifestations of this disease. Cancer continues to extract a large toll in society, both in terms of human suffering and economic cost. Cancer deaths continue to follow cardiovascular deaths as a main cause of mortality, and each year more than one million Americans develop some form of cancer, and over half a million die of this disease each year (2).

With a few exceptions, overall progress in cancer treatment has been discouraging (3), and until new therapies are developed that go beyond traditional radiotherapy and chemotherapy, this will probably remain the case. Having understood that environmental factors play a major role in the causation of cancer (4), a variety of preventive measures become increasingly important as attempts are made to alter cancer disease patterns. The workplace remains a significant source of exposures, as do certain personal habits such as cigarette smoking and exposure to sunlight.

CARCINOGENESIS

The term *cancer* refers to many dozens of distinct and separate diseases that can affect virtually any tissue in the body and that share several biologic characteristics. Cancer is characterized by rapid, generally unrestrained growth by a population of cells that has been derived from a biologically altered cell, with a failure of these cells to show normal differentiation and function, and that survive and propagate for unusually long periods of time. Lung cancer is now the leading cause of cancer deaths in both men and women and other significant numbers of cases are represented by breast cancer, prostate cancer, and colon and rectal cancer, with most cancer deaths occurring in older individuals.

A substance that is capable of producing cancer is called a carcinogen, and there is a gradation regarding the certainty with which exposures may cause this disease. There are several recognized systems for the classification of carcinogenic substances, and these can refer to a wide variety of chemicals, physical agents, biologic agents, and sometimes to various industrial processes without knowing exactly what the causative agent might be (5).

Cellular Aspects of Cancer

The exact mechanism by which exposures turn normal cells into malignant cells is still incompletely understood. Some mechanistic insights are available, as are some genetic aspects of the development of cancer. For some substances there is an understanding at the cellular level as to how and why cancer may be an outcome following exposure. While cancer is clearly a dose-response disease, with more disease occurring at higher doses, it is also clear that on occasion low levels of exposure can lead to the development of some forms of cancer, and low doses may even be more potent per unit than at higher doses.

Carcinogenesis at the Cellular Level

At the present time our understanding of the process of carcinogenesis remains incomplete. With work going back some six decades, it is clear that the development of cancer is not a simple process, and that multiple steps and several alterations of DNA may be required before cancer develops. The earliest animal models looked at the issues of initiation, which was defined as the inciting of an irreversible change occurring in a cell's genetic material, and promotion, which was looked upon as interactions that by themselves would not cause cancer to develop but that would accelerate the subsequent steps after initiation that ultimately result in clinical malignancy (6).

The changes in the genetic material are characterized by alterations of DNA, and the issues of mutagenicity, teratogenicity, and carcinogenicity are closely linked. All involve alterations of genetic material, and often substances may have the ability to produce multiple different outcomes. A surrogate for carcinogenicity, laboratory models looking at mutations, were widely evaluated as predictors of the cancer-causing ability of materials. Additional understandings that have developed have caused scientists to recognize that there is a multistep process in the development of cancers, and further complicating matters is that there are many anticancer interactions as well (7). Certain materials lessen the effects of carcinogens or mutagens, and the body's natural defense mechanisms, such as its immunologic system, deal with cell alterations on a regular basis.

Additional developments in the field of molecular biology have further clarified the multistep nature of carcinogenesis (8). Studies of RNA viruses have revealed that some, when they insert their genetic material into host genomes, can cause malignant transformation. These pieces of information were called oncogenes. It also became clear that precursor forms of these oncogenes, called proto-oncogenes, were commonly found in human and animal cells, and might well play a role in normal cell function. The transformation of proto-oncogenes into oncogenes could now alter cell cycle activities and affect the differentiation and growth patterns of cells. There are many such examples of these oncogenes and of how they are affected by materials in the general environment (9).

Another kind of gene important in the matter of carcinogenesis is the tumor suppressor gene, or antioncogene. Such suppressor genes normally function to help regulate cell growth and stimulate normal cell differentiation. When they become inactivated they fail to perform these functions and increase the likelihood of future neoplastic transformation. The most commonly identified example is the *p53* gene, located on chromosome 7. Mutations of the *p53* gene are commonly identified in a wide variety of cancers including those of the colon, lung, liver, esophagus, breast, and other tissues (10).

Increasingly, genotoxic agents are being identified in the workplace (11), and the mechanisms by which genetic change may take place is being investigated (12).

Carcinogen Metabolism

Carcinogens can act differently in terms of how they can damage DNA. Some carcinogenic agents, such as radiation or bis(chloromethyl)ether, damage DNA directly, but many compounds require metabolic activation to be transformed into a compound capable of effecting DNA. The enzymes primarily responsible for this metabolic activation are those of the cytochrome P-450 system (13). Other enzymes involved include *N*-acetyltransferase, epoxide hydrolase, and glutathione S-transferase. Basically, these enzymes take foreign compounds and make them more polar, usually allowing them to be more readily excreted by the body. In the process, however, they often create reactive electrophiles, which can more readily bind with DNA in the formation of adducts, which ultimately may cause cellular mutations.

There are considerable differences among the metabolic activation functions seen in various species, and even among different individuals (14). Humans can vary several thousand times in their levels of a common enzyme, aryl hydrocarbon hydroxylase, one of the enzymes of the cytochrome P-450 system that is active in metabolizing polycyclic aromatic hydrocarbons (PAHs). High levels of this enzyme, which more readily transform PAHs, are associated with an increased risk of lung cancer, presumably because more reactive species are created. While clearly reflecting a variety of genetic factors, differences can also result from exposures that can induce enzyme activity, such as cigarette smoking, diet, and alcohol. Because of these differences in activation, some caution should be given to interspecies extrapolation from animal evidence to humans. However, there is still considerable value in using animal models in predicting potential hazards for humans. Also, it should be recognized that these personal differences imply that some individuals are at greater risk than others because of their inherent genetic factors and other environmental influences. Such information, however, should never be used to deny individuals employment, but should provide guidance for minimizing exposure. Assessment of individuals' ability to metabolize potential carcinogens, or their history of other exposures, can give guidance to the medical surveillance and monitoring of such individuals (15).

Other Considerations of Carcinogenesis Theory

The following subsections discuss a variety of other issues relevant to understanding the development of cancer in humans.

Latency

Latency refers to the period of time between the first exposure to a carcinogen and the development of a malignancy. Technically, this would more likely refer to the clinical detection of such malignancies, which may in reality exist for many years prior to their becoming clinically apparent. Every disease has a latency period, some as short as minutes, but when it comes to carcinogenic exposure one is usually dealing with decades, although in some instances only a few years may transpire. Many human carcinogens are said to follow the "20-year rule," where the onset of an increase in malignancy rates is seen two decades after the onset of exposure, although the exposure can be of short duration. For some situations, such as malignancies arising from radiation or benzene, the time course may be much shorter, sometimes even less than 5 years. It also appears that the excess carcinogenic risk for most materials will last throughout an individual's lifetime, even after exposure ceases.

This concept of latency has implications for the surveillance of workers who are at risk for developing malignancies because of certain exposures. Surveillance programs should be established with consideration of the latency required for the development of the cancers of concern, and should focus attention on this time period, perhaps after establishing a baseline at some earlier interval. Some screenings are mandated by law, and others make good sense, although the real impact of surveillance and early detection is much less important than primary prevention.

Threshold

Another concept relevant to the issue of carcinogenesis is that of a threshold. For many nonmalignant diseases there clearly appears to be a threshold of exposure that must be crossed before disease is seen in individuals. This threshold may vary among individuals, but there does seem to be for many occupational diseases levels of exposure that do not appear to put individuals at any increased risk. However, this does not apply to the issue of carcinogenic exposure, where the widely accepted principle is that for carcinogens there is no threshold and that while the risk with lower exposures diminishes, there is essentially no safe level of exposure to a carcinogen below which cancer will not occur.

The matter of a threshold can be looked at in several ways. At any given time, a single mutation in a single cell caused by a single exposure to a carcinogenic material may give rise, ultimately, to a malignancy. This would argue against the concept of any threshold with regard to consideration of a carcinogenic material. However, it should also be noted that there are individual variations in risk, and that there are subcellular repair mechanisms when damage occurs to DNA. It may be argued that when individuals have well-functioning repair mechanisms, and such systems are not overloaded, the body has some defenses against the development of malignancy. However, with aging these defenses seem to become less efficient, and there also appear to be circumstances where massive exposures can overwhelm the ability of an individual to fight off a carcinogenic insult. There may also be special risk to younger individuals; children appear to have more rapidly growing tissue that may well put them at risk for a greater likelihood of developing malignancies than adults.

As a rule, regulations adopt the view that thresholds do not exist and that legally allowable workplace levels should not be considered safe.

Synergism

Another concept that should be considered is that of multiple factor interactions. While regulations generally look at carcinogens on a case-by-case basis, it has been well established that multiple exposures to carcinogenic substances can greatly increase the risk for individuals in developing certain kinds of cancers. First documented with regard to the combination of asbestos and cigarette smoking in the production of greatly increased numbers of lung cancer, such synergistic or multiple-factor interactions have been documented for a variety of carcinogenic substances acting together. There are also now increasing examples of antagonistic actions where the effect of carcinogenic exposure can be lessened by simultaneous exposure to anticarcinogenic agents, such as may be found in certain food products. There are some situations where this multiplicative action is noted, and others where something less, and closer to additive effects, may be found. Relevant to these issues, there is now more interest and research support for studying the effects of mixtures of chemicals than the traditional approach, which looks at chemicals one substance at a time.

Chemoprevention

Ideally, it would be possible to have humans take in substances that would delay or reverse the cancer-causing ability of carcinogens. Research has documented epidemiologically that certain populations ingesting certain products, such as green tea, have a lower risk of developing some kinds of cancers. Several mechanisms have been put forward, and some seem to have merit and biologic plausibility. However, after initial enthusiasms for the use of vitamin supplements, for example, studies in which at-risk populations are given vitamin A or C have not shown that such supplementation markedly affects cancer outcome, and some studies have even suggested an increased risk after such intake. More research is needed to better understand this multifaceted aspect.

Testing and Evaluation of Carcinogens

The identification of potential human carcinogens comes via several routes: human epidemiologic studies, evaluations done in animal models, in vitro testing systems, and analysis of structure–activity relationships.

Epidemiologic studies have the highest potential for definitively answering the question of human carcinogenicity since such studies are based on human exposures. It should be recognized, however, that epidemiologic studies are difficult and expensive to carry out, and the findings may be difficult to interpret due to a variety of issues including confounding, poor exposure data, and other difficulties.

The quality of epidemiologic studies is evaluated by many organizations when decisions are to be made regarding if a material is, or is not, a human carcinogen. Recognizing that there are difficulties in doing this, and also making use of the other test modalities that are available, agencies may decide on the basis of these various test results to differentially classify the strength with which they feel a material is a carcinogen. This is detailed below.

Animal studies are generally carried out following standard protocols, using two species of rodents and both males and females, and often at several dosage levels of a suspected carcinogen. The National Toxicology Program, run under the auspices of the National Institute for Environmental Health Sciences, uses such standard protocols in setting up animal experimentation. Animals are sacrificed at prescribed periods of time and the number and types of tumors are noted, as well as their locations. On the basis of these animal studies, often involving only several hundred animals, findings may be extrapolated to humans, given the understanding of the imprecisions of exact translation of information between species (16). It should also be recognized that high doses are generally given to animals, often exceeding levels to which humans are exposed, but given the relative small number of animals used this allows for a better likelihood of determining the carcinogenic nature of a material.

In vitro testing involves the use of cultured tissue, often bacteria, but sometimes also human cultures, which may be grown in traditional cell culture, or sometimes by organ culture technique. Possible carcinogens are added into these systems, and various end points that reflect DNA damage are monitored. The best known of these in vitro tests, the Ames test, utilizes mutant strains of *Salmonella typhimurium,* and genetic alterations in these bacteria are then recorded. Although they are less directly applicable to humans than epidemiologic or animal data, they have certain advantages including the rapidity with which testing can be done, and their relatively low cost (17).

Lastly, there is some ability to predict the possible carcinogenicity of materials based on their structure. Certain carcinogens have known structures, and certain parts of those structures appear to be the operative areas. Other compounds with similar structures are looked upon with suspicion given that they appear to have the same potential abilities. Such assessments are then generally further evaluated with increasingly more extensive testing.

Tables 23.1 and 23.2 list the International Agency for Research on Cancer (IARC) established and strongly suspected human occupational carcinogens, and examples of occurrence.

As noted above, agencies that are concerned with identifying carcinogens review all data that may be available regarding particular compounds and reach judgments based on the totality of the information. Regulatory agencies like the Occupational Safety and Health Administration (OSHA) may do this, as would the National Institute for Occupational Safety and Health (NIOSH) in terms of making their recommendations to OSHA. Internationally, agencies such as the IARC categorize potential carcinogens into various groups. Group 1 includes those chemicals or industrial processes that are well established as human carcinogens based on sufficient evidence, usually from epi-

TABLE 23.1. *Established human occupational carcinogens [International Agency for Research on Cancer (IARC) group 1]*

Industrial processes	
Aluminum production	
Auramine manufacturing	
Boot and shoe manufacturing and repair	
Coal gasification	
Coke production	
Furniture and cabinetmaking	
Iron and steel founding	
Isopropyl alcohol manufacturing (strong acid process)	
Magenta manufacturing	
Painting	
Rubber industry	
Underground hematite mining with radon exposure	
Chemicals and mixtures[a]	
Exposures	Examples of occurrence
Aflatoxins	Grains, peanuts
4-Aminobiphenyl	Rubber industry
Arsenic and arsenic compounds	Insecticides
Asbestos	Insulation, friction products
Benzene	Chemical industry
Benzidine	Rubber and dye industries
Bis(chloromethyl) ether and chloromethyl methyl ether	Chemical industry
Chromium (VI) compounds	Metal plating, pigments
Coal tar pitches	Coal distillation
Coal tars	Coal distillation
Erionite	Environmental (Turkey)
Mineral oils	Machining, jute processing
Mustard gas	Production, war gas
β-Naphthylamine	Rubber and dye industries
Nickel compounds	Nickel refining and smelting
Radon and its decay products	Indoor environments, mining
Shale oils	Energy production
Soots	Chimneys, furnaces
Talc containing asbestiform fibers	Talc mining, pottery manufacturing
Vinyl chloride	Plastics industry

[a]Other chemicals and mixtures, including chemotherapeutic agents, tobacco, and others, have been classified in group 1.

From Vainio H, Wilbourn J. Identification of carcinogens within the IARC monograph program. *Scand J Work Environ Health* 1992;18[suppl]:64.

demiologic studies. Group 2, which is then further subdivided, includes chemicals and processes that are probably (group 2A) or possibly (group 2B) carcinogenic to humans. Those materials in group 2A reflect limited evidence of carcinogenicity in humans but sufficient evidence of carcinogenicity in animal experiments, while group 2B reflects limited evidence in humans without sufficient evidence in animals, or sufficient evidence in animals but without any existing in humans. IARC policy recommends treating group 2 chemicals as if they present a carcinogenic risk to humans. Group 3 includes agents that are not classified, usually because there is insufficient evidence of any type to make a judgment, and group 4 includes agents that are thought probably not to be carcinogenic to humans. Of more than 700 chemicals, industrial processes, or personal habits that have been evaluated by IARC, more than 50 have been placed in group 1 and some 250 or so are now in group 2. This type of classification and the results of IARC evaluations, are looked at by many other organizations including the National Toxicology Program, NIOSH, OSHA, and the American Conference of Governmental Industrial Hygienists (ACGIH).

TABLE 23.2. *Strongly suspected human occupational carcinogens (IARC group 2A)*

Industrial processes	
Petroleum refining (certain exposures)	
Insecticide application (nonarsenicals)	
Chemicals and mixtures[a]	
Exposures	**Examples of occurrence**
Acrylonitrile	Plastics industry
Benz[a]anthracene	Coal distillation
Benzidine-based dyes	Dye industry
Benzo[a]pyrene	Coal and petroleum-derived products
Beryllium and Be compounds	Be extraction, electronics
Cadmium and cadmium compounds	Battery and alloy manufacturing
Creosotes	Wood preservatives
Dibenz[a,h]anthracene	Coal distillation
Diesel engine exhaust	Motor vehicles
Diethyl sulfate	Petrochemical industry
Dimethylcarbamoyl chloride	Dimethylcarbamoyl chloride manufacturing
Dimethyl sulfate	Chemical industry
Epichlorhydrin	Resin manufacturing
Ethylene dibromide	Fumigant, gasoline additive
Ethylene oxide	Sterilizing agent
Formaldehyde	Building materials
4, 4′-methylene bis(2-chloroaniline) (MBOCA)	Resin manufacturing
N-nitrosodiethylamine	Solvent
N-nitrosodimethylamine	Solvent
Polychlorinated biphenyls	Electrical equipment
Propylene oxide	Chemical industry
Silica, crystalline	Glass and porcelain manufacturing
Styrene oxide	Chemical industry
Vinyl bromide	Plastics industry

[a]Other chemicals and mixtures, including chemotherapeutic agents, tobacco, and others, have been classified in group 2A.

From Vainio H, Wilbourn J. Identification of carcinogens within the IARC monograph program. *Scand J Work Environ Health* 1992;18[suppl]:64.

MOLECULAR EPIDEMIOLOGY OF CANCER

The field of toxicology is changing rapidly and the molecular basis of cancer, and its implications for clinical medicine, are becoming better understood all the time. Clearly, future developments in this area will be of increasing significance (18).

Traditionally, evidence of carcinogens or their metabolites have often been directly measured in biologic media such as blood or urine. Examples include benzene, phenols, and exposure to benzidine-based dyes. Such markers of exposure will be added to in many ways in the future. One such way is that more recently developed assays look at the mutagenicity of urine. In addition, there are now direct measurements that are possible that look at the interaction between carcinogens and an individual's DNA. Measurements of DNA-carcinogen adducts can be done with such techniques as the ^{32}P-postlabeling technique or various immunoassays (19). Other investigators are looking at RNA adducts or protein adducts to better understand the interactions between carcinogenic exposure and the development of malignancy. One aspect of such testing that may prove to be especially useful is the ability to measure specific adducts from the potential carcinogen of interest, and not have confounding effects by other exposures such as cigarette smoke.

In addition to these measurements of exposure, there may be markers of risk that also can be developed from molecular biology. These may come in several ways, such as the ability to measure relative metabolic capacity for carcinogens, markers that may impair the repair of damaged DNA, and other markers of cancer-prone states. Such measurements will have particular effects on the ethical issues of workplaces, with the ultimate goal to be making workplaces safer, rather than screening workers for potential employment.

Lastly, there may be some markers of effect that can be looked at. The ability of carcinogens to reach target tissue and cause genetic change can be evaluated with such cytogenetic abnormalities as sister chromatid changes and the creation of micronuclei. These tests have been available for several decades, and such testing has been done in various working populations exposed to a wide range of carcinogens including benzene, styrene, vinyl chloride, asbestos, and ethylene oxide. While they may point to an increased risk for cancer in the population, such tests are not yet adequately standardized or developed to be able to use them as clinical tests for exposed individuals. With some of the new developments in the identification of the human genome, and the availability of rapidly assessing pieces of DNA through polymer chain reactions or other tests, there will undoubtedly be additional developments in studying the interactions of carcinogens and the development of cancer in humans (20). While the promise is still there for such developments, one should not overlook those techniques already well accepted for the screening of individuals at an increased risk for cancer, such as the Papanicolaou (Pap) smear, a test widely used for the early detection of malignancies of various types.

WORKPLACE REGULATION OF CARCINOGENS

The generic carcinogen standard, "Identification, Classification, and Regulation of Potential Occupational Carcinogens," embodies OSHA's approach to the regulation of carcinogens in the workplace (21). This document sets forth a standardized methodology for interpreting test data on carcinogenicity and classifying chemicals according to these test data. It then allows for the regulation of chemicals judged to be carcinogens. While this is the approach that can be taken in theory, the actual regulation of carcinogens has been through the use of earlier consensus standards and other recognitions of carcinogenic potential, rather than through this mechanism.

A fundamental issue with the management of carcinogens is how strictly they should be regulated. One viewpoint suggests that any carcinogen should be regulated as strictly as possible, while another perspective is that with differing potencies of carcinogens there should be more stringent regulations applied to those considered more potent. These kinds of discussions and philosophical differences lead to consideration of cost-benefit analysis and judgments regarding allowable amounts of carcinogens in the workplace. It should be recognized that while OSHA may regulate carcinogens, no level should be considered safe, and that the amount of carcinogen allowed in workplaces will ultimately determine the carcinogenic risk for workers due to these types of exposures.

While OSHA has the responsibility for workplace regulation, other agencies, such as the Environmental Protection Agency and the Consumer Product Safety Commission, deal with similar issues relating to carcinogens in other settings.

MEDICAL SURVEILLANCE FOR CARCINOGENS

The oversight of working populations is one continuing aspect of work in occupational medicine. When populations are known to be exposed to carcinogens, it becomes justifiable to regularly monitor individuals in these populations. Sometimes this is required by law, and OSHA has required such monitoring for many carcinogens. In addition, there are federal requirements to maintain medical records for 30 years following cessation of employment with a particular employer, allowing for future epidemiologic studies. In addition, there are times when it is unappreciated that workers may be exposed to carcinogenic substances, and some routine review of a population, or its health outcomes, can point the way to the discovery of new carcinogens.

For known carcinogens the basic principles of medical monitoring follow along with any intervention aimed at improving health outcomes (15). For some carcinogenic outcomes it appears as if the current state of monitoring, such as the use of routine chest x-rays for populations exposed to lung carcinogens, may not be especially useful. Studies are currently underway looking at additional modalities such as combining sputum cytology, computed tomography (CT) scans, or other testing to be able to detect cancer at a more curable stage than is usually the case. Other carcinogenic outcomes, such as leukemia, bladder cancer, and colon cancer, are more easily evaluated, although there may be an issue of a high rate of false positives, or the need for extensive additional testing to rule in or rule out the presence of cancer. Given the new avenues opening because of genomic research, the methodologies and modalities used to screen populations, and ultimately treat them, may soon change for the better.

PRACTICAL ASPECT OF CARCINOGENIC EXPOSURE

Physicians working in occupational medicine may be asked questions regarding the relationship of exposure to chemicals and the possible or definitive cause of cancers. A commonly asked question, and perhaps the most easily answered, is if a particular substance is a carcinogen. At the present time there are several sources of data available to answer this, and these include reviewing the IARC Monographs on the Evaluation of Carcinogenic Risk to Humans (5), data from the annual reports of the National Toxicology Program, NIOSH publications, and other databases. These databases have resulted from consensus reviews, and do not rely on single papers or data found in isolation in the scientific literature. They also take into account the role of animal studies.

Another set of frequently asked questions addresses exposure to chemicals. Workers may ask if a substance with which they have been working is a carcinogen. Available to all American workers, by law, are Material Safety Data Sheets (MSDSs), and these should help answer the question. In addition, physicians working in the field of occupational medicine will have ready access to information, such as that noted immediately above, which can then answer a worker's question.

If a worker has been exposed, the rest of the discussion should address several points. The worker should be counseled about avoiding additional further exposure, and reporting this problem of exposure to proper individuals. Ideally, measures would then be taken to replace the carcinogen, enclose the process in which it is used, or, as a last resort, lead to the use of personal protective equipment. Depending on the nature and amount of the workers' exposure, they might do well to be advised of future monitoring, depending on the type of carcinogen, the disease that it is known to cause, and the timeframes involved. Lastly, other advice should be given to workers such as the avoidance of potential cofactors in the development of malignancy, such as cigarette smoking.

Another frequently asked question is if a particular exposure led to the development of an individual's cancer. Often, this question arises in the context of litigation. The answer given may, in part, depend on the context in which information is sought, and the use to which that information will be put. It is always difficult to answer this question for an individual patient utilizing information that has arisen from epidemiologic or animal data (22).

In the legal setting, the question is usually if it is more likely than not (above 50% likely) that an individual's specific cancer was caused by exposure to a specific carcinogen. For many types of cancers there are no known causes, while for other types of cancers there are many known causes, and an individual worker may have had several exposures. This issue becomes particularly difficult when there are multiple exposures to carcinogens documented to cause specific types of cancer. For example, workers in a steel mill or foundry are likely to have been exposed to asbestos and silica, both recognized as lung carcinogens, and they may also have been cigarette smokers. How these factors get sorted out will clearly vary from legal jurisdiction to jurisdiction. For all such cases, there are a number of principles that need to be recognized when making such a judgment, such as an appropriate latency period, a true history of exposure, and an accurate diagnosis of the malignancy involved (see above).

While it is clear that considerable numbers of people in the general population get cancer, it remains a legal rather than strictly medical question when a cancer is being studied for a relationship with work, even though it may be commonly found in the population as well. Some jurisdictions have badly misapplied epidemiologic considerations when looking at issues of relative risk. Also, there are now both federal and various state rulings that require there to be an appropriate scientific chain of evidence in making certain statements.

CANCER CLUSTERS

Sometimes a cluster of unusual cancers, by cell type, age, or location, will develop in a population and generate interest in identifying possible new sources of malignancy. Two that are well known are the development of an extremely rare cancer, hemangiosarcoma of the liver, among workers exposed to vinyl chloride, and the development of small cell carcinomas among workers exposed to bis(chloromethyl)ether.

In the first instance, workers at a vinyl chloride facility were found to have an unusually large number of cases among a modest-sized workforce. The relationship was appreciated by the local occupational physician, a part-time visiting surgeon, and his reporting this to NIOSH led to more extensive evaluation and documentation of this special relationship (23). As a result of this relationship and a desire to reduce such cases in the future, regulations were passed that limited exposure to vinyl chloride to one part per million, and led to the enclosing of most operations. Rather than force companies out of business, as had been predicted, two beneficial outcomes resulted. First, no new cases developed among workers who began in the era of enclosed workplaces. Second, millions of pounds of chemical, which had previously been lost into the atmosphere, were recaptured and the cost of building the enclosures was easily recouped.

In the other situation, suspicion fell upon bis(chloromethyl)ether as a cause of lung cancer when 13 cases of lung cancer occurred in one small department of a chemical production facility, the average age of the workers being in the mid-40s, and 12 of the 13 cases were of the small cell cancer type. This unusual presentation by cell type percentage, coupled with the early age at onset, led to the recognition of this material as a carcinogen. Steps were quickly taken to reduce exposure, and future disease risk was greatly reduced.

When assessing clusters one should consider the usual issues involved, such as cell type, tissue location, age, latency, and a commonality of occupational exposure history. Steps should then be taken to reduce, or better yet eliminate, such exposures in the future (24,25).

It must be recognized that proper determination of a cancer cluster can be very difficult. Cancer is common in the general public, and some cancers especially so. It is easier to identify a true cluster from a particular exposure when the type of cancer is rare, but much more difficult when the cancer is common. Also, if the numbers, both the numerator and denominator of the population, are small, then there is great statistical instability. Proving a true cluster can then become more difficult. Further complicating the issue may be the lack of recognized biologic causality. A good example of the difficulty in assessing clusters is in the area of several types of cancer (e.g., leukemia, brain tumors, breast cancer) thought to arise following exposure to sources of nonionizing radiations (e.g., cell phones, high tension power lines, etc.).

SUMMARY

Occupational cancers have been, and continue to be, a serious problem in workplaces. Given what is already known, it is imperative that workers be protected by reducing or eliminating exposure, and workers should be educated about potential carcinogenic risks at their work sites. This should be done in conjunction with reduction or elimination of other carcinogenic hazards, such as cigarette smoking. The best principles of occupational medicine, namely getting a good history of exposure, monitoring workplaces, undertaking appropriate medical surveillance, and educating workers, are all extremely important when dealing with potential carcinogens, given the outcome of exposure in many cases. Unfortunately, given the long latency from onset of exposure to the development of disease we can expect to see many occupational cancers in the future, but with proper attention to the reduction of exposure over time occupational cancers should greatly diminish.

REFERENCES

1. Pott P. *Chirorgical observations relative to the cataract, the polypus of the nose, the cancer of the scrotum, the different kinds of ruptures and the mortification of the toes and feet.* London: Hawes, Clark and Collins, 1775.
2. *Cancer facts and figures 2001.* Atlanta: American Cancer Society, 2001.
3. Bailar JS, Smith EM. Progress against cancer? *N Engl J Med* 1986;314:1226.
4. Higginson J. Importance of occupational and environmental factors in cancer. *J Toxicol Environ Health* 1980; 6:941.
5. International Agency for Research on Cancer. *IARC monographs on the evaluation of carcinogenic risks to humans, suppl. 7.* Overall evaluations of carcinogenicity: an updating of IARC monographs volumes 1 to 42. Lyon, France: IARC, 1987.
6. Drinkwater NR. Experimental models and biological mechanisms for tumor promotion. *Cancer Cells* 1990; 2:8.
7. Farber E. The multistep nature of cancer development. *Cancer Res* 1984;44:4217.
8. Harris CC. Chemical and physical carcinogenesis: advances and perspectives for the 1990s. *Cancer Res* 1991;51[suppl]:5023s.
9. Bishop JM. Molecular themes in oncogenesis. *Cell* 1991;64:235.
10. Hollstein M, et al. p53 mutations in human cancers. *Science* 1991;253:1233.
11. Keshava N, Ong TM. Occupational exposure to genotoxic agents. *Mutat Res* 1999;437:175.
12. Major J, Jakab MG, Tompa A. The frequency of induced premature centromer division in human populations occupationally exposed to genotoxic chemicals. *Mutat Res* 1999;445:241.
13. Gonzales FJ, Crespi CL, Gelboin HV. DNA-expressed human cytochrome P450s: a new age of molecular toxicology and human risk assessment. *Mutat Res* 1991; 247:113.
14. Pelkonen O. Carcinogen metabolism and individual susceptibility. *Scand J Work Environ Health* 1992;18 [suppl]:17.
15. Ordin DL. *Surveillance, monitoring, and screening in occupational health in public health and preventive medicine,* 13th ed. Norwalk, CT: Appleton & Lange, 1992.

16. Goodman DG. Animal testing of carcinogens. *Occup Med State of the Art Rev* 1987;2:47.
17. Santella RM. In vitro testing for carcinogens and mutagens. *Occup Med State of the Art Rev* 1987;2:39.
18. Wogan GN. Markers of exposure to carcinogens. *Environ Health Perspect* 1989;81:9.
19. Perera F, Weinstein IB. Molecular epidemiology and carcinogen-DNA adduct detection: new approaches to studies of human cancer causation. *J Chronic Dis* 1982; 35:581.
20. Hemminki K. Use of molecular biology techniques in cancer epidemiology. *Scand J Work Environ Health* 1992;18[suppl]:38.
21. Occupational Safety and Health Administration. Identification, classification, and regulation of potential occupational carcinogens. *Fed Reg* 1980;45:5015.
22. Brennan T, Carter RF. Legal and scientific probability of causation of cancer and other environmental disease in individuals. *Health Polit Policy Law* 1985;10:33.
23. Creech JL Jr, Johnson MN. Angiosarcoma of liver in the manufacture of polyvinyl chloride. *J Occup Med* 1974; 16:150.
24. Frumkin H, Kantrowitz W. Cancer clusters in the workplace: an approach to investigation. *J Occup Med* 1987; 29:949.
25. Fleming LE, Ducatman AM, Shalat SL. Disease clusters in occupational medicine: a protocol for their investigation. *Am J Ind Med* 1992;22:33.

24

Cardiovascular Disorders

Daniel E. Forman and Paul P. Rountree

Cardiovascular disease is highly prevalent in the United States with high cumulative mortality and morbidity, and enormous impact in the occupational setting. This chapter focuses on general risks for cardiovascular disease (CVD) as well as risks pertaining particularly to occupational settings. We also review related issues of risk stratification, emphasize testing as one modality to quantify cardiovascular status, and discuss strategies to modify cardiovascular risks, both generally and those oriented to the workplace.

SCOPE OF THE PROBLEM

While age-adjusted mortality of CVD has declined over the last decade, the overall aging of the American population provides a basis in which CVD remains the predominant cause of morbidity and mortality in the U.S. While the estimated prevalence of coronary heart disease (CHD) is only 34% of men and 29% of women aged 45 to 54, it rises to 51% of men and 48% of women aged 55 to 64, to 65% of both men and women aged 65 to 74 years, and to 71% of men and 79% of women aged 75 and older (1). In 1997, CVD was the primary diagnosis for more than 6.1 million inpatients (1), and accounted for more than 45% of all deaths (2). The occupational implications are staggering, with cost estimates for cardiovascular disease in 1992 of approximately $108.9 billion, including costs of medication, lost productivity, and physician, hospital, and nursing home services (3).

Cardiovascular disease is a comprehensive term, referring to a spectrum of interrelated cardiac and vascular disease processes. CHD refers to blockages in epicardial arteries, but vascular abnormalities are typically diffuse, extending beyond the heart and impacting with high likelihood of peripheral arterial disease (PAD) and cerebrovascular disease. Similarly, CVD corresponds to myocardial infarction (MI) or cardiac injury that occurs when coronary arteries occlude (depriving myocardial tissue of vital blood), as well as to heart failure or ventricular pump dysfunction that occurs after MI and/or ventricular stiffening (often caused by CHD and/or hypertension) and aggravating neurohormonal responses. Arrhythmias often arise from the substrate of myocardial injury, heart failure, and associated myocardial fibrosis. Therefore, while cardiac risk factors were once primarily associated with CHD, recent insights regarding the interconnections among CVDs now illuminate broader correlation between cardiac risk factors and a spectrum of CVDs (CHD, MI, PAD, cerebrovascular disease, heart failure, and even arrhythmias).

RISK FACTORS AND CVD PATHOPHYSIOLOGY

In general, cardiac risk factors have an aggregate effect on vascular performance, resulting in diminished endothelial synthesis of nitric oxide and related susceptibility to central vascular stiffening (translating into high afterload pressures), peripheral vascular stiffening (translating into high blood pressure), and the formation of unstable atherosclerotic lesions. These vascular manifestations correspond to foreseeable myocardial responses including ventricular hypertrophy and myocyte apoptosis as the heart strains with the higher work demands associated with high afterload resistance. Moreover, myocardial vulnerability to ischemic injury and diastolic filling impairments both increase as vital blood supply is threatened by atherosclerosis and reduced coronary flow reserve (reduced maximal coronary vasodilation) as well as by the added work demands created by high afterload pressures. Related issues of myocardial stiffening, fibrosis, ventricular remodeling (i.e., vulnerability to left ventricular hypertrophy as well as to left ventricular dilation), and myocardial dysfunction are likely, with progressing liability for heart failure (systolic and diastolic heart failure) and arrhythmias. Similar vascular changes in the vessels perfusing the brain correspond to greater vulnerability to strokes, and vascular changes in peripheral vessels correspond to claudication and diminished peripheral circulation.

Among a list of widely recognized modifiable risk factors are smoking, diabetes, hypertension, hypercholesterolemia, sedentary lifestyle, obesity, and excessive salt ingestion. In a growing list of novel risk factors, hyperhomocystinemia and low-grade systemic inflammatory states have been well described. The metabolic syndrome is a hazardous constellation of abdominal obesity, atherogenic dyslipidemia [elevated triglycerides, low high-density lipoprotein (HDL), a subtype of low-density lipoprotein (LDL) with small particle sizes], hypertension, and insulin resistance. Other more intractable risk factors include advanced age, male gender, and family history (4). Because of the wide prevalence of CVD in Western societies, screening for risk factors and stratifying for cumulative CVD risk are prudent as cardiovascular instability may be modified by preemptive medical (pharmacologic, lifestyle, and workplace) interventions.

The occupational setting has often served as the base from which to provide preventive medical services. Benefits include ready access to large groups of people, greater ability to ensure follow-up study of abnormalities noted during screening measures, and financial and administrative support of the organization. All of these considerations can enhance participation and better ensure adherence to the behavioral changes necessary to reduce cardiovascular risks.

GENERAL CVD RISK FACTORS

Blood Pressure

Both diastolic and systolic hypertension are clearly associated with increased of cardiovascular instability, with risk increasing with the extent of blood pressure elevations (5). The higher the level of blood pressure, the more likely that various CVDs will develop, primarily through acceleration of atherosclerosis. If untreated, about 50% of hypertensives will die of CHD or heart failure, about 33% of stroke, and 10% to 15% of renal failure (6). Furthermore, cardiovascular risks associated with hypertension are compounded by coexisting risk factors. For example, a 55-year-old man with a systolic blood pressure of 160 mm Hg, who is otherwise at low risk, would have a 13.7% chance of a vascular event in the next 10 years. However, a man of the same age with the same blood pressure and additional risks of hypercholesterolemia, cigarette smoking, glucose intolerance, and left ventricular hypertrophy (LVH) would have a 59.5% risk of a cardiovascular event (7). Both diabetes and hypercholesterolemia often add disproportionate risk for hypertensive adults, raising the consideration that insulin resistance may play a prominent part of the underlying pathophysiology, and highlighting the fact that hypertensives often contend with a greater risk than that imposed by their blood pressure alone (6).

Despite its severe consequences, hypertension is often undertreated. Of the estimated 50 million Americans with hypertension, almost a third evade diagnosis and only a fourth receive effective treatment (8). Blood pressure control programs in work settings have proved beneficial in early recognition, appropriate follow-up, and greater compliance with treatment regimens (9). Data from the National Survey of Worksite Health Promotion Activities revealed that blood pressure screening occurred at 55.4% of private sector work sites queried (10). Such programs have also proved to be cost-effective (11). Successful occupational endeavors include special events, group classes or workshops, and on-site/off-site treatment and follow-up. Optimally, blood pressure screening should be part of a comprehensive health promotion program (12). Numerous nonprofit health organizations, such as the American Heart Association, provide opportunities for both educational material and staff to implement on-site programs (13).

Cigarette Smoking

Cigarette consumption constitutes the single most important modifiable risk factor for CVD and the leading preventable cause of death in the U.S. (14). It has been demonstrated that compared with nonsmokers, those who consume 20 or more cigarettes daily have a twofold to threefold increase in total CHD (15). Moreover, even as few as one to four cigarettes daily increases cardiovascular risks of CHD, sudden death, aortic aneurysm, PAD, cerebrovascular disease, and thromboembolic risks.

Given the serious correlation of smoking to cardiovascular and other health risks, programs facilitating smoking cessation seem highly indicated. Furthermore, as policies to restrict smoking in public areas gain momentum, more organizations are sponsoring smoking cessation programs. A random sample of a nationwide survey of work-site health promotion activities revealed that smoking cessation programs were offered at 35.6% of all work sites (16). Many different approaches to encourage people to stop smoking have been attempted, but success rates among the different strategies are similar. A recent meta-analysis of 20 controlled studies of work site smoking cessation identified the following factors as those contributing to the highest quit rate: programs that included a group component, programs that were not overly complicated, and programs that shared company and employee time. The work site appears to be especially effective in assisting heavier smokers in quitting (17). Nonetheless, many people who stop smoking do so on their own, without the benefit of a formal program (18), and the occupational physician may be helpful in such instances by providing general education and tacit reinforcement.

Cholesterol

While a causative role of LDL cholesterol in the development of CHD has been recognized for many years, the impact of acute LDL cholesterol fluctuations and the swift benefits of cholesterol reductions have only recently become widely appreciated (19). Correspondingly, cholesterol reduction has become a growing health care priority. The Third Report of the Expert Panel on Detection, Evaluation, and Treatment of High Blood Cholesterol in Adults [Adult Treatment Panel (ATP) III] constitutes the National Cholesterol Education Program's (NCEP) updated clinical guidelines for cholesterol testing and management. The report corroborates the fundamental role of cholesterol in CHD pathophysiology, and refers to a multitude of research from experimental animals, laboratory investigations, epidemiology, and genetic forms of hypercholesterolemia demonstrating that elevated LDL cholesterol is a major cause of CHD (20). Furthermore, the report refers to multiple recent clinical trials, which show unequivocally that LDL-lowering therapy reduces risk for CHD (20).

Like the preceding NCEP therapeutic cholesterol-lowering guidelines, ATP III targets LDL as the primary goal of therapy, but emphasizes a new concept of global risk as an index by which to guide cholesterol-lowering goals. The conception of calculating risk utilizes a 10-year risk score derived from the Framingham Heart Study (21) based on specific risks of age, LDL cholesterol, HDL cholesterol, blood pressure, diabetes, and smoking (Fig. 24.1). The rationale for using a risk score is that it enables the intensity of therapy and severity of risk to be better matched. One key consequence of this strategy is that more young individuals register high-risk scores with an associated mandate for cholesterol reduction. In addition, rationale for primary prevention is accentuated for those with high aggregate risks.

Once a risk score is determined, the LDL goal is established. For persons with CHD or CHD equivalents [diabetes, global risk score 20%, ankle brachial ratio <0.9, and prior history of a transient ischemic attack (TIA), stroke, or PAD] and baseline LDL cholesterol ≥130 mg/dL, therapeutic LDL goals are <100 mg/dL (as compared to ≤100 mg/dL in prior guidelines). Initially therapeutic lifestyle changes (TLCs) and control of other risk factors are recommended, but for most patients LDL-lowering medications are also required to achieve LDL cholesterol <100 mg/dL. If baseline LDL levels are 100 to 129 mg/dL, TLCs are also recommended as initial therapy, and also with consideration of LDL-lowering medications to achieve LDL <100 mg/dL. If baseline LDL cholesterol is <100 mg/dL, TLC is once more emphasized, but further LDL-cholesterol reduction is not indicated.

For persons without CHD but with multiple risk factors (two or more) and 10-year risk >20%, the LDL goal is <100 mg/dL. If baseline LDL is ≥130 mg/dL, TLC is initiated and maintained for 3 months. If LDL remains high (≥130 mg/dL) consideration of LDL-lowering medication is recommended. For those with multiple risk factors (two or more) but a 10-year risk of only 10% to 20%, the goal of cholesterol reduction is only <130 mg/dL. LDL-lowering therapy is recommended only if 3 months of TLCs fails to reduce LDL to <130 mg/dL. For those with two or more risk factors but only a 10% 10-year risk, LDL-lowering drug therapy is only recommended if LDL remains ≥160 mg/dL after TLCs. For those with only one risk factor or none, LDL-lowering drug therapy is only recommended if LDL remains ≥190 after 3 months of TLC. Added emphasis on risk reduction is focused on individuals with metabolic syndrome.

Guidelines for TLCs include reducing saturated fats to <7% of calories ingested per day and cholesterol to <200 mg/day. Nonpharmacologic options to lower LDL cholesterol include eating plant stanols/sterols (2 g/day) and increased viscous (soluble) fiber (10–25 g/day). Weight reduction, increased physical activity, and adherence to lifestyle changes are also emphasized.

Occupational physicians potentially play a key role in promoting the importance of cholesterol modifica-

Age	Points
20-34	-9
35-39	-4
40-44	0
45-49	3
50-54	6
55-59	8
60-64	10
65-69	11
70-74	12
75-79	13

Total Cholesterol	Points				
	Age 20-39	Age 40-49	Age 50-59	Age 60-69	Age 70-79
<160	0	0	0	0	0
160-199	4	3	2	1	0
200-239	7	5	3	1	0
240-279	9	6	4	2	1
≥280	11	8	5	3	1

	Points				
	Age 20-39	Age 40-49	Age 50-59	Age 60-69	Age 70-79
Nonsmoker	0	0	0	0	0
Smoker	8	5	3	1	1

HDL (mg/dL)	Points
≥60	-1
50-59	0
40-49	1
<40	2

Systolic BP (mmHg)	If Untreated	If Treated
<120	0	0
120-129	0	1
130-139	1	2
140-159	1	2
≥160	2	3

Point Total	10-Year Risk %
<0	< 1
0	1
1	1
2	1
3	1
4	1
5	2
6	2
7	3
8	4
9	5
10	6
11	8
12	10
13	12
14	16
15	20
16	25
≥17	≥ 30

A

FIG. 24.1. A: Estimate of 10-year risk for men (Framingham Point Scores). *(Continued on next page)*

Age	Points
20-34	-7
35-39	-3
40-44	0
45-49	3
50-54	6
55-59	8
60-64	10
65-69	12
70-74	14
75-79	16

Total Cholesterol	Points				
	Age 20-39	Age 40-49	Age 50-59	Age 60-69	Age 70-79
<160	0	0	0	0	0
160-199	4	3	2	1	1
200-239	8	6	4	2	1
240-279	11	8	5	3	2
≥280	13	10	7	4	2

	Points				
	Age 20-39	Age 40-49	Age 50-59	Age 60-69	Age 70-79
Nonsmoker	0	0	0	0	0
Smoker	9	7	4	2	1

HDL (mg/dL)	Points
≥60	-1
50-59	0
40-49	1
<40	2

Systolic BP (mmHg)	If Untreated	If Treated
<120	0	0
120-129	1	3
130-139	2	4
140-159	3	5
≥160	4	6

Point Total	10-Year Risk %
<9	1
9	1
10	1
11	1
12	1
13	2
14	2
15	3
16	4
17	5
18	6
19	8
20	11
21	14
22	17
23	22
24	27
≥25	≥ 30

FIG. 24.1. *Continued:* **B:** Estimate of 10-year risk for women (Framingham Point Scores). (From Executive summary of the third report of the NCEP panel on detection: evaluation and treatment of high blood pressure in adults [ATP III]. *JAMA* 2001;285[19]:2486–2497.)

tion, and providing opportunities for cholesterol screening as well as LDL cholesterol-lowering strategies. The growing emphasis on primary prevention and the related concepts of aggregate risk are also important to publicize and endorse in the workplace. Related issues of diet and exercise could also be advocated, with programs reinforcing these behaviors in the workplace and home.

Sedentary Lifestyle

Physical fitness also helps to reduce CVD (22–24). Even minimal increases in physical activity improves cardiovascular fitness among sedentary people and helps reinforce indirect cardiovascular benefits such as smoking cessation, blood pressure reduction, weight loss, and reduced arrhythmias. Although the precise amount of physical activity required to promote cardiovascular fitness is a matter of debate, sessions of 20- to 30-minute duration three times per week are routinely recommended (with the assumption that one exercises to about 75% of one's age-predicted maximal heart rate (220 – age) for the exercise period). The current best estimate is that approximately 7% to 8% of adults participate three or more times a week for 20 minutes or more in an activity that requires 60% or more of VO_2 max (25). The occupational setting provides a convenient opportunity to promote physical activity as a part of the workday as well as during leisure time at home.

However, while occupational physicians play a potentially beneficial role in promoting exercise training, they also may help identify adults with multiple cardiovascular risks for whom exercise might be initially destabilizing. This subgroup includes those with cardiac risk factors, past medical histories of CVD, or symptoms suggestive of CHD (26) (e.g., chest pain, severe shortness of breath, palpitations, dizziness). Stress testing is most commonly used to detect adults with underlying ischemia who would likely benefit from medications, revascularization, and/or monitored exercise (cardiac rehabilitation) before exercising independently. Stress testing also helps detect individuals with abnormal hemodynamic exercise responses (hyper- or hypotensive exercise responses) and/or arrhythmic exercise responses. But while exercise stress tests are useful in identifying patients who have such baseline risks, stress testing is not recommended as routine assessments for all people considering an exercise training program (27).

Additional Risk Factors

Other risk factors contribute to CVD in a list that continues to grow, corresponding in part to accelerating insights regarding cardiovascular pathophysiology and the key factors underlying CVD. Diabetes mellitus, obesity, salt-over-ingestion, hyperhomocystinemia, and inflammatory states are among the CVD risk factors for which detection and modification could be augmented by effective occupational health programs.

Diabetes and insulin resistance are particularly consequential cardiovascular risk factors. Three quarters of all deaths among diabetic patients result from CHD (28), and patients with diabetes have three- to fivefold increases in future cardiovascular events compared to nondiabetics (29). Both the major arteries and the microvascular circulation are affected with abnormal endothelial function and high propensity to atherosclerosis (30). Ventricular mural stiffening is also common, with increased likelihood of diastolic filling abnormalities and heart failure. The insulin-resistance syndrome, a constellation including hyperinsulinemia and glucose intolerance accompanied by hypertriglyceridemia, low HDL, and predominantly small dense LDL particles, also correlates with high risk of atherothrombosis (31).

Surprisingly, improved glycemic control among diabetic and insulin-resistant adults has not been definitively associated with improved outcomes. Therapeutic benefit is mostly targeted to exercise, avoidance of obesity, and aggressive control of other risk factors (32).

Obesity is associated with substantially increased cardiovascular risk, independent of physical activity (33). Some argue that CVD risks associated with obesity are primarily related to coexisting conditions that commonly exist (such as glucose intolerance, insulin resistance, hypertension, physical inactivity, and dyslipidemia). Nonetheless, even modest weight gain in mid- to late adulthood correlates with increased coronary disease among men and women, and recent studies also demonstrate that waist-to-hip ratio, an index of abdominal obesity, is an independent marker of vascular risk in women and men (34). Weight control is therefore targeted as a major goal of preventive cardiology, usually in conjunction with exercise recommendations (34).

Salt ingestion diminishes vascular endothelial production of nitrous oxide and normal vascular relaxation (35,36), which compounds risks of hypertension as well as high afterload pressures. Average sodium intake in the U.S. is 150 mmol/day, which is equivalent to 3.5 g of sodium or 8.7 g of sodium chloride. National guidelines recommend limiting average daily salt consumption to 100 mmol/day (equivalent to 2.3 g of sodium or 5.8 g of sodium chloride) (37). The Dietary Approaches to Stop Hypertension (DASH) trial was a feeding study that enrolled 459 adults with systolic blood pressures of less than 160 mm Hg and diastolic blood pressures of 80 to 95 mm Hg (38). A fruit and vegetable diet (rich in fruits and vegetables and providing high amounts of fiber, potassium, and magnesium) and a combination diet (rich in fruits and vegetables along with low-fat dairy foods, with reduced total fat, saturated fat, and cholesterol content) were contrasted with a control diet. Furthermore, three different levels of daily salt consumption (142, 107, and 65 mmol) were analyzed for each group. The gradient of blood pressure reduction observed across the diets indicates that some aspects of the fruit and vegetable diet reduced blood pressure, and that additional features of the combination diet reduced it even further. Moreover, at each level of decreased salt intake in each of the diets, there were significant, stepwise reductions in blood pressures. The reduction in blood pressure occurred within 2 weeks and was sustained for the next 6 weeks. Of additional importance, adherence to the modified diets was excellent (38).

Widespread adoption of the DASH combination diet (8 to 10 servings of fruits and vegetables and 2.7 servings of low-fat dairy products per day) could potentially shift the population distribution of blood pressure downward, reducing the occurrence of blood-pressure–related CVD (39). In fact, it is projected that a population-wide reduction in blood pressure of the magnitude observed in the DASH trial would reduce incident CHD by an estimated 15% and stroke by approximately 27% (40).

A large series of cross-sectional and retrospective studies indicate a positive relationship between mild to moderate homocystinemia and atherosclerosis, yet prospective studies exploring the relationship of elevated homocysteine and CHD have yielded mixed results. Therefore, the benefits of homocysteine-lowering therapy remain controversial.

Homocysteine metabolism requires an adequate supply of folate, vitamin B_6, vitamin B_{12}, and riboflavin, and levels of these vitamins correlate inversely with levels of circulating homocysteine (41). Normal levels of fasting plasma homocysteine are considered to be between 5 and 15 μmol/L, whereas moderate, intermediate, and severe hyperhomocystinemia refer to concentrations between 16 and 30, between 31 and 100, and >100 μmol/L, respectively (42). A prospective study of more than 80,000 women (followed for 14 years) showed significant reduction in CHD among those consuming higher levels of folate and vitamin B_6 (43,44) and led to hypotheses that folate and vitamin B_6 may play an important role in CVD prevention (45,46).

In light of the apparent relationship of plasma homocysteine to CVD risk and the estimated influence of folic acid on homocysteine levels, it has been suggested that a 359 μg/d increase in folic acid intake in men and 280 μg/d increase in women could potentially prevent 30,500 and 19,000 vascular deaths annually in men and women, respectively (47). Nonetheless, the clinical benefits of such interventions remain unknown in the absence of any prospective, controlled intervention trials.

Inflammation plays a key physiologic role in all phases of atherosclerosis such that a cascade of proinflammatory cytokines (e.g., interleukin-1 and tumor necrosis factor) underlies the formation of fatty streaks and progression to more complex and unstable atherosclerotic lesions (48). Several markers of low-grade systemic inflammation have proven useful for cardiovascular risk prediction including the nonspecific acute-phase reactants (C-reactive protein) (49).

Modifying inflammatory states may reduce cardiovascular risk. Efficacy of statins and aspirin to reduced CVD has been attributed, in part, to their inflammation-modifying effects, i.e., reducing inflammation that otherwise undermines plaque stability (50,51).

Occupational health caregivers could have significant impact by addressing each of these cardiovascular risk factors, and particularly by constructing a work environment that incorporates salient lifestyle priorities. CVD wellness can be promulgated in the cafeteria with meals minimizing salt, unhealthy lipids, and processed sugars, and high in fruits, nuts, and homocysteine-lowering vitamins (folate is commonly found in whole grain foods, green leafy vegetables, fruits, and legumes). Smoking cessation, weight reduction, and fitness can be emphasized and facilitated with on-site equipment and programming. Blood pressure and lipid screening can be reinforced, as can medication and therapeutic compliance. Preventive pharmacologic options, such as aspirin and lipid-lowering agents, can also be promoted, along with encouragement and/or referring workers to primary caregivers.

Education is also key, not only in terms of specific risks and the potential to intervene, but the notion of cumulative risk that increases with age, a positive family history, or prior cardiovascular events. Individuals with multiple risk factors can be steered to stress testing if they are considering an exercise-training program, and to appropriate medical referrals.

OCCUPATIONAL AGENTS THAT CAUSE OR AGGRAVATE HEART DISEASE

Workers in a variety of job settings, such as dry-cleaning establishments, explosives factories, and rayon production, are at risk of CVD as a result of their work. Carbon disulfide, nitrates, and carbon monoxide are firmly established as causative factors. Heart disease, however, is so prevalent in Western society that occupational factors are often overlooked in clinical management. This section reviews well-documented occupational hazards to the cardiovascular system and proposes guidelines for the clinical evaluation and placement of workers exposed to these hazards.

The clinician may be faced with work situations that are hazardous to the cardiovascular system. The clinician should evaluate the symptoms or disease experienced by workers, and refer for further treatment those with CVD. The following examples are based on experiences in providing occupational medical services to small businesses:

- A truck driver complains of headaches whenever he remains in the cab of his truck for over an hour. He does not smoke, and the problem only seems to occur during the winter months.
- An owner of an automobile repair shop experiences palpitations toward the end of the workday. He had been using cleaning solvents in an unventilated area of the shop.

In these two situations the work setting has a pronounced effect on the manifestation of heart disease. The cases demonstrate that carbon monoxide and solvents, in particular, can affect the heart. Although occupational cardiotoxins are relatively few in number (compared, for example, to pulmonary toxins or neurotoxins), the effects of these agents may be life threatening.

In the evaluation of chest pain, especially angina, inquiry is best directed toward the activity associated with the onset of the discomfort, especially if it occurs at work. Symptoms that occur during or immediately after work may be due to agents such as carbon monoxide, methylene chloride, or perhaps overexertion. Extremes of temperature (heat or cold) may also precipitate symptoms in some people, inducing vasospasm (from cold) or cardiac overexertion as the heart beats more vigorously to dissipate high core temperatures (high ambient heat). In the assessment of work-related cardiovascular disorders, it is helpful to consider associated signs and symptoms. Light-headedness and dizziness, for example, can occur as a result of solvent exposure from methylene chloride, which is metabolized to carbon monoxide.

Physical and laboratory evaluations are consistent with routine medical practice. Occupational cardiovascular disorders differ from nonoccupational types primarily in their etiologies, but clinical manifestations and management are similar. Routine diagnostic studies are utilized that are pertinent to the circumstances and symptoms pertinent to the workplace. For example, a 24-hour ambulatory electrocardiogram (ECG) monitor is appropriate for a worker symptomatic with palpitations.

To formulate these assessments, a thorough occupational history is essential. If an occupational agent is suspected of causing or aggravating a cardiovascular disorder, special attention can be directed to its specific toxicity. A review of the medical literature and industrial hygiene sampling may be necessary to form a refined opinion. A full discussion of all the agents suspected of cardiotoxicity is beyond the scope of this chapter but is provided elsewhere (52–54). Some common examples are described here.

Carbon Monoxide

Workers exposed to automobile exhaust, furnaces, the incomplete combustion of carbonaceous material, and methylene chloride may experience adverse health effects of carbon monoxide. Examples of such workers include mechanics, fork truck operators, foundry or steel workers, firemen, and others. Individuals with coronary artery disease (CAD) are especially sensitive to the effects of carboxyhemoglobin, the substance formed when carbon monoxide combines with hemoglobin, since it increases the likelihood of cardiac ischemia (55).

Carbon monoxide exposure may lead to chest pain secondary to myocardial ischemia as well as more subtle symptoms of headaches, light-headedness, and dizziness. Headaches described in the truck driver scenario at the beginning of this section were due to carbon monoxide from a faulty exhaust system. A carboxyhemoglobin of 12% is significant evidence of carbon monoxide toxicity in a nonsmoker. Increases in carboxyhemoglobin (up to 25%) have been associated with ECG abnormalities, and greater vulnerability to cardiac rhythm disturbances, supraventricular and ventricular extrasystoles, and atrial fibrillation.

In fact, a dose-response relationship generally exists between carboxyhemoglobin and a variety of symptoms, with the more serious manifestations occurring at higher levels of exposure. Individuals with CHD are more likely to develop symptoms even at low levels of carboxyhemoglobin, i.e., even levels as low as 3% to 5% (56). One study of Los Angeles freeway drivers demonstrated exacerbation of symptoms when ambient levels of carbon monoxide increased on the highway (57). Another longitudinal study has suggested that CO exposure results in an increased risk of morbidity and mortality (58).

Therefore, it is highly prudent to consider carbon monoxide exposure among adults with known CHD or CHD symptoms. For example, can a person who has recently suffered an MI return to work as a tollbooth operator or clerk at an underground garage? Proper clinical assessment should include an exercise ECG as well as ambient measurements of carbon monoxide levels. In some cases, it may be of value to propose a trial period of observation. The approach suitable for each situation depends on a number of factors, including availability of other positions and income replacement benefits. Unfortunately, no specific guidelines are available, mandating thoughtful and practical considerations for each individual.

Solvents

Solvents refer to substances, usually liquid, that are used as cleaning agents. Examples include routine household products, such as paint thinner, and industrial materials used in degreasing operations, such as trichloroethylene or methylene chloride. Associated cardiovascular risks include arrhythmias. Both halogenated and nonhalogenated compounds have been associated with sudden death. Trichloroethylene, for example, has been implicated in sudden death apparently through the induction of ventricular arrhythmias. Another type of solvent, fluorocarbons, was associated with palpitations in the course of workers preparing frozen sections from surgical specimens. In contrast, methylene chloride has the unique property of converting to carbon monoxide in vivo. Methylene chloride exposure can also result in central nervous system narcosis independent of its carbon monoxide effects, and induce respiratory depression (56,59).

Clinical evaluation of workers with symptoms of palpitations or irregular rhythms should include consideration of solvent exposures. A thorough evaluation focuses on nonoccupational as well as occupational factors and typically includes the use of a 24-hour ambulatory ECG monitor and industrial hygiene sampling.

Job placement for the patient with arrhythmias can be problematic, especially if alternative positions are unavailable. The owner of the repair shop described earlier in this section was suffering from solvent toxicity. Nonetheless, he had just purchased his business and did not want to give it up.

Carbon Disulfide

Carbon disulfide, a substance used in the viscose rayon industry, has been associated with increased rates of atherosclerosis (60). It is hypothesized that this adverse effect involves a decrease in fibrinolytic activity. Carbon disulfide is also used in chemical laboratories and in the manufacture of carbon tetrachloride. Cross-cultural studies of Japanese, Finnish, Belgian, and American workers confirm that carbon disulfide is associated with atherosclerosis, but only in populations consuming Western diets. A Japanese study, for example, showed no unusual increase in CHD but a marked elevation in retinal hemorrhages (25%) compared to a Finnish group (4%). No difference was seen among unexposed Japanese and Finnish workers. Another study of male textile workers showed a significant and positive linear trend in LDL cholesterol and diastolic blood pressure (61). These results may suggest another means by which carbon disulfide may influence ischemic heart disease.

Clinical evaluations of a person suspected of having carbon disulfide exposure might include urinary measurement of metabolites (positive iodine-azide reaction) in addition to routine diagnostic measures.

Nitro Compounds

Occupational exposure to nitroglycerin and other aliphatic nitrates has been associated with angina-like pain, MI, and cardiovascular death in workers from the explosives industry (62). Nitroglycerin and ethylene glycol dinitrate are absorbed through the skin and are associated with anecdotal occurrence of sudden death, particularly after being away from work for a brief period of time. This timing is assumed to be due to rebound coronary spasm as a result of withdrawal of nitrates. However, other studies demonstrate that increases in mortality among occupational cohorts primarily occurred months to years after exposure, raising the possibility that additional pathogenic processes may also exist. Still, the issue remains controversial; a retrospective cohort mortality study from Scandinavia analyzed more than 5,000 workers exposed to nitroglycerin, dinitrotoluene, and controls, and did not show increased cardiovascular disease risk (63). In general, clinical evaluation of workers exposed to nitrates might include determination of serum methemoglobin, in addition to standard diagnostic studies.

Other Agents

Arsine or arsenic poisoning induce acute ECG changes, and chronic arsenic exposure is associated with peripheral vascular insufficiency, pediatric heart disease, and increased CAD mortality. Cobalt exposure is associated with myocardiopathy especially among heavy beer drinkers (due to the effects of the alcohol and/or dietary deficiencies (64). Cadmium and lead have cardiotoxic effects. A comprehensive review of suspected cardiotoxins and other agents that have been considered potentially harmful is beyond the scope of this chapter.

ASSESSING WORK CAPABILITIES AND/OR EXERCISE-TRAINING CAPACITIES AMONG WORKERS FOLLOWING A MAJOR CARDIAC EVENT

Over 1.5 million Americans suffer an MI each year, and upward of 190,000 people undergo coronary artery bypass graft (CABG) surgery. Prevalence of peripheral arterial disease, cerebrovascular disease, heart failure, and arrhythmia are similarly widespread, and the capacity of patients to return to work after a CVD hospitalization presents challenges to the clinician. In general, over 80% of people who suffer an MI or undergo CABG surgery return to their original positions. The major adverse medical prognosticators for failure to return to work include left ventricular dysfunction and persistence of ischemia (65), but for most adults the ability to resume occupational activities depends more on comorbid, social, and psychological factors (Table 24.1) (66,67). In fact, nonmedical factors typically present the greatest impediment for people to resume occupational activities (68). In a review of 893 men who underwent a CABG, the major factor involved in return to work was the type of job (69). Another study failed to demonstrate significant changes in employment following CABG (70), i.e., those who worked prior to surgery tended to work thereafter. The investigators commented that there was little apparent financial incentive for people to return to work. In a different study, age played an important role in determining who returned to work; 73% of adults aged 30 to 49 years returned to work, compared with only 56% of those aged 50 to 54 years and 7% of those aged 60 to 64 years (71).

TABLE 24.1. *Factors involved in returning to work after a major cardiac event*

Medical
Severity and extent of CHD
Effort angina/post-CABG chest wall or leg pain
Physical capacity
Psychological
Pre-event and post-event anxiety/depression/coping styles/personality
Sociodemographic, economic, and cultural
Age, gender, education level
Disposable income, pension/retirement/disability benefits
National customs
Economic conditions
Individual's history and perception of prior work
Type of work/physical environment
Employment history
Physical demands of job/perceived stress on job
Job satisfaction
Work limitations prior to event
Availability of previous job/job change/retraining
Individual's perception of health and risk to life
Attribution of MI/CHD to previous job
Individual's perception of self
Self-confidence
Influence of/and constraints on others
Family
Employer's reluctance to rehire
Union practices or fears
Government/legislation
Physician advice
Individual's expectations and predictions

CABG, coronary artery bypass graft; CHD, congestive heart disease; MI, myocardial infarction.

Adapted from Davidson DM. Return to work after cardiac events: a review. *J Cardiac Rehabil* 1983;3:60; and Kavanagh T, Matosevic V. Assessment of work capacity in patients with ischaemic heart disease: methods and practices. *Eur Heart J* 1988;9[suppl L]:68.

One's level of self-assessed "disability" may affect the ability to return to work. Even low physical capacity, for example, may not interfere with one's ability to handle routine household chores, such as shopping, maintenance, and certain leisure activities (72). An Italian investigation of 118 patients who underwent valvular or CABG surgery showed that the most predictive aspect of poor psychological outcome was hypochondriasis, anxiety, and depression. Psychological factors play a very important role in return to work after a cardiac event, and assessment and sensitivity to these factors is a key part of management by the occupational caregiver (73).

Clinical Assessment of Work Capabilities

The physician overseeing an occupational medicine program is likely to be asked to evaluate a patient's work capabilities following a major cardiac event and/or a worker with multiple cardiac risk factors. A thorough analysis includes a review of the disorder, including medical records and diagnostic studies, and a related job analysis. The patient's current status is pertinent, with consideration of symptoms, physical findings, and laboratory testing, including an exercise stress test. Clinical perspectives need to be oriented to CHD, with emphasis that even among individuals who have recovered from strokes, peripheral arterial disease, or other manifestations of CVD, coronary heart disease remains the leading cause of subsequent mortality and morbidity.

History/Physical Examination

A review of the nature of the MI or CABG surgery is necessary with attention to residual ischemia, ejection fraction, history of heart failure, or arrhythmias. A review of prior cardiac-related problems (including PAD and cerebrovascular disease), medications, and symptoms such as exertional chest pain or shortness of breath, orthopnea, claudication, ankle swelling, palpitations, or dizziness can help assess level of improvement. An inquiry into tolerance for routine activities is necessary to gauge the patient's potential to resume occupational responsibilities safely.

The physical examination should be directed to signs of congestive heart failure, such as ankle swelling, pitting edema, hepatomegaly, jugular venous distention, or an S_3 gallop at the myocardial apex. The character of the pulse should be assessed for regularity to determine the presence of altered rhythms or ectopy.

Based on the evaluation and a review of records from the hospitalization, the need for additional ancillary testing can be determined. ECGs, chest x-rays, and exercise stress testing are important considerations. Likewise, echocardiography may be helpful to evaluate left ventricular systolic function, left ventricular dilation (worse prognosis), and valvular flow abnormalities. Situations vary as to whether the occupational physician or attending physician conducts these tests, and good communication among the occupational physician, attending physician, and business enterprise is essential.

Exercise ECG Stress Testing

A symptom-limited exercise ECG stress test is considered the most sensitive predictor of future reinfarction and death when the test is performed approximately 6 weeks after an acute MI (44). The test is also useful in guiding functional capacities/stability in revascularized patients or any worker with multiple risk factors, particularly among those undertaking a physically demanding job and/or an exercise training program as part of their daily work routine. Nonetheless, it is also important to emphasize that the work environment is not only associated with potential physical stresses, but also emotional stress may correlate with potential cardiovascular instability. Therefore, stress testing may also be useful in patients with CVD risks even if they anticipate a sedentary job or lifestyle.

Despite the less quantifiable nature of stress-associated occupational risks, the limits of occupational physical demands are typically guided by exercise ECG data. For example, among people aged 50 to 59 years who can generate 8 to 9 METs—a MET is the energy expenditure at rest equivalent to approximately 3.3 mL/kg body weight/min—of energy within 3 months of an uncomplicated acute MI, concerns about mild physical work are minimal (74). Furthermore, exercise ECG stress testing provides useful information regarding exercise capacity (low capacity correlates to poor prognosis overall), arrhythmias, ischemia, hemodynamic stability, and/or shortness of breath. Energy expenditure in METs can then be compared to standard references to approximate the individual's physical capacity (Table 24.2). In addition, it is important to refer patients with ECG abnormalities that obscure ischemic exercise-associated ECG changes to nuclear or echocardiographic stress testing for adequate diagnostic sensitivity (e.g., abnormal ECG waveforms due to left ventricular hypertrophy, left bundle branch block, or digoxin effects).

The following are caveats regarding the use of Table 24.2:

1. Figures represent *overage* oxygen uptake values, which may vary depending on the *pace* at which the person performs the activity and previous training and work efficiency.
2. Figures were obtained during continuous *steady-state* work, whereas most occupational duties are *intermittent* in nature.
3. Figures were obtained based on oxygen uptake for leg exercise predominantly, which may not accurately reflect cardiac demands of positions with low somatic oxygen requirements but high myocardial demands due to psychological stress. Examples include positions such as air traffic controllers, taxi drivers, and some executive roles.

TABLE 24.2. *Approximate metabolic cost of certain physical activities*

Cost (in METs)	Occupational	Recreational
1.5–2.0	Desk work, auto driving, typing, electric calculating, machine operation	Standing, walking (strolling 1.6 km/hour), flying, motorcycling, playing cards, sewing, knitting
2–3	Auto repair, radio and TV repair, janitorial work, typing (manual), bartending	Level walking (3.2 km/hour), level bicycling (8.0 km/hour), riding lawn mower, billiards, bowling, skeet, shuffleboard, woodworking (light), powerboat driving, golf (power cart), canoeing (4 km/hour), horseback riding (at a walk), playing piano and other musical instruments
3–4	Bricklaying, plastering, wheelbarrow (45.4-kg load), machine assembly, driving a trailer truck in traffic, welding (moderate load), cleaning windows	Walking (4.8 km/hour), cycling (9.7 km/hour), horseshoe pitching, volleyball (6-man noncompetitive), golf (pulling bag cart), archery, sailing (handling small boat), fly fishing (standing with waders), horseback (sitting trot), badminton (social double), pushing light power mower, energetic musician
4–5	Painting, masonry, paperhanging, light carpentry	Walking (5.6 km/hour), cycling (12.9 km/hour), table tennis, golf (carrying clubs), dancing (foxtrot), badminton (singles), tennis (doubles), raking leaves, hoeing, many calisthenics
5–6	Digging garden, shoveling light earth	Walking (6.4 km/hour), cycling (16.1 km/hour), canoeing (6.4 km/hour), horseback (posting trot), stream fishing (walking in light current in waters), ice or roller skating (14.5 km/hour)
6–7	Shoveling 10 loads/minute (4.5 kg)	Walking (8.0 km/hour), cycling (17.7 km/hour), badminton (competitive), tennis (singles), splitting wood, snow shoveling, hand lawn mowing, folk (square) dancing, light downhill skiing, ski touring (4.0 km/hour) (loose snow), water skiing
7–8	Digging ditches, carrying 36.3 kg, sawing hardwood	Jogging (8.0 km/hour), cycling (19.3 km/hour), horseback (gallop), vigorous downhill skiing, basketball, mountain climbing, ice hockey, canoeing (8.0 km/hour), touch football, paddleball
8–9	Shoveling 10 loads/minute (6.4 kg)	Running (8.9 km/hour), cycling (20.9 km/hour), ski touring (6.4 km/hour), squash racquets (social), handball (social), fencing, basketball (vigorous)
9–10	Shoveling 10 loads/minute (7.3 kg)	Running (9.6–16 km/hour), ski touring (8 km/hour),handball (competitive), squash (competitive)

Adapted from Fox SM, Naughton JP, Haskell WL. Physical activity and the prevention of coronary heart disease. *Ann Clin Res* 1971;3:404.

Job Analysis

At the minimum, the physician should request a job description, especially if high physical activity or stress is typical. Physical work can be classified into *static* and *dynamic,* which present different hemodynamic challenges. A heavy static load, for example, results in a pressure load on the heart, whereas heavy dynamic work produces a volume load (75). Energy requirements of the job may also need to be assessed, as well as the presence of temperature or psychological stress. In some settings, simulated work testing such as a weight-carrying test or a repetitive weight-lifting test can be used in conjunction with a routine exercise ECG to enhance the assessment of work capabilities. Simulated testing offers more objective data and can aid in stimulating confidence in the patient for assuming occupational activities.

CARDIAC REHABILITATION

Cardiac rehabilitation, a composite of prescribed physical activity and associated teaching, is accepted treatment for many patients with cardiovascular disease (67) or multiple CVD risk factors. Benefits include improvement in physical capacity, psychosocial attributes, and lipoprotein patterns. The goals of cardiac rehabilitation also include reduced cardiovascular complications, reduced risk factors in general, and improved health judgments.

While exercise training is generally promoted for all adults as primary and secondary prevention, there are circumstances in which monitored exercise such as cardiac rehabilitation is especially prudent. Patients recently recovered from an MI or revascularization, patients newly diagnosed with CHD (on medical therapy), severely debilitated CVD patients, patients with low ejection fractions, and patients with hemodynamic complexities are among the many who might benefit. However, cardiac rehabilitation not only provides medical surveillance as patients initiate and advance exercise, but also emphasizes teaching and supports that facilitate lifestyle modification, medication compliance, and lifelong cardiovascular safety habits.

Cardiac rehabilitation also provides opportunity for patients to gain better appreciation of their ability to perform physical work within a reasonable level of safety. Monitoring the physiologic responses to a simulated work environment may catalyze confidence and early return to work.

Automatic External Defibrillators

The Occupational Safety and Health Administration reported that from 1991 to 1993, 15% of workplace deaths were due to sudden cardiac arrest (SCA) (76), usually from ventricular fibrillation. These numbers will likely increase in years to come as more people are surviving initial hospitalizations for CHD, MI, and heart failure, but with high risks of subsequent precipitous ventricular arrhythmia.

Without intervention, survival following SCA decreases rapidly (77). Several studies have reported that for each minute of untreated cardiac arrest, the probability of successful rhythm conversion decreases by 7% to 10% (78,79). Conversely, survival rates as high as 90% have been reported when the collapse-to-defibrillation time is within 1 minute (80,81). Consequently, the American College of Occupational and Environmental Medicine (ACOEM) supports the establishment of programs by employers to use automated external defibrillators (AEDs) to manage sudden cardiac arrest in workplace settings. AEDs are highly automated devices that are simply attached to a victim's chest, with automated software then assessing the heart rhythm and administering a life-sustaining electric shock if needed (82).

It is recommended that each workplace establish an AED team with CPR and AED skills reinforced at least annually (83,84). Other areas in which medical direction is important include provision of the written authorization required in most locations to acquire an AED, establishing initial and continued AED training, and performing case-by-case review of each episode that the AED is used. Additional medical coordinating responsibilities include establishment and integration of the AED program with a quality control system, compliance with local regulatory requirements, and ensuring proper interface with the emergency medical services. Furthermore, it is recommended that all employees be informed about the medical emergency response plan, including the proper means for notifying trained internal and community emergency responders.

AEDs are ideally placed in locations throughout a workplace that will allow initiation of resuscitation and use of the AEDs (the "drop-to-shock" interval) within 5 minutes of recognized cardiac arrests. Estimating time needed for transport can help determine if the proposed locations for AEDs in the work site are appropriate.

Venous Thromboembolism (VTE)

For many years there has been speculation about the relationship between prolonged sitting posture, such as occurs with air travel, and the risk of venous thrombosis (85,86). "Shelter deaths," coined by Simpson (87) during World War II, occurred after prolonged sitting in air raid shelters during the London blitz. Studies on flight passengers have similarly contributed to the belief that extended quiet sitting carries a risk for venous thrombotic episodes (88). Intuitively, professions entailing long periods of immobility would be expected to increase rates of deep vein thrombosis (DVT) and associated incidence of pulmonary emboli. However, there is no consensus that extended quiet sitting carries increased risk for healthy young adults. This is aptly demonstrated by comprehensive studies reporting no increased risk of venous thromboembolic events among flight crew members (89).

In contrast, individuals with risk factors of venous stasis, thrombophilia, and venous wall injury (Virchow's triad) are at increased risk of thromboembolism after extended sitting. An expert panel convened by the World Health Organization (WHO) summarized the weight of evidence, and suggested that "a link probably" exists between air travel and venous thrombosis; such a link is likely to be small, and mainly affects passengers with additional risk factors (e.g., age >40, previous thrombotic episode, thrombophilic abnormalities, malignancy, pregnancy, congestive heart failure, recent surgery, chronic venous insufficiency, hormone therapy) (90). Similar associations may exist for other forms of travel, but there are insufficient data upon which to make recommendations.

REFERENCES

1. American Heart Association. *2000 heart and stroke statistical update.* Dallas: American Heart Association, 2000.
2. Murray C, Lopez A. *The global burden of disease.* Cambridge, MA: Harvard School of Public Health, 1996.
3. Gunby P. Cardiovascular diseases remain the leading cause of death. *JAMA* 1992;267:335.
4. Ridker PM, Genest J, Libby P. Risk factors for atherosclerotic disease. In: Braunwald E, Zipes DP, Libby P, eds. *Heart disease.* Philadelphia: WB Saunders, 2001: 1010–1039.
5. MacMahon S, et al. Blood pressure, stroke, and coronary heart disease. Part 1: Prolonged differences in blood pressure: prospective observational studies corrected for the regression dilution bias. *Lancet* 1990;335 (8692):765–774.
6. Kaplan NM. Systemic hypertension: mechanisms and diagnosis. In: Braunwald E, Zipes DP, Libby P, eds. *Heart disease.* Philadelphia: WB Saunders, 2001:941–971.
7. O'Donnell CJ, Kannel WB. Cardiovascular risks of hypertension: lessons from observational studies. *J Hypertens Suppl* 1998;16(6):S3–S7.
8. The Sixth Report of the Joint National Committee on prevention, detection, evaluation, and treatment of blood pressure. *Arch Intern Med* 1997;157:2413–2446.
9. Erfurt J, Foote A. Cost effectiveness of work-site blood pressure control programs. *J Occup Med* 1984;26:892.
10. Fielding J. Frequency of health risk assessment activities at U.S. worksites. *Am J Prev Med* 1989;5:75.
11. Fielding J. Effectiveness of employee health improvement programs. *J Occup Med* 1982;24:907.
12. Department of Health and Human Services. *Healthy people: national health promotion and disease prevention objectives.* Washington, DC: DHHS, 406.
13. American Heart Association. *Heart at work.* Dallas: AMA, 1984.
14. Centers for Disease Control. *The health consequences of smoking: nicotine addiction.* A report of the surgeon general. Rockville, MD: CDC, 1988.
15. Willitt W, et al. Relative and absolute excess risks of coronary heart disease among women who smoke cigarettes. *N Engl J Med* 1987;317(21):1309.
16. Fielding J, Piserchia P. Frequency of worksite health promotion activities. *Am J Public Health* 1989;79:16.
17. Fisher K, Glascow R, Terborg J. Worksite smoking cessation: a meta-analysis of long-term quit rates from controlled studies. *J Occup Med* 1990;32:429.
18. Fiore M, et al. Methods used to quit smoking in the United States: do cessation programs help? *JAMA* 1990; 263:2760.
19. Stulc T, Ceska R. Cholesterol lowering and the vessel wall: new insights and future perspectives. *Physiol Res* 2001;50(5):461–471.
20. Executive summary of the Third Report of The National Cholesterol Education Program (NCEP) Expert Panel on Detection, Evaluation, and Treatment of High Blood Cholesterol in Adults (Adult Treatment Panel III). *JAMA* 2001;285(19):2486–2497.
21. Wilson P, et al. Prediction of coronary heart disease using risk factor categories. *Circulation* 1998;97: 1837–1847.
22. McCunney R. The role of fitness in preventing heart disease. *Cardiovasc Rev Rep* 1985;6:776.
23. Manson J. The primary prevention of myocardial infarction. *N Engl J Med* 1992;326:1409.
24. Harris S. Physical activity counseling for healthy adults as a primary preventive intervention in the clinical setting. *JAMA* 1989;261:3590.
25. Powell K, et al. The status of the 1990 objectives for physical fitness and exercise. *Public Health Rep* 1986; 101:15.
26. McCunney R. Are exercise programs needed prior to a fitness program? *Occup Health Saf* 1984;53:23.
27. Balady G, et al. Recommendations for cardiovascular screening, staffing, and emergency policies at health/fitness facilities. *Med Sci Sports Exerc* 1998;30: 1009–1018.
28. Gu K, Cowie C, Harris M. Mortality in adults with and without diabetes in a national cohort of the U.S. population 1971–1993. *Diabetes Care* 1998;21:1138–1145.
29. Kannel W, McGee D. Diabetes and glucose tolerance as risk factors for cardiovascular disease: the Framingham Study. *Diabetes Care* 1979;2:120–126.
30. Wautier J, Guillausseau P. Diabetes, advanced glycation endproducts, and vascular disease. *Vasc Med* 1998;3: 131–137.
31. Reaven G. Banting Lecture 1988. Role of insulin resistance in human disease. *Nutrition* 1997;13:64–66.
32. Liu S, et al. A prospective study of dietary intake of carbohydrate, glycemic load, and risk of myocardial infarction in U.S. women. *Am J Clin Nutr* 2000;71: 1455–1461.
33. Manson J, et al. A prospective study of obesity and risk of coronary heart disease in women. *N Engl J Med* 1990;322:882–889.
34. Clinical guidelines on the identification, evaluation, and treatment of overweight and obesity in adults: executive summary. *Am J Clin Nutr* 1998;68:899–917.
35. Fujiwara N, et al. Study on the relationship between plasma nitrite and nitrate level and salt sensitivity in human hypertension: modulation of nitric oxide synthesis by salt intake. *Circulation* 2000;101(8):856–861.
36. Cubeddu LX, et al. Nitric oxide and salt sensitivity. *Am J Hypertens* 2000;13(9):973–979.
37. The sixth report of the Joint National Committee on prevention, detection, evaluation, and treatment of high blood pressure. *Arch Intern Med* 1997;157(21): 2413–2446.
38. Appel LJ, et al. A clinical trial of the effects of dietary patterns on blood pressure. DASH Collaborative Research Group. *N Engl J Med* 1997;336(16):1117–1124.
39. Stamler J. Dietary salt and blood pressure. *Ann NY Acad Sci* 1993;676:122–156.
40. Cutler JA. Progress in life-style intervention for preven-

tion and treatment of high blood pressure. *Ann Epidemiol* 1995;5(2):165–167.
41. Stampfer MJ, Malinow MR. Can lowering homocysteine levels reduce cardiovascular risk? *N Engl J Med* 1995;332(5):328–329.
42. Malinow M, Boston A, Krauss R. Homocyst(e)ine, diet, and cardiovascular disease: a statement for healthcare professionals from the nutrition committee, American Heart Association. *Circulation* 1999;99:178–182.
43. Koehler KM, et al. Association of folate intake and serum homocysteine in elderly persons according to vitamin supplementation and alcohol use. *Am J Clin Nutr* 2001;73(3):628–637.
44. Verhoef P, Stampfer MJ, Rimm EB. Folate and coronary heart disease. *Curr Opin Lipidol* 1998;9(1):17–22.
45. Selhub J, et al. Association between homocysteine concentrations and extracranial carotid-artery stenosis. *N Engl J Med* 1995;332:286–291.
46. Koehler KM, et al. Some vitamin sources relating to plasma homocysteine provide not only folate but also vitamins B-12 and B-6. *J Nutr* 1997;127(8):1534–1536.
47. Boushey CJ, et al. A quantitative assessment of plasma homocysteine as a risk factor for vascular disease: probable benefits of increasing folic acid intakes. *JAMA* 1995;274(13):1049–1057.
48. Libby P. The molecular basis of the acute coronary syndromes. *Circulation* 1995;91:2844–2850.
49. Ridker P, et al. C-reactive protein and other markers of inflammation in the prediction of cardiovascular disease in women. *N Engl J Med* 2000;342:836–843.
50. Ridker P, et al. Inflammation, pravastatin, and the risk of coronary events after myocardial infarction in patients with average cholesterol levels. Cholesterol and Recurrent Events (CARE) Investigators. *Circulation* 1998;98: 839–844.
51. Ridker P, et al. Inflammation, aspirin, and the risk of cardiovascular disease in apparently healthy men. *N Engl J Med* 1997;336:973–979.
52. Rosenman K. Cardiovascular disease and environmental exposure. *Br J Ind Med* 1979;36:85.
53. Fine L. Occupational heart disease. In: Rom W, ed. *Environmental and occupational medicine.* Boston: Little, Brown, 1983:359–365.
54. Petronio L. Chemical and physical agents of work-related cardiovascular diseases. *Ear Heart J* 1988;10 [suppl L]:26.
55. Rosenman K. Environmentally related disorders of the cardiovascular system. In: Upton A, ed. *Medical clinics of North America: 74.* Philadelphia: WB Saunders, 1990:361–375.
56. Speizer F, Wegman D, Ramirez A. Palpitation rates associated with fluorocarbon exposure in a hospital setting. *N Engl J Med* 1975;292:624.
57. Goldsmith J, Aronow W. Carbon monoxide and coronary heart disease: a review. *Environ Res* 1975;10:236.
58. Riitta-Sisko K. Cardiovascular diseases among foundry workers exposed to carbon monoxide. *Scand J Work Environ Health* 1994;20:286–293.
59. Leikin J, et al. Methylene chloride: report of five exposures and two deaths. *Am J Emerg Med* 1990;8:534.
60. Davidson M, Feinleib M. Carbon disulfide poisoning: a review. *Am Heart J* 1972;83:100.
61. Egland G. Effects of exposure to carbon disulphide on low density lipoprotein cholesterol concentration and diastolic blood pressure. *Br J Ind Med* 1992;49:287.
62. Hogstedt C, Axelson O. Nitroglycerine-nitroglycol exposure and the mortality in cardiocerebrovascular diseases among dynamite workers. *J Occup Med* 1977; 19:675.
63. Stayner L, et al. Cardiovascular mortality among munitions workers exposed to nitroglycerine and dinitrotoluene. *Scand J Work Environ Health* 1992;18:34.
64. Seghizzi P, et al. Cobalt myocardiopathy: a critical review of the literature. *Science of the Total Environment* 1994;150:105.
65. DeBusk R, Blomguist C, Kouchoukos N. Identification and treatment of low risk patients after acute myocardial infarction and coronary bypass graft surgery. *N Engl J Med* 1986;314:161.
66. Davidson D. Return to work after cardiac events: a review. *J Cardiac Rehabil* 1983;3:60.
67. Wenger N, et al. Cardiac rehabilitation as secondary prevention. Clinical practice guideline No. 17. Rockville, MD: U.S. Department of Health and Human Services, Public Health Service, Agency for Health Care Policy and Research and the National Heart, Lung, and Blood Institute, 1995.
68. Franklin B. Getting patients back to work after myocardial infarction or coronary artery bypass graft surgery. *Phys Sports Med* 1986;14:183.
69. Rimm A, et al. Changes in occupation after aorta coronary vein bypass operation. *JAMA* 1976;236:361.
70. Barnes G, et al. Changes in working status of patients following coronary bypass surgery. *JAMA* 1977;238: 1259.
71. Walter P. Return to work after coronary artery bypass surgery. *Eur Heart J* 1988;9[suppl L]:61.
72. Neill W, Branch L, Jong GD. Cardiac disability: the impact of coronary heart disease on patients' daily activities. *Arch Intern Med* 1985;145:1642.
73. Cay E, Walker D. Psychological factors and return to work. *Eur Heart J* 1988;9[suppl L]:74.
74. Balady G, et al. Exercise prescription for cardiac patients. In: Franklin B, ed. *ASCM guidelines for exercise testing and prescription.* Philadelphia: Lippincott Williams & Wilkins, 2000:165–199.
75. Sheldhal I, Wilkd N, Tristani F. Exercise prescription for return to work. *J Cardiopulmon Rehabil* 1985;5:567.
76. Antmann M. Ten frequently asked questions about automatic external defibrillators. *Occup Hazards* 1999;61 (9):85–87.
77. Cummins R, Ornato J, Theis W. Improving survival from sudden cardiac arrest: the "chain of survival." *Circulation* 1991;83:1832–1847.
78. Eisenberg M, et al. Cardiac arrest and resuscitation: a tale of 29 cities. *Ann Emerg Med* 1990;19:179–186.
79. Sedgwick M, Dalziel L, et al. Performance of an established system of first responder out-of-hospital defibrillation: the results of the second year of the Heartstart Scotland Project in the "Utstein Style." *Resuscitation* 1993;26:75–88.
80. Hossack K, Hartwig R. Cardiac arrest associated with supervised cardiac rehabilitation. *J Cardiac Rehabil* 1982;2:402–408.
81. Eisenberg M, et al. Survival rates from out-of-hospital cardiac arrest: recommendations for uniform definitions and data to report. *Ann Emerg Med* 1990;19:1249–1259.
82. Weisfeldt M, et al. American Heart Association report on the public access defibrillation conference: automatic external defibrillator task force. *Circulation* 1995;92:2740–2747.
83. Guidelines 2000 for cardiopulmonary resuscitation and

emergency cardiovascular care. International consensus on science. *Circulation* 2000;102[suppl]:1–384.
84. Weisfeldt M, et al. Public access defibrillation: a statement for healthcare professionals from the American Heart Association Task Force on Automatic External Defibrillation. *Circulation* 1995;92:2763.
85. Egermayer P. The "economy class syndrome": problems with the assessment of risk factors for venous thromboembolism. *Chest* 2001;120:1047.
86. Cruickshank J, Gorlin R, Jennet B. Air travel and thrombotic episodes: the economy class syndrome. *Lancet* 1988;2:497.
87. Simpson K. Shelter deaths from pulmonary embolism. *Lancet* 1940;2:744.
88. Ferrari E, et al. Travel as a risk factor for venous thromboembolic disease: a case-control study. *Chest* 1999; 115:440.
89. Kraaijenhagen R, et al. Travel and risk of venous thrombosis. *Lancet* 2000;28:1492.
90. Arfvidsson B. Risk factors for venous thromboembolism following prolonged air travel: coach class thrombosis. *Hematol Oncol Clin North Am* 2000;14:391.
91. Kavanagh T, Matosevic V. Assessment of work capacity in patients with ischaemic heart disease: methods and practices. *Eur Heart J* 1988;9[suppl L]:68.
92. Fox M, Naughton P, Haskell W. Physical activity and the prevention of coronary heart disease. *Ann Clin Res* 1971;3:404.

25

Neurotoxic Disorders

Robert G. Feldman and Chang-Ming Joseph Chern

Certain chemicals found in the workplace can cause biologic responses in nervous tissues at critical levels of exposure and absorption (Table 25.1) (1). Clinical manifestations of neurotoxic effects of these neurotoxicants reflect the specific anatomic structures and cellular elements of the nervous system that are affected. Central nervous system (CNS) effects occur when a toxic chemical or its metabolites cross the blood–brain barrier (BBB) and reach particular neuronal systems (1,2). When access of certain chemical molecules to the CNS is prevented, neurotoxic effects are limited to the peripheral nervous system (PNS). The clinical expressions of the effects of exposure to neurotoxic substances and subsequent damage to cell membranes, myelin sheaths, axonal transport mechanisms, or mitochondrial structures and functions may resemble the clinical features of common nontoxic neurologic syndromes. The same underlying target anatomic structures are affected in both processes.

Documentation of the presence of a suspected toxic substance in the environment in which a subject may have been exposed is of utmost importance. The coexistence of underlying systemic diseases (e.g., diabetes) or a history of previous chemical exposures may influence the patient's response to the immediate exposure circumstances. The mere presence of a substance known to be capable of producing neurotoxic effects does not mean that each exposed person will be affected to the same extent. Individual susceptibility as well as duration and intensity of exposure are major factors that determine the development of neurotoxic symptoms.

Neurologic effects of toxic exposure may be direct or indirect, reversible or irreversible, depending on the specific substance, the nature and duration of exposure, and the selective vulnerability of particular target elements of the PNS and CNS. Although a clinical diagnosis of neurotoxicity can be made based on subjective complaints (symptoms) and objective findings on neurologic examination (signs), confirmation of neurologic dysfunction requires neurophysiologic, neuropsychological, neuroimaging, neuropathologic, and biochemical methodologies (biologic markers).

SYSTEMATIC APPROACH TO DIAGNOSIS

A systematic approach to differentiating a neurotoxic syndrome from a nonneurotoxic illness begins with a good occupational and environmental history. Clinical, neurophysiologic, and neuropsychological data for each exposed subject in a suspected contaminated area are needed in the confirmation or exclusion of a neurotoxic disorder. Monitoring of personal air space and ambient air levels and testing samples of urine and blood for biologic markers of exposure are helpful in assessing current levels of suspected toxic contaminants in the suspected exposure locale and to determine an individual's body burden. Such evidence helps to determine causal relationships between a specific exposure event and toxic effects.

One systematic approach for clinical assessment of possible neurotoxic disease in individuals as well as in groups is the Boston University Environmental Neurology Assessment (BUENA) (Table 25.2) (1). It has been used in evaluating workers suspected of having been exposed to various neurotoxicants, and it has been employed during the health hazard evaluations of members of communities in which hazardous pollutants were found in drinking water sources (3,4). This protocol lists specific essential questions to be answered, elaborating an algorithm (Fig. 25.1) (1) to a greater level of detail for documenting observations and detecting as many confounding variables as possible to reach diagnostic conclusions. The clinical diagnosis of a patient is arrived at through an intellectual process that evaluates and integrates all the available information in a system-

TABLE 25.1. *Neurotoxic chemicals: sources of exposure and clinical features*

Neurotoxic chemical	Sources of exposure	Clinical features
Metals		
Arsenic	Pesticides, pigments, antifouling paints, electroplating industry, seafood, smelters, semiconductors	*Acute:* Encephalopathy, Mee's lines seizures, renal failure *Chronic:* Peripheral neuropathy, encephalopathy, hyperkeratosis
Lead	Solder, lead shot and bullets, illicit whiskey, insecticides, calcium supplements, autobody industry, storage battery manufacturing and reclamation, foundries, smelters, lead-based paints, lead water pipes	*Acute:* Encephalopathy, constipation, abdominal pain, porphyria *Chronic:* Encephalopathy and peripheral neuropathy
Manganese	Iron, steel industry, welding rods, metal-finishing operations, fertilizers, manufacturers of fireworks, matches, manufacturers of dry cell batteries	*Acute:* Mood changes, hallucinations, emotional lability *Chronic:* Parkinsonism
Mercury	Scientific instruments, electrical equipment, amalgams, electroplating industry, photography, felt making	*Acute:* Headache, emotional lability, nausea, respiratory tract irritation, fever, tremor, renal failure *Chronic:* Ataxia, tremor, encephalopathy, social withdrawal, peripheral neuropathy, gingivitis
Tin	Canning industry, solder, electronic components, polyvinyl plastics, fungicides	*Acute:* Memory defects, seizures, disorientation *Chronic:* Encephalomyelopathy
Solvents		
Carbon disulfide	Manufacturers of viscose rayon, preservatives, textiles, rubber cement, varnishes, electroplating industry	*Acute:* Encephalopathy *Chronic:* Peripheral neuropathy, parkinsonism
n-Hexane and methyl-*N*-butyl ketone	Paints, lacquers, varnishes, metal-cleaning compounds, quick-drying inks, paint removers, glues, adhesives	*Acute:* Narcosis *Chronic:* Peripheral neuropathy
Perchloroethylene	Paint removers, degreasers, oil extraction agents, dry cleaning industry, textile industry	*Acute:* Narcosis *Chronic:* Peripheral neuropathy, encephalopathy
Toluene	Rubber solvents, cleaning agents, glues, paints, paint thinners, lacquers gasoline, aviation fuel	*Acute:* Narcosis *Chronic:* Ataxia, encephalopathy
Trichloroethylene	Degreasers, varnishes, electronics manufacturing industry, spot removers, process of caffeine extraction, dry cleaning industry	*Acute:* Narcosis *Chronic:* Encephalopathy, cranial (trigeminal and facial nerve) neuropathy
Insecticides		
Organophosphates	Agricultural industry, chemical manufacturing	*Acute:* Cholinergic crisis *Chronic:* Ataxia, paralysis, peripheral neuropathy
Carbamates	Agricultural industry, chemical manufacturing, flea powders, home gardening products (e.g., Sevin)	*Acute:* Cholinergic crisis characterized by sweating, lacrimation, urinary retention *Chronic:* Tremor, peripheral neuropathy

Modified from Feldman, 1999, with permission.

atic manner. This approach formalizes techniques as they are used in the everyday practice of medicine, where the goal is to assess impairments of an individual within the environment. In this context, differing from the traditional epidemiologic study, the clinician takes the position that even a small probability of serious illness must not be dismissed, and therefore warrants a thorough assessment.

This process should be the same whether used in the day-to-day practice of clinical medicine or in the

TABLE 25.2. *Boston University Environmental Neurology Assessment (BUENA)*

I. *Are the data sufficient to identify any or all complaints as being caused by a neurotoxin?*
   A. *List complaints* and relate them on a time line identifying all possible chemical exposures, episodes, and their sources (work, home, hobby).
      1. Identify symptoms and functional changes expressed, experienced, or observed by others; list examples of mood, anxiety, sleep disturbances, and effect on quality of life.
      2. Cite time of onset, duration, and intensity of all complaints. Characterize symptoms as to worsening or remitting in relation to exposure and away from exposure sources (e.g., workweek, weekend, time of shift, on vacation).
      3. Evaluate subject's family/genetic health, special sensitivities, and possible congenital factors.
   B. *List all substances* and how they are used (at workplace, home, hobbies).
      1. Obtain chemical names (not trade label names), material safety data sheets, and other identifying data concerning each chemical substance.
      2. Review workplace information available (e.g., OSHA mandated material safety data sheets and employer training program materials; employer's medical records and exposure records, which, if kept by employer, must be made available under OSHA rules. Review, if available, the following: employer's TSCA 8c and 8e reports to EPA, employer's community right-to-know reports to local officials re: hazardous materials made, used, or sorted on site).
   C. *Obtain environmental and industrial hygiene air or drinking water samplings measures* to prove the presence of suspected or other chemicals in the alleged sources. *Current levels* are important, and levels taken in relationship to occurrence of complaints is essential.
   D. *Obtain urine andor blood samples from the suspected exposed andor affected* individuals and from known unexposed control patients of similar age and occupation, especially at time of complaints, to *establish body burden of chemical.*
   E. For suspect chemicals, *develop information on dose-response relationships, animal studies, toxicologic and epidemiologic studies.*

II. *Are the complaints substantiated by clinical neurologic physical examination; standardized neuropsychologic and neurophysiologic tests; and appropropriate blood and urine analyses?* Also, are the complaints corroborated by epidemiologic, toxicologic, animal studies; by NIOSH or OSHA or EPA studies of the workforce or community; by employer studies and reports to EPA or OSHA (e.g., TSCA 8c and 8e reports)?

III. *Are the findings due to a primary neurologic disease or other medical condition?*

IV. *Are the findings on examination explained by any other causal factors* identifiable in past medical history, previous and/or current unrelated exposures to substances from sources other than the one under consideration, or due to a primary neurologic disease or other medical condition?
   A. Time line of past jobs, residences
   B. Time line of past medical history

V. *Analyze individual cases for confirmatory studies;* group data for cluster analysis and/or population statistical study.

VI. *Identify and critically review previously published andor reported case reports, case control studies, population studies, and animal studies concerning the alleged neurotoxins and relate documentation to case data.*

VII. *Estimate the damage consequences for the subject:* disease, anxiety, loss of consort, functional impairments, need for special education or counseling or medical surveillance, need for medical therapeutic measures, job disability, loss of earnings, etc.

VIII. *Reevaluate after reasonable absence from all neurotoxic exposure* to assess course of progression, recovery, or persistent impairment and/or disability.

EPA, Environmental Protection Agency; NIOSH, National Institute for Occupational Safety and Health; OSHA, Occupational Safety and Health Administration; TSCA, Toxic Substances Control Act.

From Feldman, 1999, with permission.

special circumstances of evaluating individuals suspected of neurotoxic disease who may be involved in litigation. Knowledge of physiologic, anatomic, and behavioral concepts and principles accumulated from experience and derived from a database of previously published reports and conventionally accepted clinical norms known to the examiner serves as a frame of reference for evaluating these abnormalities and formulating a diagnosis and possible causal explanation for the reported symptoms.

SYMPTOMATIC APPROACH TO NEUROTOXIC SYNDROMES

Symptoms of neurologic dysfunction (e.g., motor weakness, sensory loss, or altered mental status) can

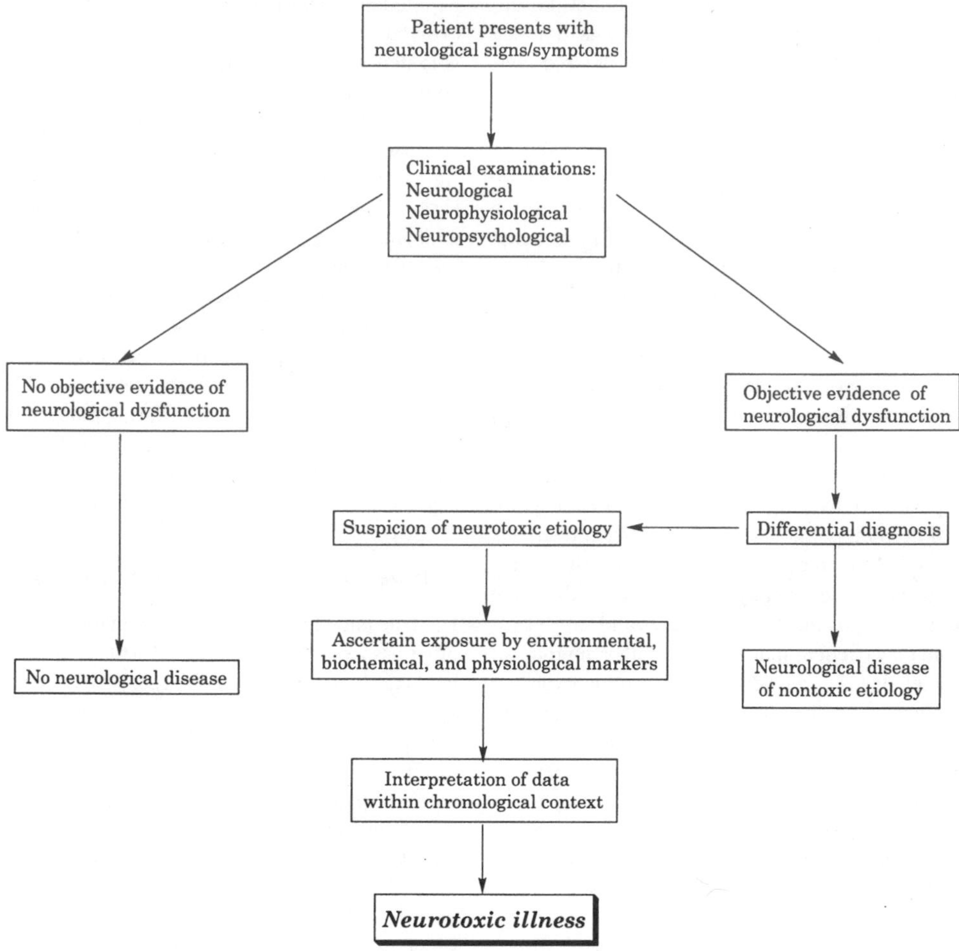

FIG. 25.1. Algorithm for differential diagnosis.

be seen in neurotoxic syndromes as well as in non-neurotoxic illnesses. For example, ataxia and tremor similar to that seen in degenerative diseases of the cerebellum (Friedreich's ataxia) also result from exposure to toluene, mercury, and acrylamide. Spinal cord lesions such as those seen in neurosyphilis, vitamin B_{12} deficiency, and multiple sclerosis (in which the posterior columns are affected) can be caused by triorthocresylphosphate poisoning (5). Spasticity, impotence, and urinary retention, commonly associated with a diagnosis of multiple sclerosis, have been seen following leptophos poisoning and exposure to dimethylaminopropionitrile (6). Parkinsonism, the clinical features of which closely resemble those of idiopathic Parkinson's disease (IPD) including disturbances of posture with rigidity and tremor, can be the result of the toxic effects of chemicals that act on neurons in the substantia nigra and striatum [e.g., carbon monoxide, carbon disulfide, manganese, and methyl-4-phenyltetrahydropyridine (MPTP)] (1,7–12). Peripheral neuropathy occurs in association with diabetes and nutritional deficiency, as well as in persons exposed to certain chemicals (e.g., *n*-hexane and carbon disulfide).

Central Nervous System Symptoms

Encephalopathy is the term used to describe disturbances of function of the brain itself. The exact localization of damage, however, whether it is cerebral cortex, basal ganglia, limbic system, or white matter, is usually not specified. The clinical manifestations of the toxic encephalopathies include cognitive disturbances of attention, problem-solving abilities, and memory function, and, at times, psychotic-like behavior. Other common CNS symptoms include headache, changes in mood and affect, altered consciousness, and motor disturbances (1).

Headache

Headache, a common neurologic complaint, arises from distention, traction, or irritation of intracranial pain-sensitive structures, such as medium- to large-sized blood vessels, dura, falx, meninges, and mucous membranes of the sinuses. Increased intracranial pressure associated with brain swelling (cerebral edema), elevated blood pressure, or chemical irritation of the membranes can cause headache. Although headache is a nonspecific symptom, the differential diagnosis must include all possible etiologies including exposure to toxic substances. Concomitant symptoms of dermal, pulmonary, or other systemic effects may corroborate an exposure to particular chemicals.

Headache is frequently associated with acute higher level exposures to metal fumes and solvent vapors and may occur simultaneously with symptoms of light-headedness and/or dizziness. Chronic exposure to low levels of chemicals is also associated with headache, but in such cases the relatively insidious onset of the headache may forestall an association with an exposure. Headache due to chemical exposure typically resolves after removal of the patient from the source of exposure, although some patients report that their headaches persist even after cessation of exposure.

Headache due to cerebral edema occurred in two men who worked in an electroplating plant using solutions of nickel chloride, nickel sulfate, and hypophosphate (1). Their work involved mixing the solution and then heating it to drive the reaction. When the temperature reached 150°F, the solution spontaneous decomposed, resulting in evolution of toxic fumes into the work environment. This event was first recognized when the two workers noted an unpleasant odor. Shortly after the incident both workers began to experience an itching sensation on the exposed skin of their arms and face. Several hours later, each developed severe headaches, nausea, and vomiting. Investigation revealed that the ingredients of the solution were in error. The usual mixture contained 70 gallons of water, 5 gallons of nickel chloride and nickel sulfate, and 14.5 gallons of hypophosphate. On this occasion the 14.5 gallons of hypophosphate had been inadvertently replaced with 14.5 gallons of hydrogen peroxide. Visual field testing showed increased blind spots consistent with the appearance of papilledema. The acute and intense exposure to nickel evolved in the accident had resulted in the characteristic itch and the subsequent cerebral edema and accompanying severe headache. Computed tomography (CT) scans in each man revealed small ventricles, consistent with cerebral edema. The cerebrospinal fluid pressures were 200 mm in case 1 and 170 mm in case 2. Nickel concentrations in 24-hour urine were 27.3 and 45 μg/L in case 1 and 8 μg/L in case 2. Both men were chelated with penicillamine (250 mg q.i.d.) to reduce their body burdens of nickel. Within 4 to 5 days after instituting chelation, improvement in the headaches began, with complete recovery by the end of the month. The output of nickel in case 1 prior to chelation was 1.4 μg per day; during the first week of chelation, it was 4.2 μg per day. Prior to chelation, case 2 had 0.4 μg/day and his average output for 4 days of chelation was 4.0 μg per day.

Disturbances of Personality, Mood, and Affect

Acute and chronic exposures to many chemicals are often associated with increased irritability, emotional lability, depression, and fatigue. These nonspecific symptoms may go unrecognized until other symptoms emerge and result in the exposed individual seeking medical attention. Family members and co-workers may report changes in personality and affect in the exposed subject, but these are often ignored or at best mistakenly associated with job stress or other life factors. Changes in mood and affect are often the first to emerge and thus are often entirely reversible with cessation of exposure. In other cases changes in mood and affect may persist after a severe acute or chronic exposure; in such cases, these symptoms are often accompanied by changes in cognitive function (1).

Cognitive Disturbances

Acute exposures to many chemicals can cause transient changes in cognitive functioning, and thus many occupational accidents attributed to human error may in fact be due to impaired alertness, judgment, or psychomotor ability. Changes in mental functioning due to intoxication often go unrecognized by the exposed worker or may be attributed to other causes such as stress or aging, particularly when associated with chronic exposures. Impaired cognitive performance can be documented using sophisticated measures of behavioral function included in formal neuropsychological assessment batteries.

Chronic exposure to a variety of neurotoxicants at levels that do not produce overt acute disturbances of functioning can cause insidious development of behavioral disturbances, mood changes, and a variety of cognitive disturbances. Clinical manifestations range from early, subtle changes in mood and affect to overt disturbances of memory and an inability to carry out activities of daily living that often bring the worker to the attention of a physician. These symptoms may also appear as sequelae to an acute exposure episode associated with overt clinical manifestations. However, as these symptoms are not specific to toxic encephalopathy, other conditions such as neurodegenerative or metabolic encephalopathy must be carefully excluded based on laboratory findings and formal neuropsychological test results (5–7).

Altered Consciousness

Central nervous system manifestations of neurotoxicity vary depending on the types and conditions of exposure to neurotoxicants, including concentrations of the chemicals and duration and route of exposure. Acute exposure may cause drowsiness, somnolence, dizziness, or loss of consciousness, resulting from neurodepression. However, in acute organic solvent exposure, these are preceded by neurostimulation with euphoria, lack of inhibition, interrupted speech, and unsteady walking in a preliminary phase. If exposure continues, it leads to the phase of clinical neurodepression. Exposure to high concentrations of organic solvent vapors in closed and poorly ventilated locations leads to loss of consciousness and asphyxia. The resulting anoxia can cause death in a few minutes.

Motor Disturbances

Disturbances of motor function associated with CNS damage due to exposure to neurotoxicants is common and may include tremor, dysmetria, slowness of movement (bradykinesia), and rigidity. Parkinsonism may develop following exposure to certain neurotoxicants, including carbon monoxide, carbon disulfide, manganese, and MPTP. The amino acid β-*N*-methylamino-L-alanine (BMAA), which is found in high concentrations in the cycad seed kernel used to make cycad flour, has been suggested as the underlying cause for parkinsonism-amyotrophic lateral sclerosis (ALS) dementia complex in Guam (8). Cell death may be mediated by BMAA activation of glutamate receptors and induction of apoptosis. The parkinsonian features of these disorders (e.g., bradykinesia, cogwheel rigidity, shuffling gait, tremor, and postural reflexes) closely resemble those of IPD leading to the suspicion that Parkinson's disease or parkinsonism may be caused by environmental agents (7–11). However, the two are associated with different neuropathologic changes. The only neurotoxicant documented to cause neuropathologic changes closely resembling those of idiopathic PD is MPTP. The major neuropathologic loci responsible for the parkinsonian features associated with exposure to neurotoxicants other than MPTP are the globus pallidus for carbon monoxide, striatum and pallidum for manganese, and pallidonigral degeneration for carbon disulfide. In addition, Lewy bodies, typical of idiopathic Parkinson's disease, cannot be found in these patients, unless a patient with Parkinson's disease has these superimposed exposures. Patients with MPTP-induced parkinsonism respond to the full array of antiparkinsonian agents in a manner quite analogous to that seen in Parkinson's disease, including the side effects of the antiparkinsonian medications, whereas patients with other exposures do not (1). Positron emission tomography (PET) scan has been used successfully to differentiate parkinsonism caused by manganese exposure from IPD (1,11).

Peripheral Nervous System Symptoms

The PNS consists of nerves with cell bodies located in the spinal cord. The axons of peripheral neurons (fibers) extend distally and follow a predictable distribution to the extremities. The motor fibers that innervate skeletal muscle originate in large neurons in the anterior gray matter of the cord and join other fibers to form the ventral root. Sensory nerve fibers originate in the unipolar cells of the dorsal root ganglia. Information from the extremities is brought to the dorsal root ganglia by the afferent fibers of these sensory nerves. The diameter of various fibers is dependent on the quantity of myelin that covers them. The largest fibers convey impulses most rapidly; the smaller fibers, which contain less myelin, conduct more slowly. The smallest fibers, however, conduct impulses most slowly and are considered unmyelinated fibers.

Nerve fibers are held together in bundles by connective tissue and are supplied with nutrients by blood vessels. The sensory fibers and the ventral root fibers of the motor neurons travel together to skeletal muscles and skin as bundles of fibers that collectively form a sensorimotor nerve.

The autonomic nervous system includes the parasympathetic and sympathetic divisions. Its fibers are distributed to smooth muscle, including that of bronchial tubes, blood vessels, and glands to permit regulation of heart rate, vasodilation, bronchial constriction, and gland secretions.

Disorders of peripheral sensory nerves are manifested clinically by a decrease in the ability to perceive sensation, spontaneous sensations (tingling), and painful sensations (dysesthesia). Reflex activity, such as that which follows tapping a knee tendon or ankle tendon, occurs when both sensory and motor fibers are able to conduct an impulse from the periphery to the spinal cord and back to the antagonist muscle group. Dysfunction of this pathway reduces or eliminates the reflex response and is a sign of a peripheral nerve disorder.

When widespread and bilateral peripheral nerve damage results from toxic causes, the condition is referred to as polyneuropathy. The deficits in function may be motor, sensory, sensorimotor, or autonomic; they may be proximal, distal, or generalized in distribution. When the small thinly myelinated and unmyelinated fibers are affected, the condition is referred to as *small-fiber neuropathy.* In this condition, the sensations of pain and temperature are markedly disturbed with a relative preservation of motor power and sensory functions of touch-pressure, vibration, and joint sensation, since these functions are carried by larger myelinated fibers.

In *large-fiber neuropathy,* there is weakness as well as loss of sensation of position, vibration, and touch-pressure. Toxic damage to myelin or the axon can result in large-fiber neuropathy. When a toxic substance primarily affects the axon, the conduction velocity is less affected than is the amplitude of the response. This preservation of conduction velocity reflects the ability of the unaffected myelinated fibers to still conduct information about the occurrence of stimulus rapidly even though the number of fibers contributing to the magnitude of the response is reduced as reflected in the small amplitude. Damage to the myelin may be incomplete, and recovery may ensue when exposure is stopped. Recovery may occur after damage to the axons, but the regeneration process is relatively slow and in many cases the reinnervation process is incomplete as many of the sprouting fibers never reach their original targets. Destruction of the nerve cell results in irreversible deficits in function.

Numbness, Tingling, and Weakness in the Extremities

Numbness, tingling, weakness, and reduced reflexes are indicators of peripheral neuropathy. LeQuesne (12) pointed out the importance of understanding the pathophysiology of a suspected toxic effect when reviewing clinical neuropathies. In neuropathy caused by *n*-hexane and methyl *n*-butyl ketone, for example, motor nerve conduction velocity is usually reduced, but in some cases, it may be perfectly normal. Neurotoxic damage from hexacarbon solvents usually causes axonal degeneration, but sufficient secondary changes in the myelin may explain an overall reduction in conduction velocity. In acrylamide neuropathy, motor nerve conduction velocity may also be either normal or show little change. Similarly, sensory nerve action potentials may be normal, but reduced in amplitude. Although acrylamide has a selective destructive action on large-diameter fibers, organophosphate insecticides do not affect these fibers, and thus conduction velocity is not affected either. In triorthocresylphosphate (TOCP) neuropathy in baboons, reduced amplitude of muscle action potential is noted without apparent effect on conduction velocity. The appropriate electrophysiologic technique should be selected in order to obtain the specific evidence needed to confirm a diagnosis. Speed of conduction is affected in demyelinating neuropathies, while amplitude of the nerve action potential is essential in ascertaining the presence of axonal neuropathies.

Complaints of numbness and tingling or weakness are early signs of peripheral neuropathy and often prompt an individual to seek a neurologic evaluation. The development of clinical features of peripheral neuropathy is insidious, occurring after several months of exposure to a neurotoxic substance. The myelin sheath and axon are the targets of neurotoxic chemicals. PNS symptoms occur after exposure to certain metals (lead, arsenic, and thallium) and solvents (methyl *n*-butyl ketone and *n*-hexane). The degreasing solvent trichloroethylene (TCE) has a predilection for cranial nerves, especially the trigeminal nerve, producing loss of sensation over the face (13).

Segmental demyelination is associated with exposure to lead, which affects the myelin sheath, with relative sparing of the axon. Numbness and tingling of the fingers and toes are the initial symptoms, followed by motor weakness. Detection of a demyelinating neuropathy in the early stages can be facilitated by nerve conduction velocity studies and allows for a significant degree of recovery if exposure is immediately ended or significantly reduced. Demyelinating neuropathy is associated with slowed sensory and motor nerve conduction velocities and distal motor latencies with relatively normal amplitudes since the number of fibers innervating the target has not been reduced. Recovery is rapid once remyelination begins and is usually complete in mild to moderate neuropathies.

Axonal degeneration results from disruptions of axonal transport and/or metabolic imbalances of the entire neuron. Accumulation of neurofilaments adjacent to a node of Ranvier and secondary demyelination is a common pathologic finding on nerve biopsy studies of patients exposed to certain neurotoxicants (e.g., *n*-hexane and carbon disulfide). Axonal degeneration develops distally and proceeds proximally to the cell body and in severe cases can result in death of the neuron. Unlike segmental demyelination, nerve conduction velocities and distal motor latencies are usually normal but amplitudes are relatively reduced as the number of fibers innervating the target is reduced. Muscles innervated by affected fibers show stages of atrophy associated with denervation. Recovery is slow and often incomplete.

While the symptoms and signs of peripheral nerve disease are either consistent with axonal or demyelinating processes, or a combination of the two, the cause of the neuropathy cannot be determined solely on clinical grounds. However, the selective toxicities of various chemicals for axonal or Schwann cell targets may point to a particular neurotoxicant exposure. For example, arsenical neuropathy initially presents as losses of sensation in the feet and hands. Dysesthesias are common. Position and vibration sensations are usually impaired, and there is reduced perception to painful stimuli. Motor impairment is gradual in its onset, involving the small muscles of the feet and hands. The site of toxicity is intracellular, causing axonal change, and fragmentation of myelin occurs after axonal degeneration takes place. Sensory fibers are affected before motor fibers, and distal sections before proximal portions. Once axonal damage and secondary myelin degeneration have occurred, there is little chance of regeneration and clinical recovery (1).

Case Study: Combined Central and Peripheral Nervous System Symptoms

The features of solvent encephalopathy are illustrated by the case of a 42-year-old optician who had worked for 5 years developing new procedures and techniques in the production of optical surfaces. He heated TCE and toluene in an ultrasonic cleaner in order to clean the optical surfaces. He frequently left the tops off the solvent containers and often leaned over the ultrasonic cleaner and breathed in the solvent vapors. Sometimes he did not leave this room, where he worked alone, for 2 to 3 days at a time. At the end of 5 years, he began to notice memory problems and concentration difficulties. In addition, he felt he had a decreased attention span, problems with recall, tremors in both hands, numbness and tingling in all extremities, and emotional lability. While driving home from work, he found it necessary to pull over to the side of the road to sleep and would be unable to recall the length of time he had been there. He was evaluated clinically and with a neuropsychological test battery for his memory and concentration difficulties. This clinical examination revealed obviously decreased attention span and memory deficits. An electroencephalogram (EEG) showed excessive amounts of bilateral theta (slow waves) activity. Neuropsychological testing revealed significant depression, memory deficits variable psychomotor speed, and slightly impaired verbal fluency. In addition to the cognitive disturbances documented by neuropsychological testing, his clinical neurologic examination had also revealed evidence of PNS dysfunction characterized by diminished sensation to vibration in the toes and over the lower extremities below the knees. He consistently interpreted pinprick as being dull except over his face. In addition, he had diminished proprioception in the feet and diminished graphesthesia in his palms. Nerve conduction velocity studies demonstrated slowed motor conduction velocities suggestive of peripheral neuropathy. Sensory conduction velocities were slowed and amplitudes were reduced, indicating an axonal neuropathy. The clinical and laboratory findings in this patient demonstrate the behavioral as well as the PNS findings that can result from exposure to organic solvents.

CLINICAL NEUROLOGICAL EXAMINATION

Mental Status

The neurologic examination begins with an assessment of the patient's ability to comprehend language, follow directions, solve problems, perform coordinated motor functions, and to perceive and identify sensations presented in various modalities. The patient's mental status is evaluated by screening tests of speech and language, and by tests of attention, memory, and cognitive performance. Formal neuropsychological tests are usually required and are performed as part of the series of diagnostic tests.

Motor Control, Strength, and Posture

A careful examination of motor function provides information about the functioning of the cerebral cortex and its connections through the subcortical, brainstem, cerebellar, and spinal cord pathways to the effector muscles that produce intended actions. A lesion or dysfunction in the motor cortex will result in weakness of the contralateral limbs, while basal ganglia dysfunction is reflected in abnormal muscle tone and impaired speed of response. Midbrain and brainstem structures control coordination of cranial nerve functions such as conjugate eye movement, articulation of speech, and swallowing. Impaired cerebellar functioning may result in ataxia and unsteadiness of gait appearing as unsteadiness of the trunk or simply as tremor of the outstretched extremities and head. Rhythmic instability of a maintained posture, tremors, result from cerebellar and vestibular dysfunction, appearing during action (action tremor), or as a result of basal ganglia dysfunction, and appearing during rest (resting tremor) and disappearing during action. Loss of muscle tone and total paralysis indicates disease in the lower motor neurons. In such instances, muscle atrophy occurs as well. Spinal cord function is best measured through combined sensory and motor examinations. The loss of sensation to pain and temperature on one half of the body to the midline from a segment below the cervical spinal cord level is consistent with a lesion in the anterior spinal cord on the opposite side as the sensory loss. Nerve fibers carrying position and light touch sensations travel in structures in the posterior columns or dorsal portion of the spinal cord on the same side of the body as the sensory receptor, so that the site of a lesion is ipsilateral to the clinical findings. Weakness in the arm and leg result from a lesion in the spinal pathways on the same side, if a lesion exists below the foramen magnum. Observations of gait, posture, muscle tone, fine motor control, and coordination are recorded. Motor and sensory functions of peripheral and cranial nerves are tested. Spinal cord reflexes and various special reflexes of upper motor neuron and basal ganglia systems are evaluated.

Sensation and Reflexes

Loss of pain and temperature occurs on the side of the body opposite to the affected spinal cord spinothalamic pathways that convey these sensations brought to them over afferent peripheral nerves. Bundles of fibers consisting of motor axons arise in the anterior horn cells of the lower motor neurons in the spinal cord ventral horn and transcending long distances from the spinal cord to the individual muscles these fibers innervate. The motor fibers connect with the muscle cells at the neuromuscular junction. The nerve trunk carries sensory fibers back into the spinal cord. These afferent fibers bring information from the sensory receptors in the skin, muscles, and joints to the spinal cord. There, after synapsing in the dorsal root ganglion, pin and temperature sensation is conducted by long fibers ascending in the ventral spinal thalamic tracts. Light touch, position, and vibration sensations are carried in the dorsal columns of the spinal cord. A complete lesion in a peripheral nerve denervates the muscle in a similar fashion as would occur with lower motor neuron disease, but the latter would be accompanied also by sensory loss in the distribution of the affected peripheral nerve.

Reflex testing is used to determine the intactness and functional continuity of afferent and efferent nerve pathways. Reflex activity involves the CNS and PNS. CNS reflexes are manifested by behavioral responses such as a startled head turning response to a sound in one ear or the effect of body posture when the vestibular reflexes are stimulated by the placement of cold water in one ear. A light placed on the eye results in a constriction of the pupil after the light stimulus has traversed the cornea and lens to the retina; the impulse then travels by way of the optic nerve, optic chiasm, and lateral geniculate ganglion and connects with the parasympathetic nuclei. From there the efferent pathways from the midbrain travel via the fibers of the pupillary constructor muscles and cause contractions in response to the light stimulation, completing this reflex loop.

Tendon reflexes are elicited by tapping, thus stretching the tendons at the biceps, triceps, gastrocnemius, and quadriceps muscles. Both symmetry and intensity of reflexes are important in determining neurologic impairment and the spinal root levels affected. Asymmetric reflexes must be explained. Bilateral reduction in reflexes in the lower extremities as compared to the upper extremities suggests the possibility of peripheral nerve disease. Increased reflexes in the extremities suggests a release of upper motor neuron control and therefore the possibility of a CNS lesion. The concomitant signs of an abnormal posture of response, such as the up-going toe (Babinski sign) when the bottom of the foot is stroked, is similarly indicative of a release of upper motor neuron control. The Babinski sign may be unilateral when there is a contralateral cerebral lesion, or ipsilateral with a corticospinal pathway lesion.

NEUROPSYCHOLOGICAL ASSESSMENT

When a patient experiences CNS behavioral effects of toxic agents such as changes in mental status, formal neuropsychological testing can aid in the diagnosis. Complaints of irritability and problems with attention and memory due to toxic encephalopathy are difficult to differentiate from those associated with other nontoxic disorders of CNS functioning. An appropriately trained neuropsychologist can provide valuable information about the integrity of specific cognitive domains including memory, fine motor skills, and reasoning ability. This can be very helpful in the differential diagnosis of senile dementia and chronic solvent encephalopathy in older workers (14).

The application of formal neuropsychological testing in assessing effects of subtle neurotoxicity offers a number of advantages. Specific, standardized rules for administering and scoring these tests exist. Results can be analyzed in terms of published normative scores based on age, sex, and education. These tests have been validated and found reliable in both research and clinical settings, allowing clear interpretation of results by independent neuropsychologists. Batteries of tests can be designed for clinical diagnosis of encephalopathy in individual patients and for screening large groups of workers. Skill areas assessed by these tests include attention (including vigilance, as well as ability to hold and manipulate information), motor skills, reaction time, concept formation (reasoning), language, visuospatial abilities, and mood and personality (2).

The most commonly used criterion for inclusion of a test in a battery is its confirmed ability to detect the effects of exposure to a particular neurotoxic substance. Since the mean differences between data obtained from the studies of exposed and nonexposed groups in research populations may be quite small, they may not always be applicable to the study of individual patients. In clinical situations, it is generally more appropriate to select neuropsychological tests that assess as many functions as possible. The battery is designed to cover a wide area of functions and to deal with as many manifestations of neurotoxic encephalopathy as possible (2).

Perhaps the most difficult situation arises with respect to estimating the severity of past exposure. Evaluation of deficits often occurs at a time when body burden of the suspected substance is no longer elevated or environmental levels can no longer be ascertained. Obtaining an occupational environmental history to estimate the extent of exposure (duration and intensity) is of the utmost importance. Essential to this inquiry are questions about the patient's current and previous occupations, job tasks, places of residence and employment, and hobbies.

ELECTRODIAGNOSTIC TESTS

Tests of Central Nervous System Functioning

Electroencephalography (EEG)

Bioelectrical potentials arising from neurons of the cerebral cortex and modulated by thalamus and the reticular activating system are transmitted via complex synaptic networks throughout the cerebral hemispheres. The electromagnetic fields associated with this constant neurologic activity can be recorded from electrodes placed on the scalp. Sensitive electronic equipment amplifies and displays the patterns of mixed frequencies, amplitudes, and their topographic distributions over the cranium. The resulting EEG provides real-time monitoring of electrophysiologic activity of the brain during the duration of the sampling. The EEG has been shown to have predictable patterns during normal waking, drowsing, and sleeping states. Mixtures of fast and slow frequencies appear in the frontal, temporal, and occipital areas. Abnormalities in the normal symmetry, amplitude, frequencies, and patterns of the EEG are associated with impairment in brain function. Paroxysmal quality in the waveforms, associated with sharp, spiked discharges, indicates epileptic activity. Diffuse slowing of the background rhythm with disappearance of normal resting frequencies suggests metabolic or toxic encephalopathy. Increased amounts of slow wave activity occur during exposure to neurotoxicants that have CNS effects. Marked asymmetry of amplitude or frequency suggests a lateralized pathologic process. A concentration of sharp, slow, or paroxysmal waves in a particular area may indicate an underlying focal, structural lesion, such as a tumor, cerebrovascular infarct, stroke, or old trauma (1).

The EEG tracing pattern typically returns to normal after the patient is removed from exposure to CNS neurotoxicants. Although the EEG findings may correlate well with behavior during acute encephalopathy, they are not well correlated with the persistent dysfunctions that remain after cessation of exposure. Abnormalities in the EEG are indicators of the physiologic state of the brain only at the time of recording, and the patterns are not specific to any particular causal substance. As with all laboratory tests, the significance of the EEG report depends on correlation with other clinical information and examinations. In the differential diagnosis of neurotoxic syndromes and nonneurotoxic, neurologic disease, the EEG is most helpful when an abnormality is seen during or in proximity in time to exposure, since the EEG becomes normal in reversible encephalopathy when the patient is away from the suspected neurotoxic environment. The persistence of an EEG disturbance long after exposure ceases should raise questions about the cause not being neurotoxic, unless there had been severe encephalopathy with marked pathology (1).

Evoked Potential Testing

Electrical cortical potentials (i.e., responses) are produced by the stimulation of specific afferent pathways and are recorded from the surface of the brain through the skull and the scalp utilizing electrodes and highly sensitive amplifying electronic equipment. The sensory evoked potentials consist of visually evoked potentials, brainstem auditory evoked potentials, and somatosensory evoked potentials.

Visual evoked potentials (VEPs) assess the functional integrity of the components of the optic system pathway including the optic nerve and chiasm, the optic tract, the geniculate nuclei, and the calcarine cortex, all of which are involved in transmitting the visual evoked response after a stimulus has been applied at the retina. Because the optic pathways decussate at the chiasm, the bioelectric response posterior to the chiasm contains transmitted impulses from both eyes when one eye is not covered during stimulation. Therefore, care must be given to the technique used in eliciting a visual evoked response. Two types of VEPs are elicited in the laboratory setting: In flash VEPs (F-VEPs), the more simplistic of the two tests, the patient's perception of the presence of light is recorded. It is useful in testing uncooperative subjects and children to see if the light signal is getting into the brain. Pattern shift VEPs (PS-VEPs), the more sensitive of the two parameters, are elicited by presenting to the subject a checkerboard pattern that flickers on and off at a rate of 2 Hz. Each eye is tested separately. In both forms of VEPs the latency between stimulus and response is approximately 100 ms, recordable over the occipital region and termed the P100 peak. Both forms can be used to assess a patient exposed to neurotoxicants (1,15).

Brainstem auditory evoked potentials (BAEPs) arise following presentation of an auditory stimulus (e.g., clicking sound) to one ear while input to the other ear is masked with white noise. Recording electrodes are placed over the earlobes and the vertex of the head. Activation of the auditory (8th cranial) nerve occurs over about 10 ms, generating a complex waveform visible by oscilloscope, which relates to specific sites along the auditory pathway (15). Wave I reflects activation of the acoustic nerve; waves II and III reflect activation of structures in the pontomedullary region; the sources of waves IV and V are less clearly defined, but appear to be related to functions of the upper pons and low mid-brain. The absolute latencies of each wave are recorded but interpeak latencies of waves I to III, III to V, and I to V are more consistent and reproducible, and therefore are utilized in clinical testing. BAEPs have been useful in studies of neurodegenerative diseases of the brainstem, and demyelinating processes, such as multiple sclerosis, and for detecting the effects of exposure to neurotoxic chemicals such as toluene (1,16, 17,18).

Somatosensory evoked potentials (SSEPs) are recorded from scalp electrodes placed over the sensory cortex after activation of the peripheral sensory or mixed nerve. The stimulus is conveyed centrally in peripheral nerve fibers to dorsal columns in the spinal cord producing a propagated potential that is then projected to the contralateral cortex. The absolute latencies can be influenced by limb length and the presence of peripheral neuropathy, and therefore the technique is important in obtaining reliable measures. SSEPs are usually tested in both upper and lower extremities, and interpeak latencies are more consistent and can help to localize pathology along the path of the peripheral nerve through the spinal cord, brainstem, and thalamus to the cortex. Since many neurotoxicants affect peripheral nerves, it is commonly the distal-most sites of sensory conduction that are slowed and affect the cortically evoked SSEPs in patients exposed to neurotoxicants. Therefore, it is uncertain whether SSEPs offer any advantage over standard nerve conduction velocities, except for studies of conduction through the spinal cord posterior columns, and in instances where proximal nerve blocks or asymmetrical problems are being considered in the differential diagnosis.

Tests of Peripheral Nervous System Functioning

Electrodiagnostic studies are used to evaluate peripheral nerve function. Measures of peripheral nerve conduction depend on the ability of sufficient nerve fibers to conduct a stimulus. The conduction characteristics of a fiber are determined by its axonal diameter and the thickness of its myelin sheath. Electrically, the fastest firing fibers (those with the most myelin) determine the measurable conduction velocity and response to a supramaximal stimulus. In moderately affected fibers, the conduction velocity is decreased; in severely affected fibers, a full block of conduction occurs. If conduction is completely blocked, no information is transmitted beyond the site of demyelination. Although remyelination of damaged peripheral nerve fibers can occur, recovery of nerve conduction is usually associated with decreased conduction velocities. Incomplete remyelination of some fibers may in turn account for persistent abnormalities in clinical function such as weakness and abnormal sensation.

Modern electronic equipment has provided a way to study physiologic function of the PNS. Transcutaneous electrical stimulation of a particular nerve can result in contraction of the muscle to which it conducts the induced impulses. The twitch of the responding muscle can be recorded by electrodes attached to the skin over the muscle or by inserting a recording needle electrode into the muscle belly. The muscle action response is conveyed by wires from the electrodes to an amplifier system and then, as an electrical potential, is displayed on a screen or printed out by a permanent recording device. Although many studies in the occupational medical and epidemiologic literature have not followed the strictest conventions, recent work reflects efforts to use standardized techniques so that interstudy comparisons can be made. The reader is referred to current textbooks of electromyography for appropriate methodology and use of control values.

Nerve Conduction Studies

The conduction characteristics of a nerve fiber are determined by the nerve cell body and axon, its axoplasm, and its myelin sheath. Transcutaneous electrical stimulation of a particular nerve results in initiation of an action potential. Action potentials are transmitted from the electrodes to an amplifier system and displayed on an oscilloscope screen, or printed out on a permanent recording device. Appropriately applied tests of nerve conduction and muscle activity can help to localize sites of impaired function whether in the individual nerve, nerve root, plexus, or motor neurons. In addition, degrees of impairment correspond to the proportion of abnormally conducting myelinated nerve fibers, whether the amplitude or speed is more affected and whether sensory or motor fibers are more involved; subsequently, on serial studies, patterns of recovery or persistence of abnormality facilitate the prognosis after neurotoxic peripheral nerve damage. These tests can also provide information about the pathophysiologic bases for neurologic findings, such as axonal, demyelinating, myopathy, or neurogenic atrophy.

A peripheral nerve is composed of axons of many neurons groups together in bundles consisting of thousands of individual nerve fibers of various sizes. The thicker the myelin sheath, the larger the fiber diameter. The amount of myelin surrounding each nerve axon determines the speed of conduction of that axon: the less myelin, the slower the conduction time; the more myelin, the faster the conduction time. The fastest firing nerve fibers deliver impulses earlier than do the slower fibers, which conduct the later-arriving impulses. A recordable complex nerve action potential involves all of the conducted nerve action potentials of the various component fiber sizes in that nerve. The proportion of larger fibers, and therefore faster firing fibers, determine the faster speeds of an evoked and conducted compound nerve impulse, traveling between the point of stimulation and the site of the response recording (15).

The delay between the stimulus point closest to the muscle and an observed motor response is called the *distal motor latency,* reported in milliseconds. It is determined by stimulating the nerve at two points (S1 and S2) and recording these response times. The difference between these two times is the residual or distal latency and includes the time it takes for the propagation of the muscle action potential including neuromuscular transmission. This parameter reflects the functional integrity of the neuromuscular junction as well as the nerve. If the number of properly conducting larger fibers is reduced because of demyelination, as occurs in lead neuropathy, the latency between the stimulus and the recorded response will be prolonged. A prolonged latency reflects the later-appearing responses of the remaining smaller and more slowly conducting fibers innervating the muscle (15).

Conduction velocities are measures of the speed at which an action potential is conducted by a nerve fiber. *Motor conduction velocity* is expressed in meters per second and is determined by dividing the distance between a more proximal stimulation site (S2) and the recording site (R) (expressed in millimeters) by the difference in the motor response latencies for the proximal stimulation site (S2) and a more distal stimulation site (S1), expressed in milliseconds. To measure *sensory conduction,* the distal portion of a nerve is stimulated transcutaneously, and then the evoked potential at a proximal site of the same nerve is recorded. *Sensory conduction velocity* is also expressed in meters per second and is determined by dividing the distance between the recording sites R1 and R2 (expressed in millimeters as D2) by the difference in the latencies recorded at these two points (expressed in milliseconds as T1 – T2) (15).

When some axons of a nerve are damaged, the induced impulse is conducted only by the undamaged axons. The resultant action potential shows an overall reduction in its amplitude (expressed in microvolts); in severe cases the action potential may be absent. Decreased sensory and motor amplitudes are associated with exposure to neurotoxicants such as *n*-hexane and carbon disulfide (15).

There are three additional electrophysiologic parameters that offer information about the integrity of central connections of peripheral nerve fibers: the F-wave, the H-reflex, and the blink reflex. The *F-wave* is a long latency muscle action potential obtained following supramaximal stimulation of motor axons. It is generally accepted that the F-wave is elicited by antidromic stimulation of the anterior horn cell at the axonal hillock. The F-wave is therefore always preceded by an M-wave. F-waves are routinely performed in the same procedure as the motor nerve conduction study, using a slower sweep speed and a higher gain and stimulating the distal stimulation site. Ten impulses are delivered. The shortest latency potential is identified and selected as the F-wave for latency measurement. A prolonged or absent F-wave is considered abnormal.

The *H-reflex* is the electrical equivalent of a monosynaptic stretch reflex. It is obtained by selectively stimulating the 1a fibers, which recruit the anterior horn cell or cells and generate a late response in the muscle, usually obtained before the direct motor response or M-wave. The H-reflex can be obtained by stimulating the posterior tibial nerve at the popliteal fossa. The response is recorded from the muscle, between the two heads of the gastrocnemii muscles. Minimal and maximal amplitude responses are obtained and the latency is measured from stimulus artifact to takeoff of the potential deflections. H-reflexes can also be obtained in the forearm muscles, most notably the flexor carpi radialis muscle.

The electrically or percussion induced *blink reflex* tests the circuitry carried by the afferent fibers of the fifth cranial nerve and its synapse directly with the ipsilateral efferent seventh cranial nerve fibers, and indirectly with both contralateral and ipsilateral seventh cranial nerve nuclei after a central (late) response. The blink reflex is elicited by stimulation of the supraorbital branch of the fifth nerve as it enters through the supraorbital foramen. On the ipsilateral side, both direct and indirect responses are seen. The direct (RI) has a latency of about 10.5 ms and is mono- or biphasic in configuration. The indirect (R2 ipsilateral) has a variable latency of about 30.5 ms and is polyphasic. On the contralateral side, only an indirect, long latency (R2 contralateral) polyphasic response is seen with a latency of about 30.5 ms (1,15). Blink reflexes have been used to document exposure to trichloroethylene (19).

Electromyography (EMG)

The integrity of the motor neuron, its axon, and the muscle cell it supplies (i.e., the motor unit) can be assessed by an EMG examination. Denervation of motor units is necessary before the muscle cells begin to develop abnormal spontaneously discharging potentials; an EMG will detect a reduced number of motor units as evidence of denervation of the motor units. As toxic neuropathy develops and neuromuscular clinical signs emerge, greater EMG changes are recordable. A pattern of muscle action potentials recorded from a muscle in conjunction with a full volitional contraction will reveal the relative drop out of units when there has been denervation and therefore loss of connection between the motor neuron, its axon, and the muscle fiber it supplies. Denervated muscle fibers exhibit spontaneous bioelectric discharges, called *fibrillations,* and can be recorded from a needle electrode inserted into the muscle when it is at rest. *Polyphasic potentials* are recorded from a previously denervated muscle that has become reinnervated; fibrillations may or may not be present depending on whether or not active denervation is occurring and how much regeneration has taken place (1,15).

Fibrillations and Positive Waves

When a muscle fiber is denervated, the acetylcholine receptors spread all across the muscle fiber to attract new innervation to the denervated muscle fiber from adjacent nerves. The muscle fiber thus becomes more sensitive to the free acetylcholine and is depolarized and repolarized spontaneously as these neurotransmitter molecules reach it. Each single depolarization is electrically detected as a single muscle fiber action potential recorded as a fibrillation or a positive wave. These discharge in a very rhythmic manner and usually start and stop abruptly. As the muscle is reinnervated, both fibrillations and positive waves decrease in numbers and eventually disappear when the reinnervation is successfully completed.

Motor Unit Action Potentials

Following denervation, reinnervation is usually accomplished by collateral sprouting with the denervated muscle cells (fiber) seeking new nerve sprouts from adjacent nerves. This reinnervation alters the motor unit in two ways: on the one hand, the motor unit now contains more muscle fibers; on the other hand, the newly acquired muscle fibers are asynchronous with those of the host unit and indeed among themselves. The newly formed end plates may not be stable in the beginning and many of them never reach maturity. Their respective muscle fibers either die or attract innervation from another source. This process of acquiring new muscle fibers and forming new end plates begins in the first 2 months after nerve injury and results in a prolongation of the motor unit potential duration and an increase in the number of the phases of the discharge potential. The duration is prolonged simply because there are more fibers to depolarize, and the increase in the number of phases is due to the lack of synchronization between the host fibers and the newly acquired fibers.

NEUROIMAGING

Neuroimaging techniques provide objective data concerning structural and functional integrity of the brain. These highly sophisticated computerized radiologic methodologies can be used to demarcate the outlines of the cerebral hemispheres and ventricular systems and to differentiate between cerebral cortex and white matter structures. Changes in cerebral blood flow and glucose metabolism are also measurable with these techniques. Although the sensitivity of neuroimaging technologies in the detection of neurotoxic effects is limited, there have nevertheless been reports of clinical correlations between images obtained with CT scans, magnetic resonance imaging (MRI), single photon emission computed tomography (SPECT), and PET associated with exposures to various neurotoxicants.

Computed tomography can be used in the differential diagnosis of encephalopathy to rule out other etiologies of the clinical manifestations such as Alzheimer's disease, ischemic stroke, hemorrhage, and tumors. CT scans have been used to document the morphologic effects of the cerebral edema associated with exposures to lead (20). The CT scan of a 19-year-old man with a 5-year history of toluene abuse revealed cerebral atrophy and bilateral lesions of the basal ganglia and cingulate gyrus (21). The T1-weighted MRI images of the young man revealed hypointense areas in the basal ganglia and cingulate gyrus; these same areas appeared as hyperintensities on T2-weighted images.

The MRI findings in a 20-year-old woman exposed to carbon monoxide showed areas of high signal intensity on T2-weighted images of the globus pallidus; these same areas appeared hypointense on T1-weighted images (22). In contrast, the MRI of a welder exposed to manganese revealed hyperintense signals in the basal ganglia on T1-weighted images, while the T2-weighted images were normal (23). The severity of cerebral white matter involvement seen on MRI following chronic toluene exposure correlates with changes in neuropsychological performance (24). Associations have been made between MRI changes and exposure to organolead in gasoline and to inorganic mercury (25,26).

The results of studies using SPECT scans to measure regional cerebral blood flow in assessing neurotoxic effects in humans has been equivocal. Triebig et al. (27) reported results of SPECT, CT, and MRI findings in patients with toxic encephalopathies associated with solvent exposures. The results of these studies did not reveal significant correlations and were thus considered inconclusive. It was thought that chronic low-dose exposure produces physiologic disruption measured by neuropsychological testing, without showing measurable effects on brain structures. In contrast, the SPECT scan of a 52-year-old woman who developed ataxia and clumsiness associated with exposure to manganese revealed significant reductions in the right caudate and in the thalamus bilaterally. A follow-up SPECT scan performed 1-year after cessation of exposure revealed that the blood flow to these regions had returned to normal in this patient.

A PET scan utilizing 18-S-2-deoxyglucose in a 31-year-old man exposed to tetrabromoethane, a halogenated aliphatic hydrocarbon, showed significant decrease in uptake in multiple areas of the brain, while not showing any abnormalities on CT or EEG. However, neurobehavioral assessments did reveal deficits in learning ability, memory, and psychomotor speed, which seem to relate to the deficits seen on PET scan. The 6-fluorodopa PET scans of workers exposed to manganese do not reveal reduction in dopamine uptake, in stark contrast to those of patients with IPD, suggesting that this technology can be useful in the differential diagnosis of parkinsonism and Parkinson's disease (1,11).

The clinical utility of magnetic resonance spectroscopy (MRS) in the assessment of neurotoxic exposure has not been fully elucidated. MRS can be used to detect changes in brain levels of *N*-acetylaspartate (NAA), a marker of neuronal viability; lactate, a marker of anaerobic respiration; as well as levels of choline, creatinine, γ-aminobutyric acid (GABA), myo-inositol, glutamate, and glutamine. As this technology becomes more widely used by clinicians, it may prove to be particularly sensitive to the affects associated with exposures to certain chemicals (28).

BIOLOGIC MARKERS OF EXPOSURE

A *biologic marker* is an indicator of an alteration in cellular structure, biochemical processes, and/or nervous system functioning that can be ascertained through a biologic sample. In the practice of clinical neurotoxicology, biologic markers can represent the severity of various effects and possibly reflect stages of progression of clinical disease following exposure. There are three types of biologic markers that are useful in making a diagnosis of neurotoxic illness (29,30):

1. *Biologic markers of exposure* are measures of the internal dose (quantity absorbed and retained) and the biologically effective dose (concentration causing an effect). Both parameters are determined by basic pharmacologic principles including absorption, tissue perfusion, metabolism, and excretion, and individual variations (e.g., gender, age, metabolic enzyme activity levels, and physiologic functioning including blood flow, membrane permeability, respiratory rate, and nervous system accessibility).
2. *Biologic markers of effect* are measurable biochemical and/or physiologic alterations within the critical organ (e.g., nervous system) that can be associated with an established or potential health impairment or disease. Markers of clinical disease can be any qualitative or quantitative change from a baseline or expected level of appearance or performance resulting from a given chemical exposure (29,30). Biologic markers of effect include markers of early biologic effects (e.g., slowing of nerve conduction velocities; neuropsychological tests) and altered cellular structure (e.g., nerve biopsy revealing evidence of demyelination; abnormal neuroimaging findings).
3. *Biomarkers of susceptibility* are indicators of increased (or decreased) risk for toxic effects. These parameters can influence the measurement and interpretation of other biologic marker data along the continuum from exposure to disease. A biologic marker of susceptibility reflects an individual's level of sensitivity to the effects of a particular chemical. Some individuals have a lower threshold to exposure effects than do others; a preexisting disease state or concurrent condition may affect the metabolism of certain neurotoxicants, thus increasing the internal dose or the biologically effective dose. Biologic markers of susceptibility include genetically determined mechanisms of absorption, tissue biochemistry, and excretion; immunoreaction; low organ reserve capacity; or other identifiable factors that can influence the effect of the neurotoxic substances (29,30).

Clinical Relevance of Biologic Marker Data

For biologic markers to be clinically useful, certain practical issues regarding collection of the appropriate sample should be considered. Can the biologic marker be readily detected in a specific specimen? Is the sample size adequate for detection of the biologic marker? (Many laboratories require minimal sample sizes for certain biologic markers.) Was the sample collected at the appropriate time in relation to the exposure circumstances (e.g., at the end of the work shift)? Have the appropriate sampling methodologies been employed including using correct sample collection, storage, and transport devices? Relevant reference values (e.g., biologic exposure indices) have been established for many of the common chemicals considered to be neurotoxic (31).

It is also important to recognize that different chemicals may have similar detoxification pathways resulting in the common detectable metabolic products. Thus, the sensitivity and specificity of a biologic marker must be considered when interpreting the findings. The *sensitivity* of a biologic marker refers to its ability to detect low levels of exposure to a particular chemical. In contrast, the *specificity* of a biologic marker refers to its ability to differentiate those who have been exposed to a specific chemical from those who have not. For example, a patient's blood level of trichloroethanol is a highly sensitive indicator of trichloroethylene exposure but it is not a specific biologic marker of exposure to this chemical as exposure to perchloroethylene and other chlorinated hydrocarbons (e.g., 1,1,1-trichloroethane) is also associated with elevated blood levels of trichloroethanol.

The ability of a biologic marker to accurately define an exposure and/or an effect is determined not only by its sensitivity and specificity, but also by the characteristics of the population to which the test is being applied. Workers who are simultaneously exposed to several different chemicals are at risk for additive and/or synergistic effects. Biologic markers of exposure such as blood levels of metabolites may not accurately predict risk of effect among workers who are simultaneous exposed to several chemicals. In such cases the physician should ascertain biologic markers of effect as well as biologic markers of exposure, as the former may reveal abnormalities associated with the synergistic effects of concurrent exposures.

KNOWN CHEMICAL EXPOSURES AND POSSIBLE TOXIC EFFECTS

Diagnosis of neurotoxic syndromes is easy when a known exposure event can be associated with circumstances in which the culprit neurotoxicants are known. For example, in the presence of battery smelting, exposure to lead is probable; in a petroleum refinery, a "knockdown" from hydrogen sulfide exposure could be expected; a machinist will probably encounter degreasing solvents such as *n*-hexane and/or trichloroethylene. Thus, it is reasonable when the presence of certain neurotoxicants is known that toxic effects of exposure should be expected and may be detected in potentially and actually exposed persons.

Lead

Overt manifestations of lead-related encephalopathy include ataxia, confusion, convulsions, fatigue, and mood changes. As cases of severe acute lead intoxication become less frequent, increasing attention has been focused on the subclinical manifestations of lead exposure. Exposure to inorganic lead has resulted in characteristic changes in behavior and cognitive functioning in patients with blood lead levels less than 70 μg/100 mL. As lead levels rise about 40 μg/100 mL, short-term verbal memory skills have been found to be consistently impaired. The Occupational Safety and Health Administration (OSHA) lead standard requires that workers receive a medical evaluation at a blood level of 40 μg/100 mL. Studies of subclinical and asymptomatic lead poisonings have shown that workers with blood lead levels in the range of 40 to 60 μg/100 mL not only show neurologic abnormalities but also have symptoms when asked. Although studies of adults with blood lead levels greater than 90 μg/100 mL have shown inconsistent results, available evidence suggests that lead exposure in this range can lead to impairment in affect, attention, psychomotor function, verbal concept formation, short-term memory, and visuospatial abilities. Mood disorders resulting in apathy, irritability, and diminished ability to control anger are apparently common. Although overt encephalopathy with cerebral edema is a common manifestation among children exposed lead, extremely high blood levels (>500 μg/100 mL) may be associated with overt encephalopathy and seizures in adults as well (32–40).

Lead exposures occur in occupational and nonoccupational settings. The removal of lead paint from older housing has been promoted by public health officials to protect children and older persons form lead poisoning. However, the processes of deleading these older homes often results in occupational and nonoccupational exposures among persons involved in the abatement process (40). Protection against increased lead intake is facilitated by the proper use of adequate exhaust ventilation systems, protective clothing, and respirators. Periodic biologic monitoring for increased body burdens is performed among occupationally exposed workers to determine the need to remove them from exposure until their lead levels recede. Despite these safety measures, inexperienced workers continue to be exposed to high concentrations of lead, resulting in clinical manifestations of CNS and PNS dysfunction.

Case Study: Lead Exposure

A 35-year-old man with no previous history of seizures experienced a generalized convulsion. His history revealed that he had been working as a deleader, removing lead paint from interior walls with sanding machines, burning equipment, and chemical solvents for the past 6 months. He admitted that he did not wash his hands before eating and that he only sporadically wore a mask or gloves and never used a respirator. He had experienced frequent headaches and stomach discomfort during the 3 months preceding the seizure. He had also experienced an unintentional weight loss of 3.6 to 4.5 kg. Physical examination after recovery from the convulsion was normal. The hematocrit was 20%, and the hemoglobin 9.1 g/100 mL; moderate basophilic stippling was present on red blood cell smear. The man's occupation raised a suspicion of lead poisoning, and his blood lead level was measured and found to be 600 μg/100 mL of whole blood. Chelation therapy brought the blood level down to 76 μg/100 mL by the seventh day. The worker was instructed to avoid further contact with lead (40).

Nerve conduction studies documented subclinical effects of lead on the PNS among demolition crew workers involved in the dismantling of old steel subway bridges. These workers used acetylene torches to cut lead painted steel beams. Conduction velocities were significantly reduced in these workers compared with demolition workers not involved in the steel cutting process and with unexposed controls. The demolition workers not involved in the cutting process who worked downwind of the cutters also had conduction velocities slower than unexposed controls. Thus, the severity of the neuropathy as evidenced by conduction velocity slowing was found to correlate with job activity and current blood lead levels.

Manganese

Of the neurotoxic effects of metals, manganese is especially known for its acute behavioral manifestations. Neurotoxicity of manganese was recognized after manganese miners developed irritability, nervousness, and emotional lability. Some experienced visual and auditory hallucinations, whereas others had compulsive, repetitive, and uncontrollable actions. In fact, this initial phase of agitation in workers exposed to manganese ore was described as "manganese madness," which heralded the prodromal phase of chronic manganese poisoning. Following or concomitant with these symptoms, signs suggesting a disturbance in basal ganglia also appeared. This intermediate phase of poisoning is further discussed in the section on motor disturbances. The final established phase exhibits muscular rigidity, fine tremors, and cock walk. Spasmodic laughter and excessive sweating also are reported in some patients (41–44).

The acute psychosis associated with manganese poisoning appears to be related to an *N*-methyl-D-aspartate (NMDA) glutamate-receptor–mediated loss of autoreceptor presynaptic control of striatal dopamine release (45,46). The acute extrapyramidal effects of manganese may involve the irreversible oxidation of dopamine to a cyclized *ortho*-quinone, resulting in a temporary decrease in the brain levels of this catecholamine (47). The chronic effects of manganese poisoning have been attributed to the generation of free radicals and cell death via apoptosis (48,49).

Case Study: Manganese Exposure

Mena et al. (42) reported on the neurologic findings in 13 former ore miners with chronic symptoms of manganese poisoning that had persisted for up to 25 years (median: 5 years). All 13 patients reported experiencing a period of acute psychosis that included headache, auditory and visual hallucinations, compulsive behavior, impaired memory, and irritability, and that lasted for at least 1 month before the onset of extrapyramidal symptoms, which included gait disturbances, dysarthria, and tremor. Clinical neurologic examinations revealed abnormal gait (13/13), increase muscle tone (9/13), dysarthria (8/13), masked facies (8/13), hyperactive deep tendon reflexes (7/13), tremor (5/13), and cogwheel rigidity (3/13). The tremor seen in these workers was of small amplitude and high frequency, in contrast to the high-amplitude, low-frequency pill-rolling type tremor of IPD. The speech of individuals who were the least handicapped improved to near normal within 1 year after cessation of exposure, but speech problems persisted in the other workers. These authors concluded that psychosis and reversible motor disturbances emerge as the earliest clinical manifestations of manganese intoxication and that these symptoms can persist for up to 3 months. If exposure continues, the psychosis gradually subsides and the motor disturbances become more pronounced until persistent parkinsonism characterized by dystonia, awkward gait, dysarthria, masked facies, and tremor is seen.

Mercury

Mercury poisoning can occur from either inorganic or organic mercury. Signs and symptoms vary with the type of mercury or mercurial compound and the type of exposure (acute or chronic). Chronic exposure to organic mercury can produce tremor, paresthesias (tingling sensations), dysarthria (slurred speech), ataxia, decreased visual fields, and mental disturbances (50). The most notorious epidemics of organic mercury poisoning were those that occurred in Minamata, Japan in the 1950s (51). The classic triad of chronic elemental inorganic mercury poisoning includes tremor, psychological instability, and stomatitis (52–55).

Case Study: Inorganic Mercury Exposure

A 48-year-old man was exposed to vapors from elemental mercury for 3.5 years in a thermometer factory (25). His job required that he vacuum up the mercury spilled on the floors, disassemble machines containing mercury, and operate a crusher machine that separated the mercury from broken glass for reuse. An accidental laceration with glass brought him to the emergency room, where an occupational physician became involved in his case when it was learned that he had been having various symptoms during the past 2 to 3 years, which included blurred vision, ocular pain, weakness, memory loss, and occasional rage and irrational behavior, hallucinations, and paranoia. In addition, his family reported that he was angry, aggressive, suicidal, and socially withdrawn. He was chelated with penicillamine after his urine mercury level was found to be 690 µg/L. He was removed from further exposure at this time. A follow-up urine mercury level after completion of chelation therapy and cessation of further exposure was 17 µg/L.

He was reevaluated 5 months later for continuing neurologic problems and complaints, at which time nystagmus, tremor, diminished reflexes, and diminished sensation to pain were noted by the neurologist. His tremor was documented by electromyographic recording. Nerve conduction studies showed evidence of mild peripheral neuropathy. An MRI performed at this time revealed mild central and cortical atrophy with punctiform foci in the precentral gyri and subcortical white matter visible on T2-weighted images. These findings did not resemble those seen in multiple sclerosis and were considered to be consistent with diffuse and focal white matter loss associated with exposure to mercury.

Formal neuropsychological assessment of this patient revealed deficits in attention and executive function. Visuospatial and visuomotor function testing revealed problems with visuospatial analysis, coding, sequencing, and visual organization. In addition, he had difficulty with facial matching, and with memory tests, particularly those involving visuospatial materials. The patient exhibited mild problems with verbal concept formation tasks, although free speech was within expectation. The Profile of Mood States (POMS) revealed irritability, fatigue, and confusion. The neuropsychological tests of this patient suggest specific problems with cognitive flexibility, cognitive tracking, visuospatial analysis, memory for visuospatial information, affect, and personality.

Organic Solvents

Because most organic solvents contain mixtures of ingredients, it is often difficult to attribute specific behavioral changes to a specific substance. However, the predominant ingredient in a mixed solvent preparation can influence the clinical picture. For example, if toluene is the predominant ingredient, the principal health effects will reflect the contribution of this solvent and may include acute excitatory effects such as euphoria, exhilaration, and excitement, and the insidious development of persistent tremor, head titubation, and ataxia.

A broad range of neuropsychological findings have been associated with exposure to organic solvents (56–68). Workers exposed to carbon disulfide showed disturbances in speech, psychomotor functioning, dexterity, and alertness. In turn, most investigations of the effects of carbon disulfide have focused on these functions. "Pseudoneurasthenic" difficulties, including changes in mood or personality; excessive irritability; increased physical complaints such as headache, dizziness, weakness, and fatigue; and memory loss have also been related to carbon disulfide exposure. These complaints usually precede the onset of more obvious neurologic impairments such as postural changes and peripheral neuropathy. Frequently, depressive symptoms are presented (57,58).

Conclusions about neurobehavioral effects of solvents are difficult to draw. Caution must be used in the generalization of results from epidemiologic studies, since exact exposure levels and knowledge of other concomitant exposures are not always known. As a result, it may be difficult to identify one single causative agent. Many solvents and mixtures are commonly used in the workplace. Exposures to mixed solvents are a particularly common occupational hazard. Extensive studies of Scandinavian workers exposed to mixed solvents, including paints, degreasing fluids, and dry-cleaning fluids, suggest the potential for the development of neurotoxic disorders that appear to be related to the level and degree of exposure. Investigators have extensively assessed neuropsychological functioning in subjects with chronic exposure to solvents. Although findings vary somewhat among study samples, the results consistently suggest that chronic solvent exposure can be associated with cognitive changes on tests of reasoning, visual constructive abilities, short-term memory, motor coordination and speed, and attention. Exposure to paints, carbon disulfide, and mixed solvents has been found to affect a particularly large number of cognitive ability. Impairment in reaction time, psychomotor ability, and short-term memory was found in painters. Investigators have consistently identified psychiatric disorders of mood and behavior among workers with occupational exposures to solvents. These cognitive and behavioral changes have been attributed to solvent-induced diffuse brain damage. Damage to central white matter and/or supportive structures are suspected to be involved (68).

Case Study: Mixed Solvents Exposure

This case study, given in detail, follows the format of evaluation as outlined in the BUENA presented earlier in this chapter.

A 57-year-old painter presented in 1996 complaining of memory problems, disorientation, irritability, and insomnia (68). His wife recalled that his mood and affect as well as his memory problems may have been evident to her approximately 15 years earlier. The patient finally sought medical attention for severe anxiety attacks and depression in 1993 but he did not acknowledge any memory problems at that time and continued to work as a painter. The anxiety attacks and depression were controlled with medications (sertraline hydrochloride and clonazepam), but the patient's memory problems continued to progress until he was asked to resign in late 1995 when his memory deficits began to interfere with his ability to work.

Examination in 1996 revealed a well-developed and well-nourished man who was well oriented to person, place, and time. His speech was fluent and his oral comprehension, repetition, and naming were intact. He had difficulty with reciting serial 7's but he subtracted 3's correctly. He was able to spell the word "world" forward and backward. His cranial nerves were normal. Motor examination revealed normal bulk, tone, and strength in the upper and lower extremities. Deep tendon reflexes were present and normal. Plantar reflexes were flexor. Sensory examination including testing of touch, vibration, and pain and temperature sensation was normal. However, there was no hair on his lower legs in a stocking distribution. Performance on finger-to-nose, heel-to-shin, and tandem gait and hopping were normal.

Although he was symptomatic when acutely seen, biologic markers including urine hippuric acid were not obtained to document his exposure at that time. Heavy metal screen done approximately 1 year after cessation of exposure to paint and painting materials revealed a blood lead level of 13 μg/dL, a mercury level of 5 μg/L, and manganese was not detectable. CBC and thyroid tests were normal. Liver function tests including serum glutamic-oxaloacetic transaminase (SGOT) and serum glutamic pyruvic transaminase (SGPT), total bilirubin, alkaline phosphatase, albumin, and protein were normal. Lyme titer was also negative.

Follow-up examination 2 years later showed that the patient was oriented to person, time, and place but now he required cuing from his wife to aid in his recall of some information. His conversational speech was fluent, and there was no indication of dysarthria. He was able to read the notes that he used to recall specific items that he wanted to talk about with the neurologist. His recall for recent events was labored but notably improved since he was first seen in 1996. His memory for past events was intact. He continued to have difficulty remembering visual information and he reported that he continues to get lost when driving to and from unfamiliar places. He had trouble acquiring new information. He stated that his wife had bought him a new toothbrush and that despite having asked her on numerous occasions what color it was, he could not remember. His visual memory impairment was described in his wife's observation that he had difficulty with object assembly tasks; he could still take things apart but could not remember how to put them back together. The patient stated that he had begun riding a bicycle for exercise and reported that he had no trouble finding his way around his neighborhood. However, when asked exactly when he started this exercise program he could not remember. His mood and affect were improved but he continued to need medication (fluoxetine hydrochloride and lorazepam) for anxiety, frustration, and reactive depression. Gait, posture, and muscle bulk were normal.

Work History

The patient began working as a painter at 16 years of age, when he quit high school. He worked for the same company from age 16 to 21 (1954–1959), during which time he mainly spray-painted the exteriors of gasoline storage tanks. When necessary, he would also assist the metal alloy welders who were making repairs to the inside of the tanks and would also spot-prime and paint the completed repairs. He did not use a respirator; his only protection from the paint fumes was to breathe through a rag he wrapped around his face.

At age 21 years he married his current wife and moved to Rhode Island, where he worked for an independent contractor painting the interiors and exteriors of residential housing. From age 22 to 24 (1959–1962) he worked for a second contractor painting interiors of university dormitories and academic buildings with a variety of oil-based paints. At age 24 (1962) he began working for union contractors. He had more steady work as a union painter and spent most of the remainder of his career working for a single union contractor, painting mainly the interiors of grocery stores and office buildings. He frequently painted the inside of poorly ventilated walk-in–type refrigerators in grocery stores. To protect the employees and customers of the grocery stores from being sickened by the paint fumes, the job foreman would often close the door, thus forcing the patient and his co-workers to paint in an unventilated area without respirators for periods of up to 2 hours. The patient and his co-workers often experienced nausea, dizziness, and staggering gait while painting in these confined spaces. Although none of them ever lost consciousness, their symptoms were often severe enough to necessitate leaving the refrigerator for relief.

Exposure History

The patient had used oil-based paints for most of the jobs he had worked on because the contractors he worked for did not believe that the water-based latex paints were of equal quality. Several years before he was forced to retire because of disability, the union contractor he was working for switched to latex paint. Materials Safety Data Sheets (MSDSs) provided by this employer indicated that the patient and his coworkers had been exposed to lead, titanium dioxide, creosote, and mixed solvents including ammonia, chlorine bleach, various alcohols (e.g., isopropanol and methanol) methyl ethyl ketone, methyl isobutyl ketone, formaldehyde, carbon tetrachloride, methylene chloride, ethylene glycol, propylene glycol, hexylene glycol, nitroethane, cyclohexanone, acetone, xylene, toluene, benzene, and petroleum naphthas. The patient frequently used painter's naphtha, a petroleum derivative containing a mixture of C_5-C_{11} hydrocarbons (also known as VM and P naphtha or benzine) to clean off his hands, arms, and face at the end of each work shift.

Neurophysiologic Diagnosis

The EEG of this patient done in 1996 was characterized by excessive theta activity. Low- to medium-voltage sharp activity was noted in the posterior (occipital) area. A moderate amount of beta (fast) activity was also seen superimposed over the background activity. Response to photic driving was normal. Frank epileptiform activity was not seen. Nerve conduction studies were not performed on this patient, who also had no clinical evidence of peripheral neuropathy.

Neuroimaging

Magnetic resonance imaging studies were made 6 months after the patient first sought medical attention for his cognitive deficits in 1996. The neuroimaging findings were considered to be indicative of global and symmetric volume loss, predominantly involving the white matter. Symmetry and the general cerebral architecture were intact except for subtle findings related to a generalized volume loss. The sulcal markings were wider than would be expected for the patient's age. The amount of volume loss observed at the base of the brain was similar to that seen in the frontal and parietal lobes. White matter tracts were symmetrical but qualitatively thinned throughout the brain. The cortical ribbon in the supratentorial neocortex was uniform and normal in signal throughout, but thinner than would be expected for a patient of this age. T1-weighted coronal images revealed medial temporal lobes to be normal in signal and configuration. The hippocampal formations are of normal architecture and signal. The basal ganglia and brainstem were normal in appearance. In particular, the amygdalae were not atrophied. On T1-weighted midsagittal images the cerebellum appeared moderately atrophied, but this was not disproportionate to that seen in the cerebral cortex. These abnormal MRI findings were in stark contrast to the normal findings on CT scans performed 8 years earlier in 1988. This dramatic change in neuroimaging findings can be chronologically related to the patient's clinical progression, which had reached maximum severity at the time of the second neuroimaging study.

Neuropsychological Diagnosis

Neuropsychological assessment in 1996 revealed a full-scale IQ of 93 (Verbal IQ = 96; Performance IQ = 91). Impaired performance was noted on tests of verbal (California Verbal Learning Test) and nonverbal memory (delayed reproduction of Rey-Osterreith complex figure). Performance on tests of attention and executive function (Trails A and B and Wisconsin Card Sort Test) was impaired as well. Visuomotor coordination (Grooved Pegboard Test) was also below expectation. Tests of mood and affect revealed anxiety and depression. Tests of language function including confrontation naming (Boston Naming Test) were within normal limits.

A second neuropsychological assessment done 1 year later (1997) revealed a full-scale IQ of 90 (Verbal IQ = 92; Performance IQ = 88). His performance was impaired on tests of attention and executive function (Trails A and B and Wisconsin Card Sort Test). His scores on tests of visuospatial planning and organization (copy of Rey-Osterreith complex figure; Hooper Test of Visual Organization) were below expectation. Deficits in visuomotor coordination (Grooved Pegboard Test) were also noted. Remote memory was intact, but his performance on tests of verbal (California Verbal Learning Test) and nonverbal memory (delayed reproduction of Rey-Osterreith complex figure) remained below expectation. Language functions including spontaneous speech and confrontation naming (Boston Naming Test) were intact. The findings of this follow-up assessment demonstrated a persistent impairment of cognitive function and support the diagnosis of chronic toxic encephalopathy. Such static deficits on serial neuropsychological testing and the preservation of language function are not seen in progressive dementing processes such as Alzheimer's disease and multiinfarct dementia, both of which are associated with marked worsening of performances on serial neurobehavioral assessments (6).

Clinical Diagnosis

The clinical diagnosis is chronic toxic encephalopathy associated with exposure to mixed solvents, based on the exposure history revealing chronic occupational exposure to mixed solvents at very high air concentrations during periods of painting in confined spaces such as walk-in refrigerators. In addition, the emergence and stabilization of the patient's symptoms can be chronologically related to his exposure circumstance and show stabilization after cessation exposure as demonstrated by the *time-exposure-symptom line* and further supports the diagnosis. Furthermore, the medical history and laboratory data do not reveal any findings such as hypothyroidism or abnormal liver or renal functions that could account for the clinical manifestations. The pattern of deficits on neuropsychological test results and neuroimaging findings are inconsistent with Alzheimer's disease or any other idiopathic dementing process, further supporting the diagnosis of chronic toxic encephalopathy.

REFERENCES

1. Feldman RG. *Occupational and environmental neurotoxicology.* Philadelphia: Lippincott Williams & Wilkins, 1999.
2. White RF, Feldman RG, Proctor SP. Neurobehavioral effects of toxic exposures. In: White RF, ed. *Clinical syndromes in adult neuropsychology: the practitioner's handbook.* New York: Elsevier, 1992:1–51.
3. Feldman RG, Ricks NL, Baker EL. Neuropsychological effects of industrial toxins: a review. *Am J Ind Med* 1980;1:211.
4. Feldman RG, White RF, Travers PH. Neurobehavioral effects of toxicity due to metals, solvents, and insecticides. *Clin Neuropharm* 1990;13:392–412.
5. Taranova NP. Intensity of 14C-2-acetate incorporation into guinea pig brain and spinal cord phospholipids and cholesterol under normal conditions and following triorthocresylphosphate poisoning. *Biull Eksp Biol Med* 1978;85(4):427–429.
6. Kreiss K, Wegman DH, Niles CA, et al. Neurological dysfunction of the bladder in workers exposed to dimethylaminopropionitrile. *JAMA* 1980;243:741–745.
7. Feldman RG, Ratner MH. The pathogenesis of neurodegenerative disease: neurotoxic mechanisms of action and genetics. *Curr Opin Neurol* 1999;12:725–731.
8. Spencer PS, et al. Guam amyotrophic lateral sclerosis-parkinsonism-dementia linked to a plant excitant neurotoxin. *Science* 1987;237:517.
9. Bleecker ML. Parkinsonism: a clinical marker of exposure to neurotoxins. *Neurotoxicol Teratol* 1988;10:475.
10. Feldman RG. Manganese as possible ecoetiologic factor in Parkinson's disease. *Ann NY Acad Sci* 1992;648: 266–268.
11. Wolters E, Huang CC, Clark C, et al. Positron emission tomography in manganese intoxication. *Ann Neurol* 1989;26:647–651.
12. LeQuesne PM. Electrophysiological investigation of toxic neuropathies. In: Juntunen J, ed. Occupational neurology. *Acta Neurol Scand* 1982;66[suppl 92]:75.
13. Feldman RG, et al. Blink reflex measurement of effects of trichloroethylene exposure on the trigeminal nerve. *Muscle Nerve* 1992;15:490.
14. White RF. Differential diagnosis of Alzheimer's disease and solvent encephalopathy in older workers. *Clin Neuropsychol* 1987;1:153–160.
15. Kimura J. *Electrodiagnosis in diseases of nerve and muscle: principles and practice.* Philadelphia: FA Davis, 1989.
16. Chiappa K. Evoked potentials. In: Chiappa K, ed. *Clinical medicine,* 2nd ed. New York: Raven Press, 1992.
17. Metrick SA, Brenner RP. Abnormal brainstem auditory evoked potentials in chronic paint sniffers. *Ann Neurol* 1982;12:553–556.
18. Otto DA, Fox DA. Auditory and visual dysfunction following lead exposure. *Neurotoxicol* 1993;14:191–208.
19. Feldman RG, Chirico-Post JA, Proctor SP. Blink reflex latency after exposure to trichloroethylene in well water. *Arch Environ Health* 1988;43:143–148.
20. Pappas CL, Quisling RG, Ballinger WE, et al. Lead encephalopathy: symptoms of cerebellar mass lesion and obstructive hydrocephalus. *Surg Neurol* 1986;26: 391–394.
21. Ashikaga R, Araki Y, Miura K, et al. Cranial MRI in chronic thinner intoxication. *Neuroradiology* 1995;37: 443–444.
22. Gotoh M, Kuyama H, Asari S, et al. Sequential changes in MR images of the brain in acute carbon monoxide poisoning. *Comp Med Imag Graph* 1993;17(1):55–59.
23. Nelson K, Golnick J, Kom T, et al. Manganese encephalopathy: utility of early magnetic resonance imaging. *Br J Ind Med* 1993;50:510–513.
24. Filley CM, Heaton RK, Rosenberg NL. White matter dementia in chronic toluene abuse. *Neurology* 1990;40: 532–534.
25. White RF, Feldman RG, Moss MB, et al. Magnetic resonance imaging (MRI), neurobehavioral testing, and toxic encephalopathy: two cases. *Environ Res* 1993;61: 117–123.
26. Prockop LD, Karampelas D. Encephalopathy secondary to abusive gasoline inhalation. *J Fla Med Assoc* 1981; 68:823–824.
27. Triebig G, Weltie D, Valentin H. Investigations on neurotoxicity of chemical substances at the workplace: determination of the motor and sensory nerve conduction

velocity in persons occupationally exposed to lead. *Int Arch Occup Environ Health* 1984;53:189.
28. Jenkins BG, Kraft E. Magnetic resonance spectroscopy in toxic encephalopathy and neurodegeneration. *Curr Opin Neurol* 1999;12:753–760.
29. National Research Council (NRC). *Environmental neurotoxicology.* Washington, DC: National Academy Press, 1992.
30. Chern C-M, Proctor SP, Feldman RG. Exposure assessment in clinical neurotoxicology: environmental monitoring and biologic markers. In: Chang L, Slokker W Jr, eds. *Neurotoxicology: approaches and methods.* San Diego: Academic Press, 1995:695–671.
31. American Conference of Government Industrial Hygienists (ACGIH). *Documentation of the threshold limit values and biological exposure indices,* 5th ed. ACGIH, 1988.
32. Valciukas JA, et al. Lead exposure and behavioral changes: comparison of four occupation groups with different levels of lead absorption. *Am J Med* 1980;1:421.
33. Baker EL, et al. Occupational lead neurotoxicity—a behavioral and electrophysiologic evaluation: I. Study design and year one results. *Br J Ind Med* 1984;41:352.
34. Feldman RG, Travers PH. Environmental and occupational neurology. In: Feldman RG, ed. *Neurology: the physician's guide.* New York: Thieme-Stratton, 1984: 191–212.
35. Feldman RG. Effects of toxins and physical agents on the nervous system. In: Bradley WG, et al., eds. *Neurology in clinical practice,* vol 2. Stoneham, MA: Butterworth-Heinemann, 1991:1185–1209.
36. American Public Health Association (APHA). Lead poisoning. In: Weeks JL, Levy BS, and Wagner GR, eds. *Preventing occupational disease and injury*. Washington, DC: APHA, 1991:374–387.
37. Hanninen H. Behavioral effects of occupational exposure to mercury and lead. *Acta Neurol Scand* 1982;66 [suppl 92]:167.
38. Valciukas JA, et al. Behavioral indicators of lead neurotoxicity: results of a clinical survey. *Int Arch Occup Environ Health* 1978;41:217.
39. Grandjean P, Arnvig E, Beckman J. Psychological dysfunctions in lead-exposed workers: relation to biological parameters of exposure. *Scand J Work Environ Health* 1978;4:295.
40. Feldman RG. Urban lead mining: lead intoxication among deleaders. *N Engl J Med* 1978;298:1143–1145.
41. Whitlock CM, Amuso SJ, Bittenbender JB. Chronic neurological disease in two manganese steel workers. *Am Ind Hyg Assoc J* 1966;27:454.
42. Mena L, et al. Chronic manganese poisoning: clinical picture and manganese turnover. *Neurology* 1967;17: 128.
43. Cook DG, Fahn S, Brait KA. Chronic manganese intoxication. *Arch Neurol* 1974;30:59.
44. Seth PK, Chandra SV. Neurotoxic effects of manganese. In: Bondy SC, Prasad KN, eds. *Metal neurotoxicity.* Boca Raton, FL: CRC, 1988:19–33.
45. Chandra SV, Shukla GS, Srivastava RS. An exploratory study of manganese exposure to welders. *Clin Toxicol* 1981;18:407–416.
46. Cuesta de Di Zio MC, Gomez G, Bonilla E, et al. Autoreceptor presynaptic control of dopamine release from striatum is lost at early stages of manganese poisoning. *Life Sci* 1995;56(22):1857–1864.
47. Segura-Aguila J, Lind C. On the mechanism of the Mn3+-induced neurotoxicity of dopamine: prevention of quinone-derived oxygen toxicity by DT diaphorase and superoxide dismutase. *Chem-Biol Interact* 1989;72: 309–324.
48. Halliwell B. Manganese ions, oxidation reactions, and the superoxide radical. *NeuroToxicology* 1984;5(1):113–118.
49. Halliwell B. Oxidants and the central nervous system: some fundamental questions. Is oxidant damage relevant to Parkinson's disease, Alzheimer's disease, traumatic injury, and stroke? *Acta Neurol Scand* 1989;126:23–33.
50. APHA. Mercury poisoning. In: Weeks JL, Levy BS, Wagner GR, eds. *Preventing occupational disease arid injury.* Washington, DC: APHA, 1991.
51. Eto K, Oyanhei S, Itai Y, et al. A fetal type of Minamata disease: an autopsy case report with special reference to the nervous system. *Mol Chem Neuropathol* 1992;16: 171–186.
52. Kark RAP. Clinical and neurochemical aspects of inorganic mercury intoxication. In: de Wolff FA, ed. *Handbook of clinical neurology, vol 20 (64), Intoxications of the nervous system, part 1.* Amsterdam: Elsevier Science BV, 1994:367–411.
53. Jaeger A, Tempe JD, Haegy JM, et al. Accidental acute mercury vapor poisoning. *Vet Hum Toxicol* 1979;21 [suppl]:62–63.
54. Bluhm RE, Bobbitt RG, Welch LW, et al. Elemental mercury vapour toxicity, treatment and prognosis after acute intensive exposure in chloralkali workers. Part I: history, neuropsychological findings, and chelator effects. *Hum Exp Toxicol* 1992;11:201–210.
55. Zelman M, Campfield P, Moss M, et al. Toxicity from vacuumed mercury: a household hazard. *Clin Pediatr* 1991;30:121–123.
56. Pezzoli G, Canesi M, Antonini A, et al. Hydrocarbon exposure and Parkinson's disease. *Neurology* 2000;55 (5):667–673.
57. Hanninen H. Behavioral study of the effects of carbon disulfide. In: Xintaras C, Johnson BL, de Groot I, eds. *Behavioral toxicology: early detection of occupational hazards.* NIOSH publication No. 74-126. Washington, DC: U.S. Government Printing Office, 1974:73–80.
58. Hanninen H, et al. Psychological tests as indicators of excessive exposure to carbon disulfide. *Scand J Psychol* 1978;19:163.
59. Lindstrom K. Changes in psychological performances of solvent poisoned and solvent-exposed workers. *Am J Ind Med* 1980;1:69.
60. Lindstrom K. Behavioral changes after long-term exposure to organic solvents and their mixtures. *Scand J Work Environ Health* 1981;4[suppl]:48.
61. Hanninen H, et al. Behavioral effects of long-term exposure to a mixture of organic solvents. *Scand J Work Environ Health* 1976;4:240.
62. Seppalainen AM, Lindstrom K, Martelin T. Neurophysiological and psychological picture of solvent poisoning. *Am J Ind Med* 1980;1:31.
63. Elofsson S, et al. Exposure to organic solvents. *Scand J Work Environ Health* 1980;6:239.
64. Axelson O, Hane M, Hogstedt C. A case-referent study on neuropsychiatric disorders among workers exposed to solvents. *Scand J Work Environ Health* 1976;2:14.

65. Struwe G, Mindus P, Jonsson B. Psychiatric ratings in occupational health research: a study of mental symptoms in lacquerers. *Am J Ind Med* 1980;1:23.
66. Rather MH, Feldman RG, White RF. Neurobehavioral toxicology. In: Ramachandran VS, ed. *Encyclopedia of the human brain, vol 3*. New York: Elsevier, 2002: 423–439.
67. Feldman RG, et al. Long-term follow-up after single exposure to trichloroethylene. *Am J Ind Med* 1985;8:119.
68. Feldman RG, Ratner MH, Ptak T. Chronic encephalopathy in a painter exposed to mixed solvents. Harvard School of Public Health, Grand Rounds in Environmental Medicine. *Environ Health Perspect* 1999;107:417–422.

FURTHER INFORMATION

Clayton GD, Clayton FE, eds. *Patty's industrial hygiene and toxicology, Vol II: Toxicology,* 4th ed. New York: Wiley-Interscience, 1994.

This six-volume set provides an extensive encyclopedia-type reference for chemical information; usage, occupational standards, animal and human toxicology data, and exposure effects.

Chang LW, Slikker W Jr, eds. *Neurotoxicology: approaches and methods.* New York: Academic Press, 1995.

This text provides the reader with assessment protocols and methodologies that can be used in clinical settings to ascertain exposure response relationships among patients exposed to neurotoxic chemicals.

Hayes WJ Jr, Laws ER Jr, eds. *Handbook of pesticide toxicology.* New York: Academic Press, 1991.

An excellent three-volume encyclopedia-type reference for information on the toxicology of pesticides. Limited information on assessment of effects but a good source for basic information on classification, mechanisms of action, and expected clinical outcome of exposure to pesticides.

Feldman RG. *Occupational and environmental neurotoxicology.* Philadelphia: Lippincott Williams & Wilkins, 1999.

The most complete and current textbook available for the practicing neurologist interested in neurotoxicology. Provides a detailed review of the literature on 20 of the most commonly encountered toxins and toxicants found in the workplace and environment. Symptomatic, neurophysiologic, neuropsychological, and neuroimaging as well as biochemical diagnostic protocols and parameters are included to make it easy for the clinician to ascertain a causal relationship between exposure and symptoms.

Goetz CG. *Neurotoxins in clinical practice.* New York: Spectrum, 1985.

Basic information on neurotoxins as seen in a clinical setting, but lacking in depth of reference sources.

Schaumburg HH, Berger AR, Thomas PK. Toxic neuropathy. In: Schaumburg HH, Berger AR, Thomas PK, eds. *Disorders of peripheral nerves.* Philadelphia: Davis, 1992.

Good source of information for nonneurologists interested in furthering their understanding of neuropathy.

Spencer PS, Schaumberg HH, eds. *Experimental and clinical neurotoxicology,* 2nd ed. Philadelphia: Lippincott Williams & Wilkins, 2000.

An update of the extensive edited encyclopedia-type review on the classification, pathophysiology, epidemiology, and experimental information of the "classic" neurotoxins, e.g., acrylamide, n-hexane, metals (lead, mercury, aluminum, cadmium), carbon monoxide, and carbon disulfide.

26

Noise-induced Hearing Loss

John D. Meyer

Noise-induced hearing loss (NIHL) from occupational exposure was recognized as early as the 18th century, when Bernardo Ramazzini (1) described deafness in Venetian coppersmiths that arose from constant hammering. Long recognition of the hazard has not brought about comparable improvements in control. Recent estimates by the National Institute for Occupational Safety and Health (NIOSH) indicate that 30 million people in the United States work where noise exposure levels of 85 dB or greater may present a hazard to hearing (2), and the condition is currently identified as one of the ten leading work-related disorders. Hazardous noise levels are present in a variety of work environments, including military service, manufacturing, construction, transportation, and communications, as well as in leisure-time pursuits, such as music and hunting. Reduction of exposures will reduce or obviate the damage that arises from noise; occupational NIHL thus is typical of many work-related conditions in its susceptibility to preventive measures. Prevention is made more difficult, however, by the insidious nature of noise-induced damage to hearing, which occurs over a period of years to decades without the worker's awareness of harm. Primary and secondary preventive measures that emphasize control of noise at the source along with surveillance efforts to detect early evidence of hearing loss are essential, as sensorineural hearing loss is irreversible once symptomatic, and leaves the individual susceptible to further damage and disability. This chapter presents a framework for the recognition, control, and prevention of occupational NIHL.

PREVALENCE AND EPIDEMIOLOGY OF NOISE-INDUCED HEARING LOSS

Data from the 1977 National Health Interview Survey and the National Occupational Hazard Survey indicate that approximately 3.2% of those surveyed had some degree of hearing loss. The proportion of those with hearing loss increased with age; within age groups, rates were consistently greater for those who worked in industries defined as noisy (3). The Occupational Safety and Health Administration (OSHA) has estimated that mild degrees of hearing loss are present in 17% of production workers, while a further 16% have more substantial impairments of hearing. Overall more than three million workers are estimated to be affected in the manufacturing sector alone (4). NIOSH has suggested that nearly one in four workers older than 55 years who have been exposed to high noise levels (beyond 90 dB) has some degree of material impairment (5).

Although work duties across a broad range of industries present a risk to hearing, some sectors have a greater proportion of workers at risk for NIHL. In the petroleum, lumber, and food-processing industries, as much as 25% of the workforce may be exposed to levels beyond the OSHA permissible exposure level of 90 dB on an 8-hour time-weighted average. Manufacturing industries, including furniture, metals, rubber, and plastics, also present risks to human hearing if workers are not properly protected from hazardous levels of noise. Industries in which large numbers of workers are exposed to noise at or above 85 dB are shown in Table 26.1.

Similar occupations at risk are identified in surveillance reports from European sources. The Finnish Register of Occupational Diseases indicates an incidence rate for occupational hearing loss of 50.3 per 100,000 workers; this figure most closely approaches the probable true incidence of NIHL, as it is determined from mandatory reporting of cases from all physicians in the country (6). Other data sources yield lower figures, as they may be selective in their covered population or in definitions of impairment. Sur-

TABLE 26.1. *Industries with large numbers of workers exposed to noise at or above 85 dB*

Industry	Noise-exposed production workers	
	Number	As % of production workers within industrial sector
Food products manufacture	343,030	29
Fabricated metal products	336,919	29
Primary metal industries	269,270	33
Textile mill products	262,108	43
Transportation equipment	238,609	18
Industrial machinery	229,509	15
Lumber and wood products	196,489	41
Construction contractors	191,087	16
Paper and allied products	164,808	34
Printing and publishing	154,862	21

Source: National Institute for Occupational Safety and Health. *Criteria for a recommended standard. Occupational noise exposure.* Revised criteria. Washington, DC: U.S. DHHS, 1996.

veillance data based on cases reported by occupational physicians from Great Britain describes an incidence of NIHL of 2.2 cases per 100,000 working persons; it is likely that this is a substantial underestimation, since many workers do not have access to occupational health services (7). The largest numbers of occupational hearing loss cases in this scheme were reported in manufacturing workers, including metal workers, maintenance fitters, woodworking machine operatives, electricians, and vehicle assemblers.

The cumulative nature of NIHL leads to difficulty in assigning causation to exposure in a single occupation or work location. Individual workers may have had exposures to noise in a variety of occupational settings, through service in the military or reserves, or in such community work as volunteer firefighting. Continued exposure in these settings may accelerate hearing loss, and a history of current or part-time work in such settings should be obtained when evaluating individuals and work sites. Further complicating the assessment of hearing loss are the avocations and recreation in which workers engage outside of employment; hunting, recreational shooting, metalwork, and music are common activities that produce significant hearing impairment outside of the occupational setting. Lastly, the decline in acuity produced by presbycusis or age-induced hearing loss can accentuate impairment already present from noise exposure and other factors; from 25% to 40% of people older than 65 years have some degree of hearing loss.

The major risk factor for noise-induced hearing loss is prolonged unprotected exposure to levels of noise beyond 85 dB. NIOSH has estimated that the excess risk of hearing impairment after a working lifetime of exposure to an average daily noise level of 85 dB is roughly 8%; this figure jumps to 25% when average exposure increases to 90 dB (2). As noted earlier, the decibel scale is logarithmic, and therefore a 3-dB increase represents a doubling of noise intensity. Predictive models of NIHL at higher exposures indicate that hearing damage follows this scale proportionately, although other factors, such as the intermittency of noise appear to modify the extent of hearing loss in the more extreme ranges.

A number of other risk factors have also been proposed, including lipid and cholesterol abnormalities, diabetes, solvents, cigarette smoking, and thyroid abnormalities. Smoking may represent both an independent and predisposing factor for NIHL. Office workers in Japan who smoked one pack or greater per day had a relative risk for hearing loss that was twice that of nonsmokers, even when controlled for other risk factors (8). Major risk factors in a cohort of noise-exposed white males in an aerospace company were cigarette smoking, a noisy hobby such as shooting, and number of years worked at a noisy plant (9). The implication of smoking as a risk factor supports the hypothesis that that susceptibility to NIHL may be due to relative ischemia of the vasculature of the inner ear.

Non–insulin-dependent diabetes mellitus may increase the risk of severe hearing loss in those with occupational exposure to noise. Imprecise data, especially regarding the duration and severity of disease, and small sample sizes of workers with insulin-dependent diabetes mellitus (IDDM), have hampered attempts to draw a link between IDDM and NIHL (10). Patients with diabetic retinopathy, however, had no greater prevalence of sensorineural hearing impairment than controls (11). The cause of diabetes-induced hearing loss, however, is not entirely clear, but appears to be due to metabolic disturbances that affect nerve function. Despite the possibility of increased risk of NIHL among diabetic patients, scientific evidence does not appear to warrant restriction of individuals with this disorder from noisy work if appropriate measures for reducing noise exposure are followed.

Industrial solvent exposures in the workplace setting may potentiate hearing loss from noise exposure (12). Hearing deficits have been demonstrated in experimental animals exposed to toluene, styrene, xylenes, and trichloroethylene. Solvent abusers with exposure primarily to toluene have also demonstrated balance disorders and hearing impairment. Epidemiologic studies of hearing loss in solvent-exposed workers have shown more variable results, possibly because of the role of other factors, such as workplace noise, aging, and smoking. High-frequency hearing loss has been described in workers exposed to mixed solvents and noise. Several cohorts of workers exposed to solvents in the absence of noise have also been noted to have abnormalities on pure-tone audiometry or on brainstem auditory evoked response testing, indicating an effect on more central pathways of the auditory response (12).

HEALTH EFFECTS OF NOISE

Sound may be defined as mechanical energy transmitted as pressure waves through a medium, usually air, and detected by the organs of hearing—the ear and its related apparatus. Human hearing has a remarkable capability for differentiating sounds ranging from a falling leaf to the blast of armaments. Audible frequencies of sound range from 20 to 20,000 cycles per second or *hertz* (Hz), with the ear's greatest sensitivity occurring between 500 and 4,000 Hz. Normal speech lies within this range. The intensity of sound, a measure of the energy transmitted by pressure waves, is described in *decibels* (dB). At 1,000 Hz, the minimum sound pressure detectable by a healthy young adult ear is 2×10^{-5} pascals (Pa or newtons/square meter); this value is characterized as 0 dB. The dB scale is logarithmic, so that an increase of 10 dB represents a tenfold increase in sound pressure, and an increase of 3 dB indicates a doubling of intensity. Some typical values for everyday sounds and those often found in occupational settings are shown in Table 26.2.

Noise has a more subjective definition, and may be considered to be unwanted sound that disturbs or injures the hearer. All noises in general comprise an assembly of sounds over a range of frequencies and intensities. An analysis of this noise spectrum is essential in order to define the hazard, as well as to select acoustic noise control measures, including personal hearing protection. Measurements of noise in the workplace are adjusted to match the sensitivity and range of the human ear, since sound meters have the same sensitivity across all frequencies. This weighting system is referred to as the *A* scale and values thus corrected are given as "dBA" to indicate that the adjustment has taken place. The two designations are used interchangeably here, but the occupational health professional interpreting noise survey results should be aware that raw data from sound level meters must be adjusted to have meaning when results are applied to workplace situations and human exposures.

TABLE 26.2. *Typical sound levels for some common activities and machines*

Sound	Sound level (dBA)
Leaves rustling	0–10
Quiet office	40
Normal conversation	65
Busy office	60–70
Ringing alarm clock at 3 feet	80
Drill press	90
Power saw	110
Coarse grinding	115
Jackhammer	120
Jet aircraft takeoff	140

Damage to human hearing from exposure to noise can take two forms: *acute,* secondary to a loud noise such as a blast, and *chronic,* due to long-term exposure to hazardous noise levels. In addition, there are extraauditory effects of noise, which are not well defined but may present health risks.

Acute Acoustic Trauma

Exposure to brief intense levels of noise, usually from blasts or explosions, can cause acute and permanent damage to the middle and inner ear. Most cases arise from exposure to noise levels in the range from 140 to 160 dB, with military service accounting for the greatest proportion (45%) of cases (13). The most common symptoms in acute acoustic trauma (AAT) are hearing loss (95% of cases in one series) and tinnitus (70%); about one in four had bilateral damage (13). Tinnitus, rather than pain or decreased hearing acuity, appears to be the symptom most likely to prompt affected individuals to seek medical evaluation.

Clinical evaluation in AAT demonstrates conductive hearing loss from traumatic rupture of the tympanic membrane, disruption of the ossicular chain, and mechanical damage to the oval window, as well as sensorineural loss from cochlear hair cell disruption. Higher-frequency pure-tone hearing loss is more common in AAT than in chronic NIHL, with frequencies between 4,000 and 8,000 Hz most affected. A period of weeks to months may be required for hearing to stabilize; the pathologic process resulting in progression of hearing loss from AAT appears not to extend beyond a year unless other factors are present. Although audiometric results may return to baseline values, permanent damage may have occurred to the sensory cells of the inner ear, and continued exposure to noise may result in further deterioration of hearing (14).

On physical examination, the ear usually appears normal unless the tympanic membrane is ruptured, which occurs in approximately a third of cases of AAT. Weber and Rinne tests may demonstrate conductive hearing loss with lateralization of bone conduction to the unaffected side. Audiometry may indicate both conductive and sensorineural hearing loss. Paradoxically, the ear more directly exposed to the blast may not be the one that sustains the injury, since blast waves may bounce off walls and surrounding objects to cause injury to the opposite ear.

Complications following AAT include persistent perforation of the tympanic membrane, permanent hearing loss, both sensorineural and conductive, and cholesteatoma. About 10% to 20% of tympanic membrane ruptures require surgical correction, with the remainder generally healing without intervention. The patient with a perforation should be advised to keep water, foreign bodies, and other potential contaminants out of the external auditory meatus. Large perforations and those that appear not to be healing mandate referral to an otolaryngologist.

Although prevention of AAT through the use of engineering controls and personal protective equipment should be emphasized, these injuries can rarely be predicted. Where prevention fails, proper treatment depends on access to medical care. A number of treatment measures have been attempted that are based on the premise that the blast has caused metabolic disturbances in the sensory cells of the inner ear. Evaluation of the effectiveness of medications, however, is impeded by the lack of preexposure audiometric values. No convincing evidence has been noted for a variety of proposed treatments including vitamins A, B, or E, nicotinic acid, or papaverine hydrochloride (15). Therapies targeted at improving oxygenation and blood flow to the inner ear have been used more recently. Dextran has been widely used by the German military with variable results, which may have been in part due to better pretreatment thresholds in the treated subjects; controlled studies indicate a lack of efficacy of dextrans and of pentoxifylline when compared with placebo (16). Hyperbaric oxygen has also been used with some success, although clinically controlled double-blind evaluations are lacking. Most reports stress the need for early intervention if any form of treatment is to be successful.

Chronic Hearing Loss

A combination of mechanical, metabolic, and vascular factors are involved in the destructive changes that lead to NIHL. The effects of noise occur in the organ of Corti, within the cochlea of the inner ear. This structure has three outer rows and one inner row of hair cells, the sensory receptors of the ear, with the tectorial membrane suspended above them. The hair cells contain cilia, which project toward the tectorial membrane. The energy transmitted from the tympanic membrane via the ossicles to the cochlea vibrates the cilia, which convert this mechanical energy into nerve impulses transmitted through the acoustic nerve. The hair cells are highly susceptible to the mechanical trauma of loud noise. The cell bodies swell with repeated exposure to loud noise, and ultimately the hair cells are destroyed. In addition, high noise levels disrupt the vascular supply of the basilar membrane. Capillary vasoconstriction in response to loud noise may result in reduced oxygen tension and local hypoxia within the cochlea. Eventually, the organ of Corti breaks down, with separation of segments of sensory cells from the basilar membrane, leading to elimination of sensory structures and replacement by a single flat cell layer. Electron photomicrographs of the cochlea in experimental animals subjected to noise show dropout and progressive destruction of hair cells. Hair cells of the basal turn of the cochlea, which conduct sound at higher frequencies (4,000–6,000 Hz), appear to be preferentially affected, most probably because of their location in areas of high shear stress along the organ of Corti, which explains the findings of early NIHL, with hearing loss most affected in this range. Eventually, disruption of the medial and apical areas occurs as well, leading to hearing loss at a wider range of frequencies. Cochlear blood vessels, the stria vascularis, and nerve endings associated with the hair cells can also be damaged.

Pathologic abnormalities associated with NIHL are distinct from those due to presbycusis. Prolonged noise exposure is associated with disruption of the outer and inner hair cells of the organ of Corti; ultimately degeneration of nerve fibers and ganglion cells occurs. Presbycusis, by contrast, arises from changes across the entire auditory system, including loss of elasticity of the tympanic membrane, and reduction of mobility of the ossicular chain; loss or malfunction of hair cells in presbycusis occurs at higher frequencies initially (8,000 Hz) than in NIHL.

Although the risk of NIHL tends to increase with advancing age as well as with length of employment, most noise-related effects occur within the early phases of exposure to noise, with most of the damage arising within the first 10 years. Persons with sensorineural hearing loss, however, do not usually recognize early changes in their ability to hear. Nonetheless, early changes can usually be documented by audiometric monitoring. Early symptoms of NIHL reflect a person's ability to distinguish higher-pitched consonant sounds. For example, the word *fist* may sound like *fish,* and *hat* may become *has.* Speech is rendered less intelligible, as opposed to lower in volume. This latter point accounts for the lack of efficacy of hearing amplification devices in the treatment of people whose hearing is impaired due to noise exposure.

Extraauditory Effects of Noise

The nonauditory effects of environmental noise on human health, most notably hypertension, have also aroused concern. Health effects arising from ambient noise present substantial scientific challenges in study design, implementation, and analysis, particularly with respect to confounding factors, and as such have not yet attracted well-controlled epidemiologic studies. A theoretical basis exists for a proposed relationship between noise and hypertension, grounded in the stress response; as a result of noise, release of adrenocortical hormones and sympathomimetic mediators leads to increased heart rate and eventually higher blood pressure. Investigation is made more difficult, however, because the prevalence of both hypertension and presbycusis, as well as NIHL, tends to increase with age. Cross-sectional studies indicate a correlation of NIHL with high diastolic blood pressure, particularly for those with the most severe hearing loss (17). Longitudinal observation of a mining cohort has failed to show an association between noise exposure and hypertension, however (18). At this point, the relationship between the two must be considered as possible, but without substantial scientific proof.

Various hormonal responses have also been described secondary to noise; effects range from increased levels of urinary catecholamines to increased concentration of 17-hydroxycorticoids. Increased postshift urinary cortisol excretion has been noted in workers exposed to high ambient noise levels compared with those wearing hearing-protection equipment (19). These findings bolster the hypothesis that noise acts as a general stressor in the setting of normal work demands.

Exposure to noise has caused teratogenic effects on laboratory rats, including reduced fertility and enlargement of the ovaries. Results in human studies have been mixed, and may be confounded by exposures to stressors other than noise. A case-control study in Finland (20) showed no relationship between occupational noise exposure (greater than 80 dB) and risk of either premature birth or low birth weight, although only approximately 3% of the study group reported any exposure to noise at work during pregnancy. An association of noise exposure with low birth weight in a prospective cohort study was noted by the same investigators; these findings were more pronounced in women in standing work positions or performing shift work, indicating the possible contribution of other stressful factors on outcome (21).

CLINICAL EVALUATION OF HEARING IMPAIRMENT

History and Physical Examination

The physician's role in the clinical evaluation of NIHL is to obtain an objective assessment of hearing impairment, prevent further deterioration of hearing, and recommend patients for further evaluation and treatment. A particular problem in diagnosis is the insidious nature of the injury; thus the early symptoms of NIHL tend to be subtle and may not be readily recognized by the patient. Initial complaints tend to focus on clarity of sound, particularly speech, rather than its intensity. As NIHL progresses, the person's ability to distinguish softer sounds is usually disrupted first. For example, the sounds of birds and other high-frequency sounds such as voices may be difficult to discern. People with high-pitched voices, such as children, may speak in a way that presents difficulties for a person with NIHL. As noted earlier, there is difficulty with higher-pitched sibilant consonant sounds, for example distinguishing *fish* from *fist.* There will often be a complaint of inability to understand speech in a noisy room. NIHL rarely, if ever, produces profound deafness, but the condition tends to be progressive. Hearing handicaps are usually noticed when the threshold hearing level of frequencies in the normal speech range (usually from 500 to 3,000 Hz) averages more than 25 dB.

An overall health history and review of systems should be taken when evaluating suspected NIHL, as other disease entities may cause both conductive and sensorineural hearing loss. The presence of contributory diseases, including diabetes, hypertension, metabolic disorders, and autoimmune conditions, should be ascertained. Mumps, congenital rubella, and central nervous system infections, including meningitis, may affect hearing, as may a history of head injury. The physician should also inquire into past and current medications, particularly during hospitalizations. The drugs most commonly associated with deafness include furosemide and aminoglycoside antibiotics such as gentamicin. Analgesics, such as salicylates, and antihistamines, as well as tricyclic antidepressants, have also been associated with ototoxicity. Salicylates, in particular, are well known to cause reversible tinnitus. Sensorineural hearing loss may be hereditary as well, and a family history of deafness should be ascertained. A history of accompanying symptoms, particularly those referable to the inner ear, is useful in the differential diagnosis of hearing loss. Vertigo is often the first symptom of inner ear disorders, and, along with decreased acuity and high-pitched tinnitus, may indicate the possibility of an acoustic neuroma. Its presence may also suggest Meniere's disease. Vertigo, however, is seldom associated with NIHL or presbycusis.

The diagnosis of NIHL is straightforward when the physician incorporates a clear occupational history of noise exposure with the results of audiometric testing. Evaluation of occupational exposures should include an estimate of years of exposure in conjunction with any information on noise levels in the workplace. Area surveys or individual monitoring data are particularly useful in establishing the exposure history; however, these are often infrequent and may not reflect actual or long-standing exposures. In the absence of such data, a careful description of the processes and equipment used in the workplace may give the evaluating physician a reasonable estimation of exposure. A history describing personal protective equipment and other measures to reduce noise in the workplace should also be taken. Physicians evaluating the contribution of workplace noise to hearing loss should also consider nonoccupational causes, such as target shooting, motorcycle riding, hunting, loud music, and portable radios. Personal stereos with headphones, for example, can generate noise levels well beyond OSHA standards (22).

Physical examination should be targeted toward the assessment of the extent and possible contributing causes of hearing loss. Examination of the external meatus should show a canal free from cerumen impaction; if this is noted, the impaction should be removed (generally by irrigation) and audiometry deferred until another day to allow time for the minor trauma of removal to resolve. The tympanic membrane should be examined for signs of scarring or trauma; bulb insufflation may be useful in determining the presence of a persistent middle ear effusion such as that arising from chronic otitis media. A rapid assessment of hearing may be made using a whispered voice, although results of audiometry will be more informative. Performing Weber and Rinne tests with a tuning fork will assist the examiner in differentiating conductive from sensorineural hearing loss, particularly if loss is unilateral or asymmetric. The remainder of the cranial nerves should be examined, as should coordination, gait, and balance, to evaluate the possibility of neurologic disease.

Audiometry and Other Testing

Pure-tone audiometric testing, which assesses the ability to hear various standardized frequencies, is the mainstay of evaluation. During the test, tones in the frequency range between 25 and 8,000 Hz are increased in volume until the person recognizes the sound. The decibel reading at which the sound is first recognized at each frequency is recorded; this value is termed the *hearing threshold* for that frequency. Normal threshold values range from –0.5 dB to 20 dB; those at or above 25 dB are considered abnormal, and are especially important when the speech frequency ranges (500 to 4,000 Hz) are affected.

Early impairment due to NIHL tends to occur at 4,000 Hz, with relative sparing of hearing at higher frequencies (Fig. 26.1). These findings are typical of NIHL, though they are not pathognomonic, as solvent exposure in the absence of noise may cause a similar pattern. In presbycusis, the audiometric pattern has a similar decrement in the 4,000-Hz range; however, the loss tends to be greater still in the 8,000-Hz range. Audiometric findings of hearing loss due to ototoxicity are similar to those of presbycusis, while those from infections such as mumps will demonstrate equivalent hearing loss across the spectrum of pure tones. With continued exposure the *4,000-Hz notch* of NIHL will persist and deepen, eventually involving the speech frequencies in the 2,000- to 3,000-Hz range. Despite the contrast in audiometric patterns, differentiating NIHL from presbycusis can be a diffi-

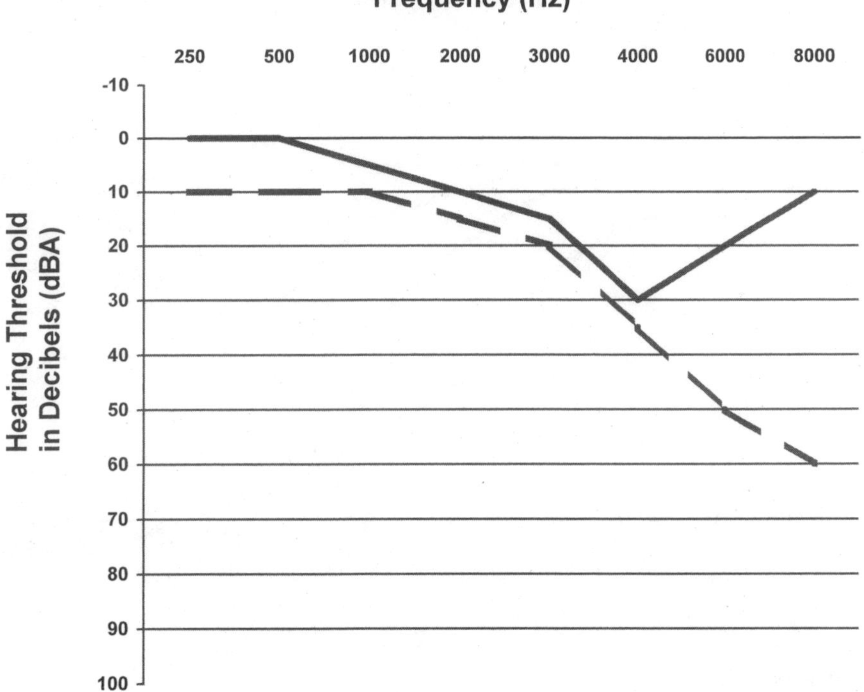

FIG. 26.1. Pure-tone audiogram showing characteristic 4,000-Hz notch of a noise-induced hearing loss (NIHL) *(solid line)* and increasing hearing threshold with higher frequencies characteristic of presbycusis *(dashed line).*

cult exercise. Moreover, presbycusis and NIHL can act concurrently to affect hearing. The combination of persistent noise exposure with aging will cause accelerated hearing loss in the higher frequency ranges, and the resultant pattern indicates the additive effects of NIHL and presbycusis (Fig. 26.2).

The finding that a pure tone presented at two unequal frequencies will be subjectively "heard" only on the side of the louder tone forms the basis of the Stenger test to detect malingering that involves a claim of unilateral hearing loss. The individual with true unilateral loss does not hear the louder tone in the damaged ear, but indicates instead that he hears the softer tone in the good ear. The malingering patient, by contrast, localizes the sound to the feigned affected ear, as would an individual with normal hearing, and therefore denies hearing any tone at all.

Other diagnostic and screening tools used to identify hearing impairment and distinguish between differing etiologies have been described. Speech discrimination testing, which assesses the ability to identify words in addition to hearing them, may provide a finer discrimination of impairment than pure-tone audiometry. The patient is presented with 50 selected monosyllabic words at the intensity level at which audiometry suggests they would be recognized. The proportion of words correctly identified is the speech discrimination score (SDS). Speech discrimination may be affected not only by sensorineural hearing loss at the cochlea but also by abnormalities of the neural pathways along the eighth nerve or in the auditory cortex, which might render easily heard sound unintelligible. Individuals with conductive hearing loss, by contrast, recognize words as long as they are presented at a sufficient volume. Shorter versions of the SDS, in which words are presented with a competing sound, have been used in workplace screening tests to identify practical difficulties in everyday communication, and as a research tool (17).

Another, more sensitive, diagnostic study used to evaluate hearing loss is the *brainstem auditory evoked potential* (BAEP), which tracks the brainstem response to auditory stimuli. This test may be especially valuable in assessing persons who report hearing loss but whose audiometric test results are equivocal, and may be particularly useful in the diagnosis of acoustic

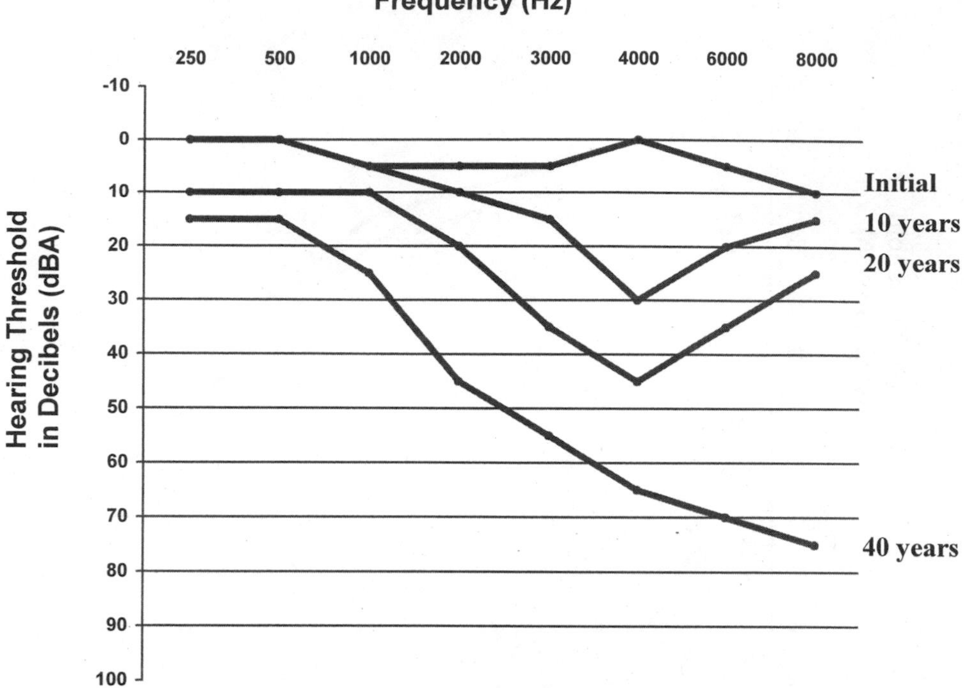

FIG. 26.2. Pure-tone audiogram showing the combined effects of noise exposure and aging. Initial pattern characteristic of NIHL at 10 years shows increasing decrement at 8,000 Hz with increasing age.

neuroma and other conditions affecting neural pathways to the auditory cortex.

Threshold Shifts and Changes in Hearing Acuity

The importance of periodic audiometric monitoring in preventing noise-induced hearing loss cannot be overemphasized. Audiometry serves as an effective tool for surveillance if used regularly and properly. Especially in the early years of noise exposure, decrements in hearing can occur without being noticed by the worker. The physician interpreting audiometric results must look for deviations from the baseline values. A *threshold shift* refers to a significant hearing decrement as documented by audiometry; these may be classified as temporary and permanent. While definitions of a threshold shift may vary, the most frequently used is the OSHA criterion of a *standard threshold shift* (STS), which refers to a 10-dB or greater change from baseline for the average of hearing thresholds at 2,000, 3,000, and 4,000 Hz in either ear. Noise-induced temporary threshold shifts (NITTSs) are changes in hearing associated with transient overexposures to noise that can be observed and documented by serial audiometry testing. These may persist for hours or even several days, depending on the magnitude and length of exposure to the noise that produced the shift. The person experiencing a NITTS notices diminished hearing acuity that is most pronounced after noise exposure. Retesting after an adequate period of auditory rest usually demonstrates a return of hearing to baseline values, unless some degree of permanent damage has occurred. Most audiometric examinations should be performed at least 14 hours after the last unprotected exposure to noise, to avoid the effect that a NITTS may have on determination of NIHL.

Repeated episodes of exposure to hazardous levels of noise may result in permanent damage to hearing that no amount of auditory rest can restore. These noise-induced permanent threshold shifts (NIPTSs) are irreversible, and serve as an important signal that noise levels are not well controlled. An employee meeting the OSHA criteria for an STS should be retested within 30 days to see if the shift persists. If the increased hearing thresholds persist, the new audiogram, reflecting the STS, is used as a new baseline to measure any further hearing decrements. The employee with a confirmed STS needs to be informed and evaluated to ensure that hearing-protection devices fit properly and are being used as directed. Confirmed threshold shifts with an average decrement of 25 Hz or greater in either ear must be recorded as an occupational illness on the OSHA log form (24) proposed changes to the OSHA record-keeping standard would mandate reporting of cases that meet the definition of an STS with a 10-dB mean decrement (25). In some cases the physician must address the contribution of presbycusis to hearing impairment. The OSHA standard includes recommended calculations to determine the contribution of age to hearing impairment (24). More recently, the validity of applying population-derived statistics to individual audiometric results has been challenged, and NIOSH, in its criteria document for a revised standard, has recommended that audiograms no longer be adjusted to account for the effects of presbycusis (2).

Table 26.3 illustrates a case of progressive, albeit subtle, changes that occurred over a 10-year period, ultimately leading to serious hearing impairment. This case exemplifies the difference between the clinical diagnosis of hearing loss and findings on screening for early signs of noise-induced hearing impairment. An STS became apparent at the third annual hearing examination, yet, because the capacity to hear and understand speech was not compromised at this early stage, no further measures were made to conserve hearing at this detectable preclinical phase. The occupational physician, in a preventive role, is charged with recognizing the vitally important role of early changes in hearing, before substantial and irreversible impairment develops.

Some additional points to remember in the evaluation of suspected NIHL include the following (26):

1. Chronic NIHL is usually *symmetric;* other otologic disorders, especially the more serious, as well as treatable, types, are often asymmetric. Localization of hearing deficits may depend on the specifics of exposure, however. Truck drivers may present with greater hearing loss in the left ear, the result of heavier exposures through the window of the truck cab.
2. NIHL usually develops gradually; other otologic disorders may progress rapidly.
3. NIHL usually causes *high-frequency* threshold shifts, while hearing loss from other sources, such as infections, may cause uniform loss across the hearing spectrum.
4. Regardless of the cause, a pure-tone threshold average in excess of 25 dB in either ear is likely to cause hearing difficulties.

Disposition and Follow-up

After reviewing diagnostic studies, especially the audiometric evaluation, the physician can formulate an opinion as to the cause of hearing loss and whether therapy may be effective. Unfortunately, treatment measures for NIHL tend to be ineffective, since the primary problem is not the amplification of sound but the distinguishing of various types of sounds. There is considerable difficulty hearing conversation in the presence of background noise and differentiating between competing sounds. Thus, amplification devices that correct other types of hearing impairment by increasing transmission of sound in the middle ear are largely ineffective. Nonetheless, the physician is wise

TABLE 26.3. *Example of annual audiometric thresholds obtained on worker who exhibited progressive noise-induced hearing loss*

	Frequency (Hz)					
Thresholds on	500	1,000	2,000	3,000	4,000	6,000
Reference	5	0	0	10	10	5
1st annual	0	0	0	10	10	10
2nd annual	5	5	0	10	15	10
3rd annual	0	5	5	15	15	15
4th annual	5	5	10	15	20	20
5th annual	0	5	15	25	30	25
6th annual	5	10	20	35	40	30
7th annual	0	10	30	45	50	40
8th annual	5	15	35	50	55	40
9th annual	10	25	40	60	70	50
10th annual	10	35	55	70	85	60
11th annual	15	40	65	80	95	80

to be aware of the need for otologic referral in evaluating hearing loss, if only to assess potentially remediable causes of hearing loss. The American Academy of Otolaryngology–Head and Neck Surgery has published guidelines for otologic referral that apply to most hearing conservation programs (27). Indications for referral include a threshold average in excess of 25 dB in either ear on testing at 500, 1,000, 2,000, and 3,000 Hz, or a mean difference in acuity between the two ears of 15 dB at lower frequencies (500 to 2,000 Hz), or a 30-dB difference at higher frequencies (3,000 to 6,000 Hz) on baseline audiometry. Referral is also recommended for findings of an average change of 15 dB at the lower frequencies or a high-frequency loss of 20 dB noted on periodic examination. In addition, an otolaryngologist should be consulted for other medical problems related to the ear that may be outside the expertise of the occupational physician, including problems with persistent ear pain, drainage, dizziness, severe persistent tinnitus, or sudden, fluctuating, or rapidly progressive hearing loss not explained by a history of noise exposure alone.

Situations may arise where the occupational physician must recommend restrictions, accommodations, or modifications that affect worker assignment in jobs involving potentially hazardous noise exposures. These actions may be needed for persons with good hearing in only one ear (severe unilateral loss); persons with moderate to severe hearing impairment that appears to be progressive in spite of efforts to control exposures; persons who continue to demonstrate progressive threshold shifts in hearing that are attributable to causes other than noise exposure; and persons with chronic otologic conditions, including chronic otitis media or otitis externa, who are unable to adequately use or wear hearing protection. Decisions on job placement in these individuals should consider the potential likelihood and severity of further injury, as well as work modifications that might reduce the hazard to the worker. Reasonable accommodations that would allow such potentially disabled employees to continue work must be considered under the Americans with Disabilities Act (see Chapter 5); elimination of job tasks with higher exposure or their reassignment to other workers may be appropriate, depending on individual circumstances.

Determination of Impairment

Evaluation of hearing impairment may be requested in cases where hearing loss has become permanent and irreversible. As with impairment and disability evaluations for other organ systems, the physician is requested to make a determination of impairment based primarily on testing results, which may be problematic in many cases. Pure-tone audiometry, as noted above, may not reflect impairment based on inability to function in areas of daily activity, including work. Modest decrements in speech recognition, for example, may be severely disabling if fine discrimination of sound is a part of an employee's work. Nonetheless, most approaches to impairment evaluation are founded on standardized testing. The American Academy of Otolaryngology has published a formula for calculating hearing impairment based on pure-tone hearing loss at various frequencies (28). These criteria have been adopted by the AMA in the *Guides to the Evaluation of Permanent Impairment* to aid physicians in the process of disability determination (29). The guidelines assign a 1.5% impairment of monaural hearing for every decibel that the average hearing level (the mean thresholds measured at frequencies of 500, 1,000, 2,000, and 3,000 Hz) exceeds a 25-dB threshold. Impairment does not begin until an average hearing loss of 25 dB has been reached, and is considered complete at a threshold average of 92 dB. Provision is made for correction for the effects of aging and presbycusis, although the literature has argued against this approach in the individual worker (2). Calculation of binaural hearing impairment, as well as whole-person impairment resulting from hearing loss, is made from tables provided in the *Guides*. Additional impairment may be assigned for the presence of tinnitus, although such a determination is necessarily subjective. Evaluation should be made without regard to the use of hearing aids or other assistive devices, as these will not permit an evaluation of the possible extent of impairment. Other approaches have been recommended based on job-specific functions; one designed for army personnel uses a mathematical model to evaluate a soldier's ability to hear when engaged in certain required or frequently performed tasks (30).

REGULATION AND CONTROL OF NOISE EXPOSURE

OSHA Regulations

A standard to help prevent NIHL in American industries was issued by OSHA in 1983 (4). This regulation requires employers to assess the level of noise in a facility, to reduce noise when it exceeds certain levels, and to provide employees with appropriate medical testing, education, training, and hearing-protection devices. The OSHA standard requires employers to implement noise control measures when levels exceed 90 dB, expressed as an 8-hour time-weighted average (TWA_8), and to establish a hearing conservation program when levels are beyond 85 dB. Revised criteria for a recommended standard were published by NIOSH in 1998 (2) based on its evaluation of the latest scientific information. The NIOSH recommendations differ from current OSHA requirements in their proposal to reduce the permissible 8-hour exposure limit to 85 dB, a level that would be protective of greater numbers of workers. In addition, they seek to reduce exposures by cutting the exchange rate at which exposure time must be halved from the current 5-dB increase to 3 dB, a figure that better reflects actual exposures. At the present time, however, these recommendations have not been promulgated in a new standard, although they represent a scientifically valid approach to hearing protection in the workplace. The elements of a hearing conservation program and the control of noise exposures in the workplace will be outlined here.

Permissible Exposure Limits and Identification of Exposed Employees

According to the current OSHA standard, the permissible daily exposure limit for noise is 90 dB TWA_8. An *exchange rate* of 5 dB for every doubling or halving of the exposure time is used to modify the permissible TWA for louder noise exposures. For example, workers are permitted only a 4-hour exposure to noise at 95 dB, and a 2-hour exposure at 100 dB. The ceiling or short-term exposure limit (STEL) is 115 dB for no more than a 15-minute period; this is the maximum value beyond which noise exposure is not permitted regardless of duration. Some European countries use an exchange rate of 3 dB for every halving of the exposure time; this is also the value recommended in the NIOSH revised criteria for a new standard. Acoustically, this approach is considered to have a firmer mathematical foundation, since, as a logarithmic measurement, an increase of 3 dB represents a doubling of sound wave pressures.

The employer is required to institute a hearing conservation program (HCP) when workers are exposed to sound levels at or above the *action level* of 85 dB TWA_8. Noise exposures in workers must be calculated without regard to the attenuation that may be provided by personal protective equipment. The fundamentals of an HCP include noise level assessment, noise control measures, audiometric monitoring, education and training, and hearing-protection devices.

Noise Level Assessment

The first step in assessing the need for an HCP is to measure the ambient noise level. An industrial hygienist or a similar professional customarily performs noise assessments. Measurements performed in the occupational setting usually consist of overall levels that are obtained either through a sound level meter or a noise dosimeter (31). OSHA requires monitoring of areas that might reasonably be expected to expose employees to noise in order to identify those who need to be enrolled in the HCP or who will need hearing protection. These measurements can also be effective in determining the amount of attenuation required of the hearing-protection devices that may be used. Moreover, noise assessments help to acquaint employees and employers with the level of noise in the facility. Generally, OSHA allows area surveys to assess individual exposure if the workforce is located in the same general area and the noise levels are relatively uniform throughout the work shift. Settings in which impulse or impact noises are present, or where workers are highly mobile, require different approaches.

When area surveys are not appropriate, individual measurements must be made with a personal dosimeter. This particular approach, although capable of yielding more accurate results, tends to be more time-consuming and complicated. Generally, an employee wears the noise dosimeter on the shirt collar throughout a work shift. Accurate measurements depend on reliable calibration of the monitoring device. In certain circumstances it is worthwhile to assess "noise at the ear," when area or personal exposure measurements are felt not to give an accurate picture of exposure. An approach to monitoring noise exposure in workers who wear communication headsets has also been introduced (32).

This first step, assessing the noise levels encountered in work, is one of the more critical determinants in evaluating the need for an HCP. Once noise levels are determined, they need to be reevaluated at intervals, especially if new processes or plant equipment are introduced into an operation. Periodic measurement may serve as a method of evaluation of the efficacy of preventive controls. It is essential that noise measurements be accurately recorded and available for review, especially by regulatory agencies such as OSHA. The occupational physician or health service should also, if possible, obtain results of noise level assessments, the date of the measurements, and whether they reflect normal operations; these data may prove useful in the clinical evaluation of noise-exposed workers.

Control Measures

In work settings where noise levels exceed 90 dB TWA_8, engineering controls should be employed as the principal measure for noise reduction. Machinery design, enclosure of noisy machinery, installation of sound-absorbent surroundings, and noise control products such as baffles or mufflers can be effective in reducing noise at its source. Improved maintenance of machinery may serve to lessen ambient noise. In most existing settings noise control measures must be retrofitted onto existing equipment, and such measures should involve participation by engineers, safety personnel, and workers who operate the machinery in order to establish their acceptability and appropriateness (2). A prospective approach to noise reduction is emphasized by the "buy-quiet" policies adopted by some corporations. This involves identification and targeting of machinery and processes for noise reduction through new equipment purchases, and inclusion of noise-level criteria in bidding and purchasing procedures (33). Despite apparent high initial costs, substantial savings may be realized by using this approach; at its most effective, it may obviate the need for many elements of a hearing conservation program, such as personal protective equipment and annual audiometric examinations, if noise levels are reduced below the action level.

Administrative procedures may also become necessary if engineering controls fail to limit noise exposures to acceptable levels. Rotation of workers from exposed to nonexposed areas and limitation of working hours in areas with hazardous levels of noise are the main methods by which these controls are effected. The exchange rate proposed by NIOSH, which halves allowable exposure time for every 3-dB increase in sound intensity, may be used as guidance for administrative reduction of noise exposures.

Hearing-protection Devices

The fundamental approach to reducing the risk of NIHL is to control noise at its source. In some cases, however, this approach is still inadequate or not feasible, so it is essential to provide hearing-protection devices. These are of three basic types: *insert,* devices placed directly into the ear canal; *semiinsert,* devices that cover entry into the ear canal; and *muffs,* which completely encapsulate the ear itself. Hearing-protection devices provide various levels of attenuation; this is usually expressed as a *noise reduction rating* (NRR) that represents the manufacturer's assessment of testing under optimum conditions. Actual efficacy of these devices in the workplace, however, is dependent on many variables, and attenuation of noise under normal working conditions may be 25% to 75% of the labeled NRR. Most hearing-protection devices provide 15- to 30-dB attenuation if they are fitted properly and used in accordance with their instructions. When insert plugs are combined with muffs, an additional 10 to 15 dB of protection can be obtained.

No single type of hearing protection can be considered the single best choice for all users; different workers choose different devices because of such factors as personal comfort and variations in the anatomic structure of their ears. Thus it is essential to offer employees a variety of hearing-protection devices, to ensure that all can comfortably wear them. During the audiometric evaluation it is worthwhile to acquaint or reeducate the employee in the proper use of the hearing-protection device.

Noise cancellation technology has received increasing interest as a possible means by which high ambient noise levels can be reduced at the ear. Such devices operate by registering immediate noise levels and blocking them by generation of a canceling waveform relayed back to the ear. Problems remain with the use of this technology in most workplace settings; it is best adapted to low-frequency noise in confined spaces, where noise usually originates from a single direction. It performs less well in work sites where higher-pitched noise, which presents a greater hazard to hearing, is transmitted from a variety of sources and directions. At the present time, its use in the workplace should be considered experimental, and noise cancellation instruments should not be used in place of more generally accepted methods of hearing protection (34).

Audiometric Monitoring

The principles of audiometric testing have been outlined above. Systematic and regular monitoring is essential to preventing NIHL. Periodic audiometric examination is a notable example of an effective screening tool that can reduce the likelihood of occupational illness, because workers with early decrements on audiometric tests usually do not describe hearing difficulties. One study of army helicopter pilots noted that nearly three out of four soldiers with abnormal audiometric test results (as reflected by a significant threshold shift) were unaware of any hearing loss (35).

Occupational physicians who participate in HCPs are often responsible for interpreting audiometric test results. Although most monitoring is performed in response to OSHA mandates, general principles of medical surveillance apply to these testing programs. Among the occupational physician's tasks are (a) to determine the acceptability of the results; (b) to assess the results for evidence of alterations in hearing, both for individuals and in aggregate; (c) to counsel workers as to the results of testing and recommend additional evaluation for hearing abnormalities; and (d) to communicate aggregate results to management, worker representatives, and others with a need to know. Physicians should ensure that the audiometric equipment is properly calibrated according to criteria of the Council for Accreditation in Occupational Hearing Conservation. These guidelines also stipulate training requirements for the person performing the audiometric test, the proper calibration of the audiometer, and the efficacy of the sound control booth. Occupational hearing tests are conducted in many settings, including in the plant, at clinical facilities, and in mobile vans. It is essential that the results be reliable and based on proper testing procedures with well-functioning equipment.

For employees covered under the OSHA standard, baseline audiometric testing is required within 6 months of hire. The OSHA standard mandates yearly audiometric examinations for employees exposed at or above the action level of 85 dB. Periodic test results must be compared to the baseline values. If any abnormalities are noted in this evaluation, the worker should be retested after a 14-hour period without exposure to noise. The presence of a standard threshold shift, even in the absence of clinical symptoms of hearing loss, should be recorded in the OSHA Log. More importantly, it should trigger a comprehensive audit of the HCP. An abnormal finding may represent a sentinel event, indicating a failure of primary noise controls or the presence of unanticipated exposures. Reassessment of ambient noise levels and the extent of compliance with the use of hearing-protection devices is indicated, both for the affected individual and for co-workers. Although there is no requirement for outside referral in the OSHA regulations, the reviewing or examining physician may find it appropriate to help workers obtain more detailed audiometric evaluations. Records of audiometric testing must be maintained by the employer for the duration of the affected worker's employment.

Although audiometric screening is effective among occupationally exposed groups, this testing has not been valuable as a screening tool in the general population because of the low prevalence of hearing loss in younger cohorts (36).

Education and Training

Under the OSHA standard, education of employees in hearing protection and the adverse effects of exposure to noise must be undertaken in workplaces where ambient noise levels exceed 85 dB. Workers should understand the means by which noise damages hearing and the consequences of prolonged unprotected exposure to high levels of noise. The importance of participation in hearing conservation programs, and the benefits of wearing hearing-protection devices and participating in annual audiometric monitoring programs should be reinforced. The insidious nature of hearing loss tends to encourage a relaxed attitude toward compliance, as the consequences are often not recognized for many years. To combat this tendency, employees and supervisors must develop the motivation and discipline to ensure the success of a long-term hearing conservation program. Employee participation in the planning and development stages can help to ensure that rewards and disciplinary procedures are appropriate and effective, and not viewed as a "top-down" effort at control by management (37). Physician participation in educational and training programs designed to acquaint managers and employees with the health implications of long-term exposure to high noise levels can be of great benefit, and sends a message that hearing conservation is taken seriously by the occupational health service and the organization. A variety of materials are available for training purposes and may be used to tailor educational programs to the specific needs of the workforce; a useful compendium of films, computer software, and videotapes is available through NIOSH (33).

REFERENCES

1. Ramazzini B. *Diseases of workers*. Trans. WC Wright. Thunder Bay, Canada: OH&S Press, 1993:261–263.
2. National Institute for Occupational Safety and Health. Criteria for a recommended standard. Occupational noise exposure. Revised criteria 1998. USDHHS publication. No. 98-126, 1998.
3. Moss AJ, Parsons VL. Current estimates from the National Health Interview Survey—United States, 1985. *Vital Health Stat* 1986.
4. Occupational Noise Exposure. Hearing conservation amendment 29 CFR 1910.95 (final rule). *Fed Reg* 1983(March 8);48(46):9737.
5. Leading work-related diseases and injuries—United States. *JAMA* 1986;255:2133.
6. Karjalainen A, Aalto L, Jolanki R, et al. Occupational diseases in Finland in 1996. New cases of occupational diseases reported to the Finnish Register of Occupational Diseases. Helsinki. Finnish Institute of Occupational Health, 1998.

7. Cherry NM, Meyer JD, Holt DL, et al. Surveillance of work-related diseases by occupational physicians in the UK: OPRA 1996–99. *Occup Med* 2000;50:496–503.
8. Nakanishi N, Okamoto M, Nakamura K, et al. Cigarette smoking and risk for hearing impairment: a longitudinal study in Japanese male office workers. *J Occup Environ Med* 2000;42:1045–1049.
9. Barone J, Peters J, Garabrant D, et al. Smoking as a risk factor in noise-induced hearing loss. *J Occup Med* 1987;29:741–745.
10. Hodgson MJ, Talbot E, Helmkamp JC, et al. Diabetes, noise exposure, and hearing loss. *J Occup Med* 1987; 29:576–579.
11. Miller JJ, Beck L, Davis A, et al. Hearing loss in patients with diabetic retinopathy. *Am J Otolaryngol* 1983; 4:342–346.
12. Johnson AC, Nylen PR. Effects of industrial solvents on hearing. *Occup Med State of the Art Rev* 1995;10: 623–640.
13. Axelsson A, Hamernik RP. Acute acoustic trauma. *Acta Otolaryngol (Stockh)* 1987;104:225–233.
14. Segal S, Harell M, Shahar A, et al. Acute acoustic trauma: dynamics of hearing loss following cessation of exposure. *Am J Otol* 1988;9:293–298.
15. Melnick W. Medicinal therapy for hearing loss resulting from noise exposure. *Am J Otolaryngol* 1984;5: 426–431.
16. Probst R, Tschopp K, Ludin E, et al. A randomized, double-blind, placebo-controlled study of dextran/pentoxifylline medication in acute acoustic trauma and sudden hearing loss. *Acta Otolaryngol (Stockh)* 1992;112: 435–443.
17. Talbott E, Findlay R, Kuller L, et al. Noise-induced hearing loss: a possible marker for high blood pressure in older noise-exposed populations. *J Occup Med* 1990; 32(8):690–697.
18. Hessel PA, Sluis-Cremer GK. Occupational noise exposure and blood pressure: longitudinal and cross-sectional observations in a group of underground miners. *Arch Environ Health* 1994;49:128–134.
19. Melamed S, Bruhis S. The effects of chronic industrial noise exposure on urinary cortisol, fatigue, and irritability. *J Occup Env Med* 1996;38:252–256.
20. Hartikainen-Sorri AL, Sorri M, Anttonen H, et al. Occupational noise exposure during pregnancy: a case-control study. *Int Arch Occup Environ Health* 1988;60: 279–283.
21. Hartikainen AL, Sorri M, Anttonen H, et al. Effect of occupational noise on the course and outcome of pregnancy. *Scand J Work Environ Health* 1994;20:444–450.
22. Catalano PJ, Levin SM. Noise-induced hearing loss and portable radios with headphones. *Int J Pediatr Otorhinolaryngol* 1985;9:59–67.
23. Deleted in proof.
24. Occupational Safety and Health Administration. Occupational noise exposure. 29 CFR 1910.95(c)(10)(i).
25. Occupational Safety and Health Administration. Occupational Injury and Illness Recording and Reporting Requirements; Final Rule. *Fed Reg* 2001(January 19); 66(13):6129.
26. Dobie RA. Noise-induced hearing loss: the family physician's role. *Am Fam Physician* 1987;36:141–148.
27. *Otologic Referral Criteria for Occupational Hearing Conservation Programs.* Alexandria, VA: American Academy of Otolaryngology–Head and Neck Surgery, 2001.
28. Ward WD. The American Medical Association/American Academy of Otolaryngology formula for determination of hearing handicap. *Audiology* 1983;22:313–324.
29. American Medical Association. *Guides to the evaluation of permanent impairment,* 4th ed. Chicago: American Medical Association, 1993.
30. Price G, Kalb J, Garinther G. Toward a measure of auditory handicap in the army. *Ann Otol Rhinol Laryngol* 1989;98:42–51.
31. Berger E, et al., eds. *Noise and hearing conservation manual,* 4th ed. Akron, OH: American Industrial Hygiene Association, 1986.
32. Van Moorhem WK, Woo KS, Liu S, et al. Development and operation of a system to monitor occupational noise exposure due to wearing a headset. *Appl Occup Environ Hyg* 1996;11:261–265.
33. National Institute for Occupational Safety and Health. Preventing occupational hearing loss: a practical guide. USDHHS publication No. 96-110. 1996. Available at: *www.cdc.gov/niosh96-110.html.*
34. Gordon RT, Vining WD. Active noise control: a review of the field. *Am Ind Hyg Assoc J* 1992;53(11):721–725.
35. Fitzpatrick D. An analysis of noise-induced hearing loss in army helicopter pilots. *Aviat Space Environ Med* 1988;59:937–941.
36. U.S. Preventive Services Task Force. *Guide to clinical preventive services,* 2nd ed. Baltimore: Williams & Wilkins, 1996.
37. Gasaway DC. *Hearing conservation: a practical manual and guide.* Englewood Cliffs, NJ: Prentice-Hall, 1985.

27

Occupational Skin Diseases

Edward A. Emmett

Occupational skin diseases are those disorders of the skin caused by or made worse by components of the workplace environment. Physicians engaged in evaluating occupational skin conditions should be familiar with their appearance, causes, methods of evaluation, diagnosis, treatment, and prevention. This chapter reviews these topics, emphasizing contact dermatitis, which accounts for approximately 90% of all occupational skin disease.

SIGNIFICANCE OF OCCUPATIONAL SKIN DISEASE

Occupational skin diseases remain among the most common occupational diseases. In the 1970s skin diseases constituted about 40% of all reported cases; now they constitute about 10%, due mainly to the dramatic rise in reported musculoskeletal conditions attributed to cumulative trauma such as carpal tunnel syndrome as well as to a modest decline in the number of cases of occupational skin diseases (1). The current annual incidence of occupational skin disease, reported to the Occupational Safety and Health Administration (OSHA), is about 5 per 10,000 full-time workers, down from about 8 per 10,000 full-time workers in the 1970s. The highest incidence in 1999 was in the agriculture forestry and fishing sector (15.5 per 10,000 full-time workers), followed by manufacturing (11.0 per 10,000 full-time workers); services (5.0); transportation and public utilities (3.6); construction (3.0); wholesale and retail trade (1.6); finance, insurance, and real estate (1.0); and mining (0.7).

The officially recorded figures appear to greatly underestimate the true prevalence of occupational skin disease. Surveys of large groups of workers in high-risk fields (e.g., physicians and nurses, metal workers, construction workers, and fish processors) consistently find 1-year prevalence rates for occupational skin disease of between 5% and 20% (2). There are many reasons for the observed underreporting of occupational skin diseases. For example, in certain states, an occupational disorder is compensable only if a skin disease is *caused* by work and not when a preexisting disease is *made worse* by work. Also, in some states there are additional requirements; in Massachusetts, problems due to work are compensable only if they cause more than 5 successive days of lost time. As a result, many skin disorders that are occupational in origin are troublesome to the worker but do not result in a lost workday, and may not come to the attention of management. Underreporting may also result if either the worker or the physician fails to associate the skin disorder with workplace activities. Finally, some workers are afraid to report a skin condition for fear of losing their jobs.

CAUSES AND TYPES OF OCCUPATIONAL SKIN DISEASE

The physician is most commonly confronted with occupational contact dermatitis, but there are many other types of occupational skin conditions, as illustrated in color plates 27.1 through 27.10.

Contact Dermatitis

Irritant and/or allergic contact dermatitis constitutes 80% to 90% of all occupational skin diseases. Irritant contact dermatitis is responsible for approximately 80% of all occupational contact dermatitis problems, although the proportion is different for different occupations depending on the pattern of chemical exposure. *Irritant reactions* are caused by substances that damage the skin at the site of contact through nonimmunologic mechanisms. Irritants, in general, are substances that cause injury to most individuals, given a sufficient concentration and time of exposure. There is a spectrum of types of irritant reactions depending on the strength of the irritant. The most severe irritants may cause corrosion (sometimes loosely referred to as chemical burns). Corrosives include strong alkalies and acids such as sodium hydroxide, triphenylphosphate, hydrochloric acid, sulfuric acid, and others. Strong alkalies are particularly damaging to the skin because the epidermis is normally slightly acid with a pH of 5.5. Irritants of medium strength cause classical irritant or toxic dermatitis. This is normally apparent shortly after the exposure, although some agents such as the antifouling agent dibutyl tin dioxide characteristically cause irritation after a delay on the order of 8 to 12 hours. Acute irritant dermatitis is characterized by erythema, swelling, and vesiculation in precise areas of contact, with a relatively sharply delineated border from unaffected skin (color plate 27.1), which, in the case of corrosion, is followed by sloughing of damaged skin. Healing then progresses to no visible evidence of past injury, hypo- or hyperpigmentation, or, with corrosion, to varying degrees of scarring depending on the depth of injury. Repeated exposure to moderately strong irritants may lead to chronic dermatitis with thickened leathery, hyperkeratotic skin (color plate 27.2).

At the other end of the irritancy spectrum is *cumulative insult dermatitis,* which is caused by repeated or prolonged exposure to weak, marginal irritants, which include mild detergents and some metalworking fluids. Cumulative insult dermatitis is not apparent until after days or weeks of exposure, but once present it is slow to resolve. Whereas standard toxicity and Materials Safety Data Sheets (MSDSs) usually identify other grades of irritants satisfactorily, standard toxicity testing does not satisfactorily identify marginal irritants, so the clinician must have a high degree of suspicion to diagnose this condition appropriately. The skin response is more chronic in nature and is characterized by erythema, scaling, fissuring, and pruritus. The affected skin is not usually clearly demarcated from normal skin. Improvement, which may be quite slow, occurs with avoidance of irritant exposure. Individuals with a personal or family history of atopy are more likely to be affected.

Allergic contact reactions require a cell-medicated hypersensitivity mechanism. Generally, a smaller number of workers are affected, although the strong sensitizer urushiol, the allergen in poison ivy and some other plants of the *Rhus* species, has sensitized approximately 60% of Americans. There are two phases in the development of allergic contact dermatitis: sensitization and elicitation. The sensitization phase takes 7 to 10 days after the first contact with the allergen. In practice, the exposure that causes sensitization may occur after the worker has worked with a substance for years without incident. Once an individual is sensitized, an allergic reaction is elicited upon reexposure to the allergen, with a characteristic delay of about 48 hours before the lesions are visible. This delayed hypersensitivity is characteristic of cell-mediated immunity. Allergic contact dermatitis often occurs as an acute vesicular reaction at definite sites of contact, although it may mimic a chronic irritant dermatitis.

Allergic and irritant skin reactions generally cannot be differentiated by their clinical appearance, as they may produce similar skin changes. Skin biopsies do not generally help to distinguish the reactions since, although it may be possible to separate an allergic from an irritant contact dermatitis during the first 24 to 48 hours after exposure, most reactions are seen after this time. Allergic contact dermatitis is definitively diagnosed through patch testing and establishing the probability of exposure. Irritant contact dermatitis is diagnosed through an appropriate history of exposure to one or more irritants and the exclusion of other diagnoses as necessary, i.e., by clinical evaluation and knowledge of the toxicity of workplace substances.

Ultraviolet radiation can react with certain chemicals on the skin to cause *photosensitivity contact dermatitis*. Topical photosensitivity reactions are of two types. In *phototoxic contact dermatitis* the irritant is activated by ultraviolet (UV) rays. Examples include coal tar products such as creosote and plant components such as psoralens. Phototoxic reactions commonly leave residual brown hyperpigmentation after they resolve. In *photoallergic contact dermatitis,* the UV converts chemical on the epidermis to an allergen so that an allergic reaction is provoked when there is simultaneous exposure to the chemical and UV.

Table 27.4 lists the irritants and sensitizers commonly encountered in selected occupations. More detail is available in several standard texts dealing with occupational skin disease (3,4) and with contact dermatitis (5).

Other Occupational Skin Diseases

Skin disorders caused by work have a number of clinical patterns, as illustrated in color plates 27.1 to 27.10. Selected conditions are briefly described here. Standard textbooks of dermatology should be consulted for more detail (6).

Occupational and Contact Urticaria

Urticarial reactions may occur as erythematous, edematous, pruritic, evanescent papules (hives) or as more extensive subcutaneous lesions (angioedema) that have their onset within seconds to minutes of exposure. The reactions may occur as a result of allergy, where there has been prior sensitization and there is a specific immunoglobulin E (IgE) mediating the response. IgE-mediated reactions occur more frequently in individuals with a history of atopy. Contact urticaria can also occur as a result of contact with certain substances (such as the food preservative sodium benzoate) that directly release histamine and other vasoactive substances from mast cells. Concomitant respiratory symptoms including asthma and laryngeal or epiglottic edema may occur if there is a combined respiratory and dermal exposure. Recently, latex allergy in health care workers has received much attention, especially because of the risk of anaphylaxis with inadvertent latex exposure in these individuals. However, there are numerous other occupational associations including reactions to dander from laboratory animal and small animal handlers, food handlers reacting to shellfish and other foods, hairdressers reacting to ammonium persulfate, and pharmaceutical workers sensitized to antibiotics. In some cases a positive radioallergosorbent test (RAST) may confirm the diagnosis, and scratch, prick, or open patch testing may also confirm some reactions. Where there is an allergic basis, the responsible allergen must be avoided. Antihistamines may control the reactions. Epinephrine administered subcutaneously is indicated for angioedema. Individuals should be advised to wear a Medic alert bracelet or other indicator of allergic sensitivity where there is a risk of anaphylaxis, particularly in the case of latex allergy.

Acne and Folliculitis

Heavy exposure to oils, greases, and other occlusive materials can exacerbate acne vulgaris, with its characteristic scattered open and closed comedones and cysts of the face and chest. This is seen quite frequently in young adults who have airborne exposure to cooking oil and when cooking in fast food restaurants. Certain chlorinated polycyclic hydrocarbons (polychlorinated naphthalenes, azobenzenes, azoxybenzenes, dibenzofurans, dioxins, and biphenyls) cause chloracne, a rare, specific type of acne. Affected individuals develop comedones, straw-colored cysts, milia, and papules, initially on the malar "crow's feet" area but then more generally on the face, neck, ear lobes, shoulders, abdomen, and genitalia. Blepharitis may occur. The condition is characteristically refractory to treatment and may take many years to resolve.

Folliculitis characterized by perifollicular papules and pustules commonly occurs under oil-soaked clothing.

Occupational Vitiligo

Occupational vitiligo consists of localized areas of depigmentation at sites where there has been contact with depigmenting chemicals. Causes include hydroquinone, monobenzyl ether of hydroquinone, and monomethyl ether of hydroquinone (these chemicals are used as rubber and plastic additives) as well as para-tertiary butylphenol and other alkyl phenols. These substances are toxic to melanocytes. Sometimes allergic contact dermatitis to these materials may be present. The areas of depigmentation may slowly repigment if there is no further contact with the depigmenting agent.

Granulomas

Foreign substances penetrating the skin may induce granulomas, palpable nodular lesions varying in size from a few millimeters to centimeters in diameter. Foreign body granulomas have been caused by silk, nylon, paraffin, plants, talc, and other substances. Allergic granulomas have been triggered by zirconium, beryllium, and tattoo pigments. Infectious granulomas are associated with sporotrichosis. Human hair can cause reactions in hairdressers; animal hair also causes granulomas (e.g., cow hair causes "milker's hand").

Occupational Skin Neoplasms

There are three principal types of skin cancer: squamous cell and basal cell carcinomas, which are derived from keratinocytes in the epidermis, and malignant melanomas, which are derived from the pigment-forming melanocyte cells. Squamous cell cancers arise in chronic sun-damaged skin as a result of repeated overexposure to solar UV radiation. They are common in outdoor workers. They may arise from, and often occur in association with, actinic keratoses. Squamous cell cancers resulting from sun exposure rarely metastasize. Squamous cell cancers of the lower lip are also common in outdoor workers, especially fishermen; these cancers pose a greater risk of local metastasis. Various carcinogenic polycyclic aromatic hydrocarbons such as those present in coal-tar products and in soot also cause cutaneous squamous cell cancers. Rarely squamous cell cancers may arise in old trauma or burn sites, especially if healing is long delayed. These non–sun-induced cancers show a much higher propensity to metastasize.

Sun exposure also causes basal cell cancers, particularly of the head and neck. Occupational arsenic exposure may cause basal cell cancers, which are often multiple and occur in non–sun-exposed areas of the body. Other cutaneous signs of arsenic such as palmar and plantar punctate keratoses and pigmentary changes are often also present.

Squamous cell and basal cell cancers may occur from exposure to ionizing radiation. Relatively high doses delivered over a short period of time and repeated lower doses over a long period may be carcinogenic.

Malignant melanoma is also associated with sun exposure, and particularly sun exposure before the age of 18, according to a number of studies. Melanomas may arise de novo in previously normal skin or may arise from dysplastic pigmented moles. Those with dysplastic moles who have a family history of these moles are at higher risk; the risk is higher still if there is a family history of melanoma. Individuals with dysplastic nevi thus need particular counseling to avoid sun exposure and to promptly report changes in any mole lesions. Certain other occupational exposures have been postulated to be associated with an increased risk of melanoma, but to date none has been definitively confirmed.

Physical Injuries

Physical injury may cause calluses at sites of repeated trauma. Such "occupation marks" are typical of a number of types of work (e.g., calluses on the necks of violinists). Sudden or acute friction may cause blistering. Other microtrauma results in a variety of superficial injury.

Fibrous glass (with a fiber diameter >3.4 μm) produces an intense itching reaction, with folliculitis and excoriations, particularly on sites of friction with clothing. In most workers the condition generally subsides within a week or two, but may last longer in a few individuals. Fibers may be identified in Scotch tape stripping of the skin or in skin scrapings. Excessive heat exposure may cause miliaria, a diffuse papulovesicular eruption usually on the trunk and intertriginous areas.

Table 27.1 lists various occupational skin diseases from mechanical and physical causes. These are discussed more completely in dermatology texts.

Occupational Raynaud's Disease and Vibration White Finger

A syndrome of reversible vascular spasm is seen in those working with hand-held vibrating tools such as jackhammers, pounding machines, riveting hammers, motor saws, and others.

In more severe cases there may be neuromuscular and arthritic symptoms and even bone degeneration. Cold provocation may reproduce the condition. Peripheral vascular function tests including plethysmography and use of Doppler devices may help in evaluating peripheral vascular function. Accelerometer measurements help establish the intensity and frequency of vibration generated by the suspect tool.

Improved chain-saw design (to decrease acceleration and reduce weight) has been effective in reducing the frequency in some workers, and a similar approach can be taken in design and selection of the other tools. The condition needs to be differentiated from primary Raynaud's disease and other secondary causes of Raynaud's phenomenon.

The earliest manifestation of this condition (stage 1) is blanching of one or more fingertips, with or without tingling or numbness, first noted in winter. In stage 2 the blanching extends beyond the tips of the fingers. In stage 3 there is extensive blanching, usually to the base of the fingers bilaterally; frequent attacks occur in summer as well as winter, and numbness may be apparent. In stage 4 extensive blanching occurs in winter and summer and the thumbs may be involved. Those with paresthesiae and neuromuscular symptoms such as weakening of grip strength are more impaired. The syndrome is progressive as long as exposure to vibration continues.

Occupational Infections of the Skin

Skin infections caused by contact with infectious agents at the workplace occur in many occupations; Table 27.2 gives a partial list. Bacteria, viruses, rick-

TABLE 27.1. *Mechanical and physical causes of occupational skin disease*

Mechanical
- Friction—calluses, abrasions, lichenification of skin (violinist's neck, knuckle pads in carpet layers), Koebner's phenomenon (development of lesions of psoriasis or lichen planus in traumatized area of skin)
- Pressure—blisters, nail dystrophy
- Vibration—vibration-induced white fingers or Raynaud's syndrome (vibrating equipment)

Physical
- Heat—burns, sweating (miliaria, intertriginous rashes)
- Cold—frostbite, Raynaud's symptoms
- Radiation—radiation dermatitis, skin cancers (x-ray exposure), photosensitivity eruptions phytophotodermatitis (eruption from contact with plant containing furocoumarin in presence of light)

TABLE 27.2. *Selected occupational skin infections*

Causal agent	Occupational association
Bacteria	
Bacillus anthracis	Wool sorters, tanners, postal workers
Brucella abortus, B. suis, B. melitensis	Meat packers, veterinarians
Erysipelothrix insidiosa (erysipeloid)	Fisherman, meat handlers
Francisella tularensis	Farmers, meat handlers, veterinarians, laboratory workers
Mycobacterium tuberculosis	Pathologists, veterinarians, farmers, meat handlers
Mycobacterium marinum	Fishermen, fish tank cleaners
Fungi	
Candida albicans and other *Candida* sp.	Food workers, health professions
Trichophyton, Microsporum	Health professions
Sporothrix schenckii	Farmers, nurserymen, gardeners
Blastomyces dermatitidis	Farmers, laborers
Coccidioides immitis	Farmers, construction workers
Actinomyces, Nocardia (mycetoma)	Agricultural workers
Viruses	
Pox virus (orf)	Sheep handlers, farmers, veterinarians
Paravaccinia virus (milker's nodules)	Milkers, farmers, veterinarians
Herpes simplex virus (hepatic whitlow)	Health professionals
Protozoa, metazoa, helminths, and arthropods	
Ancylostoma capillaria (larva migrans)	Agricultural workers, lifeguards
Schistosoma sp. (swimmer's itch)	Lifeguards at the lakes of north central U.S.
Acardiae, Glycyphagus sp. (foot mites)	Longshoremen
Pyemotes ventricosus (grain mites)	Grain handlers
Trombicula autumnalis (chiggers)	Outdoor workers
Ticks (Lyme disease)	Outdoor workers
Ticks (Rocky Mountain spotted fever)	Outdoor workers, pet handlers
Sarcoptes scabiei (scabies)	Health professionals, teachers
Caterpillar hairs	Outdoor workers

ettsia, fungi, protozoa, metazoa, helminths, and arthropods can be responsible.

Treatment is the same as for skin infections in the general population, together with an investigation of the circumstances of infection so that recommendations can be made to prevent further cases and to protect the workforce against spread of infection.

TABLE 27.3. *Questions to ask*

Where on your skin is the problem, and where did it begin?
When did the rash begin?
What kind of work do you do?
What happens to the skin condition on days off, on vacations, or when away from regular job duties?
What has been used to treat the condition?
What do you think might be the cause of the present skin problem?
Are other workers affected?
Have there been any changes in work practices?
Past history:
Other skin disorders
Previous contact allergies
Previous jobs
Hobbies
Medications

Work-aggravated Dermatitis

Many cutaneous diseases are exacerbated by exposure to irritants in the workplace. For example, workers with eczematous dermatitis who are exposed to irritants or physical injury in the workplace may experience flares of the disease. Similarly, because many skin diseases are aggravated by emotional stress, stressful working conditions may cause aggravation.

Papulosquamous diseases such as psoriasis and lichen planus are characterized by the development of new skin lesions at sites of physical or chemical injury—the so-called isomorphic response or Koebner's phenomenon. Individuals with psoriasis or lichen planus may develop new lesions at sites of physical injury from abrasions or burns. Patients with vitiligo are predisposed to develop new lesions at sites of physical or chemical injury. Counseling such patients to avoid cutaneous injury, so as to prevent further aggravation of the disease, is essential.

Such diseases present a challenge to the physician because of the work association. Affected workers are understandably inclined to attribute disease entirely to the work exposure. Some compensation authorities accept certain work-aggravated dermatoses for compensatory purposes, but this is certainly not uniform.

EVALUATION OF POTENTIAL OCCUPATIONAL SKIN DISEASE

The purposes of the evaluation of potential occupational skin disorder are to enable the worker to benefit from appropriate diagnosis, treatment, and prevention, and, if the condition is occupational, to identify preventable causes to decrease the risk of occupational disease to other workers. Prevention of continuing dermatitis in the affected worker and prevention of dermatitis in others requires an etiologic diagnosis, recognizing that there may multiple causal factors. It is not unusual for both management and the worker to want some quick answer to the worker's problem, so that both can get on with the job and with compensation claims. However, if the diagnosis is incorrect, the worker may be destined to have a chronic dermatitis that may never totally clear. The worker may wander from one industry to the next, one job to another, without a true understanding of why the skin eruption fails to clear. Therefore, the answer to many occupational skin diseases is not a simple job change but a full evaluation of the problem when it initially develops.

Evaluations of occupational skin disorders, whenever feasible, should be made by a dermatologist or trained occupational physicians; however, in practice a primary care physician is often the first consulted. Although the most common setting for the evaluation of an occupational skin disorder is the physician's office, a review of the workplace can be invaluable. In the workplace the physician can associate skin changes with certain hazardous substances with more certainty. Whatever the venue, a comprehensive history and physical examination are necessary to determine the cause of the skin eruption.

The History—Some Questions to Ask (Table 27.3)

Where on Your Skin Is the Problem, and Where Did It Begin?

Many occupational skin eruptions begin on exposed skin. If seen in its earliest stages, hand dermatitis may show a sharp cutoff at the wrist (where long-sleeved shirts protect the forearm). Similarly, facial eruptions may stop abruptly at the neck where the shirt collar begins (Fig. 27.1). However, as dermatitis progresses, it may involve contiguous areas of the skin and distant sites, a process known as autoeczematization or an id reaction. If seen during this flare stage, the eruption can be misdiagnosed as a nonspecific eczema unless one is careful to ask where the eruption began. Knowing where the rash began can also rule out an occupational disorder. For example, if one is assuming an airborne contact as a cause and the first expression of the rash was in a covered area of the chest (and not the face or hands), the case for an airborne exposure is weakened.

Not all occupational skin disorders develop in overtly exposed sites. If a worker is careful to wear gloves when handling corrosive or irritating liquids but has a habit of wiping soiled gloves on the trousers, the rash may initially develop on the thighs. A key question is to find out where the eruption began and to determine if known substances could have reached these sites.

When Did the Rash Begin?

Knowing the date of onset of the eruption helps in determining whether the eruption is related to some workplace activity such as a change in work practices or introduction of new materials.

Skin eruptions may begin insidiously, thus requiring a number of weeks or months to become obvious. Determining when the first signs of skin irritation developed can facilitate efforts to relate them as closely as possible to some workplace activity or production change.

What Kind of Work Do You Do?

The worker needs to be specific in describing the job so that the physician has a full understanding of job activities. All materials with potential for worker exposure, especially irritants or allergens, should be reviewed. Some workers may say that they work with caustic liquids, but in fact one discovers that these substances are contained in totally enclosed systems and no skin contact is possible. Other workers may neglect to mention gross exposure to low-grade irritants, compounds they think could not produce a skin rash. The physician should realize the importance of a thorough job history to avoid overlooking "trivial" exposures as a cause of the skin irritation. It is critical to establish whether the worker has the potential for a true contact with the materials in question and whether gloves or other personal protective equipment are used. Often a useful way to elicit this information is to have the worker progressively explain his tasks and work exposures over the course of a workday. It is important to inquire about the skin-cleaning methods worker's use,

TABLE 27.4. *Some occupations and risk of dermatitis*

Occupation	Irritants	Sensitizers	Contact urticaria
Agriculture (farmers, animal handlers, and keepers)	Artificial fertilizers, disinfectants and cleansers for milking utensils, petrol, diesel oil	Rubber (boots, gloves, milking machines), cement, paints, local remedies for veterinary use, wood preservatives, plants, pesticides, antibiotics and preservatives in animal feed (quindoxin, ethoxyquine), penicillin for mastitis, cobalt in animal feed	Animal hair
Artists	Solvents, clay, plaster	Turpentine, cobalt, nickel and chromate in pigments, azo dyes, colophony, epoxy-, acrylic-, formaldehyde resins	
Automobile mechanics	Solvents, oils, cutting oils, paints, hand cleansers	Chromate (primers, anticorrosives, oils, welding fumes and cutting oils), nickel, cobalt, rubber, epoxy and acrylic resins, dipentene in thinners	
Baking and pastrymaking	Flour, detergents	Citrus fruits, flour improvers, thiamine, spices (cinnamon, cardamon), essential oils, food dyes	
Bartenders	Detergents, citrus fruits	Flavoring agents	
Bathing attendants	Detergents	Antimicrobial agents, formaldehyde, essential oils	
Bookbinders	Glues, solvents, paper	Glues, formaldehyde, plastic monomers	
Building trade	Cement, chalk, hydrochloric and hydrofluoric acids, glasswool, wood preservatives, organic tin compounds	Cement (chromate, cobalt), rubber and leather gloves, additives in shale oils, glues (phenol- or urea-formaldehyde resins), wood preservatives, teak, tar, epoxy resin, polyurethanes, rubber strip seals, joining material	Animal tissues
Butchers	Detergents, meat, entrails	Nickel	
Canning industry	Brine, syrup, prawns, and shrimps	Asparagus, carrots, preservatives (hexamethylene tetramine in fish canning), rubber gloves	Fruits, vegetables
Carpenters, cabinetmakers, timbermen	French polish, solvents, glues, cleansers, wood preservatives (also phototoxic), glass fiber	Exotic woods (teak, mahogany, rosewood, etc.), glues, polishes, turpentine, nickel, rubber (handles), colophony, epoxy-, acrylic-formaldehyde-, isocyanate resins	
Chemical and pharmaceutical industry	Numerous and specific for each workplace	Numerous and specific for each workplace	
Cleaning work	Detergents, solvents	Rubber gloves, nickel, formaldehyde	
Coal miners	Stone dust, coal dust, oil, grease, wood preservatives, cement, powdered limestone	Rubber (boots), face masks, explosives, chromatic and cobalt in cement	
Cooks, catering industry	Detergents, dressings, vinegar, fish, meat and vegetable juices	Vegetables (onions, garlic, lemons, lettuce, artichokes), knife handles (exotic woods), spices, formaldehyde	Meat, fish, fruits, vegetables
Dentists and dental technicians	Soap, detergents, acrylic monomer, fluxes	Local anesthetics (tetracaine, procaine), mercury, rubber, UV-hardening acrylates acrylic monomer, disinfectants (formaldehyde, eugenol), nickel, epoxy resin (filling), methylmethacrylate, periodontal dressing (balsam of Peru, colophony, eugenol), the catalyst methyl-p-toluenesulfonate in plastics used for sealing teeth	Saliva
Dyers	Solvents, oxidizing and reducing agents, hypochlorite, hair removers	Dyes, chromate, formaldehyde	
Electricians	Soldering flux	Soldering flux, insulating tape (rubber, resin, tar), rubber, nickel, bitumen, epoxy resins, glues (phenol formaldehyde), polyurethanes	

Continued on next page

TABLE 27.4. *Continued*

Occupation	Irritants	Sensitizers	Contact urticaria
Enamel workers	Enamel powder	Chromate, nickel, cobalt	
Fishing	Wet work, friction, oils, petrol, redfeed from mackerel	Tars, organic dyes in nets, rubber boots, rubber gloves	Fish, "aquatic irritant reactions" from toxins in sea organisms
Floor layers	Solvents, detergents	Chromate (cement), epoxy resin, glues (phenol and urea formaldehyde), exotic woods, acrylates, varnish (urea formaldehyde), polyurethanes	
Florists, gardeners, plant growers	Manure, bulbs, fertilizers, pesticides	Plants (*Primula obconica,* chrysanthemum, tulips, narcissus, daffodils, alstromeria), formaldehyde, pesticides (e.g., thiuramsulfides), lichens (e.g., reindeer moss)	
Food industry, food handler	Detergents, vegetables	Rubber gloves, spices, vegetables, preservatives	Vegetables, fruit, meat, fish
Foundry work	Oils, hand cleansers	Phenol- and carbamide formaldehyde, furan-, epoxy resins, chromate (cement, gloves, bricks)	
Glaziers	Rubber, epoxy resin, joining material, exotic wood		
Hairdressers and barbers	Shampoos, soaps, permanent wave liquids, bleaching agents	Hair and eyebrow dyes, rubber, nickel, perfumes	Ammonium persulfate
Histology technicians	Solvents, formaldehyde	Formaldehyde, glutaraldehyde, organic dyes, acrylates	
Hospital personnel	Disinfectants, quaternary ammonium compounds, hand creams, soaps, detergents	Rubber gloves, formaldehyde, antibacterial agents, piperazine, phenothiazines, hand creams, nickel, glutaraldehyde, acrylic monomer, nitrogen mustard, local anesthetics	
Household work	Detergents, wet work, solvents, polishes, vegetables	Rubber (gloves), nickel, chromate, flowers and plants, turpentine (polishes), hand creams and lotions, handles of knives and irons, balsams, spices, citrus fruits	Vegetables, fruit, meat, fish, spices
Jewelers	Solvents, fluxes	Nickel, epoxy resins, enamels (chromate, nickel, cobalt)	
Laundry workers	Detergents, bleaches, solvents	Formaldehyde	
Manicurists, beauticians	Wet work	Formaldehyde, cosmetics, acrylic monomers (nails), nail polish (sulfonamide-formaldehyde plastic), perfume	
Masons	Cement, chalk, bricks, acids	Chromate and cobalt in cement, rubber and leather gloves, epoxy resin, exotic woods	
Mechanics	Solvents, detergents, degreasers, lubricants, oils, cooling system fluids, battery acid, soldering flux	Rubber, chromate, nickel, epoxy resin	
Metal workers	Cutting and drilling oils, hand cleansers, solvents	Nickel, chromate (antirust agents and dyes, welding fumes), cobalt, antibacterial agents, and antioxidants in cutting oils; chromate, cobalt, nickel may be found in cutting oil after it has been in use	
Office workers	Photocopy paper, NCR paper	Rubber (erasing rubber, mats, cords, finger stalls), nickel (clips, scissors, typewriters), copying papers, glue, feltpen dyes	

Painters	Solvents, turpentine, thinner, paints, wallpaper adhesive	Turpentine, thinner containing turpentine or dipentene (limonene), cobalt (dyes, driers), chromate (green, yellow), polyurethane-, epoxy-, acrylic resins, glues (urea- and phenol formaldehyde), varnish (colophony, urea formaldehyde), preservatives in water-based paints and glues (e.g., chloracetamide, methylol chloracetamide), putty (epoxy, acrylate, formaldehyde resins, polyurethane)	
Photography	Alkalis, reducing and oxidizing agents, solvents	Metol (*p*-aminophenol), color developers (azo compounds), chromate, formaldehyde	
Plastic industry	Solvents, styrene, oxidizing agents, acids	Low molecular raw material, hardeners, additives, dyes	
Platers	Solvents, paints	Chromate in paints and on zinc galvanized sheets, glues	
Plating industry, electroplating	Metal cleaners, alkalis, acids, detergents, heat, dust from metal blasting	Chromate, nickel, cobalt, gold, mercury, rubber gloves	
Plumbers	Oils, hand cleansers, soldering flux	Rubber (gloves, packings, tubes), nickel, chromate (cement, antirust paint), glues, hydrazine	
Printers	Solvents	Nickel, chromate, cobalt, colophony, paper finishes, glues, turpentine, azo dyes, formaldehyde, printing plates (acrylates and other chemicals), UV-hardening acrylates in printing ink, rubber gloves	
Radio, television, electronic repairmen	Soldering flux	Soldering flux (hydrazine), epoxy resin, colophony (soldering), nickel, chromate	
Restaurant personnel	Detergents, vegetables, citrus fruits, shrimps, herring	Nickel spices, vegetables, exotic wood (knife handle)	Vegetables, fruit, meat, fish
Road workers	Sand/oil mixture, hand cleansers,) asphalt (phototoxic	Cement, gloves (leather, rubber), epoxy resin, tar, chromate in antirust paint	
Rubber workers	Talcum, zinc stearate, solvents	Rubber chemicals, organic dyes, tars, colophony, chromate, cobalt, phenol-formaldehyde resin	
Shoemakers	Solvents	Leather (formaldehyde, chromate, dyes), rubber, colophony, glues (e.g., p-tert, butylphenol formaldehyde)	
Shop assistants	Detergents vegetables, fruit, meat, fish	Nickel	Fruits, vegetables
Tanners	Acids alkalis, reducing and oxidizing agents	Chromate; formaldehyde, vegetable tanning agents, glutaraldehyde, finishes, antimildew agents, dyes, resins	
Textile workers	Solvents, bleaching agents, fibers	Finishes (formaldehyde resins), dyes, mordants, nickel, diazo paper	
Veterinarians	Hypochlorite, quaternary ammonium compounds, cresol, rectal and vaginal examination of cattle	Rubber gloves, antibiotics (penicillin, streptomycin, neomycin, tylosine tartrate, virginiamycin), antimycotic agents; mercaptobenzthiazole (MBT) in medicaments (tuberculin for injection in animals can elicit reactions on the hands)	Animal hair and dander, cow placenta, animal tissues
Welders	Oil	Chromate (welding fumes, gloves), nickel, cobalt	
Woodworkers		Woods, colophony, turpentine, balsams, tars, lacquers, *Frullania,* lichens, glues, wood preservatives	

Adapted from Fregert S. *Manual of contact dermatitis,* 2nd ed. Chicago: Year Book, 1981.

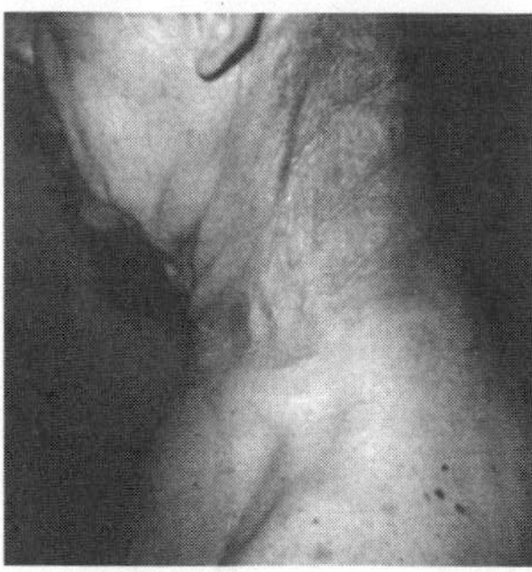

FIG. 27.1. This eruption involves the neck and stops abruptly at the face and shoulders. The distribution suggests an airborne contactant, with the face protected by the full face mask the worker was using and the trunk protected by a shirt and collar.

and about the environmental conditions during work (temperature, humidity, dustiness, etc.).

As discussed in Chapter 2, the Hazard Communication Standard stipulates that all workers in certain industries should be informed about the materials with which they work and their respective toxicity. In most cases, the first step in evaluating a potential occupational skin disease is to suggest that the worker bring in the data sheets for all substances the worker may use in the course of his or her job duties.

What Happens to the Skin Condition on Days Off, on Vacations, or Away from Job Duties?

In many cases of occupational contact dermatitis, the eruption worsens as the workweek progresses and stabilizes or lessens on weekends and vacations. However, after many months of recurrent eruptions, this pattern may change, and the skin irritation may not improve. The initial pattern of clearing following removal from certain job activities is helpful in establishing a potential link between the rash and an occupational substance.

The time relationship between exposure and reaction for contact dermatitis depends on the cause. Acute irritants cause a fairly immediate reaction, which usually resolves after cessation of exposure. Cumulative insult dermatitis may begin rather insidiously. Episodes of allergic contact dermatitis are characteristically delayed a few days after exposure, so that in a person working a normal workweek the eruption may begin to worsen around midweek, be present at the weekend, and improve somewhat on Monday and Tuesday.

What Are Your Opinions as to How Work Is Causing Your Condition?

Does the worker feel the dermatitis is exacerbated by specific work activities? It is quite appropriate to ask the worker for whatever information he or she has with regard to the skin eruption. One should exercise judgment in sorting through the information that begins to accumulate, but never overlook the fact that it is often the worker who will suggest important possibilities that must be explored.

Are Other Workers Affected?

It is useful to know whether one is dealing with an isolated case (which may suggest an allergic contact dermatitis) or with numerous cases (which may suggest an irritant contact dermatitis). One should be cautioned, however, in evaluating alleged cases, that interviews and examinations of these workers may uncover conditions not related to the present problem and/or that are nonoccupational in origin.

Have There Been Any Changes in Work Practices?

A change in the rate of production may cause workers to work more quickly and overlook safe work practices. Sometimes, a new material has been introduced into the process, and shortly thereafter a number of skin eruptions are noted. Ask about protective gear that workers are using. Sometimes appropriate gloves are available, but replacement of the gloves is not done on a regular basis. Despite their wear, gloves may be replaced only when workers feel they need to be replaced, a practice that tends to allow for cracks to appear and thus contamination of the worker's skin. Inquire about the kind of soap that is available in the workplace. Although a wide range of work materials can cause a rash, recently introduced abrasive soaps may also be responsible for skin eruptions.

Past Medical History

Other skin disorders such as psoriasis should always be considered in the differential diagnosis. Always ask about past skin problems. A palmar eruption, for example, that one is labeling as an occupational contact dermatitis in fact may be an expression of psoriasis. Idiopathic lichen planus can also be confused with occupational skin eruptions.

Atopic individuals have up to a 13-fold greater risk of developing an occupational skin problem, especially irritant reactions, than nonatopics. A history of previous atopic dermatitis rather than previous respiratory allergies is a better prognosticator of future work-related dermatitis.

Previous Contact Allergies

One should inquire about other contactants or substances that might have resulted in previous skin eruptions. Allergies to chromium and to nickel have been associated with persistent and recurrent skin eruptions that are difficult to eliminate despite apparent cessation of contact.

Previous Jobs and Present Part-time Jobs

A good occupational history of substances used in previous jobs can be helpful in evaluating the present eruption. For example, if a worker used an epoxy resin in the past (especially if there is a history of a rash during that time), one can focus on the role of the epoxy resin during the present job. A history of irritant dermatitis secondary to wet work in previous jobs can suggest that a similar problem is recurring.

One should also ask about part-time work. A physician may not uncover a cause for a skin eruption in company A, but learning that the affected employee is a part-time hair stylist in company B (where numerous opportunities for irritant exposures exist) can uncover the problem.

Hobbies

Hobbies may present opportunities for the development of contact dermatitis. An example is the use of epoxy resins and other glues in model airplane building or of pesticides and herbicides and exotic plants in gardening.

What Has Been Used to Treat the Condition?

An eruption may not clear because of inadequate therapy or because the worker is using a preparation that is itself an irritant or allergen. Preservatives in ointments or topical antibiotics such as neomycin can be allergens. A number of home, traditional, and alternative medications and herbal applications can contain irritants or sensitizers. Therefore, all medications that have been used in an attempt to treat the eruption should be reviewed in a search for a possible secondary dermatitis.

Medications

Systemic medications can occasionally explain an unusual contact dermatitis. For example, a worker became sensitized to ethylenediamine from Mycolog cream, which was used on a hand rash. The rash, which had totally cleared, recurred when the worker was prescribed aminophylline (contains theophylline and ethylenediamine) for asthma.

Physical Examination

A complete skin examination is necessary to determine the presence of other dermatologic conditions, such as psoriasis, lichen planus, or atopic eczema, that may explain the present skin condition. In the case of hand dermatitis the feet should always be examined carefully to exclude the possibility of a fungal infection of the feet with an id reaction on the hands.

A thorough skin examination will also determine the extent of the eruption, which will ultimately influence both the person's capability of returning to work and the aggressiveness of therapy. Mild local eruptions can be treated without interruption of job duties, but extensive rashes often require both time off and aggressive treatment. Determination of the distribution of the rash can aid in the diagnosis. Ninety percent of cases of occupational contact dermatitis involve the hand; potential cases without hand involvement may thus require explanation. Eruptions involving the face and hands may suggest a component of airborne contact dermatitis.

Work-site Evaluation

An optimal place to evaluate an occupational skin disease is the workplace. Planning a work-site visit requires preparation and diplomacy to be successful. Permission of management must be obtained. The purpose and likely length of the visit, and any specific requirements such as an examination area or need to review MSDSs or OSHA logs is best explained to management beforehand. The physician needs to maintain a good working relationship with management and labor and to avoid any hint of bias and to emphasize that the purpose of the visit is health related. If one loses the trust of any party, the investigation becomes more difficult and sometimes impossible.

Where possible, the physician should tour the plant with representatives of all interested groups but insist that someone familiar with both production and substances used be available to answer questions of a technical nature. It is important to have an overview of the process of production, including the various stages and potential for exposure to hazardous materials. Then one can become more specific in the evaluation of the individual worker. Ideally, one should watch the worker perform the task, especially so-called normal operations. It is also very helpful to see the normal problems that arise throughout the day. There may be no physical contact with chemicals of concern during normal operations, but when a machine breaks down, which may be often, ample opportunity for gross exposure may exist. One should note the protective gear that a worker uses, as well as personal hygiene, such as eating and smoking habits. The facilities used to wash or clean the skin should be visited, and the skin cleaning preparations and procedures noted.

After a plant tour, the physician should have a thorough understanding of the potential for certain materials to cause skin irritations. A closing meeting, where appropriate with both management and labor, should be held so that the physician can summarize impressions, ask additional questions, make appropriate recommendations, and outline any subsequent steps. Specific conclusions are not recommended about items where additional requested information may change an opinion.

The work-site evaluation also gives an opportunity to identify the potential for improvement and to identify alternative sites for job placement. In addressing workplace issues, the physician should be cognizant of the concerns of workers and management that may not have been specifically raised, such as whether medical conditions in other workers are contagious, and whether chemicals that present a skin hazard also present systemic, carcinogenic, reproductive, or other hazards.

Based on the medical office evaluation and a work-site visit, an opinion can usually be formulated as to whether an occupational skin disease exists. This opinion is based on the history, appearance, and distribution of the lesions; a review of workplace materials (including workers' hobbies); a physical examination; and, if applicable, the results of diagnostic tests. If an irritant or an allergic contact dermatitis is suspected, removal of the allergen or irritant is indicated. If the condition improves, the diagnostic accuracy of an occupational skin disorder is enhanced.

DIAGNOSTIC TESTING FOR OCCUPATIONAL SKIN DISEASE

Role of Patch Testing

Diagnostic patch tests reveal only allergic contact sensitization. Patch testing cannot be used to determine the presence of an irritant contact dermatitis, except to exclude tested allergens as causes of allergic contact dermatitis. If an allergen is believed to be the possible cause of an occupational skin disease, patch tests can be confirmatory. To ensure validity, the patch testing should be performed only by a physician who is trained and experienced in its use. Patch testing involves the standardized application of chemicals (in a nonirritating concentration) onto the skin of the patient. Either strips of cellulose disks (Al-test) or aluminum chambers (Finn Chambers) are applied to the skin, generally to the back, for 48 hours, after which the test strips are removed and the areas examined. The test sites are reevaluated again after an additional 48 hours. True allergic reactions have a fairly typical appearance; however, both false-positive and false-negative reactions can occur, and differentiation requires a great deal of observer experience.

Generally sets of allergens are tested at the same time; the most commonly used set is of common contactants, the allergens that are most commonly positive at the time. The exception is that patch testing is rarely done for poison ivy, since sensitization is so common in the U.S. population and the clinical diagnosis is reliable.

Patch testing has certain limitations. Industrial substances or unknown compounds from the work-site area cannot simply be taken and applied to a worker's back. It is essential to know that the product of chemical will not irritate human skin under the circumstances of application. Indiscriminate patch testing could also sensitize the worker to different substances to which the worker was not previously sensitized. The reader is referred to textbooks of occupational and contact dermatitis (3–5) for further discussion of the role of patch testing in diagnosing occupational skin diseases.

Skin Biopsy

Skin biopsy is rarely useful in the diagnosis or management of contact dermatitis, but may be necessary for the diagnosis of a number of other types of occupational skin disease.

Other Investigations

Other investigations that are occasionally useful include microscopic examination of skin scrapings after KOH digestion for fungi and yeasts; scrapings or microscopy of adhesive tape strippings of the epidermis for fibrous glass; cultures for skin infections; and RAST tests for specific IgE to identify possible causes for allergic urticarial reactions (e.g., in possible latex reactions).

PREVENTIVE MANAGEMENT

After determining the presence of either allergic contact dermatitis or an irritant contact reaction and its respective cause, the physician should then advise on the need to avoid future exposure to the offending substance. This may require a change of job placement or even of employer, although this does not always result in cure (see section on prognosis, below), or use of the exposure minimization techniques described in this section. In the case of allergic sensitization, the worker must be carefully instructed about other sources of the offending allergen and significant sources of cross-sensitizers.

Product or Chemical Substitution

Another substance that is less strongly irritating or allergenic may be introduced into an industrial process. Examples could include the use of a relatively nonirritating metal-working fluid to replace a formulation that was causing a high incidence of irritant reactions.

Engineering and Hygienic Controls

These controls might include the use of closed systems for mixing or transferring chemicals so that there was no need for direct handling by the workers. If airborne contact is the cause of the skin problem, the ventilation system may be altered to prevent or minimize skin contact. General housekeeping measures, especially to clean surface contamination, may greatly reduce skin exposure.

Personal Protective Measures

A range of personal protective clothing, from gloves, boots, and aprons to impervious suits, is available. To ensure effectiveness, the fabric must be impervious or at least resistant to the agent against which protection is desired. Because occlusion against the skin by gloves or other protective clothing will increase the percutaneous absorption of most chemicals, it is important that protective clothing be discarded once it is contaminated and that protective clothing be donned when the skin is relatively clean of contaminants. Sweating under gloves can irritate the skin; cotton liners or undergloves help reduce this problem. Protective barrier creams may be used on the hands and other parts of the skin including the face, but they are a poor substitute for protective clothing because the integrity of the so-called impenetrable barrier is difficult to maintain. Where a high degree of protection is not essential, barrier creams may make it easier to wash dirt and other contaminants from the skin.

Personal Hygiene

Contaminating chemicals should be remove promptly from the skin; washing facilities must be readily available if this recommendation is to be achievable. Mild soap and water is usually the best solvent and is normally available in considerable quantity compared with potential alternatives. Where workers are exposed to hazardous chemicals that may persist on skin and clothing, showering, shampooing hair, and changing clothes before leaving the work site may be indicated. Care must be taken in some situations that excessive cleansing and abrasive soaps or solvents used for cleaning are not contributing to skin damage. If frequent washing of hands and other areas is necessary, use of a mild emollient product after washing should be considered. Other personal hygienic measures, such as not smoking, eating, or drinking at the workstation, may also be relevant to reducing exposure.

Administrative Controls and Proactive Management

Individuals who have current dermatitis or a history of allergy or frequent irritation from particular work substances or conditions may need to be placed in jobs that do not entail casual exposure.

More fundamentally, some individuals are known to be at a higher risk of skin disease from certain types of work. Ideally, such individuals would not be placed in these jobs. For example atopics who become hairdressers have a higher frequency of job-related dermatitis than nonatopics. Historically, some such workers were excluded from jobs on the basis of a preemployment examination. The Americans with Disability Act of 1991 affords job protections to such individuals, as discussed in Chapter 5. Nevertheless, some careers may not be wise choices for some susceptible individuals were they in full possession of the facts at the time they made a career choice. Ideally, this issue would be discussed at the time of career selection and/or by the pediatrician, dermatologist, or allergist treating such individuals during the teenage years.

TREATMENT

Local Topical Treatment of Contact Dermatitis

Topical steroid preparations have been a mainstay of the treatment of contact dermatitis for many years. In cases of localized acute contact dermatitis, or in patients in whom even a short course of systemic steroids is contraindicated, a potent topical corticosteroid cream can be used. Potent steroids, however, should not be used on the face or intertriginous areas for periods longer than 1 to 2 weeks. In any case, if high-potency steroids are prescribed, the worker should be closely monitored; as the eruption begins to clear, lower-potency steroids should be instituted.

Wet compresses help dry acute, weeping lesions. An astringent solution such as Domeboro (aluminum sulfate and calcium acetate, 1 part to 20 of water) is applied with a moistened cloth for 20 to 30 minutes several times a day. In the case of extensive lesions, the patient can bathe in a solution of oatmeal (Aveeno).

In the case of chronic contact dermatitis, the most important component of treatment may be emollients to decrease itching and reduce scaling. Numerous lubricants are available; their effectiveness depends both on the type of lubricant and the frequency of application. Some lubricants may be applied up to 10 to 15 times a day. Patient acceptance of the lubricant product is important, some ointments are too greasy for some patients. Low- to medium-strength topical steroids such as hydrocortisone and hydrocortisone valerate are used, usually in an ointment form.

Excessive washing particularly of the hands should be avoided when there is contact dermatitis. Fissured crusted lesions readily become secondarily infected; treatment with an antibiotic ointment such as erythromycin ophthalmic ointment, oral erythromycin, or another antibiotic active against staphylococcus and streptococcus may be indicated. Painful fissures can be carefully coated with a cyanoacrylate (Krazy Glue, Super Glue), with care taken to ensure that the fingers are not glued together. Otherwise, the patient should avoid the use of Band-Aids or other adhesives directly on the skin; instead, light cotton gloves should be used to protect the hands. In the case of lesions localized to a finger, use of a cotton finger cot may be helpful.

Sedation with cyproheptadine hydrochloride (Periacten), diphenhydramine (Benadryl), or hydroxyxine hydrochloride (Atarax) may help sleepless pruritic patients. Antihistamines are most helpful for their soporific and sedating properties. Itching in contact dermatitis is usually best treated with steroids rather than with antihistamines.

Treatment of hand dermatitis warrants special attention. Although the hand represents about 5% of the total body surface, hand dermatitis can be disabling for many activities. A weeping or blistering eruption leading to painful fissures can be totally incapacitating for many tasks even if only a few fingers are affected, and therefore should be treated efficiently and aggressively.

Although corticosteroids have been widely used in treatment of contact dermatitis, their effect is nonspecific. Several new agents are appearing on the market or are under development that may have a more specific antiinflammatory effect in contact dermatitis. These include topical tacrolimus, which is demonstrably effective in atopic dermatitis. A number of such agents should come into use in the next several years.

Systemic Steroids

In severe acute eruptions characterized by extensive involvement with weeping and inflammation, oral prednisone is effective. Generally 60 mg per day initially, tapered gradually over 10 to 14 days, will clear almost all eczematous eruptions. As with high-potency topical steroids, systemic steroid therapy should not be given as a means of keeping a worker on the job when the environment is the cause of the persistent skin problems. In contrast with their effective use in acute dermatitis, systemic steroids should be used with caution in chronic dermatitis because of the difficulty of discontinuing the steroid therapy as the dermatitis recurs when the dose is reduced or suspended. The first line of treatment in these conditions should be emollients and low- to medium-strength topical steroids; in selected cases 40 mg Kenalog intramuscularly may give benefit for 3 to 6 weeks.

PROGNOSIS OF OCCUPATIONAL CONTACT DERMATITIS—PERSISTENT POSTOCCUPATIONAL DERMATITIS

It has long been recognized that severe occupational contact dermatitis carries a surprisingly poor prognosis in some individuals in that the condition persists despite treatment and the apparent removal of the triggering exposures. Persistence of dermatitis has been known to be a particular problem with chromium and nickel allergy, where it has been sometimes attributed to the presence of small amounts of these metals, which are ubiquitous in the work, home, and general environments. Most follow-up studies have found that persistence is a much greater problem in atopics, and is also associated with delays in instituting treatment.

The most complete follow-up study was that of Wall and Gebauer (7,8), who were able to follow 96% of 993 cases of occupational contact dermatitis that had occurred over an 8-year period (1980–1987) in the state of Western Australia. The follow-up period was more than 6 months in all cases and ranged up to 8 years. Seventy-five percent of the subjects were reexamined. Overall, 54% were still suffering from occupational dermatitis and/or a complication at the time of follow-up. Fifty-four percent were still in the same job; of these individuals 68% still had occupational skin disease or a complication. Forty-three percent were in a different job, but 37% of these still had occupational skin disease or a complication. Overall, 61% of subjects had lost work time, 23% had reduced income, and 60% of males and 73% of females reported interference with life and/or leisure activities. Over 10% had evolved into what the authors described as *persistent postoccupational dermatitis*. In these cases there was no apparent continuing cause for dermatitis. The most common association was with chromate allergy in men and nickel allergy in women, but a wide range of allergic and irritant reactions had preceded the persistent postoccupational dermatitis. Neither time in the job before developing dermatitis, age of the worker, nor duration of occupational skin disease appeared to predispose to the persistent dermatitis. This condition was not a phenomenon generated through workers compensation; 25% of those with persistent postoccupational dermatitis had never sought compensation, and 32% who received compensation initially no longer received it despite the continued problems.

The persistence of some cases of occupational dermatitis remains an unsolved problem. It appears to parallel conditions in other organ systems where following a severe inflammatory insult there is persistent hypersensitivity and a heightened inflammatory response to trivial insults. These conditions include persistent airway reactivity in occupational pulmonary disease and persistent nasal and sinus inflammation following severe nasal chemical insults. The current therapeutic approach (9) is to continue conventional treatment, with special care that the therapy is not exacerbating the condition through secondary irritation or allergy from a medication component, and to ensure as far as possible complete avoidance of known exposures that trigger reactions.

REFERENCES

1. Emmett EA. Occupational contact dermatitis I: incidence and return to work pressures. *Am J Contact Derm* 2002;13:30–34.
2. Smit H, Coenraads P-J, Emmett E. Dermatoses. In: McDonald JC, ed. *Epidemiology of work-related diseases.* London: BMJ Publishing Group, 1995:143–164.
3. Adams RM. *Occupational skin disease,* 3rd ed. Philadelphia: WB Saunders, 1999.
4. Marks JG, DeLeo VA *Occupational and contact dermatitis.* Philadelphia: Mosby, 1997.
5. Rietschel RL, Fowler JF. *Fisher's contact dermatitis,* 5th ed. Philadelphia: Lippincott Williams & Wilkins, 2001.
6. Freedberg TM, Eisen AZ, Wolff K, et al. *Fitzpatrick's dermatology in general medicine,* 5th ed. New York: McGraw-Hill, 1999.
7. Wall L, Gebauer K. Occupational skin disease in Western Australia. *Contact Dermatitis* 1991;24:101–109.
8. Wall L, Gebauer K. A follow-up study of occupational skin disease in Western Australia. *Contact Dermatitis* 1991;24:241–243.
9. Emmett EA. Occupational contact dermatitis II: risk assessment and prognosis. *Am J Contact Derm* 2003 (in press).

28

Psychiatric Aspects of Occupational Medicine

Stuart Gitlow and Peter J. Holland

Most medical illness isn't a simple yes or no at the outset. Blood pressure slowly rises from normal to hypertensive. A skin lesion grows and invades surrounding tissue. The thyroid-stimulating hormone (TSH) is slightly elevated but the other thyroid tests are within normal limits. While it is straightforward to identify the patient who meets criteria for posttraumatic stress disorder following a dangerous workplace trauma, it is also straightforward to identify as hypertensive the patient who presents with a pressure of 180/100. What's more difficult is to identify the patients who fall on the cusp, a cusp that exists in psychiatry as it does in other specialties. But in psychiatry there are almost never any measurements, any numbers, or any blood levels that can assist in the diagnosis. The occupational specialist must therefore be acquainted with the identification and evaluation of psychiatric symptoms likely to be found in the workplace.

The normal emotions of depression and anxiety, the normal behaviors of eating and sleeping, and the routine social activities of gambling and consuming alcohol can all go awry in response to a multitude of possible stressors. Sometimes these stressors are internal, based on our genetic composition, biology, or on now-internalized environmental stimuli of childhood. At other times, the stressors are external—a hazardous workplace, a troubled marriage, or a sick child. Generally, though, that which falls under the psychiatric rubric is often a combination of the two. Individuals with a certain genetic makeup, who have grown up learning a certain set of defense mechanisms against the difficulties of life, and who are placed within certain stressful environments may have a transition from a "normal" response to an "abnormal" response. This transition is often gradual, difficult for the individual to identify, and frequently denied as a result of both assumed and real stigmas. Sometimes the presentation is dramatic and obvious.

While treatment intensity may be varied depending on the severity of psychiatric symptoms, the patient with mild to moderate symptoms thought to be the result of workplace stress requires treatment just as does the patient with more severe symptoms thought to be the result of genetic predisposition. For the initial stages of referral and treatment, it can often be helpful to view the psychiatric status of the patient simply in terms of the patient's symptoms rather than by attempting to determine their origin.

PSYCHIATRIC ILLNESS

Within the occupational setting, the clinician is likely to encounter the full gamut of possible psychiatric illness. The most frequently observed symptoms can be divided into three groups: those affecting mood, those affecting anxiety, and those affecting perception. Substance use can produce symptoms falling within any of these symptom categories.

Mental Status Examination

Prior to discussing the symptom profiles, an approach to evaluating existing symptoms should be established. The cornerstone of psychiatric diagnosis and evaluation is the mental status examination, an assessment of a patient's mood, presentation, speech pattern, thought processes, and cognition. Although the complexity and depth of the examination depend on the nature of the problem and the expertise of the clinician, a routine approach is recommended.

Appearance is the first area of interest. Beyond the usual question as to whether patients appear to be their age, we are concerned with their hygiene, their dress, and their level of comfort with the process. Does the patient wear many rings and have black fingernail polish? Is her hair dyed several different colors? Does the patient pull his chair right next to yours, or does he pull it away to place it next to the door? Does he make good eye contact or does he look away the moment you look at him?

Speech is observed for rate, rhythm, and volume. Is there a significant delay prior to responding to questions? Is it possible to interrupt the patient? Does the patient randomly begin talking about a new topic, entirely disconnected from the previous conversation?

Mood can be described both subjectively and objectively. The patient may state that he feels fine, but easily break into tears when describing a stressful event. The patient might describe a horrible tragedy, claiming to have been saddened by the event, but smile while relating the information. An overall description of the patient's emotional expression is appropriate here as well, with an indication as to whether a broad or narrow range of expression is present.

Thought form refers to the logic of the patient's presented discussion. *Thought content* refers to the ideas presented by the patient. If the patient describes the messages that he is receiving from his television each night, he has abnormal thought content. If as he talks about this, his description varies without logic among several subjects and occasionally contains inappropriate rhyme, he has abnormal thought form. It must be determined if the patient has suicidal or homicidal ideation.

Perception is analyzed to determine if hallucinations are present. Patients should always be asked if they are experiencing the feeling that voices in their head are not their own thoughts, or if they believe they are seeing things that others can't see.

Finally, a series of questions are asked to determine the patient's level of alertness, orientation, concentration, memory, intellect, insight, and judgment, all falling into the broad category of *sensorium.*

Whenever serious psychopathology is suspected, consultation with a psychiatrist is essential. Any patient with a psychotic illness or a severe affective disorder is ideally followed at regular intervals by a psychiatrist.

Substance Use

Note that the heading for this section uses the word "use" rather than "abuse" or "dependence." Use of certain substances as prescribed or in a socially acceptable manner may well impact the patient's functional ability, or may lead to the presentation of an apparent psychiatric disorder, but such use may not necessarily fall into the abuse or dependence categories. As described in the introduction, it is essentially meaningless to attempt to determine whether the patient is using drugs or alcohol in response to perceived stress or in response to preexisting psychiatric symptoms.

Substance use disorders are diagnosed independently of quantity or frequency of use. The diagnosis is determined based on whether the patient uses despite himself. That is, is the patient harming himself, aware that he is harming himself or placing himself at substantial risk, and yet continuing to use despite that knowledge? If Mr. Smith drinks a couple of shots with his friends after work each day, and then goes home and drinks three or four beers, but all is well with his marriage, his job, and his health, he may not have a substance use disorder. In contrast, if Mr. Jones has been told of his liver abnormalities, has received one driving while intoxicated (DWI) citation, and occasionally gets into fights with peers at the bar, and yet continues to stop at the bar each Friday, he has a substance use disorder. Note that Mr. Jones drinks far less than Mr. Smith, yet it is Mr. Jones who needs medical attention most urgently. Mr. Smith will likely develop alcohol-related medical illness, but may have no difficulty stopping his alcohol intake once this takes place.

Substance use has a tendency to lead to psychiatric symptoms consistent with mood, anxiety, or psychotic disorders. This masquerade of almost any other illness, whether the substances are being used as prescribed or not, needs to be evaluated as a possible explanation of presenting symptoms. Ongoing use of alcohol, benzodiazepines such as Valium, nonbenzodiazepine sedatives such as Ambien and Sonata, muscle relaxants such as Soma, or any other drug cross-tolerant with alcohol can produce depressive symptoms over time. These depressive symptoms often include a lack of motivation and energy that quickly becomes apparent in the workplace. Patients may not recall without prompting the sleeping pill that they take each evening, or describe their use of alcohol each day unless asked. Symptoms of anxiety can also result from these medications, more typically observed with shorter-acting benzodiazepines taken several times each day. As each dose wears off, the patient feels increasingly anxious, eventually more anxious than the anxiety for which they were prescribed the sedative.

Nicotine should also be considered. The pack-a-day smoker takes in anywhere from 10 to 30 mg of nicotine each day. Smokers tend to feel significantly more anxiety during extended periods without smoking, more common now that we have tobacco-free office environments. Finally, note that the substances we are concerned with are not simply those generally thought of as psychotropics. Prescribed corticosteroids, for example, may lead to significant mood alteration, presence of hallucinations, and neurocognitive deficits.

If symptoms are suspected as being the result of prescribed medication, a discussion with the patient and the prescribing physician is warranted. The patient should be warned of the dangers of sudden cessation of sedative agents, and an appropriate taper schedule should be arranged. Such tapers can often last many months, particularly if the patient has been prescribed sedative agents for years. If, alternately, symptoms are found due to previously undiagnosed addictive disease, referral to an appropriate specialist is in order. Such illness is more likely present if patients complain of the workplace as irritating, overwhelming, or stressful to the extent that they use certain drugs, including alcohol, to reduce the subjective feeling of discomfort that results from their participation in the workplace. Remember that addictive disease is not dependent on either the quantity of use or frequency of use, but rather more on the reason for use. Nevertheless, the worker who often arrives late on Monday, or tends to miss Mondays altogether, should at least be screened for a substance-related diagnosis.

If a substance use disorder is noted, it is of little value to attempt to determine if another primary psychiatric disorder is present. This may instead be determined after a significant period of sobriety has passed. Note that a positive toxicology screen does not prove the existence of a substance use disorder. It simply indicates that a given substance was used.

Anxiety Disorders

Anxiety disorders seen in the workplace include panic disorder and generalized anxiety disorder, as well as posttraumatic stress disorder, discussed in the next section. Symptoms of panic often include perceived tachycardia, diaphoresis, shortness of breath, and chest or abdominal discomfort. Patients feel they are dying and sometimes seek medical attention. As the illness worsens, the frequency of panic symptoms increases and patients begin to avoid specific locations. Driving and shopping are the two activities frequently described as those in which panic symptoms take place, and patients therefore begin to avoid such activities. If the patient drives to work, an early sign of panic disorder would be the failure of the patient to show up in a timely manner, or at all, on days when it rains or snows. Patients might describe shopping for food only early in the morning, or late at night, when the store is likely to be least crowded. Agoraphobia, anxiety about being in a place from which escape or return home is difficult, often is present in the context of panic disorder.

Diagnosis of panic disorder is based on the presence of recurrent panic attacks followed by at least 1 month of persistent concern about the attacks, worry about the implications of the attacks, or a significant change in behavior related to experiencing the panic symptoms.

Generalized anxiety disorder (GAD) is a more generalized state of anxiety than panic disorder. In panic disorder, there are discrete episodes of severe anxiety. In GAD, there are extended periods of variable levels of worry and anxiety. Again, it is important to distinguish GAD from normal anxiety. If an individual works at a company with budgetary difficulties, where his job may realistically be in danger, and the individual has a family to support and an elderly mother to care for, ongoing levels of anxiety may be completely appropriate. While counseling can be useful in such cases, a psychiatric diagnosis of GAD accompanied by antianxiety medication may do more harm than good. In GAD, the level of anxiety and worry significantly exceeds the level appropriate given the stressors and the patient is worried about many things.

The diagnosis of GAD cannot be made until the symptoms have been present for at least 6 months. The symptoms generally include sleep difficulties, muscle tension, irritability, difficulty with concentration, fatigue, and restlessness, or a subset of these. Symptoms may be due to or worsened by substance use, medical illness, or workplace stress. Antidepressant medication has been shown to be quite effective for both panic disorder and GAD. For initial treatment, sedative agents should be avoided. Sertraline, paroxetine, escitalopram, or fluoxetine are all reasonable initial medications. Evening dosing of trazodone or mirtazapine may be helpful for sleep without causing rebound anxiety during the following day. Therapy for each of the anxiety disorders should be arranged as rapidly as possible.

Posttraumatic Stress Disorder

A cashier is held up at gunpoint while the gunman's accomplice empties the register. During the robbery, the normally capable and hardworking cashier is repetitively insulted and threatened while he thinks of his family and worries that his life is about to end.

A truck driver making a delivery is caught in the hydraulic lift at the back of his truck, calling out for help for 5 long minutes as he watches his leg being crushed before help finally arrives.

The cashier has no physical injuries, and the driver walks only with difficulty now, but both are equally subject to symptoms of posttraumatic stress disorder (PTSD). This disorder, more common in women than men, has significant components of both depression and anxiety. As with other psychiatric disorders, a patient's predisposition represents an important component to the development of PTSD. The presence of untreated anxiety or mood disorders or addictive illness increases the likelihood of PTSD developing in response to a traumatic situation. As we discussed above, this in no way alters the causality of the problem. Just as not all individuals who smoke get cancer, not all individuals who are traumatized get PTSD. Further, the quality of the exposure and the speed with which treatment is obtained are both important factors in the disease course. Patients with PTSD may shy away from telling a clinician about their trauma history unless specifically asked, both about the trauma itself and the hallmark symptoms as well.

There are situations that may produce more severe symptoms. Was the trauma extended, as it might be with an abusive supervisor, or was it brief, as it might be in an accident? Did the patient keep the situation to him- or herself for an extended period of time? Was initial treatment incomplete, or lack a behavioral intervention? Does the workplace represent a constant reminder of the traumatic event, or does participation in the workplace constitute an increased risk for a repeat of the same type of event?

Critical for diagnosis of PTSD is the traumatic event itself, in which either the patient or a nearby individual was threatened with death or serious injury, and in which the patient was helpless to solve the problem or felt simultaneously horrified and afraid. Following the trauma, the patient develops recurrent episodes of reliving the trauma, either in dreams or distressing memories, often feeling as if the trauma were actually recurring. The patient develops behavior in which he avoids certain places that remind him of the trauma. He may also begin to develop a certain expectation that his own life could end shortly, resulting in less interest in work. Motivation in general can drop off, and relationships with family and work colleagues can deteriorate. Symptoms need to be present for longer than 1 month for the diagnosis to apply. At any point earlier than that, the same symptoms may lead to a diagnosis of acute stress disorder.

Preventive treatment for PTSD should be implemented as rapidly as possible following a known trauma. Such treatment falls into two categories: exposure therapy and anxiety management education. Exposure therapy involves confrontation with the initial stressor through discussion, working through the fear elicited through a corrective process. Patients reluctant to undergo this process often improve with anxiety management instead. If PTSD symptoms have already developed, behavioral treatment combined with antidepressant medication is indicated. Antidepressants should be continued for at least 12 months, and recovery will be a gradual process. Of importance, sedative agents are not indicated and are likely to be counterproductive if prescribed.

Mood Disorders

Mood disorders can be divided into two groups: unipolar, in which patients experience depressive symptoms; and bipolar, in which patients experience both depressive and elevated symptoms. Depressive disorders also can be divided into two groups: dysthymia, in which the symptoms are generally mild to moderate, and the mood is found to be stable but low for years, often starting before adolescence; and major depressive disorders, which generally start after adolescence, are cyclic in nature, and can sometimes be seen in combination with an ongoing dysthymia. Elevated symptoms also can be divided into two groups: manic and hypomanic. The significant difference between the two is that the manic episode causes marked impairment in occupational or social functioning or includes psychotic symptoms, whereas the hypomanic episode causes neither.

Of note, psychotic symptoms may also occur in the context of severe depressive symptoms. More importantly, suicidality is not uncommon in depressive episodes. The clinician must explicitly ask the patient whether suicide has been considered as a potential option. If the patient answers in the affirmative, clinicians must then explore whether the patient has any specific intent or plan. Should answers to these questions also be affirmative, immediate safe (accompanied) referral is indicated.

Depressive disease includes lack of interest in usual activities accompanied by difficulties with sleep, energy, concentration, and appetite. Patients may feel hopeless about their future, helpless to do anything to solve the problem, and may make decisions that are not in their best interest. They often have guilt feelings based on their inability to conduct business as usual; they blame themselves and feel their family and colleagues blame them as well. Treatment with antidepressant medication accompanied with therapy is quite effective. Major depression often responds more rapidly than does dysthymia, and with a lesser dose of medication, but treatment for dysthymia is efficacious as well. ECT (electroconvulsive treatment) remains very effective and often rapid treatment for severely depressed patients. Bipolar illness is generally discovered due to episodes of mania resulting in inflated self-esteem, decreased sleep, pressure to speak (often with rapid speech patterns), a subjective feeling of racing thoughts, easy distractibility, and involvement in activities with potentially harmful outcomes. Mood stabilizers such as lithium and divalproex remain the mainstay of treatment of bipolar disorder, though several of the atypical antipsychotic agents are now being used with good results. Patients with bipolar illness often have poor compliance with medication that leads to relapse.

Psychotic Disorders

While there are many definitions of the term psychosis, we are concerned primarily with patients who present with significant disorganization, hallucinations, delusions, or catatonia. While at first glance it may appear that such patients quickly call attention to themselves and permit a rapid diagnosis and disposition, the situation can be quite variable. Patients are often reluctant to acknowledge the presence of hallucinations, certain that their delusions are reasonably derived, and quick to assure the physician that they are just fine despite their odd appearance. The physician should investigate delusions that appear outwardly reasonable. While working at an employee assistance program (EAP), I had a patient on medical leave tell me company representatives were following him. He told me that he had taken to keeping all his shades drawn at home and to driving different routes while on errands. I found during exploration of the issue that indeed the company had hired detectives to follow the employee to ascertain that he was really disabled and not merely working at another place of employment. True psychotic symptoms may be the result of bipolar disorder, depression, or substance use. They do not necessarily indicate the presence of a primary psychotic disorder such as schizophrenia. Paranoid and schizotypal personality traits may also be mistaken for signs of psychotic disorders.

Symptoms of psychosis are often divided into two groups: positive, which include all forms of hallucinations and delusions as well as acutely bizarre behavior and formal thought disorders; and negative, which include social inattention, poor grooming, lack of vocal inflections, and blocking of speech. This latter group often leads to the occupational physician being called as peers of the employee become concerned. Often the problem has developed gradually, or the symptoms are residual in nature, waxing and waning in response to medication or other factors. If the psychotic symptoms are secondary to a primary psychotic disorder, treatment tends to be lifelong with widely ranging responses. The atypical antipsychotic medications represent an extraordinary improvement over haloperidol and other traditional medications; side effects are markedly reduced and overall compliance appears to have improved significantly. While many patients are unable to work following their first psychotic break, quite a few respond to the extent that they can carry out at least a portion of their earlier tasks. The new onset of schizophrenia should not be taken as a reason for patients to permanently leave their position.

Adjustment Disorders

Significant impairment in occupational function sometimes results from adjustment difficulties to known stressors. The stressor may be work related, as when the company is being purchased by another company, resulting in significant management and structural changes. The patient might be able to function at work without significant impairment but might alternately have subjective distress with respect to the stressor that is outside of the expected response range. This is a judgment call on the part of the physician. For the diagnosis of an adjustment disorder, symptoms do not meet the criteria for another primary psychiatric disorder and are not the result of a death in the patient's immediate family. The duration of symptoms can be quite long, depending on the duration of the stressor. For example, if an employee is dealing with the stress of medical problems that are ongoing in nature, the adjustment disorder may last indefinitely. There is no time limit for the disorder. Types of stresses that can contribute to this type of disorder are discussed below.

Adjustment disorders are classified based on the predominant symptoms. Within the workplace, disorders likely to be observed are those with depressed mood, with anxiety, and with mixed anxiety and depressed mood. Disturbance of conduct is also a possibility that is easily identified.

Personality Disorders

Personality disorders or, more frequently, personality traits can often lead to a request for medical eval-

TABLE 28.1. *Personality disorders*

Paranoid—pervasive distrust and suspiciousness, with motives of others thought to be malevolent
Schizoid—detached from social relationships with a restricted range of expressed emotion
Schizotypal—acute discomfort with close relationships accompanied by perceptual difficulties and odd behavior
Antisocial—deceitful and manipulative, often failing to conform to lawful behavior
Borderline—unstable interpersonal relationships with marked impulsive behavior
Histrionic—excessively emotional and attention seeking
Narcissistic—grandiose, seeking admiration, and lacking empathy
Avoidant—socially inhibited, feels inadequate, hypersensitive to criticism; note that the colloquial use of the term *antisocial* refers more to an individual who is avoidant than to one who is antisocial
Dependent—submissive clinging behavior with fears of separation from others
Obsessive-compulsive—preoccupied with orderliness, perfection, and control of surroundings; lacks flexibility

uation in the workplace. In the presence of an enduring and stable pattern of interpersonal relationships that deviates from the norm and can be traced back to adolescence, in which the pattern is not the result of a medical or psychiatric problem, personality traits should be considered. Medication has generally not been found useful, and therapy is often difficult and protracted. Some personality types may be particularly sensitive to stressors. For example, a worker with an obsessive personality often has a rigid coping strategy for approaching new situations. If this strategy fails, the worker may lack the flexibility needed to find new solutions.

Over the years, there have been a variety of methods used to divide personality traits into groups. The current categories are found in Table 28.1.

Malingering and Emotional Factors in Physical Symptoms (Somatoform Illness)

The emotional components of many medical illnesses are well recognized by astute physicians. The occupational physician must also be able to evaluate whether a volitional component plays a role in a worker's complaint. In most clinical settings, there is a tendency to consider a worker's illness as due to either a bona fide disease or a conscious attempt to deceive the physician. This view is overly simplistic, inaccurate, and not helpful when dealing with these workers. A more useful approach is to conceptualize a continuum of diagnostic entities. Often, patients' symptoms do not fall into either extreme, but somewhere in the middle where there is an element of both conscious and unconscious motivation. It may be difficult to distinguish the degree of voluntary control a patient has over symptoms.

Occupational physicians should be familiar with the disorders noted in Fig. 28.1. At one end of the spectrum are disorders in which psychological factors affect the expression of physical illness (e.g., asthma, irritable bowel syndrome). The midrange includes somatoform disorders, which refer to the presence of physical symptoms that suggest physical disorders but for which no organic basis can be established as the cause. Evidence often suggests that the symptoms are linked to psychological dysfunction. Examples of somatoform disorders include conversion reactions, psychogenic pain, and hypochondriasis. Somatization occurs when a patient expresses psychological distress through a physical route; the patient may not even be aware of the psychological distress or feel able to control the symptoms. Successful interventions with patients suffering from somatoform disorders utilize the following techniques:

1. Establish a good patient–physician relationship. Initially, convey acceptance of the patient's problems, and then gradually shift to an exploration of the psychological variables and stress in a patient's life that may contribute to the problems.
2. Avoid placing "cure" as the goal of your interventions. Focus rather on improved functioning or coping with symptoms.
3. Encourage exercise and physical therapy.
4. Treat any concomitant depression with antidepressant drugs at full therapeutic doses.
5. Accept the long-term chronic nature of these illnesses. It is more efficient to see patients for follow-up at regular intervals regardless of whether they are symptomatic. This approach is generally more beneficial than advising a return only if symptoms recur.

At the other end of the continuum are conditions in which symptoms are under the worker's voluntary control, such as malingering and factitious disorder. In factitious disorders, the symptoms are "voluntary" in that they are deliberate and purposeful but not in the sense that they can be controlled; there is a compulsive quality to the simulation of illness. There is no apparent goal other than to assume the patient role. Often a severe personality disturbance exists. In malingering, the patient is also in voluntary control of the symptoms, but the goal is based on environmen-

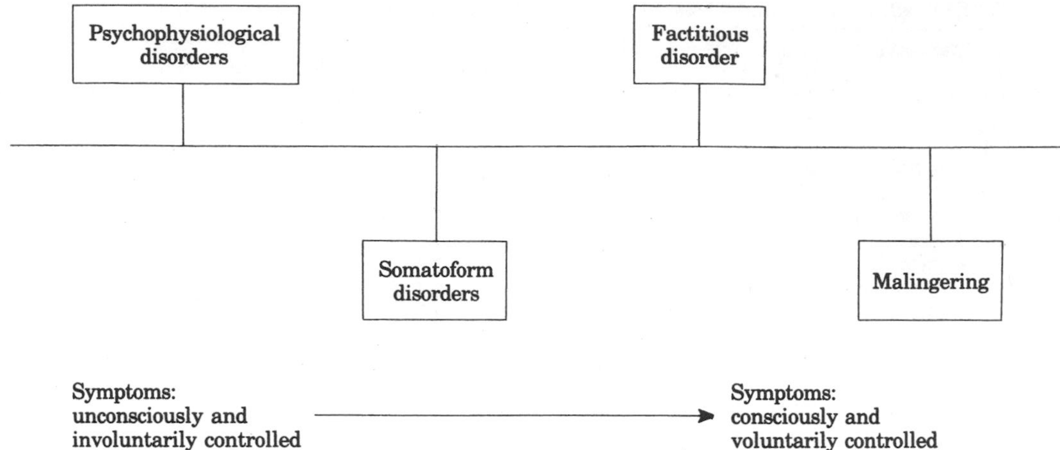

FIG. 28.1. The continuum of psychological factors influencing physical symptoms.

tal circumstances (rather than the patient's psychology). Under some circumstances, malingering may represent an adaptive behavior, such as feigning illness while a captive of an enemy during wartime. Malingering is not attributable to a mental disorder, although it is often associated with an antisocial personality.

The following are guidelines for identifying the patient who has a higher degree of voluntary conscious control of symptoms:

1. The patient has a carefully documented medical history.
2. The patient has extensive legal involvement.
3. The patient is angry and defensive during examinations.
4. The patient resists diagnostic procedures and prescribed treatment regimens.
5. The patient selectively prevents family or employer input to the evaluating doctor.
6. The patient has inconsistencies in the reporting of physical symptoms.
7. When confronted with the nonorganic nature of the complaint, the malingerer often develops a new problem.
8. Medical record appears to have been altered.
9. The patient is reluctant to accept a favorable prognosis.

Neuropsychiatric Disease Secondary to Toxic Exposure

Solvents, pesticides, and heavy metals are ubiquitous, and thus human exposure is inevitable. Workers, however, may be exposed to higher concentrations on the job. Although the exact amount required to produce symptoms is often unknown, marked variation in individual vulnerability appears to exist. Symptoms may be acute, resulting from brief, intense exposure, or chronic, secondary to many years of exposure at lower concentrations (7).

Acute intoxication syndromes depend on the particular agent; however, common symptoms include dizziness, light-headedness, and incoordination (see Chapter 25). In rare cases a florid psychosis may occur. Removal from exposure to the toxic substance usually clears the symptoms.

The chronic syndromes can be divided into three types: mild, moderate, and severe. The mild type is an organic affective disorder, a reversible syndrome of depression identical to depression from other etiologies. Noting a temporal relationship between the onset of symptoms and the exposure to the toxic substance makes the diagnosis. (The diagnosis is considered by some to be one of exclusion.) The organic affective disorder is often reversible if the offending substance is removed. The moderate type includes cognitive symptoms, such as short-term memory loss and psychomotor disturbances (slowness in response time, clumsy eye–hand coordination, or clumsy dexterity), in addition to the affective symptoms. The severe type resembles dementia. As the severity of these conditions increases, withdrawal of the toxic substance is less likely to reverse the symptoms.

Measurement of cognitive function is particularly important when the possible effects of a toxic exposure are suspected. The Mini-Mental State examination can be helpful as a screening tool but is unlikely to detect even moderate levels of disease in those with significantly above-average baseline intellectual function. When neuropsychiatric illness secondary to toxic exposure is suspected, neuropsychological testing by a psychologist trained in behavioral toxicology or neuropsychology may be helpful. Such testing can be used to assess a worker's level of psychological impairment. Serial testing can be used to measure the change in functional level.

Stress

Stress refers not to a single event or reaction but rather to a process that begins with a stressful event or series of events and ends with one's reaction to that event. The common factor seen in all stress is *change.* Stress is encountered whether the change is conceptualized as beneficial, as in promotion, or detrimental, as in being fired.

In moderate amounts, stress can be motivating and is known as "eustress." However, if the duration or intensity of the stress overloads a person's ability to manage the stress, it can lead to "distress," a spiral of emotional and physical ills. To illustrate these concepts, think of the metal spring of a watch. When stressed, the spring provides the force to keep the mechanism working. Without constant winding and stress, the watch will stop. If overwound, however, the metal becomes strained and may even break. This proper "spring tension" varies widely between individuals and also within an individual at different times.

Stressors, the factors involved in causing stress, can be divided into acute and chronic types. We have all experienced acute stress when we are traveling in a car and the vehicle in front of us makes a short and unexpected stop. The immediate release of epinephrine (the "adrenaline rush") causes the familiar "fight or flight" response that increases heart rate, blood pressure, and respiratory rate. Dissatisfying interpersonal relationships are usually responsible for chronic stress. The mechanism whereby chronic stressors exert their damage is primarily due to the increase of corticotropin-releasing factor and other mediators, which increase levels of circulating corticosteroid and increase blood pressure and heart rate, as well as possibly impairing immune response.

Occupational stress research has shown a clear relationship between stress and productivity (Fig. 28.2). All occupations have their own intrinsic characteristics including level of responsibility and degrees of authority, autonomy, and ambiguity. If one plots stress versus any of these characteristics, one finds that either extreme in characteristics can produce higher levels of stress. For example, a midlevel manager with responsibility for 20 employees (high level of responsibility) may be as stressed as an assembly line worker (low level of responsibility). Although highly ambiguous occupations can be stressful, having no occupation at all is perhaps more stressful.

A worker confronted with termination at age 45 compared to age 25 demonstrates the influence of life stage on adaptation to stressors. "Midlife crisis" also lowers one's ability to manage stress. The importance of recent life changes was first addressed by physician Adolph Meyer and more recently by Holmes and Rabe (1), who developed the Schedule of Recent Life Events. They assigned "life change units" (LCUs)

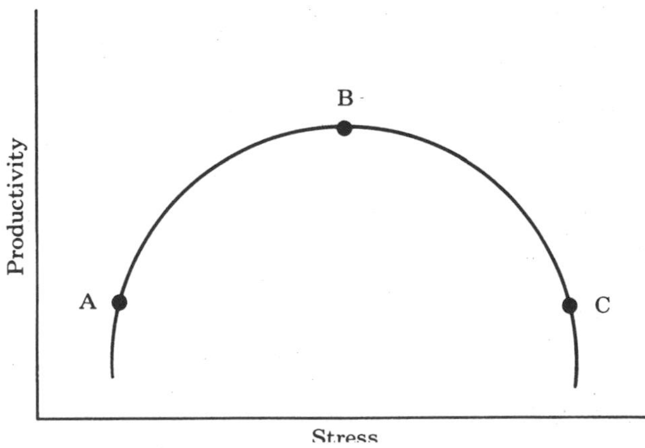

FIG. 28.2. The relationship between productivity and stress. **A:** Stress is too low; therefore, productivity is low. **B:** Optimum stress and productivity. **C:** Stress is too high; therefore, productivity is low.

and ranked them according to commonly encountered life changes. Individuals who accumulate large amounts of LCUs appear to have increased risk of suffering stress-related illness (Table 28.2).

The context in which individuals face stressors should be taken into account, as should the factor causing the adverse effect itself. Context is made up of all the external factors in a person's life, including the world economy and one's family unit, friends, and work atmosphere, both people and the physical environment. The social/psychological support that one receives from co-workers and family does much to buffer the impact of the stressor. Although every occupation has unique stressors, certain jobs are associated with high levels of stressors, including shift work, work overload or work underload, physical danger, noise and lighting, role ambiguity or conflict, high responsibility with low authority, and interpersonal conflicts.

TABLE 28.2. *The Holmes-Rabe schedule of recent life events*

Rank	Event	Value (LCU)
1	Death of spouse	100
2	Divorce	73
3	Marital separation	65
4	Jail term	63
5	Death of a close family member	63
6	Personal injury or illness	53
7	Marriage	50
8	Fired from work	47
9	Marital reconciliation	45
10	Retirement	45
11	Change in family member's health	44
12	Pregnancy	40
13	Sex difficulties	39
14	Addition to family	39
15	Business readjustment	39
16	Change in financial status	38
17	Death of close friend	37
18	Change to different line of work	36
19	Change in number of marital arguments	35
20	Mortgage or loan over $10,000	31
21	Foreclosure of mortgage or loan	30
22	Change in work responsibilities	29
23	Son or daughter leaving home	29
24	Trouble with in-laws	29
25	Outstanding personal achievement	28
26	Spouse begins or stops work	26
27	Starting or finishing school	26
28	Change in living conditions	25
29	Revision of personal habits	24
30	Trouble with boss	23
31	Change in work hours, conditions	20
32	Change in residence	20
33	Change in schools	20
34	Change in recreational habits	19
35	Change in church activities	19
36	Change in social activities	18
37	Mortgage or loan under $10,000	17
38	Change in sleeping habits	16
39	Change in number of family gatherings	15
40	Change in eating habits	15
41	Vacation	13
42	Christmas season	12
43	Minor violation of the law	11

LCU, life change units.

From Holmes TH, Rabe RH. The social readjustment rating scale. *J Psychosom Res* 1967;11:213. © 1967, Pergamon Journals, Ltd.

It is not always possible or desirable to remove stressors that confront a patient. We can, however, help patients modify their circles of individual vulnerability, context, and stressors so that overlap and thus symptoms are minimized. Substance use (alcohol, drugs, caffeine, nicotine) or chronic sleep deprivation inhibits successful treatment; their presence must be addressed.

ENGAGING THE PATIENT AS YOUR ALLY

The physician who delivers occupational health services is likely to be called on to evaluate people who may have symptoms due to stress. Necessary for any successful intervention is the establishment of the therapeutic alliance. The basic strategy is to create a nondefensive atmosphere where you can evoke a patient's willingness to work with you. The technique for achieving this outcome involves five simple but vital steps that cannot be overlooked (2):

1. *Reduce the patient's defensiveness:* A good technique for reducing the patient's defensiveness is to externalize the patient's difficulty; rephrase the problem so that it is not coming from within the patient entirely. For example, you might ask, "What are the pressures on you at this time?"
2. *Inventory the patient's stress symptoms:* Your goal is to understand how stress is affecting the patient. Ask "What do these pressures do to you?" or "How do you notice these pressures affecting you or your ability to handle life's problems?"
3. *Tap the patient's level of motivation:* It is imperative to determine whether the patient is truly interested in working on the problem before you undertake any stress management program. Ask the patient, "Are you willing to do something about it?"
4. *Review the patient's work environment:* Ask specifically about how work (i.e., job duties, physical environment, other workers) may be affecting the person. (This critical question, if over-

looked, can result in failure to understand the broad dimensions of stress-related illnesses.)

5. *Check the patient's willingness:* Ask the patient, "Are you willing to work with me on solving this problem?"

Successfully completed, these steps result in an implicit contract between you and the patient to work together toward a common goal—the reduction of stress. Five commonly used stress management techniques—time management, relaxation training, physical exercise, increasing avocational interest, and spreading out life changes—help attain this goal.

STRESS MANAGEMENT TECHNIQUES

Time Management

Structured time planning can help a patient who is overwhelmed by a task. Often, large tasks can be divided into manageable units. Have patients make up to-do lists and set priorities among the items on the list. Patients also need to decide what level of perfection is required for a particular task. Lists can be updated and priorities changed as needed.

Relaxation Training

Many people do not know how to relax because it is a skill that must be developed. For many, it is like learning to drive a stick-shift automobile. At first it is very awkward and unnatural, but with training and practice it can become smooth and comfortable.

Relaxation training can take many forms. Commonly used techniques include biofeedback, transcendental meditation, self-hypnosis, and progressive muscle relaxation. Both patient and physician must be comfortable with the technique used. For example, a computer programmer may feel uncomfortable with the idea of hypnosis but intrigued with the hardware of biofeedback.

Exercise

Exercise is one of the simplest yet most effective antidotes to stress. Studies suggest that running has antidepressant qualities (3). The better an activity is for cardiopulmonary training, the more powerful is its antistress effect. Walking, cycling, running, and swimming are all good cardiopulmonary training activities. For optimal effectiveness, an exercise program should be well integrated into a person's daily life. Although daily exercise is most desirable, 30-minute periods three times per week where one exercises to 75% of one's maximal heart rate appear to be beneficial (see Chapter 24).

Avocational Interests

Patients should be encouraged to expand their scope of gratifications. A person who depends on work as the sole source of self-esteem is heading for trouble. Placing a few of one's eggs in the family, sports, and hobby baskets will help to avoid so-called burnout.

Spread Out Life Changes

This stress reduction strategy comes directly from the Holmes-Rabe Schedule of Life Change Events. Often we have no control over major life changes, but when a choice exists, major changes should be spread over several months. Good stress management skills are good health skills; strategies rely primarily on reducing one's circle of individual vulnerability.

Group Stress Management Programs

Group stress management programs can provide employees with an awareness of how stress affects their lives. For many employees, a 4- to 8-hour program enables them to begin to make changes to a healthier style of coping with stress. These programs are primarily educational in scope and are designed to acquaint people with stress, its adverse health effects, and means of control. Those employees with a large stressor load or rigid coping styles can benefit from an individualized stress management program.

Organizational change can challenge workers' ability to adapt to that change. This kind of stress can drastically affect employee morale and productivity. One technique of assaying this type of stress is through the periodic administration of opinion surveys. Professional interpretation and analysis of such surveys can yield information pertinent to improving the situation and thus reducing stress.

SHIFT WORK

Shift work refers to either long-term night work or rotation among day, evening, and night shifts. Over 27% of male workers and 16% of female workers have jobs that require them to rotate shifts (4). Studies suggest that these workers, presumably due to a disruption in circadian rhythm, have increased morbidity and decreased work performance. Marked variability exists in people's vulnerability to the adverse effects of shift work, and vulnerability increases with

TABLE 28.3. *Guidelines on preventing the ill effects of shift work*

Weekly rotating shifts—working 4 or 5 days on a particular shift before rotating to the next
Rotate shifts in the direction of delay of rhythms (working later)
Schedule meal time ("lunchtime") halfway through a given shift
Maintain exposure to bright light during waking hours (5)
Sleep in a dark, quiet place (6)

advancing age. Workers who categorize themselves as "night people" and those who find it easy to sleep at unusual times are more likely to tolerate shift work. Although most studies can be criticized on some level, approximately 25% of workers are estimated to have significant difficulties in family, work, or social adaptation related to shift work (4) (Table 28.3).

Acute Time Shift Syndrome

Our circadian system can adapt to a phase delay of 2 hours or a phase advance of one-half hour without much disruption. Whenever a change in schedule occurs outside this limited "range of entrainment," an acute time shift syndrome may occur. During the process of readjustment to the new schedule, circadian rhythms in alertness, mood, and digestion are disrupted. Although short-lived, the most common symptoms of acute time shift syndrome, that is, "jet lag," are insomnia, gastrointestinal distress, sleepiness, and fatigue. The intensity of the reaction is determined by the degree and direction of time shift. Since it is easier to adjust to a delay in schedule than to an advance, workers adapt more readily to switching from day shift to night shift. Similarly, traveling westward across time zones (delay in time) has less potential for adverse effects than traveling eastward. Adequate hydration, avoidance of alcohol and cigarettes, and appropriate use of short-acting hypnotics to induce sleep at the "new" bedtime may speed resolution of jet lag symptoms (6). (Table 28.4 includes other measures designed to prevent jet lag.)

TABLE 28.4. *How to prevent jet lag*

Keep well hydrated
Avoid alcohol
Eat lightly on travel days
Avoid caffeine in the evening
Consider using short-acting hypnotics to help induce sleep at the "new" bedtime
Set your watch to the new time as soon as you get on the airplane

Chronic Shift Maladaptation Syndrome

Disturbance of the worker's biologic clock or circadian rhythms is responsible for a shift maladaptation syndrome, which affects wakefulness, thermoregulation, and neuroendocrine regulation. The most common effects include gastrointestinal and cardiovascular disturbances and effects on level of alertness.

Disturbances on level of alertness are the most commonly encountered consequence of shift work. Night shift or rotating shift workers are more likely to suffer from insomnia and difficulty staying awake at work. The decreased total sleep time also results in a chronically sleep-deprived condition. This disrupted sleep pattern may be related to the higher incidence of both work and off-work accidents among shift workers.

Shift workers have a higher rate of gastrointestinal complaints and peptic ulcer disease than do day workers. Disturbed eating habits combined with disrupted diurnal control of intestinal enzymes are thought to contribute to these disturbances.

Several studies indicate that shift workers have higher than expected rates of cardiovascular disease and acute myocardial infarctions in particular (4).

Those who work nights or on evening rotation are less likely to be involved in political or social organizations. With fewer friends, they tend to have hobbies that are solitary in nature. Disruptions of family life among shift workers are often more problematic than the disruptions in community and social life. Marital disharmony may result from the shift worker's relative unavailability; a myriad of difficulties in parenting can also occur.

VIOLENCE IN THE WORKPLACE

Workplace violence ranges from offensive language to homicide, with a reasonable working definition including violent acts such as physical assaults and threats of assault, all directed toward persons at work.

Homicide itself is now the third leading cause of fatal occupational injury in the United States; in 2000, there were 674 workplace homicides, accounting for 11% of the total fatal injuries. Past studies have indicated that a majority of such homicides are related to robberies. Nonfatal injuries due to assault occur at much higher incidence rates, and while police officers experience such hazards at the highest rate of any work group, social service and health workers suffer from such injuries far beyond the average rate as well. Risk factors for such injuries are listed in Table 28.5.

TABLE 28.5. *Risk factors for violent injuries in the workplace*

Contact with the public
Exchange of money
Delivery of passengers, goods, or services
Having a mobile workplace such as a taxicab or police cruiser
Working with unstable or volatile persons in health care, social services, or criminal justice settings
Working alone or in small numbers
Working late at night or during early morning hours
Working in high-crime areas
Guarding valuable property or possessions
Working in community-based settings

From National Institute for Occupational Safety and Health (NIOSH) Current Intelligence Bulletin 57. Violence in the workplace: risk factors and prevention strategies, 1996.

The Occupational Safety and Health Administration (OSHA) has developed guidelines and recommendations to reduce worker exposures to the hazards of workplace violence. There are four basic elements of which the occupational physician should be aware:

1. Management commitment and employee involvement: Physicians may assist the company in setting clear goals for worker security.
2. Work-site analysis: Identification of high-risk situations through employee surveys, workplace walkthroughs, and reviews of injury and illness data, taking into account the risk factors shown in Table 28.5.
3. Hazard prevention and control: Controls to prevent or limit violence are placed where necessary.
4. Training and education: Physicians can help educate employees regarding potential hazards and ways in which they can protect themselves and their co-workers.

A variety of controls may be used to reduce risk to employees. The physician can bring these potential controls to the attention of managers and administrators:

- Physical barriers such as bullet-resistant enclosures or shields, pass-through windows, or deep service counters
- Alarm systems, panic buttons, global positioning systems (GPSs), and radios ("open mike switch")
- Convex mirrors, elevated vantage points, clear visibility of service and cash register areas
- Bright and effective lighting
- Adequate staffing
- Furniture arranged to prevent entrapment
- Cash-handling controls, use of drop safes
- Height markers on exit doors
- Emergency procedures to use in case of robbery
- Training in identifying hazardous situations and appropriate responses in emergencies
- Video surveillance equipment, in-car surveillance cameras, and closed circuit TV
- Liaison established with local police

Sexual harassment may also be viewed as a workplace mental health hazard. Such harassment includes unwelcome sexual advances, requests for sexual favors, and other verbal or physical conduct of a sexual nature when the response to this conduct might affect another individual's employment or work performance. Harassment also exists when an intimidating, hostile, or offensive workplace environment results.

The victim may be either male or female, as may be the harasser. The victim may not be the person directly targeted, but may be any other employee affected by the conduct of the harasser. The conduct of the harasser must be not welcome. Victims of such harassment may turn to their EAP or their occupational physician both for assistance and for an independent third-party assessment of the situation, particularly when they feel harassed by a supervisor.

REFERENCES

1. Holmes TH, Rabe RH. The social readjustment rating scale. *J Psychosom Res* 1967;11:213.
2. Personal communication, William Hollister, M.D., University of North Carolina, Chapel Hill.
3. Mellion M. Exercise therapy for anxiety and depression. *Postgrad Med* 1985;77:3.
4. Moore-Ede MC, Richardson GS. Medical implications of shift-work. *Annu Rev Med* 1985;36:607–617.
5. Van Cauter E, Turek F. Strategies for resetting the human circadian clock. *N Engl J Med* 1990;322:18.
6. Nicholson AN, et al. Sleep after transmeridian flights. *Lancet* 1986;2:1205.
7. Flodin U, et al. Clinical studies of psycho-organic syndromes among workers with exposure to solvents. *Am J Ind Med* 1984;5:287.

FURTHER INFORMATION

American Psychiatric Association. *Diagnostic and statistical manual of mental disorders (DSM-IV-TR).* Washington, DC: APA, 2000.

Baker E. Organic solvent neurotoxicity. *Annu Rev Public Health* 1988;9:223.

Baker EL, Fine LJ. Solvent neurotoxicity: the current evidence. *J Occup Med* 1986;28:126.

Benson H. *The relaxation response.* New York: Morrow, 1975.

Bureau of Labor Statistics. National Census of Fatal Occupational Injuries, 2000. Washington, DC: BLS, 2001.

Collijan MJ, Pennebaker JW, eds. *Mass psychogenic illness.* Hillsdale, NJ: Erlbaum, 1982.

Drugs that cause psychiatric symptoms. *Med Lett* 1986;28:81.

Fiedler N, Maccia C, Kipen H. Evaluation of chemically sensitive patients. *J Occup Med* 1992;34:5.

Florence D, Miller T. Functional overlay in work-related injury. *Postgrad Med* 1985;77:8.

Gabbard GO. *Treatments of psychiatric disorders,* 3rd ed. Washington, DC: American Psychiatric Publishing, 2001.

Gamino L, Elkins G, Hackney K. Emergency management of mass psychogenic illness. *Psychosomatics* 1989; 30:4.

Harris JS. Stressors and stress in critical care. *Crit Care Nurse* Feb. 1984.

Lande R. Malingering. *J Am Osteopath Assoc (United States)* 1989;89(4):483–488.

McLean A. *Work stress.* Series on occupational stress. Reading, MA: Addison-Wesley, 1979.

Meja S. Post-traumatic stress disorder: an overview of three etiological variables and psychopharmacological treatment. *Nurse Pract* 1990;August 15:41.

Moore-Ede MC, Richardson GS. Medical implications of shift-work. *Annu Rev Med* 1985;36:607–617.

Siebenaler MJ, McGovern P. Shiftwork consequences and considerations. *AAOHN J* 1991;39:12.

29

Allergy and Immunology

Jack E. Farnham and Donald Accetta

Allergic reactions to occupational vapors, mists, gases, fumes, and dusts are merely one way in which the immune system interacts with the xenobiotic agents in the workplace. Other manifestations are autoimmune reactions, deficiency diseases, and malignancy. This chapter presents a brief overview of the immune system, discusses common occupational allergic diseases, and considers the evaluation and management of each, including latex allergy, sinusitis, and fungal diseases. An overview of immunotoxicology with the usefulness and limitations of related immunologic tests is presented. In addition, current views on idiopathic environmental intolerance (multiple chemical sensitivity) are summarized.

OCCUPATIONAL ALLERGIC DISEASES

Occupational allergic diseases include allergic contact dermatitis, allergic respiratory diseases (allergic rhinitis, asthma, bronchitis, hypersensitivity pneumonitis, and bronchopulmonary aspergillosis), and anaphylaxis. Of more than 400,000 cases of occupational illnesses annually (1), about 20,000 are due to allergic contact dermatitis, which result mostly from contact with epoxy, *Rhus* oleoresin, chromates, nickel, and rubber products. These are fully described in Chapter 27, and are not discussed further here.

Occupational allergic respiratory diseases comprise about 65,000 cases annually. In addition to the discussion in this chapter, these diseases are also discussed in Chapter 21.

Occupational latex hypersensitivity is increasingly diagnosed especially in health care and emergency personnel, and number about 13,000 cases annually. Occupational anaphylaxis, in contrast, only occurs in approximately 200 patients annually.

IMMUNE SYSTEM OVERVIEW

The basic functions of the immune system are protection of the body from agents of external intrusion and maintenance of internal homeostasis and surveillance. A unique array of unconnected organs, freely mobile cells, and several types of acellular communicating agents accomplish these functions.

The primary organs include the thymus and bone marrow; secondary organs are the spleen, lymph nodes, and lymphoid tissue along the interface between the body and the external environment [oropharynx, bronchial walls, and gastrointestinal (GI) and genitourinary (GU) tracts].

The cellular elements of the immune system arise from a common bone marrow–derived pluripotent stem cell that gives rise to the lymphoid and myeloid series. Some lymphoid stem cells are processed in the neonatal thymus and develop into T lymphocytes. T lymphocytes may be facilitators of the immune reaction (T helper or Th cells) or inhibitors of the immune reaction (T suppressor or Ts cells). Other lymphocytes bypass the thymus and are processed in the bursal equivalent tissues (bone marrow, lymph nodes, appendix, tonsils, and other GI and GU associated tissues) to become B lymphocytes. Upon antigenic stimulation B lymphocytes transform into plasma cells, which produce specific antibodies. T and B lymphocytes and plasma cells are involved in specific immunity and respond only to recognized antigens. Still other lymphocytes develop into natural killer (NK) cells.

Myeloid stem cells develop into macrophages, mast cells, Langerhans cells, and polymorphonuclear leukocytes (PMNs), consisting of eosinophils, basophils, and neutrophils. The NK and PMN cells are involved in nonspecific immunity and can interact with much foreign material.

The acellular components of the immune system consist of antibodies, complement, and the cytokines. Antibodies are proteins formed from B-lymphocyte–derived plasma cells in the immunoglobulin (Ig) classes A, D, E, G, and M. IgE is the antibody responsible for most allergic reactions, IgM is formed initially after exposure to most foreign proteins, and IgG is stimulated after exposure to bacteria, viruses, and toxins. Complement is a serum enzyme system consisting of at least 19 separate proteins. The functions of complement are to mediate inflammation, opsonize antigenic material, and inflict membrane damage to pathogens. The cytokines are intercellular messengers secreted by T lymphocytes and some other tissue cells; they consist of interleukins, interferons, and colony-stimulating factors among others.

Outline of Immune Function

Environmental and genetic factors acting at the time of macrophage processed antigen presentation to naive T lymphocytes determine the development of two types of helper cells (Th1, Th2) or Ts cells (2). Th1 cells liberate interferon, interleukin-2, and tumor necrosis factor, which lead to autoimmune diseases or cell-mediated hypersensitivity. Th2 cells liberate interleukin-4 (among others lymphokines), which leads to stimulation of B cells to transform into plasma cells, which produce allergic antibodies involved in the immediate hypersensitivity reactions (allergy) (3). Ts lymphocytes function to suppress these reactions instituted by Th1 and Th2 cells.

Circulating immunoglobulin antibodies attach to receptor sites on mast cells and remain there until specific antigens are attracted to them. When the specific antigen cross-links with two antibody molecules on the mast cell surface, there is a disruption of the surface membrane; internally contained histamine, leukotrienes, and other vasoactive amines are then released, causing the allergic inflammatory reaction.

Host Immune Status

The immune system of any given individual may be normal, in a state of hyperactivity, or in a state of hypoactivity. In these various states, the source of antigenic insult determines the type of immune disease that may result. As shown in Table 29.1, if an individual has a hyperactive immune system, an external antigen will cause a hypersensitivity reaction (allergy). If the antigen comes from an internal source, an autoimmune reaction may occur. In contrast, if the individual has a hypoactive immune state, an external antigenic challenge could lead to an infection or immunodeficiency disease. Internal antigens (mutations or tumor cells) in such a person could lead to failure of surveillance and the development of neoplasia.

An update on the immune system (4) and a series of review articles on advances in immunology was published beginning in the July 4, 2000, issue of the *New England Journal of Medicine* and appears in the first issue of each month.

Hypersensitivity Types

Proposed in 1975, the Gell and Coombs classification of hypersensitivity reactions still remains a general guide for types of immune responses (5). The four types of reactions are based on the presence or absence of humoral antibodies, the type of antibodies involved, whether or not complement is required to drive the reaction to completion, the target organ, and the cell types involved. Although the four types are described separately, they may occur in combination simultaneously.

Type I (allergic or anaphylactic) reactions require IgE antibody attached to mast cell receptors before antigen introduction. When the antigen cross-links with the specific antibody, the resulting reaction causes a release of histamine, serotonin, and other vasoactive amines from the mast cell. These chemical mediators induce the allergic reaction seen in allergic rhinitis, asthma, and anaphylaxis.

Type II reactions usually require IgG antibodies directed against antigen located on target cell surfaces (often red blood cells). Complement may be needed to drive the antigen antibody reaction, resulting in target cell destruction (immune hemolytic anemia, transfusion reaction, and some types of autoimmune disease).

TABLE 29.1. *Immune system*

Immunogen source	Hyperactive	Normal	Hypoactive
External	Hypersensitivity	N	Immune deficiency
Internal	Autoimmunity	N	Neoplasia

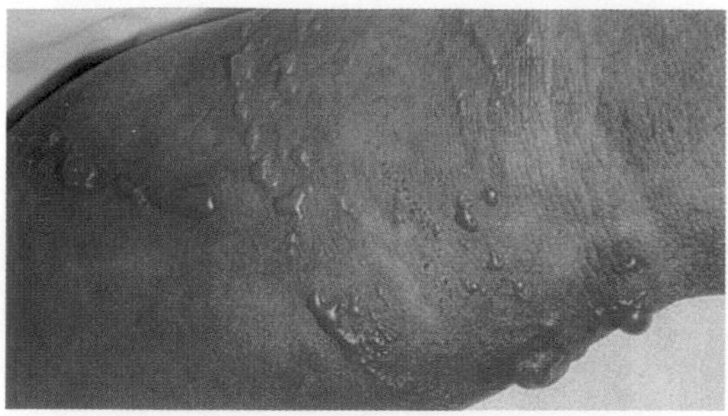

Color Plate 27.1. Eczema. An acute blistering irritant contact dermatitis to ethylene oxide is seen here (National Institute for Occupational Safety and Health, NIOSH).

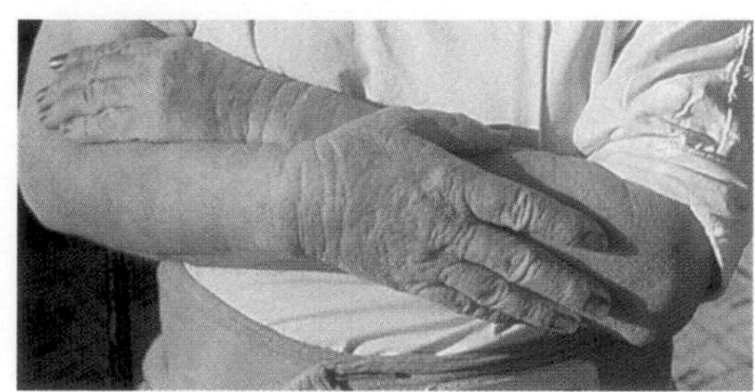

Color Plate 27.2. Eczema. These leathery-appearing hands are representative of chronic irritant dermatitis in a worker who uses kerosene to clean his hands (NIOSH).

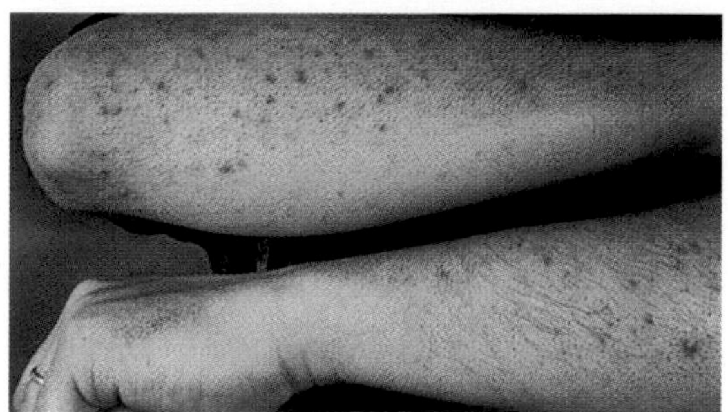

Color Plate 27.3. Acneiform. This car mechanic's forearms exhibit folliculitis from exposure to grease and lubricating oils (NIOSH).

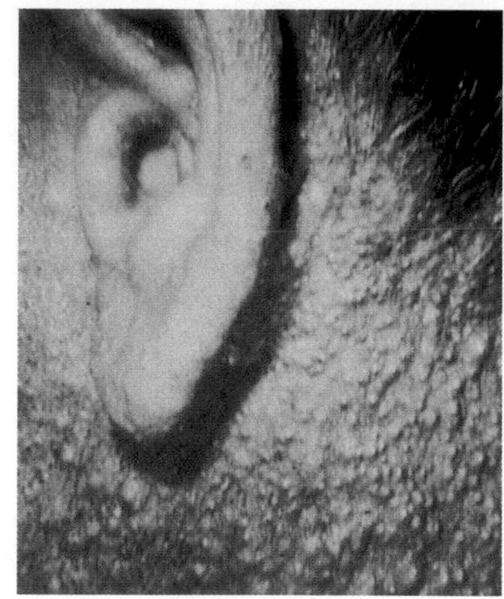

Color Plate 27.4. Acneiform. Exposure to certain halogenated aromatic chemicals by this worker led to this acne-like eruption, chloracne. It may be accompanied by systemic toxicity. (From *Cutis* 1974;13:588.)

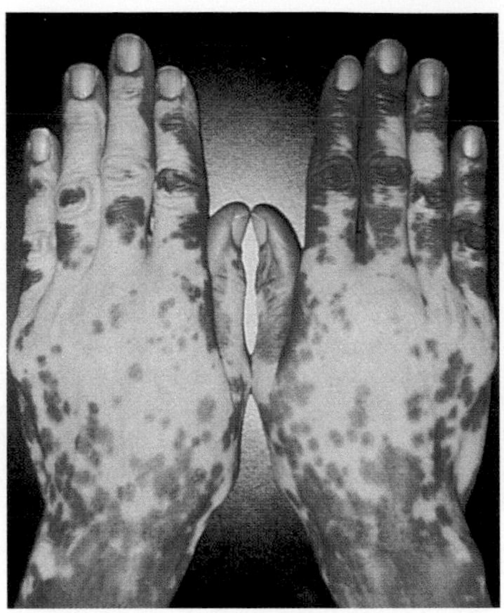

Color Plate 27.5. Depigmentation. Depigmentation of hands of this hospital worker was the result of contact with phenolic germicidal detergent (NIOSH).

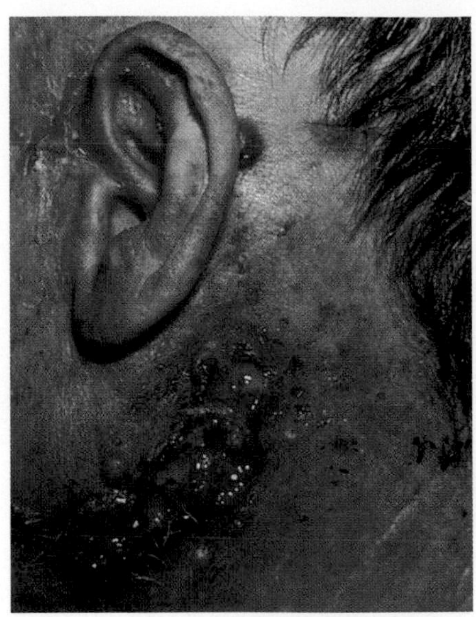

Color Plate 27.6. Tumors. Malignant tumors, such as this squamous cell carcinoma, can result from years of occupational exposure to both sunlight and coal tar (a carcinogen) (NIOSH).

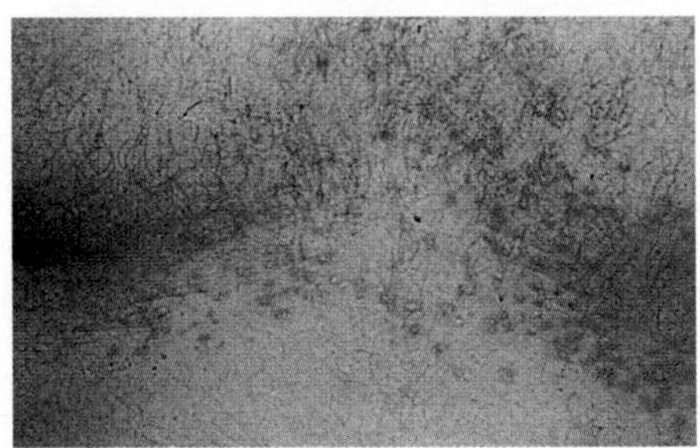

Color Plate 27.7. Miliaria. Excessive heat, leading to blockage of sweat ducts, can result in this bothersome eruption (NIOSH).

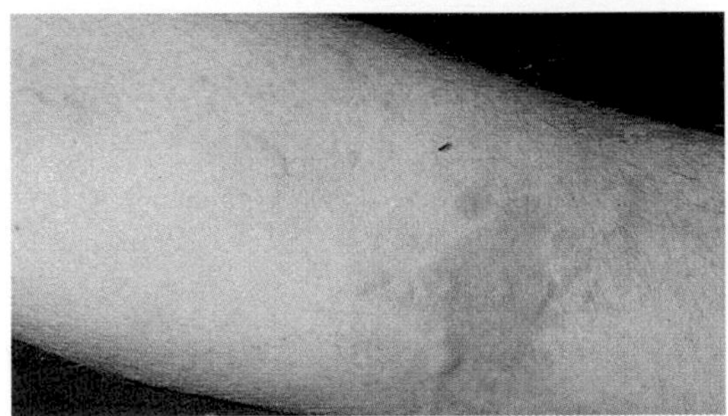

Color Plate 27.8. Urticaria. Urticarial lesions develop on skin contact with gypsy moth caterpillar. This worker in a forestry laboratory also had asthmatic attacks when in close proximity to this caterpillar. (Courtesy of Dr. Shama.)

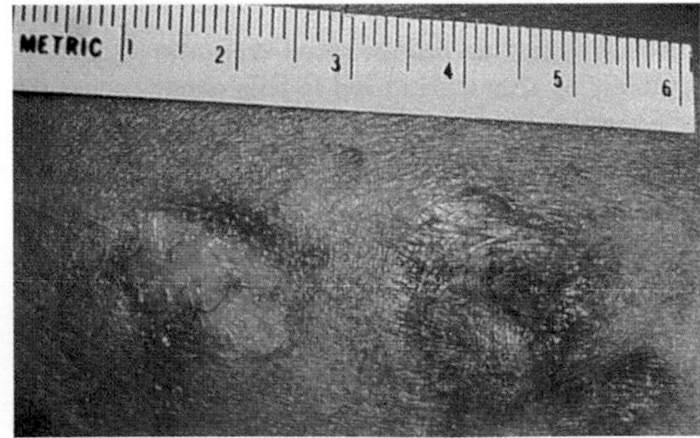

Color Plate 27.9. Granulomas. A chronic inflammatory allergic reaction to skin contact with beryllium can lead to granuloma formation (NIOSH).

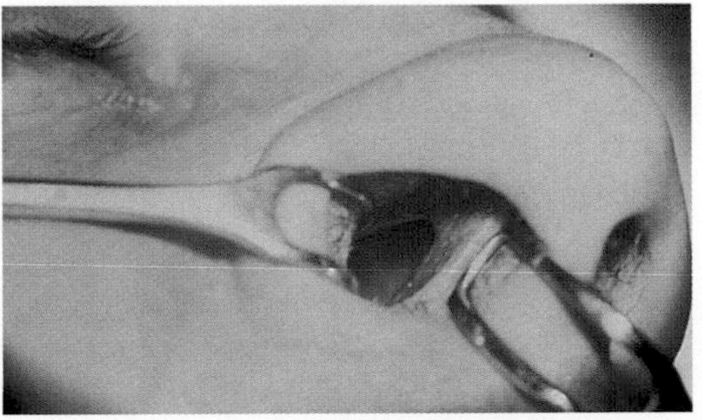

Color Plate 27.10. Ulcerations. Exposure to aerosolized chromic acid may result in painless ulceration of the nasal mucosa and septum (NIOSH).

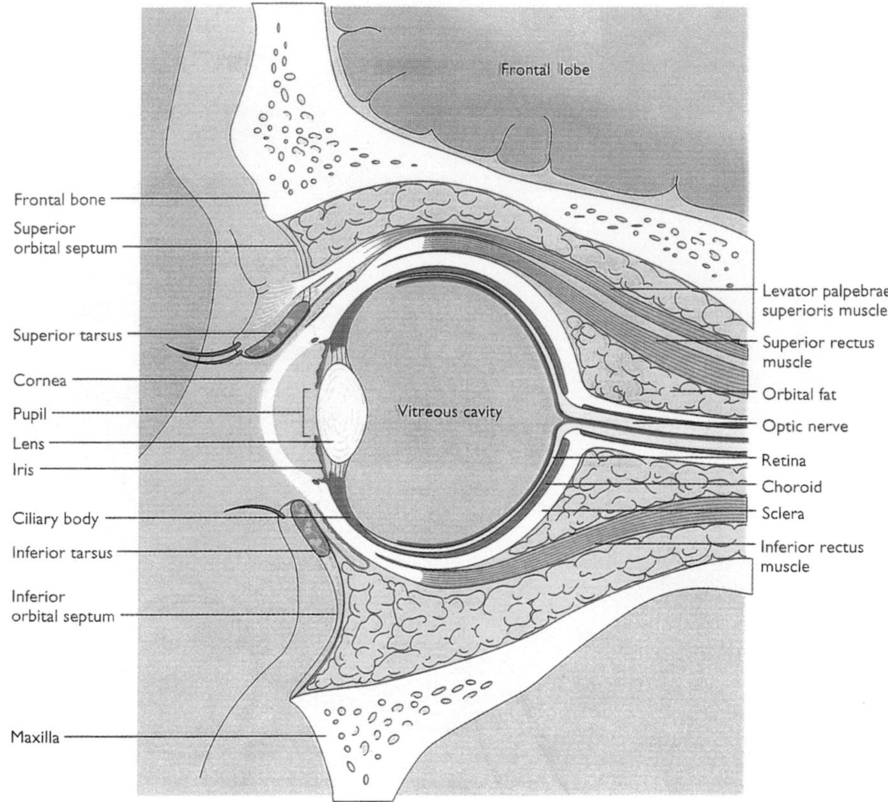

Color Plate 34.1. Sagittal section of the eye and orbit. (From Trobe J. *The physicians guide to eyecare.* San Francisco: Foundation of the American Academy of Ophthalmology, 1993, with permission.)

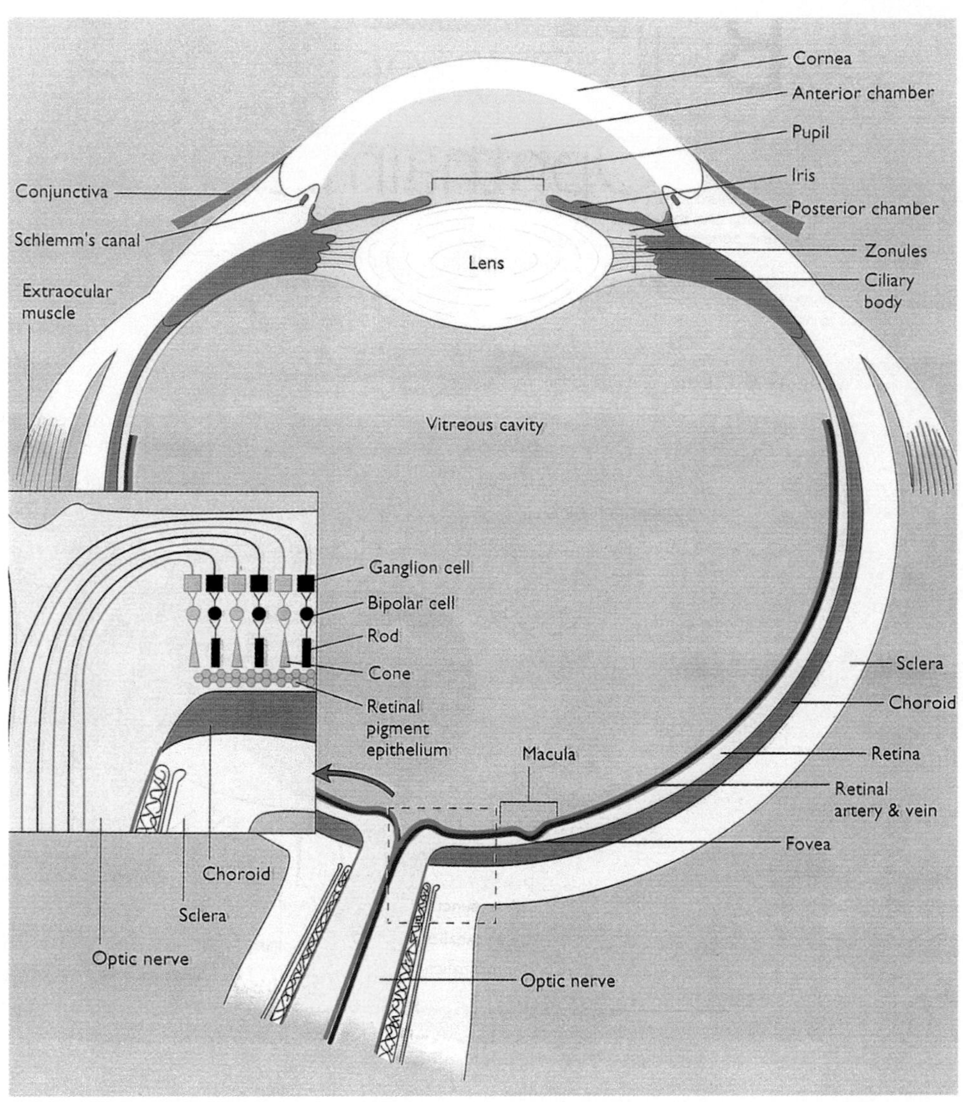

Color Plate 34.2. Cross section of the eye. (From Trobe J. *The physicians guide to eyecare.* San Francisco: Foundation of the American Academy of Ophthalmology, 1993, with permission.)

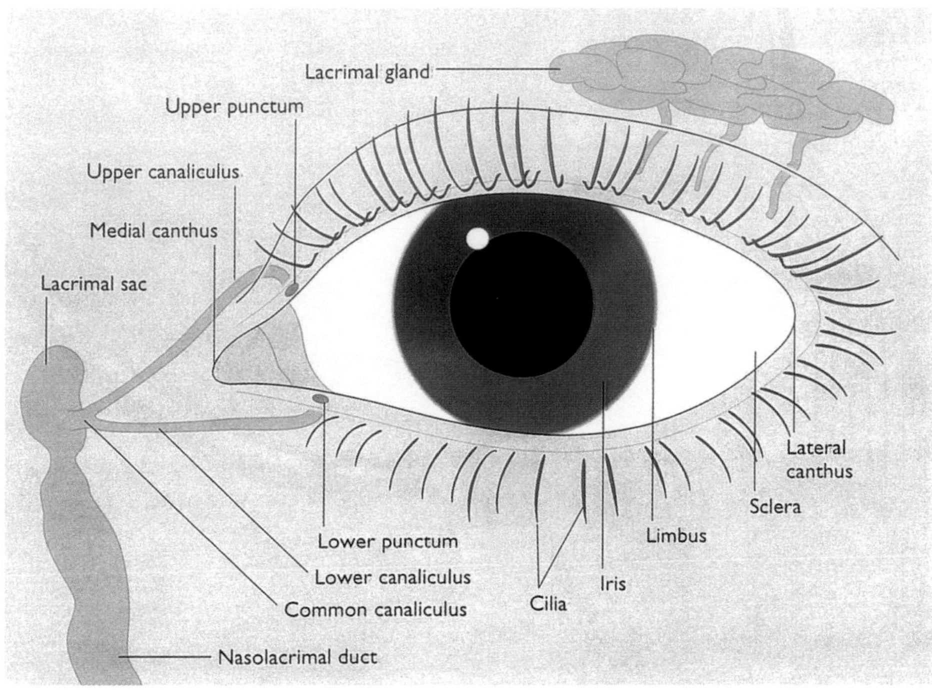

Color Plate 34.3. External eye and lacrimal system. (From Trobe J. *The physicians guide to eyecare.* San Francisco: Foundation of the American Academy of Ophthalmology, 1993, with permission.)

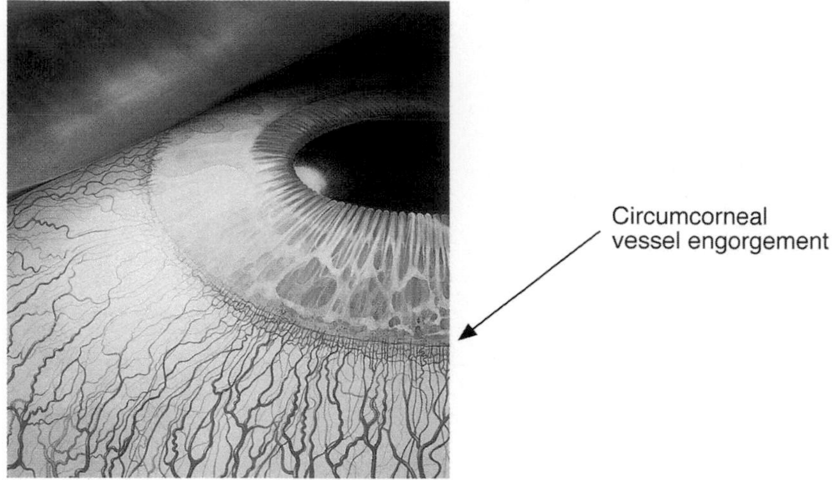

Color Plate 34.5. Ciliary flush. (From Bradford CA, ed. *Basic ophthalmology for medical students and primary care residents,* 7th ed. San Francisco: American Academy of Ophthalmology, 1999, with permission.)

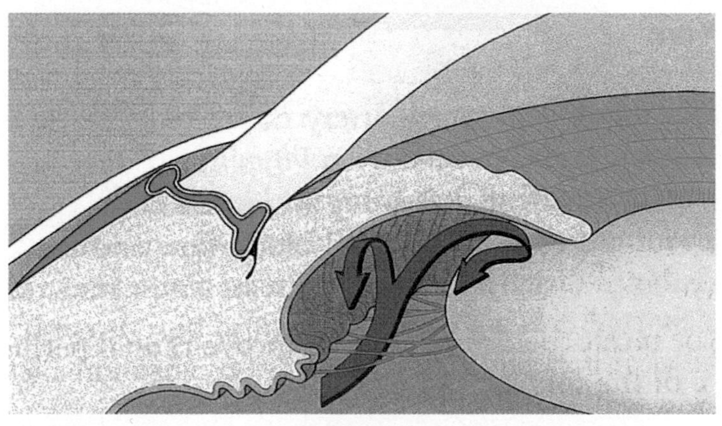

Color Plate 34.6. Iris bombe in acute angle closure glaucoma. (From Wilson FM. *Practical ophthalmology.* San Francisco: American Academy of Ophthalmology, 1996, with permission.)

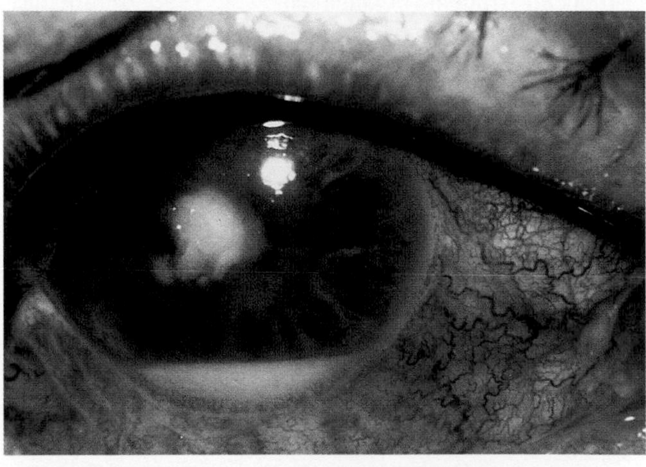

Color Plate 34.7. Hypopyon—layering of white blood cells in up to 50% of the inferior anterior chamber, associated with a corneal ulcer external disease and cornea. (From a slide-script shown by the American Academy of Ophthalmology, 1988.)

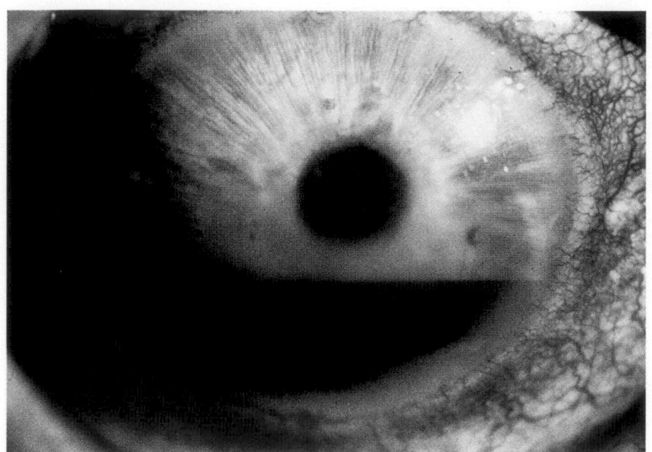

Color Plate 34.8. Hyphema. Gross accumulation of red blood cells in anterior chamber in the inferior one half. (From *Eye trauma and emergencies: a slide script program.* San Francisco: American Academy of Ophthalmology, 1985, with permission.)

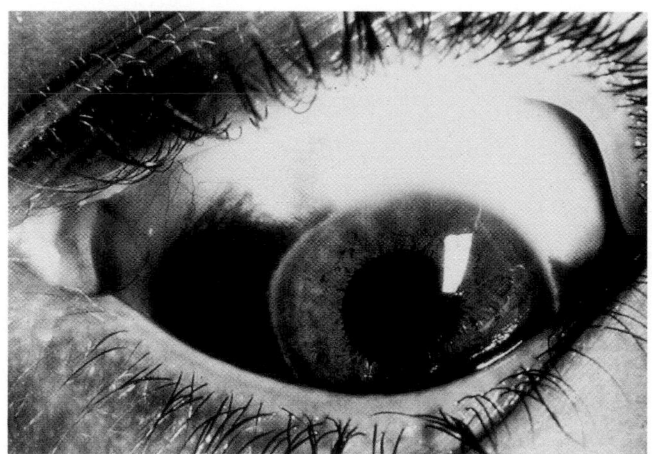

Color Plate 34.9. Subconjunctival hemorrhage: nontraumatic. (From Tredici TJ. Ophthalmology in aerospace medicine. In: DeHart RL, Davis JR, eds. *Fundamentals of aerospace medicine,* 2nd ed. Baltimore: Williams & Wilkins, 1995, with permission.)

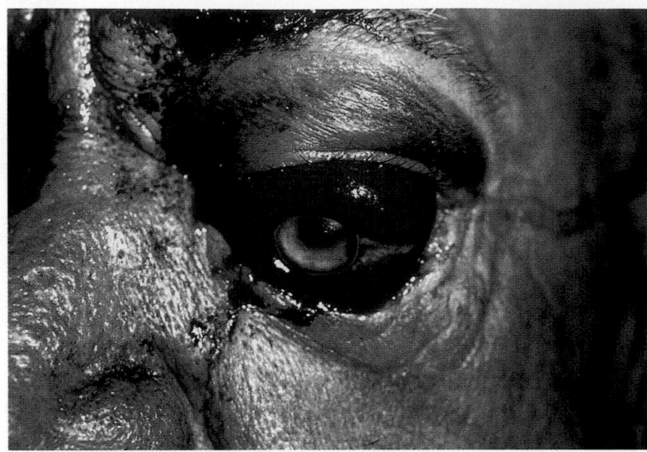

Color Plate 34.10. Proptosis, subconjunctival hemorrhage, microscopic hyphema secondary to blunt trauma to orbit. (From *Eye trauma and emergencies: a slide script program.* San Francisco: American Academy of Ophthalmology, 1985, with permission.)

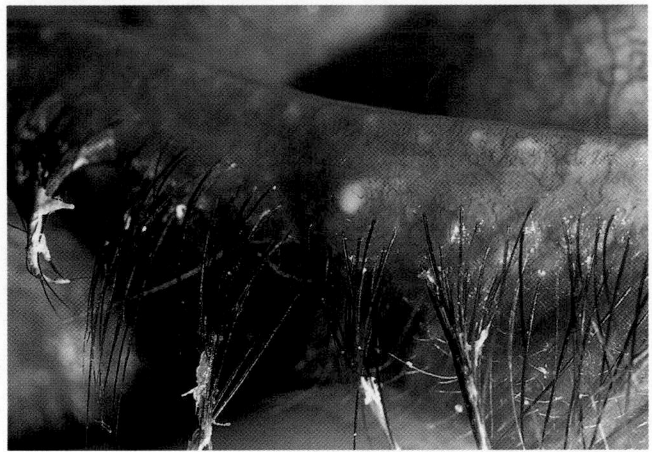

Color Plate 34.14. Acute hordeolum on stye infection of the hair follicle or associated glands of lens or moll. (From a slide-script shown by the American Academy of Ophthalmology, 1994.)

Type III (immune complex) reactions occur when excessive antigen causes a precipitation of antigen-antibody (usually IgG or IgM) complex along the vascular endothelium, resulting in the subsequent attraction of PMNs that cause local damage; complement is required for this to occur. Examples of this type of reaction are hypersensitivity pneumonitis and some autoimmune diseases.

Type IV (delayed hypersensitivity) reactions require previously sensitized lymphocytes but no humoral antibodies or complement. Antigenic stimulation of lymphocytes causes release of lymphokines (interleukins and interferons). The lymphokines attract macrophages and leukocytes, which result in allergic contact dermatitis and granulomatous diseases such as tuberculosis.

Since the last edition of this book, new research has suggested that there are additional types of reactions such as a type V (secretory) and perhaps a new type combining some of the original ones.

ALLERGIC REACTION IN DETAIL

The hypersensitivity reaction consists of two stages: the sensitizing stage and the shocking stage. The sensitizing stage occurs when the individual is initially exposed to the antigen and requires months to years for the specific IgE antibody to bind to the mast cells. The shocking stage takes only a few seconds to minutes and occurs upon reexposure to the specific antigen. Upon reexposure to the same or similar antigen, the antigen binds to the IgE, triggering the mast cell to degranulate and release numerous preformed mediators (e.g., histamine). Leukotrienes and other inflammatory mediators are newly formed and also released during the degranulation process and in the hours after degranulation. Inflammatory cells are recruited into the area and further accentuate the inflammatory reaction. Typical symptoms of the allergic reaction are itchy eyes and nose, nasal congestion, sneezing, coughing, wheezing and/or pruritus, urticaria, and eczema. Thus, the reaction may occur immediately, producing only an immediate hypersensitivity reaction, or may be delayed for several hours (late-phase allergic reaction). Frequently a dual (immediate and late) reaction occurs. It is the late or delayed reaction, occurring during the evening or nighttime hours, that can create confusion and difficulty in evaluating the person with a suspected occupational allergy. Further confusing the situation is the fact that the late-phase reaction, once initiated, can continue for hours, days, or even weeks with only minimal or even no further exposure to the inciting antigen.

Evaluating the Worker for a Suspected Allergy

Assessing the atopic potential of a worker is important for a number of reasons. Some occupational diseases are more likely to occur in the allergic person (e.g., allergic people who are animal handlers) than in nonallergic workers. The latency period before symptoms develop is much shorter in the atopic person. Taking an allergy history is similar to taking any comprehensive history, although several areas are stressed. The timing of symptoms (including any seasonal variation) is important, although it may be misleading, for example, in a late-phase reaction (see previous section). A family history of atopic disease (eczema, allergic rhinitis, asthma, hives, allergy to foods and medications) is significant because allergic diseases are genetically determined. Itching of mucous membranes, although rarely mentioned by the patient, is often a major complaint in the atopic patient.

In the review of systems, one should search for concomitant diseases that might mimic allergy. For example, chronic sinusitis is a very common disease in both atopic and nonatopic individuals. Many persons with this disease have only vague complaints of fatigue, nasal discharge or stuffiness, or a chronic cough. Sinusitis has been clearly shown to exacerbate preexisting asthma. Diagnosing sinusitis requires a high index of suspicion for the disease because its manifestations are often quite protean. Once the infection resolves, nasal and chest symptoms previously attributed to an allergy may disappear or subside. In addition, the review of systems should involve queries about hay fever, intermittent or recurrent dyspnea, chronic cough, any prior diagnoses of asthma, bronchitis or allergy, and repeated infections (especially in the skin and respiratory tract).

In performing the physical examination, one should search for manifestations of atopic diseases, such as eczema, changes in the nasal membranes, and asthma. The person with chronic sinusitis may have severe nasal stuffiness, tenderness when the cheeks and forehead are palpated, halitosis, and frequently a thick, discolored nasal discharge. Eczematous changes in the skin, particularly in the popliteal, antecubital, postauricular, and palmar areas, indicate an atopic tendency. The presence of nasal polyps may indicate an underlying atopic condition (Sampter's triad—nasal polyposis, asthma, and aspirin hypersensitivity). Classic textbooks of medicine often associate specific coloration of the nasal mucosa with certain diseases. This is of little or no practical help in diagnosing allergic rhinitis, however. Wheezing may be absent on the physical examination of asthmatic individuals. Clubbing of the fingers is rarely present in asthma unless accompanied by other lung diseases.

Skin testing remains the gold standard in determining the presence of specific IgE antibody. A wide variety of antigens are available and the procedure is quick, relatively inexpensive, and easy to perform. Interpreting the tests, however, requires a physician to correlate the test results with the history and physical examination; a positive skin test signifies only the presence of IgE and is not diagnostic of an allergic disease.

The chief disadvantages of skin testing are the potential for anaphylaxis; expertise is required to perform, grade, and interpret the test; and the presence of severe skin disease in some people prohibits skin testing.

Laboratory studies are often inconclusive. An elevated eosinophil count is frequently present in a patient with asthma or eczema. The IgE level is not a good screening test for atopy, and a normal IgE level should not exclude the diagnosis of allergy. An extremely elevated eosinophil count or IgE level should prompt a search for alternative diseases (such as bronchopulmonary aspergillosis).

Alternative to skin testing are the radioallergosorbent test (RAST) and the enzyme-linked immunosorbent assay (ELISA), which is currently used most frequently. In these tests, an allergen is bound to a solid-phase support system, the patient's serum is added, and, if antigen-specific IgE is present, it binds to the solid phase. Radioactive or enzyme-labeled anti-IgE is then added and radioactive counts or colorimetric changes are measured. The major advantages of these tests are the ease of testing and absence of anaphylaxis. Some workplace chemicals cannot be skin tested, but RAST and ELISA testing can detect antibodies. The major disadvantages are lack of sensitivity (about 20% less sensitive than skin testing), the limited number of antigens available, and cost. Like skin testing, an elevated RAST or ELISA is a marker of exposure, not of disease.

Other laboratory tests employed in diagnosing asthma include spirometry (Chapter 21) and peak flow measurements (see discussion of occupational asthma, below).

Nasal smear cytology for eosinophils is often a help in diagnosing allergic rhinitis and allergic nasal conditions. This requires a technician experienced in interpreting thin mucus smears for cell types.

X-rays are usually of little benefit in the workup of allergic diseases, with the exception of sinus x-rays or computed tomographic (CT) scan of the sinuses. The best test for chronic sinusitis and nasal polyps is CT scan of the sinuses. Chest x-rays are of value only in ruling out other types of diseases of the lungs that are masquerading as asthma.

OCCUPATIONAL RESPIRATORY DISEASES

Occupational allergic respiratory diseases include allergic rhinitis and allergic rhinosinusitis, occupational allergic asthma, hypersensitivity pneumonitis, and allergic bronchopulmonary aspergillosis.

Occupational rhinitis and rhinosinusitis may be irritative or allergic in nature. Irritation of the nasal mucosa occurs from physical (e.g., talc, coal dust) and chemical (e.g., aldehydes) agents. Allergic reactions result from exposures to high or low molecular weight antigens. Most high molecular weight antigens are naturally occurring substances, such as dust mites, fungal spores, animal danders, and food substances. These antigens react with IgE antibodies present on the mast cells to result in a typical allergic reaction. The low molecular weight antigens such as organic chemicals (isocyanates, acid anhydrides, aldehydes) and inorganic chemicals (chromium, platinum) cause allergy through IgE-IgG human serum albumin hapten complexes or poorly understood mechanisms. All antigens, whatever their molecular weight, cause sensitization (antibody formation after a latent period).

Symptoms of occupational rhinitis are similar to those of spontaneous allergic rhinitis, that is, nasal congestion, sneeze, rhinorrhea, lacrimation, and itchy eyes. These usually appear in the workplace and clear shortly after leaving, unless an isolated late reaction occurs 6 to 8 hours after leaving the workplace. Examination usually reveals pale, boggy nasal turbinates with serous drainage. Rhinometry shows airway obstruction; nasal smear and nasal lavage show increased eosinophils and leukotriene levels. Permanent removal from the offending environment is required for a lasting relief, although antihistamines, decongestants, and nasal steroids may temporarily control the symptoms.

Occupational asthma is bronchial inflammation, airway hyperresponsiveness, and reversible bronchospasm caused by irritants and sensitizers in the workplace. It may be of new onset or aggravation of preexisting asthma. Typical symptoms are chest tightness, dyspnea, cough and wheezing; in some cases cough is the only manifestation. According to Centers for Disease Control (CDC) statistics, there has been a 75% increase in self-reported asthma of all types from 1960 to 1995 and a 46% increase in mortality from 1977 to 1995 (6). The prevalence of asthma in general in the United States is estimated to be 17 million cases; assuming that occupational asthma represents 5% to 15% of this total (average 10%) this would mean that an estimated 1.7 million cases are occupational in nature.

Host Factors

In an occupational cohort, only 5% to 15% of workers in the same environment and exposed to the same agents develop occupational asthma, because host risk factors predispose certain workers to becoming ill. These risk factors are (a) atopy [the state of being allergic, i.e., the presence of elevated IgE levels and a specific human leukocyte antigen (HLA) type], (b) bronchial hyperreactivity, and (c) cigarette smoking.

Classification

Occupational asthma may have irritant, pharmacologic, and immunologic pathogenesis. Brooks et al. (7) have described two types of irritant asthma: Reactive airways dysfunction syndrome (RADS) results from a single massive exposure to irritants in nonatopic workers with no prior history of asthma; chronic low-dose exposure to irritants may result in a slowly developing but persistent chronic irritant asthma (8). Although no sensitizing mechanism has been discovered, reexposure to the offending irritants may exacerbate this chronic irritant asthma.

Pharmacologic agents are represented by three groups of chemicals: the β-adrenergic blocking agents such as toluene diisocyanate (which causes bronchospasm by blocking β-adrenergic receptors in the bronchi); direct histamine releasers such as cotton fibers and narcotics; and anticholinesterase chemicals found in insecticides (inducing asthma by allowing acetylcholine concentration to increase). The remainder of this section deals only with immunologic occupational asthma; Chapter 21 discusses other causes.

Antigenic Molecular Weight

Immunologic occupational asthma is related to workplace antigens that are capable of causing sensitization, i.e., subsequent reexposure to minute concentrations causes sudden and often severe asthma exacerbations. These antigens are classed according to molecular weight, greater than or smaller than 40,000 daltons.

The high molecular weight antigens usually involve the IgE class I mechanism and are found in materials from plants, animals, and foods. Plant sources include fungal spores, grain dust, cereal dust, flour dust (wheat), green coffee bean, tea, green tobacco leaf, and vegetable gums, in addition to tree, grass, and weed pollens. Animal exposure occurs from dander, pelt, saliva, urinary proteins, scales, and feathers. Workers who have contact with animals include animal handlers, researchers, farmers, livestock workers, and veterinarians. These exposures may be complicated by pets at home. Inhalation sensitivity in the food industry can occur from exposure to eggs, mushrooms, shellfish, garlic, and many other foodstuffs. Occupational asthma to enzymes such as trypsin, chemotrypsin, and papain occurs in the pharmaceutical industry. The enzyme from *Bacillus subtilis* causes asthma in sensitized detergent industry workers. Most high molecular weight antigens can be detected by skin or RAST/ELISA testing.

The low molecular weight antigens are a varied group of agents that fall into three subdivisions: therapeutic drugs, organic chemicals, and inorganic chemicals. The first two groups generally cause asthma by means of the antigen human serum albumin (HSA) hapten interacting with antibody (usually IgG, occasionally IgE). Some of these can be evaluated by RAST/ELISA in vitro testing, and a few by skin testing.

Therapeutic agents capable of causing allergic occupational asthma include antibiotics, other pharmaceuticals, and miscellaneous therapeutic agents. The β-lactam antibiotics (penicillins, cephalosporins), the tetracyclines, and the sulfonamides, among others, are the most common causes of sensitivity. Other pharmaceuticals, such as methyldopa (Aldomet), psyllium, cimetidine, albuterol (Salbutamol), pentamidine, ipecac, and ethylene oxide, are capable of triggering allergic asthma. Miscellaneous agents such as piperazine and chloramine have also been implicated in immunologic asthma.

The major low molecular weight organic chemicals known or suspected of causing immune-mediated occupational asthma are abietic acid (colophony), acid anhydrides, aldehydes, isocyanates, and plicatic acid (western red cedar).

Abietic acid is the principal ingredient in colophony, which is produced from distillation of pine resin. Colophony is used as soldering flux (particularly in the electronics industry) and can be inhaled, causing suspected (but not proven) sensitization. It is possible that pine allergy may be a predisposing factor. Some workers are sensitized by inhaling pine dust, although there is no greater incidence of atopy in these workers.

Acid anhydrides are composed of several highly reactive low molecular weight compounds, notably phthalic anhydride (PA) and trimellitic anhydride (TMA). PA causes allergic rhinitis and asthma through anhydride–HSA hapten–specific IgE antibody (type 1). TMA causes not only occupational asthma (type I) but also hypersensitivity pneumonitis (type III), late respiratory systemic syndrome (cough, dyspnea, fever, myalgia-arthralgia) through a TMA–HSA hapten–specific IgG or IgA (not IgE) (type I), and TMA pulmonary disease–anemia syndrome (cough, dyspnea, and hemoptysis) through TMA–HSA hapten–specific IgG.

Aldehydes (formaldehyde and glutaraldehyde) are airway irritants in most workers but can be sensitizers to a few through the IgE or IgG mechanism.

Isocyanates, along with acid anhydrides, are highly reactive compounds that cause sensitization in 5% to 10% of exposed workers. Allergen-specific IgE or IgG-HSA–type reactions have been reported, but generally occupational asthma from isocyanates is believed to be multifactorial (pharmacologic, immunologic, and irritative).

Plicatic acid, which is present in western red cedar wood dust, can cause occupational asthma through a variety of pharmacologic, irritant, and specific and nonspecific immunologic mechanisms. It is not believed to be an IgE-type allergen. Immediate, isolated, late, and dual asthmatic reactions can occur, which seem to implicate an immunologic basis. Much study is ongoing in an attempt to clarify this.

Inorganic chemicals, particularly the salts of chromium, cobalt, nickel, aluminum, platinum, and vanadium, can cause occupational asthma; however, the mechanisms are unclear at the present time. Similar to the situation with red cedar, an underlying immunologic mechanism is implicated.

Phases of the Asthmatic Response

Because of the complex mechanisms involved in the causation and manifestations of asthma, the duration may vary between the exposure and actual onset of symptoms. Currently, three phases of the asthmatic are recognized: immediate, isolated late, and dual.

The immediate-phase reaction occurs within seconds to minutes after exposure to the offending antigen. It is caused by the release of histamine, prostaglandins, leukotrienes, and platelet-activating factors. Fifty percent of cases exposed to high molecular weight antigens will respond immediately, in contrast to only 10% of cases exposed to low molecular weight antigens.

About 6 to 8 hours after an initial exposure an isolated late-phase reaction may occur, with no immediate reaction preceding. These responses are usually caused by leukotriene release and inflammatory cell infiltration. Forty percent of these isolated late reactions are caused by low molecular weight antigens; only 2% result from exposure to high molecular weight antigens. These reactions occur when the worker is at home or away from the workplace, resulting in much confusion as to the exact cause of the attack. Further confusing the situation is that the late-phase reaction, once initiated, can continue for hours, days, or even weeks with only minimal or no further exposure to the inciting allergen. Thus, removing the worker from the suspected allergen for one or two shifts may not be sufficient to determine if the exposure is causing the symptoms. The suggested trial period is a minimum of 2 weeks.

The dual response includes both immediate and late phases. These responses occur with almost equal frequency (48% to 50%) in high and low molecular weight antigenic exposure.

Evaluation of Occupational Asthma

The purpose of a complete evaluation is to establish whether asthma indeed exists and, if so, whether it is related to the workplace. Initially, a general complete history with emphasis on allergy and occupational factors is extremely important. This history would include a review of the job description and the Material Safety Data Sheets, if available. A complete physical examination and routine laboratory workup are necessary to rule out any underlying diseases. Becklake (9) presents a logical, stepwise workup to ascertain criteria for the presence of an asthma, allergy, and workplace relationship.

To establish the presence of bronchospasm, the clinician must be given a history of dyspnea, wheeze, and cough. Physical examination revealing wheezing is ideal, but often this is not present because asthmatics may be completely asymptomatic during the office evaluation. Pulmonary function tests at this point should show a decrease in the forced expiratory volume in 1 second (FEV_1) and perhaps a decrease in forced expiratory flow of 25% to 75%.

To establish the presence of bronchial hyperresponsiveness, a history of episodic dyspnea, wheeze, and cough is needed. If baseline spirometry demonstrates an obstructive pattern, bronchodilator (such as albuterol) inhalation should show a 20% or greater increase in FEV_1. However, if the baseline spirometry is normal, a methacholine challenge test should result in a 20% drop in FEV_1. If no significant change occurs in the FEV_1, using these procedures, then no significant bronchial hyperresponsiveness exists.

To establish the presence of atopy, there should be an atopic family history or a history of previous allergies in the patient. More likely than not, skin tests to common antigens should be positive and a RAST may be helpful. Increased levels of total IgE and elevated total eosinophil counts are likewise helpful in diagnosing allergies.

To establish the work-relatedness of airway obstruction, a history of relation of symptoms to work with cessation of symptoms when away from work is valuable. Pre- and postshift peakflow rate (PFR) diaries both at work and at home are helpful. The PFR should be recorded before, during, and after work. The physician should stress to the patient the importance of keeping the PFR diary on holidays and vacations as well as documenting any change in pulmonary function that occurs away from work.

To establish the presence of specific sensitization, skin testing is sometimes possible in cases of high molecular weight agents. Skin tests, however, afford little or no value when low molecular weight agents are involved. At times, a specific IgE RAST may be helpful for certain chemicals. Inhalation challenge testing using specific agents is considered the gold standard among all tests for occupational asthma. Specific inhalation challenge testing, however, should be carried out only under conditions of close medical supervision in a specially designed inhalation unit at a medical center and with emergency care available. Overnight observation of the patient is suggested because of the possibility of an isolated late reaction.

Malo (10) suggests a questionnaire, skin or RAST testing, and pre– and post–work shift spirometry by the pulmonologist, allergist, or occupational medicine physician. Only if a 20% drop is seen in the FEV_1 at the end of the work shift does Malo recommend proceeding with repeated workplace and nonworkplace PFRs, workplace inhalation tests if feasible, or specific inhalation challenge in a medical center under a specialist's supervision.

Peak Flowmeter Measurements

Peak flow measurement is a low-cost, effective way to help diagnose and monitor a worker's airway disease. Many peak flowmeters currently available provide sufficiently reproducible readings in a given patient to assist the physician in diagnosis and treatment of suspected bronchospastic lung disease. However, since the peak flow is effort dependent, a patient may not perform the test properly or may use it for secondary gain.

The physician should become familiar with one or two types of meters. Criteria used in selecting a particular meter include availability, cost (an adequate meter can be purchased for about $30), an easily readable scale, and durability.

Using a peak flowmeter is simple and easily mastered by almost all patients after minimal (5–10 minutes) training. Training must be conducted by an individual knowledgeable in the peak flow maneuver and the reading and charting of values. The patient should be observed while performing three peak flow measurements, but one should chart only the best (not the average) reading. Changes in medications and symptoms, as well as any changes in work schedule or duties, should also be noted on the chart. Ideally, the worker should take the first reading on arising and every 2 hours thereafter until bedtime. If the individual is taking a β-adrenergic inhaler, all readings should be consistently taken before he or she uses the inhaler. Practically, however, it is probably sufficient to perform readings upon awakening and at preshift, midshift, end of shift, and bedtime. It is important to assess any important changes in readings (generally 20% change or greater) over the course of a day, as well as any significant differences among the different days of the workweek, weekends, and vacations.

When the peak flow chart is reviewed, the physician should correlate the readings with the patient's symptoms and physical findings. A marked discrepancy between these factors suggests poor effort or technique in performing the maneuver. Fluctuations in the range of $\pm 10\%$ are usual when comparing readings taken at the same time on different days. Too little variability suggests that the patient is not performing peak flow readings well.

Even with all the caveats noted above, peak flowmeters are a useful tool for the occupational medicine physician. In addition, the readings can provide useful feedback information for the patient in judging the degree of impairment and the need for medication.

Treatment of Occupational Asthma

The goals of treatment are the same for all types of asthma: to maintain pulmonary function as close to normal as possible, to maintain a normal lifestyle, and to prevent exacerbations.

In occupational asthma, more than any other type of asthma, the patient must be removed from the offending environment as soon as possible. With continued exposure to the offending agent, more and more bronchial damage develops and irreversible changes occur in the airways. This damage appears to be related to duration and dose, further emphasizing the need for early removal from the workplace. Removal of the offending agent by process substitution measures may be possible, but this should not delay interruption of exposure. A respirator is not a suitable alternative in cases of allergy.

If occupational asthma symptoms are present during or after removal from the workplace, then pharmacologic treatment of asthma as outlined by the National Heart, Lung, and Blood Institute guidelines is needed (11). Treatment is based on the classification of severity in four steps: mild intermittent asthma, mild persistent asthma, moderate persistent asthma, and severe persistent asthma.

Return to Work

Returning the occupational asthma patient to work requires much deliberation on the part of the occupational physician, with each case being considered individually. Under Americans with Disabilities Act (ADA) guidelines, workers initially cannot be denied any job they are qualified to do as long as they are aware of the risk factors (see above). It is the occupational physician's duty to advise the worker of these risk factors and consequences before exposure.

Acute asthma or exacerbation of chronic asthma of any type requires removal from exposure until pulmonary symptoms and function return to the patient's norm, with or without treatment. Return to the workplace then becomes a difficult decision.

If the asthma is caused by irritants, then an industrial hygiene consultation is necessary to ensure environmental controls are able to eliminate or reduce the irritant to tolerable levels. The worker may then return to work using person protective equipment [PPE, a National Institute for Occupational Safety and Health (NIOSH)-approved respirator] if necessary. The worker should be reevaluated at frequent intervals and removed permanently from the workplace if symptoms recur or pulmonary function deteriorates.

In cases of immunologic occupational asthma, the worker must be permanently removed from the exposure. If administrative and environmental controls are possible to eliminate the exposure (this is usually not possible), then a trial return to the original job is feasible. Frequent reevaluation of the worker is mandatory and any indication of deterioration of lung function demands immediate permanent withdrawal.

It is important to note that workers with occupational asthma may be impaired but they are not disabled and usually can be reassigned to an alternative job. This may mean a change in financial and administrative status, however. Controversial aspects of impairment and disability are beyond the scope of this chapter.

Hypersensitivity Pneumonitis (Extrinsic Allergic Alveolitis)

Hypersensitivity pneumonitis occurs when inhaled antigens in the home or work environment cause an immunologic inflammatory reaction (type III, immune complex reaction) in the bronchioles, alveoli, and lung interstitium. The most frequent allergens are thermophilic actinomycetes, which are found in warm, humid environments (such as soil, hay, or forced heating and cooling systems) in which the water has stagnated. Other causes of hypersensitivity pneumonitis include chemicals such as isocyanates and trimellitic anhydride. The prevalence of the disease is about 7% to 15% of exposed individuals.

Hypersensitivity pneumonitis (HP) can occur in an acute, subacute, or chronic form. The acute form appears as a flu-like illness 4 to 6 hours after heavy intermittent exposure. Symptoms abate after a few hours to a few days if exposure is avoided. Pulmonary function tests show a restrictive pattern. Hypoxemia and decreased diffusing capacity are found. The chest x-ray may be normal or show granular or nodular infiltrates. The subacute and chronic forms occur with continued exposure. Progressive dyspnea, decreased exercise tolerance, productive cough, and weight loss develop gradually. Pulmonary function tests show a severe restrictive pattern. The chest x-ray findings are typical of diffuse interstitial fibrosis.

On physical examination, the lung auscultation reveals dry, crackling rales throughout the lungs that are more prominent at the bases. Wheezing generally does not occur, but if present, makes the differentiation between HP and occupational asthma quite difficult. Asthma may coexist with HP, especially in the atopic patient.

There is no single pathognomonic test for HP. Specific precipitating (IgG) antibodies to offending substances are helpful in making the diagnosis and are present in over 90% of individuals with the disease, but there are several points to remember. First, these antibodies are only a marker to exposure, not disease. Second, since the sensitivity of the test varies among commercial laboratories, negative tests in the context of strong clinical evidence suggesting the disease do not exclude the diagnosis. In addition, not all patients demonstrate antibodies to the same antigen and many patients have multiple precipitating antibodies. Finally, antibody levels begin to fall once exposure is terminated, although this fall in antibody levels does not correlate with disease remission or progression. Thus, the patient with severe, chronic HP may have no detectable precipitating antibodies. Since skin testing only detects IgE antibodies, it provides little or no help in confirming the diagnosis.

In treating the acute episodes, corticosteroids are often used to hasten recovery. There is no evidence that long-term corticosteroid usage protects against lung damage from chronic exposure. Avoidance of the offending antigen is the most important treatment. Masks, dust filters, and attention to the heating and air conditioning systems are all important. The patient may need to change occupations depending on the degree of modification required to make the worker's environment safe and the specific antigen involved.

Acute Bronchopulmonary Aspergillosis

Acute bronchopulmonary aspergillosis (ABPA) is severe asthma associated with an elevated serum IgE and total eosinophil count. The condition results from colonization of the lower-respiratory tract with *Aspergillus fumigatus* spores (rarely other fungi). In addition to periodic episodes of severe bronchoconstriction, the patient demonstrates transient pulmonary infiltrates on x-ray and has thick, brown sputum plugs. Skin testing shows an immediate reaction to the fungal spores, with a late reaction appearing in about 4 hours in some patients. Serum precipitating IgG antibodies are also present. Damage to the bronchial walls occurs from the action of IgE and IgG *Aspergillus* antibody. This leads to central bronchiectasis and granulomas through type I, II, and IV reactions. Long-term use of corticosteroids is required for control.

NATURAL RUBBER LATEX (NRL) ALLERGY

Since the early 1980s, it has been recognized that products containing latex and natural rubber can cause immediate and delayed hypersensitivity reactions. Severe anaphylactic reactions and deaths have been reported. The prevalence of NRL allergy in the general population ranges from less than 1% to as high as 9% in various studies (12). However, certain groups are at higher risk for NRL allergy (Table 29.2). Several studies have suggested that the most important risk factor is the degree of exposure. For example, among health care workers, those with the highest incidence of latex allergy are those who use and change gloves frequently. There is no correlation with age or sex.

TABLE 29.2. *Groups at higher risk for developing NRL allergy*

Health care workers
Workers in the rubber industry
Children with spina bifida (up to 60%)
Individuals who use latex gloves and who have a hand dermatitis
Prior history of atopy (especially allergies to food such as avocado, chestnut, banana, kiwi)
Individuals who have had multiple surgeries

Types of reactions include local or generalized eczema or urticaria, rhinitis, conjunctivitis, bronchospasm, and anaphylaxis. The type of reaction is often correlated with the route of exposure. For example, latex exposure of the skin may cause a dermatitis, aerosolized particles from the latex gloves may produce rhinoconjunctivitis or bronchospasm, and latex exposure intraoperatively and during dental procedures can cause anaphylaxis as a result of the direct exposure of mucous membranes to the latex. Any worker with unexplained skin rash who has regular and frequent exposure to latex or rubber should be suspected of having latex hypersensitivity. NRL allergen is readily absorbed from the skin and mucosal surfaces. Reactions usually begin within 30 minutes of exposure, although delayed reactions occurring hours after the exposure can also occur.

Once a worker is suspected of having a NRL allergy, the presence of NRL antibodies in the serum should be sought. At the present time, there are several diagnostic tests available: CAP RAST (Pharmacia Upjohn), AlaSTAT (Diagnostic Products), and HY-TEC-EIA (HYTEC). Since each product has about a 25% false-negative response, a negative test in a patient with a history suggestive of a latex allergy should prompt further investigation. Consideration should be given at this point to referring the patient to an allergist who has experience in evaluating and treating latex allergic patients. Further evaluation might include having the person wear a latex glove for 15 minutes, following by 20 minutes of observation looking for findings suggesting a positive response (such as urticaria). This glove-use test should be carried out with extreme caution (if at all) in a patient suspected of having bronchospastic or anaphylactic reactions due to NRL, and should be done only if the physician has experience in recognizing and

TABLE 29.3. *Treatment of the latex-allergic person*

Avoid unnecessary latex exposure.
Use nonlatex gloves exclusively.
Wear a medical bracelet stating that the person is "ALLERGIC TO LATEX AND NATURAL RUBBER."
Be trained in the usage of and carry an injectable epinephrine kit (Epipen).
Work in a low latex environment.

treating anaphylaxis. Outside the U.S., there are now several standardized skin test reagents available but none has yet been approved for commercial usage by the Food and Drug Administration (FDA). Once these are available, however, the ability to objectively verify NRL allergy will be greatly enhanced.

The treatment of the patient who has latex allergy (Table 29.3) is avoidance of NRL proteins. Total avoidance is generally unnecessary and in any case it is extremely difficult or impossible to do because rubber- and latex-containing products are ubiquitous. Rather, what is generally recommended is a "latex-safe" environment. A latex safe environment is one in which the ambient concentration of NRL proteins is low. In a health care facility this is generally most easily accomplished by having all non-NRL sensitive workers use only nonlatex (preferable) or at least nonpowdered latex gloves. The sensitized worker should use nonlatex gloves exclusively.

At the present time, premedication of the sensitized person with oral steroids and other medications prior to significant NRL exposure (for example prior to a dental visit or surgery) is questionable. Avoidance remains the best method of protection.

SINUSITIS

Acute and chronic sinus infections are common illnesses in both the allergic and nonallergic populations. Individuals who have acute sinusitis generally pose few difficulties in diagnosis since they usually present with the typical symptoms of stuffiness, facial pain, and purulent nasal discharge, often accompanied by fever. The diagnosis of chronic sinusitis, however, requires a high index of suspicion since the patient often complains of vague symptoms such as fatigue, headaches, cough, nasal congestion, and/or a nasal discharge (which may be clear or purulent). Many individuals with chronic sinusitis are suspected of having "allergies." Sinusitis has also been shown to exacerbate asthma. In addition, the cough due to asthma can sometimes be difficult to distinguish from that due to a postnasal drip secondary to the sinus infections. Acute

TABLE 29.4. *Treatment of sinusitis*

Acute sinusitis
- Antibiotic: amoxicillin, trimethoprim/sulfamethoxazole for 10–14 days, azithromycin (Zithromax)[a]
- Consider: oral decongestants
  - Nasal decongestants (no longer than 2–3 days)
  - Nasal steroid spray
  - Saline nasal lavage (½ tsp table salt + 8 oz boiled, cool tap water)
- Encourage hydration (6–8 glasses of water daily)

Chronic sinusitis
- Antibiotic: amoxicillin,[b] trimethoprim/sulfamethoxazole,[b] amoxicillin-clavulanate (Augmentin), cefuroxime axetil (Ceftin), loracarbef (Lorabid), a quinolone such as levofloxacin (Levaquin), for 21–30 days
- Consider: oral decongestants
  - Nasal decongestants (no longer than 2–3 days)
  - Nasal steroid spray
  - Saline nasal lavage (½ tsp table salt + 8 oz boiled, cool tap water)
- Encourage hydration (6–8 glasses of water daily)

[a]If no significant improvement within 1 week of initiating antibiotic, reconsider the diagnosis or switch to a broad-spectrum antibiotic (see chronic sinusitis).

[b]If the diagnosis is reasonably certain and the patient has not improved, switch to a broad-spectrum antibiotic.

sinus infections generally require 10 to 14 days of an antibiotic; chronic sinus infections are much more difficult to resolve and frequently require far longer courses of treatment. While narrow-spectrum antibiotics such as amoxicillin or trimethoprim/sulfamethoxazole should be considered when treating a chronic sinus infection, often a more broad-spectrum drug is needed and should be considered if there is no significant improvement in 5 to 7 days. A recommended approach to treating acute and chronic sinusitis is outlined in (Table 29.4). If the diagnosis is in doubt, a coronal sinus CT scan rather than routine sinus x-rays should be considered since the latter will miss up to 20% of significant sinus infections. Referral to an allergist or otolaryngologist for further evaluation should be considered if the infection does not resolve after aggressive treatment or frequently reoccurs.

FUNGAL DISEASES

Of all the microbiologic agents, the fungi present particular problems, not only because of their ubiquity (greatest source of aeroallergens worldwide), but also because of their ability to cause hypersensitivity, infection, and toxicity. Fungal growth in the workplace is enhanced by dampness (standing water and high relative humidity), warm temperature, poor air circulation, and darkness. Source control requires attention to all these factors.

Hypersensitivity reactions result from the antigenic material released from fungal spore walls, mycelial walls, and submicronic airborne particles. All four types of hypersensitivity reactions defined above can occur in the following patterns from fungal exposure: type I, immediate hypersensitivity (occupational rhinitis and asthma); type III, immune complex reactions (hypersensitivity pneumonitis) if spores are small and exposure is very intense; and a combination type I-II-IV reaction in ABPA.

Although fungal infections are usually limited to immune-suppressed workers, overwhelming exposure to the spores of *Histoplasma* and *Cryptococcus* may cause infections in otherwise healthy people.

Mycotoxins are a result of fungal metabolites that contaminate foods, particularly nuts, corn, rice, and other grains. These metabolites are toxic to animals and humans ingesting the contaminated foodstuffs. *Aspergillus flavus* produces aflatoxin, which is a powerful hepatocarcinogen. Trichothecenes are formed from *Fusarium, Trichoderma,* and *Cephalosporium* fungi and cause diarrhea, multiple hemorrhages, skin inflammation, and death if contaminated wheat is ingested. At present, no cases of mycotoxicity from inhalation have been reported.

ANAPHYLAXIS

Anaphylaxis refers to a (potentially) life-threatening, acute IgE-mediated reaction that results in the release of large amounts of mediators. An anaphylactoid reaction produces physical findings and symptoms indistinguishable from those of an anaphylactic reaction, but without demonstrable IgE involvement (Table 29.5).

Symptoms may be limited to one organ system or involve multiple organs. Once the reaction begins, it may rapidly progress and become fatal. Nonfatal reactions resolve within 1 or 2 days.

TABLE 29.5. *Common cause of anaphylactic and anaphylactoid reactions*

Food
Food additives
Antibiotics
Other drugs
Allergenic extracts
Diagnostic agents
Blood products (human, animal)
Local anesthetics
Insect sting
Latex
Exercise
Temperature extremes (heat, cold)

Clinical manifestations of anaphylaxis present in three forms: mild systemic reactions, moderate systemic reactions, and severe systemic reactions. Mild systemic reactions are characterized by peripheral tingling, a warm sensation throughout the body, fullness in the mouth and throat, nasal congestion, sneezing, facial swelling, and pruritus. Moderate systemic reactions usually involve respiratory distress (wheezing, dyspnea, hoarse voice, cough), anxiety, generalized hives, or angioedema. Severe systemic reactions are characterized by severe respiratory distress and inability to talk, cyanosis, swollen tongue, abdominal cramps, diarrhea, vomiting, hypotension, shock, and loss of consciousness.

Treatment consists of a rapid assessment since delay in therapy can result in a fatal outcome. Epinephrine 1:1,000, 0.3 to 0.5 mL subcutaneously, is the treatment of choice. Diphenhydramine (25–75 mg) intramuscularly may be given in addition to the epinephrine. (In patients with only skin rash, the physician may elect to use only the diphenhydramine.) If the reaction is the result of a medical injection or an insect sting (see below), a tourniquet should be applied above the injection site if possible. The patient should be observed for at least 30 minutes after symptoms subside and be told to contact his or her physician if symptoms reoccur over the next several hours. If symptoms progress or do not begin to subside quickly, one should consider transporting the patient by ambulance to an emergency facility for vasopressors, with fluid therapy and airway management if needed. After the acute episode, the patient should be referred to an allergist for further evaluation.

Patients who are taking a beta-blocking drug may experience less effectiveness from epinephrine and a more severe or prolonged anaphylactic episode. Injection of glucagon has been advocated in such patients.

Allergy to insect stings is reported to be the cause of 40 to 60 deaths annually, although the actual number may be higher. A study of factory workers found that 5% had a history of significant reaction to an insect sting in the past (13). Outdoor workers such as agricultural workers or utility linemen may also experience reactions at a higher prevalence. The symptoms of insect sting anaphylaxis are no different from those outlined above. Although most cases of insect sting anaphylaxis occur soon after the sting, there have been several reports of late reactions, more than 24 hours following the sting.

Treatment of large local reactions to an insect sting consists of elevation of the limb, ice applied to the sting site, and oral antihistamines. One should consider a short course of prednisone for massive local reactions (reactions extending more than two joints beyond the sting site). Any patient who has had a generalized reaction should be assumed to be at risk for a serious anaphylactic reaction and, therefore, treated according to the protocol outlined above. In addition, any patient who has had a generalized reaction (including generalized hives) should be referred for an allergy evaluation. Insect venom immunotherapy is safe and extremely effective in preventing further systemic reactions. Also, any patient suspected of being venom allergic should be trained in the use of an emergency treatment kit containing epinephrine. Epi-Pen and Epi-Pen, Jr. can be obtained from Dey Laboratories (Napa, California). Demonstration kits for health professionals are available.

IMMUNOTOXICANTS

Immunotoxicology is the study of toxic effects of xenobiotics on the cellular and acellular components of the immune system. The multiplicity of chemical and biologic agents in the home and workplace and their complex interactions within the immune system make this field confusing and difficult to assess.

Although the majority of immunotoxicants have a suppressive effect, some may stimulate the immune mechanism, resulting in allergy or autoimmunity, while others may cause uncontrolled cellular proliferation and altered host defense mechanisms.

Regarding immunostimulation, some metals (nickel, platinum, and beryllium) are capable of causing asthma (type I), pulmonary hypersensitivity syndromes (type III), and allergic contact dermatitis (type IV). Isocyanates can cause asthma (type I) and anhydrides can cause asthma (type I), pulmonary disease–anemia syndrome (type II), hypersensitivity pneumonitis (type III), and delayed-type hypersensitivity (type IV). Therapeutic drugs (especially β-lactam antibiotics), food additives (sulfides and MSG), and pesticides (pyrethrum) are all capable of immunostimulation resulting in anaphylactic reactions (type I). Fossil fuel combustion products such as diesel exhaust particles may act as adjuvants to stimulate IgE production and eosinophilic inflammation (type I) leading to asthma (14).

The low molecular weight compounds may bind with serum albumin to form haptens against which T and B cells misdirect antibodies, resulting in autoimmune destruction of autologous tissue. Dieldrin pesticide is associated with immune hemolytic anemia, hydrazine with lupus-like syndrome, monomeric vinyl chloride with scleroderma-like changes, and heavy metals (such as gold) with immune complex glomerulonephritis. Most of these autoimmune reactions are reversible upon removal of the offending chemicals.

The majority of immunotoxicants are suppressive, either dampening the whole immune apparatus or acting at specific points. For instance, benzene, although capable of general bone marrow suppression, specifically causes the reduced synthesis of IgG and IgE antibodies. Polychlorinated biphenyls (PCBs) depress both humoral (B cell) and delayed-type (T cell) immunity while the polycyclic aromatic hydrocarbon 7,2-dimethylbenz (a) anthracene (DMBA) causes long-lasting immune suppression, mostly affecting the B cells. Urethane suppresses NK cell activity, allowing neoplastic cells to grow unchecked.

Many airborne pollutants, such as formaldehyde, ozone, asbestos, oxidant gases, and environmental tobacco smoke, depress nonspecific resistance to bacteria and viruses by suppressing macrophage, phagocytic, and enzymatic activity.

Microbiologics such as bacteria (thermophilic actinomycetes) and fungi *(Aspergillus)* can stimulate immune hypersensitivity lung reactions. Viruses (human immunodeficiency virus) can destroy T-cell clones, thus permitting opportunistic infections *(Pneumocystis carinii)* and unusual neoplasia (Kaposi's sarcoma).

Physical agents such as heat, cold, and vibration promote urticaria and angioedema through nonspecific immune aberrations.

IMMUNE TESTING

The multitude of chemicals, complex interactions of the immune system, and confusing array of symptoms require a logical system of testing (in addition to a complete history and physical examination) to ensure that all major possibilities are investigated. The subcommittee on immunotoxicology of the National Research Council's Committee on Biological Markers has proposed a tiered testing approach (15).

Tier I (used in all people exposed to immunotoxicants) includes measurements of humoral antibody (such as pneumococcal or polio), total levels of the specific immunoglobulins (IgG, IgM, IgA, IgE) and isotope-specific antibody titration (ELISA), complete blood counts and differentials, lymphocyte enumeration and typing (T and B cells, T-cell subsets, and plasma cells), and measurements of delayed-type hypersensitivity (*Candida,* purified protein derivative, mumps, tetanus) and antibody titers (e.g., antinuclear antibody).

Tier II tests are only carried out in people with significant abnormalities in tier I. These tests include the induction of primary antibody response to injected protein or polysaccharide antigens, stimulation of lymphocyte proliferation with specific mitogens, additional T- and B-cell marker determinations, and measurement of cytokines (interleukins and interferons).

Tier III tests (limited to people with abnormalities in tier II) consist of tests for NK cell function (such as nonspecific killing of tumor cells in culture) and biopsy of lymphatic tissue, spleen, or bone marrow.

It should be pointed out that flow cytometry requires close attention to quality control and must be carried out precisely in specialized immunologic laboratories. All tests should correlate with the history and physical examination, and care should be taken to allow for individual ranges of variation. Indiscriminate use of biomarker assays may lead to misdiagnosis and erroneous associations.

Because of the complexity of techniques and multiple factors affecting the final laboratory results, it is important to have tier testing done and interpreted by certified immunologists at well-established, university-recognized immunotoxicologic laboratories.

IDIOPATHIC ENVIRONMENTAL INTOLERANCE (MULTIPLE CHEMICAL SENSITIVITY)

In 1989, the Ontario (Canada) Ministry of Health defined Multiple Chemical Sensitivity as:

> A chronic (i.e., continuous over three months) multi-system disorder, usually involving symptoms of the CNS and at least one other system. Affected persons are frequently intolerant to some foods and react to some chemicals and environmental agents, singly or in combinations at levels generally tolerated by the majority of people. Affected individuals have varying degrees of morbidity, from mild discomfort to total disability. Upon physical examination, the patient is usually free from any abnormal or objective physical findings (16).

McClellan (17) lists five points that he considers necessary to make the diagnosis: (a) at least three organ systems are involved, with a plethora of symptoms; (b) symptoms result from extremely low doses; (c) symptoms may start localized and then spread; (d) patients are more vocal about their symptoms; and (e) patients are more disabled than anticipated.

In 1996, a World Health Organization Workshop on Multiple Chemical Sensitivity recommended that the term "multiple chemical sensitivity" (MCS) be discontinued. Among other organizations, the American College of Physician (ACP), American Academy of Asthma, Allergy, and Immunology (AAAAI) (18), American College of Asthma, Allergy, and Immunology (ACAAI), American Medical Association (AMA) (19), and American College of Occupational Environmental Medicine (ACOEM) (20) have concurred. A new name was recommended: idiopathic environmental intolerance (IEI). The term MCS makes an unsupported judgment about causation; there may not be multiple chemicals involved, and there is no objective evidence of hypersensitivity by immunologic parameters.

The patient with IEI is generally a woman in her 40s who is usually well educated (often at least 2 years of college education). The individual patient may manifest a variety of symptoms, including extreme sensitivity to odors, fatigue, headache, inability to concentrate, paresthesias, and other symptoms involving the central nervous, respiratory, and GI systems. The initiating event is usually a well-defined (but frequently unmeasured and/or undocumented) exposure to a petrochemical, pesticide, or generally innocuous environmental substance. Thereafter, symptoms may be triggered or exacerbated by almost any other natural or manmade substance often at extremely low (frequently unmeasurable) levels of exposure. The physical examination is generally unremarkable and fails to disclose any objective evidence of disease, even though the patient may complain of severe discomfort. Sometimes the patient may present with extremely bizarre symptoms that cannot be objectively verified upon physical examination. Standardized laboratory testing (including standard immunologic tests) also fail to disclose any significant evidence of organic disease. Indeed, the diagnosis of IEI rests on the fact that there is no other organic disorder that can explain the patient's symptoms. Physicians who are proponents of MCS often attempt to offer as proof of organic disease many tests, which upon close scrutiny will be found to have no standardized normal ranges and/or have not been shown to have any clinical significance. Since there are no objective physical or laboratory findings, the diagnosis is based on the person's history alone. In an attempt to control the symptoms, patients and their physician impose severe limitations on work and social activities. At this point, individuals often become prisoners of their symptoms, leading to extreme social isolation, loss of income, and a frustrating search for adequate and compassionate medical care.

In addition to the physical symptoms, many patients with IEI/MCS complain of confusion, diffi-

TABLE 29.6. *Evaluation of the patient with IEI*

Listen to the patient's symptoms with an open mind.
Be empathetic but maintain scientific objectivity, especially when the complaints and symptoms cannot be objectively measured or are out of proportion to physical findings.
Perform a physical examination that addresses the patient's complaints.
Order only those tests necessary to rule out diseases suggested by the history and examination.
Order tests only if they have been standardized, and you are familiar with the interpretation of the results.
Realize that the obvious diagnosis may not be the best diagnosis.
Treat all diagnosable medical and psychological problems.
Create a treatment plan that encourages physical activity and social interaction, and has as its goal that the person will continue to be a functioning member of society.
Educate the patient and present an air of optimism when discussing the long-term prognosis.
If indicated, refer to a specialist who is familiar with this entity and do it early in the evaluation.
Do not abandon common sense.

culty in concentrating, and other psychiatric complaints. Physicians who care for these patients frequently make a diagnosis of organic brain disease due to chemical poisoning. The intellectual deficits, which are quite worrisome for the patients, frequently cannot be verified using standard psychological tests. A number of studies, however, have demonstrated that these patients meet the criteria for the diagnosis of depression, anxiety, or panic disorders. In fact, the emotional component seems to be the only common thread among patients claiming to suffer from MCS/IEI.

At this time, and until appropriate scientific studies are conducted and published in peer reviewed journals, MCS/IEI remains an unproven belief system with no well-defined objective findings or diagnostic criteria.

A recommended approach to evaluating and treating patients with presumed MCS/IEI is listed in Table 29.6 (adapted from the position statement of the ACOEM). Position statements have also been presented by the AMA and AAAAI (18). For a more complete discussion of MCS/IEI, see Sparks (21).

REFERENCES

1. Bureau of Labor Statistics, U.S. Department of Labor, 1999.
2. Romagnani S. Human Th1 and Th2 doubt no more. *Immunol Today* 1991;12:256–257.
3. Jelnik DF. Regulation of B lymphocyte differentiation. *Ann Allergy Asthma Immunol* 2000;84:375–386.
4. Delves PJ, Roitt IM. Advances in immunology: the immune system. *N Engl J Med* 2000;343:37–49; 2000; 343:108–117.
5. Coombs RRA, Gell PGH, eds. *Clinical aspects of immunology.* Philadelphia: Lippincott, 1975:761.
6. Mannino DM, Homa DM, Pertowski CA, et al. CDC surveillance for asthma—U.S., 1960–1995. *MMWR* 1998;47(1):1–27.
7. Brooks SM, Weiss MA, Bernstein IL. Reactive airways dysfunction syndrome. *Chest* 1985;88:376–384.
8. Albert WM, Brooks SM. Advances in occupational asthma. *Clin Chest Med* 1992;13:281–302.
9. Becklake MR. Features used to establish the clinical diagnosis of occupational asthma. *Chest* 1990;98[suppl]: 165S.
10. Malo JL. The case for confirming occupational asthma. *J Allergy Clin Immunol* 1993;91:967.
11. *Guidelines for the diagnosis and management of asthma,* vol 14. Expert panel report 2. Bethesda, MD: National Heart, Lung, and Blood Institute, 1997.
12. *www.latex-allergy.org,* a useful site to find practical information on latex allergy, such as where to obtain common household and medical products which are latex free.
13. Golden DB, March DG, Kagey-Sobotka A, et al. Epidemiology of insect venom sensitivity. *JAMA* 1989;262: 240–244.
14. Casillas AM, Hiua T, Li N, et al. Enhancement of allergic inflammation by diesel exhaust particles. *Ann Allergy Asthma Inmunol* 1999;83:624–629.
15. Golstein B, et al. *Biomarkers in immunology*. Committee on Biological markers, National Research Council. Washington, DC: National Academy Press, 1992.
16. Report of the Ad Hoc Committee on Environmental Hypersensitivity Disorders. Office of the Minister of Health, Toronto, Canada, 1989:17–18.
17. McClellan RK. Biological intervention in the treatment of patients with multiple chemical sensitivity. *Occup Med State of the Art Rev* 1987;2:663.
18. *www.aaai.orgprofessionalphysicianreferenceposition-statementsdefaults.stm.* This site contains a position statement on IEI/MCS discussing the scientific basis for the Academy's position.
19. American Medical Association Council on Scientific Affairs. Multiple chemical sensitivity syndrome. *JAMA* 1992;268:3465.
20. *www.acoem.org,* ACOEM's position paper on IEI/MCS presents a reasonable approach when faced with issues concerning IEI/MCS.
21. Sparks PJ, ed. Multiple chemical sensitivity/idiopathic environmental intolerance. *Occup Med State of the Art Rev* 2000;15(3).

FURTHER INFORMATION

Banks DE, Wang ML, eds. Occupational asthma. *Occup Med State of the Art Rev.* 2000;15(2).
An up-to-date overview of latest thinking in occupational asthma.
Bardana EL, Montanaro A, O'Halloran MT. *Occupational asthma.* Philadelphia: Hanley and Belfus, 1992.

A text covering all types of occupational asthma, particularly strong on immune mediated types. Also has discussion of sick building syndrome and MCS.

Bernstein IL, et al., eds. *Asthma in the workplace,* 2nd ed. New York: Marcel Dekker, 1999.

A comprehensive text-reference that details the pathophysiology and step-by-step evaluation and treatment of occupational asthma with particular emphasis on immunologic laboratory tests.

Burns LA, Meade BJ, Munson AE. Toxic response of the immune system. In: Amdur, Doull, Klassen, eds. *Casarett and Doull's toxicology,* 5th ed. New York: McGraw-Hill, 1996.

A detailed account of current knowledge of this specialized field. The text is a standard teaching and reference work in toxicology.

DeShazo RD, Smith DL, eds. *Primer on allergic and immunologic diseases,* 3rd ed. *JAMA* 1992;260:2785.

A state-of-the-art update. Many articles, particularly those covering the traditional areas of allergy, are suitable for the generalist.

Middleton E, Reed CE, et al., eds. *Allergy principles and practice,* 5th ed. St. Louis: Mosby Year-Book, 1998.

A two-volume reference work that is a standard text in the field of clinical allergy and immunology.

30

Arm Pain in the Workplace

Nortin M. Hadler

The experience of discomfort in the upper extremity is commonplace (1), as each year some 30% of us will be forced to cope with it for at least 1 week. Often these symptoms are exacerbated by usage of the affected limb or limb region so that performance in any setting is rendered less instinctive. Nonetheless, nearly all of us can find the personal resources to cope effectively until the symptoms subside spontaneously. There are occasions, however, when such coping becomes counterintuitive, and guidance is sought. In the context of the workplace, the manifestation can be work incapacity and the readily available resource is the medical department.

This chapter focuses on the plight of individuals with regional musculoskeletal illnesses of the upper extremity. They can identify no forceful physical insult as a precipitant and have incurred no damage to the integument. Rather, their illness occurs in the course of activities that are customary and customarily comfortable. Regional musculoskeletal illnesses comprise the vast majority of disorders of the upper extremity. However, the clinician must be prepared to discern the patient whose upper extremity symptoms follow no traumatic insult yet are not likely to reflect a regional musculoskeletal illness. Table 30.1 lists a number of red flags. In the presence of any of these clues, appropriate referral is advisable. Referral is also advisable for some forms of regional musculoskeletal illnesses. But these are exceptional and will be pointed out when we come to the particular entities.

There are three categories of regional musculoskeletal illness of the upper extremity: illness that relates to osteoarthritis, illness as a consequence of neuropathy, and soft tissue illnesses. All three are common, and can be recognized with confidence on the basis of history and physical examination. There is a body of information for each category upon which sound advice can be based.

REGIONAL MUSCULOSKELETAL ILLNESS THAT CAN BE ASCRIBED TO OSTEOARTHRITIS

Osteoarthritis refers to progressive changes in the biochemistry and anatomy of a joint eventuating in compromise in its structure and function. A dearth of inflammatory changes is characteristic of the pathology. Involvement of the articulating structures of the axial skeleton is common in adults, such as osteoarthritis of the great toe presenting as a bunion. Elsewhere involvement is less predictable and seldom generalized, so that patients with osteoarthritis of the hip need not be afflicted in the knee. There is always

TABLE 30.1. *Upper extremity symptoms and/or signs that suggest a systemic etiopathogenesis*

Clinical clue	Diagnostic specter
Pain with ambulation	Angina
Pain with respiration	Pleural/diaphragmatic inflammation
Cramping with usage	Peripheral vascular disease
Writhing with pain	Aortic dissection
Erythema of tendon or joint or swelling of tendon or joint or bilaterality of symptoms or cutaneous pathology or Raynaud's phenomenon	Systemic rheumatic diseases

discordance between the pathoanatomy and symptoms. In fact, discordance with symptoms is a hallmark of osteoarthritis; many patients with impressively damaged joints are totally asymptomatic and vice versa. Furthermore, spontaneous regression of the symptoms—but not the anatomic damage—is the rule.

Osteoarthritis of the proximal joints of the upper extremity, the glenohumeral joint and elbow, is distinctly unusual and need not concern us. In the working-age adult, such involvement is generally consequent to trauma or to extraordinary usage such as is entailed in professional baseball pitching. Osteoarthritis of the hands is common. The process afflicts all of us as we age but is most frequent and more advanced in postmenopausal women. Those most severely afflicted are likely to remember similar affliction in their mother and grandmother. Osteoarthritis of the hands is readily recognized on examination. There is degeneration of the joint spaces associated with exuberant lateral growth of cartilage-covered osteophytes. However, not all hand joints are involved. There is a predilection for the distal interphalangeal joints leading to decreased motion, malalignment, and osteophytes known as Heberden's nodes. The proximal interphalangeal joints are similarly involved but to a lesser degree. Here the excrescences are termed Bouchard's nodes. No other joint in the hand or wrist is involved by osteoarthritis, with one important and insufficiently recognized exception—the first carpometacarpal joint at the base of the thumb.

For most women osteoarthritis of the hands is, to some degree, a cosmetic concern. Occasionally, an involved joint is inflamed, even slightly erythematous. But this is usually intermittent and seldom is pharmacologic suppression of the inflammation warranted. The principal compromise to which these women are at risk relates to a power pinch. The forces of pinching are transduced to the base of the thumb, to a first carpometacarpal joint that is often damaged, fixed in flexion to some degree, and tender. The symptoms can be reproduced readily; a contribution to the discomfort by the tendons that course across this joint can be excluded by stabilizing the carpometacarpal joint and demonstrating pain free excursion of the overlying tendons when the interphalangeal joint is moved. Osteoarthritis of the first carpometacarpal joint is a far more common cause of discomfort at the base of the thumb in women beyond middle age than is carpal tunnel syndrome or tendinitis. Management of this discomfort is to readjust tasks to obviate the need for a power pinch. A classic intervention for workers who do a lot of writing is to provide them with a pen that has a hefty diameter; the pen can be cradled in the length of the thumb and index finger so that pinching is no longer necessary.

NEUROPATHIC SYNDROMES

Cervical radiculopathies are common and present with pain that, whether localized or radiating, is not exacerbated by limb motion. Often, motion at the neck exacerbates the symptoms. The cervical radiculopathies are discussed in Chapter 22.

Entrapment neuropathies of the upper extremities are far less frequent than cervical radiculopathies. Most are rare indeed. Entrapment neuropathies all share the features listed in Table 30.2, but they do so with varying sensitivity and specificity.

The most common entrapment neuropathy is carpal tunnel syndrome with an incidence that approximated one case per thousand adults per year (2,3) prior to the past decade. In the past decade there have been epidemics of individuals whose complaint of upper extremity discomfort eventuated in the "carpal tunnel syndrome" label and in empirical interventions on that basis. If these individuals were disabled workers whose putative carpal tunnel syndrome was deemed a compensable injury, their prognosis was particularly dismal (4). In an object lesson in circular reasoning, policy makers and the lay press have felt compelled to hang the label "carpal tunnel syndrome" over the workforce, warning all to seek medical advice for upper extremity discomfort, particularly if that discomfort harkens to the symptoms of carpal tunnel syndrome.

Who has carpal tunnel syndrome? Two community-based surveys quantify the prevalence of symptoms suggestive of carpal tunnel syndrome and the

TABLE 30.2. *Classical clinical features of an entrapment neuropathy*

Dysesthesias are localized to the sensory distribution of the nerve.
Discomfort and parasthesia are more prominent at rest than with usage. Dysesthias often interrupt sleep and may cause the patient to move the limb.
Sensory fibers are more susceptible to insult than motor fibers. Therefore, atrophy is a late sign and an indication for surgical intervention.
A Tinel's sign is frequently present; tapping the nerve at the site of entrapment elicits dysesthias in the sensory distribution of the nerve.
Electrodiagnostic studies provide the gold standard for diagnosis.

coincident prevalence of electrodiagnostic abnormalities (5,6). In both surveys, nearly 20% of the adults had recently experienced or were experiencing symptoms of carpal tunnel syndrome. Of these, nearly 20% had delayed median conductivity. Can it be that 5% of people are suffering from carpal tunnel syndrome and only 1 in 50 of them find their way to diagnostic labeling each year? Some have argued so (7). I doubt it. Rather, numbness, even nocturnal numbness, is yet another one of the intermittent and remittent symptomatic regional musculoskeletal disorders with which we must all cope if we are to remain well. It is reasonable to ascribe classic symptoms of carpal tunnel syndrome to having "slept on it funny" or the like. Such a construction is far more likely to be rewarded by spontaneous regression of symptoms (8) than medicalization is to be rewarded by specific effective therapy.

However, medicalization is the reflex in contemporary culture, even when it comes to workplace health. The classic symptoms of carpal tunnel syndrome are now common knowledge and workers are encouraged to be proactive in seeking care. This has dramatically altered the prior probability that any patient with hand or arm symptoms, even classic symptoms, actually has median neuropathy. The predictive value of the classic features of carpal tunnel syndrome, if electrodiagnostic studies are used as the gold standard for diagnosis, are so marginal as to render them useless as screening tools (9). Electrodiagnostic studies leave much to be desired in that they are difficult to perform well, are uncomfortable, and are of limited sensitivity for radiculopathies and for all entrapment neuropathies other than carpal tunnel syndrome. Even when carpal tunnel syndrome is the issue, one needs to be wary of minimal conduction delay as a basis for diagnosis given the considerable variability in the normal population. Furthermore, conductivity by the median nerve is inversely proportional to age and body mass index, particularly in women, further compromising the specificity of the finding of a conduction delay.

It follows that the astute clinician, even one familiar with the sensory innervation of the upper extremity, faces considerable uncertainties when evaluating a patient with complaints of dysesthesias or pain not exacerbated by motion. Any evidence of muscle atrophy is a reason for consultation. However, even in the presence of classic features (Table 30.2), reassurance and expectant observation is likely to be more beneficial than leaping to diagnostic inferences and pursuing empirical interventions. With persistence of symptoms, and certainly with any hint of atrophy, the guidance of a perspicacious expert should be sought. Finally, given the prior probabilities, surgical intervention for entrapment neuropathy without atrophy is a recourse of desperation. This remedy should be applied infrequently and only when the diagnosis is substantiated by unequivocal electrodiagnostic abnormality. Even then, the alleviation of symptoms and the abrogation of work incapacity are inconsistent outcomes, particularly in the population whose putative carpal tunnel syndrome is considered a compensable injury (10,11). Critical thinking is necessary if we are to extricate the American worker from the cumulative trauma disorder quagmire from which we are now emerging (vide infra).

SOFT TISSUE REGIONAL MUSCULOSKELETAL ILLNESSES OF THE UPPER EXTREMITY

Soft tissue illnesses represent the bulk of the regional musculoskeletal illnesses of the upper extremity. However, medicine seems wedded to the exercise of labeling these illnesses as soft tissue "syndromes," taking advantage of an extensive literature littered with the inventive terminology of generations of clinicians. These labels—tendinitis, fasciitis, fibrositis, epicondylitis, tendovaginitis, tenosynovitis, etc.—are the issue of noncritical thinking. They are obfuscating malapropisms and should all be expunged from our thinking, our literature, and consequently, the lay mind. Remember that we are considering the plight of patients with upper extremity pain who lack any objective sign of inflammation (Table 30.1). Furthermore, there is no specific pathology to be demonstrated by any imaging or biochemical technique available today! Why then do we insist on applying labels that sound ominous, imply inflammation, or imply damage? These patients have localized discomfort, often localized tenderness, and often exacerbation with motion of the painful region. Furthermore, their prognosis is excellent even though the symptoms can take months to remit. Instead of "tendinitis" or "epicondylitis," why not tell them they have localized arm pain that will remit in time. Such a diagnosis takes advantage of our ability to exclude more worrisome causes, and our ability to prognosticate based on accumulated clinical experience. Furthermore, we can suggest motions that might circumvent exacerbation. The design of tasks should be based on a science that demonstrates them to be comfortable when we are well and accommodating when we experience our next regional musculoskeletal illness. Other interventions, based on extrapolations from biomechanical principles or other leaps of inference, are elective trade-offs in nuisance and expense and should be offered as such.

Acetaminophen is the analgesic with the most compelling benefit/risk ratio. Over-the-counter nonsteroidal antiinflammatory drugs (NSAIDs) are a close second given the fact that toxicity is vanishingly rare in the working-age adult who is otherwise well. There is no advantage to be gained from prescription NSAIDs. This holds for the newer agents in view of the marginal data supporting improved safety, the absence of surveillance for long-term toxicity, and their expense. There is no role for opiates given the lack of a demonstrably favorable benefit/risk ratio. Prescribed physical modalities lack a convincing benefit/cost ratio.

Regional Musculoskeletal Illnesses at the Shoulder

The shoulder region is the most frequent target for regional illness of the upper extremity. The approach to the patient is straightforward. If the patient can comfortably reach the occiput and the interscapular region with the involved hand, the shoulder pain is referred and the differential diagnosis includes the entities displayed in Table 30.1 and cervical radiculopathies. If motion at the shoulder is impaired, one must next exclude a process involving the true shoulder (glenohumeral) joint. The diagnostic maneuver is to have the patient stand with the arm dependent and the elbow flexed. Passive internal rotation isolates the glenohumeral joint and should be gliding and pain free. If this arc of motion is impaired or painful, rheumatologic or orthopedic consultation is in order to exclude inflammatory monoarthritis, reflex sympathetic dystrophy, avascular necrosis, etc. Very few patients with pain and impaired shoulder motion will manifest compromise in this arc of glenohumeral motion.

For most, the pain reflects a disorder of the soft tissues around the shoulder. Typically, external rotation in abduction is most difficult. It has become tradition to try to turn a complaint of "shoulder pain" into a syndrome. Certainly there must be subsets that differ in the fine details of presentation and for which treatment and prognosis might be specific. Orthopedists and rheumatologists rely on categorizations handed down through the generations. These have now been put to systematic testing and hold up very poorly (12,13). The simple fact is that many of the signs long held to be specific for particular pathologic states are not reproducible. Furthermore, much of the pathology inferred from nuances in the examination is readily demonstrable in the asymptomatic shoulders of age- and gender-matched people, or for that matter in the patient's contralateral shoulder. Shoulder region pain is shoulder region pain; further characterization as to intensity and duration is reasonable but little else.

Perhaps some of the old clinical saws are worth repeating in the context of the treatment of regional shoulder pain, or perhaps not. After all, the supporting data are tenuous (14). Many feel that there is clinical utility in discerning the sites of maximum tenderness about the shoulder because infiltration of such areas with nonabsorbable corticosteroid preparations has been shown to be palliative in controlled trials. However, the intervention should be reserved for acute involvement and should seldom be repeated. The data for antiinflammatory pharmaceuticals or physical therapy is less compelling.

Regional Musculoskeletal Illnesses of the Elbow

The commonest elbow illness is to experience discomfort with motion that lateralizes to the muscle mass about one or the other epicondyle. Hence, the heuristic label of "epicondylitis." Usually, there is tenderness to deep palpation. More specific signs involve the elicitation of discomfort when the lateral muscle masses are contracted against resistance. Flexion of the supinated wrist against resistance is the sign of "medial epicondylitis"; either supination of the forearm or extension of the pronated wrist against resistance is the sign of "lateral epicondylitis." Not only are the signs diagnostic, they suggest advice that can be palliative, i.e., patterns of usage to be avoided until the illness subsides, which it will, over the course of weeks. Intralesional steroid instillation has fleeting benefit at best (15).

Regional Musculoskeletal Illnesses of the Wrist

Discomfort about the wrist is an extremely common experience; well over 25% of us can be brought to a level of awareness that facilitates recall of prolonged or recurrent episodes. Overt swelling or erythema are distinctly unusual and call into question the diagnosis of regional illness. Rather, there is tenderness localized to one or another compartment, usually of the dorsum of the wrist, and exacerbation in discomfort when that compartment is stressed. An appropriate diagnostic label for this presentation is "benign localized discomfort" since the prognosis is so favorable and syndrome diagnoses for regional disorders of the wrist are no more valid than for regional disorders elsewhere in the arm (16). Benign localized discomfort is managed conservatively with reassurance, and consideration of the fashion in which dexterity can be maintained while avoiding stressing the involved region. The prognosis is excellent, although, as is the case for most regional musculoskeletal illnesses, weeks or even months may pass before the region can be again stressed without discomfort.

Regional Musculoskeletal Illnesses of the Hand

The hand is remarkable for the fashion in which it serves us without discomfort. There are few regional illnesses—far fewer than proximally. Some of us will develop a nodule, usually in a flexor tendon. Occasionally the nodule impedes the glide through a fibrous tether that anchors that tendon in the hand. Motion of the finger served by the tendon can be impeded, until the nodule suddenly pops through the tether, a "trigger finger." Triggering usually subsides spontaneously, although infiltration with corticosteroid preparations can be useful in the face of persistence.

Dupuytren's contractures are at least as common as trigger fingers. In this condition, there is hyperplasia and hypertrophy of the palmar fascia with fibrotic nodule formation manifesting the biochemical hallmarks common to wound healing (17). There is an impressive genetic component to predisposition (18) as well as associations with inflammatory diseases, such as rheumatoid arthritis, and metabolic diseases, such as diabetes (19). The data suggesting associations with integumental fibrosis elsewhere (soles, knuckle pads, penile shaft, etc.) are more compelling than any association with physical exposures, including physical exposures in the workplace (20). Although painless, the process is progressive and disfiguring, and can interfere with finger extension. At that point, surgery offers a remedy.

WHEN IS A REGIONAL MUSCULOSKELETAL ILLNESS OF THE UPPER EXTREMITY AN INJURY?

The plight of individuals with regional musculoskeletal illnesses of the upper extremity is the focus of this chapter. There is always a component of work incapacity in the illness, inasmuch as regional musculoskeletal illness challenges the comfort if not the effectiveness of usage of the involved region. Therefore, there is always some risk of disability. Furthermore, particularly for the soft tissue illnesses, usage may exacerbate discomfort.

During the mid-1980s the entire regulatory and insurance establishment in the United States, much of the ergonomics establishment, and even the occupational medical establishment came to accept two inferences based on this description of regional illness of the upper extremity: (a) since the pain is exacerbated by usage, usage must be causal; and (b) the regional pain is a manifestation of underlying damage, so that the "illness," in fact, is a work-related injury that is a consequence of repetitive motion. These injuries are encompassed by the rubric "cumulative trauma disorders" (CTDs). CTDs became compensable, and redress through litigation and regulation was necessary. As a consequence, workers with regional musculoskeletal symptoms who sought medical care no longer did so as patients; they assumed the status of claimants under workers' compensation insurance. Out of the turmoil that has followed has grown an appreciation that both inferences were wrong (21) and that their premature introduction has proven harmful.

The legislated redress for worker health and safety is designed to prevent trauma and to provide redress for tissue damage. If we use discomfort as a surrogate for damage, the legislated redress can backfire. The worker who hurts is drawn into the contest of causation. The pain becomes the evidence for hazard, and the persistence of pain becomes prerequisite to carry forth the argument. Likewise, when pain is the cause of disability, persistence of pain is necessary to carry forth the argument. In either contest, the hurting workers are poorly served, because they can't get well if they have to prove illness! To the contrary, they are at risk for getting sicker. They can become angry, beleaguered, desperate claimants willing to grasp at any straw, even multiple unproven surgical interventions, in defense of their claim. This is the vortex that has enveloped the industrial backache for decades (1), and now threatens to confound our predicaments of arm pain even to the extreme of subjecting workers to multiple empirical surgical interventions (22) and provoking pervasive somatization disorders (23). This vortex is one of the major pitfalls of the format for disability determination that the West inherited from the Prussian statutes of 100 years ago. Other countries have experimented with alternatives. But compassionate, major reform is long overdue to provide more efficient redress for the illness of work incapacity, whether a consequence of damage or of discomfort.

Regional musculoskeletal illnesses of the upper extremity or axial skeleton are important targets for improved worker comfort and workplace healthfulness. These predicaments, like stress and unhappiness, color all our lives at some time both in and out of the workplace. Outside the workplace, confounding burdens of social deprivation and psychosocial stress, not of physical demands, render the discomfort memorable and so intolerable that one is driven to seek help from a health care provider (24,25). Similar inferences pertain to regional disorders in workers (21). If all one seeks is an association between the physical demands of tasks and the disabling arm pain, that's all one can find—though anything but consistently, and seldom is the association robust. Fortunately, modern science is no longer bound to this preconception. If one seeks associations with the physical demands of tasks and with aspects of the psychosocial context of work, the former pales next to the latter. The cutting edge of clinical investigation is probing the elements of the psychosocial context of work that compromise one's ability to cope with the next episode of regional musculoskeletal pain (26).

There are lessons that apply directly to the clinic (27), one patient at a time. But it is in the workplace where salutatory reform is feasible. We need to complain when our own coping mechanisms are exhausted; interpersonal relationships, fiscal and other rewards, information and misinformation, personal psychosocial confounders, and, yes, even ergonomics are relevant variables. Compassionate micromanagement should be the response to our plea—not contests, gauntlets, and ill-conceived medical and ergonomic interventions. The rallying cry is for enlightenment of labor, management, and the individual worker.

REFERENCES

1. Hadler NM. *Occupational musculoskeletal disorders,* 2nd ed. Philadelphia: Lippincott Williams & Wilkins, 1999.
2. Stevens JC, Sun S, Beard CM, et al. Carpal tunnel syndrome in Rochester, Minnesota, 1961 to 1980. *Neurology* 1988;38:134.
3. Vessey MP, Villard-Mackintosh L, Yeates D. Epidemiology of carpal tunnel syndrome in women of childbearing age: findings in a large cohort study. *Int J Epidemiol* 1990;19:655.
4. Carmona L, Faucett J, Blanc PD, et al. Predictors of rate of return to work after surgery for carpal tunnel syndrome. *Arthritis Care Res* 1998;11:298.
5. Ferry S, Silman AJ, Pritchard T, et al. The association between different patterns of hand symptoms and objective evidence of median nerve compression. *Arthritis Rheum* 1998;41:720.
6. Atroshi I, Gummesson C, Johnsson R, et al. Prevalence of carpal tunnel syndrome in a general population. *JAMA* 1999;282:153.
7. Ferry S, Pritchard T, Keenan J, et al. Estimating the prevalence of delayed median nerve conduction in the general population. *Br J Rheumatol* 1998;37:630.
8. Nathan PA, Keniston RC, Myers LD, et al. Natural history of median nerve sensory conduction in industry: relationship to symptoms and carpal tunnel syndrome in 558 hands over 11 years. *Muscle Nerve* 1998;21:711.
9. Hadler NM. Carpal tunnel syndrome: diagnostic conundrum. *J Rheum* 1997;24:418.
10. Katz JN, Fossel KK, Simmons BP, et al. Symptoms, functional status, and neuromuscular impairment following carpal tunnel release. *J Hand Surg* 1995;20A: 549.
11. Carmona L, Faucett J, Blanc PD, et al. Predictors of rate of return to work after surgery for carpal tunnel syndrome. *Arthritis Care Res* 1998;11:298–305.
12. de Winter AF, Jans MP, Scholten RJPM, et al. Diagnostic classification of shoulder disorders: interobserver agreement and determinants of disagreement. *Ann Rheum Dis* 1999;58:272.
13. Winters JC, Groenier KH, Sobel JS, et al. Classification of shoulder complaints in general practice by means of cluster analysis. *Arch Phys Med Rehabil* 1997;78:1369.
14. Green S, Buchbinder R, Glazier R, et al. Systematic review of randomised controlled trials of interventions for painful shoulder: selection criteria, outcome assessment, and efficacy. *BMJ* 1998;316:354.
15. Price R, Sinclair H, Heinrich I, et al. Local injection treatment of tennis elbow hydrocortisone, triamcinolone, and lignocaine compared. *Br J Rheumatol* 1991;30:39.
16. Buchbinder R, Goel V, Bombardier C, et al. Classification systems of soft tissue disorders of the neck and upper limb: do they satisfy methodological guidelines? *J Clin Epidemiol* 1996;49:141.
17. Badalamente MA, Hurst LC. The biochemistry of Dupuytren's disease. *Hand Clin* 1999;15:97.
18. Burge P. Genetics of Dupuytren's disease. *Hand Clin* 1999;15:63.
19. Arkkila PE, Kantola IM, Viikari JS. Dupuytren's disease: association with chronic diabetic complications. *J Rheumatol* 1997;24:153.
20. Liss GM, Stock SR. Can Dupuytren's contracture be work-related? Review of the evidence. *Am J Ind Med* 1996;29:521.
21. Hadler NM. Comments on the "Ergonomics Program Standard" proposed by the Occupational Safety and Health Administration. *J Occup Environ Med* 2000;42: 951.
22. Himmelstein JS, Feurstein M, Stanek EJ, et al. Word-related upper extremity disorders and work disability: clinical and psychosocial presentation. *J Occup Environ Med* 1995;37:1278.
23. Helfenstein M, Feldman D. The pervasiveness of the illness suffered by workers seeking compensation for disabling arm pain. *J Occup Environ Med* 2000;42:171.
24. Macfarlane GJ, Hunt IM, Silman AJ. Role of mechanical and psychosocial factors in the onset of forearm pain: prospective population-based study. *BMJ* 2000; 321:676.
25. Urwin M, Symmons D, Allison T, et al. Estimating the burden of musculoskeletal disorders in the community: the comparative prevalence of symptoms at different anatomical sites, and the relation to social deprivation. *Ann Rheum Dis* 1998;57:649.

26. Torp S, Riise T, Moen BE. The impact of psychosocial work factors on musculoskeletal pain: a prospective study. *J Occup Environ Med* 2001;43:120.
27. Hadler NM. Rheumatology and the health of the workforce. *Arthritis Rheum* 2001;44:1971.

FURTHER INFORMATION

Hadler NM. *Occupational musculoskeletal disorders,* 2nd ed. Philadelphia: Lippincott Williams & Wilkins, 1999.

A comprehensive and practical treatise on the scope of the impact of all the regional musculoskeletal disorders. The predicament suffered by each of us before we seek professional guidance, our fate should we choose medical care, the ramifications should we seek recourse under workers' compensation insurance, and the process of disability determination are all analyzed. In this monograph one can find a greatly expanded treatment of the topic of this chapter. Furthermore, the monograph treats other regional illnesses, including those of the axial skeleton and lower extremity, in a similarly comprehensive fashion.

31

Infectious Disease

Alain Couturier

The incidence of disease, including that of many infectious diseases, has been recorded for centuries. The field garnered increased attention during the industrial revolution, although it was not until the late 19th century that clear cause-and-effect relationships between health and the workplace were understood (1). Throughout the 1800s, many physicians observed that workers in certain professions tended to have similar diseases, and that infections and disease seemed to spread within groups in which close contact or living quarters were present. Likewise, with the growth of factories it was noted that diseases tended to spread among the workers (2).

The potential for blood-borne transmission of hepatitis B was actually demonstrated among factory workers who became infected following smallpox vaccination as early as 1885 (3). Much of this spread of disease was deemed due to "bad air or humor," however, as the link between pathogens and disease was not yet established.

The recognition of infectious disease in the workplace started with recognition in the early 1900s that health care workers exposed to patients with tuberculosis incurred a higher incidence of the disease than the general population (4,5). In addition, more reports came in the 1930s and 1940s regarding transmission of disease linked to measles, mumps, polio, and yellow fever vaccines (3). However, even with sound data supporting this fact, preventative measures against exposure were still long in coming.

Significant improvements in sanitation throughout many parts of the world has decreased the incidence of work-related occupational infection, but numerous workplace infections still occur.

In addition to the initial recognition of disease spread, as this field grew focus was also placed on acute injuries, as the majority of jobs entailed physical labor or manufacturing. Today, however, over 70% of jobs are in nonmanufacturing sectors, such as the service or health care industry, or professional services. While injuries still occur on the job, the focus of occupational medicine has significantly shifted toward exposure to environmental and man-made hazards and diseases, and their potential to cause acute or chronic disease (2). The study of occupational infectious disease is now a multifaceted specialty that deals with infectious disease acquired in the workplace, taking into account how disease is communicated and spread, along with consideration of measures that can be taken to prevent or reduce the risk of disease contraction.

Any agent that can be spread through the environment and that causes infection and clinical disease in an occupational setting is of concern (6).

Such agents may be bacterial, viral, fungal, protozoan, or helminthic. Transmission of infectious agents can occur through direct or indirect contact. Direct transmission can occur through three primary routes. The most common is through direct contacts, such as skin to skin or skin to mucous membrane touching, or droplet spread of contaminated fluid onto the mucous membranes of the nose or mouth, or the conjunctiva. Droplet spread is typically limited to about 1 m in distance. A second direct route is parenteral, which may take the form of percutaneous needle sticks or transfusion of contaminated fluid. Exposure of susceptible skin to an infectious agent, such as through a bite, laceration, or compromised skin, is a third route. Indirect routes include airborne, vector-borne, and vehicle-borne transmission. Airborne transmission is the most common indirect route, and typically involves the dissemination of infectious agents through aerosols that enter a host through the respiratory tract. Airborne transmission occurs via suspensions of small particles (1–5 mm) in the air that often can be carried great distances; this route is distinct from droplet transmission, which is considered direct and typically occurs over a short distance. Vector-borne transmission describes disease carried by insects or animals. Vehicle-borne transmission occurs when an intermediate object transports an infectious agent into a suitable port of entry into the host.

Such vehicles may include food, and biologic products such as blood, plasma, tissues, or fomites. It is not necessary that the agent multiply or develop in or on the vehicle for transmission to occur (7).

Factors that go into determining the potential of the infectious agent to pose an occupational risk include the characteristics of the agent, its propensity to cause disease, the potential methods of transmission, and the ability of the agent to survive environmental conditions. The characteristics of agents involved in spread through the environment vary with the method of transmission. Regardless of the method of transmission, it is necessary for a minimum number of organisms to survive transport through the environment to reach and enter a susceptible host. For example, agents that are transmitted by direct person-to-person contact must be able to survive only minimal stressful environmental conditions, whereas agents spread through indirect contact often have evolved to survive adverse conditions. Some agents can survive for months or years under relatively hostile conditions. For those agents for which humans are the only known reservoir, the longer the time between the likelihood of contact between two susceptible hosts, the greater the resistance that the agent must have to environmental conditions such as heat, drying, ultraviolet light, or dilution by airflow. Some agents have the capacity to infect a nonhuman host such as animals, birds, or an insect vector. Such nonhuman hosts may play an important role in maintenance of the agent in the environment.

In the past, the greatest risk of infectious disease was related to exposure to animals or unsanitary working conditions. The advent of animal vaccination has greatly diminished the incidence of infections acquired through them. Likewise, improvement in sanitary conditions has lessened the incidence of infection. Furthermore, globalization and the increase in travel by workers to underdeveloped countries is increasing the risk again due to contact with unsanitary conditions and exposure to new pathogens. This chapter provides an overview of common infectious diseases found in the workplace, occupations at risk, and preventative measures.

OCCUPATIONS AT RISK

A risk for contraction of infectious disease exists in many occupations (Table 31.1) (8). The type of infections for which workers are at risk is largely dependent on the type of work they do. Occupations at risk tend be those in which workers have close or frequent contact with other humans and animals. One of the highest risk occupations for exposure to infectious disease is health care. Since infectious disease is now largely passed by human contact, the health care industry is a prime setting for disease transmission. Health care is one of the fastest growing and largest industries in the United States. Hospitals employ about 50% of all health service personnel, approximately 20% work in nursing homes and personal care settings, and the remainder work in outpatient care settings (9). Although the majority of injuries experienced by health care workers are musculoskeletal in nature, infectious diseases have a high incidence rate

TABLE 31.1. *Occupations at risk for infectious disease*

Agricultural workers
Miners
Animal handlers
Packing house workers
Animal husbandry workers
Personal care workers
Butchers
Pest control workers
Cannery workers
Primate handlers
Cattle breeders
Public safety and emergency response workers
Construction workers
Ranchers
Dairy farmers
Research laboratory workers
Day-care workers
Sewer workers
Excavators
Sheepherders
Fishermen
Slaughterhouse workers
Forestry workers
Stockyard workers
Geologists
Trappers
Health care workers
Travelers
Hunters
Veterinarians
Livestock handlers
Weavers
Lumberjacks
Zookeepers
Meat and poultry workers

that is significant. Those who work in the health care industry are not only exposed to a variety of infections from patients, but they also often have close contact with patients in whom the risk of transmission is high. Likewise, health care workers may spread their own infections to patients. Typical routes of infection include direct contact, airborne spread, fecal-oral transmission, transmission via fomites, and percutaneous sticks, cuts, or abrasions. Other areas of risk for health care workers and many other occupations include pathogens that are passed through skin or oral routes and that are transmitted by direct contact, food handling, bite wounds, or breaks in the mucosal surface. Diseases passed by these routes include conjunctivitis, skin infections, and a variety of gastrointestinal disturbances.

Occupational Safety and Health Administration (OSHA) initiatives are intended to protect health care workers from blood-borne pathogens and tuberculosis. They mandate immunization, surveillance, and postexposure protocols and procedures. Routine infection control policies and procedure that health care workers follow are also extremely important. These policies include isolation precaution, appropriate handling of material, disinfection and sterilization practices, waste disposal practices, immunization, and proper handwashing procedures, all of which work together to protect the worker and patients. However, it is important to note that there are many infections that are not unique to the health care setting or that may not follow a recognized exposure event.

TABLE 31.2. *Vaccine preventable diseases*

Cholera
Plague
Diphtheria
Pneumococcal disease
Hepatitis A
Polio
Hepatitis B
Rabies
Influenza
Rubella
Japanese encephalitis
Tetanus
Lyme disease
Tick-borne encephalitis
Malaria
Typhoid
Measles
Typhus
Meningococcal disease
Varicella
Mumps
Yellow fever
Pertussis

Other industries likewise employ a variety of methods intended to prevent spread of infectious disease. Such methods may include administrative controls, engineering controls, personal protective equipment, hand washing, and appropriate handling of material. Vaccines exist for many common infectious diseases, and workers should obtain the appropriate vaccines based on their exposure risk (Table 31.2) (10).

Following is an overview of the more commonly seen infectious diseases. These descriptions are grouped by the primary route of transmission, although it should be noted that some of these diseases have more than one potential route.

BLOOD-BORNE PATHOGENS

Blood-borne pathogens are typically spread through direct contact. Throughout the general population, many are spread through sexual contact or intravenous drug use, but exposure in the workplace typically occurs through percutaneous sticks, spray of droplets onto mucous membranes or compromised skin, or via a parenteral route. The implementation of universal precautions when handling potentially infectious materials and the increase in vaccinations have helped to decrease the incidence of disease spread, but have not eliminated the problem.

Human Immunodeficiency Virus

Human immunodeficiency virus (HIV) is a retrovirus that progressively damages the immune system, eventually leading to AIDS. The hallmark of the disease is a severe quantitative depletion of $CD4^+$ helper T lymphocytes. This depletion leaves the infected individual susceptible to opportunistic infections. The virus was first recognized in 1981, and by 1997 the Centers for Disease Control (CDC) had documented 52 confirmed cases of occupational HIV transmission (11). HIV exposure is a definite risk for health care, laboratory, and home health care workers. Occupational transmission can occur through percutaneous, mucous membrane, or skin exposure. Most documented cases of occupational transmission were caused by percutaneous injuries with sharps. However, there are a few well-documented reports of infections in health care workers following mucous membrane or extensive skin exposures. The majority of documented HIV seroconversion in health care workers has resulted from direct exposure to blood. Source materials of infection include blood, fluid containing visible blood, or potentially infectious body fluids or tissue such as urine. Exposure to tears, sweat, or nonbloody urine or feces is not considered an HIV exposure. Overall about 18,000 cases of HIV have been reported in health care workers; most are thought to result from non–work-related exposures (12). Following infection with HIV, it may take several years to develop full-blown AIDS.

Throughout the health care and research fields, the use of universal precautions and personal protective equipment has minimized exposure to HIV; however, when an event occurs, postexposure prophylaxis should be considered. The seroconversion rate following a needle stick with HIV-positive blood is generally estimated to be about 0.3%; the rate is 0.1% after mucous membrane splash, and less than 0.1% for a cutaneous splash on compromised skin (13). After exposure to HIV through blood or body fluids, surveillance for seroconversion should be continued for a minimum of 6 months, according to CDC guidelines. Based on case-control studies, the efficacy of azidothymidine (AZT) in the reduction of risk of HIV in health care workers is about 80% (3). If the risk of transmission is believed to be high, a three-drug regimen using zidovudine, lamivudine, and a protease inhibitor is recommended. At present, there is no vaccine for HIV.

Hepatitis B Virus

The hepatitis B virus (HBV) is a hepadna virus that is transmitted through blood or body fluids such as wound exudates, semen, cervical secretions, and saliva. It was the first blood-borne disease recognized to pose an occupational risk through a preponderance of cases among pathologists, lab workers, and blood bank workers. Occupations at risk are those with exposure to blood or fluids. Dentists, physicians, lab workers, dialysis workers, cleaning service, and nurses have the highest prevalence. The staff of institutions and child-care programs, and workers in facilities for the mentally handicapped are also at increased risk. Modes of occupational transmission include percutaneous or mucous membrane exposure to blood or fluids. The virus can also be spread by transfusion and sharing or reusing of needles.

Person-to-person transmission can occur in settings involving interpersonal contact over extended periods of time. The virus is not transmitted by the fecal oral-route. The risk of transmission is 1% to 6% with HBe antigen-negative blood, and is estimated to be 22% to 40% for HBe antigen-positive blood (3).

The incubation period for acute infection is 45 to 160 days, with an average of 90 days.

Infection with the virus can result in a wide spectrum of presentations ranging from asymptomatic seroconversion to a fulminant fatal hepatitis.

One third of HBV infections are asymptomatic. Typically those infected may show a subacute illness with nonspecific symptoms such as anorexia, nausea, vomiting, abdominal discomfort, and malaise; some may have extrahepatic symptoms, and others will have clinical hepatitis with jaundice. These symptoms may last weeks to months. Chronic HBV infection occurs in 2% to 6% of infected adults (3). The risk of chronic infection is inversely related to age at the time of exposure. The risk of developing hepatocellular carcinoma in this group is 5% to 15% (12). Persons chronically infected are the primary reservoirs of the disease.

The estimated prevalence of HBV by serologic evidence in the American population is thought to be about 5%. A serologic antigen test is used to diagnose HBV infection. If the infection is self-limited, the hepatitis B surface antigen (HBsAg) disappears before serum anti-HBs can be detected.

Since 1985, the rate of infection has decreased by 90% in health care workers (12). This decrease is attributed to the widespread adoption of preventive immunization, universal precaution, and personal protective equipment. OSHA requires that the hepatitis B vaccine be offered to all health care workers who are exposed to blood and body fluids in performing their job duties. This protection should also be offered to individuals who are not health care workers per se but are also at risk, such as hospital housekeeping or maintenance personnel who have contact with infected material or encounter needle sticks from improperly disposed sharps. The HBV vaccine involves a series of three injections, and postvaccination testing is helpful if performed within 1 to 6 months of completing the vaccination series. Antibody titers decline in about 60% of immunized individual over a 12-year period. Some individuals fail to seroconvert after the three-shot series, or subsequently convert after a second series of three doses. Two highly effective and safe vaccines are used in the U.S., which have 90% to 95% efficacy. The vaccine is injected into the deltoid muscle; gluteal injection is associated with failure to develop antibody. At present there is no recommendation for administration of a routine booster dose after the initial HBV vaccine series.

For inadvertent exposure, the decision to give prophylactic treatment depends on whether the HBsAg status of the person who was the source is known and the hepatitis B immunization status of the exposed person. Postexposure immunoprophylaxis with either

HBV vaccine or hepatitis B immune globulin can prevent infection. In the event of infection with HBV, tests for hepatitis B early antigen (HBeAG) and HBV DNA are useful in the selection of candidates to receive antiviral therapy and to monitor the response to treatment. No specific therapy for acute HBV infection is available. In chronic infection interferon-α has been demonstrated to induce a long-term remission in 25% to 40% of patients treated (14). Lamivudine is also licensed for use in adults.

Hepatitis C Virus

The Hepatitis C virus (HCV) is a flavivirus, and is responsible for most cases of transfusion-related hepatitis. Infection is spread primarily by parenteral exposure to blood and blood products. Household contacts or heterosexual activity may account for up to 10% of cases. Health care workers are at risk for occupational exposure through percutaneous sticks or direct membrane exposure. All persons with HCV antibody or HCV RNA in their blood are considered to be infectious. The incubation period averages 6 to 7 weeks, with a range of 2 weeks to 6 months. The signs and symptoms of hepatitis C infection are usually not distinguishable from those of hepatitis A or B infection. The acute disease is mild and insidious in onset. Jaundice occurs in approximately 25% of infected individuals. Abnormalities in liver function tests are generally less pronounced than in those with HBV infection. Infection can lead to chronic hepatitis in 60% to 70% of those infected, and persistent infection in 75% to 85% of cases (14). The disease usually develops slowly over decades. Cirrhosis develops in 10% to 20% of patients, and hepatocellular carcinoma is a late risk, developing after cirrhosis.

The incidence of HCV has been on the rise, particularly in health care personnel. The prevalence in the U.S. population is estimated at 1.8% (14). The estimated prevalence in health care workers is thought to be between 1% and 5%, and HCV in health care workers may account for about 10% of all cases (12). Serum alanine aminotransferase (ALT) levels begin to rise several weeks after initial infection and remain elevated after acute symptoms resolve. The risk of HCV transmission from a needle stick has been found to be roughly 4%, using the anti-HCV test, or 10% using the more sensitive but less available RNA polymerase chain reaction (PCR) test for follow-up (12). Most cases of transmission to health care workers occur because of accidental needle sticks or a sharps cut. Treatment is interferon alone or in combination with ribavirin. Interferon alone results in sustained response in 15% to 25% of patients treated, while combination therapy results in a sustained response in about 40% (14).

AIRBORNE INFECTIONS

Both bacterial and viral pathogens can be carried by air. To be transmitted in the air, particles must be aerosolized, small, and viable in the air. Particles are typically on the order of 1 to 5 mm. Some common diseases that workers may be exposed to include tuberculosis, influenza, pertussis, measles, and upper respiratory infections caused by agents such as respiratory syncytial virus (RSV) and parainfluenza virus (PIV). Many bacteria and viruses that are spread by direct contact may also be spread through airborne respiratory secretions.

Tuberculosis

Tuberculosis (TB) is caused by *Mycobacterium tuberculosis* and is characterized by primary caseous lesions in the lungs, and may include disseminated caseous lesions of the meninges, bone, gastrointestinal tract, larynx, skin, pleura, and peritoneum. Active disease may be the result of primary or secondary infection; typically more severe disease occurs with secondary infection. The primary infection may be self-limiting, in which case the site of infection is walled off. Secondary infection may occur in the lungs or other areas if the immune system is unable to contain the initial infection; however, the time course of secondary infection is highly variable. Active TB presents with symptoms of cough, weight loss, and malaise.

Diagnosis of TB can be made through a skin test or chest radiograph. The skin test consists of a subcutaneous injection of purified protein derivative (PPD), which is read after 48 hours. Current CDC guidelines for interpretation are shown in Table 31.3 (12). One drawback to the PPD test is that it only indicates previous exposure; it does not designate active infection. In suspected cases of TB, a chest radiograph should be taken.

At one time, the rate of transmission had dropped dramatically. However, due to laxity in public health measures and the AIDS epidemic, the incidence of TB has increased significantly in the last decade. Health care workers and staff in institutional settings have the highest risk of exposure. OSHA estimates that over 5 million workers are exposed to TB (15). These workers should undergo skin testing annually and adhere to isolation procedures for potentially in-

TABLE 31.3. *Guidelines for determining a positive tuberculin skin test reaction*

Induration ≥5 mm and <10 mm	Induration ≥10 mm and <15 mm	Induration ≥15 mm
HIV-positive persons	Recent arrivals (<5 yr) from high-prevalence countries	Persons with no risk factors for TB
Recent contacts with TB case	Injection drug users Residents and employees[a] of high-risk congregate settings: prisons and jails, nursing homes and other health care facilities, residential facilities for AIDS patients, and homeless shelters Mycrobacteriology laboratory personnel	
Fibrotic changes on chest radiograph consistent with old TB	Persons with clinical conditions that make them high risk: silicosis diabetes mellitus, chronic renal failure, some hematologic disorders (e.g., leukemias and lymphomas), other specific malignancies (e.g., carcinoma of the head or neck and lung), weight loss of >10% of ideal body weight, gastrectomy, jejunoileal bypass	
Patients with organ transplants and other immunosuppressed patients (receiving the equivalent of >15 mg/d prednisone for >1 mo)	Children <4 yr of age or infants, children, and adolescents exposed to adults in high-risk categories	

[a]For persons who are otherwise at low risk and are tested at entry into employment, a reaction of >15 mm induration is considered positive.

fectious TB patients in hospitals, outpatient, or institutional settings. The baseline prevalence of past TB infection in health care workers has been estimated at 1% to 28% (16). After exposure to TB a range of 4% to 70% have been reported to have a positive PPD test, with a yearly conversion rate of 0.1% to 5% (16,17).

Recent skin test converters should be evaluated for isoniazid [isonicotinic acid hydrazide (INH)] prophylaxis after a chest radiograph is taken to rule out active disease.

Prophylactic INH is typically given for 6 months in adults, 9 months in children, and 12 months in HIV-infected individuals. Individuals with multidrug resistant (MDR) strains of TB are of increasing concern and have shown resistance to INH and rifampin. Patients who are HIV positive or who have AIDS with low CD4 lymphocytes can have atypical presentations of TB. A vaccine is available, but is not routinely recommended for prevention in the U.S.

Influenza

Influenza is a viral infection that may be transmitted by large airborne droplets or by aerosolization of small particles. Inculcation is typically 1 to 5 days. Individuals are most contagious in the first 3 days of illness; the virus is shed prior to the onset of symptoms and for 7 days thereafter. The influenza virus may cause a broad range of symptoms, which range from pharyngitis and malaise to secondary pneumonia and concomitant mortality. Vaccination is recommended for health care workers, who are most at risk for occupational exposure. The optimal time for vaccination is mid-October to mid-November. Zanamivir and Oseltamivir are also now available for use. Recent research has shown that the flu vaccine may reduce overall rates of respiratory illness and absenteeism compared to placebo, justifying its use on a cost-effectiveness basis, in healthy workers.

Pertussis

Pertussis (whooping cough), caused by *Bordetella pertussis,* can be a life-threatening infection in infants, but routine childhood immunization has eliminated much of the morbidity and mortality in young children. The pertussis vaccine is not given to children older than 7 years; immunized adolescents and adults can be susceptible to infection and serve as a reservoir of infection to children since vaccine immunity wanes with time. The traditional pertussis vaccine for children is not used in adults due to a high frequency of side effects. Health care and child-care workers are at risk for exposure. Over the past 5 years the number of reported cases has increased. In adults, pertussis presents as a mild atypical respiratory illness, without the characteristic whooping cough, although a paroxysmal cough may be present. The cough typically persists over a 1- to 2-week period. Specific testing is needed to diagnose adults with pertussis, such as a nasopharyngeal culture for *B. pertussis* on Bordet-Gengou or Regan-Lowe media and direct-fluorescent antibody testing. PCR and enzyme-linked immunosorbent assay (ELISA) for antibodies are more accurate. For an individual who is symptomatic, a nasopharyngeal swab specimen is cultured and the individual should be isolated within reason and started on an antibiotic regimen. After a 5-day treatment with antibiotics, the individual may return to work if asymptomatic. Following exposure, prophylactic treatment consists of a 14-day course of erythromycin (adults 500 mg p.o. q.i.d. × 14 days) or trimethoprim-sulfamethoxazole (DS 1 tablet 850 mg p.o. b.i.d., 800 mg–160 mg [tab]) b.i.d. started within 3 weeks of exposure. The treatment dose and prophylactic dose are the same. Isolation precautions to control droplet spread should be instituted.

Measles

Measles is an acute viral disease characterized by fever, conjunctivitis, coryza, cough, and a red blotchy rash. The rash begins on the face and then becomes generalized, lasting 4 to 7 days. Pneumonia and encephalitis are potential complications. The disease is transmitted by large airborne respiratory droplets, with an incubation period of 5 to 21 days. The virus sheds from the nasopharynx during the prodrome and for 3 to 4 days after the rash appears. The rash may take longer to resolve in immunocompromised individuals. During an outbreak, vaccination within 72 hours after exposure without prior serologic testing is recommended to any adult who has not received two doses of vaccine, regardless of age or serologic status. The vaccine has an efficacy of 95% with one dose and 99% with two doses.

FECAL-ORAL INFECTIONS

Fecal-oral transmission most commonly refers to transmission of infectious agents via contaminated food or water. Prevention and control includes strict hygienic standards such as hand washing and appropriate personal protective equipment. Workers with acute gastrointestinal illness (e.g., vomiting, diarrhea, nausea, fever, and abdominal pain) should be excluded from work that involves personal contact or contact with food. Return to work is appropriate after the symptoms resolve. Observance of standard contact precaution such as hand washing when in contact with other people, food, or after the use of the bathroom would minimize the risk of transmission.

Gastrointestinal Infection

Gastrointestinal infections can occur through contact with infected individuals, consumption of contaminated food, water, or beverages, or exposure to contaminated objects or environmental surfaces. *Salmonella, Shigella, Clostridium,* and a variety of *Enterococcus* often cause such infections. Workers at risk include those who come in direct contact with an infected animal or contaminated water or food. Laundry, food handlers, and health care workers have been noted to be at increased risk for these types of infection.

Hepatitis A Virus

Hepatitis A virus (HAV), a picornavirus, is a common infection transmitted by the fecal-oral route. Exposure typically results in an acute self-limited illness with fever, malaise, jaundice, anorexia, and nausea. These symptoms usually last several weeks. Prolonged or relapsing disease for as long as 6 months can occur. Fulminant hepatitis is rare but may occur with underlying liver disease. Infection also can be asymptomatic, and as a result is often not reported.

Many occupations are at risk for this infection, including military personnel, health care workers, day-care workers, food handlers, staff workers in institutions for the developmentally delayed and/or handicapped, and those working in prisons and jails. Sources of infection include close personal contact, child-care centers, international travel, and food-borne or water-borne outbreak. Outbreaks caused by transmission in hospitals have been reported. Often the source of exposure cannot be determined. In underdeveloped countries, infection with HAV is considered a common childhood disease. However, in developed countries infection typically occurs at an older age.

HAV is one of most frequently reported vaccine-preventable diseases. In 1998, 23,000 cases were reported to the CDC (14). More than one third of the U.S. population has the antibody to HAV, which is similar to the prevalence among health care workers (35–54%) (3). Two inactivated HAV vaccines are available in the U.S. for active immunization. Vaccination is recommended for persons at risk of occupational exposure and for those who travel abroad. The vaccine is 94% to 100% effective in preventing clinical hepatitis. An immune serum globulin provides passive protection from the virus. Treatment is supportive. Immune globulin given within 2 weeks of exposure is more than 85% effective in preventing symptomatic infection.

INFECTIONS ACQUIRED BY DIRECT CONTACT

Infections transmitted by direct contact include infections of the skin, hair, or eyes, and a variety of gastrointestinal disturbances. Direct contact may include actual skin to skin or skin to mucous membrane touching, contact with a contaminated fomite, or may involve droplet spread. The blood-borne pathogens can be transmitted in this manner through droplet spread.

The family of herpes simplex viruses (HSVs) may also be transmitted in this manner. Fungal infections may spread from person to person and via fomites as well. Skin breaks, lesions, and rashes, regardless of cause, may present an occupational health hazard. Skin breaks present an entry route for a variety of infectious agents in addition to blood-borne pathogens. Careful hygienic practices and universal precautions when handling potentially infectious material are the best means of preventing spread.

Conjunctivitis

Many types of viruses or bacteria can cause conjunctivitis, such as *Haemophilus influenzae, Streptococcus pneumoniae,* enterovirus, adenoviral pharyngitis, conjunctival fever, or chlamydia. Epidemic keratoconjunctivitis (EKC) is spread by direct contact with infected eye secretions. The incubation time for adenoviral conjunctivitis averages 5 to 12 days. The virus is typically in a communicable form late in the incubation period up to 14 days after onset of symptoms, although viral shedding may be prolonged beyond 14 days. Thorough hand washing and high-level disinfection can help prevent the spread of conjunctivitis. Individuals with conjunctivitis should avoid direct or close contact with others while symptoms are present.

Herpes Viruses

HSV-I and -II are transmitted through direct contact. HSV-I is most likely to be of risk in an occupational setting. A higher than average occurrence exists in the health care field. Dentists and medical health care workers are at risk from oral secretions and can develop herpetic whitlow in the periungual skin of the hand. HSV goes through remission and can become dormant in the dorsal root ganglion. Treatment consists of both oral and topical acyclovir.

Varicella

Varicella, or chickenpox, is an acute viral disease characterized by sudden onset of fever, mild constitutional systems, and skin eruption. The rash occurs in crops, and is maculopapular for a few hours and then vesicular for 3 to 4 days, leaving scabs. Varicella-zoster virus is spread from person to person by the airborne route or direct contact with vesicular fluid or respiratory secretions, or by articles freshly soiled by these fluids.

Varicella infection is most severe in adults, with a fatality rate of 30 per 100,000 in the U.S. (12). Viral pneumonia is a frequent complication of varicella infection. Herpes zoster, or shingles, is a localized outbreak of skin vesicles, and results from reactivation of varicella virus, which lies dormant in the dorsal root ganglia years after the primary chickenpox infection. Varicella virus is highly contagious, especially in the early stages of cutaneous eruption; herpes zoster has a lower rate of transmission. Both can cause chickenpox in seronegative contacts. If infected, an individual is contagious for 1 to 2 days prior to the onset of the rash, at which time the virus can be spread to nonimmune or immunocompromised individual. Nonimmune pregnant mothers who develop chickenpox near term can also transmit varicella to the newborn. Overall, premature or low birth weight infants and individuals with immune suppression or malignancy are at greatest risk for infection. For these reasons the CDC has recommended that individuals who have been exposed not return to work for 10 to 21 days following exposure. The American Academy of Pediatrics has recommended a similar time period of 8 to 21 days. Most adults have developed immunity to varicella. Of adults with a negative or uncertain history, about 71% to 93% are seropositive (12). However, prior infection and antibody development is not 100% protective against reinfection with chickenpox or herpes zoster. The varicella vaccine is recommended for those who have no history of chickenpox and have tested negative for varicella antibodies.

Mumps

Mumps is a viral illness that affects the salivary (parotitis) and other glands. Teens are of greatest risk for contraction of this disease. In postpubertal teens, orchitis occurs in 20% to 30% of male cases, and oophoritis in 5% of female cases; sterility is a rare complication (18). Other complications include aseptic meningitis, encephalitis, and pancreatitis.

Mumps is spread by contact with saliva or other respiratory secretions. Virus can be present in saliva for 6 to 7 days prior to observable parotitis, with an incubation period of 12 to 15 days. Infection is asymptomatic in about one third of cases. Individuals are considered immune if they have had previously physician-diagnosed mumps, received one dose of vaccine after age 1, or have serologic evidence of immunity. The vaccine is reported to be 95% effective.

Rubella

Rubella (German measles) is a mild febrile illness. A diffuse punctate, maculopapular rash is noted in over half of all cases. Encephalitis and arthralgia/arthritis are occasional complications seen in adults. Transmission occurs through direct contact and nasopharyngeal droplets. The incubation periods ranges from 12 to 23 days, with the rash appearing at 14 to 16 days. Shedding of the virus occurs for 1 week before the 5 to 7 days after the appearance of the rash. Individuals are contagious during the rash eruption.

A live attenuated virus vaccine elicits an antibody response in 98% to 99% of recipients. Rubella is most important because of its teratogenic effect on the developing fetus. Congenital rubella syndrome occurs in up to 90% of infants born to women infected during the first trimester. Fetal risk falls to 10% to 20% by the 16th week of gestation and does not have a significant risk level after the 20th week. Rubella during pregnancy is associated with intrauterine fetal death, spontaneous abortion, and congenital malformations resulting in deafness, cataracts, glaucoma, microphthalmia, mental retardation, cardiac defects, or insulin-dependent diabetes. Pregnancy is not a contraindication to vaccination, and women are counseled to avoid pregnancy for 3 months following administration of the vaccine (10).

Meningococcus

Meningococcus is caused by *Neisseria meningitidis* and may lead to a wide spectrum of disease, including sepsis, meningitis, and pneumonia. *N. meningitidis* can be found asymptotically in the nasopharynx. Three distinct groups exist. Group A is found in sub-Saharan Africa and the Asian subcontinent. Currently, serogroups B and C cause 90% of epidemic cases in the U.S. Infection is ubiquitous, and disease occurs commonly in children and young adults, frequently among newly aggregated adults in crowded conditions. Infection transmission occurs by intimate, direct contact with oropharyngeal secretions of infected individuals.

Lice and Scabies

Lice *(Pediculus humanus, P. capitis, P. pubis,* or *P. corporis)* and ectoparasite scabies *(Sarcoptes scabiei miti)* can be transmitted person to person. Scabies is a skin infection caused by a burrowing mite, and usually involves the interdigital space of the hand and flexor surface of the wrists. The rash runs in tracks and can cause an intense itch 2 to 6 weeks after exposure. Microscopic evaluation of tissue scraping with 10% potassium hydroxide confirms the infection. Scabies is readily spread by direct skin-to-skin contact. A scabicide prescription is recommended for treatment. Permethrin cream 5% is the current topical medication of choice. Lice are ectoparasites that are transmitted from person to person by direct contact and by contact with clothing, where they can live for up to a week.

Diagnosis is confirmed by finding the adult lice or nits on hair or clothing of infested persons. Head lice are spread by head-to-head contact with infected persons, and body lice may be spread by manual contact with the clothing of infested persons, necessitating the use of gloves for such activities. Lice stay alive while on the host; when away from the host, their survival time ranges from 1 to 2 days. It typically takes 10 days for eggs to hatch. Treatment includes application of permethrin 1%, Marathon 0.5%, and lindane 1% lotion to the affected areas.

BITE WOUNDS

Bite wounds from animals or humans can also lead to infections or blood-borne pathogen transmission. Treatment with broad-spectrum antibiotics covers most potential pathogens. Amoxicillin-clavulanate, ciprofloxacin, or cloxacillin may be used for prophylaxis or treatment. If the bite wound bleeds, the individual who did the biting may be exposed to the blood. A potential for the transmission of blood-borne pathogens exists from a bite where the biter has bleeding gums or open mouth lesions.

Zoonoses

Zoonoses describe diseases that are naturally transmitted between vertebrate animals and humans. This definition is sometimes extended to include those diseases transmitted by insects, such as arboviruses. Most zoonoses occur in the general population, and are not limited to work environments. Little firm data exist on rates of infection, as not all states require reporting.

Occupations at risks include zoologic workers, farmers, veterinarians, research laboratory workers, and animal control workers. Some common organisms include *Staphylococcus aureus,* streptococcal species, and anaerobes that can cause local infection at the site of inoculation. Such diseases are often transmitted directly, such as through a bite, droplet, or aerosol spray. In some instances, the infectious agent is amplified or developed in the nonhuman host prior to transmission. The most common zoonoses are brucellosis, rabies, Q fever, tularemia, Lyme disease, toxoplasmosis, cryptosporidiosis, and arboviruses causing encephalitis. A risk also exists for transmission of leptospirosis, anthrax, Hanta, viral hemorrhagic fever, and spongiform encephalitis, although these are more rare. Personal protective equipment and appropriate animal vaccination should be used where possible to prevent transmission of zoonoses. For illnesses transmitted via insect vectors, prevention of bites from ticks, flies, and fleas by use of appropriate repellents and personal protective clothing while working in endemic areas limits the acquisition of these illnesses.

Brucellosis

Brucellosis can be caused by several different species of *Brucella* such as *B. suis, B. Melitensis,* and *B. abortus.* Brucellosis can cause a wide array of syndromes that include nonspecific fever, rigor, malaise, anorexia, and arthralgia. Spleen and liver suppurative complications can also occur.

Osteoarticular complications are common and may present as sacroiliitis, osteomyelitis, tenosynovitis, arthritis, or bursitis. Granulomatous hepatitis, meningitis, endocarditis, pulmonary lesion, epididymitis orchitis, and colitis may occasionally occur. The infections can be derived through direct cutaneous contact, inhalation, or conjunctive inoculation from animal tissue or placenta, or through ingestion of unpasteurized milk products. A wide variety of animals harbor the organisms, including goats, sheep, camel, cattle, pigs, dogs, buffalo, and yaks. Workers at risk include those who directly handle potentially infected animals, such as ranchers, farmers, veterinarians, abattoir workers, hunters, butchers, researchers, and laboratory workers. Treatment includes a combination therapy of tetracycline and an aminoglycoside or rifampin. Prevention through animal control programs include improved sanitary conditions for swine, cattle vaccination, and serologic testing of cattle herds with the elimination of infected cattle. These preventive methods have significantly reduced the incidence of the disease in the U.S.

Rabies

Rabies is a rhabdovirus that causes an acute viral encephalomyelopathy, which presents as headache, fever, malaise, and other localized sensory changes, progressing to delirium, convulsions, and death. The route of infection is typically from saliva from a bite from zoometric sources or person to person.

The most common animal carriers include skunks, raccoons, rabbits, coyotes, bats, beavers, foxes, cattle, dogs, and cats. Percutaneous or mucous membrane contact with saliva, respiratory secretions, corneal tissue or tears, cerebrospinal fluid, or urinary sediment, especially with a bite, skin break, or percutaneous injury, is considered high risk. Prophylaxis is highly recommended following a bite, scratch, or stick with potentially infected material, or if mucous membranes or broken skin is splashed with infected fluid. Prophylaxis consists of immediate administration of human rabies immune globulin, 20 IU/kg, with half infused into the wound and the other half given intramuscularly, and initiation of the rabies vaccine series. Rabies vaccination consists of one dose injected into the deltoid muscle on days 1, 3, 7, and 14, followed by one dose anytime from day 28 to 35. If the recipient has previously been immunized, only two booster doses of vaccine are needed after exposure. Preexposure prophylaxis is indicated for veterinarians, animal researchers, and laboratory personnel. Approximately 40% of all cases have no identifiable source of exposure. Rabies in the U.S. occurs infrequently but is almost always fatal. The incubation period is 3 to 8 weeks, but can be as short as 9 days or as long as several years. The rabies virus may be present in a variety of human fluids, most commonly in saliva and respiratory secretions. Cerebrospinal fluid, brain tissue, skeletal muscle, skin, and peripheral nerve tissue also are frequent sites for virus isolation. The virus can be found in these types of tissue during the first 5 weeks of illness.

Q Fever

Coxiella burnetii can cause Q fever. Q fever may present as a nonspecific febrile illness, pneumonia, osteomyelitis, endocarditis, or hepatitis. Many animals are known to harbor the organism, but the most common animal reservoirs are cattle, goats, and sheep. The placentas of infected animals have large numbers of the organism. Other routes of infection include direct contact with infected animals, laboratory contact, or ingestion of contaminated milk. Simply working or living in a rural environment may put individuals at an increased risk of inhalation-related disease. Workers who have been associated with Q fever include farmers, dairy workers, sheep workers, abattoir workers, veterinarians, research and lab workers, and meat handlers.

Tularemia

The tularemia etiologic agent is *Francisella tularensis,* a gram-negative pleomorphic bacillus. Clinical disease may present in several syndromes and varies with the site of inoculation. Most of the time it is an ulcer at the site of inoculation with local lymphadenopathy. The bacteria are found in hundreds of animals species. Disease transmission most commonly occurs due to direct contact with or a bite from an infected animal, inhalation, and/or contact with infected animal tissue, or through the bite of an infected insect. Insect vectors vary according to geographic locale, but ticks, biting flies, and mosquitoes may transit the organism. Inhalation of aerosolized particle during slaughtering of infected animals, or in the laboratory doing routine microbiologic handling or through direct contact with contaminated water or mud, may transmit the disease. Workers at risk include hunters, trappers, skinners, meat handlers, sheep shearers, farmers, laboratory workers, and veterinarians. Treatment involves aminoglycosides. Prevention is best accomplished by limiting exposure to potentially infected animals. When exposure is unavoidable, proper barrier precaution with personal protective equipment such as masks, gloves, and goggles should be worn. Outdoor workers in endemic areas should be encouraged to wear appropriate clothing and repellents to avoid mosquito and tick bites.

Lyme Disease

Lyme disease is caused by *Borrelia burgdorferi,* which is transmitted by a tick bite and causes a characteristic rash, fever, arthralgias arthritis, carditis, or neurologic abnormalities. People at risk are those who work outside in endemic areas. Amoxicillin and doxycycline are both effective treatments. Currently there is a vaccine available.

Toxoplasmosis

Toxoplasmosis is caused by *Toxoplasma gondii,* whose definitive host is the cat and whose intermediate hosts include birds, sheep, goats, swine, cattle, and chickens. The acute disease in humans may be asymptomatic or may produce a nonspecific mononucleosis-like illness with fever, lymphadenopathy, and lymphocytosis. In immunocompromised humans it may result in chorioretinitis or cerebritis. Women who acquire the infection during pregnancy may have a chance of passing the infection on to the fetus. Workers at risk include those who work with meat or with cats, abattoir workers, butchers, pet store personnel, cat breeders, and veterinarians. Treatment involves pyrimethamine and sulfadiazine or clindamycin. Prevention involves meticulous attention to hand washing. Women who are pregnant should be advised to avoid cat litter boxes or cats with an unknown feeding history. Litter boxes should be changed daily.

Leptospirosis

Leptospirosis is caused by a number of serovariants of spirochete such as *Leptospira interrogans.* The clinical symptoms are varied but usually include nonspecific constitutional symptoms of fever, headache, myalgia, and nausea.

Severe illness is characterized by conjunctivitis, jaundice, meningitis, and renal failure. The organism has been found in rodents, swine, dogs, cats, raccoons, and cattle. Human contact with contaminated food and inhalation of infectious aerosols have also been implicated as modes of transmission. Workers at risk include those involved with animal husbandry, veterinarians, dairy farmers, abattoir workers, meat handlers, farmers, laboratory personnel, farm field workers, miners, sewer workers, fishery workers, and military troops. Treatment usually involves doxycycline.

Prophylactic weekly doxycycline has proven effective for military personnel during high-risk activities. Prevention of disease can be achieved by limiting direct contact of workers to livestock, rodents, and other animals, as well as by avoiding exposure to contaminated environments by providing personal protective equipment such as gloves boots and aprons, and disinfecting contaminated work areas. Livestock vaccination programs my also be effective in reducing the incidence of disease.

ANTHRAX

Anthrax is caused by *Bacillus anthracis* and can results in a cutaneous or pulmonary infection. Cutaneous anthrax is characterized by a black eschar ulcer on the skin. Outbreaks have been described in industrialized countries due to the importation of contaminated animal products, especially goat hair. Reservoirs include large herbivores such as agricultural animals, and the bacteria may be found in contaminated soil where animals graze.

Transmission occurs through direct contact with infected animals, or inhalation of spores. Occupations at risk include those who handle or who are around livestock. Control and prevention include vaccination programs, improvements in industrial dust control, and disinfections of imported animal fibers.

ENVIRONMENTAL INFECTIONS

A variety of occupations may expose workers to infectious agents found in the environment. Diseases exist that spread through contact with the environment, and can be inhaled, or inoculated through the skin. Direct inoculation from different organisms can cause infection or illness. Such infections can occur from a bite, or through breaks in the skin. Infection can be prevented through the appropriate use of personal protective equipment.

Environmental infections may also refer to diseases obtained in an artificial or indoor environment. Exposure to microbiologic aerosols indoors is a significant problem. About one third of indoor air problems in buildings are related to contamination. Contamination can occur from fungi, bacteria, and viruses, as well as toxins produced by any of these. Buildings may foster the growth, amplification, and dissemination of these agents, and our understanding of this process is still evolving. Problems caused by environmental infectious agents include hypersensitivity, inhalation fever, and infections. Infections include legionellosis, tuberculosis, and various bacterial, viral, or fungal forms.

TRAVEL-RELATED INFECTIONS

The significant increase in travel over the last decades has raised concern for both businesspeople and companies (see Chapter 13). Individuals who travel both domestically and internationally may be exposed to infectious diseases, and may knowingly or unknowingly become carriers. Persons from industrialized nations who travel to underdeveloped countries where a threat exists of acquiring infectious illnesses should take specific precautions. A risk exists for exposure both to unsanitary conditions and to new pathogens for which acquired or passive immunity does not exist.

Preventive medical care before traveling should be encouraged to minimize the opportunity for transmission of infectious disease. The risk of specific exposures should dictate the precautionary measures that are warranted. A detailed itinerary, anticipated length of stay, and estimated likelihood of exposure are important to review, because both recreational and business activities may expose travelers to risk factors of illnesses and injury. A publication is available from the CDC that is frequently updated with specific recommendations for countries and locations of concern. In addition, at the time of the preventive medical appointment, vaccinations and education about how to avoid infectious illnesses and exposures can be given. Many insurance companies in the U.S. do not provide medical coverage for care obtained outside of the country; however, some companies now have coverage for employees who travel abroad.

The most common mode of disease transmission in travelers is through ingestion of contaminated food or water. Usually these infections are self-limiting and last only 3 to 4 days; however, early self-treatment with a short course of fluoroquinolone, in combination with loperamide, may shorten the symptoms. Other agents such as amebae, cyclospora, or cryptosporidium may occasionally cause persistent diarrhea in travelers. A vaccine is available for those who might anticipate exposure to hepatitis A.

Another common route of disease transmission in travelers is through insect bites, particularly in tropical and subtropical climates. The most common are those caused by mosquito-borne transmission such as yellow fever, malaria, and Japanese encephalitis. Yellow fever is a mosquito-borne viral illness endemic to central Africa and South America for which a vaccine is available. Malaria is a febrile flu-like illness that can present in a 3- or 4-day cycle, or that can cause more severe disease, including cerebral, pulmonary, and renal failure. Precautions against malaria include preventive vaccination or treatment of the illness with mefloquine, primaquine, or chloroquine. Japanese encephalitis virus can occur in Southeast Asia and the Indian subcontinent. The most common agents are *Plasmodium vivax* and *Plasmodium ovale.* Those at risk should obtain a three-dose series of inactivated vaccine prior to travel.

Risk of susceptibility to airborne pathogens can be reduced or prevented by updating immunizations, including influenza, pneumococcal, and measles-mumps-rubella (MMR) vaccines. Those going to sub-Saharan Africa, Nepal, portions of India, or Saudi Arabia should consider a meningococcal vaccine.

LABORATORY-RELATED INFECTIONS

Infectious disease can be transmitted in laboratories in academic, hospital, industrial, or government settings. Exposure can occur from agents or organisms being studied or used in the course of research, from recombinant viruses or organisms, from hazards in human- or primate-derived materials, from zoonoses, and from shared equipment. However, lab workers are most at risk for contraction of infectious agents spread through direct contact or airborne transmission. Those who work directly with infectious agents in public health and hospital settings have laboratory-related infection rates of 2.7 per 1,000 and 4.0 per 1,000, respectively (19).

The most commonly reported laboratory-acquired infections are brucellosis, Q fever, typhoid, hepatitis, tularemia, chlamydia, tuberculosis, dermatomycosis, Venezuelan equine encephalitis, psittacosis, and coccidioidomycosis. A potential exists for transmission of simian immune deficiency virus, Hanta virus, Sabia virus, spongiform encephalopathies, and systemic lupus erythematosus, although these are rare. Typical routes of infection include needle sticks, aerosol spray from syringes, lacerations from sharps or broken glassware, conjunctival exposure mouth pipetting, and equipment failure. However, laboratory-related infections have a documented accident in less than 20% of cases (20).

Many laboratory-related infections can be prevented. It is important for laboratories to conduct a hazard assessment and to develop a prevention plan. Much potential for exposure can be limited by a combination of administrative, engineering, and work practice controls. Decontamination of surfaces, proper labeling, use of gloves and lab coats, use of masks and isolation work in hoods when appropriate, and proper disposal of sharps and contaminated materials will reduce the risk. Vaccination against infectious agents may be warranted. A plan for postexposure evaluation and treatment should also be generated.

CONCLUSION

Occupational infection disease remains a significant concern. Despite improvements in sanitation, awareness of the issue, and preventative measures such as vaccines and protective equipment, several diseases continue to be a problem. Not only have many infectious diseases not been eradicated, but some are actually rising in incidence. Employers and workers need to be aware of what types of occupational exposure are present, and to take preventative measures against transmission.

REFERENCES

1. Felton JS. History of occupational infectious diseases. In: Couturier A, ed. *Occupational and environmental infectious diseases.* Beverly, MA: OEM Press, 2000:4.
2. Rom WN. The discipline of environmental and occupational medicine. In: Rom WN, ed. *Environmental and occupational medicine,* 3rd ed. Philadelphia: Lippincott-Raven, 1998:3.
3. Sepkowitz KA. Nosocomial hepatitis and other infections transmitted by blood and blood products. In: Mandell, ed. *Principles and practice of infectious diseases,* 5th ed. Churchill Livingstone, 2000:3039.
4. Sepkowitz KA, Schluger NW. The occupational risk of tuberculosis care. In: Rom WN, ed. *Environmental and occupational medicine,* 3rd ed. Philadelphia: Lippincott-Raven, 1998:797.
5. Felton JS. History of occupational infectious diseases. In: Couturier A, ed. *Occupational and environmental infectious diseases.* OEM Press, 2000:7.
6. Centers for Disease Control and Prevention. Case definitions for infectious conditions under public health surveillance. *MMWR* 1997;46(RR-10):2.
7. Osterholm MT, Hedberg CW, Moore KA. Epidemiologic principles. In: Mandell, ed. *Principles and practice of infectious diseases,* 5th ed. Churchill Livingstone, 2000:163–164.
8. Kelafant GA. Occupations at risk. In: Couturier A, ed. *Occupational and environmental infectious diseases.* Beverly, MA: OEM Press, 2000:597–631.
9. Rogers B. Health hazards in nursing and health care. *Am J Infect Control* 1997;25:248–261.
10. Kessler ER, Dickerson D. Vaccine-preventable diseases in occupational medicine. In: Couturier A, ed. *Occupational and environmental infectious diseases.* Beverly, MA: OEM Press, 2000:143–147.
11. Stansbury LG, Couturier AJ. Occupational HIV infection. In: Couturier A, ed. *Occupational and environmental infectious diseases.* Beverly, MA: OEM Press, 2000:427.
12. Swinkler M. Occupational infections in health care workers. In: Couturier A, ed. *Occupational and environmental infectious diseases.* Beverly, MA: OEM Press, 2000:604.
13. Gerberding JL. Prophylaxis for occupational exposure to HIV. *Ann Intern Med* 1996;125:497–501.
14. *AAP 2000 Red Book: Report of the Committee on Infectious Diseases,* 25th ed. American Academy of Pediatrics, 2000:293.
15. Meyer JD. Occupational tuberculosis. In: Couturier A, ed. *Occupational and environmental infectious diseases.* Beverly, MA: OEM Press, 2000.
16. Bowden K, McDiarmid M. Occupationally acquired tuberculosis: what's known. *J Occup Med* 1994;36:520–524.
17. Sbarbaro J. Tuberculosis: yesterday, today, and tomorrow (editorial). *Ann Intern Med* 1995;122:955–956.
18. Benenson A, ed. *Control of communicable diseases manual.* Washington, DC: American Public Health Association, 1995.
19. Dieckhaus KD, Garibaldi RA. Occupational infections.
20. Stave GM. Occupational infections in laboratory workers. In: Couturier A, ed. *Occupational and environmental infectious diseases.* OEM Press, 2000:591.

32
Hepatic Disorders

Ross S. Myerson

ROLE OF THE LIVER IN DETOXIFICATION OF FOREIGN SUBSTANCES

Occupational liver diseases are caused by a variety of biologic, chemical, and physical agents. Biologic agents involved in occupational settings are primarily confined to the viral hepatitides, which are considered elsewhere in this text. Physical agents include ionizing radiation, heat (heat stroke), and vibration.

This chapter addresses liver disease induced by chemical agents. The liver is the organ that is mainly responsible for the detoxification and elimination of foreign substances from the bloodstream. By virtue of the portal circulation, the liver is the initial site for action on ingested toxins. However, xenobiotics absorbed through inhalation and the skin also rapidly make their way to the liver via the hepatic artery. Thus, the liver serves to detoxify chemicals regardless of their route of entry into the body. The liver performs this function through its unique ability to detoxify chemicals and drugs through complex biochemical reactions. These chemical reactions are many times facilitated by enzyme systems that include mixed function oxidases (MFOs) otherwise known as cytochrome P-450 enzymes systems. Many potentially foreign substances are lipid soluble and must be made more water soluble in order to be excreted by the kidney. This is often accomplished by oxidation, hydrolysis, or conjugation. Phase I reactions serve to make compounds more polar through hydrolysis, oxidation, or reduction. Phase II reactions serve to conjugate the foreign compound with another functional group, which usually results in a less toxic, more easily excreted compound. Most hepatotoxic agents produce liver injury only after biotransformation to an active metabolite through the action of these enzyme systems (1).

CLASSIFICATION OF HEPATOTOXINS

Chemical hepatotoxins are most commonly classified into two broad categories based on their presumed mechanism of action. Table 32.1 lists examples of some common hepatotoxins categorized by mechanism of action.

Intrinsic Hepatotoxins

Intrinsic hepatotoxins are agents that are either directly or indirectly toxic to the liver. Their toxicity is a predictable and inherent property of the chemical structure of the compound or its metabolite and is, in general, dose dependent. More often than not, intrinsic hepatotoxins require biotransformation to an active metabolite prior to causing injury to hepatocytes or their cellular organelles. Direct intrinsic hepatotoxins produce hepatic injury through the direct destructive action of the toxin on the hepatocyte. Direct toxic actions include peroxidation by free radicals and covalent binding of toxins or their metabolites to tissue molecules. Some of the most widely known occupational liver toxins including yellow phosphorus, carbon tetrachloride, and other haloaliphatics are direct intrinsic hepatotoxins. Direct hepatotoxins most often lead to cell necrosis or steatosis.

Indirect intrinsic hepatotoxins produce liver injury by disruption and interference with specific cellular metabolic processes or components responsible for cellular structural integrity or secretory activity. Hepatic injury by indirect hepatotoxins may result in necrosis, steatosis, or a combination of the two. They can also produce cholestatic injury through interference with bile excretion or bile duct injury.

TABLE 32.1. *Hepatotoxins and their compounds*

Type of hepatotoxin	Compounds
Intrinsic direct hepatotoxins	Carbon tetrachloride, 1,1, 2, 2-tetrachloroethane, paraquat, white phosphorus
Intrinsic indirect hepatotoxins	Aflatoxin B_1, ethanol, bromobenzene, methylenedianiline, acetaminophen
Idiosyncratic (immunologic)	Halothane, phenytoin
Idiosyncratic (metabolic)	Isonaizid, valproate

Idiosyncratic Hepatotoxins

Agents that produce liver injury as a result of an individual susceptibility (as opposed to an intrinsic property of the agent) are considered idiosyncratic hepatotoxins. There are two types of intrinsic hepatotoxicity: one is the result of an immunologic (allergic) response, and the other is a result of a metabolic aberration. Toxins that produce an immunologic response act like other allergens in that a sensitization period is usually required (1 to 5 weeks). Toxic manifestations are not necessarily dose dependent and demonstrate other hallmarks of hypersensitivity such as an eosinophilic or granulomatous inflammatory infiltrate, fever, and rash. Common agents that can produce idiosyncratic allergic hepatotoxicity are medicinal agents such as halothane, penicillin, streptomycin, and chlorpromazine. Metabolic-based idiosyncratic reactions are less well understood but are hypothesized to occur as a result of an individual variation in enzymatic biotransformation of the offending agent. This type of toxicity does not demonstrate any predictable latency period. Liver toxicity associated with isoniazid is one of the more common examples of this type of toxic reaction.

HEPATOTOXIC INJURIES

Hepatotoxic injuries vary in nature. Acute injuries may result in outcomes that range from mild transient elevation of liver enzymes to massive necrosis and death. Chronic exposures to toxins can result in subacute disease that may or may not progress to chronic disease. Persistent exposures can lead to chronic disease that may become apparent only after significant tissue damage has accumulated.

Acute Hepatotoxic Injury

Acute hepatotoxic injury usually results from a significant exposure occurring over a relatively short period of time. Most acute hepatotoxic injuries involve a cytotoxic injury. Morphologic patterns of injury are variable and include necrosis, steatosis, cholestasis, fibrosis, cirrhosis, and carcinogenesis. In some cases, cellular injury can involve two or more of these patterns. Many hepatotoxins cause a combination of necrosis and steatosis.

Necrosis

Necrosis of hepatocytes is felt to result from injury to plasma membranes and cellular organelles (mitochondria, lysosomes, rough and smooth endoplasmic reticulum). It may occur in a zonal or nonzonal pattern. Zonal necrosis is identified by the zone of the liver lobule in which it occurs. Zone 3 (centrolobular, perivenular) is the most common and characteristic of a wide number of compounds including carbon tetrachloride (CCl_4), chloroform, acetaminophen, halothane, and others. Zone 1 (periportal) lesions are less common and are associated with agents such as allyl alcohol and esters, white phosphorus, and ferrous sulfate. A few agents can induce both zone 1 and 3 necrosis and include aflatoxins, trinitrotoluene, and possibly arsenic. Necrosis in zone 2 (midzone) most commonly results from extension of the necrotic processes underway in zone 1 or 3. Most agents that produce a zonal necrosis are intrinsic hepatotoxins. Necrosis from idiosyncratic toxins (mostly drugs), is usually nonzonal and appears as panacinar degeneration and spotty necrosis. Halothane toxicity, which is idiosyncratic in nature, is an exception to this general rule and produces zonal necrosis.

Steatosis

Steatosis refers to fatty changes in the liver and is often an early indicator of hepatotoxicity. The presumed mechanism for this change is interference with egress of triglycerides from, or oxidation of fatty acids by, hepatocytes; increased rate of flow of fatty acids from fat depots; or a combination of both factors. Steatosis may be microvesicular or macrovesicular in nature. Steatosis associated with occupational hepatotoxins (CCl_4, tetrachloroethane, trichloroethylene, and others) is more often macrovesicular.

Cholestasis

Cholestasis refers to cessation or alteration of bile flow. This can result from hepatocanalicular injury, canalicular injury, necrosis of bile ducts, or necrosis and scaring of septal ducts. It is more commonly seen as a result of drug-induced idiosyncratic reactions. However, it has been attributed to occupational exposure to chemicals such as methylenedianiline, dinitrophenol, and paraquat. Cholestasis is suspected when tests reveal elevation of serum bilirubin or alkaline phosphates.

Subacute Hepatotoxic Injury

The most common form of subacute hepatotoxic injury is subacute hepatic necrosis. This entity was seen in workers in the munitions industry during both world wars and was attributed to exposure to TNT, tetrachloroethane, dinitrobenzene, and PCB-chloronaphthalene mixtures. It was histologically characterized by necrosis, fibrosis, and regeneration. The clinical onset included anorexia, nausea, and vomiting accompanied by hepatomegaly and jaundice. Some individuals followed a dramatic course culminating in death in 2 to 3 weeks from massive hepatic necrosis. Others had a more benign course over several months with eventual recovery.

Chronic Hepatotoxic Injury

Chronic hepatotoxic injury can manifest itself in a number of ways including cirrhosis, hepatoportal sclerosis, hepatic porphyria, and neoplastic changes. Cirrhosis is a chronic, irreversible condition in which the normal hepatic architecture is replaced by fibrous tissue and regenerating nodules. It is most often seen as a sequela of long-standing alcohol abuse or chronic viral infection. Cirrhosis is associated with occupationally induced subacute hepatic necrosis, discussed earlier in this chapter. Cirrhosis has also been associated with chronic and repeated exposures to a number of hepatotoxins including arsenicals, dimethylnitrosamine, carbon tetrachloride, and mixtures of other chlorinated hydrocarbons (2,3). However, with the exception of CCl_4, evidence for cirrhosis as a consequence of acute occupational hepatotoxic exposure is lacking.

Hepatoportal Sclerosis

Hepatoportal sclerosis is a fibrous lesion that causes obstruction of branches of the portal vein. It has been associated with exposure to vinyl chloride and arsenic and may be a precursor of vinyl chloride–induced angiosarcoma (4).

Porphyria Cutanea Tarda

Porphyria cutanea tarda is the most common type of porphyria in humans. Like hemachromatosis, it causes increased iron stores in the liver. It is characterized by chronic photosensitivity with resultant skin fragility and the appearance of lesions (vesicles and bullae) most frequently seen on the dorsum of the hands, forearms and face. It has been reported in workers in a plant involved in the manufacture of 2,4,5-trichlorophenoxyacetic acid (2,4,5-T) and 2,4-dichlorophenoxyacetic acid (2,4-D) where process contamination by dioxin (TCDD) was the most likely cause (5).

Cancers of the Liver

Cancers of the liver in humans have been described in association with a number of agents including chronic viral infections (hepatitis B and C), chronic alcohol ingestion, contraceptive steroids, aflatoxin B_1, inorganic arsenic, and vinyl chloride. In 1974 a U.S. company reported three cases of hepatic angiosarcoma (HAS), a rare form of liver cancer, in workers with a common exposure to vinyl chloride. The following year, a study reported 75 cases of hepatic angiosarcoma associated with exposure to vinyl chloride (6). Subsequently, there have been many other published reports establishing a firm link between vinyl chloride and HAS. A worldwide registry of vinyl chloride–related HAS has been maintained since 1974. As of 1993, 173 deaths had been reported (7). HAS has also been reported in vintners with long-term exposure to inorganic arsenicals and patients with psoriasis treated with Fowler's solution (arsenic trioxide). In addition to HAS, vinyl chloride is associated with hepatocellular carcinoma (HCC) and has been found to cause other liver abnormalities including parenchymal damage, periportal and capsular fibrosis associated with hepatomegaly, and portal hypertension. There is ample evidence that HCC can be induced in animals by a number of chemical and botanical toxins. However, in the occupational setting, only vinyl chloride has a proven association. In the U.S. and Western Europe, the overwhelming majority of HCC cases are associated with excessive ethanol ingestion or chronic viral hepatitis. In Asia and Africa, where HCC is a leading cause of cancer mortality, chronic viral hepatitis and dietary intake of aflatoxin B_1 are the significant exposures.

OCCUPATIONAL AND ENVIRONMENTAL EXPOSURES TO HEPATOTOXINS

Exposure to hepatotoxins can occur in a variety of settings including the workplace, home, and outside environment. Exposure in any of these settings can lead to acute, subacute, and chronic injury. In the occupational setting, inhalation is the primary route of exposure; however, many hepatotoxins are readily absorbed through the skin and can contribute substantially to total worker exposure (8). Table 32.2 lists some of the more common hepatotoxins, their industrial uses, and most common hepatotoxic manifestations.

Hepatotoxins in the Workplace, Environment, and Home

A large number of agents commonly encountered in occupational settings can be toxic to the liver. These include inorganic chemicals, halogenated aliphatic organic compounds, halogenated aromatic compounds, organochlorine pesticides and herbicides, and nitrogen-bearing compounds (nitroaliphatic and nitroaromatic). Nonhalogenated aliphatic hydrocarbons for the most part either do not cause hepatic injury or are considered only trivial hepatotoxins (9). Hepatotoxic environmental exposures most often occur through contamination of food and/or water. A large number of consumer products including medications (acetaminophen, aspirin), pesticides, automotive products (antifreeze, carburetor cleaners), painting products, adhesives, and cleaning products contain a variety of hepatotoxic chemicals.

Inorganic Compounds and Metals

While not a major source of hepatotoxic compounds, a number of metals and metalloids have been shown to be experimental hepatotoxins in animal models. Of these compounds, only arsenic and hydralazine have been a significant cause of occupational liver injury. Arsenic has been a known cause of chronic liver disease found in agriculture workers using arsenical pesticides. Hydrazine used in the development of rocket fuels has been associated with elevated levels of alanine aminotransferase (ALT) and steatosis in jet fuel workers (10).

Halogenated Aliphatic Organic Compounds

This group of compounds comprises the most widely known hepatotoxins. Their toxicity varies from compound to compound and ranges from the highly toxic carbon tetrachloride to the trivially toxic 1,1,1-trichloroethane. Liver injury induced by these compounds usually consists of zone 3 necrosis and steatosis. There are also reports of cirrhosis in work-

TABLE 32.2. *Compounds and their toxic endpoints*

Class of compound	Examples	Uses	Most common toxic end points
Inorganic elements and compounds	Arsenic	Agriculture	Steatosis, cirrhosis
	Phosphorus	Fireworks, matches	Subacute, hepatic necrosis
	Beryllium		Mid-zone necrosis, granulomatous lesions
	Hydralizine	Rocket fuels	Elevation of liver enzymes, steatosis, focal necrosis
	Iron and copper		
Nonhalogenated aliphatic hydrocarbons	Ethanol	Alcoholic beverages	Steatosis, alcoholic hepatitis, cirrhosis
	Toluene	Multiple industrial applications	No or trivial hepatic injury: case reports of steatosis and necrosis in glue sniffers; some case reports of hepatomegaly
	Zylene	Multiple industrial applications	No or trivial hepatic injury: case reports of mild steatosis
Halogenated aliphatic hydrocarbons (high toxicity)	Carbon tetrachloride	Solvents, multiple industrial applications	Hepatic necrosis, steatosis, cirrhosis
	Tetrachloroethane		
	Chloroform		
	Vinyl chloride		Angiosarcoma, hepatocellular carcinoma
Halogenated aliphatic hydrocarbons (moderate toxicity)	1, 1, 2-trichloroethylene, trichloroethylene		Mild steatosis
Halogenated aliphatic hydrocarbons (low or trivial toxicity)	Tetrachloroethylene, 1, 1, 1-trichloroethane		Case report of steatosis and mild liver injury

ers exposed to these compounds in a variety of industries (11). CCl_4 is the prototype of this group. Once widely used as a solvent, degreaser, and fumigant, this compound was commonly encountered in both industry and the home. The discovery of its hepatotoxic properties in humans has led to its withdrawal from most commercial products and a dramatic decrease in its industrial uses. CCl_4 causes a characteristic zone 3 hepatic necrosis, leading to rapid destruction of the hepatic parenchyma, leading to liver failure (12). The laboratory picture commonly includes marked elevation of aspartate aminotransferase (AST) and ALT. CCl_4 also affects other organ systems and can lead to renal failure and cardiac failure. The less toxic compounds of this group such as 1,1,1-trichloroethane were widely used as substitutes for the more toxic compounds, but their use has more recently decreased as a result of environmental concerns and the development of even safer and environmentally friendly compounds.

Halogenated Aromatic Compounds

This group of compounds includes the polychlorinated biphenyls (PCBs), polybrominated biphenyls (PBBs), chlorinated dibenzo-p-dioxins, and dibenzofurans and chlorophenols. PCBs comprise a group of synthesized organochlorine compounds with remarkable chemical stability and flame resistant and insulating properties that led to their extensive use in the electric utility industry and as heat exchange and hydraulic fluids. They were used extensively in the U.S. until the 1970s, when concern over their toxicity in laboratory animals and persistence in the environment led to governmental restrictions on their manufacturing and distribution. However, the heavy use of PCBs prior to the restrictions led to worldwide environmental contamination of varying degrees and concerns over PCB bioaccumulation in the food chain (13).

PCBs and their structurally related dioxin and dibenzofurans, are potent inducers of the cytochrome P-450 system. There is evidence that they may induce hepatocellular carcinomas in animals (14). The majority of PCB-attributed liver disease was recorded during and before World War II. Most of the exposures were to PCB-chloronaphthalene mixtures. The clinical picture included anorexia, nausea, edema of the face and hands, and jaundice. Liver findings in patients were described as "acute yellow atrophy," which was characteristic of a massive necrosis (zone 3). The evidence that PCBs by themselves cause occupational liver disease is weak. Studies of PCB-exposed workers have shown some evidence of alteration of liver enzymes levels; however, liver function parameters such as albumin, bilirubin, and prothrombin times were unaffected (15,16). Dioxin and dibenzofuran compounds are structurally related to PCBs and exhibit similar effects on the liver. Like PCBs there is no firm evidence that they cause occupational liver disease, although a follow-up study after a significant environmental contamination incident in Seveso, Italy, in 1975 suggested an increase incidence of cholangiocarcinoma in those exposed (17).

Organochlorine Pesticides and Chlorphenoxy Herbicides

This group of chemicals includes a large number of commercially available products that have had extensive use in agriculture and other applications. Examples of these compounds include DDT, lindane, chordane, chlordecone (Kepone), and heptachlor.

The organochlorine pesticides present similar problems with environmental persistence and bioaccumulation as discussed above for PCBs. The majority of these compounds show no convincing evidence of significant hepatotoxicity in humans. However, there continues to be controversy regarding the hepatic effects of Agent Orange (a mixture of 2,4-D and 2,4,5-T and containing dioxin). Chlordecone (Kepone) has been associated with minor hepatic injury characterized by steatosis and dysfunction (18).

Nitroaliphatic and Nitroaromatic Compounds

Nitroaliphatic compounds display a spectrum of hepatotoxic potential in animals. 2-Nitropropane has been associated with hepatic necrosis, and there is some evidence that it may be carcinogenic (19). Elevated aminotransferase levels, focal necrosis, and microvesicular steatosis have been described in a group of workers exposed to dimethylformamide (20,21). Methylenedianiline is an epoxy resin–hardening agent that has been associated with cholestatic injury in occupationally exposed workers (22).

Trinitrotoluene (TNT) is the best known of the nitroaromatic occupational hepatotoxins. It caused severe and often fatal liver disease in munitions workers during both world wars.

Potentiation Related to Alcohol and Other Chemical Interactions

In the industrial world, most chemical exposures are not to a single chemical agent, but rather to a mix of various substances used in a particular manufacturing process. Furthermore, often workers are exposed to other substances outside the workplace such as alcohol, drugs, and pesticides. It has been long known that ethanol potentiates the toxicity of carbon tetrachloride and that alcoholics are more likely to develop hepatic injury after exposure to CCl_4 than nondrinkers (23). Isopropanol, methanol, 2-butanol, and acetone have been found to have potentiating properties similar to ethanol (24). The likely mechanism for this potentiation is alcohol induction of hepatocyte cytochrome P-450 systems with enhanced metabolic conversion of CCl_4 to its toxic metabolite. Trichloroethylene also potentiates the toxicity of CCl_4; however, the mechanism for this is unknown. Drugs can also interact with or potentiate the effects of workplace exposure. Common examples are isoniazid enhancement of acetaminophen toxicity and phenobarbital enhancement of halothane toxicity (25,26). There has been much interest in investigating possible hepatotoxicity from exposure to solvent mixtures. Multiple studies have been done in a variety of industrial and exposure settings. These studies have had mixed results, with some studies demonstrating an increased frequency of liver pathology in those exposed (27,28), while other studies have demonstrated few findings or findings confounded by age and/or alcohol ingestion (29,30).

A PRACTICAL GUIDE TO THE PREVENTION OF, AND MEDICAL SURVEILLANCE FOR, OCCUPATIONAL LIVER DISEASE

The first step in preventing occupational liver disease is to substitute and replace hepatotoxic agents with nonhepatotoxic agents whenever possible. In the last two decades, significant progress has been made in the elimination and substitution of many of the more common hepatotoxic chlorinated hydrocarbons that had been widely used in a variety of industrial applications. Solvent-based cleaning and degreasing operations have increasingly been changed to aqueous-based systems. This trend is encouraging and has resulted in a reduction in the prevalence of acute occupational hepatotoxicity. Beyond elimination and substitution of toxic agents, engineering controls to reduce exposure is an important measure to prevent and/or reduce hepatotoxic exposures. Finally, it must be emphasized that when an individual presents with a possible work-related liver disorder, removal from exposure should be considered early on and may provide both preventative and diagnostic benefits.

Medical Monitoring of Workers Exposed to Hepatotoxins

The surveillance of workers with potential exposure to hepatotoxins presents a challenge for the occupational health professional. The ideal medical surveillance test would be one that has both high sensitivity and specificity. However, there is still a lack of tests that meet this criterion and that are practical to implement in the occupational health setting. Thus, for the most part we are constrained to using biochemical and functional tests for liver disease. Biochemical tests include standard serum transaminase measures as well as serum and urine bilirubin. In addition, tests of synthetic liver function and clearance tests are available to the clinician.

Biochemical Tests

These tests are the most commonly used measures to detect liver disease. The ones most commonly used in workplace medical surveillance are AST, ALT, serum alkaline phosphatase (ALP), serum lactate dehydrogenase (LDH), and γ-glutamyl transpeptidase (GGT). Transaminases are released from hepatocytes following cell injury or death. These tests are more sensitive than specific, and may be useful in detecting early stages of both toxic liver injury and nontoxic liver disease (viral hepatitis, extrahepatic obstructive conditions). Furthermore, in the occupational health setting, it is most likely that one will be dealing with an asymptomatic population with a significant number of individuals who drink alcohol to varying degrees. Thus, transaminase screening frequently identifies individuals with elevated transaminase levels that could be due to a variety or combination of factors. In these cases, the occupational health clinician will have to evaluate the total picture, which includes workplace exposures, exposures outside the workplace, nonoccupational medical conditions, and the use of alcohol. Elevations of other transaminases such as ornithine carbamoyl transferase (OCT) and sorbitol dehydrogenase (SD) may help in ruling out certain enzyme elevations that may be due to other tissues (heart, skeletal muscle, or kidney). Transaminase levels are not a sensitive measure of steatosis and are of little value in conditions where fatty change is not accompanied by hepatocellular injury or necrosis.

Bilirubin

Serum bilirubin is typically elevated when there is significant parenchymal liver injury. It is the pigment most likely to be elevated in patients with toxic liver injury. Nevertheless, compared with transaminases, it is considered an insensitive measure of chemical liver injury and thus is of limited value in the occupational setting. Hyperbilirubinemia may be either conjugated or unconjugated. Unconjugated hyperbilirubinemia is commonly seen in Gilbert's disease, hemolytic disorders, and congestive heart failure. Measurement of bilirubin has greatest utility in providing a measure of the severity of hepatocellular or cholestatic injury when following a diagnosed condition.

Synthetic Liver Function and Clearance Tests

Measurement of serum albumin and prothrombin time are commonly done to assess the liver's synthetic function. However, neither is a sensitive measure of liver injury and has little or no value in medical surveillance for exposure to hepatotoxins. Clearance tests measure the ability of the liver to excrete substances and can be sensitive and specific in the detection of liver disease. These tests can measure clearance of exogenous substances (indocyanine green, antipyrine) or endogenous substances (serum bile acids).

Indocyanine green clearance has been used to detect subclinical injury in vinyl chloride workers, and antipyrine clearance has been used in a variety of occupational settings including working exposed to chlordecone and chlorinated solvents.

Physical Examination and Structural Studies

Physical examination is useful in detecting hepatomegaly. However, hepatomegaly usually occurs after there has been a prolonged or significant hepatotoxic exposure. Thus, physical examination is not a sensitive screening tool. Likewise, radiologic and ultrasound studies have not been found to be useful screening tools in the workplace setting. Liver biopsy is the gold standard in establishing the most specific diagnosis possible. However, liver biopsy is highly invasive and carries some significant risks of complications. Thus, it is never used as a screening tool and is reserved for those cases where tissue diagnosis is required. It must be remembered that even with a biopsy-proven histologic diagnosis, the work-relatedness of an individual's liver pathology may remain in question.

REFERENCES

1. DeLeve LD, Kaplowitz N. Mechanism of drug-induced liver disease. *Gastroenterol Clin North Am* 1995;24:787.
2. Paganini-Hill A, Glazer E, Henderson BE, et al. Cause-specific mortality among newspaper web pressmen. *J Occup Med* 1980;22:542–544.
3. Thiele DL, Eigenbrodt EH, Ware AJ. Cirrhosis after repeated trichloroethylene and 1,1,1-trichloroethane exposure. *Gastroenterology* 1982;83:926–929.
4. Popper H, Thomas LB. Alterations of liver and spleen among workers exposed to vinyl chloride. *Ann NY Acad Sci* 1975;246:172.
5. Poland A, Smith D, Matter C, et al. A health survey of workers in a 2,4-D and 2,4,5-T plant. *Arch Environ Health* 1971;22:316.
6. Creech JL Jr, Johnson MN. Angiosarcoma of the liver in the manufacture of polyvinyl chloride. *J Occup Med* 1974;16:150.
7. Lee FI, Smith PM, Bennett B, et al. Occupationally related angiosarcoma of the liver in the United Kingdom, 1972–1994. *Gut* 1996;39:312–318.
8. Daniell W, Stebbins A, Kalman D, et al. The contributions to solvent uptake by skin and inhalation exposure. *Am Ind Hyg Assoc J* 1992;53(2):124–129.
9. Zimmerman HJ. *Hepatotoxicity: the adverse effects of drugs and other chemicals on the liver,* 2nd ed. Philadelphia: Lippincott Williams & Wilkins, 1999.
10. Peterson P, Bredahl E, Lauritsen O, et al. Examination of the liver in personnel working with liquid rocket propellant. *Br J Ind Med* 1970;27:141.
11. Dossing M, Skinhoj P. Occupational liver injury: present state of knowledge and future perspective. *Int Arch Occup Environ Health* 1985;56:1–21.
12. Pond SM. Effects on the liver of chemicals encountered in the workplace. *West J Med* 1982;137:6:506–514.
13. Kimbrough RD. Human health effects of polychlorinated biphenyls (PCBs) and polybrominated biphenyls (PBBs). *Annu Rev Pharmacol* 1987;27:87.
14. Norback DH, Weltman RH. Polychlorinated biphenyl induction of hepatocellular carcinoma in the Sprague-Dawley rat. *Environ Health Perspect* 1985;60:97–105.
15. Chase KC, Wong O, Thomas D, et al. Clinical and metabolic abnormalities associated with occupational exposure to polychlorinated biphenyls (PCBs). *J Occup Med* 1982;24(2):109–114.
16. Emmett EA, Maroni M, Jefferys J, et al. Studies of transformer repair workers exposed to PCBs II. Results of clinical laboratory investigations. *Am J Ind Med* 1988;14:47–62.
17. Stone R. New findings point to cancer. *Science* 1993;261:1383.
18. Guzelian P. Comparative toxicology of chlordecone (Kepone) in humans and experimental animals. *Annu Rev Pharmacol* 1982;22:89.
19. Harrison R, Letz G, Pasternak G, et al. Fulminant hepatitis after occupational exposure to nitropropane. *Ann Intern Med* 1987;107:466.
20. Redlich CA, Beckett WS, Sparer J, et al. Liver disease associated with occupational exposure to the solvent dimethylformamide. *Ann Intern Med* 1988;108:680.
21. Redlich CA, West AB, Fleming L, et al. Clinical and pathological characteristics of hepatotoxicity associated with occupational exposure to diethylformamide. *Gastroenterology* 1990;99:748.
22. McGill DB, Matto JD. An industrial outbreak of toxic

hepatitis due to methylenedianiline. *N Engl J Med* 1974;291:278.
23. Cornish HH, Adefuin J. Ethanal potentiation of halogenated aliphatic solvent toxicity. *Am Ind Hyg J* January–February, 1966.
24. Cornish HH, Adefuin J. Potentiation of carbon tetrachloride toxicity by aliphatic alcohols. *Arch Environ Health* 14:447–449.
25. Nomura F, Hatano H, Ohnish K. Effects of anticonvulsant agents on halothane-induced liver injury in humans subjects and experimental animals. *Hepatology* 1986;6:952.
26. Murphy R, Swartz R, Watkins PB. Severe acetaminophen toxicity in a patient receiving isoniazid. *Ann Intern Med* 1990;113:399.
27. Brodkin CA, Danielle W, Checoway H, et al. Hepatic ultrasonic changes in workers exposed to perchloroethylene. *Occup Environ Med* 1995;52(10):679.
28. Dossing M, Arlein-Soborg P, Peterson LM, et al. Liver damage associated with occupational exposure to organic solvents in house painters. *Eur J Clin Invest* 1983; 13:151.
29. Kurppa K, Husman K. Car painters exposure to a mixture of organic solvents. *Scand J Work Environ Health* 1982;8:137.
30. Rees D, Soderlund N, Cronje R, et al. Solvent exposure, alcohol consumption, and liver injury in workers manufacturing paint. *Scand J Work Environ Health* 1993;19 (4):236.

33

Case Report: Discovery of Occupational Disease

William E. Wright

A patient relates that he thinks he has lung cancer, just like a number of other men with whom he works.

A doctor caring for a patient observes that the man was exposed to high levels of a chemical when a large volume of it spilled years ago. The patient's co-worker, who helped clean up the spill, is found to have an identical cancer.

A man has developed difficulty urinating and asks his doctor whether she thinks that this condition is caused by his work.

Physicians are often introduced to workplace concerns through questions from their patients. Sometimes the questions are directly related to work (e.g., "Doctor, do you think my hypertension is caused by my work?"). Sometimes clues related to work are provided by the patient's history (e.g., "My wheezing started after I took on the new job"). Sometimes a patient inadvertently suggests that unusual factors or work may be responsible (e.g., "Why me? Why should I have this cancer since I never smoked?").

Work as a cause of illness may also be suggested by co-workers, worker representatives, or legal counsel. Physicians should be prepared to address their patients' questions and concerns by determining whether work conditions are likely to have affected the illness. They should also share with others concerns about confirmed or likely associations of work and illness. One way to share these concerns is through a case report.

This chapter provides a framework for identifying occupational diseases and preparing case reports. The approach consists of a clinical diagnostic tool, the occupational history, and a series of questions, the answers to which help organize the data for decision making. To attribute an illness accurately to a workplace substance or process, the questions should be answered thoroughly. Consultation may be needed with others who have specialty training in occupational medicine, clinical toxicology, or a related discipline. A review of pertinent medical literature is usually necessary and can help formulate an opinion that may serve as the basis of a case report.

Patients and society expect physicians to recognize occupational disease and, more recently, cumulative trauma, and be able to determine the cause and share their findings. The physician's role is not only in assessing traditional or new occupational illnesses, but also in evaluating the occupational contribution, if any, to common musculoskeletal disorders, cumulative trauma, and stress-related symptoms. While physicians are frequently faced with evaluating whether work has caused or aggravated illnesses (1), their inquiry is usually hampered by insufficient information. The clinician may lack adequate information on exposure to industrial materials, group data on health outcomes, access to working populations for study, and sufficient time and resources for epidemiologic studies to test for suspected associations between work and illness.

In addition to these obstacles, there are other factors that may interfere with identifying new associations of work and illness. The small number of physicians trained in occupational medicine contrasts with the large potential for patients to develop occupational diseases. Many thousands of chemical substances are commonly used in the United States, and hundreds of new ones are introduced each year (1). Our knowledge about the toxic properties of many of these substances is limited. Only a small proportion of the materials in use are covered by occupational health standards. The development of new commercial materials is proceeding at a pace beyond the capability to evaluate their toxicity adequately. The large number and wide variety of substances used and the continual changes in industrial technology create a situation in which new work-related illnesses will occur. Despite these obstacles, the physician has the responsibility of benefiting society by recognizing previously unrecognized health problems associated with exposure to workplace materials.

Identifying the cause of these illnesses is essential to their primary prevention through implementation of appropriate changes in the workplace. Health effects of many workplace materials are uniquely preventable with approaches of material containment, substitution, elimination, and personal protection. In addition to prevention, the benefits of recognizing the occupational components of illness include providing more effective treatment, enhancement of health and productivity at work (1a), assisting patients in obtaining appropriate workers' compensation benefits, and fulfilling the physician's legal obligation to report the occurrence of occupational disease. In the case of newly recognized or suspected associations of work and illness, publication of case reports can stimulate others to perform more formal evaluations to test and further define the association.

How can the physician identify new occupational diseases or unusual manifestations of traditional occupational afflictions and share this information with others? Historically, physicians generated a case report of an occupational disease when the disease had been unusual, the number of cases had been large, or the association between the exposure and the disease had been strong. Identification of additional occupational ailments can be enhanced by routinely considering occupational exposures as possible causes in clinical evaluations, by considering the worker to be an important source of information, and by applying a logical and methodical approach to investigate work and health interactions. With a basic knowledge of epidemiology and common occupational diseases, the physician can employ a methodical approach to assess possible interactions of work and illness. The occupational history is the cornerstone of the approach to recognition of occupational disease and generation of case reports.

OCCUPATIONAL HISTORY

The occupational history is the clinical tool used to elicit and organize information about the workplace for any thorough diagnostic evaluation. Descriptions of the occupational history have been published in the medical literature and are highlighted in Chapter 20. A basic occupational history includes the following:

1. Description of current and recent work, including longest held job and years worked in each position.
2. Report of any exposure to chemicals, dusts, or fumes, including type, intensity, and duration; and information from manufacturers, employers, and Material Safety Data Sheets (MSDSs). A request for exposure monitoring data, if available, is recommended.
3. Relationship of symptoms to periods away from work (e.g., weekends, holidays, vacations, or other absence) and to changes in work schedule.
4. Description of any change in work activities, production quotas, work processes, or other work routine preceding or coinciding with the development of symptoms.
5. Occurrence of similar symptoms or illness in coworkers.
6. The patient's opinion regarding the relationship of illness to work and reasons supporting the opinion.
7. History of use of substances in avocational activities and their relationship to symptoms or illness.
8. Contact with workplace or work-site visit.

The description of recent and longest held jobs, a screening question about exposures, and attention to the temporal relationship between the patient's chief complaint and work activities are suggested as part of a brief, routine survey provided to every patient (Fig. 33.1) (2,3). Use of the mnemonic WHACS (*W*hat do you do? *H*ow do you do it? *A*re you concerned about any of your exposures on and off the job? *C*o-workers or others exposed? *S*atisfied with your job?), which has been used to assist with the occupational history (3a), incorporates an important inquiry about job satisfaction, which is critical in the presentation, course, prognosis, and employee perceptions about their condition. For illnesses likely to have a long latency between exposure to a hazardous substance and clinical presentation (e.g., cancer and chronic diseases), a complete chronologic occupational history is often needed.

CLINICAL DIAGNOSTIC EVALUATION

The clinical diagnostic evaluation, which includes the occupational history, provides a starting point for decisions regarding the relation of work to illness. The following steps, expressed as questions to be addressed, can be used to evaluate a case or group of cases for which a diagnosis of occupational disease is entertained. An outline of this approach is shown in Table 33.1.

What Is the Medical Condition?

An accurate diagnosis is essential. The physician must establish the presence of disease in accordance

1. Name ______________________ Date ________
2. Current position (job) ______________________
   Type of business ______________________
   Description of work activities ______________________
   ____
3. Are you exposed to or do you work with any chemicals, dusts, or fumes? Yes __ No __ Don't know __
4. Do any co-workers have medical complaints similar to yours? Yes __ No __ Don't know __
5. Do you think you have a medical problem related to or aggravated by your work? Yes __ No __ Don't know __
6. Have you ever worked with any of the following materials?

Asbestos	___	Plastics	___
Solvents	___	Radiation	___
Petroleum products	___	Lead	___
Vehicle or engine exhaust	___	Mercury	___
Degreasers	___	Other metals	___
Paints	___	Welding, brazing, soldering	___
Glues	___	Insulation	___
Grease and oil	___	Other dusts	___
Pesticides	___	Other gases	___
Silica	___	Noise	___

7. Have you ever done any of the following types of work?

Plumbing or pipefitting	___
Shipyard work	___
Building construction	___
Mining	___
Forge or foundry work	___
Chemical plant work	___

8. Have you worked in any other environments or with any other materials about which you are concerned? Yes ___ No ___
   If yes, describe: ______________________
   ____
9. Do you have any hobby activities that involve use of or exposure to dusts, chemicals, or fumes? Yes ___ No ___
   If yes, describe: ______________________
   ____
10. Starting with your first job, list your complete occupational history. Include summer jobs and part-time jobs.

Dates (month/yr.) From	To	Employer	Job	Exposures

FIG. 33.1. Taking an occupational history requires using traditional techniques of medical interviewing with prompts, follow-up questions, and interpretation by the physician. No form can provide a complete occupational history and yet be a convenient length for use with all patients. The form shown here covers the essential elements of the occupational history; questions numbered 1–6, 9, and 10 cover the outline of the brief, routine survey that can easily be applied to all patients. The form can be shortened or expanded to suit the user's needs.

with standard diagnostic practices. If no actual disease is noted, a report of the presence of a constellation of symptoms or physiologic or laboratory abnormalities may be sufficient. When dealing with several cases, diagnostic criteria should be uniformly applied.

Where feasible, diagnoses should be reviewed and confirmed. Assuring the uniformity of diagnoses is important because criteria for diagnoses can change as the understanding of the pathologic process evolves. For example, the association of asbestos ex-

TABLE 33.1. *Summary of the evaluation of work-related disease*

Determine the diagnosis accurately:
- Uniformity of diagnosis among cases
- Standard diagnostic practices or clearly defined case definition

Describe working conditions (occupational history)
Review toxicity of materials (literature review)
Evaluate information on dose and response:
- Consider dose-response relationships from epidemiologic studies
- Consider factors that modify exposure
- Consider exposure to analogous substances

Consider plausible alternative explanations
Review aggregate data related to the hypothesis that materials at work caused the illness:
- Features that substantiate the proposed relationship
- Alternative explanations and their likelihood
- Type of cause considered to be present (e.g., de novo, aggravation, predisposition)

posure with malignant mesothelioma was first noted in a number of people, most of whom had been exposed to asbestos (4). Malignant mesothelioma is now widely considered to be primarily of occupational origin, although as many as one third of patients lack specific exposure to asbestos. However, earlier in this century, pathologists debated whether primary tumors of the pleura occurred at all, and pathologists still differ on the criteria that should be used to diagnose the tumor with certainty (5).

Case reports of clusters of tumors of unusual types or at unusual anatomic sites have led to identification of occupational carcinogens. One example is the first report of an occupational cancer in 1775 by Pott (6), who noted that scrotal cancer occurred with an unusually high frequency among chimney sweeps. Contemporary examples include identification of the extremely rare tumor angiosarcoma of the liver in some workers at a plant where vinyl chloride was polymerized into polyvinyl chloride resins (7), and oat-cell carcinoma of the lung in a group of men who worked with bis-chloromethyl ether manufacturing ion exchange resins (8). In addition to peculiar cancers, clusters of workers with unusual symptoms, such as difficulty in urinating among foam workers exposed to a newly introduced catalyst, dimethylaminopropionitrile (9), and clusters of people with unusual illness, such as aspermia in workers exposed to the nematocide dibromochloropropane (10), in groups sharing work experiences have led to case reports of new relationships between exposure and disease.

Some medical conditions may be more likely to be related to workplace factors than others. A way to increase the possibility of identifying occupational disease for case reports is to use the sentinel health event (SHE) approach described by Rutstein and associates (11,12). A SHE is a condition already known to have occupational causes that contributes to unnecessary disease, disability, or untimely death. Such conditions, when they occur in a practice setting, warrant special scrutiny of occupational factors. When used by practitioners, this approach has been shown to assist with identification of occupational diseases. This area is covered in detail in Chapter 20.

What Are the Working Conditions, Including Level and Degree of Exposure to Materials?

The occupational history should be taken in sufficient detail to identify the type, intensity, and duration of exposure to materials. If specific exposure information is not known, description of work activities and processes may be an adequate substitute. A good example of this is seen in a case report of pulmonary alveolar proteinosis in a cement truck operator (14). The author lacked air monitoring to quantify exposure, but used quantitative factors such as duration and frequency of exposure along with qualitative information such as verbal accounts of dust obscuring vision, the worker being covered with dust, and photographs of conditions to document significant exposure to dust.

Additional information obtained from an occupational health nurse, physician, industrial hygienist, plant engineer, or supervisor at the work site can assist in characterizing the working conditions. Industrial hygiene monitoring data for similar jobs should be reviewed, if available. Manufacturers of substances may be able to provide information on chemical formulations and toxicity. A visit to the work site and observation of work activities can be extremely valuable in determining the character and extent of exposure to certain materials.

A number of texts on industrial processes are useful for understanding work activities, potential for exposures, and chemical or physical agents that should be considered as potential causes of disease (15–19). As a result of the Hazard Communication Standard, companies should have MSDSs on file that describe materials used and their toxicity. Review of MSDSs can yield clues for further investigation. One should recognize that a file of MSDSs may not cover all substances that are used in industrial processes, and that potential health effects of combined exposures, reactants, by-products, and contaminants may not be addressed. MSDSs only cover known toxicity; additional effects not listed on the MSDSs may occur, which may serve as the basis for a case report.

Based on Current Knowledge, Can the Exposure, in Any Quantity, Cause the Disease?

Although obtaining the answer to this question may be time consuming, the process is straightforward and depends on a review of current information in the literature. In addition to the standard medical texts on occupational medicine, the physician should become familiar with other available references that provide specific information regarding toxicity of materials (20–24).

A number of government agencies provide information on commercial substances and their effect on health. For example, the National Institute for Occupational Safety and Health (NIOSH) has regional offices that can provide current information. Criteria documents, medical advisories, and other bulletins are periodically published by NIOSH and are readily available to physicians upon request. The Agency for Toxic Substances and Disease Registry (ATSDR) has developed a series entitled "Case Series in Environmental Medicine." This material, which describes an initial case, is followed by an overview of key considerations, such as toxicology and biologic monitoring. In addition, state governments and chemical manufacturers' associations can be sources of valuable information.

The *Index Medicus* and National Library of Medicine computerized literature searches (e.g., MEDLINE, TOXLINE) are becoming routine tools in this stage of the information-gathering process. A number of these databases are now available for access through personal computers at home, as well as at medical libraries and academic centers.

One should note that of many case reports related to occupational health issues that have attracted media attention (7–10), little or no relevant information was available on the toxicology of the suspected chemicals. In the case of dibromochloropropane (10), however, animal evidence of testicular toxicity could have been used as a basis for further evaluation or more cautious use. Some computerized literature services, such as TOXLINE, offer information on animal studies, significant results from which should not be ignored. But in the case of dimethylaminopropionitrile (9), no industrial material was recognized to have the observed clinical effect in animals or humans (i.e., sacral autonomic neuropathy producing urinary bladder dysfunction).

Based on Current Information, Is the Level of Exposure Sufficient to Cause the Disease?

When evaluating new substances or unrecognized effects of low exposure to familiar materials, this question usually cannot be answered with a desirable level of accuracy. In other situations, it is important to consider what is known about the relationship between exposure and response. Characteristics of exposure, such as intensity, duration, and route, and personal characteristics, such as cigarette smoking, alcohol consumption, age, genetic susceptibility, intercurrent disease, and coexposures, may interact to influence the ultimate effect on health.

Sometimes, simply relating timing of exposure and effects gives convincing evidence about sufficiency of exposure and work-relatedness. Several recent case reports lacking quantitative information on exposure emphasized that symptoms occurred at work or during work with a particular substance but did not occur on days off. This approach, which emphasizes a hallmark of occupational disease, was critical in linking epistaxis and dermatitis to the use of glutaraldehyde for cold sterilization (25,26), asthma to the use of alkyl cyanoacrylate adhesives (27), allergic rhinitis to handling psyllium (28), and dermatitis to a non–bisphenol A epoxy used in preparation of tissue for electron microscopy (29).

The human body has the capacity to detoxify materials without recognizable ill effects. At some levels of exposure, homeostatic mechanisms allow transport, metabolism, and excretion of materials without discernible disruption of biochemical or physiologic function and without apparent clinical effects. For a clinical effect to become apparent due to exposure to a hazardous substance, the level of exposure must be sufficient to overwhelm homeostatic mechanisms and disrupt metabolic pathways so that damage occurs at the target tissue. In the case of alteration of genetic material as a target tissue for development of cancer, the damage must also be allowed sufficient time to be expressed. Unfortunately, adequate exposure information is not often available, and some plausible estimate is necessary. Toxicologic information related to the effect of dose on target organs is also usually unavailable. Results of animal studies may be available in some cases, but the validity of extrapolating results to humans is often subject to a variety of opinions. For example, a report linking stillbirth in a laboratory worker to use of the solvent *N*-methyl-2-pyrrolidone noted concordance of this effect in animal data (29a).

Epidemiologic studies can be of considerable value in assessing the contribution of exposure to illness in individual patients if the studies demonstrate a dose-response relationship and if the working conditions of the patient under consideration resemble those described in the study. Investigations limited to only dichotomous exposure information (e.g., Exposed? Yes or No), job title, or employment in an industry without quantitation are more difficult to use. If the level of exposure under consideration seems insufficient to cause disease, it is also possible that the character of the exposure has not been accurately defined or personal characteristics of the patient have magnified the effect. In addition, some materials may affect the body through pathogenetic mechanisms, such as activation of the immune system, in which a graded response to increasing dose may not be apparent (e.g., as happens with industrial exposure to beryllium).

One should also be aware that even though levels of exposure are below recommended standards, the exposure still may not be safe. As new information becomes available, the American Conference of Governmental Industrial Hygienists (ACGIH) and regulatory bodies such as the Occupational Safety and Health Administration (OSHA) can be expected to revise the current recommendations and standards, and historically such revisions have usually lowered the threshold limit values.

Are There Any Factors that Modify the Exposures in Some Way?

Apparently harmless industrial processes can sometimes be modified by work practices or personal habits to lead to occupational disease. For example, the high temperature of burning cigarettes has been recognized to alter fluoropolymers into harmful fumes that produce flu-like polymer fume fever (30). The occurrence of osteosarcoma of the jaw in painters of clock dials early in the 20th century resulted in part from the work practice of using the tongue to point the tip of the paintbrushes laden with radium (31). Personal techniques of job performance, hand washing, and preparation and consumption of food in a contaminated area should also be considered in assessing possible occupational exposures. One case report related an unusual exposure to carmustine from faulty equipment. The effects of the exposure may have been enhanced by prolonged contact with clothing that the drug had penetrated (32). Another report related Reactive Airways Dysfunction Syndrome to a leak of aerosolized pentamidine (32a). The pace of work and energy demands may also be important with some exposures, since mouth breathing, breath holding, and rapid, deep respirations may increase exposure to dusts and chemicals. Use of personal protective equipment may also modify exposure, but consultation with the worker and with an industrial hygienist may be necessary to assess whether the protective equipment being used is providing effective protection.

Is the Agent Similar to Any Other Recognized Hazards?

A report of three cases of hematologic malignancy sharing exposure to 1,3-dichloropropene pointed out that the chemical structure is similar to that of dibromochloropropane and vinyl chloride, two recognized carcinogens (33). One clue to the presence of a potential toxic effect of a substance is whether its chemical structure is similar to that of other substances with recognized toxicity. An analysis of the threshold limit values for chemical exposures set by the ACGIH emphasized that about one quarter of the chemicals for which exposure values were published were based on chemical analogy (1).

Although a review of the chemical structure is one way to assess a substance's potential for human toxicity, there are pitfalls in using this approach. The similarity of effects of organophosphate compounds on the nervous system, for example, appears to be due to the similarity in the active site of a number of otherwise dissimilar compounds. Another example is that among di-isocyanates that affect the respiratory system, the relevant similarity of structure also appears to be in the active site rather than in the entire molecule. Additional examples include toluene and xylene, which share the aromatic ring of benzene but apparently not its carcinogenicity. Undoubtedly, other chemical and physical features of chemicals, including polarity, molecular size, physical form, and metabolic pathways for activation or degradation, have important roles in determining potential for toxic effects. Metabolic conversion is recognized to be important in activating polycyclic aromatic hydrocarbons to carcinogenic epoxides that bind DNA and in degrading methylene chloride into carbon monoxide, which may be responsible for some of the acute toxic effects of this compound.

Can Other Conditions or Factors Provide a Plausible Alternative Explanation for the Findings?

The history should be explored for the occurrence of other exposures during hobby or home activities that might be related to the condition under consideration (34). A report relating a case of toxic epidermal necrolysis to work with plastic resins is a good example of an issue that is sometimes considered in attributing an illness to a workplace material (35). The authors dealt with complexities of the workplace (mixed exposures, pyrolysis products) as well as the possibility that intercurrent infectious disease or medical treatment caused the observed illness. In assessing the relevance of work to the occurrence of similar conditions in a group of cases, the differential diagnosis should be explored sufficiently to be sure that the conditions cannot be explained by coincident occurrence of different disease processes in each person (e.g., evaluating several people with neuropathy, alcohol consumption, diabetes mellitus, arteritis, trauma, or heavy metal poisoning, instead of a shared exposure, may account for the development of some of the cases). In addition, cigarette smoking, which is a common occupational and avocational exposure, can have an independent effect in causing disease that may be mixed with the effects of other substances (see Chapter 40).

If Current Information Does Not Support the Hypothesis that the Exposure Caused the Disease and No Viable Alternative Exists, How Should the Data Be Interpreted?

Several features of a disease are often emphasized in case reports to substantiate a claim that the exposure of interest is related to the disease under consideration. Occasionally, available data can be used to estimate the likelihood of the number of observed cases in the exposed population. Presentation of figures of disease incidence was used in Figueroa and associates' (8) report of oat-cell carcinoma of the lung in chloromethyl methyl ether workers to emphasize the unusual nature of the case's occurrence. Other factors noted in case reports that are used to support claims of causality include (a) the exposure of interest precedes the occurrence of disease by a reasonable period of time; (b) the people proved or presumed to be the heaviest exposed are the ones to develop the disease, the first to develop the disease, or the ones to develop the most severe form of the disease; (c) signs and symptoms improve coincident with removal or reduction of exposure; (d) the exposure is relevant to the chronic disease under consideration because past high exposure was associated with severe acute illness; and (e) only chance provides a recognized viable alternative explanation. Most of these arguments are supported by information obtained from a thorough occupational history.

The diagnosis of an occupational illness is often one of exclusion; that is, the diagnosis is made after ensuring that other well-known causes for the disorder are not present. However, the occurrence of disease in only one or several of a group of people who have shared exposure to a material should not detract from reporting a suspected association; not only are working conditions highly variable, but also people often react quite differently when exposed to the same material (see Chapter 40). As an analogy, even in infectious diseases, attack rates are usually far less than 100% (36).

GUIDELINES FOR PREPARING THE CASE REPORT

Detailed descriptions of methods for preparation of medical research papers and reports have been published. If, after a review of the case material using the steps suggested in this chapter, the physician believes that a new occupational illness or syndrome has been identified, the following guidelines, based on the format outlined by Huth (37), can be used to prepare the case report (Table 33.2).

Type of Case

First, decide on the type of case to be reported. Case reports in occupational medicine that contribute most to new and useful knowledge are usually one of three types.

TABLE 33.2. *Summary of case report preparation*

Decide on type of case to be reported:
- Unique case
- Previously unrecognized effect of a material
- Unexpected course of an illness

Decide on the format of the presentation:
- Use journal's guidelines to determine specific form
- General outline for the single case:
  - Introduction
  - Description of case
  - Discussion
  - Conclusion
- Considerations for reports of multiple cases:
  - More detailed section on methods
  - Tables or figures for presenting data

The Unique Case

Reporting of a unique illness resulting from an exposure may require extensive review of the literature to support the claim of uniqueness. In cases in which the pathophysiology of the condition is investigated using sophisticated medical technologies, the report may be best presented as a research paper rather than a case report (37).

New Association of an Illness with Exposure to a Material or Other Stressor (Mechanical or Psychological)

Many associations of illness with exposure to materials are likely to be coincidental. Support for the argument that a causal association exists may depend on either defining a plausible pathogenic mechanism or providing statistical evidence consistent with a low probability of a chance association (see Chapter 40). The coincidental occurrence of illness and exposure may still be an important factor in many cases. Symptoms that occur only with exposure or on workdays but not on days off, or allergic symptoms that occur after a period adequate for sensitization, lead to a strong presumption that some workplace factor is important in occurrence of illness. The proportion of people exposed to the material who experience the health effect carries weight if it is high. A recent example is a report of seven people in a workplace in which an undiluted glycol ether solvent, 2-butoxyethanol, was used. All seven had acute irritant symptoms and six of the seven experienced delayed onset of eruptive cherry angiomas (37a).

Unexpected Course of an Illness

Unexpected improvement or deterioration of a patient's condition coincidental with exposure to a material may provide hints about the pathogenesis of the illness and about the metabolic fate and effects of the material. Support of the argument that a cause-and-effect relationship exists depends on excluding plausible alternative explanations, including chance, to the extent possible.

Unique or Unusual Circumstances of Exposure

Sometimes materials can produce occupational disease because of unusual circumstances of exposure. One of the case reports already cited focused on exposure to an antineoplastic drug that was probably enhanced by prolonged skin contact (32). Another case report focuses on respiratory effects of unexpectedly aerosolized pentamidine (32a). Pyrolysis of chemicals with cigarettes producing polymer fume fever represents another unusual circumstance (30). There are other examples of unique or unusual circumstances. A case report noted that when a material (phenoxyethanol), which could reasonably be expected to produce central nervous system depression, was used as an anesthetic for fish in a way that produced skin contact, serious chronic neurotoxicity ensued (38). A case of sensory neuropathy was reported in a man who took home a workplace degreasing agent (1,1,1-Trichloroethane) and used it without personal protective equipment (38a). Another recent example in this category is a report of chronic beryllium disease in users of alloys containing only 2% beryllium in a setting with no documentation of exposure beyond the OSHA PEL (38b).

Clarification of Pathophysiology

Some case reports are produced because new or more sophisticated testing is available to define the disease or mechanisms of illness. Examples are found in two case reports of Schwartz and associates in which reactions to psyllium dust (28) and permanent wave solutions (39) were studied by using challenge tests and measuring nasal as well as lower-airway resistance. Another report focuses on laryngoscopic confirmation of vocal cord dysfunction, distinct form suspected asthma, thought to result from exposure to workplace irritants (39a).

Format of the Presentation

The journal to which the case report is submitted will determine the format to a large extent. The journal's guidelines will specify whether an abstract, summary, conclusion, or other special sections are required. In addition, the following format is usually sufficient and provides a concise framework for the case report.

Introduction

The introduction includes several paragraphs explaining how the case came to the author's attention, describing the illness and the material of interest or work setting in general terms to clarify the focus of the report, and stating why the case is of special interest.

Description of the Case

This section can be handled as a narrative account of the occurrence of illness, with flashbacks to prior events, illnesses, or work history that are relevant. The sequence of presentation of clinical and occupational information may vary depending on the author's preference for developing the narrative (e.g., chronologic versus presenting illness, course, and flashbacks) and on the nature of the case. The clinical evaluation and the details of the occupational history that provide a clear and coherent account of the workplace, job activities, and character and extent of exposure can be provided in this section. Any factors that may have modified the exposure to the material should be covered as well.

Other Considerations

Reports of multiple cases may require attention to additional detail or special sections. Case definition, uniformity of the cases, and methods used for case finding and for confirmation of the diagnoses and work histories may be addressed in the section describing the cases or in a separate section describing methods. Tables and figures may be used to illustrate the associations. For example, a case series of three workers exposed to trichloroethylene included a figure demonstrating symptoms corresponding to levels of urinary trichloroacetic acid (40). The discussion section should address similarities among the cases and exclude, to the extent possible, plausible alternative diagnoses or explanations for the occurrence of the cases.

Discussion

This section provides the argument regarding the uniqueness of the case and the logical explanation of why the case is worth reporting. The literature reviewed and its support or conflict with the proposed association should be presented here. Information about the toxicology of the material of interest or about analogous materials should be presented. Critical analysis of the likelihood of associations being causal should be developed. An account of attempts to identify similar cases in the population at risk could also be included here. A conclusion can be placed at the end of this section or can be presented separately according to the journal format. The conclusion should cover the possibilities for further studies, the implications of the discovery for clinical medicine and public health, the opportunities for prevention, and the anticipated effects of preventive intervention for the population at risk.

Notes on Causation

A cause can be defined as an exposure to a substance that, if the exposure is modified, alters the rate of disease occurrence in populations. In occupational medicine, a case report may suggest either that a material presumed to be safe has adversely affected health or that an acknowledged hazard has resulted in a previously unrecognized effect. The reports are not definitive statements of cause. The case report, by the nature of the data on which it is based, involves a degree of uncertainty that can only be resolved by more extensive analytic studies.

Opinions among physicians vary regarding criteria considered valid to establish a causal relationship. For some, the term *cause* indicates a clear and generally accepted relationship between exposure and illness, for which no alternative explanation exists. This approach to formulating opinions regarding causes, however, may be considered restrictive and may lead to overlooking possible new associations. Even in medicolegal settings, cause is implied if exposure to an agent is considered to be more likely than not (i.e., 51% likely or more) to have caused the disease, based on available medical and epidemiologic data. Case reports, which are suggestions of causal relationships, are expected to have a lower level of certainty than might be required in other settings. This latitude in thinking is necessary to allow hypotheses to be tested so that new associations can be recognized. Clearly each situation should be evaluated based on careful consideration of the aggregate information, including all supportive and nonsupportive elements.

Hazardous substances can alter the rate of occurrence of disease in several ways. For example, a hazardous agent may be the sole cause of a unique disease. More commonly, an occupational illness does not have a unique clinical presentation or course that distinguishes it from a nonoccupational disease. What distinguishes an occupational disease is neither its histopathology nor its clinical, radiographic, or laboratory features, but its *etiology*, an occupational agent. Hazardous materials may cause disease de novo, alter a biologic function without apparent clinical effect, bring to light an existing subclinical condition, predispose individuals to develop a disease, or aggravate a preexisting disease. One should consider the range of adverse health effects that can result from exposure to materials. After presentation of the case report, universal acceptance of the proposed relationship between the illness and the agent will depend on confirmation by more refined epidemiologic studies.

One characteristic of case reports is that the number of cases reported may not include all cases that may have occurred. Furthermore, since the number of people at risk of developing the illness from the exposure may be unknown or poorly defined, the actual incidence rates or prevalence may not be obtainable. The case report, however, can provide useful information that can serve as the basis for investigating and preventing illness in other people exposed to the same agent.

REFERENCES

1. Peters JM. Occupational health: working yourself sick. In: Kane RL, ed. *The challenges of community medicine.* New York: Springer, 1974.
1a. McCunney RJ. Health and productivity: a role for occupational health professionals. *JOEM* 2001;43:30.
2. Guidotti TL. Taking the occupational history. *Ann Intern Med* 1983;99:641.
3. Goldman RH, Peters JM. The occupational and environmental health history. *JAMA* 1981;246:2831.
3a. Blue AV, et al. Medical students' abilities to take and occupational history: use of the WHACS mnemonic. *JOEM* 2000;42:1050.
4. Wagner JC, Slegg CA, Marchand P. Diffuse pleural mesothelioma and asbestos exposure in the North Western Cape Province. *Br J Ind Med* 1960;17:260.
5. Wright WE, et al. Malignant mesothelioma: incidence, asbestos exposure, and reclassification of histopathology. *Br J Ind Med* 1984;41:39.
6. Pott P. Cancer scroti. *The chirurgical works of Percivall Pott.* London: Hawkes, Clark and Collins, 1775: 734–736.
7. Creech JL Jr, Johnson MN. Angiosarcoma of liver in the manufacture of polyvinyl chloride. *J Occup Med* 1974; 16:150.
8. Figueroa WG, Raszkowski R, Weiss W. Lung cancer in chloromethyl methyl ether workers. *N Engl J Med* 1973; 288:1096.
9. Kreiss K, et al. Neurological dysfunction of the bladder in workers exposed to dimethylaminopropionitrile. *JAMA* 1980;243:741.
10. Whorton MD, et al. Infertility in male pesticide workers. *Lancet* 1977;2:1259.
11. Rutstein DD, et al. Sentinel health events (occupational): a basis for physician recognition and public health surveillance. *Am J Public Health* 1983;73:1054.
12. Mullen RJ, Murthy LI. Occupational sentinel health events: an up-dated list for physician recognition and public health surveillance. *Am J Ind Med* 1991;19:775.
13. Fontus HM, Levy BS, Davis LK. Physician-based surveillance of occupational disease. Part II: Experience with a broader range of diagnoses and physicians. *J Occup Med* 1989;31:929.
14. McCunney RJ, Godefroi R. Pulmonary alveolar proteinosis and cement dust: a case report. *J Occup Med* 1989;31:233.
15. Burgess WA. *Recognition of health hazards in industry—a review of materials and processes.* New York: John Wiley & Sons, 1995.
16. Considine DM, ed. *Chemical and process technology encyclopedia.* New York: McGraw-Hill, 1974.
17. Cralley LV, Cralley LJ, eds. *Industrial hygiene aspects of plant operations, vol 1: process flows.* New York: Macmillan, 1982.
18. Cralley LJ, Cralley LV, eds. *Industrial hygiene aspects of plant operations, vol 2: unit operations and product fabrication.* New York: Macmillan, 1984.
19. *Encyclopedia of occupational health and safety,* vols 1–2, 3rd ed. Geneva: International Labour Organization, 1983.
20. Key MM, et al., eds. *Occupational diseases—a guide to their recognition.* Public Health Service, NIOSH publication No. 77-181. Washington, DC: U.S. Department of Health, Education and Welfare, 1977.
21. Harbison RD. *Hamilton and Hardy's industrial toxicology,* 5th ed. St. Louis: Mosby, 1998.
22. Mackison FW, et al., eds. *Occupational health guidelines for chemical hazards. NIOSHOSHA,* vol 1–3. Department of Health and Human Services, NIOSH publication No. 81-123, 1978.
23. Bingham E, Cohrssen B, Powell CH. *Patty's toxicology,* vols 1–9, 5th ed. New York: John Wiley & Sons, 2001.
24. Lewis RJ. *Sax's dangerous properties of industrial materials,* 8th ed. New York: Van Nostrand Reinhold, 1992.
25. Wiggins P, McCurdy SA, Zeidenberg W. Epistaxis due to glutaraldehyde exposure. *J Occup Med* 1989;31:854.
26. Fowler JF. Allergic contact dermatitis from glutaraldehyde exposure. *J Occup Med* 1989;31:852.
27. Nakazawa T. Occupational asthma due to alkyl cyanoacrylate. *J Occup Med* 1990;32:709.
28. Schwartz HJ, Arnold JL, Strobl KP. Occupational allergic rhinitis reaction to psyllium. *J Occup Med* 1989;31: 624.
29. Dannaker CJ. Allergic sensitization to a non-bisphenol A epoxy of the cycloaliphatic class. *J Occup Med* 1988; 30:641.
29a. Solomon GM, et al. Stillbirth after occupational exposure to *N*-Methyl-2-pyrrolidone. *JOEM* 1996;38:705.
30. Wegman DH, Peters JM. Polymer fume fever and cigarette smoking. *Ann Intern Med* 1974;81:55.
31. Rowland RE, Stehney AF, Lucas HF Jr. Dose-response relationships for female radium dial workers. *Radiat Res* 1978;76:368.
32. McDiarmid M, Egan T. Acute occupational exposure to antineoplastic agents. *J Occup Med* 1988;30:984.
32a. Stanbury M, et al. Reactive airways to dysfunction syndrome in a nurse exposed to pentamidine. *JOEM* 1996;38:330.
33. Markovitz A, Crosby WH. Chemical carcinogenesis: a solid fumigant, 1,3-dichloropropene, as possible cause of hematologic malignancies. *Arch Intern Med* 1984; 144:1409.
34. McCunney RJ, Russo PK, Doyle JD. Occupational illness in the arts. *Am Fam Physician* 1987;36:145.
35. House RA, et al. Work-related toxic epidermal necrolysis? *J Occup Med* 1992;34:135.
36. Monson RR. *Occupational epidemiology,* 2nd ed. Boca Raton, FL: CRC, 1990.
37. Huth EJ. *How to write and publish papers in the medical sciences.* Philadelphia: ISI, 1990.
37a. Raymond LW, et al. Eruptive cherry angiomas and irritant symptoms after one acute exposure to the glycol ether solvent 2-Butoxyethanol. JOEM 1998;40:1059.
38. Morton WE. Occupational phenoxyethanol neurotoxicity: a report of three cases. *J Occup Med* 1990;32: 42.
38a. House RA, et al. Paresthesias and sensory neuropathy due to 1,1,1-Trichloroethane. *JOEM* 1996;36:123.
38b. Balkissoon RC, et al. Beryllium copper alloy (2%) causes chronic beryllium disease. *JOEM* 1999;41:304.

39. Schwartz HJ, Arnold JL, Strobl KP. Occupational allergic rhinitis in the hair care industry: reactions to permanent wave solutions. *J Occup Med* 1990;32:473.

39a. Perkner JJ, et al. Irritant-associated vocal cord dysfunction. JOEM 1998;40:136.

40. McCunney RJ. Diverse manifestations of trichloroethylene. *Br J Ind Med* 1988;45:122.

FURTHER INFORMATION

Huth EJ. *How to write and publish papers in the medical sciences.* Philadelphia: ISI, 1990.

Written by the editor of the *Annals of Internal Medicine,* this book covers many of the dimensions of medical writing. This excellent reference includes guidance on many fundamentals, such as preparation of tables, figures, and references and conducting a search of the literature.

Rutstein DD, et al. Sentinel health events (occupational): a basis for physician recognition and public health surveillance. *Am J Public Health* 1983;73:1054.

This article introduces a list of diagnoses that can be used by practicing physicians for occupational health surveillance. Diseases on the list serve as warning signals that an occupational relationship may be likely and should be considered. Some details of the sentinel health events approach are also covered in Chapter 20.

Vanderbroucke JP. In defense of case reports and case series. *Ann Intern Med* 2001;134:330.

This article addresses recent criticism of the value of case reports in the face of demands of modern evidence-based medicine. Claims have been made that the new ideas from case reports often are not sustained on further research, the clinical presentations in case reports may contain misleading elements, and case reports emphasize the bizarre. The author defends case reports as having a high sensitivity for detecting novelty, providing new ideas in medicine, and serving medical progress. Suggestions are made for focusing the case report and clarifying why the observations are important.

SPECIFIC CASE REPORTS

The case reports referenced in this chapter can be used as models. Some of the more instructive reports are listed below by type of illness and exposure to help the reader identify reports of interest:

1. Unusual illnesses attributed to specific chemicals
   A. Oat-cell carcinoma—bis-chloromethyl ether (8)
   B. Angiocarcinoma—vinyl chloride (7)
   C. Difficult urination—dimethylaminopropionitrile (9)
   D. Aspermia—dibromochloropropane (10)
   E. Eruptive cherry angiomas—2-butoxyethanol
2. Unusual illness attributed to mixed exposures
   A. Pulmonary alveolar proteinosis—cement dust (14)
   B. Toxic epidermal necrolysis—plastic resins (35)
3. Common illnesses attributed to specific chemicals
   A. Asthma—alkyl cyanoacrylate (27)
   B. Dermatitis—glutaraldehyde, non–bisphenol A epoxy (29)
   C. Epistaxis—glutaraldehyde (25)
   D. Neuropathy, cognitive impairment—2-phenoxyethanol (38)
   E. Rhinitis—psyllium (28)
   F. Stillbirth—*N*-methyl-1-2-pyrrolidone (29a)
4. Common illnesses attributed to mixed exposures
   A. Rhinitis—permanent wave solutions (39)
   B. Asthma type symptoms (vocal cord dysfunction) due to irritants (39a)
5. Unusual circumstances of exposure
   A. Spill, prolonged skin contact with an antineoplastic drug (25)
   B. Exposure modified by pyrolysis in cigarettes (30)
   C. Unusual ingestion of materials (31)
   D. Prior chemical spill (33)
   E. Undiluted use of glycol ether solvent (37a)
   F. Unprotected use of a workplace solvent at home (38a)
   G. Chronic beryllium disease with low alloy work (38b)

34

Occupational Ophthalmology

Bernard R. Blais, Thomas J. Tredici, and John Williams, Sr.

Vision is a key ingredient for most jobs, and occupational physicians are expected to advise companies about relevant visual skills. Eye injuries have accounted for a large percentage of industrial accidents during the past century. The vast majority could have been prevented by the adoption of appropriate protective eyewear. The basic principles of industrial ophthalmology were developed almost 100 years ago but unfortunately were never thoroughly implemented. Over 50 years ago the text on *Industrial Ophthalmology* (1) described the state of the art in eye safety, and research established vision standards that are still in use today.

This chapter provides a brief review of the anatomy and physiology related to vision, screening examinations, the treatment of the "red eye," the analysis of eye hazards, and the prevention of eye problems.

BACKGROUND

Epidemiology of Occupational Eye Injuries

An estimated 2.4 million people suffer eye injuries each year. Between 40,000 and 60,000 of these injuries are associated with severe vision loss (2). In addition to the traumatic cases, millions more visit physicians in emergency rooms or clinics each year for less serious acute eye conditions, such as a nonpurulent conjunctivitis. Reports concerning the incidence of occupational eye injuries are somewhat inconsistent and discussion about the true extent is ongoing. Pizzarello (3) reported a dramatic change in the patterns of eye injuries over the past 50 years as the manufacturing sector has eroded and the workplace has changed. Liggett et al. (5) found in inner city of Los Angeles that only 8% of eye injuries occurred at work. Most injuries were sustained at home or on the street. Schein et al. (6) reported that 48% of injuries seen in an urban emergency room occurred at work. Statistics from *Prevent Blindness America* estimate that there are 2.4 million eye injuries each year, and approximately 250,000 (about 10%) of these occur at the job (3).

Role of the Occupational Physician

The occupational physician and nurse should screen workers and advise workers and employers regarding visual skills. They examine and may also treat numerous causes of "red eye" disorders (Table 34.1A), foreign body injuries, and similar eye problems. The physician's most important responsibility is to distinguish between vision-threatening conditions and those that are minor. Serious disorders, listed in Table 34.1B, require early recognition and prompt referral to an ophthalmologist for ideal management.

TABLE 34.1A. *Red-eye disorders—non–vision threatening*

Stye
Chalazion
Blepharitis
Conjunctivitis
Tear deficiency—dry eyes
(Most) corneal abrasions

Adapted from Young SE. *Managing the red eye—a slide script program.* San Francisco: American Academy of Ophthalmology, 1988.

TABLE 34.1B. *Red-eye disorders—vision threatening*

Corneal infections
Scleritis
Hyphema
Iritis
Acute glaucoma
Orbital cellulitis

Adapted from Young SE. *Managing the red eye—a slide script program.* San Francisco: American Academy of Ophthalmology, 1988.

Equipment Necessary for Screening and Treatment (7)

Examination Equipment (7)

The following equipment and supplies are important for the evaluation of the patient with an eye complaint.

1. Reclining chair or table and cart
2. Red lens
3. Amsler grid
4. Visual acuity card, distant and near
5. Visual screener
   a. Titmus model 2a or 2c
   b. Stereo optical model 2000, 2500, 3500
6. Direct ophthalmoscope
7. Pocket light—penlight or Finoff transilluminator tip, attached to the ophthalmoscope handle
8. Binocular loupe or slit lamp

Treatment Materials (7)

1. Ophthalmic solutions should be in eye drop bottles, well labeled, sterile, and with colored tops. These solutions should be used for eyes only. Some medications may irritate the eyes, but this does not preclude their use. Fluorescein strips are also important.
2. Distilled sterile water, dextrose 5% in half-normal saline, or normal saline in 1-L containers, with associated tubing, may be necessary for irrigation of cul-de-sacs in chemical injuries.
3. Anesthetics, preferably proparacaine HCL 0.5%
4. Antibiotics, such as sulfacetamide 10% solution and ointment, bacitracin eye ointment, Polysporin eye ointment, erythromycin eye ointment, tetracycline eye ointment
5. Supplies:
   a. Sterile hypodermic needles (25g, 26g, or 27g)
   b. Sharp point Bard-Parker No. 15 blade
   c. Golf club spud
   d. Dental burr (kept clean and free of rust)
   e. Small pickup forceps (Paufigues or Bishop Harmon's)
   f. Ophthalmic needle holder
   g. Tying forceps × 2
   h. Demarres lid retractors (two adult)
   i. Sutures for closure of lacerations around the lids and ocular adnexae: 5-0 and 6-0 plain catgut or chronic; 5-0, 6-0, 7-0, 8-0 silk, nylon, or prolene.
   j. Sterile eye pads; an eye pad should be placed with anchoring tape (adhesive or plastic tape) from forehead to cheek
   k. Fox shields (or cone made of x-ray film) for eye protection.

ANATOMY AND PHYSIOLOGY OF THE EYE AND ORBIT

Vision occurs peripherally at the eye and centrally in the brain. The retina receives electromagnetic energy (photons) and converts them into electrical signals that are relayed to the brain and interpreted as vision (8).

The *bony orbits* (see color plate Fig. 34.1) afford protection and support for the globe while allowing maximum exposure for vision. The globe acts as an external sensor, gathering information and relaying it to neural paths. Extraocular muscles (except the inferior oblique muscle) originate from a fibrous ring, the annulus of Zinn, located at the orbital apex in close approximation to the optic nerve. For this reason inflammation of the optic nerve (retrobulbar neuritis) may cause pain with motion of the eye. "Blowout" fractures of the orbital floor may result in double vision (diplopia), especially with upward gaze. The thinnest bones are in the medial wall, and orbital cellulitis may ensue if fracture of this delicate bone allows communication with the ethmoid sinus or nasal cavity. Hemorrhage into the orbit following injury may displace the globe, causing proptosis, immobility, and diplopia. An accumulation of fluid in the body (edema) is manifested as puffy eyelids, while dehydration or starvation causes the eyes to sink deeply into the orbit.

The *globe* (see color plate Fig. 34.2) has three coats or layers: the sclera, for support and protection; the uvea, for nutrition; and the retina, containing light-sensitive neuronal elements. The extraocular muscle tendons are contiguous with the sclera and merge into it. An anterior bulge, the cornea, measures approximately 12 mm in diameter. The transition between the opaque sclera and the clear cornea is called the limbus.

The *cornea* is composed of collagen fibers and is transparent to visible radiation. Collagen fibers extend in regular layers of parallel fibers. An endothelial pump mechanism keeps the cornea continuously dehydrated. There are no blood vessels or pigmented cells present in the corneal stroma. The cornea is thinnest in the center and thickens toward the edge. Oxygen supplied to and metabolized in the cornea is derived from three sources: the aqueous humor, the perilimbal vascular supply, and the tear film bathing the epithelial cells. Capping this oxygen source, as by placing some types of contact lenses over the surface, reduces oxygen tension at the corneal epithelium.

The eye is approximately a 60-diopter (D) refracting system (9). The cornea is the most powerful component of the ocular refracting system because it separates elements of the greatest difference in indices of refraction (air/cornea). Approximately 45 D of total refraction is due to the cornea, while 15 D is due to the unaccommodated lens. Small changes in the corneal radius can cause substantial changes in refraction, and attempts are often made to alter corneal curvature to change refraction, such as with the use of contact lenses (orthokeratology), newer surgical procedures (radial keratotomy), or more recently by excimer laser lamellar keratectomy, also known as photorefractive keratectomy (PRK) and LASIK.

The *uvea,* inside the scleral coat, is the pigmented vascular portion of the eye and consists of the choroid posteriorly and the ciliary body and iris anteriorly. The uveal tract contains melanin pigment. The iris color is a function of the degree of pigmentation. Brown eyes are heavily pigmented, whereas blue or green eyes have a sparsely pigmented iris. The outer half of the retina is nourished by the choroid's abundant vascular supply. Anteriorly, the choroid, along with the anterior extensions of the retina, becomes the ciliary body, which is composed of smooth muscle lying in circular, longitudinal, and radial directions. More than 70 ciliary processes extend centrally toward the lens. The ciliary muscle, innervated by the parasympathetic nervous system, supplies the contractile forces necessary for accommodation, which allows one to see clearly close up. Aqueous humor, derived from blood plasma, is produced by diffusion and secretion in the epithelium of the ciliary process.

The *iris* is a thin, circular disk that controls the amount of light entering the eye and affects the depth-of-field of the eye's optical system. The iris divides the anterior segment into an anterior and posterior chamber. The *aqueous humor,* formed in the ciliary process, enters the posterior chamber, bathes the lens, flows through the pupillary opening into the anterior chamber, continues through the trabecular meshwork, and into Schlemm's canal, flows into the aqueous veins, and returns to the general circulation. A delicate balance of the sympathetic and parasympathetic tone of the autonomic nervous system controls the pupil. The sympathetic system innervates the dilator of the iris, while the parasympathetic system innervates the sphincter. This mechanism regulates the amount of light that enters the eye, which is proportional to the square of the pupillary diameter. In brightest daytime illumination the pupil can constrict to 1.5 mm. In darkness in can open to 8 mm in diameter. Even with maximum dilation, sufficient light may not be present to stimulate retinal receptors in darkness. After 30 minutes in darkness, however, another mechanism, adaptation, is triggered and increases light sensitivity many thousand times. This is called "night" or scotopic vision.

The *lens,* approximately 9 mm in diameter and 4 mm in thickness in an unaccommodated state, is held in place by zonular fibers inserted into the lens capsule and into the valleys between the processes on the ciliary body. In young individuals the lens is quite malleable. Its elastic capsule deforms the lens to view near objects clearly. When accommodation occurs, an increase in the refractive power is manifest on the lens as it becomes more spherical. This is accomplished by constriction of the circular muscle of the ciliary body through parasympathetic innervation. The zonular fibers slacken and the inherent elasticity of the lens capsule allows it to become more spherical, thus increasing its dioptric power. In the young this can be as much as 15 D over the amount of refractive power in the resting state of the lens. At age 40, approximately 5 D of accommodative power remains. When this drops to 4 D the individual is said to be presbyopic. Most reading is accomplished at 0.33 m where it is necessary to have 3 D to see clearly. One requires a 20% to 25% reserve of accommodation, however, to prevent symptoms of presbyopia. Only 1 D of accommodative power remains by age 65. The stimulus for accommodation is probably the blurred retinal image. The eye is in focus for monochromatic yellow only, being hypermetropic for red and myopic for blue (10).

The *retina* is the innermost photosensitive layer and is protected and nourished by the choroid (see color plate Fig. 34.2). The outer half of the retina is nourished by the choroid. From the internuclear layer to the inner limiting membrane, the retinal vessels nourish the retina. The neurosensory retina is composed of ten layers. The light-sensitive elements are the rods and cones. The rods serve vision at low levels of illumination (scotopic vision), whereas the cones are effective both for medium and high levels of illumination (mesopic and photopic vision) and for color vision. The cones are mainly concentrated in the fovea centralis. The center of an avascular area, known as the macula, is located 15 degrees temporal to the optic disk. The macular area is 1.5 mm in diameter and subtends 5 degrees at the nodal point. The fovea centralis, where form vision is most acute, measures approximately 0.3 mm in diameter and subtends an arc of 54 minutes, or approximately 1 degree. In the center of this area visual acuity can be as high as 20/10, whereas at the macula, or 2.5 degrees from the center of the fovea, the visual acuity has dropped to 20/50. The other retinal system, the rod receptors, is mainly useful in low illumination rods are more sensitive than the cones and are better for motion detection. The rods reach a maximum density in the retina at 15 to 20 degrees from the fovea centralis; therefore, looking 15 degrees off center maximizes one's scotopic vision.

To facilitate color vision, the cones have three different photosensitive pigments, one absorbing primarily in the blue wavelength at 445 nm, one in the green wavelength at 535 nm, and one in the red wavelength at 570 nm. Absorption at these wavelengths in varying amounts gives the human eye its color vision capabilities (8). All retinal nerve fibers combine into the optic nerve and leave the globe at the disk. No receptors are manifest here; thus, a functional "blind spot" is formed. The optic disk, or blind spot, is located 15 degrees nasal from the fovea and covers an area 7 degrees in height and 5 degrees in width. Because the functioning retina of the other eye covers one blind spot, we are unaware of its existence unless the unilateral visual field is being mapped. The optic nerves extend through the optic foramina, decussate at the chiasm, and continue as optic tracts to the lateral geniculate body. From the lateral geniculate body, the optic radiations fan out over the temporal and parietal lobes, eventually reaching the occipital lobe and concentrating in the posterior calcarine fissure of Brodmann's area 17. Decussation of the nerve fibers allows us to have corresponding points in each retina, which facilitates stereoscopic vision, the highest order of depth perception obtainable.

The *vitreous,* a clear, colorless, gel-like structure, fills the posterior four fifths of the globe, and is firmly attached to the ciliary epithelium in the area of the ora serrata and surrounding the optic disk. The vitreous is composed of 99.6% water with proteins and salt comprising the remainder. The proteins form scaffolding, which are fine fibrils (microfibrils seen only in the electron microscope on tissue preparation) composed of collagen. The spaces between the microfibrils are filled with hyaluronic acid and form the molecular network in the vitreous. The complaint of vitreous floaters is universal and usually is innocuous. Floaters are probably due to collapse of the protein/collagen scaffolding, which causes thickening and casts a shadow on the retina. More ominous floaters are red blood cells following a hemorrhage into the vitreous. The complaint of a dark floating membrane that may obscure vision should be investigated for the possibility of a retinal detachment.

The *adnexa* of the eye include the extraocular muscles, the eyelids, and the lacrimal apparatus (see color plate Fig. 34.3). Six extraocular muscles are attached to each globe, and because of the strong desire for fusion and the maintenance of single binocular vision, both foveae are maintained on the object of regard by both reflex and voluntary action. This is accomplished by the yoke muscles of each eye, which are driven by Hering's law of equal and simultaneous innervation to each muscle. If dysfunction occurs in either the nervous arc organization or in the muscles, binocularity is lost, causing strabismus and diplopia. The elevators of the globe are the superior recti and inferior oblique muscles. The depressors are the inferior recti and superior oblique muscles, and the horizontal rotators are the medial and lateral recti muscles. The actions of the muscles are described with the eye in the primary position of gaze. The actions of these muscles change depending on the position of the globe.

A thin, three-layered, precorneal tear film covers the corneal epithelium. The thin, outer, oily layer is derived from the meibomian glands of the tarsal plate. The middle aqueous layer is derived from the lacrimal glands, and the inner mucoid layer arises from the goblet cells of the conjunctiva. The external oily layer helps to retard evaporation of the tears and produces a smooth and regular anterior optical surface to the cornea. Ordinarily, a large part of the tear film evaporates each minute, with only the remainder passing through the lacrimal passages. This evaporation causes the tears to become slightly hypertonic, producing an osmotic flow of water from the anterior chamber through the cornea to the tear film. The lacrimal gland (see color plate Fig. 34.3) is situated in a bony fossa of the frontal bone just posterior to the superior and temporal rim of the orbit. It secretes the aqueous portion of the precorneal tear film layer. Accessory lacrimal glands, located in the conjunctiva, also can secrete tears. Tears drain through a small punctum, or opening, in the innermost edge of the upper and lower lids medially. These openings lead into a common canaliculus, then into the lacrimal sac, and finally into the nasolacrimal canals exiting under the inferior turbinate in the nose. Obstruction in any part of this system prevents normal drainage from the conjunctival sac, and a chronic conjunctivitis and dacryocystitis can result. Excess tearing interferes with visual capabilities, but a dry eye due to lack of tears also interferes with visual efficiency.

The *eyelids* provide protection for the cornea and the remainder of each eye by reflexive, involuntary closing. The lids blink involuntarily six to eight times per minute, thus evenly distributing and smoothing the precorneal tear film to enhance the optical qualities of the cornea. The eyelids are closed by action of the orbicularis oculi muscle, which is innervated by the seventh cranial nerve, and are opened by the levator palpebrae superioris muscles, which are innervated by the oculomotor nerve (cranial nerve III), assisted by Müller's muscle, which is innervated by the sympathetic nervous system. The lids are composed of several layers: the outer skin, which is the thinnest on the body and contains no subcutaneous fat; a muscle layer, formed by the orbicularis oculi muscle; the tarsal plate and the tarsal conjunctiva. This is a fibrous plate lending shape to the lids and containing the meibomian glands, which secrete the oily portion of the precorneal tear film, and the conjunctiva, inside the lid and proximal to the cornea. The oily secretion of the tarsal glands is spread over the lid edges. When the lids are tightly closed, a watertight seal is formed. The lids have an abundant vascular supply so that they heal quite rapidly even when severely injured. The ducts of the meibomian gland are located at the inner edge of the ducts from the glands of Moll, and the hair follicles are on the outer, or skin, edge of the lid. When the duct of the meibomian gland becomes occluded, the oily secretion remains in the tarsal plate, leading of stagnation of the oily material with subsequent foreign body reaction, forming a small granuloma or chalazion.

OCCUPATIONAL DISORDERS

The initial assessment of patients with acute and subacute eye problems should focus on detecting indications of potentially serious ocular pathology, termed *red flags,* and determining an accurate diagnosis. In the absence of red flags, work-related eye complaints can be safely and effectively handled by occupational or primary care providers. The focus is on monitoring for complications, facilitating the healing process, and the return to work in a modified or full-duty capacity.

Red flags, for these purposes, are defined as a sign or symptom of a potentially serious condition indicating that further consultation, support, or specialized treatment may be necessary. The term *red flags* as utilized by Payers looking for causality is not applicable to this discussion. Payers generally used the term to earmark a potentially fraudulent case.

Yellow flags indicate psychosocial or other barriers to recovery.

Algorithms for patient management have been written in the American College and Occupational and Environmental Medicine (ACOEM) *Occupational Medicine Practice Guidelines* (11).

The history of ocular injury may be obtained from the patient, first responder(s), or others involved or associated with an event. The specific work activity may provide clues about the extent of damage. Hammering or welding activities, for example, may suggest a penetrating wound to the globe. The focused occupational history should elicit the following information about presenting symptoms:

- Date and time of onset
- Nature of onset (very gradual, increasing, acute)
- Mechanism: how the patient thinks it happened

For acute trauma:

- Where? Location of the accident
- When? Time and date
- Who? The individual involved
- What? A detailed description of accident circumstances including force and load
- Sources of history
  - Patient
  - First responder(s)
  - Other personnel involved or associated with accident
  - Site of accident

Such information, coupled with a careful examination, directs the management of the injury (12,13). If the victim used personal protective equipment, the fact should be mentioned. If chemical exposure was involved, available information should be obtained.

For potential chemical exposure:

- What chemical? Description of Material Safety Data Sheets (MSDSs) (2) information
  - Type of chemical (alkali, acid, solvent)
  - Type of exposure (liquids, solids, fumes)
  - Dose of exposure
  - The pH of the material
  - The concentration of the material
  - The solubility of the material
  - The contact time
    - Emergency medical care by the first responder(s)
    - Product manufacturer
    - Availability of chemical data

Specific chemical data may be obtained from MSDSs, the Regional Poison Control Center, or from the Internet. It is also helpful to record emergency care delivered by the first responder.

OCULAR EXAMINATION AFTER INJURY TO THE EYE

The occupational physician should evaluate an eye complaint with a visual acuity chart, a penlight, a tonometer, fluorescein dye, topical anesthetic drops, slit lamp (Biomicroscope), and an ophthalmoscope. Many contemporary clinics have a Titmus or stereo optical visual screener, an air puff tonometer, and a slit lamp. A systematic approach to the examination should be utilized, beginning with the inspection of the face, orbital area, lids, and ending with the close view of the eyeball. The preferred method for examination of the eyeball includes the use of the slit-lamp biomicroscope and the ophthalmoscope.

If an ophthalmology consultation is required the patient should be made comfortable and the injured eye protected from further injury by application of a Fox shield (or equivalent) and a patch over the other eye in cases of an open globe injury.

The New Standardized Classification of Ocular Trauma *[Birmingham Eye Trauma Terminology (BETT)]* is the acceptable current terminology. This new classification (Fig. 34.4) has been endorsed by the American Academy of Ophthalmology, the board of directors of the International Society of Ocular Trauma, the United States Eye Injury Registry, and numerous other groups. When the system was published in 1997 (14), it was reasonably expected that it eventually would become the standardized international language of ocular trauma. Ophthalmologists were urged to use this terminology in clinical practice and research. It is mandated by several medical journals. Definitions in medical dictionaries are tailored toward general medical use and cannot be effectively applied to ocular trauma. The new system always uses the entire globe as the tissue of reference; therefore, the type of the injury is described unambiguously without the need to indicate the tissue involved. When a tissue is specified, it refers to wound location, not to injury type. A corneal penetrating injury thus involves an open globe injury with the wound being in the cornea. The system provides unambiguous definitions of each term (Table 34.2) and a complete classification of injury type (Fig. 34.4). Some injuries remain difficult to classify. For instance, an intravitreal BB pellet is technically an intraocular foreign body (IOFB) injury. However, since this is a blunt object that requires a huge impact force if they enter, not just contuse, the eye, there is an element of rupture involved. In such situations, an ophthalmologist should either describe the injury as "mixed" (i.e., rupture with an IOFB) or select the most serious type of the mechanisms involved.

The American Academy of Ophthalmology (AAO) specifies nine diagnostic steps to be used to evaluate a patient with a red eye (12,15–17):

1. Determine whether the visual acuity is normal or decreased (see Appendix), using a Snellen or preferred early treatment diabetic retinopathy study (ETDRS) chart. A visual acuity exam must be completed as a minimum prior to treatment except in chemical injuries where immediate irrigation is mandated. In this case the visual acuity is determined after the irrigation is complete.

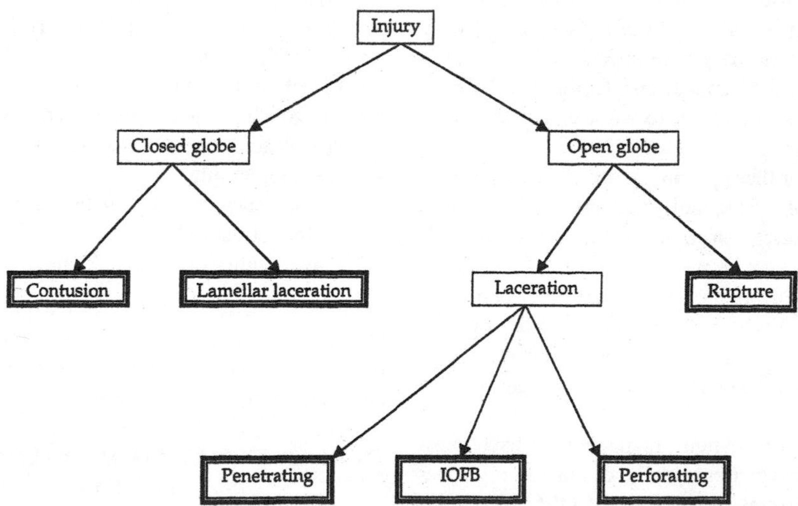

FIG. 34.4. Ocular trauma classification system. Birmingham eye trauma terminology(BETT). The double-framed boxes show the diagnoses that are commonly used in clinical practice. (From Kuhn F, Morris R, Witherspoon C, et al. *Ophthalmology* 1996;103:240–243, with permission.)

TABLE 34.2. *Birmingham Eye Trauma Terminology (BETT) glossary of terms*

Term	Definition and Explanation
Eyewall	**Sclera and cornea:** *though technically the eyewall has three coats posterior the limbus, for clinical and practical purposes violation of only the most external structure is taken into consideration.*
Closed globe injury	**No full-thickness wound of eyewall**
Open globe injury	**Full-thickness wound of the eyewall**
Contusion	**There is no (full-thickness) wound:** *the injury is due to either direct energy delivery by the object (e.g., choroidal rupture) or the changes in the shape of the globe (e.g., angle recession).*
Lamellar laceration	**Partial-thickness wound to the eyewall**
Rupture	**Full-thickness wound of the eyewall, caused by blunt object:** *since the eye is filled with incompressible liquid, the impact results in momentary increase of the intraocular pressure (IOP). The eyewall yields at its weakest point (at the impact site or elsewhere; example: an old cataract wound dehisces even though the impact occurred elsewhere); the actual wound is produced by an inside-out mechanism).*
Laceration	**Full-thickness wound of the eyewall, caused by a sharp object:** *the wound occurs at the impact site by an outside-in mechanism.*
Penetrating injury	**Entrance wound:** *if more than one wound is present, each must have been caused by a different agent.*
	Retained foreign objects: *technically a penetrating injury, but grouped separately because of different clinical implications.*
Perforating injury	**Entrance *and* exit wounds:** *both wounds caused by the same agent.*

2. Decide by inspection what pattern of redness is present and whether it is due to subconjunctival hemorrhage, conjunctival hyperemia, ciliary flush, or a combination of these.
3. Detect the presence of conjunctival discharge and categorize it as to amount—profuse or scant—and character—purulent, mucopurulent, or serous.
4. Detect opacities of the cornea, including large keratic precipitates or irregularities of the corneal surface such as corneal edema, corneal leukoma (a white opacity caused by scar tissue), and irregular corneal reflection. Examination is done using a penlight or transilluminator.
5. Search for disruption of the corneal epithelium by staining the cornea with fluorescein and lack of corneal epithelium integrating by staining with rose Bengal.
6. Estimate the depth of the anterior chamber as normal or shallow; detect any layered blood or pus, which would indicate either hyphema or hypopyon, respectively, or a corneal ulcer with hypopyon or hyphema.
7. Detect irregularity of the pupils and determine whether one pupil is larger than the other. Observe the reactivity of the pupils to light to determine whether one pupil is more sluggish than the other or is nonreactive.
8. Determine whether the intraocular pressure is high, normal, or low by performing tonometry if clinically indicated, for example, if acute angle-closure glaucoma is suspected. (Tonometry is omitted when there is an obvious external infection or lack of integrity of the globe.)
9. Detect the presence of proptosis, lid malfunction, or any limitations of eye movement.

Evaluation of the "Red Eye"

"Red eye" refers to hyperemia of the superficially visible vessels of the conjunctiva, episclera, or sclera. Hyperemia, or engorgement of the conjunctival blood vessels, can be caused by disorders of these structures or of adjoining structures including the cornea, iris, ciliary body, and ocular adnexa. The onset and duration of the redness, and clinical course, should be noted to help distinguish the causative agents (Table 34.3). The patient's complaints may reveal the cause of the red eye. Table 34.4 relates the symptoms and the causes of these disorders.

TABLE 34.3. *Causative agents for red eye*

Trauma
Chemicals
Infection
Allergy
Systemic conditions

From Young SE. *Managing the red eye—a slide script program.* San Francisco: American Academy of Ophthalmology, 1988.

TABLE 34.4. *Symptoms of red eye*

Symptom	Referal advisable if present	Acute glaucoma	Acute iridocyclitis	Keratitis	Bacterial conjunctivitis	Viral conjunctivitis	Allergic conjunctivitis
Blurred vision	Yes	3	1 to 2	3	0	0	0
Pain	Yes	2 to 3	2	2	0	0	0
Photophobia	Yes	1	3	3	0	0	0
Colored halos	Yes	2	0	0	0	0	0
Exudation	No	0	0	0 to 3	3	2	1
Itching	No	0	0	0	0	0	2 to 3

Note: The range of severity of the symptom is indicated by 0 (absent) to 3 (severe).

A *scratchy* or *burning sensation* suggests lid, conjunctival, or corneal disorders, including foreign bodies, in-turning eyelashes, and dry eyes. Patients with conjunctivitis may describe mild irritation but do not have severe pain. *Localized lid pain* or tenderness is a common presenting complaint of a stye or an acute chalazion of the lid. *Deep, intense aching pain!*[1] is not localized but may reflect corneal abrasions, iritis, keratitis, ulcer, iridocyclitis, or acute glaucoma, as well as sinusitis or tension headaches (12,13). A *halo effect!* around lights is commonly reported in acute glaucoma. Individuals who have corneal edema associated with contact lens wear may also experience halo vision. Colored halos or rainbow-like fringes seen around a point of light from corneal edema often results from an abrupt rise in intraocular pressure and are a dangerous symptom associated with a red eye. Other acute or subacute symptoms may provide helpful information in the differential diagnosis of the red eye (12,13,17) (Table 34.4). *Blurred vision!* often indicates serious ocular disease. Blurred vision that improves with blinking suggests a discharge or mucus on the ocular surface. *Photophobia!* is an abnormal sensitivity to light. It may occur either alone or secondary to corneal inflammation. Photophobia suggests problems arising from the anterior segment of the eye, such as corneal abrasions, iritis, and acute glaucoma. Patients with conjunctivitis have normal light sensitivity. *Exudation,* also called mattering, is a typical result of conjunctival or eyelid inflammation and does not occur with iridocyclitis or glaucoma. Patients with exudates often complain that their lids are "stuck together" on awakening. A *corneal ulcer!* is a serious condition that may or may not be accompanied by an exudate. *Mucoid discharge* is generally related to allergic conditions. *Watery discharge* may occur with viral conditions, and a *purulent discharge* is related to bacterial conditions. *Itching* is a nonspecific symptom, but usually indicates allergic conjunctivitis. Acute onset of spots, floaters, or flashes of light, or a *curtain drawn across the eye* is suggestive retinal detachment.

[1]An exclamation point (!) after a symptom or sign indicates a danger signal.

Diagnostic Steps

Patients who complain of a red or painful eye (Table 34.3) should be examined to detect any of several conditions (12,13). *Conjunctivitis* is manifested by hyperemia of the conjunctival blood vessels; the cause may be bacterial, viral, allergic, or irritative; the condition is common, and often not serious. *Episcleritis* is an inflammation (often sectorial) of the episclera, the vascular layer between the conjunctiva and the sclera. It is an uncommon problem, without discharge, and is not serious. It may be allergic, and is occasionally painful. *Scleritis* is an inflammation (localized or diffuse) of the sclera. It is uncommon, often protracted, and is usually accompanied by pain. It may indicate serious systemic disease such as a collagen-vascular disorder. It is potentially serious to the eye. *Subconjunctival hemorrhage* is an accumulation of blood in the potential space between the conjunctiva and the sclera. It is rarely serious. A *pterygium* is an abnormal growth consisting of a triangular fold of tissue that advances progressively over the cornea, usually from the nasal side. It is usually not serious. Localized conjunctival inflammation may be associated with pterygia. Most cases occur in tropical climates. Surgical excision is indicated if the pterygium encroaches on the visual axis. On the cornea, *herpes simplex keratitis!* is an inflammation caused by a virus. It is common, potentially serious, and can lead

TABLE 34.5. *Signs of red eye*

Sign	Referall advisable if present	Acute glaucoma	Acute iridocyclitis	Keratitis	Bacterial conjuncti-vitis	Viral conjuncti-vitis	Allergic conjuncti-vitis
Ciliary flush	Yes	1	2	3	0	0	0
Conjunctival hyperemia	No	2	2	2	3	2	1
Corneal opacification	Yes	3	0	1 to 3	0	0 or 1	0
Corneal epithelial disruption	Yes	0	0	1 to 3	0	0 or 1	0
Pupillary abnormalities	Yes	Middilated, nonreactive	Small, may be irregular	Normal or small	0	0	0
Shallow anterior chamber depth	Yes	3	0	0	0	0	0
Elevated intraocular pressure	Yes	3	−2 to +1	0	0	0	0
Proptosis	Yes	0	0	0	0	0	0
Discharge	No	0	0	Sometimes	2 or 3	2	1
Preauricular lymph-node enlargement	No	0	0	0	0	1	0

Note: The range of severity of the sign is indicated by −2 (subnormal) to 0 (absent) to 3 (severe).

to corneal ulceration. *Abrasions and foreign bodies* may be associated with hyperemia. In the anterior chamber, *acute angle-closure glaucoma!* is an uncommon form of glaucoma due to sudden and complete occlusion of the anterior chamber angle by its tissue. It is serious. The more common chronic open-angle glaucoma causes no redness of the eye. *Iritis or iridocyclitis!* is a serious inflammation of the iris, alone or with the ciliary body, often manifested by ciliary flush (see color plate Fig. 34.5). In the adnexa, disease may affect the eyelids, lacrimal apparatus, and orbit. It includes dacryocystitis, styes, and blepharitis. Red eye can also occur secondary to lid lesions (such as basal cell carcinoma or squamous cell carcinoma), thyroid disease, and vascular lesions in the orbit. Abnormal lid function can result in a red eye. Lesions such as Bell's palsy, thyroid ophthalmopathy, and others allow ocular exposure. These are potentially serious.

Inflammation of the conjunctiva and cornea produces only a few clinical signs (12,16,17). Some of these, such as hyperemia of conjunctival vessels, edema, and conjunctival papillae, are nonspecific and may not be helpful in determining the etiology of inflammation. The signs and symptoms of various disorders overlap to some extent. Several signs and symptoms signal danger, although many conditions can cause a red eye (12,13,15,17). The presence of one or more of these danger signals should alert the physician that the patient has a disorder requiring an ophthalmologist's attention. Table 34.5 summarizes the significant signs of red eye, Table 34.4 summarizes the symptoms, and Table 34.6 provides the differential diagnosis.

TABLE 34.6. *Differential diagnosis of red eye*

Acute angle-closure glaucoma: an uncommon form of glaucoma due to sudden and complete occlusion of the anterior chamber angle by iris tissue; serious. The more common chronic open-angle glaucoma causes no redness of the eye.

Iritis or iridocyclitis: an inflammation of the iris alone or of the iris and ciliary body; often manifested by ciliary flush; serious.

Herpes simplex keratitis: an inflammation of the cornea caused by the herpes simplex virus; common, potentially serious; can lead to corneal ulceration.

Conjunctivitis: hyperemia of the conjunctival blood vessels; cause may be bacterial, viral, allergic, or irritative; common, often not serious.

Episcleritis: an inflammation (often sectorial) of the episcleral, the vascular layer between the conjunctiva and the sclera; uncommon, without discharge, not serious, possibly allergic, occasionally painful.

Signs Detected in the Evaluation of the Red Eye (Table 34.5)

Reduced visual acuity! suggests serious ocular disease, such as an inflamed cornea, iridocyclitis, or glaucoma. It never occurs in simple conjunctivitis unless there is associated corneal involvement. A *ciliary flush!* is an injection of the deep conjunctival and episcleral vessels surrounding immediately the limbus cornea (see color plate Fig. 34.5). It is seen most easily in daylight and appears as a faint violaceous ring in which individual vessels are indiscernible to the unaided eye. Ciliary flush is a danger sign often seen in eyes with corneal inflammations, iridocyclitis, or acute glaucoma. It is a manifestation of inflammation of the anterior segment of the eye. Usually ciliary flush is not present in conjunctivitis. *Conjunctival hyperemia* is an engorgement of the larger and more superficial bulbar conjunctival vessels. A nonspecific sign, it may be seen in almost any of the conditions causing a red eye. *Corneal opacification!* in a patient with a red eye always denotes disease. These opacities may be detected by direct illumination with a penlight, or they may be seen with a direct ophthalmoscope (with a plus lens in the viewing aperture) outlined against the red fundus reflex. Several types of corneal opacities may occur including *keratic precipitates!,* cellular deposits on the corneal endothelium, usually too small to be visible without a magnification and focal illumination. These occasionally form large clumps, and may result from iritis or from chronic iridocyclitis. A diffuse haze obscuring the pupil and iris markings may be characteristic of *corneal edema.* It is frequently seen in acute glaucoma. Localized opacities may be due to keratitis or ulcer.

Corneal epithelial disruption! occurs in corneal inflammations and trauma. It can be detected in two ways:

1. Position yourself so that you can observe the reflection from the cornea of a single light source (e.g., window, penlight) as the patient moves the eye into various positions. Epithelial disruptions cause distortion and irregularity of the reflection.
2. Apply fluorescein to the eye. Areas denuded of epithelium will stain a bright green with a blue filter.

To identify the disruption of integrity of any layer of corneal epithelium:

1. Use the position described above.
2. Apply rose Bengal vital stain. Defective epithelium will stain a reddish-purple color.

A *pupillary abnormality!* may be noted in an eye with iridocyclitis. Typically the affected pupil is somewhat smaller than that of the other eye, due to reflex spasm of the iris sphincter muscle. The pupil is also distorted occasionally by posterior synechiae, which are inflammatory adhesions between the lens and the iris. In acute glaucoma, the pupil is usually fixed, mid-dilated (about 5 to 6 mm), and slightly irregular. Conjunctivitis does not affect the pupil.

Inspection of the *anterior chamber* in terms of (a) its depth, and (b) the contents of the anterior chamber, is extremely important and correlates well with the symptoms and signs previously obtained (15). In the case of narrow angle glaucoma, the edema of the cornea is associated with an *iris bombe!* (see color plate Fig. 34.6) where the anterior surface of the iris almost touches the cornea and where the anterior chamber is extremely shallow. An ancillary finding in these cases is an increase in intraocular pressure averaging 40 to 60. The content of the anterior chamber is significant as it correlates with the other findings of the conjunctiva and cornea. In cases of a uveitis (purulent cyclitis) the presence of protein and cells in the anterior chamber is classical. When the number of cells develop sufficiently that they precipitate, a *hypopyon!* (see color plate Fig. 34.7) will be present. A hypopyon is associated with layering of cells in up to 50% of the inferior anterior chamber inferior. A *hyphema!* (see color plate Fig. 34.8) is an accumulation of red blood cells secondary to trauma in the anterior chamber generally in the inferior half, but it can occupy the entire anterior chamber. One can see the difference between subconjunctival hemorrhage (see color plate Fig. 34.8) and microscopic hemorrhage with severe subconjunctival hemorrhage in Fig. 34.9 (see color plate Fig. 34.9). The determination of a microhyphema requires the use of a slit lamp. When there is an associated increase in intraocular pressure, the blood will be forced into the cornea, causing blood staining of the cornea.

Shallow anterior chamber depth! in a red eye (especially related to acute ocular pain, nausea, and sometimes vomiting) (see color plate Fig. 34.6) should always suggest acute angle-closure glaucoma. Anterior chamber depth can be estimated through side illumination with a penlight. Intraocular pressure should be measured. *Elevated intraocular pressure (glaucoma)!* accompanies iridocyclitis. The pressure is unaffected by most common causes of red eye. *Proptosis!* (see color plate Fig. 34.10) is a forward displacement of the globe. Proptosis of sudden onset suggests serious trauma, orbital infection, or tumor. The most common cause of chronic proptosis is thyroid disease. Orbital mass lesions also result in proptosis and should be considered. Proptosis may be accompanied by conjunctival hyperemia or limitation of eye movement. Standing behind a seated patient and looking downward to compare the positions of the two corneas most easily detects a small amount of proptosis. Acute orbital proptosis secondary to trauma is an ophthalmologic emergency (red flag) as it causes severe pressure on the eyeball with markedly elevated intraocular pressure, which can lead to central retinal artery occlusion. Pressure must be relieved within 10 minutes or the patient may have no light perception due to the lack of blood supply through the central retinal artery. Discharge may be an important clue to the cause of conjunctivitis. Preauricular node enlargement can be a prominent feature of some unusual varieties of chronic granulomatous conjunctivitis, known collectively as Parinaud's virus oculoglandular syndrome and conjunctivitis. Usually, such enlargement does not occur in acute bacterial conjunctivitis.

Red Eye Differential Diagnosis (12,13,17)

The red eye can be generally categorized in four classes: conjunctivitis, iritis, keratitis (corneal inflammation or foreign body), and acute glaucoma (Table 34.6). The changes in vision, type of discharge, presence or absence of pain, pupillary size, presence of conjunctival injection, pupillary response to light, intraocular pressure, appearance of the cornea, and the anterior chamber depth assist in the determination of the diagnosis (Table 34.5).

Slit-lamp Biomicroscopy

The slit-lamp examination is a standard of practice when examining the eye. First designed in 1911 by Gullstrand, it featured an oblique (condensed) illumination and a magnifying system (Fig. 34.11). With refinements this system is utilized in current slit lamps (17). Detail is seen by the viewer with reflected light. Substances that do not reflect light, such as tears or aqueous humor, are not visible; they are termed "optically empty." Structures that transmit light but can be seen in the beam are termed "reluctant," for example, the cornea, lens, vitreous. Structures that do not transmit light are opaque. The examiner must use special techniques for illumination and focusing that enhance the examination. The methods include (a) diffuse illumination, (b) direct or focal illumination (the most useful and important type of slit-lamp illumination whereby tissues such as the cornea are seen as an optical section or a block of tissue known as a parallelepiped), (c) retroillumination, where the area is being illuminated by reflected rays (e.g., corneal foreign body, corneal ulcer), and (d) indirect illumination. The use of the slit-lamp biomicroscope has been established as a competency for occupational health physicians by the ACOEM.

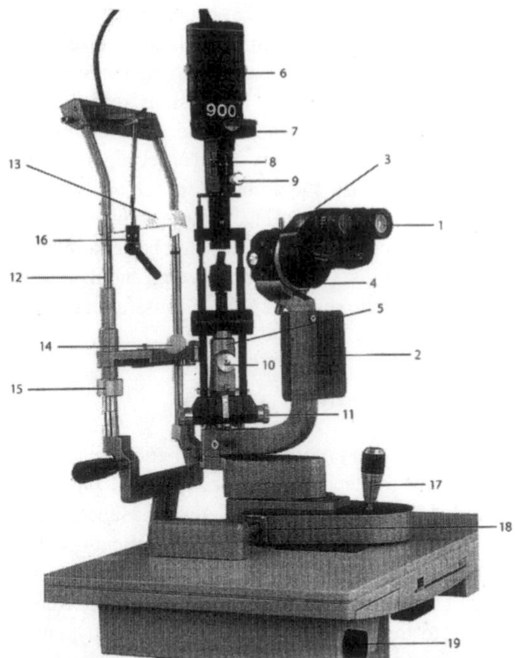

FIG. 34.11. Slit lamp—Hoog Strict 900. Part 6—collimated light system. Part 3—binocular microscope. (From Wilson FM. *Practical ophthalmology: a manual for beginning residents.* San Francisco: American Academy of Ophthalmology, 1996, with permission.)

LABORATORY DIAGNOSIS

Most mild cases of conjunctivitis are managed without laboratory assistance (12,13,17). This represents a compromise with ideal management but is justified by the economic waste of obtaining routine smears and cultures in such a common and benign disease. Most clinicians prescribe broad-spectrum topical ophthalmic antibiotic treatment. Cases of presumed bacterial conjunctivitis that do not improve after 2 days of antibiotic treatment should be referred, as a red flag, to an ophthalmologist for confirmation of the diagnosis and appropriate laboratory studies. In cases of hyperpurulent conjunctivitis, when copious purulent discharge is produced, conjunctival cultures should be done and an ophthalmologic consultation made because of possible gonococcal cause. Gonococcal hyperpurulent conjunctivitis is a serious, potentially blinding disease. In doubtful cases, smears of exudate or conjunctival scrapings can confirm clinical impressions regarding the type of conjunctivitis. Generally, the amount of exudate in an ocular infection is very small especially in corneal ulcers and this task should be left to the ophthalmologist with his microsurgical techniques. Typical findings include polymorphonuclear cells and bacteria in bacterial conjunctivitis. Cultures for bacteria and determinations of antibiotic sensitivity are also useful in cases resistant to therapy.

TREATMENT

Conditions that require no treatment or may be appropriately treated by most occupational physicians include blepharitis, stye and chalazion, subconjunctival hemorrhage, conjunctivitis, superficial corneal, and conjunctiva foreign body. Cases requiring prolonged treatment, or those in which the expected response to treatment does not occur promptly, should be referred to an ophthalmologist. For further details, see ACOEM *Occupational Medicine Practice Guidelines,* Chapter 17 (11).

Blepharitis (19)

Response to the treatment of blepharitis, or inflammation of the eyelid, is often frustratingly slow, and relapses are common (Figs. 34.12 and 34.13). The mainstays of treatment are:

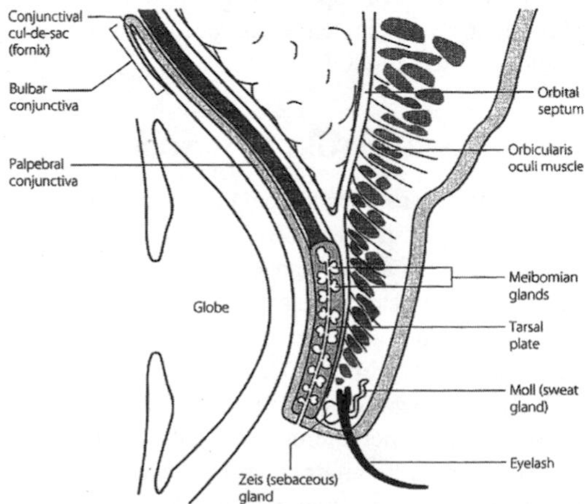

FIG. 34.12. Cross section of the eyelid. (From Wilson FM. *Practical ophthalmology: a manual for beginning residents.* San Francisco: American Academy of Ophthalmology, 1996, with permission.)

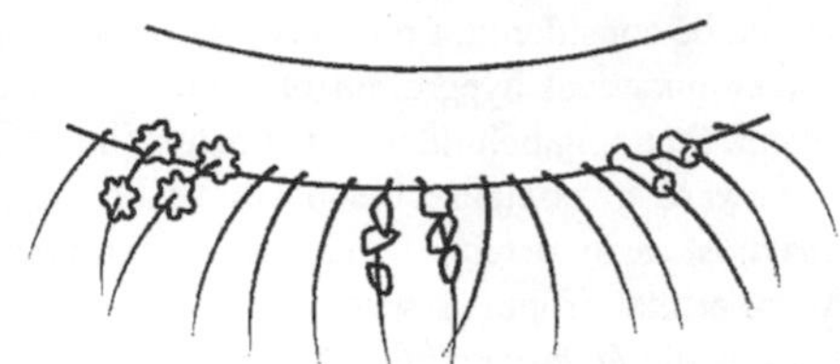

FIG. 34.13. Classes of eyelash discharges in blepharitis. (From Wilson FM. *Practical ophthalmology: a manual for beginning residents.* San Francisco: American Academy of Ophthalmology, 1996, with permission.)

- Eradication of staphylococcal infection with frequent applications of appropriate antibiotic eye drops or ointment.
- Treatment of scalp seborrhea with antidandruff shampoos to prevent the spread of seborrhea to the eyes.
- Cleansing of the lids to alleviate seborrheic blepharitis.

Stye and Chalazion (17,19)

A stye, or hordeolum, is an acute inflammation of the eyelid that may be characterized generally as an external swelling (involving the hair follicle or associated glands of Zeis or Moll) (see color plate Fig. 34.14) or an internal swelling (involving the meibomian glands). An external hordeolum occurs on the surface of the skin at the edge of the lid. An internal hordeolum presents on the conjunctival surface of the lid (see color plate Fig. 34.14). A chalazion is a chronic granulomatous inflammation of a meibomian or hair follicle gland that may develop spontaneously or may follow a hordeolum. The fat from the ruptured fat-producing glands acts as a tissue foreign body.

Styes are initially treated with hot compresses and topical antibiotics. Because most chalazia are sterile, antibiotic therapy is of no value, but hot compresses may be useful for early lesions. Incision with curettage of the chronic granuloma is indicated when lesions do not resolve spontaneously or with medical therapy. A persistent or recurring lid mass should undergo biopsy because it may be a rare meibomian gland carcinoma or a squamous cell carcinoma of the conjunctiva, rather than a benign chalazion.

Subconjunctival Hemorrhage (17,19)

In the absence of blunt trauma, hemorrhage into the subconjunctiva (see color plate Fig. 34.9), the potential space between the conjunctiva and the sclera, requires no treatment and, unless recurrent, no evaluation. Causes include a sudden increase in ocular venous pressure, such as occurs with coughing, sneezing, vomiting, or vigorous rubbing of the eye. Many subconjunctival hemorrhages occur during sleep. If recurrent, an underlying bleeding disorder should be considered (see color plate Fig. 34.9). Massive subconjunctival hemorrhage secondary contusion injury of the orbit needs further diagnostic evaluation.

Conjunctivitis (17,19)

Bacterial conjunctivitis is treated with frequent antibiotic eye drops as well as antibiotic ointment applied at bedtime. Cool compresses may give some relief. There is no specific medicinal treatment for viral conjunctivitis, although patients should be instructed in proper precautions to prevent contagion. Corticosteroids have no place in the treatment of infectious conjunctivitis. Eye drops containing a combination of antibiotics and corticosteroids are seldom indicated for the treatment of ocular inflammation. Steroids should be prescribed only by the ophthalmologist.

Foreign Bodies of Cornea/Conjunctiva (17,19)

1. Use of a slit lamp is recommended; otherwise loupes and flashlight are helpful.
2. Use proparacaine HCl 1% ophthalmic solution for anesthesia is the topical anesthetic of choice.
3. Attempt to remove the object with wet (sterile saline) cotton swab. If unsatisfactory, use a TB syringe and 25-gauge needle or "eye spud."
4. If unable to remove the object readily refer patient to an ophthalmologist.
5. If treatment is satisfactory, generally apply a broad-spectrum ophthalmic antibiotic.
6. Recheck patient in 24 hours to determine integrity of epithelium by fluorescein stain and slit lamp, after documenting the patient's visual acuity.
7. If the area is not healing or showing evidence of healing, refer to an ophthalmologist.

Occupational Eye Infections

Few infections are directly and primarily caused by occupational hazards. A classic condition, originally described as *shipyard's conjunctivitis* (20), was first reported in the U.S. in 1938 (21). In 1941, an epidemic involving 25,000 persons was reported in Hawaii (20,22). The disease spread rapidly to shipyards on the west coast of the U.S. in 1941 to 1942 and was called epidemic keratoconjunctivitis (EKC) (22). EKC was not caused by the occupation of a shipyard worker, but was due to transfer of the infectious disease among workers by direct or indirect contact.

Infections may also be acquired by exposure to blood-borne pathogens (22,23). Acquired immune deficiency syndrome (AIDS) can develop from eye exposure after splatter from contaminated tissue and/or blood. Blood-borne pathogens are not caused by the duties of medical workers, but may result from the spread of infectious products from afflicted individuals. Some infectious diseases of the eye are not unique to the duties of individuals but rather are acquired from tropical conditions found in the area of employment. Examples include onchocerciasis (23), leishmaniasis (24), and trachoma (25).

Epidemic Keratoconjunctivitis

The epidemiology of this disease has been well established, particularly in Eastern countries where subclinical infection is common. Only 5% of adults in the U.S. have antibodies, but the prevalence rises to 30% in Japan and 60% in Taiwan (20). Sporadic cases are common. Apart from the epidemic previously described, the most dramatic incidence in Western countries occurs in industrial plants where the disease periodically affects a considerable portion of workers. Outbreaks appear from time to time in hospitals (26), families (27), children (28), and in ophthalmologic clinics, perhaps due to the use of unsterilized tonometers, eyedroppers, or by finger-to-eye transmission (29–34). Males are affected more frequently than females.

Blood-borne Pathogens

Blood-borne pathogen regulations (29 CFR 1910.1030) (35,36) apply to occupational exposures from blood and other potentially infectious materials (including but not limited to semen; vaginal secretions; cerebrospinal fluid; synovial, pleural, pericardial, peritoneal, or amniotic fluid; saliva in dental procedures; and any body fluid visibly contaminated with blood). These materials may include pathogenic microorganisms present in human blood that can cause disease in humans. A partial list of pathogens include hepatitis B virus (HBV) and human immunodeficiency virus (HIV). Other examples include hepatitis C, malaria, syphilis, babesiosis, brucellosis, leptospirosis, arboviral infections, relapsing fever, Creutzfeldt-Jakob's disease, human T-lymphotropic virus type 1, and viral hemorrhagic diseases. An exposure to a blood-borne pathogen includes eye, mouth, or other mucous membrane, nonintact skin, or parenteral contact with blood or other potentially infectious materials.

The regulation intends to prevent exposure incidents through appropriate administrative controls and personal protective equipment (35,36). As an example, an applanation tonometer must be thoroughly cleansed and sterilized after being used on an individual with HIV. The use of such a contaminated instrument may transmit the virus. Personal protective equipment appropriate to a procedure must be available.

SCREENING FOR EYE DISORDERS IN THE WORKPLACE

How to Evaluate Vision for Various Jobs

Visual skills are one of the most universal and frequent factors affecting job performance (1,37–39).

Accident-free work and visual test requirements have been related, and minimum requirements or standards can be expected of any employee (1,37). One author, after comparing visual performance and safety, reported a 106% increase in accidents with extreme deviation from the standard, 43% with moderate deviation, and 31% with negligible deviation (37).

Visual standards (1,3,38–41) have been established by (a) observational methods, which outline types of testing to be used and levels of performance required for specific jobs based on direct and expert observation of the job, and (b) statistical methods, which evaluate facts that determine which tests and what minimum levels of test performance most adequately identify the worker who is potentially better on a specific job.

Jobs differ in visual demands, and variations are both qualitative and quantitative (42). For example, a crane operator must see clearly at a distance of 60 to 100 feet in order to set down a load accurately and within a narrowly prescribed area. In contrast, electronics assembly obliges a worker to see clearly material that is close to the eyes in order to fit together an intricate system of small parts and wires. The crane operator has less need to differentiate close detail.

Vision screening tests may be related to an analysis of job tasks (40) that is ideally performed on-site (e.g., in the factory or office). The distance and size of critical details of the task should be assessed, along with the need for color discrimination; depth perception; body, head, or eye postures; field of vision; eye movement requirements; and the contrast and illumination at the job site. A plant walk-through enables the physician to scrutinize plant illumination and visual requirements of specific jobs. Analysis of workplace visual requirements requires a broad knowledge of visual abilities and limitations (problems of accommodation, convergence, presbyopia, coordination, muscle balance, etc.), lighting, physical factors, and the host of eye hazards of a particular operation (41). Such analysis fulfills the regulatory requirements of the American with Disabilities Act (ADA) 1990 (43) and the Occupational Safety and Health (OSH) Act 29 CFR 1910.130 (44). The visual survey is best accomplished as a cooperative venture among the occupational physician, the consulting eye specialist, and plant management representatives.

Others have used a statistical basis to recommend visual standards (42,45). Large numbers of employees, assigned to diverse jobs and exhibiting all degrees of ability and achievement, have been tested and classified on the basis of job success into categories ranging from "definitely superior" to "definitely inferior." The visual skills of superior performers were compared with other workers. Analysis of these data suggested visual-performance requirements for the jobs. Twelve vision tests were found to be most useful for job efficiency (1,45,46). Patterns revealed by combinations of these vision tests were also significant. It was noted that groups of jobs shared visual requirements, providing the concept of visual job "families" (42). Visual demands for the majority of industrial jobs fall into one of six job families (1,45,46), described in Tables 34.7 through 34.12. The visual requirements of Bausch & Lomb Ortho-Rater test scores of each of the six job families are given in Tables 34.7 to 34.12 as Column A. Kuhn, based on her extensive experience (1935-1950), devised minimum visual standards for use by medical directors and consultants. They are the same main groups, but they are expressed in clinical terms and differ occasionally (listed in Tables 34.7 to 34.12 as Column B). The profile and group numbers in Tiffin (42), Novak (46), and Kuhn (46a) do not agree but the family names do, and therefore they have only been used in Tables 34.7 to 34.12. (It is important to always remember that these are minimum requirements.) The sketches are presented with the knowledge that they are not complete descriptions of the groups (42,46,46a). In some cases the essential job task may fall into two or more of these families and the most stringent of the standards would apply.

Visual screening has been defined by numerous organizations. Graduated visual stimuli should be employed to allow quantitative determination of acuity (e.g., Snellen chart). Screening tests may also determine contrast sensitivity, ocular alignment, color vision, and visual fields. Common methods of ocular (vision) testing include the use of test batteries. Snellen charts represent only one measurement of the ability of the eyes to discriminate high-contrast black and white

TABLE 34.7. *Visual job family: clerical and administrative profile*[a]

Column A	Column B
Corrected distance acuity both eyes 20/29	
Corrected distance acuity each eye 20/33	Corrected distance acuity, 20/40 each eye
Corrected near acuity both eyes 20/25	
Corrected near acuity each eye 20/29	Corrected near acuity 20/30 each eye
Far vertical <2Δ across LH and 1½Δ RH, lateral 6.5Δ EP[1] and 6.5 XP[1]	Whether individual has normal distance muscle balance or normal depth perceptions is not of importance
Near vertical LH 1½Δ and RH 2Δ, lateral 5 EP[1] and 13Δ XP[1]	Normal muscle balance for near
Color pass	Color discrimination is not important unless individual is working with colored file cards or colored materials
Stereo N/A	

[a]This standard covers those jobs primarily concerned with paperwork. All types of clerical jobs and those administrative occupations that are of the desk work type are included.

LH, left hyperphoria; RH, right hyperphoria; EP, esophoria; XP, exophoria; N/A, not applicable; Δ, prism diopters.

TABLE 34.8. *Visual job family: inspection and close machine work profile*[a]

Column A	Column B
Corrected distance acuity both 20/33	
Corrected distance acuity each eye 20/40	Corrected 20/40 each eye distance acuity (actually degree of distance acuity important only for safety reasons not for work requirements)
Corrected near acuity both 20/25	
Corrected near acuity each eye 20/29	Corrected near acuity, 20/30 each eye (20/25 may be essential at times)
Far vertical½ LH <2Δ and RH 1½Δ, lateral 6.5Δ EP and 6.5Δ XP	Distance muscle balance not important
Near vertical LH 1½Δ and RH <2Δ, lateral 5.0 EP[1] and 13Δ XP[1]	Normal near muscle balance
Color pass normal	Normal color discrimination if inspection includes color evaluation
Stereo <83 seconds	

[a]This standard covers jobs involved in the inspection of small parts for surface defects. Also involved are jobs of the machine operating type in which the work is done at close range (such as sewing machine operator). Assembly jobs involving very small parts (such as watches, radio tubes, and so forth) also fall in this category.

LH, left hyperphoria; RH, right hyperphoria; EP, esophoria; XP, exophoria; Δ, prism diopters.

TABLE 34.9. *Visual job family: operator of mobile equipment profile*[a]

Column A	Column B
Corrected distance acuity both 20/25	
Corrected distance acuity each eye 20/29	Corrected distance acuity, 20/30 each eye
Corrected near acuity both 20/33	Degree of near acuity depends on whether individual needs to handle orders or make recordings (bifocals are contraindicated on crane operators)
Corrected near acuity each eye 20/40	Corrected near acuity each eye 20/40
Far vertical LH <2Δ and RH 1½Δ, lateral 6.5 EP and 6.5 XP	
Near vertical LH 1½Δ and RH <2Δ	Normal muscle balance for distance
Color pass	Normal color discrimination
Stereo <83 seconds	Normal distance depth perception

[a]This standard covers jobs requiring the operation of moving vehicles (truck driver, crane operator, high lift operator, and so forth).

LH, left hyperphoria; RH, right hyperphoria; EP, esophoria; XP, exophoria; Δ, prism diopters.

TABLE 34.10. *Visual job family: machines operators' profile[a]*

Column A	Column B
Corrected distance acuity both 20/29	
Corrected distance acuity each eye 20/33	Corrected distance acuity, 20/40 each eye
Corrected near acuity both 20/29	
Corrected near acuity each eye 20/33	Corrected near acuity, 20/30 each eye
Far vertical LH <2Δ and RH 1½Δ, lateral 6.5Δ E and 6.5x	
Near vertical LH 1½Δ and RH <2A, lateral 5.0EP[1] and 13Δ XP[1]	Normal muscle balance
Color pass	Color not of importance unless special requirement
Stereo <83 seconds	Normal depth perception

[a]This standard covers those jobs involving the operation of machines in which the operating parts of the machines are within arm's length (such as lathes, drill presses, spinning machines, and so forth).

LH, left hyperphoria; RH, right hyperphoria; EP, esophoria; XP, exophoria; Δ, prism diopters.

TABLE 34.11. *Visual job family: laborers' profile[a]*

Column A	Column B
Corrected distance acuity both 20/29	
Corrected distance acuity each eye 20/33	Corrected distance acuity, 20/50 each eye—or 20/60, 20/40
Corrected near acuity both 20/33	Degree of near acuity not important unless individual has to read orders, then should have corrected 20/30 each eye
Corrected near acuity each eye 20/40	
Far vertical N/A, lateral N/A	Distance muscle balance not important
Near vertical N/A, lateral N/A	Near muscle balance not important
Color N/A	Color not important (unless some special danger requires recognition of green-red signals)
Stereo N/A	Depth perception not important

[a]This standard involves jobs of the relatively unskilled type (porters, janitors, guards, hand truckers, and so forth).

LH, left hyperphoria; RH, right hyperphoria; EP, esophoria; XP, exophoria; N/A, not applicable; Δ, prism diopters.

TABLE 34.12. *Visual job family: mechanics and skilled tradesmen profile[a]*

Column A	Column B
Corrected distance acuity both 20/29	
Corrected distance acuity each eye 20/33	Corrected distance acuity, 20/30 each eye
Corrected near acuity both 20/25	
Corrected near acuity each eye 20/29	Corrected near acuity 20/25 each eye
Far vertical LH <2Δ and RH 1½Δ, lateral 6.5E and 6.5X	
Near vertical LH 1½Δ and RH <2Δ, lateral 5.0 EP1 and 13ΔXP1	Normal near muscle balance
Color pass	Normal color appreciation (if colors are used during operation)
Stereo <83 seconds	Normal depth perception

[a]This standard involves jobs of the mechanical type (such as radio mechanic, diesel mechanic, machine fixer, and so forth). Also included are skilled trades (such as carpenter, plumber, millwright, electrician, and so forth).

LH, left hyperphoria; RH, right hyperphoria; EP, esophoria; XP, exophoria; Δ, prism diopters.

detail, generally about 85% at some standard distance, generally 6 meters or 20 feet (central visual acuity). Often, the distance at which the work must be performed is not considered when evaluating the results. The significance of any test depends on job requirements, and individual correlation is necessary.

Careful diagnostic appraisal of near vision (near-point acuity, near-point accommodation, near-point of convergence, lateral and vertical phorias, and others) is important for job applicants requiring exact visual perception when working at distances of 16 inches or less. This is especially true for employees over 40 years of age when presbyopic symptoms/signs develop. Estimates of intraocular tension, and ophthalmoscopic findings are related more specifically to health rather than to eye efficiency. In time, these processes may cause a change in visual acuity and visual fields. In some jobs speed of vision and recovery from glare may be important.

Visual tests can be time consuming and require considerable space. Binocular testing instruments are commonly used by industry to discover visual defects and appraise visual skills [Stereoptical Co. Inc. model Optec 2000C vision test, 2000, 25000; Titmus Optical Inc., model 2A and 2C, Armed Forces Tester (now Stereoptical Co. model 3500 vision tester)]. Such equipment is portable, durable, and designed to optimize accuracy and speed. These test batteries can detect substandard visual qualifications, but the results do not provide a diagnosis, and follow-up procedures may be necessary. Employees who appear to have limitations of visual skills that are likely to affect their work should be referred to a competent professional who has knowledge of visual requirements of the job for which the employee is being considered.

A clinically "normal" pair of eyes may be inadequate for unusual job demands. For example, 8 inches is an abnormal work distance. An individual with normal vision might not be able to function optimally at that distance. Occupational lens additions may enhance performance.

Other factors that may require consideration include dark adaptation (important for truck drivers, night flyers, soldiers, welders, etc.), form field (important in aviation and as safety factor), external gross pathology, and fundus pathology (very low vision may require further study to determine the possibility of serious pathology, such as congenital amblyopia or an optic atrophy). More detailed knowledge of near visual function may be necessary for specific occupations (e.g., blueprint work, inspection, hosiery looping, etc.) where the near point of accommodation and ductions play an important role in efficiency.

Environmental Surveillance Programs

Medical surveillance (47) includes detailed physical examinations of exposed individuals in order to detect a specific effect. Some environmental hazards may be associated with changes in visual functions resulting in abnormalities on screening. Solvent exposure, for example, has been associated with changes in the retina and optic nerve, resulting in an acquired change in decreased contrast sensitivity and acquired color vision defects, starting first with yellow-blue and proceeding to red-green.

ADA Issues: Performance of Essential Functions with or without Accommodation

The ADA of 1990 (43) and its provisions are discussed in Chapter 5. Many federal agencies have published visual standards, and contradictions may exist between regulatory requirements. ADA guidelines require that workers perform the essential visual functions with or without accommodation, without significant increased risk, and without direct threat to themselves and others. Not all regulations fulfill this mandatory requirement. The U.S. Supreme Court opinions provide legal guidance (39).

Role of Ergonomics

Eye complaints occur in 50% to 90% of workers who use video display terminals (VDTs) (18,48–51). Such problems result from visual inefficiencies or from eye-related symptoms caused by a combination of individual visual abnormalities and poor visual ergonomics. Problems occur whenever visual demands exceed the abilities of the individual (50). Visual symptoms can usually be resolved with ergonomic

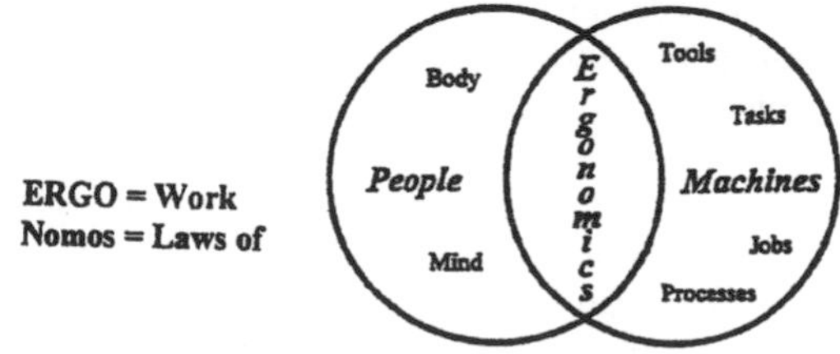

FIG. 34.15. Ergonomics—science of designing the workplace machines and work tasks with capabilities and limitations of the human being in mind. (From Blais BR. Basic principles of industrial ophthalmology, sports and industrial ophthalmology. Pizzarella, ed. *Ophthalmol Clin North Am* 2000;13(2), with permission.)

modification and the provision of appropriate visual care to the worker (Fig. 34.15). Factors that influence visual performance may include the individual's vision, task visibility, and both psychological and physiologic factors (40,41). Motivation, intelligence, and general health are not discussed in this chapter, but can significantly influence visual performance.

Safe, efficient, and comfortable job performance depends on visibility and visual capability (40). Enhanced visibility eases performance of tasks. Numerous factors (40) influence the ability to see detail. These include luminance, contrast, spectral nature of light, size and intensity of surrounding field, region of retina stimulated, distance and size of object, time available to see object, glare, foggy/steamy atmosphere, refractive error, pupil size, age, attention, intelligence, boredom, ability to interpret blurred images, general health, and emotional state (52,53).

Prevention and Control

Administrative controls and safe work practices help to prevent dissemination of infectious agents from person to person. Members of medical departments are at risk for conditions such as EKC and AIDS. Occasionally nonmedical staff may be utilized to clean body secretions or blood products containing the AIDS virus, and similar safe practices must be employed.

Personal protective equipment for the eyes and face, in accordance with the Occupational Safety and Health Administration (OSHA) 29 CFR 1910.132, must be worn by individuals potentially exposed to hazardous conditions (44). The use of disposable latex gloves and eye and face protection is mandated in situations where medical personnel might have exposure or transmit infectious products from person to person. Such equipment may include type C spectacles with full side shield, type D spectacles with detachable side shield, type E spectacles with nonremovable lens, type H cover goggles with indirect ventilations, as dictated by the American National Standards Institute (ANSI) Z87.1-1998 (54). In cases involving potential exposure to AIDS, personal protective equipment is mandated and directed in 29 CFR 1910.1030.35. Exposure from splattering or generation of droplets would necessitate the use of eye protection noted above and a mask or ANSI Z87.1 type N face shield. (54)

Employee education and training, as mandated by OSHA regulations (29 CFR 1910.132) (44), provide information about potential hazards and their prevention through the use of the appropriate personal protective equipment. No individual likely to be exposed to hazards should be allowed to work in such an environment without appropriate education and training and personal protective equipment as required.

Preventive Strategies and Tactics

The primary prevention of work-related disorders depends on the reduction or elimination of exposure to causal factors (11). In the past emphasis has been placed on physical risk factors such as lighting, terminal design, and posture. Other issues, such as workers' job satisfaction and interpersonal relations with supervisors, also have a strong relationship to visual and ergonomic complaints. Primary prevention of complaints may depend on minimizing physical, personal, and psychosocial stressors.

Secondary prevention aims to reduce disability and hasten recovery after a health concern has been identified (11). It involves a partnership with the worker. The cornerstones of this process include two-way communication, exploration of myths and misconceptions, management of expectations, bilateral or trilateral planning, and management of the episode and the situation. Modified or temporary work is an important way to keep workers on the job and it prevents social isolation and deconditioning.

Tertiary prevention efforts limit recurrences in a patient. Job tasks and the person-job fit should be evaluated (11). Task modification or workstation changes may be necessary. Repetitions, abnormal postures, and other ergonomic problems should be addressed. If the individual cannot return to the job as originally designed due to an impairment, reasonable accommodation should be considered. If no accommodations are possible, job transfer or retraining may be indicated.

Beyond Prevention: Promotion

Preventive ophthalmology has been emphasized both as an academic discipline and as an institutional commitment in the U.S. Major industries are fostering these efforts to contain medical program costs (55). The Public Health Service of the Department of Health and Human Services has created the Office of Disease Prevention and Health Promotion to enhance morale and to improve productivity. Initially data collection can be used to identify medical, health, and eye problems particular to a given industry or plant. Sources of information may include preexisting medical screening, injury prevention, and on-the-job initial medical care. Such an approach reinforces ongoing activities and may identify untapped resources of people, materials, and equipment within a company or plant. Prevention efforts may be integrated with traditional public health programs and prevention of ocular injury efforts such as those associated with the National Society to Prevent Blindness (NSPB) [now called Prevent Blindness America (PBA)]. A qualified and enthusiastic individual, given clear responsibility, can develop these activities.

GENERAL REQUIREMENTS ON PERSONAL PROTECTIVE EQUIPMENT

OSHA 29 CFR 1910.132 (44) has listed general requirements for personal protective equipment (PPE). PPE should not be used as a substitute for engineering out hazards, work practice, and/or administrative controls, such as the following:

Static Shielding of Equipment

Barrier or deflector screens of transparent plastics can provide a clear view of a work process while protecting workers from grinding fragments, accidental sprays, or specific optical irradiations. Cutters, grinders, and fixed-location tools have long been safeguarded by properly designed static shielding. Similarly, cathode ray or television tubes have a radiation barrier glass over the surface exposed for viewing.

Static Shielding of Personnel

Physicians are familiar with the principle of static shielding in radiology offices. Technicians or radiologists step into separate cubicles or behind leaded glass while x-ray films are exposed. Similarly, in large molten steel pours, workers now control the operation from shielded booths that protect against heat and accidental splashes. Static shielding may be suspended from the ceiling, mounted on the floor, or constructed as a separate control area.

If employees provide their own PPE, the employer is responsible to ensure its adequacy. Equivalent requirements exist for shipyards (28 CFR 1916.152), marine terminals (29 CFR 1917.96), long shoring (29 CFR 1918.108), and construction (29 CFR 1926.95).

Employees should understand that lives may depend on the use of PPE. The use of such equipment should be combined with hazard awareness and training. It should be emphasized that PPE does not eliminate a hazard. When equipment fails, exposure will occur. Equipment must be properly fitted and maintained in a clean and serviceable condition to reduce the possibility of failure (56).

Contact Lenses at Work

Individuals should not be disqualified from a job because of contact lens use. Such lenses may be used under a full-face respirator. Although contact lenses provide some protection, they do not fulfill the requirements of ocular safety standards. Industrial safety eyewear for specific hazards is identified in ANSI Z87.1 (54) and should be worn over the contact lens (56–62).

Developing a PPE Program

The following items must be included when developing a PPE program (44):

1. Hazard assessment guidelines
2. Identifying hazards
3. Identifying personal eye and face protection equipment
4. Identifying individual exposed to the identified hazards
5. Assigning PPE to individuals
6. General training prior to initiating work
7. Retraining
8. Program review and evaluations

Hazard Assessment Guidelines

To assess the need for eye and face protective equipment, the practitioner should conduct a walk-through survey of the area to identify sources of hazards to the eyes and faces of workers. General hygiene and compliance with rules about the use of personal protective equipment, such as safety glasses, can be noted. The OSHA log can give valuable information about eye injury patterns. Safety equipment, such as eye wash booths, can be inspected. During the walk-through survey one should specifically observe (44) basic hazard categories:

1. Impact
2. Heat
3. Chemical
4. Dust
5. Optical radiation
6. Contusion

Specific causes of eye injuries and some workplace operations where they exist include the following (63):

Dusts or powders, fumes, and mists: sources include scaling, light grinding, spot welding, and woodworking, but can also include very small flying particles and chemical exposures.

Flying objects or particles: sources include caulking, chiseling, grinding, hammering, and metal working; these activities cause the majority of eye injuries.

Injurious gases, vapors, and liquids: workers handling acids or caustics or doing welding are subject to these hazards.

Splashing metal: sources include babbitting, casting of hot metal, and dripping in hot metal baths.

Thermal and radiation hazards such as glare, ultraviolet, and infrared rays: sample sources are welding, brazing, metal cutting and furnaces, heat treating, high-intensity lights, etc. Sources of high temperatures can cause facial burns, eye injury, or ignition of protective equipment, etc.

Lasers: a recent addition to the list of eye hazards; laser beams can present dangerous and unusual exposures, and various types of laser beams require different methods of eye protection.

Electrical hazards: sample sources are arcing and spark.

Ergonomic stresses: muscular and visual.

Identification of Personal Eye and Face Protection Equipment

Appropriate protective equipment for the eye and face is required by OSHA (29 CFR 1910.133) (64). Eye and face protection is required where there is reasonable probability of preventing injury with such equipment. Other standards—ANSI Z136.1 (65) and Z136.3 (66)—address the prevention of laser burns using similar engineering controls or personal protective goggles. All employees should acquire PPE appropriate for their activities or processes and it should be conveniently available. Employees should be required to use such equipment. No unprotected personnel should be subjected to hazardous environment conditions. These same stipulations should apply to supervisors, management personnel, and visitors while they are in hazardous areas.

Efficacy

A study of patients who presented to the Massachusetts Eye and Ear Infirmary emergency services with ocular injuries in 1985 was reported by Schein et al. (6). All injuries were included except those due to contact lens use. Only 66% of those injured at work reported that protective eyewear was provided at the job site. Of those suffering severe injury, only one third reported that protective eyewear was available. Among those injured at work, 10% stated they were wearing protective eyewear at the time of injury, and none of these injuries was severe. Ruptured globes were the most common severe injury occurring at work. In approximately one third of the cases, a history of previous eye injury was obtained. Schein et al. illustrated the type of eyewear worn at the time of injury for the study population: 70% were wearing no glasses, 10% wore safety glasses (of which 2% had side shields), 6% wore regular glasses, and 3% wore contact lenses. One third of the subjects whose regular glasses were broken at the time of trauma suffered severe injury.

A 1980 Bureau of Labor Statistics study (67) noted about 60% of workers who suffered eye injuries were not wearing eye protective equipment. When asked why they were not wearing face protection at the time of the accident, workers indicated that face protection was not normally used for practice in their type of work, or it was not required for the type of work performed at the time of the accident.

The U.S. Eye Injury Registry's 1996 report on 10,964 cases for the period 1988–2001 revealed that 62.5% of injured patients wore no protection, 2.7% wore regular street-wear spectacles, 1.5% wore safety eye and face protection, and 0.3% wore sun spectacles. The Food and Drug Administration regulation requires that all street-wear eyeglasses and sunglasses sold to the general public be shatterproof resistant.

Types of Hazards vs. PPE

PPE is a part of the job in some industries (such as face shields for welding) but is considered a last resort, temporary type of protection for most. The elimination of hazards in the environment, rather than PPE, is optimal (44).

OSHA 29 CFR 1910.133 (64) mandates the ANSI Z87.1 Eye and Face Protection (54) regulations; a table correlates the basic types of eye hazards with the specific general type of spectacle and/or face shield required for the hazard. Although not mandated by OSHA, similar requirements should be implemented when eye hazards exist in hobbies, at home, in school, in sports, or in workplaces where there is a reasonable probability of preventing injury with the use of such equipment (56).

The ANSI Z87.1 (54) tables on protective devices are representative only of eye and face protective devices commonly found at the time of the writing of the standard. Protective devices do not need to take the exact forms shown, but must meet the requirements of the standard. In Figs. 34.16 through 34.24,

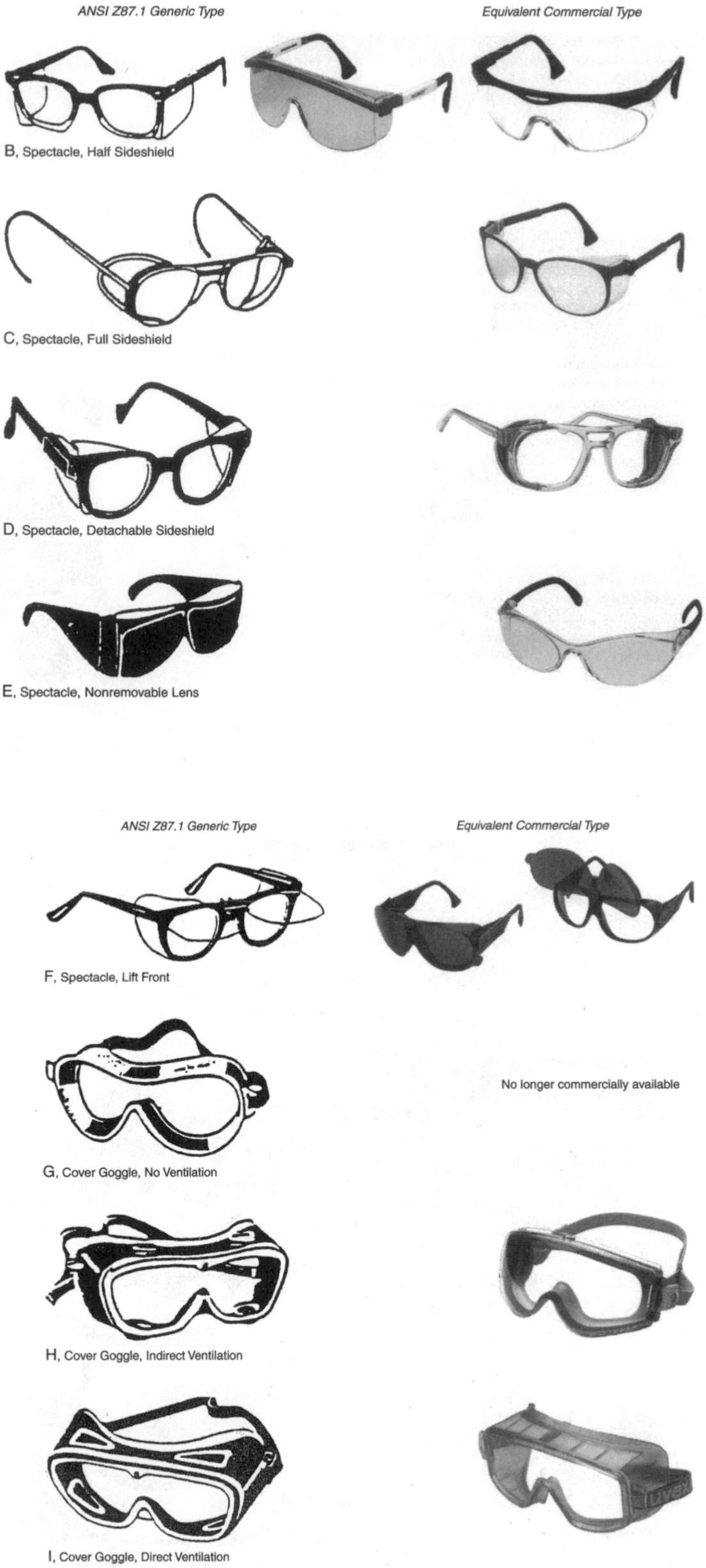

ANSI Z87.1 Generic Type

Equivalent Commercial Type

B, Spectacle, Half Sideshield

C, Spectacle, Full Sideshield

D, Spectacle, Detachable Sideshield

E, Spectacle, Nonremovable Lens

ANSI Z87.1 Generic Type

Equivalent Commercial Type

F, Spectacle, Lift Front

G, Cover Goggle, No Ventilation

No longer commercially available

H, Cover Goggle, Indirect Ventilation

I, Cover Goggle, Direct Ventilation

FIG. 34.16. Impact source hazard. (From Blais BR. Basics of industrial ophthalmology. *Ophthalmol Clin North Am* 2000;13, with permission.)

Continued on next page

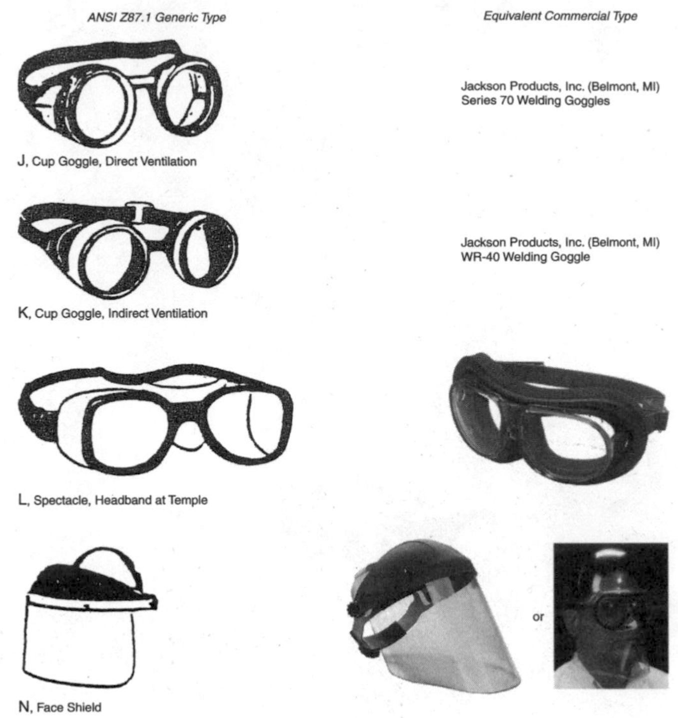

FIG. 34.16. *Continued.*

FIG. 34.17. Heat source hazard. (From Blais BR. Basics of industrial ophthalmology. *Ophthalmol Clin North Am* 2000;13, with permission.)

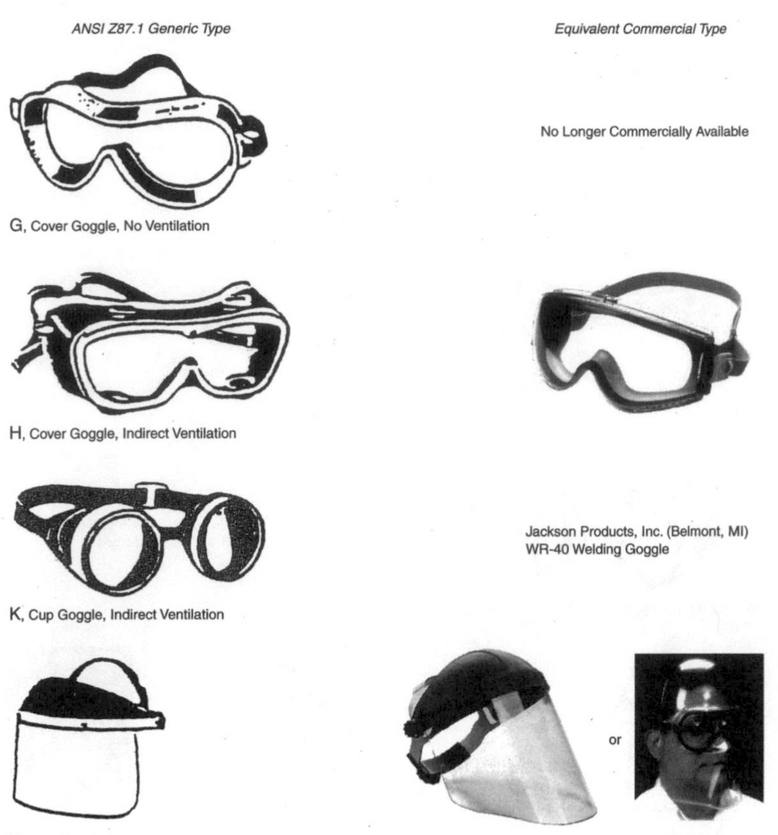

FIG. 34.18. Chemical source hazard. (From Blais BR. Basics of industrial ophthalmology. *Ophthalmol Clin North Am* 2000;13, with permission.)

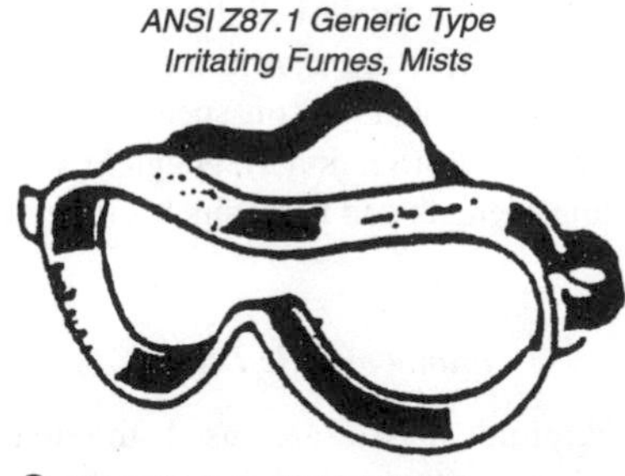

FIG. 34.19. Chemical source hazard. (From Blais BR. Basics of industrial ophthalmology. *Ophthalmol Clin North Am* 2000;13, with permission.)

the generic types from ANSI Z87.1 (54) are shown under the specific classes of hazards, and the generic protective devices are compared with current nonprescription safety equivalent devices. Blais (39) submitted a new organization of existing ANSI Z87.1 tables information that enables the user to identify the specific type of lens mandated by 29 CFR 1910.133 (64).

Selection of safety glasses is especially critical for individuals with a loss of accommodation (presbyopia) or for those who must use contact lenses in the workplace. A presbyopic lens should provide for the lack of accommodation so the user can perform visual tasks efficiently and effectively. The occupational presbyopic lens should attempt to mimic the normal accommodative process and provide physiologic amplitude of accommodation. The provider should prescribe lenses to allow the performance of essential tasks comfortably with good visual and body ergonomics.

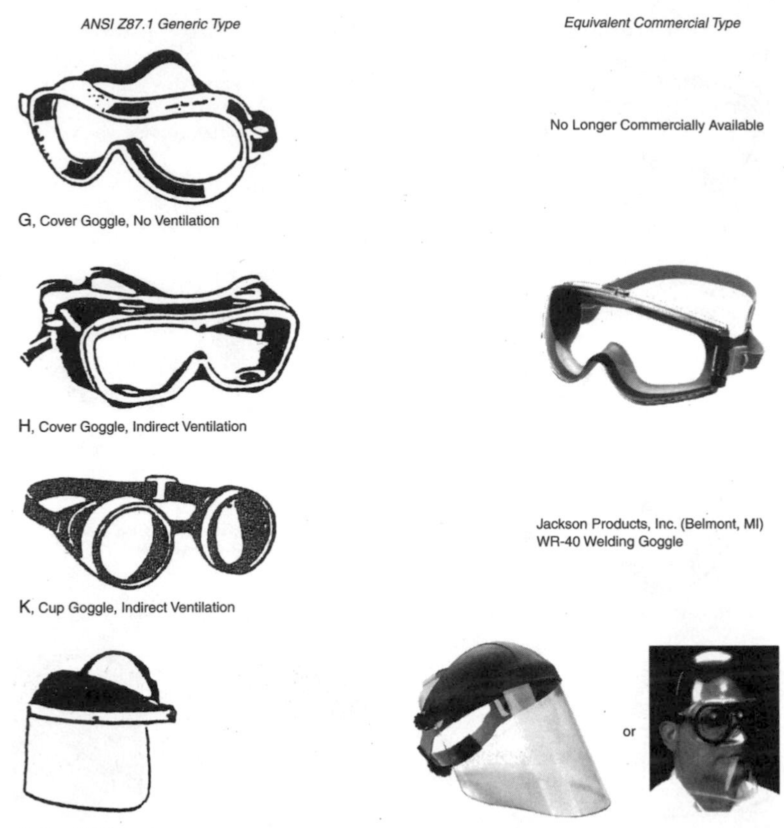

FIG. 34.20. Dust source hazard. (From Blais BR. Basics of industrial ophthalmology. *Ophthalmol Clin North Am* 2000;13, with permission.)

Special-purposes Lenses

Requirements regarding special-purpose lenses are outlined in ANSI Z87.1(a)-1991 (54). Such lenses should meet all requirements of the standard except for the transmittance requirements in Table 1 of 29 CFR 1910.133 (64). They may be used at the discretion of the individual responsible for the eye safety program.

General

Special-purpose lenses provide eye protection while performing visual tasks that require unusual filtering of light. Examples include, but are not limited to, didymium-containing, cobalt-containing, uniformly tinted and photochromic lenses, and lenses prescribed by an eye specialist for particular vision problems. However, many such lenses offer inadequate ultraviolet and/or infrared protection. Caution should be exercised in their use. For each application (13,68), the responsible individual should ensure that the proper ultraviolet, infrared, and visible protection is provided. Spectral transmittance data shall be available to buyers upon request. Both viewing areas of a protector must meet the transmittance matching requirements of the standard on spectacles (63) (Section 8), face shields (Section 9), goggles (Section 10), and welding helmets and hand shields (Section 11).

Photochromic Lenses

Photochromic lenses are used throughout the world, and over 500 million lenses have been sold (39). The photochromic lens is a common type of special purpose lens that darkens when exposed to sunlight, and that fades when removed from the sunlight. This lens is frequently used to provide comfortable vision for a wide range of ambient illumination. In

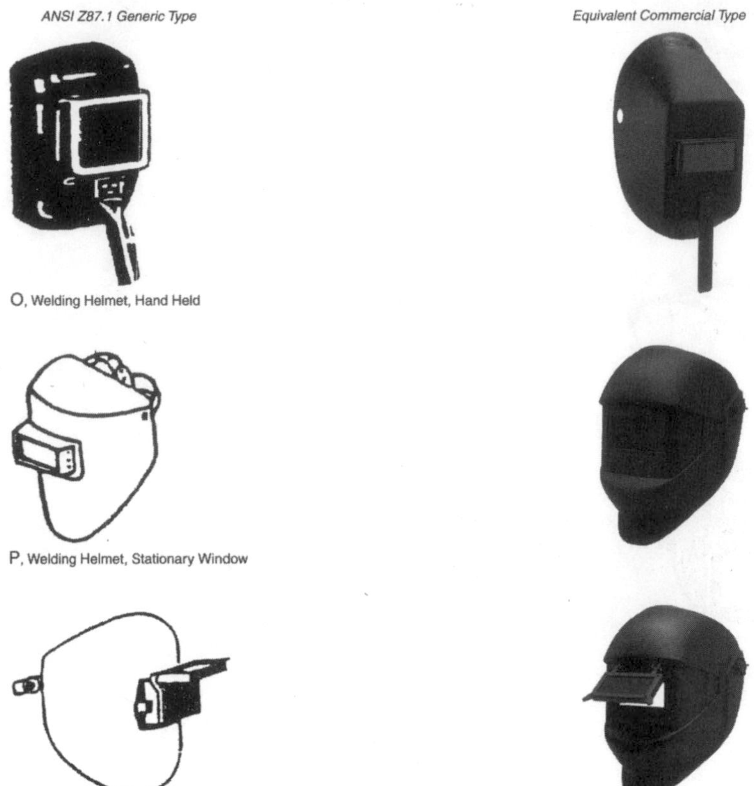

FIG. 34.21. Optical radiation source hazard—electric arc welding. (From Blais BR. Basics of industrial ophthalmology. *Ophthalmol Clin North Am* 2000;13, with permission.)

daylight, outdoors, when the photochromic lenses darken to function as sunglasses, they protect the eye dark adaptation process. Those who wear sunglasses in sunlight adapt to dark environments up to twice as fast as those who do not. In transient conditions, such as coming in from lighter outdoor conditions to darker indoor conditions, photochromic lens use can provide better, more stable, and more comfortable vision under the broad variety of work conditions. Since the fading process is gradual, photochromic lenses should be used with care in operations requiring critical acuity, or fast reaction to visual stimuli, particularly in operations where the wearer passes from outdoors to indoors in the course of the job (for example, a forklift operator passing from outdoors to indoors).

Corning, the manufacturer of glass items, has hundreds of millions of man-years of experience with the use of photochromic eyeglasses without any reported safety problems. Transitions Optical, Inc. offers a polycarbonate lens with new percentages for clearing and darkening. Transitions from Advanced Quantum Technologies are appropriate for persons who need a versatile technologically advanced lens that quickly adjusts to changing light conditions, moving from virtually clear indoors to a dark tint outdoors. They are scratch resistant, compatible with antireflective coatings, and can be designed as single or multifocal, including progressive addition lenses and occupational lenses (special lenses for specific tasks—double segs). Although photochromic lenses absorb ultraviolet light, they should not be used as a substitute for the proper protector in hazardous optical radiation environments.

Limitations (39,69)

In general, lenses having low luminous transmittance should not be worn indoors, except when needed for protection from optical radiation, since indoor light levels tend to be only adequate. Care should be exercised in conjunction with wearing such lenses for driving vehicles with tinted windshields or for night driving.

ANSI Z87.1 Generic Type

Equivalent Commercial Type

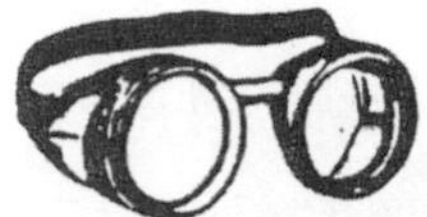

J, Cup Goggle, Direct Ventilation

Jackson Products, Inc. (Belmont, MI)
Series 70 Welding Goggle

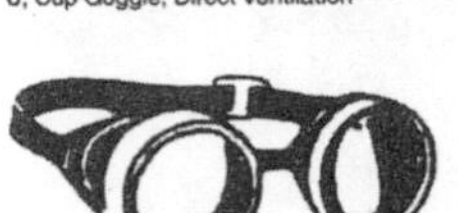

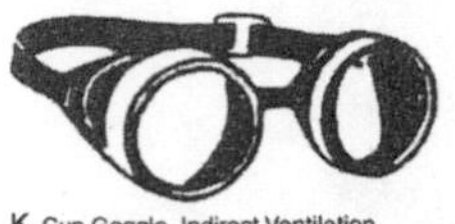

K, Cup Goggle, Indirect Ventilation

Jackson Products, Inc. (Belmont, MI)
WR-40 Welding Goggle

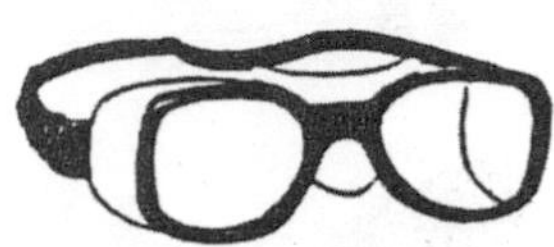

L, Spectacle, Headband Temple

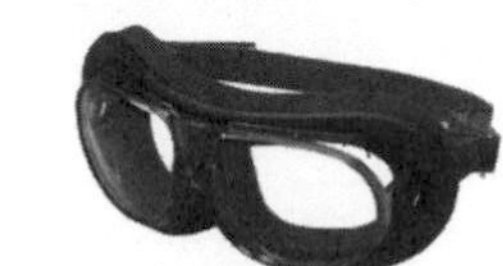

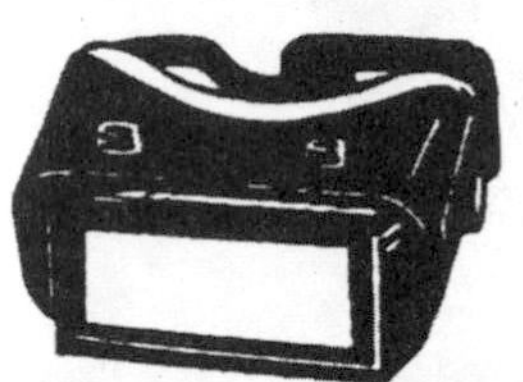

M, Cover Welding Goggle, Indirect Ventilation

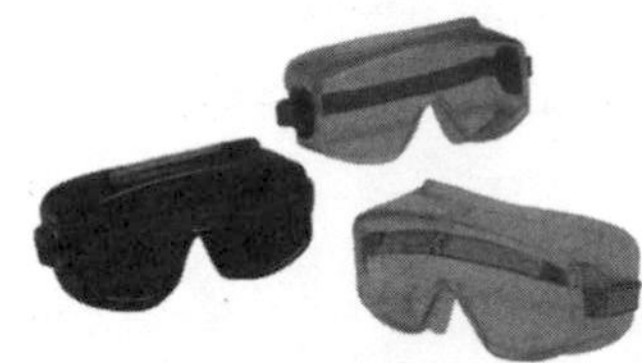

ANSI Z87.1 Generic Type

Equivalent Commercial Type

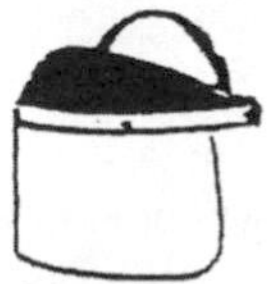

N, Face Shield

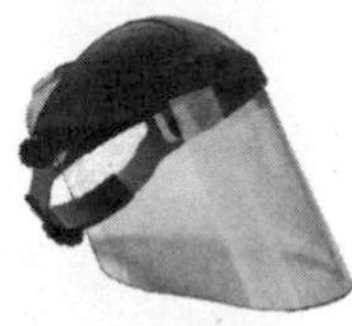

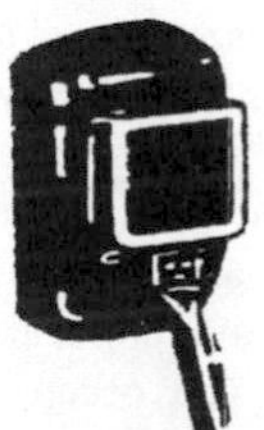

O, Welding Helmet, Hand Held

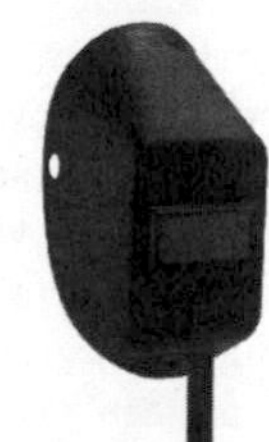

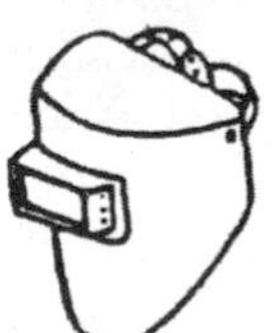

P, Welding Helmet, Stationary Window

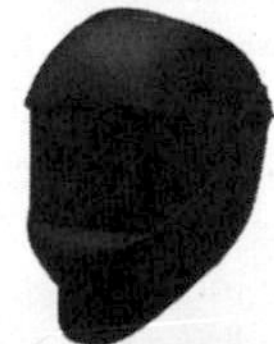

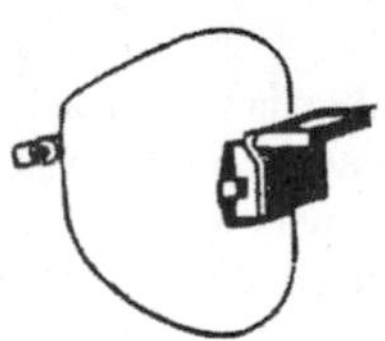

Q, Welding Helmet, Lift Front

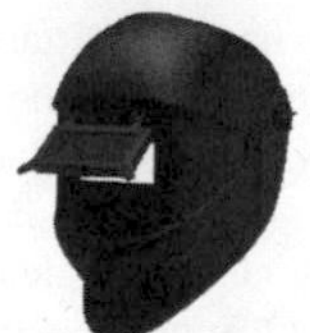

FIG. 34.22. Optical radiation source hazard—welding gas, cutting, torch brazing. (From Blais BR. Basics of industrial ophthalmology. *Ophthalmol Clin North Am* 2000;13, with permission.)

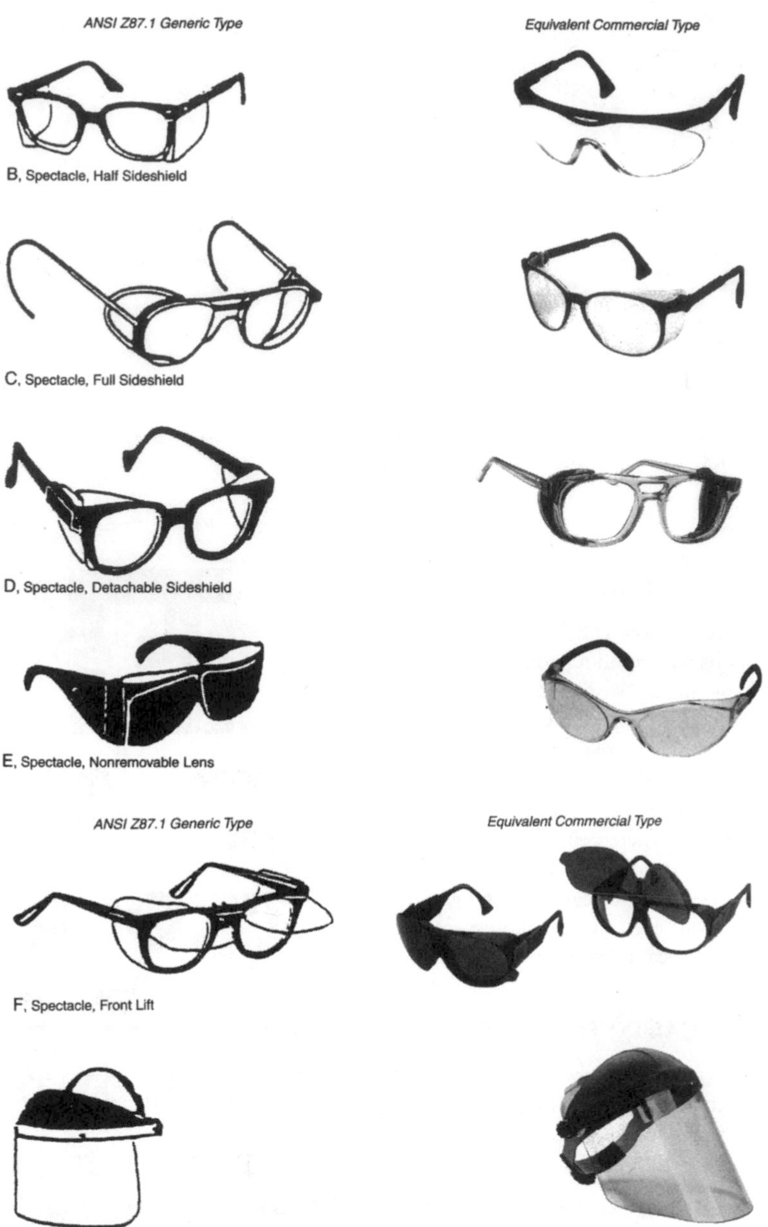

FIG. 34.23. Optical radiation source hazard—torch soldering. (From Blais BR. Basics of industrial ophthalmology. *Ophthalmol Clin North Am* 2000;13, with permission.)

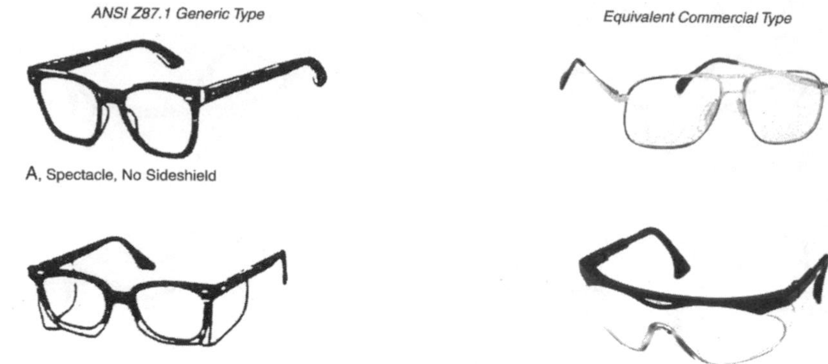

FIG. 34.24. Glare source hazard. (From Blais BR. Basics of industrial ophthalmology. *Ophthalmol Clin North Am* 2000;13, with permission.)

SUMMARY

In the past 50 years, no occupational medicine texts have been published providing composite information about vision in the workplace (68). Much work remains to be done to generate visual standards for all occupations. Such information will allow individuals to perform their tasks safely and efficiently, without problems resulting from muscular or visual ergonomic abnormalities. There continues to be a significant shortfall in the training of employees, employers, first responders and professionals in the prevention and diagnosis of eye injuries, and especially in the treatment of chemical injuries of the eyes.

APPENDIX: CLINICAL INSTRUMENTATION

In addition to the equipment needed for a standard ophthalmologic evaluation, the following tools are required for the functional evaluation:

Standardized Visual Acuity Charts

If performed, they should utilize standardized tests with continuous text.

Standardized Letter Chart

The typical letter chart shaped like a capital A (Fig. 34.25) (69) is now replaced by a chart shaped like a capital V (Fig. 34.26) (70). The Ian Bailey and Jan Lovie chart (70,71) log out was designed with the use of Sloan letters, which subsequently was utilized by the National Eye Institute in the early treatment of diabetic retinopathy and known as the ET-

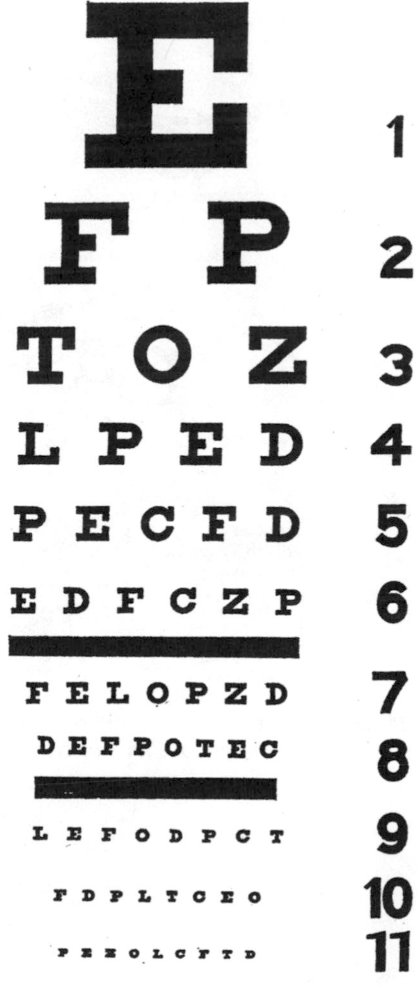

FIG. 34.25. The Snellen vision test chart.

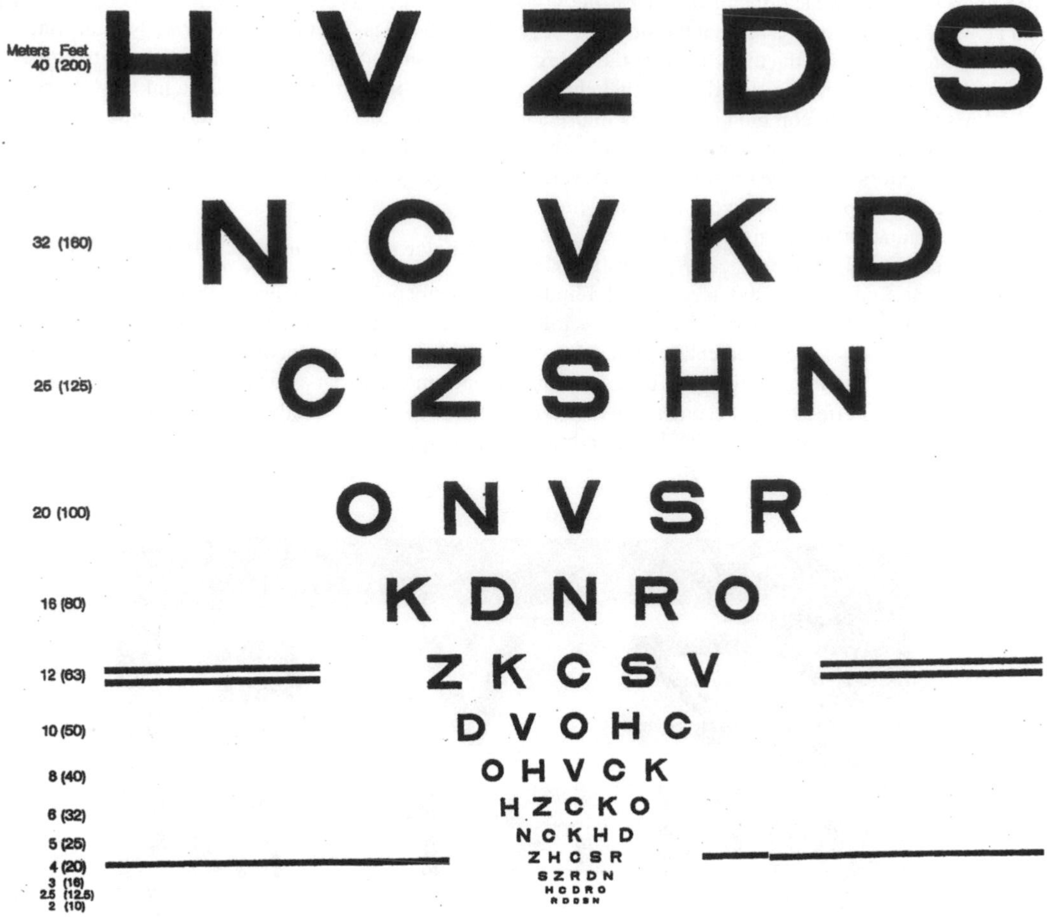

Meters (Feet)	
40 (200)	H V Z D S
32 (160)	N C V K D
25 (125)	C Z S H N
20 (100)	O N V S R
16 (80)	K D N R O
12 (63)	Z K C S V
10 (50)	D V O H C
8 (40)	O H V C K
6 (32)	H Z C K O
5 (25)	N C K H D
4 (20)	Z H C S R
3 (16)	S Z R D N
2.5 (12.5)	H C D R O
2 (10)	R D O S N

FIG. 34.26. Bailey–Lovie–ETRS eye test chart.

DRS chart (72). The basic principle of measuring visual acuity with the letter test is that the smallest letters that can be read satisfactorily provide the index of visual acuity. However, currently available charts fail in this respect. The common practice is to use a single or two-letter task for low acuity levels and eight or ten letters in a row for high acuity levels. Furthermore, the spacing between adjacent letters and between adjacent rows rarely has any systematic or logical relationship to letter size. When testing visual acuity around the 20/200 level (legal blindness), the choice of letter chart is particularly important. On traditional A-shaped charts, which have no lines between 20/100 and 20/200, the descriptor "20/200 or less" effectively becomes "less than 20/100" so that patients with 20/125 would be recorded as "20/200." On the newer ETDRS charts, "20/200 or less" is more appropriately interpreted as "less than 20/160." If only an older printed chart is available, the patient can be brought to 10 ft, so that "less than 20/160" can be interpreted as "less than 10/80." The patient with 20/125 (20/63) is then appropriately reported as "better than 20/200" (73).

Choice of Criterion and Rounding-off Values

The recorded visual acuity value can be influenced by the choice of completion criterion and by rounding. Most clinicians record visual acuity in line increments and consider a line read if more than half of the letters are read correctly (e.g., three of five on an ETDRS type chart) (73). A suffix such as −1 or +2 may

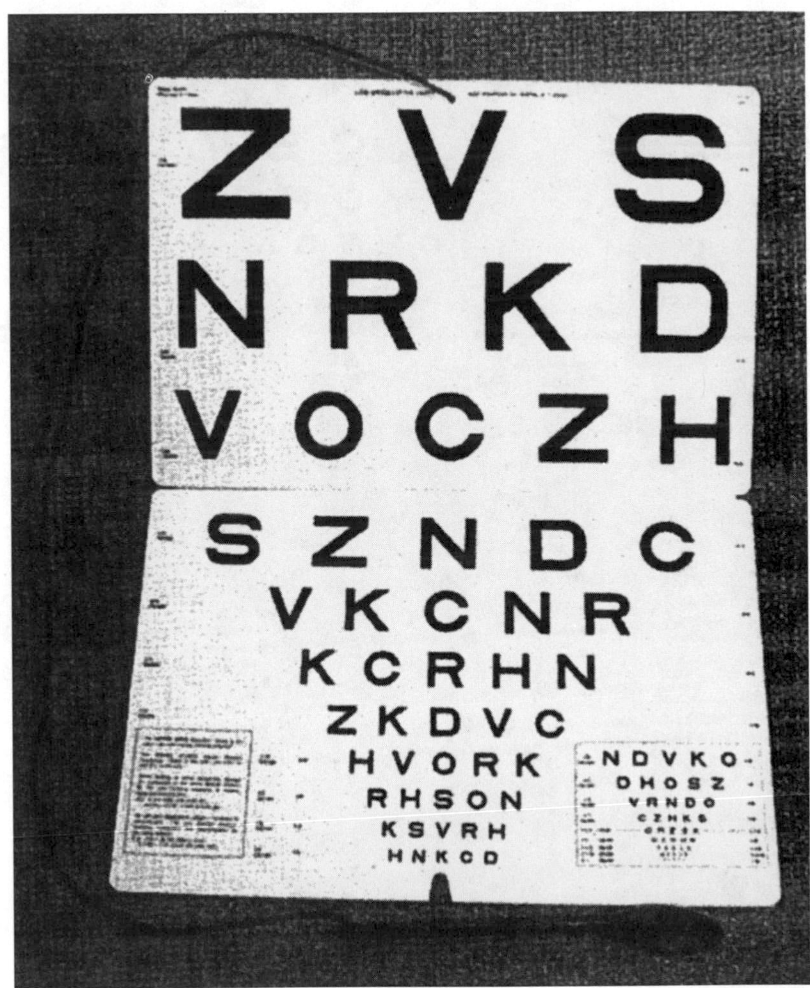

FIG. 34.27. Colenbrander one-meter chart.

be added to indicate one letter messed or two letters read on the next line. These suffixes are most meaningful if the number of letters on each line is constant. On most charts the test-retest confidence limits are about ±2 letter increments or about one-half line increment (73). For routine clinical use, where the patient generally reads each line only once, rounding to line values is common practice. It is appropriate, since the rounding errors are of the same order as the confidence limits. The lighting of the charts should be at least 7 foot-candles without glare.

In the clinical measurement of visual acuity with letter charts, it is not uncommon to use nonstandard testing distances. This procedure becomes necessary when the acuity of the examinee is not sufficient to permit reading of the largest letters on the chart at the standard distance; the viewing distance is then reduced. Nonstandard viewing distances are also used when the layout of the examination room does not readily lend itself to viewing the chart from the standard distance. The use of a vision screener manufactured by Titmus Optical or Stereo Optical Company limits these problems.

For vision worse than 20/400, the Colenbrander one-meter chart (Fig. 34.27) (74) should be utilized. Count fingers (CF) and hand motions (HM) at a given distance are old terms that can no longer be utilized for quantitative evaluation of vision. The terms should be replaced on chart review where complete data may not be available (75). If no better information is available:

CF feet should be interpreted as ___/200
CF meters should be interpreted as ___/60
HM feet should be interpreted as ___/1,000
HM meters should be interpreted as ___/300

For example:

CF 3′ → 3/200, HM 5′ → 5/1000

Benjamin (76) has a detailed description of principles and applications of visual acuity.

REFERENCES

1. Kuhn HA. *Eyes and industry.* St. Louis, CV Mosby, 1944.
2. Leopold. *Am J Ophthalmol* 1957;43(2):93.
3. Pizzarello L. Eye safety and the economic impact of eye injuries during the last century in the United States. *Sports Ind Ophthalmol* 1999;12(3):298.
4. Transaction American Academy of Ophthalmology (TAAOO), January/February 1944, Business Meeting of the Joint Industrial Ophthalmology Committee, p. 105.
5. Liggett PE, Pince KI, Barlow W. Ocular trauma in an urban population. *Ophthalmology* 1990;97:581.
6. Schein OD, Hibbard PL, Shingleton BJ. The spectrum and burden of ocular injury. *Ophthalmology* 1988; 95:300–305.
7. Tredici TJ. Lecture notes, management of eye injuries, 2001.
8. Tredici TJ. Ophthalmology in practice of aerospace medicine. In: DeHart R, Davis J, eds. *Fundamentals of aerospace medicine and otolaryngology.* 2nd ed. Baltimore: Williams & Wilkins, 1995.
9. Duke Elder SS. *System of ophthalmology, vol V. Ophthalmic optics information.* London, Henry Kempler, 1970:81.
10. Moses RA, Hart WA Jr. *Adler's physiology of the eye: clinical applications.* St. Louis: CV Mosby, 1989: 561–562.
11. Harris JS, ed. *Occupational medicine practice guidelines.* Beverly, MA: OEM Press, 1998.
12. Berson FG. *Basic ophthalmology for medical students and primary care residents,* 6th ed. San Francisco: American Academy of Ophthalmology, 1993.
13. Bradford CA. *Basic ophthalmology,* 7th ed. San Francisco: American Academy of Ophthalmology.
14. Kuhn F, Morris R, Witherspoon CD, et al. *Ophthalmology* 1996;103:240–243.
15. Trobe JD. *Physicians guide to eyecare.* San Francisco: American Academy of Ophthalmology, 1993.
16. *Basic and clinical science course, section 8: external disease in cornea.* San Francisco: American Academy of Ophthalmology (updated annually).
17. Wilson FM. *Practical ophthalmology.* San Francisco: American Academy of Ophthalmology, 1996.
18. Coe JV, Cuttle K, McClellan WC, et al. *Visual display units: a review of potential health problems associated with their use.* Wellington, New Zealand: Department of Health Regional Unit, 1980.
19. *Managing the red eye—a slide script program.* San Francisco: American Academy of Ophthalmology, 1988. London, England.
20. Duke Elder SS. *System of ophthalmology.* 1965;8(pt 1):353. London, England.
21. Hobson. *Am J Ophthalmol* 1938;21:1153.
22. Holmes. *Hawaii Med J* 1941;1:11.
23. Duke Elder SS. *System of ophthalmology.* 1965;8(pt 1):406. London, England.
24. Duke Elder SS. *System of ophthalmology.* 1965;8(pt 1):398. London, England.
25. Duke Elder SS. *System of ophthalmology.* 1965;8(pt 1):260. London, England.
26. Leopold. *Am J Ophthalmol* 1957;43(2):93.
27. Dawson J. *Am J Hyg* 1960;72:279.
28. Dawson J, Darrell. *N Engl J Med* 1963;268:1031.
29. Pellitteri, Fried. *Am J Ophthalmol* 1950;33:1596.
30. Pillat. *Wien Klin Wochenschr* 1953;65:41.
31. Thygson P. *Am J Ophthalmol* 1957;43(2):98.
32. Jawetz, et al. *Am J Ophthalmol* 1953;40(2):200.
33. Dawson J, et al. *N Engl J Med* 1963;268:103.
34. Dawson J, et al. *Am J Hyg* 1960;72:279.
35. OSHA 29 CFR 1910.1030. *Fed Reg* 1991(December 6);56(235):64–175.
36. OSHA Instruction CPL, 2-2.44 C, Enforcement Procedure for the Occupational Exposure to Blood-Borne Pathogens under 29 CFR 1910.1030, March 6, 1992.
37. Tiffin J, Wirt ED. Determining visual standards for industrial jobs by statistical method. *Am Acad Ophthalmol Otolaryngol* 1945;58:4.

38. Stump NF. How inefficient vision causes industrial accidents. *Optometric Weekly* July 4, 1946.
39. Blais BR. Basic principles of industrial ophthalmology, sports and industrial ophthalmology. Pizzarella, ed. *Ophthalmol Clin North Am* 2000;13(2):309–343.
40. North RV. *Work and the eye.* Oxford: Oxford University Press, 1993.
41. Koven AL. The right eyes for the right job. *TAAOO* 1947–1948;52:46–50.
42. Tiffin J. *Visual skills and vision tests, industrial psychology.* New York: Prentice Hall, 1943.
43. Americans with Disabilities Act (ADA), 1990.
44. OSHA 29 CFR 1910.132. Personal Protective Equipment. OSHA 3077.1994, rev. Washington, DC: Occupational Safety and Health Administration, 1994.
45. Tiffin J. *Visual skills and vision tests, industrial psychology.* New York: Prentice Hall, 1952.
46. Novak JF. *Are the eyes right for the job? Industrial and traumatic ophthalmology.* Symposium of the New Orleans Academy of Ophthalmology. St. Louis: Mosby, 1964.
46a. Kuhn HA. *Eyes and industry.* St. Louis: CV Mosby, 1950.
47. Confer RG, Confer TR. *Occupational health and safety: terms, definitions, and abbreviations.* Boca Raton, FL, Livis, 1994.
48. Pitts DG. Visual display terminals, visual problems, and solutions. In: Pitts DG, Kleinstein RN, eds. *Environmental vision.* Boston: Butterworth-Hermann, 1993.
49. Blais BR. *Visual ergonomics of the office workplace, health and safety.* 1999(July/August);31–38.
50. Sheedy JE. *Vision and computer displays,* 2nd ed. Walnut Creek, CA: Vision Analysis, 1991.
51. Collins MJ, Brown B, Bowman KJ. Visual discomfort and VDTs, Centre for Eye Research, Department of Optometry, Queensland Institute of Technology, 1988.
52. Riggs LA. Visual acuity. In: Graham CH, ed. *Vision and visual perception.* New York: John Wiley & Sons, 1965:321–349.
53. Westheimer G. Visual acuity. *Adler's physiology of the eye: clinical application,* 8th ed. St. Louis: CV Mosby, 1987:415–428.
54. ANSI Z87.1A-1991. New York: American National Standards Institute, 1991.
55. Keeney A. *The eye and the workplace: special considerations.* In: Tasman W, Jaeger E, eds. Duane's clinical ophthalmology. Philadelphia: Lippincott, 1995:199.
56. Blais BR. A century of progress in eye safety. Presented at the American Academy of Ophthalmology, October 29, 1996.
57. Blais BR. Visual ergonomics of the workplace. Presented at the American Occupational Health Conference, May 23, 1994.
58. Blais BR. Contact lenses in industry: the ongoing discussion. Chemical Health and Safety, published by the American Chemical Society, July/August 1997, p. 22–26.
59. Blais BR. Are contact lenses a direct threat as defined by the Americans with Disabilities Act? Chemical Health and Safety, published by the American Chemical Society, July/August 1997.
60. Blais BR. Does wearing of contact lenses in the workplace pose a direct threat. *OEM Rep* 1998;12(3):17–31.
61. Blais BR. Chemical eye injuries. In: *Best safety directory,* vol 1. Old Wick, NJ: A.M. Best, 1998:204–208.
62. Blais BR. Does wearing of contact lenses in the workplace pose a direct threat. *Occup Environ Med Rep* 1998;12(3):17–31.
63. Keller JJ. *Head, body, and foot protection.* Government and Industry Standard Cross References 64M. Neenah, WI: OSHA, 1998:6.
64. OSHA 29 CFR 1910.133. *Eye and face protection.* Parts 1900–1910, 1994 rev. Washington, DC: Occupational Safety and Health Administration, 1994.
65. ANSI Z136.1. *Safe use of lasers.* New York: American National Standards Institute, 1993.
66. ANSI Z136.1. *Safe use of lasers in health facilities.* New York: American National Standards Institute, 1993.
67. Bureau of Labor Statistics. Report 597. Washington, DC: Bureau of Labor Statistics, 1980.
68. Holmes C, Joliffe H. *Guide to occupational and other visual needs,* vols 1 and 2. Los Angeles: Silver Lake Lithographers, 1958 (vol 1); St. Louis: Vision-Ease Corp., 1968 (vol 2).
69. Sloan LL. New test charts for the measurement of visual acuity at far and near distances. *Am J Ophthalmol* 1959;48:807–813.
70. Bailey IL, Lovie JE. New design principles for visual acuity letter charts. *Am J Optom Physiol Ophthalmol* 1976;53:740–745.
71. National Academy of Sciences, National Research Council, Committee on Vision. Report of Working Group 39. Recommended standard procedures for the clinical measurement and specification of visual acuity. *Adv Ophthalmol* 1980;41:103.
72. Ferris FL, Kassov A, Bresnick GH, et al. New visual acuity charts for clinical research. *Am J Ophthalmol* 1982;94:91–96.
73. Colenbrander A. Measuring vision and vision loss. In: *Duane's clinical ophthalmology,* vol 5. 2002, CO-01.
74. *Precision vision.* LaSalle, IL: Colenbrander Low Vision Test Systems, 2000.
75. Mansfield JS, Legge GE, Bane MC. Psychophysics of reading. XV. Font effect in normal and low vision. *Invest Ophthalmol Vis Sci* 1996;37:1492–1501. The MNREAD Acuity Chart (Lighthouse Low Vision Products, Inc., Long Island City, New York).
76. Benjamin WJ. *Borish's clinical refraction.* Philadelphia: WB Saunders, 1998.

FURTHER INFORMATION

American Medical Association. *Guide to the evaluation of permanent impairment,* 4th ed. Chicago: AMA, 1993.

American Medical Association. *Guide to the evaluation of permanent impairment,* 5th ed. Chicago: AMA, 2000.

American Medical Association. *Physicians current procedural terminology (CPT).* Chicago: AMA, 2003.

Colenbrander A. The visual system. In: Cachiarella L, Anderson GBJ, eds. *Guides to the evaluation of permanent impairment,* 5th ed. Chicago: AMA Press, 2000.

Colenbrander A. Measuring vision and vision loss. In: *Duane's clinical ophthalmology,* vol 5. Philadelphia: Lippincott Williams & Wilkins, 2001:1–27.

Duke-Elder SS. *System of ophthalmology, vol 5, ophthalmic optics information.* London: Henry Kempler, 1970:81.

Fox SL. *Industrial and occupational ophthalmology.* Springfield, IL: Charles C Thomas, 1973.

Kephart NC. An example of increased production through an industrial vision program. *Opt J Rev* September 15, 1948.

Low Vision Test Chart. One side: Letter chart from 50M to 1M, representing acuity values from 1/50 (20/1000, 0.02) to 1/1 (20/20, 1.0); 1M cord attached. Other side: standardized reading segments (10M to 0.6M) for reading rate measurements; diopter ruler included. Available in English, Spanish, Portuguese, German, French, Dutch, Swedish, Finnish. From Precision Vision, 944 First Street, LaSalle, IL 61301. Fax: 1-(815)-223-2224.

Resnick L, Carris LH. *Eye hazards in industrial occupations.* New York: National Committee for the Prevention of Blindness, 1924.

Snell AC. The need for more realistic ophthalmic service in industry. *NYS J Med* 1942;42:1435.

TAAOO, Announcements, Industrial Ophthalmology, March/April 1943, p. 315.

TAAOO, Supplement, June 1944.

TAAOO, December 1946.

The Rehabilitation Act of 1913. 29 U.S.C. 701-796.

The use of contact lenses in an industrial environment. A joint statement of the American College of Occupational and Environmental Medicine and the American Academy of Ophthalmology. Arlington Heights, IL: ACOEM, 1997.

Wood CA, ed. *The American encyclopedia and dictionary of ophthalmology.* Chicago: Cleveland Press, 1913.

U.S. District Court Stipulation of Settlement. Keith RE, Kimble B, et al. v. Dr. George Hayes et al., May 2, 1992.

35

Use of Molecular Genetics in Occupational Medicine

Peter G. Shields

The genetic basis of disease and disease risk is the focus of many research laboratories. Such efforts have wide-ranging clinical importance and their introduction into the workplace is rapidly coming. The lessons learned through molecular genetics will impact on medical decision making, worker protection, risk assessment processes, and other parts of the occupational medicine practice. Genetic biomarkers are being developed that reflect a spectrum of effects from internal exposure to disease and prognosis (Fig. 35.1). The ethical, legal, and social implications of genetic testing are profound. Significant efforts are underway to ensure the proper uses of such testing, although many potential problems are only now being elucidated. These efforts cannot be separated from the research, development, and incorporation of genetic testing into the workplace. This chapter reviews some of the more commonly used molecular genetic methods of value in occupational practice and research.

Occupational disease is caused by the interactions of exposure to exogenous agents, inheritable susceptibilities that determine the response to those agents, and endogenous processes that act independently of exposure. Each of these is important and dictates, for example, why one worker will develop an illness in response to a small exposure while another does not in spite of a large exposure. Genetic testing can be useful in several clinical areas (Table 35.1). It might predict which workers are at risk for specific diseases, identify who needs additional workplace protection, and suggest maximal allowable exposures, ethical, legal, and social issues notwithstanding. It also may be useful for finding an occupational etiology for a disease in an individual worker or provide prognostic information. However, the primary goal for biomarkers is to prevent disease, and the secondary goal is to facilitate early detection of disease.

Some currently available tests provide direct information about DNA sequence, structure, and expres-

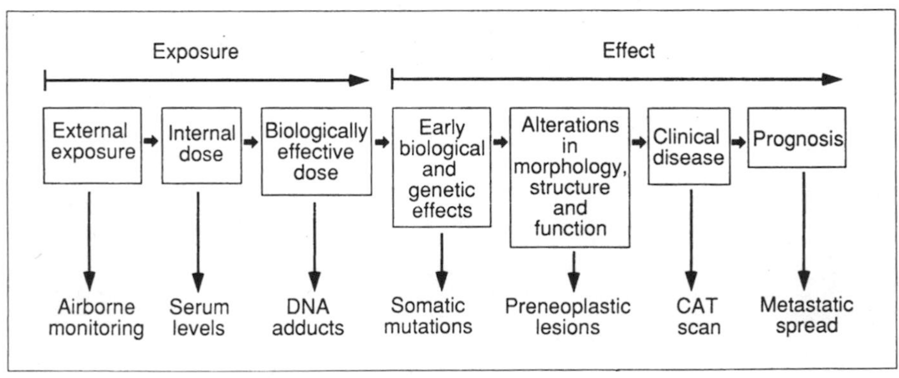

FIG. 35.1. Biomarkers of exposure and effect.

TABLE 35.1. *Clinical applications of genetic tests in occupational medicine*

Disease risk
Markers of inherited susceptibility
Genetic variation causing impaired metabolic activation or excretion of toxins
Genetic variation causing defects in the repair of DNA, cell cycle control or programmed cell death
Markers of acquired susceptibility
Formation of DNA adducts
Integration of viral DNA
Mutations in critical genes
Mutations in noncritical genes
Hypermethylation of gene promoter region
Altered gene expression
Clastogenic abnormalities
Antibodies to DNA adducts
Altered protein or mRNA expression patterns
Preclinical disease
Markers of cellular alteration
Altered morphology of cells
Altered phenotypic expression of cells
Clonal proliferation of cells
Altered gene expression
Antibodies to gene products
Altered protein or mRNA expression patterns
Clinical disease
Markers of cellular alteration
Altered morphology of cells
Altered phenotypic expression of cells
Immunohistochemical staining
Clonal proliferation of cells
Altered gene expression
Antibodies to gene products
Altered protein or mRNA expression patterns
Markers of prognosis
Pathological diagnosis
Immunohistochemical staining
Altered gene expression
Cytogenetic abnormalities
Altered protein or mRNA expression patterns

mRNA, messenger RNA.

sion of specific gene products. Other tests determine the phenotypic expression of a gene indirectly reflecting a genotype. Newer technologies may focus on genes (e.g., genotyping, DNA sequencing) or phenotypes (e.g., microarrays). For example, serum cholesterol testing reflects the phenotypic expression of several genes that determines the risk of heart disease. It is important to realize that phenotypes might not always accurately reflect genetic function because of exogenous influences, e.g., lifestyle factors also affect serum cholesterol levels.

The importance of molecular genetics is exemplified by the Human Genome Project (1). This federally funded program, conceived in 1986 and formally established in 1990, is coordinated by the Department of Energy and the National Institutes of Health. Its goal has been largely achieved, although now the challenge is to use the information in meaningful ways. To achieve this goal, significant amounts of research focus on technology development, including improvement of molecular genetic techniques, bioinformatics, and research training. The Human Genome Project, in recognition of the potential problems of such an effort, also sponsors programs directed toward an understanding of the ethical, legal, and social implications of such research and policy options to address them.

BACKGROUND

Molecular genetics is the study of genes and gene structure. There are over 100,000 human genes located on 46 chromosomes. Genes are composed of deoxyribonucleic acid (DNA) sequences that provide a written language for genetic function. DNA is double stranded and joined by nucleotide base pairing. An important property of DNA strands is that they bind to complementary copies of each other (guanine binds to cytosine and adenine to thymine). The genetic sequences are transcribed by enzymes that make complementary copies of messenger ribonucleic acid (mRNA). The mRNA is then translated into proteins that perform the basic cellular functions.

The genetic language that codes for the amino acid sequence in proteins is organized in triplets called codons. Each codon dictates which amino acid is to be incorporated into proteins and in what sequence. Not all of a gene and not all of a chromosome codes for amino acids, however. Genes are composed of exons, which are transcribed, and introns, which are not. They also contain transcribing regions that decide when and how much a gene is transcribed. Genes are the basic building blocks of heredity, controlling diverse body cellular functions such as determining hair color, height, and facial characteristics. This diversity is controlled through variations in DNA sequence. Any variation that occurs in more than 1% of the population is considered a polymorphism. Genetic polymorphisms might result in only one base change that fundamentally alters structure (e.g., sickle cell disease), or it may be reflected in all or part of gene being deleted. It is estimated that genetic polymorphisms occur approximately every 500 bases.

As most diseases ultimately relate back to altered cell function, the basis is frequently in genetic dysfunction such as point mutations (exchanging one base for another), base deletions, or gross chromosomal aberrations (loss of part of a chromosome or exchanging parts of a chromosome). A recently characterized and common mechanism for gene inactivation is hypermethylation of the promoter regions of genes. Mutations and hypermethylation in genes might result in a decrease in necessary protein production or altered gene transcription that can lead to a variety of diseases including cancer, hormonal disturbances, rheumatologic problems, etc. Exogenous exposures such as viruses and chemicals also cause mutations and hypermethylation. Here, dysfunction is acquired and not inherited. Finally, genetic dysfunction through mutational mechanisms can be acquired through endogenous mechanisms such as oxidative damage by chemicals released from neutrophils, errors during cell replication, and others. In fact, endogenous mutations are estimated to occur millions of time per day in any person but are efficiently repaired by the body.

MOLECULAR GENETIC ASSAYS

Our technology is expanding more rapidly than our ability to apply these technologies to biomedical research and the clinic. Several recently developed genetic tests are widely available (Table 35.2). Some of

TABLE 35.2. *Selected examples of molecular genetic assays*

DNA analysis

Single nucleotide polymorphism (SNP): There are a variety of assays that can detect an SNP, but all are based on the polymerase chain reaction. Small fragments of DNA are amplified from small amounts of DNA that can be coupled to other procedures or used by themselves to detect the presence of a gene or mutation. Then the genetic variant is identified by restriction fragment length analysis and gel electrophoresis, fluorescent labeling of probes that bind to DNA when a specified variant is present, fluorescent labeling of DNA, and gel electrophoresis via an automated DNA sequencer, denatured high-performance liquid chromatography, Maldi-TOF (time of flight) mass spectroscopy, and microarray.

Southern blot analysis: DNA is subjected to restriction enzyme digestion and the resulting DNA fragments are separated by gel electrophoresis. The fragments are transferred to a membrane that is probed for a specific gene sequence. The presence and size of the fragment are then detected.

Screening for mutations in genes: There are a variety of methods based up differences in DNA migration depending on the variant. Examples include denatured high-performance liquid chromatography and single-strand conformation polymorphism (SSCP) analysis where the DNA is run on a matrix that is sensitive to the DNA structure and conformation where differing variants migrate differently.

DNA sequencing for sequence or mutations: Using the polymerase chain reaction, DNA is used as a template for the amplification of complementary strands of DNA with fluorscently labeled nucleotides but also where 2, 3′-dideoxynucleotides are incorporated into the DNA, which causes the reaction to stop. The location of these labeled nucleotides reveals the genetic sequence when the are resolved electrophoretically.

DNA sequencing by microarray technologies for mutations: The polymerase chain reaction is used to amplify tumor DNA. The DNA is then fragmented and fluorescently labeled. The labeled products are hybridized to a microarray chip that has probe cells for wild type and mutant. The degree of binding to the cells is read by a fluorescent reader and reported out as a score for binding to the wildtype or mutant sequence.

Carcinogen-DNA adduct detection: Several methods are available. The ^{32}P-postlabeling assay is where DNA is enzymatically digested to individual nucleotides. An enzyme is used to radiolabel the nucleotides, which are then resolved and quantitated by thin layer chromatography. Other methods include mass spectroscopy, immunoassays, and laser-induced fluorescence.

Chromosomal assays: Each of the 46 chromosomes are isolated from cultured cells and identified. Deletions, additions, and translocations are detected by specific markers. Sister chromatid exchanges are used to detect abnormal DNA replication using nonspecific markers. Micronuclei are observed in cells where extra genetic material occurs outside the nucleus.

RNA analysis

Northern blot analysis: RNA is resolved by gel electrophoresis and then transferred to a membrane that is probed for a specific gene sequence. The presence and size of the fragment are then detected. The amount of RNA can be quantitated to reflect gene transcription.

cDNA microarrays: cDNA is enzymatically amplified using RNA as the template. Thus, all RNA in the sample are amplified. The fragments are fluorescently labeled and then hybridized to a microarray chip where each probe cell is for a known sequence for a particular gene. The degree of binding is detected by a fluorescence scanner, and the amount of fluorescence indicates the amount of RNA present in the sample.

Real-time polymerase chain reaction (PCR): The polymerase chain reaction is used with fluorescently labeled probes that have a quencher. The probes are matched to known genes. As the reaction occurs in real time, the quencher is released and the probe become fluorescent. As the reaction occurs, the amount of fluorscence is graphed by time and number of cycles. The number of starting copies is back-extrapolated.

these are described below. These assays can detect mutations, determine susceptibilities through genetic polymorphism detection, use biochemical methods to detect carcinogens bound to DNA, and measure abnormal or altered gene products and others.

The majority of molecular genetic tests used today begin with the polymerase chain reaction (PCR). There are emerging technologies that will eliminate this need, but none has been sufficiently validated for use in the clinical setting. PCR, in fact, is among the most important recent advances in molecular genetics. The reaction is the amplification of small amounts of DNA to make lots of DNA, which are then available for subsequent analyses. PCR is facile and inexpensive. It has been used in forensic medicine for DNA fingerprinting from a single hair follicle or blood stain (2); for mutation detection in single sperm cells to assess teratogenicity rates (3); and for amplification of DNA from paraffin embedded tissue blocks (4), serum (5), or ancient DNA (6). It also forms the basis for microarray technology (7,8). PCR relies on a temperature stable enzyme (*Taq* polymerase) that can replicate DNA when using gene- and site-specific primers that begin the reaction. While PCR is generally used for DNA amplification, it also can be used for RNA amplification using a different enzyme (reverse transcriptase) (9). The major limitations for PCR lie in its sensitivity that allows for contamination by unwanted DNA from other sources. It also is critical to choose primers carefully to ensure specificity and prevent amplifying the wrong gene.

There are many applications for PCR. It is being used directly without other techniques for diagnosing viral infections [e.g., HIV in lymphocytes (10), hepatitis B virus in liver and serum (11), and papilloma virus in uterine cervix (12)]. It can be used to amplify mutated and structurally altered regions of a given gene [e.g., translocation of chromosomes by determining the breakpoint cluster region for the *bcr-abl* oncogene for the diagnosis of chronic myelogenous leukemia (13)]. Other applications involve the identification of single base mutations or genetic polymorphisms by designing primers that anneal only if matched to the unique sequence [e.g., oligo-specific PCR for the identification of polymorphisms in the *N*-acetyltransferase gene predictive of cancer risk in workers exposed to aromatic amines (14)]. PCR also is combined with other techniques whereby PCR amplification products can be subjected to restriction enzyme digestion to identify genetic polymorphisms or mutations [e.g., restriction fragment length polymorphism (RFLP) analysis for cytochrome P-450 genetic polymorphisms (15)] or used for hybridization with mutation-specific probes [e.g., oligonucleotide hybridization for the detection of Ras mutations (16)]. Another important application is the use of PCR to amplify sufficient quantities of DNA fragments for nucleotide sequencing. This method allows for the determination of specific sequences from unknown genes or for the detection of mutations (17).

Genotyping to determine genetic variation (e.g., color of hair, metabolic activity, DNA repair) can be done by using different types of detection methods following PCR. This genetic variation can happen via single nucleotide polymorphisms (SNPs) or multiple base pair insertions or deletions. A common way is to utilize RFLP analysis. RFLP enzymes identify short specific DNA sequences, cutting the DNA at those sequences into uniquely sized fragments that can be separated electrophoretically. Restriction enzymes recognize palindromic sites where the sequence on each strand is identical with each other (when read in $5'$ to $3'$ direction). RFLP enzymes are only useful when a palindromic site exists. In other cases, the variant may be determined using single-strand conformational polymorphism analysis. If the variant results in the insertion or deletion of a base or bases, then electrophoretic methods that separate fragments based on size can be used. The fortunate property of DNA, where each strand is complementary and annealed by nucleic acid base-pairing (guanine to cytosine and adenine to thymine) can be taken advantage of to identify specific genetic sequences. Under experimental conditions the two complementary DNA strands can be separated and reannealed. Single-stranded probes of short DNA fragments can be used to identify a specific genetic sequence by exposing DNA to the probe. Using oligo-specific hybridization, a radioactive or fluorescently labeled probe marker will bind to the matched DNA. Two probes are used in tandem that are matched to one variant or the other. This unique property allows for Southern blot analysis of DNA (18), which subjects DNA to restriction enzyme digestion, separation of the resulting fragments by electrophoresis, and then probing the fragments for the genetic sequence and measuring the lengths of the fragments. The method also is used for Northern blot analysis of mRNA (19), which is almost identical with Southern blot analysis except that RNA is used instead of DNA.

Several new methodologies exist for high throughput genotyping. These include microarrays that can determine 2,000 SNPs following 24 different PCR assays, real-time PCR that allows for detection of SNPs without gel electrophoresis, matrix-assisted laser desorption/ionization time of flight (Maldi-TOF) mass spectroscopy (20), denatured high-performance liquid chromatography (21), capillary gel electrophoresis and fluorescence detection (22), and pyrosequencing (23).

DNA sequencing can be used to determine the actual genetic code. This may be used for identifying an inherited code (e.g., sequence of entire gene or SNPs) or mutations in tumors. The dideoxy-mediated chain termination method was among the first established and allows for the determination of a nucleic acid sequence of a gene (24). For example, a PCR fragment is amplified and four dideoxy reactions are carried out for each of the four nucleotides. The amplified product, radiolabeled nucleotides, 2,3′-dideoxynucleotides and a polymerase are mixed so that the 2,3′-dideoxynucleotide is randomly incorporated into the DNA. Based on the location of the dideoxynucleotide incorporation, the DNA sequence can be determined after electrophoretic separation. More recent high throughput methods rely on microarray technology following PCR (7) or capillary electrophoresis.

There are many types of DNA damage that can be detected using molecular genetic methods, such as carcinogen-DNA adduct detection. Chemicals or their reactive metabolites can bind to DNA, resulting in promutagenic lesions. The combination of the chemical and the nucleotide is an adduct. The measurement of DNA adducts allows for the distinction between the measurement of chemicals in the environment and exposures inside the body and in target organs, because the former is not always indicative of the latter. DNA adducts reflect the biologically effective dose of an exposure, resulting from the competition of exposure, absorption, activation, detoxification, and DNA repair. Thus, the measurement of DNA adducts reflects both exposure and inherited susceptibilities. Elevated levels of DNA adducts have been correlated with cigarette use (25), occupational exposures to polycyclic aromatic hydrocarbons (26), and air pollution (27).

Several methods are currently available for the measurement of DNA adducts, although all remain research tools. These include the ^{32}P-postlabeling assay that uses hydrolytic enzymes to reduce DNA to individual nucleotides and then uses another enzyme to radiolabel the nucleotides (28). Any adducts that are present are then resolved chromatographically and quantitated by measuring the radioactivity incorporated into the nucleotide. This assay can be used as a screening method to detect unknown adducts (28) or can be combined with purification techniques to identify specific compounds such as adducts formed from polycyclic aromatic hydrocarbons (29) and *N*-nitrosamines (30). Several important immunologic methods are available for the detection of DNA adducts. Using procedures such as enzyme-linked immunosorbent assays (ELISA) or radioimmunoassays, adducts for polycyclic aromatic hydrocarbons can be measured (31–33). More recent methods utilize improved mass spectroscopy (34) and fluorescence detection.

Several methods are available to analyze the gross structure of chromosomes in metaphase and prophase of mitosis. Chromosome aberrations can be observed by identifying each of the 23 chromosomal pairs for completeness and number (35). Common uses of such analyses include the detection of trisomy 21, which is diagnostic for Down syndrome, and detection of a translocation between chromosomes 9 and 21, which is diagnostic for the chronic myelogenous leukemia and the Philadelphia chromosome. The availability of specific chromosomal markers now makes this method more specific. Another gross chromosomal change detectable in human cells includes the sister chromatid exchange (36). In this case, sister chromatids of one chromosome are switched, which can be can be counted using nonspecific markers and correlated with exposures to tobacco and certain chemicals. A method of detecting DNA damage that does not require cell culture and examination of chromosomes during mitosis is the detection of micronuclei (37). Small chromosomal fragments are sometimes found to exist outside the nucleus. This assay is rapid, relatively inexpensive, and quantitative, so that its potential is greater as a screening test in humans for mutagenic exposures. It can be used for white blood cells and epithelial cells (bladder, lung, oral mucosa).

Microarray technology can be used for nucleotide sequence detection, SNP analysis, and aberrant gene expression using RNA (8). These methodologies begin with PCR, followed by enzymatic fragmentation of the PCR product and fluorescent labeling. Then the labeled product is hybridized to a microarray chip. The chip contains thousands or pads or cells that have bound short DNA sequences. The fragmented PCR products that have the identical sequence to the permanently bound sequence will bind to the chip. The chip is then scanned with a fluorescent reader, which informs the investigator of the amount of binding and hence the amount of labeled product. These technologies, because of the large amount of information that can be obtained, pose formidable data handling and bioinformatics issues.

CLINICAL APPLICATIONS OF GENETIC TESTING—SELECTED APPLICATIONS

While most genetic assays are being used in the research setting, several studies demonstrate how such research might be applied to workers' health. However, there are many clinically available tests for various nonoccupational settings, such as the detection of blood clotting disorders, cardiovascular disease risk, and human leukocyte antigen (HLA) typing. In general, the type of testing described herein is recently developed or applied to occupational cohorts. Research results should be carefully interpreted with regard to the study design and any methodologic limitations associated with the assay.

A potentially important clinical application of genetic testing will be the prediction of occupational lung disease in persons with decreased production of α_1-antitrypsin (38). Absence of two functional copies of this gene leads to the development of premature emphysema, which is worsened by concurrent exposure to tobacco smoke. The absence of one of two copies might lead to a partial deficiency and an inability for natural lung defense mechanisms to work properly when challenged by pulmonary irritants, allergens, or inflammatory agents. This gene is polymorphic, with over 7% of the population carrying a defective gene. The presence of an inheritable abnormality is demonstrable by PCR and oligonucleotide hybridization. If studies indeed identify an increased genetic risk, then industrial hygiene and medical surveillance might change.

Several genetic polymorphisms for drug and carcinogen metabolism have suggested that some workers might be at increased risk for occupational cancers. For example, the *N*-acetyltransferase enzyme is responsible for activating and also detoxifying aromatic amines and heterocyclic amines, depending on the organ and compound, and may place workers at increased risk of bladder cancer (39–41). The activity of this gene can be directly measured by administering isoniazid, dapsone, or caffeine, and measuring urinary metabolites (42). Another example is the genetic polymorphism for cytochrome P-4502D6. This gene is responsible for *N*-oxidation of many medications (tricyclic antidepressants, antiarrhythmic agents, beta-blocking antihypertensive agents, and others). The activity can be assessed in individuals by administration of dextromethorphan (cough medicine) or debrisoquine. Rapid metabolizers (approximately 90% of Americans) are at increased risk of lung cancer compared to poor metabolizers. Cigarette smokers who are homozygous for the active gene have a relative risk of 7.9 for lung cancer, which increases to 18.4 with concurrent exposure to asbestos or polycyclic aromatic hydrocarbons (43).

Recent advances in PCR amplification and DNA sequencing have led to findings that chemicals can cause specific point mutations in DNA that may be "fingerprints" of that exposure (mutational spectra). This type of testing might be useful in learning the etiology of cancer in an individual. The determination of mutations present in the *p53* tumor suppressor gene, which is the most commonly mutated gene in cancer, has been used to suggest a particular chemical etiology. Persons who develop hepatocellular carcinoma in regions where aflatoxin is a common dietary contaminant, believed to be etiologically linked to this cancer, have a typical G to T transversion in codon 249 (44). This type of transversion is also demonstrable in vitro and is not found in persons with the same tumor but residing in non–aflatoxin-contaminated areas (45). For lung cancer, it has been observed that the *p53* mutations detected in persons who smoke can display different patterns compared to smokers who also are uranium miners and exposed to radon (4). Cigarette smoking is associated with a greater frequency of *p53* mutations (46).

Specific and nonspecific genetic markers of exposure might be useful for assessing industrial hygiene safeguards and indirectly assessing the inherited predispositions to DNA damage. Sister chromatid exchanges, micronuclei, and chromosomal aberrations are observed more frequently in persons exposed to radiation (47), benzene workers (48), cytostatic drugs (49), and vinyl chloride (50).

The detection of infectious agents in vivo and in environmental samples has been an important application for molecular genetics, in some cases entirely replacing culture techniques. Genital infections such as papilloma viruses, gonorrhea, and chlamydia can be screened using PCR and genetic probes. Hepatitis B virus can be detected in serum or liver DNA, in some cases even when serologies are negative.

Cancer screening may be enhanced in persons known to be at increased risk. Using specific probes, mutated *ras* oncogenes can be detected in the stool in persons with colon cancer (51); this technique also is being applied in sputum, urine, and other body fluids. Increased production of Ras p21 proteins, detectable in the blood by immunoassays, has been observed in persons who develop lung cancer with preexisting asbestosis or silicosis, in some cases predating the diagnosis of lung cancer (52). Smokers more commonly have abnormalities in gene promoter hypermethylation (53) that can silence critical cancer susceptibility genes.

IMPLICATIONS FOR GENETIC TESTING IN THE WORKPLACE

Advances in technology will improve the accuracy, decrease the cost, and increase the speed of genetic testing. Further studies will elucidate mechanistic relationships of genetics to disease, while epidemiology will assist in the identification of relevant assays for human risk. Ultimately, the institution of any clinical test depends on its reliability, sensitivity, specificity, predictive value, and cost. Quality control and quality insurance of critical parts of genetic testing are necessary (54).

The ethical, legal, and social implications of the use of genetic assays has stimulated much debate, especially in the workplace. Employers and medical providers are mandated to avoid discriminatory practices, as addressed in part by the Americans with Disabilities Act (55). Additional legislation related to inherited risks may be required. Other forms of discrimination, such as might occur in the insurance industry remains to be adequately addressed (56). The odds of never developing a disease in spite of having a specific genetic trait must be considered in the context of other commonly used actuarial predictors (e.g., cholesterol level, hypertension). Separately, the stigmatization of having a specific genotype needs to be addressed in a number of different forums. Providing results of genetic testing can avoid wrongful stigmatization, if accurate risks are presented clearly. Further, due to the large diversity in human genotypes (polymorphisms of individual nucleotides occurs approximately every 500 bases), there can no longer be one genotype that is considered "normal"; rather, there are common and less common types. The potential harmful effects of genetic testing must be considered in light of the many potential benefits. Strategies for disease prevention can focus on persons most at risk, thereby enabling programs to be cost-effective and enhance chances for success. Chemoprevention trials might be directed toward persons with the best-defined risks. Industrial hygiene measures could be designed to protect the workers at greatest risk, or vary according to the characteristics of a particular workforce (different ethnic groups may have different risks so that allowable exposure limits might justifiably be very different in different countries). Finally, medical surveillance projects might identify which workers require more or less surveillance, depending on genotype and exposure. Significant efforts, such as those funded by the Human Genome Project (1), are now addressing many of the potential problems and benefits of genetic testing.

The risk assessment process relies on epidemiologic studies and mathematical modeling to predict risk in populations. However, for many hazardous exposures, adequate epidemiologic evidence is not available so that extrapolations from laboratory animal studies are required. The use of such studies has been problematic because of study design (e.g., use of maximally tolerated doses) and inherent differences between laboratory animals and humans. Even when epidemiologic studies are available, they are generally unable to distinguish persons with different sensitivities to a particular hazard. Further, as the carcinogenic process is significantly complex and multistaged, greater emphasis needs to be directed toward risk assessment methods that are biologically, physiologically, and genetically based. The use of genetic studies also might better identify which laboratory animal studies more closely approximate human responses. Molecular epidemiologic studies, such as the measurement of DNA adducts in exposed populations, might help better approximate risk by including the degree of DNA damage in risk assessment models.

The use of genetic testing for evaluation of disease risk, diagnosis, and prognosis will be incorporated into many parts of our lives. It is important to note that the prevalence of genetic disease is not increasing, in contrast to those diseases caused by infectious agents, so that there should not be a negative economic impact to society of genetic testing. In fact, there might be a reduction in the cost of health care and a positive influence on the workforce if preventable genetic diseases are appropriately addressed. The prevention of discriminatory practices, education, and dissemination of information and the best uses of such testing are still evolving.

REFERENCES

1. U.S. Dept. of Energy and Office of Health and Environmental Research. Human Genome: 1991–92 Program Report. Washington, DC: U.S. Dept. of Energy, 1992.
2. Erlich HA, ed. *PCR technology: principles and applications for DNA amplification.* New York: WH Freeman, 1991.
3. Zhang L, Cui X, Schmitt K, et al. Whole genome amplification from a single cell: implications for genetic analysis. *Proc Natl Acad Sci USA* 1992;89:5847–5851.
4. Vahakangas KH, Samet JM, Metcalf RA, et al. Mutations of p53 and ras genes in radon-associated lung cancer from uranium miners. *Lancet* 1992;339:576–580.
5. Martin M, Carrington M, Mann D. A method for using serum or plasma as a source of DNA for HLA typing. *Hum Immunol* 1992;33:108–113.
6. Paabo S. Amplifying ancient DNA. In: Innis MA, Gelfand DH, Sninsky JJ, et al., eds. *PCR protocols: a guide to methods and applications.* San Diego: Academic Press, 1990:159–166.

7. Ahrendt SA, Halachmi S, Chow JT, et al. Rapid p53 sequence analysis in primary lung cancer using an oligonucleotide probe array. *Proc Natl Acad Sci USA* 1999; 96:7382–7387.
8. Ramaswamy S, Golub TR. DNA microarrays in clinical oncology. *J Clin Oncol* 2002;20:1932–1941.
9. Kawasaki ES, Clark SS, Coyne MY, et al. Diagnosis of chronic myeloid and acute lymphocytic leukemias by detection of leukemia-specific mRNA sequences amplified in vitro. *Proc Natl Acad Sci USA* 1988;85: 5698–5702.
10. Hewlett IK, Laurian Y, Epstein J, et al. Assessment by gene amplification and serological markers of transmission of HIV-1 from hemophiliacs to their sexual partners and secondarily to their children. *J Acquir Immune Defic Syndr* 1990;3:714–720.
11. Kato N, Yokosuka O, Omata M, et al. Detection of hepatitis C virus ribonucleic acid in the serum by amplification with polymerase chain reaction. *J Clin Invest* 1990;86:1764–1767.
12. Manos MM, Ting Y, Wright DK, et al. Cancer cells: molecular diagnostics of human cancer. In: Furth M, Greaves M, eds. *Cancer cells: molecular diagnostics of human cancer,* 7th ed. New York: Cold Spring Harbor Press, 1989:209–214.
13. Kurzrock R, Shtalrid M, Gutterman JU, et al. Molecular diagnostics of chronic myelogenous leukemia and Philadelphia-positive acute leukemia. In: Furth M, Greaves M, eds. *Cancer cells: molecular diagnostics of human cancer,* 7th ed. New York: Cold Spring Harbor Press, 1989:9–13.
14. Blum M, Demierre A, Grant DM, et al. Molecular mechanism of slow acetylation of drugs and carcinogens in humans. *Proc Natl Acad Sci USA* 1991;88:5237–5241.
15. Kawajiri K, Nakachi K, Imai K, et al. Identification of genetically high risk individuals to lung cancer by DNA polymorphisms of the cytochrome P450IA1 gene. *FEBS* 1990;263:131–133.
16. Rodenhuis S, Van de Wetering ML, Mooi WJ, et al. Mutational activation of the K-ras oncogene: a possible pathogenetic factor in adenocarcinoma of the lung. *N Engl J Med* 1987;317:929–935.
17. Pawson T, Olivier P, Rozakis-Adcock M, et al. Proteins with SH2 and SH3 domains couple receptor tyrosine kinases to intracellular signalling pathways. *Philos Trans R Soc Lond B Biol Sci* 1993;340:279–285.
18. Southern EM. Detection of specific sequences among DNA fragments separated by gel electrophoresis. *J Mol Biol* 1975;98:503–517.
19. Maniatis T, Fritsch EF, Sambrook J. *Molecular cloning: a laboratory manual.* New York: Cold Spring Harbor Press, 1982.
20. Bray MS, Boerwinkle E, Doris PA. High-throughput multiplex SNP genotyping with MALDI-TOF mass spectrometry: practice, problems, and promise. *Hum Mutat* 2001;17:296–304.
21. Matyas G, De Paepe A, Halliday D, et al. Evaluation and application of denaturing HPLC for mutation detection in Marfan syndrome: identification of 20 novel mutations and two novel polymorphisms in the FBN1 gene. *Hum Mutat* 2002;19:443–456.
22. Moretti TR, Baumstark AL, Defenbaugh DA, et al. Validation of STR typing by capillary electrophoresis. *J Forensic Sci* 2001;46:661–676.
23. Fakhrai-Rad H, Pourmand N, Ronaghi M. Pyrosequencing: an accurate detection platform for single nucleotide polymorphisms. *Hum Mutat* 2002;19:479–485.
24. Sanger F, Nicklen S, Coulson AR. DNA sequencing with chain-terminating inhibitors. *Proc Natl Acad Sci USA* 1977;74:5463–5467.
25. Phillips DH, Hewer A, Martin CN, et al. Correlation of DNA adduct levels in human lung with cigarette smoking. *Nature* 1988;336:790–792.
26. Savela K, Hemminki K, Hewer A, et al. Interlaboratory comparison of the 32P-postlabelling assay for aromatic DNA adducts in white blood cells of iron foundry workers. *Mutat Res* 1989;224:485–492.
27. Perera FP, Hemminki K, Gryzbowska E, et al. Molecular and genetic damage in humans from environmental pollution in Poland. *Nature* 1992;360:256–258.
28. Randerath E, Agrawal HP, Weaver JA, et al. ^{32}P-postlabeling analysis of DNA adducts persisting for up to 42 weeks in the skin, epidermis, and dermis of mice treated topically with 7,12-dimethylbenz[a]anthracene. *Carcinogenesis* 1985;6:1117–1126.
29. Shields PG, Bowman ED, Harrington AM, et al. Polycyclic aromatic hydrocarbon-DNA adducts in human lung and cancer susceptibility genes. *Cancer Res* 1993;53:3486–3492.
30. Shields PG, Povey AC, Wilson VL, et al. Combined high performance liquid chromatography/^{32}P-postlabeling assay of N7-methyldeoxyguanosine. *Cancer Res* 1990;50:6580–6584.
31. Van Schooten FJ, Hillebrand MJ, Van Leeuwen FE, et al. Polycyclic aromatic hydrocarbon-DNA adducts in lung tissue from lung cancer patients. *Carcinogenesis* 1990;11:1677–1681.
32. Perera F, Mayer J, Jaretzki A, et al. Comparison of DNA adducts and sister chromatid exchange in lung cancer cases and controls. *Cancer Res* 1989;49:4446–4451.
33. Perera FP, Hemminki K, Young TL, et al. Detection of polycyclic aromatic hydrocarbon-DNA adducts in white blood cells of foundry workers. *Cancer Res* 1988;48: 2288–2291.
34. Goldman R. Quantitation of benzo[alpha]pyrene-DNA adducts by postlabeling with 14C-acetic anhydride and accelerator mass spectrometry. *Chem Biol Interact* 2000;126:171–183.
35. Bender MA, Awa AA, Brooks AL, et al. Current status of cytogenetic procedures to detect and quantify previous exposures to radiation. *Mutat Res* 1988;196: 103–159.
36. Latt SA. Microfluorometric detection of deoxyribonucleic acid replication in human metaphase chromosomes. *Proc Natl Acad Sci USA* 1973;70:3395–3399.
37. Heddle JA, Hite M, Kirkhart B, et al. The induction of micronuclei as a measure of genotoxicity: a report of the U.S. Environmental Protection Agency Gene-Tox Program. *Mutat Res* 1983;123:61–118.
38. Lappé M. Ethical issues in genetic screening for susceptibility to chronic lung disease. *J Occup Med* 1988; 30:493–501.
39. Cartwright RA, Glashan RW, Rogers HJ, et al. Role of N-acetyltransferase phenotypes in bladder carcinogenesis: a pharmacogenetic epidemiological approach to bladder cancer. *Lancet* 1982;2:842–845.
40. Evans DA. N-acetyltransferase. *Pharmacol Ther* 1989; 42:157–234.

41. Ladero JM, Kwok CK, Jara C, et al. Hepatic acetylator phenotype in bladder cancer patients. *Ann Clin Res* 1985;17:96–99.
42. Weber WW, Hein DW. N-acetylation pharmacogenetics. *Pharmacol Rev* 1985;37:25–79.
43. Caporaso N, Hayes RB, Dosemeci M, et al. Lung cancer risk, occupational exposure, and the debrisoquine metabolic phenotype. *Cancer Res* 1989;49:3675–3679.
44. Hsu IC, Metcalf RA, Sun T, et al. Mutational hotspot in the p53 gene in human hepatocellular carcinomas. *Nature* 1991;350:427–428.
45. Ozturk M. p53 mutation in hepatocellular carcinoma after aflatoxin exposure. *Lancet* 1991;338:1356–1359.
46. Kure EH, Ryberg D, Hewer A, et al. p53 mutations in lung tumours: relationship to gender and lung DNA adduct levels. *Carcinogenesis* 1996;17:2201–2205.
47. National Research Council. *The effects on populations of exposure to low levels of ionizing radiation (BEIR III).* Washington, DC: National Academy Press, 1990.
48. Sarto F, Cominato I, Pinton AM, et al. A cytogenetic study on workers exposed to low concentrations of benzene. *Carcinogenesis* 1984;5:827–832.
49. Sorsa M, Yager JW. Cytogenetic surveillance of occupational exposures. In: Obe G, Basler A, eds. *Cytogenetics: basic and applied aspects.* New York: Springer-Verlag, 1987:345–360.
50. Au WW. Monitoring human populations for effects of radiation and chemical exposures using cytogenetic techniques. *Occup Med* 1991;6:597–611.
51. Sidransky D, Tokino T, Hamilton SR, et al. Identification of ras oncogene mutations in the stool of patients with curable colorectal tumors. *Science* 1992;256:102–105.
52. Brandt-Rauf PW, Smith S, Hemminki K, et al. Serum oncoproteins and growth factors in asbestosis and silicosis patients. *Int J Cancer* 1992;50:881–885.
53. Palmisano WA, Divine KK, Saccomanno G, et al. Predicting lung cancer by detecting aberrant promoter methylation in sputum. *Cancer Res* 2000;60:5954–5958.
54. Blomeke B, Shields PG. Laboratory methods for the determination of genetic polymorphisms in humans. *IARC Sci Publ* 1999;133–147.
55. Orentlicher D. From the Office of the General Counsel. Genetic screening by employers. *JAMA* 1990;263:1005, 1008.
56. Harper PS. Insurance and genetic testing [see comments]. *Lancet* 1993;341:224–227.

36

The Human Genome Project and Occupational Medicine Practice

Amy J. Behrman and Judith Green-McKenzie

> Based on science, medicine has followed and partaken of its fortunes, so that in the great awakening which has made [it] memorable among centuries, the profession received a quickening impulse more powerful than at any period in its history... There seems to be no limit to the possibilities of scientific medicine...with the colossal advance of the past fifty years.
>
> William Osler, Address to the Canadian Medical Association, 1902

This chapter, new to the textbook, addresses a tremendous recent achievement in genetics that is likely to impact the future practice of occupational medicine (OM) on multiple levels. The Human Genome Project (HGP), having beaten all its target dates, has achieved a (nearly) complete, validated, publicly accessible sequence of the human genome. In addition, the HGP has produced complete genomic sequences of a number of nonhuman species with enormous research value, a rapidly expanding library of human polymorphisms, and new technologies that will carry genetics and medicine into new frontiers of knowledge. The HGP follows and builds on the explosively paced genetic discoveries of the past five decades. Indeed, Osler's words may be more accurately applied to our new century than to his own.

BACKGROUND OF THE HUMAN GENOME PROJECT

The HGP is best understood in the context of the science that preceded it. A prehistory of the HGP began in 1953 with the elucidation of the paired-nucleotide, double-helical structure of DNA by James Watson and Francis Crick (1). The concepts and details of RNA transcription from DNA templates and protein translation from messenger RNA (mRNA) templates followed over the next 15 years. In 1972, Paul Berg's group (2) created the first recombinant DNA molecule, heralding molecular biologists' ability to create pure preparations of specific DNA sequences and precipitating an ethical debate on the use of recombinant constructs, which seems almost quaint in light of today's capabilities and issues.

DNA sequencing efforts began immediately, but were slow and laborious until dideoxy chain-termination techniques were developed in the late 1970s (3). Concomitantly, the techniques of restriction endonuclease digestion and mapping were refined to the point that researchers suggested the possibility of mapping the human genome with overlapping restriction fragments as early as 1980 (4). In the mid-1980s, automation of DNA sequencing techniques (5) and the development of polymerase chain reaction (PCR) techniques (6) accelerated scientists' abilities to identify, replicate, and sequence substantial lengths of DNA.

Nevertheless, the effort and cost involved in identifying, mapping by linkage analysis, and sequencing individual genes for human disorders with even the most obvious mendelian inheritance were substantial, and progress was tantalizingly slow. Momentum built in the United States and Europe during this decade to develop a comprehensive human genome map utilizing the new knowledge and technologies described briefly above. In 1988, the U.S. Department of Energy (DOE) and the National Institutes of Health

(NIH) agreed to collaborate on the HGP under the leadership of James Watson.

HISTORY OF THE HGP

The HGP began in 1988 with the pragmatic realization that the technology for actually sequencing the 3 billion base pairs of the human genome would be developed rapidly, but did not yet exist. The estimated time course to completion at that time was 15 years given expected technologic advances. The first "Five-Year Plan" of the HGP, published in 1990, included the following goals: (a) developing preliminary genetic maps of the human genome; (b) developing physical maps of the chromosomes; (c) mapping and fully sequencing simple laboratory organisms such as *Saccharomyces cerevisiae, Caenorhabditis elegans, Escherichia coli,* and *Mycoplasma capricolum;* (d) investing in sequencing technologies; and (e) proactively researching potential ethical, legal, and social issues (ELSIs) expected to arise from the HGP (7). The unprecedented dedication of 3% to 5% of the HGP budget to ELSI research reflected early recognition by HGP leaders of the negative social potential embedded in genomic promise. Equally unprecedented, the HGP involved laboratories from many countries around the world from its inception. The majority of the work was eventually done in four U.S. labs and one United Kingdom lab (the "G5").

In 1992, Craig Venter left the NIH and the HGP to start a private genomics company after vigorous debate with James Watson regarding patent issues and HGP discoveries. At this time Francis Collins succeeded Watson as director of the HGP. Under Collins's leadership (8), the HGP and its international partners agreed in 1996 to make all sequence data freely accessible in public databases on an ongoing basis within 24 hours of validation. This commitment to public domain was termed the "Bermuda Principle" after the location of the meeting.

During this period, the HGP achieved an accelerating series of interim goals: Complete physical maps of two human chromosomes were completed by French and U.S. labs (9). There was a tenfold increase in the number of positionally mapped human genes known to cause single-gene disorders. A physical map of the human genome with 15,000 markers was published (10). The genomes of several single-cell organisms were fully mapped and sequenced. A complete set of complementary DNAs (cDNAs) for the mouse genome was created, and technologies continued to improve with DNA microarray "chips" becoming widely available (see New Genomic Technologies and the Status of the HGP, below).

The HGP pace continued to gather speed in the late 1990s (11). The NIH funded six groups to attempt large-scale human genome sequencing as well as a new project to map human single nucleotide polymorphisms (SNPs). Celera, a new private company headed by Craig Venter and not bound by the Bermuda Principle, announced plans to complete human genome sequencing in 3 years using a different strategy of sequencing without prior positional mapping. Even this ambitious time frame was beaten, with both the HGP group and Celera announcing working drafts of the human genome in June 2000 with simultaneous publication in February 2001 (12,13).

RECENT FINDINGS OF THE HGP (14)

Both draft sequences are over 90% complete, and they show great agreement for the overlapping sequences. The 16 sequencing centers that contributed data to the HGP draft provided sevenfold coverage of the genome, so that a substantial portion (over 30%) of the sequence is free of gaps and ambiguities. The entire sequence should be available with this degree of reliability by 2003.

The human genome sequence is not yet fully complete, and the functional genomic research that must follow, and will surely occupy scientists for many decades to come, has barely begun. Nevertheless, the HGP has already yielded a plethora of insights into human genome structure and function. First, and most surprisingly, the total number of genes appears to be only about 30,000, which is a third of that previously estimated for humans and only twice that of *C. elegans*. Although the genome consists of over 3 billion base pairs, only 2% appears to code for proteins, and more than 50% consists of highly repetitive "junk DNA" sequences that do not have regulatory or coding function. Humans apparently generate most translation products via "alternative splicing" of mRNA so that the number of protein products actually is in the range of 100,000. The mechanisms controlling alternative splicing are poorly understood but are separate from those controlling posttranslational modifications such as methylation and glycosylation.

Human genes are enriched for GC base pairs, and are clustered randomly along chromosomes, separated by long stretches of AT-rich, noncoding DNA. Other sequenced species have more uniform distributions of genes along their chromosomes. The average human gene is 3,000 base pairs in size, but may range to over two million base pairs. At the time of this writing, function is known for only half of the human genes that have been sequenced. The HGP data and the research technologies associated with it should lead to vastly better understanding of multiple gene interactions as well as the functions of individual genes and their encoded products.

NEW GENOMIC TECHNOLOGIES AND THE STATUS OF THE HGP

Existing research strategies will continue to be used to explore the human genome and the multitudes of new questions raised by the information pouring from HGP-related studies. These strategies include gene amplification, DNA sequencing, probing for specific sequences with blot techniques, the investigation of nonhuman homologs of human genes, and the elucidation of DNA adduct formation and repair (see Chapter 35).

The HGP is also stimulating the development of new research technologies. New technologies and exponentially expanding databases (14) of genome structure and function (for humans and nonhuman species) are fueling both *genetic research* (the elucidation of the structure, control, and products of individual genes) and *functional genomic research* (the study of gene function in the context of the other genes, gene products, and regulatory processes that affect expression and variation) (15,16). A partial review of newer technologies may assist the reader in assessing current and future applications to medical practice:

DNA Microarrays

DNA microarrays (or DNA "chips") are fields of single-stranded DNA that may comprise tens or hundreds of thousands of oligonucleotides or cDNA strands. The chips themselves are small wafers, usually glass, and the DNA fragments bound to them can be "downloaded" in arrays based on known sequence so that each tethered DNA probe sits in a defined location. The array is then bathed in a solution of the labeled nucleic acid mixture that is to be probed. The nucleic acids being assayed could be derived from sources as diverse as a clone of tumor cells, an uncharacterized infectious pathogen, or the blood of a patient seeking information on inherited disease susceptibility. The nucleic acid fragments in solution are labeled with fluorescent or radioactive tags that can be read by standardized instruments after washout of nonhybridized material. The location of the labeled sequences on the microarray after hybridization identifies those gene fragments or transcripts as homologous to known probes. Conditions of hybridization can be varied to meet the needs of the experiment or test based on temperature, pH, electrical field, or other variables. In essence, microarray technology is a refinement of classic nucleic acid hybridization methods such as Southern or Northern blotting, reinterpreted in the context of DNA sequence information from the HGP.

DNA microarrays can be used in several ways (15,17). Most simply, they can qualitatively identify specific sequences. More than 2 million SNPs have been mapped across the human genome (7). Most genetic variation in humans appears to be due to SNPs, and many of these are likely to be associated with specific diseases. Microarrays can rapidly identify individual SNPs or other structural alleles known to cause inherited illnesses such as sickle cell disease or cystic fibrosis. Since microarrays are ideally suited for identifying multiple target sequences or patterns of genes, they can also identify markers known to increase the risk of, or susceptibility to, diseases of multigene etiology such as diabetes, certain malignancies, coronary artery disease, and Alzheimer's disease. Similarly, DNA microarrays are ideally suited to screen for an individual's potential risk for many possible diseases at once. Microarrays can also be used to rapidly identify pathogens, to screen for drug-resistance plasmids, or to identify clones of tumor markers associated with differential responses to chemotherapy agents.

Expression Profiles

A second major use for DNA microarrays is to identify "expression profiles," which are quantitative measurements of mRNAs (or cDNA copies of mRNAs) from tissue samples. With this technology, scientists can begin to explore regulatory pathways and functional genomics. The levels and pattern of mRNA production for specific genes and gene groups give a snapshot of cellular function at a single point in time. These levels and patterns can be followed sequentially to study developmental and disease states. Sets of co-regulated genes or "regulons" (15) may be identified, which will enhance the simpler concept of gene cascades in the control of normal development and pathophysiology. Expression profiles can also be used to study drug responses or lifestyle interventions at the level of the genome in different individuals (7,15,17) or populations.

Protein Arrays

A fascinating sequel to genomics research with microarrays is the parallel exploration of the "proteome," the fluctuating profile of protein expression in individuals. Proteins reflect the regulation and transcription of mRNAs, but may be even more diverse and potentially easier to study. The details of their posttranslational modifications, regulation, and functions are well beyond the scope of this chapter. However, it is clear that "protein chips" consisting of defined arrays of antibodies embedded in small surfaces can be used to probe for protein products just as DNA arrays can be used to probe for oligonucleotides, mRNAs, or cDNAs. Protein arrays could be used to look for multiple protein products, coexpressed protein products, and protein synthesis responses to drugs, toxins, or diseases just as DNA microarrays measure nucleic acids in these ways. This technology is likely to accelerate our understanding and utilization of the proteins, which are the ultimate products of the human genome (18).

Informatics

The exponentially proliferating data from the HGP on gene sequences, products, functions, and regulation pose a huge bioinformational challenge. The HGP leadership has committed to immediate public data access, although privately generated data may be restricted to varying extents (8,15). The HGP-derived databases can be analyzed in conjunction with other genetic/genomic databases of humans and nonhuman species, many of which are accessible by direct Internet links from the HGP Web site (19). However, even more powerful tools will be needed to integrate sequence, genetics, gene expression, homology, regulation, function, and phenotypic data in forms that are organized, accessible, and searchable (15) to support genomic research in the immediate future. It is not clear to what extent patent issues and privacy concerns will impact information availability, nor whether ELSI developments can be linked to these databases in a useful manner. It is clear that clinicians as well as researchers will have stay continually educated regarding the basic science, clinical applications, and ELSI potential of the HGP.

CLINICAL MEDICINE AND THE POTENTIAL IMPACT OF THE HGP

Standard medical practice is already influenced by genetic knowledge, and the HGP will accelerate this process. Classical genetics has identified a large number of human diseases with mendelian inheritance consistent with single-gene etiologies, most of which are relatively rare and many of which may have conveyed a selective advantage to heterozygotes. Examples include the thalassemias, cystic fibrosis, spinal muscular atrophy, muscular dystrophy, sickle cell anemia, retinoblastoma, hemochromatosis, and phenylketonuria. Prenatal and neonatal genetic screening for gene carriage is routinely available for screening and diagnosis of these conditions.

More common, adult-onset conditions such as diabetes, hypertension, vascular disease, emphysema, and allergy, which have more complex polygenic etiologies, are only beginning to be amenable to genomic testing. The burgeoning understanding of human gene sequence and function from the HGP, together with more powerful techniques such as microarrays to screen multiple gene sequences and transcripts, will bring genetic/genomic testing to the forefront of clinical medicine over the next decade (7). Examples of current and pending genomic testing capabilities in internal medicine are given below.

Primary Screening

Most adult diseases are the result of complex interactions between lifetime environmental exposures and genes, or gene combinations, that confer an increased risk (20). Genomic screening is being studied for many diseases with such complex etiologies including early-onset Alzheimer's disease (21), some breast cancers (22), nonmelanoma skin cancers (23), lung cancer (24,25), and diabetes (26).

It is important to realize that screening for gene products is already available for many more common adult-onset diseases. Simple lab tests already in daily clinical practice, such as lipid profiles and human leukocyte antigen (HLA) screening, measure the products of genes known to be associated with an increased risk of common diseases such as coronary artery disease, asthma, and inflammatory arthritides. They are genetic tests in a very real sense. Nevertheless, the ability to screen patients directly for genes that convey an increased risk for developing these diseases will give clinicians and their patients the earliest opportunities to intervene with dietary changes, lifestyle modifications, and drug therapies. Patients or populations with genomic risk for specific diseases may also benefit from increased surveillance for early diagnosis and treatment. However, ELSIs, including insurance access, discrimination, and social stigmatization, may adversely affect the same patients and populations (see HGP and Ethical, Legal, and Social Issues in the Workplace, below).

Genomic Surveillance in Primary Care Medicine

HGP-derived tests may also enable clinicians to facilitate secondary prevention by monitoring for genomic changes that indicate early disease in patients or populations at risk. Recently published studies have addressed genetic testing for early detection of colon cancer (27), lung cancer (28), and mutation loads due to environmental carcinogens (29). DNA microarrays are likely to increase the sensitivity of surveillance as well as screening tests by combining the predictive value of multiple gene sequences and/or gene expression profiles

Diagnosis, Prognosis, and Pharmacogenetics

Currently, some of the most widely used genomic tests are those used to characterize malignancies with respect to expression profiles that define specific diagnoses even in atypical presentations (30,31) and identify tumors with good or poor prognoses (32,33). Collins and McKusick (7) estimate that by 2020, it is likely that every tumor will have a known "molecular fingerprint," and nonmalignant diseases may be similarly subcategorized to guide counseling and treatment. Molecular diagnosis is therefore likely to play an ever-increasing role in the management of common as well as rare diseases. In this institution, the volume of molecular diagnostic testing has increased sixfold over the past 5 years (R. Wilson, personal communication).

Expression profiling (or "fingerprinting") will also identify patients (with malignant or nonmalignant diseases) who will most benefit from specific therapies or be most at risk for adverse drug reactions from specific therapies. That is, more complete knowledge of the human genome and its range of variations will allow clinicians to design therapies tailored to individual patients with specific diseases (34). This new field, termed *pharmacogenetics,* is likely to drive drug development and drug response monitoring through the coming decades. Reports have described genotypes less likely to respond to tacrine therapy in Alzheimer patients (35), more likely to develop thromboses on oral contraceptives (36), and more likely to develop nucleoside toxicity during HIV treatment (37). Many more drugs and vaccines may also be developed from human gene products, as some hormonal therapies are now (34). In 10 years, the majority of new drugs may be designed based on HGP data and associated clinical studies.

OCCUPATIONAL MEDICINE AND THE IMPACT OF THE HGP

The potential impact of new clinical tests derived from ongoing HGP research will present special opportunities and issues for OM physicians. The clinical practice of OM depends on (a) screening for susceptibility to occupational injury and illness, (b) surveillance or monitoring for exposure, (c) designing and implementing interventions to minimize hazardous exposures, (d) early diagnosis of occupational syndromes, and (e) treatment of occupational illnesses. All of these practice components are likely to expand as genomic testing and pharmacogenetics evolve over the next decade. In addition, when health insurance is provided primarily through the employer, as in the U.S., the employer acquires an interest in identifying genetic risk factors for disease and injury. The employer may hope to decrease costs by encouraging risk-reduction interventions—or by excluding high-risk persons from insurance or even employment. HGP-related ELSIs are therefore inevitable in OM practice (see HGP and Ethical, Legal, and Social Issues in the Workplace, below).

Preemployment Screening

Preemployment health screening has been recommended for decades as a means to increase workers' health, to decrease their risk of chronic disease, and to decrease employer costs. Most preemployment health screening tests over the last century have not been based in molecular genetics, although proxy genetic tests such as family history and blood counts have been widely used. However as early as 1938, Haldane (38) hypothesized that genetic factors might explain why some workers appeared more susceptible to toxic occupational exposures than others. He suggested that workplace genetic screening could improve public health by excluding vulnerable individuals from hazardous environments. Genetic testing technology was not available to Haldane, but his rationale was utilized to justify genetic screening beginning in the 1960s and 1970s (39–41). Since that time, genetic testing has been part of the employment screening armamentarium, although the predictive value and validity of these tests in reducing illness and costs is often questionable. Variable penetrance, incomplete understanding of gene–gene interactions, and the unpredictability of complex environmental exposures strongly limit the usefulness of occupational genetic screening outside research protocols at this time (see HGP and Occupational Epidemiology, below).

The range, sophistication, and predictive value of genetic and genomic testing for the workplace will increase in the near future (42). OM physicians will need to maintain up-to-date knowledge of (a) the biologic bases of the tests, (b) whether the tests have actually been linked to susceptibility phenotypes, (c) whether workplace screening is likely to decrease adverse medical outcomes, and (d) which interventions are available to protect susceptible workers. Some genetic tests currently or recently under investigation for susceptibility to workplace hazards are summarized in the Table 36.1.

The HGP is likely have its greatest immediate impact on primary care by genomic testing (i.e., multigenic profiling and expression profiling) to identify risks for common polygenic diseases such as coronary artery disease, diabetes, and hypertension. Similarly, it is likely to have its greatest immediate impact on OM screening by enhanced susceptibility testing for common polygenic conditions such as occupational allergies, occupational asthma, DNA-repair deficiencies, and connective tissue variants linked to musculoskeletal injuries. These examples are all multifactorial conditions where workplace engineering controls and protective equipment could be designed and targeted to reduce hazardous exposures for those at risk. It is even possible that expression profiles linked to behavioral characteristics may be utilized in preemployment evaluations (50), although the ELSIs would be even more problematic.

Genomic Surveillance and OM Monitoring

Genetic testing can be used like other biomarkers to screen for damage from hazardous exposures before the development of symptoms or disease states. The HGP will enhance this capability by furthering our understanding of clinically relevant sequence changes and DNA adduct formation. Recently, the detection of *k*-ras in workers with adenocarcinoma and exposure to asbestos has been reported. DNA adducts clearly have the potential to serve as surveillance tools (52–54) and are likely to become more useful as HGP sequence and microarray data enable us to understand which adducts are most reliably linked to adverse clinical outcomes (25,28).

The HGP will also allow researchers, and eventually clinicians, to detect expression profiles indicative of clinically relevant toxicity. HGP-derived expression profiles may be more sensitive and specific than nongenetic biomarkers (55). That is, just as pharmacogenomics is expected to lead to highly individualized therapeutic interventions and exquisitely sensitive monitoring of adverse drug reactions, the same types of expression profile and protein profile techniques should allow us to monitor individual reactions to toxins and perhaps infectious agents (56). One could think of this as "toxigenomics."

HGP and the Diagnosis and Treatment of Occupational Diseases

As expression profiles and DNA adducts may allow surveillance for predisease states indicative of

TABLE 36.1. *Examples of genetic and genomic screening tests in occupational medicine (OM)*

Marker(s)	Susceptibility hazard	Disease	Validated yet in workplace	Reference
HLA-DPbetaGlu69	Beryllium	Berylliosis (CBD)	No	43,44
Vitamin D receptor (VDR-B)	Lead	Hypertension	No	45
Delta-aminolevulic acid dehydratase (ALAD1, ALAD2)	Lead	Hypertension, heme synthesis	No	45,46
α_1-antitrypsin (A1AT)	Particulates	Chronic obstructive pulmonary disease	No	47
G6PD	Environmental oxidants	Hemolysis	No	48
Pseudocholinesterase variants	Organophosphates	Organophosphate toxicity	No	40
Cytochome P-450 polymorphisms	Aromatic hydrocarbons, etc.	Hepatic injury	No	48
PMP 22	Ergonomic stresses	Carpal tunnel syndrome	No	49

occupational toxicity (see above), they may also allow early diagnosis of occupational malignancies, such as bladder cancer, lung cancer, and skin cancer, and nonmalignant occupational diseases, such as fibrosing lung diseases, hepatotoxicity, and allergies. The rationale is the same as for nonoccupational diseases (7,30–33), but OM physicians may have special opportunities to make early diagnoses and therapeutic interventions in occupationally and environmentally defined risk groups.

Pharmacogenomics should likewise be as productive for OM as for other clinical fields. In the next two decades, OM physicians should expect to see vast improvements in drug efficacy and safety as chemotherapeutics, chelating agents, antitoxins, antibiotics, antivirals, vaccines, and other medications are targeted to individual workers' needs and genetic profiles—as well as to individual tumor or pathogen sensitivities (57).

HGP AND OCCUPATIONAL EPIDEMIOLOGY

In 1976, Milton Terris coined the term "second epidemiologic revolution" (58). The first epidemiologic revolution started with population-based studies of infectious diseases. Terris considers the second epidemiologic revolution to have started in the 1940s with investigations of noninfectious agents. These agents, primarily workplace toxins, included cigarette smoke, asbestos, vinyl chloride, bischloromethyl ether, and radiation. As a result of knowing the effects of these exposures, worker populations could be ranked by risk in groups. Surveillance and prevention programs in the workplace became possible. Irving Selikoff has noted that the third epidemiologic revolution is upon us. Molecular biology is the hallmark of the third epidemiologic revolution. Discoveries resulting from the application of molecular biology techniques, and more specifically from the application of HGP discoveries, will allow the stratification of workers into risk groups depending on their genomic makeup and the hazards to which they are exposed (58). More and more tests will allow for identification of genetic traits that may be associated with increased susceptibility to toxic exposures (48).

Enthusiasm for these potential advances must be tempered by the consideration that the science and technology behind these advances is not flawless. Research on studied markers has been mostly descriptive. Studies have shown associations between markers and exposures, effects or susceptibilities, but they have not provided a probability determination at either the individual or population level. The assessment of the probability of cancer given particular markers will require more prospective studies, nested case-control studies, studies using banked specimens, and integration of animal and human studies. There is also a need for further consideration of the paradigm of a continuum between exposure and disease. Not all markers will be specific for a particular exposure, but they may be predictive of cancer or inflammatory risk. The relationships between markers and diseases need further consideration (58).

Environmental health research must consider how the availability of genomic information might be used in early detection, intervention, and prevention programs. The National Institute of Environmental Health Sciences' Environmental Genome Project (EGP), launched in 2000, focuses on common sequence variations in environmental-response genes. Certain genetic polymorphisms affect metabolism of drugs and xenobiotics and thus seem to have important implications for human health. The EGP aims to identify such polymorphisms and clarify how polymorphic variation affects individual response to environmental exposures. Individuals with specific polymorphisms may not develop disease but may be at increased risk of developing disease if certain environmental exposures are present. These "susceptibility genes" may have different levels of penetrance (59).

Few biologic markers have met the ultimate test of being able to predict disease occurrence (60) (Table 36.1). As noted, individuals differ in their response to chemicals, medications, smoking, alcohol, ionizing radiation, and other environmental exposures. Genetic variability in human populations can affect entry, absorption, activation, and detoxification of environmental toxins. Because much of human disease results from a combination of environmental exposures and genetic variation, genomic technologic advances will affect disease prevention and allow clinicians to identify individuals and groups who are most at risk and direct early intervention efforts to them. Understanding specific relationships between genetic variation and response to environmental exposure is important for understanding disease causation and for developing effective disease prevention strategies (59).

OM specialists conduct biologic monitoring for occupational exposures. Recent applications of molecular biology and genetic screening promise to advance biologic monitoring from identifying simple associations between exposure and disease to gaining insight into previously unknown mechanisms and prevalence of diseases. Meaningful utilization of HGP data in OM research and practice will require linking that genomic information with exposure histories and outcomes. Defining exposures and outcomes for a study population has always been problematic in occupational epidemiology. Exposure histories are complicated by diverse confounding exposures and multiple sources of potential bias. Outcomes may be difficult to quantitate, including increased absences, decreased productivity, exacerbation of preexisting diseases, and injuries and illnesses to self or others.

In the context of epidemiologic research on low-penetrance genes, it is important to make the distinction between "susceptibility genes" and "disease genes."

As more is learned about how genetic factors influence our responses to environmental exposures, there may be a tendency to pathologize genotypic differences on the basis of perceptions of disease risk (59).

Another important consideration in interpreting tests is that if a test has a high sensitivity and specificity, but the disease prevalence is low, one will expect a high false-positive rate and a low positive-predictive value. In this circumstance, many people who test positive for the condition will not actually have it. Depending on the interpretation, this could lead to needless anxiety and potential exclusion from employment. OM professionals will need to be able to interpret and understand the results of these tests in the context of specific workplace factors, as the use of such tests may give rise to discrimination or restriction of a person's liberty to pursue one's chosen career (61).

The debate lies not so much with the technology but in how it is used. Single-gene disorders do exist (e.g., Alzheimer's disease and Huntington disease), which impact one's health and ability to perform at work. However, for complex disorders, the presence of a specific gene will indicate only one risk factor among many. Expressivity may be variable and penetrance incomplete. Carriers may never develop the disease linked to their genes, and people may also compensate for an increase in susceptibility by reducing the hazard (62).

HGP AND ETHICAL, LEGAL, AND SOCIAL ISSUES IN THE WORKPLACE

The vision of genetically based, individualized preventive medicine is exciting and could make profound contribution to human health. This remarkable achievement comes with a price, however. From its inception (7), the HGP leadership recognized the need to guard against abuse of genomic technology, especially among populations at highest risk, such as workers. There was the concern that the collection of genetic information might result in denial of employment or insurance on the basis of genetic susceptibility to an occupational agent (59). Employers might not want to hire or train workers they feared might become prematurely unable to work. Another concern is that worker selection and job placement may supplant protective environmental controls and stricter standards for permissible exposure limits (PELs) (63), as employers may eliminate workers by not hiring them, rather than eliminating the hazard or providing protective equipment (61). Many employers are concerned about the spiraling cost of health insurance and the possibility of genetic susceptibility to illness caused by exposure to workplace toxins (59). Employees may decline genetic testing for fear of employment discrimination, loss of primary medical insurance, and lack of privacy in the workplace. To prevent misuse of information, there is a need for solid legal and ethical systems to be in place. Legislative and regulatory strategies are needed to address these concerns, particularly when health insurance and employment are intertwined.

Laws addressing genetic discrimination in the workplace have been in existence for half a century. In 1955, the first law was passed in North Carolina prohibiting employers from discriminating against workers with sickle cell trait. A few years later, four other states passed laws prohibiting the same as well as discrimination against other carriers of other traits. In 1989, Oregon made it unlawful for employers to subject employees or prospective employees to many medical tests, and in 1991 Wisconsin prohibited workplace discrimination as well as employer access to genetic tests and provided privacy protections for employees. Similarly, in 1996, New Jersey prohibited employment discrimination based on genetic information. Many states, however, have been silent on genetic testing. Most jurisdictions are not prohibited from requiring genetic testing. Confidentiality of medical records is also an issue. There is concern about unregulated gathering and banking of data from genetic testing (58).

On the federal level, the Americans with Disabilities Act (ADA) and Health Insurance Portability and Accountability Act of 1996 (HIPAA) offer limited protection from discrimination but do not prohibit employers and insurers from gaining access to genetic information. HIPAA applies primarily to employer-based health insurance coverage. It provides that genetic information should not be used as a preexisting condition in the absence of diagnosis of the condition related to such information. It does not provide any privacy protection, however, nor does it protect the worker from higher insurance rates by the insurer. The ADA potentially offers protection from discrimination. However, the ADA focus is not protection of an employee's right to privacy. Although the ADA prevents employers from making preemployment medical inquiries, it does not prevent employers from obtaining medical information, including genetic information, after a conditional offer of employment. Employers can require a preplacement medical exam, which may include a physical examination and blood tests (including genetic tests). They may also require a general release of individual's medical records. Although an employer is prohibited from discriminating on the basis of a disability, it is difficult for the individual to prove that a lack of promotion, for instance, was due to having a disability or an undesirable genetic state. At present, there is no uniform protection against the use of, misuse of, and access to genetic information in the workplace. Even if employers do not use genetic testing, they may still have access to workers' medical records and thus the ability to know or guess if these individuals have genetic predispositions and/or susceptibilities to disease. It is important that the legal system address these issues. The ELSI component of the HGP will become more important to OM practice as more genomic screening becomes available.

HGP AND IMPLICATIONS FOR THE FUTURE

HGP research is likely to advance our understanding of disease mechanisms and lead to the availability of safer, more effective therapeutics. There will be potential for mass genetic screening with identification of workplace susceptibilities and predisposition to disease in essentially healthy people. This raises ethical and moral issues, which will inevitably impact OM practice.

Legal and ethical issues will continue to arise from the ability to identify genetic markers for susceptibility to work-induced diseases. Can employers demand tests of potential or current employees? Should employers deny jobs to those who are genetically at increased, but not absolute, risk for disease? Do laws prohibiting disability-based job discrimination protect workers with these traits? Do these tests allow early detection after exposure? If so, will the availability of these tests encourage employers to remove susceptible workers rather than to prevent exposures to occupational hazards?

The primary legislative approach to addressing genetic information in the workplace has been the prohibition of employment discrimination. Some laws try to prohibit both access to and use of genetic test results. Other laws provide for use of test results if the information is job-related. Some state laws allow genetic testing by employers in order to determine an employee's susceptibility to workplace toxins, although cleaning up the workplace would enhance safety for all employees and alleviate the needed for genetic testing of individuals (48).

Proposed legislation to protect individual privacy may inadvertently curtail important epidemiologic studies employing genetic markers to examine gene–environment interactions (64). However, these legal and ethical issues must be worked out if workers are to benefit from the HGP. OM physicians will need to stay abreast of ongoing developments in genomic research in order to serve their patients and influence policy.

REFERENCES

1. Watson JD, Crick FHC. Molecular structure of nucleic acids. *Nature* 1953;171:737–738.
2. Jackson DA, Symons RH, Berg P. A biochemical method for inserting new genetic information into SV40 DNA: circular SV40 DNA molecules containing lambda phage genes and the galactose operon of *E. coli. Proc Natl Acad Sci USA* 1972;69:2904.
3. Sanger F, Nicken S, Coulson AR. DNA sequencing with chain-terminating inhibitors. *Proc Natl Acad Sci USA* 1977;74:5463–5467.
4. Botstein D, White RL, Skolnick M, et al. Construction of a genetic linkage map in man using restriction fragment length polymorphisms. *J Hum Genet* 1980;32(3): 314–331.
5. Smith LM, Sanders JZ, Kaiser RJ, et al. Fluorescence detection in automated DNA sequence analysis. *Nature* 1986;321(6071):674–679.
6. Saiki RK, Scharf S, Faloona F, et al. Enzymatic amplification of beta-globin genomic sequences and restriction site analysis for diagnosis of sickle cell anemia. *Science* 1984;230(4732):1350–1354.
7. Collins FS, McKusick VA. Implications of the Human Genome Project for medical science. *JAMA* 2001;285 (5):540–544.
8. Collins FS, Galas D. A new five-year plan for the U.S. Human Genome Project. *Science* 1993;262:43–46.
9. Foote S, Vollrath D, Hilton A, et al. The human Y chromosome: overlapping DNA clones spanning the euchromatic region. *Science* 1992;258(5079):60–62.
10. Hudson TJ, Stein LD, Gerety SS, et al. An STS-based map of the human genome. *Science* 1995;270(5244): 1945–1954.

11. Collins FS, Patrinos A, Jordan E, et al. New goals for the U.S. Human Genome Project: 1998–2003. *Science* 1998;282:682–689.
12. Venter JC, et al. The sequence of the human genome. *Science* 2001;291:1304–1351.
13. International Human Genome Sequencing Consortium. Initial sequencing and analysis of the human genome. *Nature* 2001;409:860–921.
14. *www.ornl.govhgmisprojectinfo.html.*
15. Lockhart DJ, Winzeler EA. Genomics, gene expression, and DNA arrays. *Nature* 2000;405(6788):827–836.
16. Collins FS, Guyer MS, Chakravarti A. Variations on a theme: cataloging human DNA sequence variation. *Science* 1997;278(5343):1580–1581.
17. Shoemaker DD, et al. Experimental notation of the human genome using microarray technology. *Nature* 2001;409:922–927.
18. Service RF. High-speed biologists search for gold in proteins. *Science* 2001;294:2074–2077.
19. *www.ornl.govhgmislinks.html.*
20. Peltonen L, McKusick VA. Dissecting human disease in the postgenomic era. *Science* 2001;291:1224–1229.
21. Verlinsky Y, et al. Preimplantation diagnosis for early-onset Alzheimer disease caused by V717L mutation. *JAMA* 2002;287:1018–1021.
22. Wooster R, et al. Identification of the breast cancer susceptibility gene BRCA2. *Nature* 1995;378:789–792.
23. Nelson HH, Kelsey KT, Mott LA, et al. The XRCC1 Arg399Gln polymorphism, sunburn, and non-melanoma skin cancer: evidence of gene-environment interaction. *Cancer Res* 2002;62:152–155.
24. Fan R, et al. The p53 codon 72 polymorphism and lung cancer risk. *Cancer Epidemiol* 2000;9:1037–1042.
25. Duell EJ, et al. Polymorphisms in the DNA repair genes XRCC1 and ERCC2 and biomarkers of DNA damage in human blood mononuclear cells. *Carcinogenesis* 2000;21:965–971.
26. Yamagata K, et al. Mutations in the hepatocyte nuclear factor-4 (alpha) gene in maturity-onset diabetes of the young (MODY 1). *Nature* 1996;384:458–460.
27. Traverso G, et al. Detection of APC mutations in fecal DNA from patients with colorectal tumors. *N Engl J Med* 2002;346:311–320.
28. Kim DH, et al. P16(INK4a) and histology-specific methylation of CpG islands by exposure to tobacco smoke in non-small cell lung cancer. *Cancer Res* 2001; 61:3419–3424.
29. Burnouf D, et al. Molecular approach in cancer epidemiology: early detection of carcinogen-induced mutations in a whole genome. *Int J Mol Med* 2000;5: 15–20.
30. Alizadeh AA, et al. Distinct types of diffuse large B-cell lymphoma identified by gene expression profiling. *Nature* 2000;403:503–510.
31. Perou CM, et al. Distinctive gene expression patterns in human mammary epithelial cells and breast cancers. *Proc Natl Acad Sci USA* 1999;96:9212–9217.
32. Golub TR, et al. Molecular classification of cancer: class discovery and class prediction by gene expression monitoring. *Science* 1999;286:531–537.
33. Ross DT, et al. Systematic variation in gene expression patterns in human cancer cell lines. *Nat Genet* 2000; 24:227–235.
34. Collins FS. Medical and societal consequences of the human genome project. *N Engl J Med* 1999;341:28–37.
35. Poirer J, et al. Apolipoprotein E4 allele as a predictor of cholinergic deficits and treatment outcome in Alzheimer disease. *Proc Natl Acad Sci USA* 1995;92: 12260–12264.
36. Martinelli I, et al. High risk of cerebral-vein thrombosis in carriers of a prothrombin-gene mutation and in users of oral contraceptives. *N Engl J Med* 1998;338: 1793–1797.
37. Cote HCF, et al. Changes in mitochondrial DNA as a marker of nucleoside toxicity in HIV-infected patients. *N Engl J Med* 2002;346:811–820.
38. Haldane JBS. *Heredity and politics.* London: Allen and Unwin, 1938.
39. Murray TH. Ethical issues in human genome research. *FASEB J* 1991;5:55–60.
40. Billings P, Beckwith J. Genetic testing in the workplace: a view from the USA. *Top Genet* 1992;8:198–202.
41. Omenn GS. Predictive identification of hypersusceptible individuals. *J Occup Med* 1982;24:369–374.
42. Ishibe N, Kelsey KT. Genetic susceptibility to environmental and occupational cancers. *Cancer Causes Control* 1997;8:504–513.
43. Amicosante M et al. Beryllium binding to HLA-DP molecule carrying the marker of susceptibility to berylliosis glutamate beta 69. *Hum Immunol* 2001;62(7): 686–693.
44. Lombardi G, et al. HLA-DP allele-specific T cell responses to beryllium account for DP-associated susceptibility to chronic beryllium disease. *J Immunol* 2001; 166(5):3549–3555.
45. Lee BK, et al. Associations of blood pressure and hypertension with lead dose measures and polymorphisms in the vitamin D receptor and delta-aminolevulinic acid dehydratase genes. *Environ Health Perspect* 2001;109 (4):383–389.
46. Alexander BH, et al. Interaction of blood lead and delta-aminolevulinic acid dehydratase genotype on markers of heme synthesis and sperm production in lead smelter workers. *Environ Health Perspect* 1998;106(4): 213–216.
47. Mittman C, Barbela T, Lieberman J. Alpha 1-antitrypsin deficiency as an indicator of susceptibility to pulmonary disease. *J Occup Med* 1973;15:33–38.
48. Mohr S, Gochfeld, Pransky G. Genetically and medically susceptible workers. *OM: State of the Art Rev* 1999;14:595–611.
49. Agnall E. Genetic liability: is there a predisposition to injury? *Safety and Health* 2001;30–35.
50. Gilger JW. Contributions and promise of human behavioral genetics. *Hum Biol* 2000;72:229–255.
51. Nelson HH, et al. k-ras mutation and occupational asbestos exposure in lung adenocarcinoma: asbestos-related cancer without asbestosis. *Cancer Res* 1999;59: 4560–4573.
52. Perera FP, et al. Molecular and genetic damage in humans from environmental pollution in Poland. *Nature* 1992;360:256.
53. Shields PG, et al. Polycyclic aromatic hydrocarbon DNA adducts in human lung and cancer susceptibility genes. *Cancer Res* 1990;50:6580–6584.
54. Perera FP, et al. Detection of polycyclic aromatic hy-

drocarbon-DNA adducts in white blood cells of foundry workers. *Cancer Res* 1988;48:2288.
55. Schneider J, et al. p53 protein, EGF receptor, and anti-p53 antibodies in serum from patients with occupationally derived lung cancer. *Br J Cancer* 1999;80:1987–1994.
56. Nebert DW. Pharmacogenetics and pharmacogenomics: why is this relevant to the clinical geneticist? *Clin Genet* 1999;56:247–258.
57. Osdemir V, Shear NH, Kalow W. What will be the role of pharmacogenetics in evaluating drug safety and minimizing adverse effects. *Drug Safety* 2001;24:75–85.
58. Samuels SW, Upton AC, eds. *Genes, cancer, and ethics in the work environment.* Solomons Island, MD; Beverly Farms, MA: Ramazzini Institute/OEM Press, 1998.
59. Christiani DC, et al. Applying genomic technologies in environmental health research: challenges and opportunities. *J Occup Environ Med* 2001;43:526–533.
60. Schulte PA, Perrara FP, eds. *Molecular epidemiology: principles and practices.* New York: Academic Press, 1993.
61. Rawbone R. Future impact of genetic screening in occupational and environmental medicine. *J Occup Environ Med* 1999;56:721–724.
62. Deitchman S. Occupational medicine and molecular biology. *Lancet* 1994;l34:1427.
63. Rothstein MA. *Genetic secrets: protecting privacy and confidentiality in the genetic era.* New Haven: Yale University Press, 1997.
64. Wilcox AJ, et al. Genetic determinism and overprotection of human subjects (letter). *Nat Genet* 1999;2211: 362.

FURTHER INFORMATION

HGP Publication and Commentaries

Nature February 15, 2001.
Science February 16, 2001.

In addition to the first publication of the human genome, these issues contain multiple reviews of the historical, scientific, political, economic, and ethical issues raised by the HGP as well as related research regarding positional and functional mapping.

Human Genome Project information and related links: *www.ornl.govhgmislinks.html.*

This site provides background information, references, and links for physicians, scientists, and lay education as well as direct access to the HGP sequence data and related genomic databases such as GenBank and Online Mendelian Inheritance in Man (OMIM).

Technology Reviews

Friend SH, Stoughton RB. Microarrays. *Sci Am* 2002;286 (2):44–53.
Ezzel C. Proteomics. *Sci Am* 2002;286(4):40–47.

These reviews of current technology are well illustrated and suitable for patient and provider education.

37

Industrial Hygiene

J. Torey Nalbone and James P. McCunney

The physician who practices occupational medicine needs to have a working knowledge of many related disciplines, including epidemiology, toxicology, and industrial hygiene. The industrial hygienist especially can offer valuable assistance to the physician who is asked to consider the health risks associated with certain work settings. The industrial hygienist, usually a graduate-level professional, can help in many areas, but most often in the following:

1. Determining the need for medical surveillance or special examinations of workers exposed to particular materials (see Chapter 41).
2. Evaluating whether exposure to an occupational or environmental hazard may have contributed to the development of an occupational illness.
3. Determining the presence of potential offending agents and the adequacy of ventilation systems in outbreaks of illness, such as indoor air pollution (see Chapter 53).
4. Complementing the efforts of a physician who has completed a preliminary plant walkthrough (see Chapter 4).
5. Evaluating the presence of physical hazards in the workplace.

This chapter presents an overview of industrial hygiene, and discusses the types of hazards found in the workplace, their means of detection, and guidelines for interpretation of the results.

Industrial hygiene is concerned with identifying, preventing, and controlling occupational exposures that result in illness injury. Although it is a new field, it has accumulated a wealth of knowledge about the inner workings of the workplace. Conversely, important findings uncovered by astute physicians have steered the industrial hygienist in the right direction when searching for the offending agent. The relationship has proved valuable for both parties. A physician who suspects lead poisoning, for example, can ask an industrial hygienist to review the workplace for a source of lead. Joint efforts on behalf of the industrial hygienist and physician can reduce the time needed to reach an assessment. Ideally, the industrial hygienist's thorough knowledge of the workplace will be combined with the physician's knowledge of disease to minimize workplace hazards and prevent occupational illnesses.

The American Industrial Hygiene Association states that the hygienist "anticipates, recognizes, evaluates and controls those environmental factors or stresses" to protect the health of the worker and the community. Thus, the profession of industrial hygiene has as its main goals the anticipation, recognition, evaluation, and control of workplace health hazards. *Anticipation* is relatively new to the general principles of industrial hygiene and takes into account the experience the profession has had over the years. This experience in specific jobs, occupational settings, and industrial processes allows the industrial hygienist to specifically identify hazards that should be considered in the worker's exposure. *Recognition* of a hazard requires knowledge of both the processes and hazards of the materials used in the processes. A thorough grasp of these matters is essential as the foundation for a health hazard investigation. Reviewing the various hazardous materials used will reveal potential air contaminants. In addition, reviewing the process can also uncover air contaminants that may be released as an intermediate or as a decomposition product in the chemical reaction. Some decomposition products may be more hazardous than the raw materials.

After the type of air contaminant that may be released is determined, a sampling strategy can be developed that will provide the information needed to *evaluate* the hazards. Selecting a sampling strategy depends on the information that is sought. The data obtained from the monitoring of a person performing a process are then compared to exposure guidelines. For example, the Occupational Safety and Health Administration (OSHA) permissible exposure limit (PEL) for the air contaminants of concern may be used. This approach will determine whether the person is overexposed to any air contaminants and by how much.

If an overexposure exists or if there is a desire to reduce employee exposure, a *control* measure is then determined to bring the air contaminant concentration below the exposure guideline or to the desired level. Control methods typically employed are administrative, engineering or requiring the use of personal protective equipment. Another way to view these options is that we can reduce exposure by controlling the contaminant at the source, modifying the pathway that the contaminant travels, or isolating and protecting the worker. This hierarchy is followed to remove the contaminant or reduce the contaminant's concentration, and then, when all other mechanisms are inadequate or not feasible, to place protective equipment on the worker.

Administrative controls are implemented by either chemical substitution or by modifying the amount of time a worker is exposed to a particular job or substance. If a less hazardous material is introduced into the process and as a result the airborne exposure to a particular substance is eliminated, the hazard is controlled at the source. An engineering control, either actively or passively, reduces the exposure after it leaves the source. Noise barriers and local exhaust ventilation systems that effectively remove the contaminant are examples of how control can be exercised *at the pathway* of the contaminant or hazard. Finally, having people use personal protective equipment such as hearing or respiratory protection or work inside an enclosure will control the exposure *at the person.* This method of exposure control should be considered only during the installation of more permanent engineering controls, when the infrequency of exposure makes engineering impractical, or when available resources (economical or technologic) are not available, and thus other control measures cannot be considered.

Any of these methods will control or limit the exposure because the contaminant does not reach the person or its concentration is reduced. Ideally, the most desirable approach would be to eliminate the hazard altogether, for example, by replacing the material with a nonhazardous material. Controlling the hazard at the person by using respiratory protection is the least desirable approach because it is dependent on the person's work habits. An enclosure is preferable because it is independent of the worker's habits.

TYPES OF HAZARDS

The hazards found in the workplace can be divided into five types: gases/vapors, dusts, fumes/mists, physical agents, and biologic agents. An understanding of these hazards can be helpful to the physician because routes of entry of the contaminant, applicable personal protective equipment, and appropriate sampling methods will be determined by the type of hazard. In some instances, many types of hazards are present simultaneously. This situation not only makes evaluation more difficult for the industrial hygienist but also presents the physician with a more complicated array of factors to consider in diagnosing an occupational health problem.

Gases and Vapors

Gases are substances that are normally in the gaseous state at room temperature; in contrast, vapors are the gaseous state of substances that are normally in the liquid state at room temperature. For example, carbon monoxide is a common gas found in the workplace that is produced as a result of incomplete combustion (e.g., propane-powered forklift trucks, gasoline-powered engines, kerosene heaters). Trichloroethylene, in contrast, is normally a liquid but becomes vaporized when heated in a vapor degreaser. The main route of entry into the body for both gases and vapors is through inhalation. Some industrial chemicals, such as 1,1,2-trichloroethane, that are typically considered inhalation hazards also present a significant exposure risk when absorbed through the skin. If the cutaneous route contributes to the exposure of the individual, the designation "skin" will appear next to the name of the substance in either the American Conference of Governmental Industrial Hygienist's (ACGIH) Threshold Limit Value (TLV) book or OSHA's permissible exposure limits (1).

Dusts

Many types of dust are found in the workplace, including nuisance-type dusts, toxic dusts, and pneumoconiosis-producing dusts. Dusts can be generated by a variety of means. For example, the handling or dumping of a crushed solid like limestone creates dust that, although considered a nuisance dust, will result in exposure to the lungs in most people. The use of lead oxide in the manufacture of automobile batteries creates a toxic lead dust exposure. Foundries that use green sand molds to make metal castings have the potential for crystalline silica dust exposures (pneumoconiosis-producing) in work areas involving molding, shakeout, and grinding.

The contaminant dust size depends on the material used and the respective process involved. Large dust particles that can be seen with the eye (50 μm or more in size) may coexist with respirable-sized dusts (<10 μm in size). The upper respiratory tract, however, traps most of the large dust particles, whereas the respirable dusts reach the alveoli. For most substances suspended in air, the hazard is a function not only of the mass concentration but also of the particle size. For many years the ACGIH has included the particle-size consideration in its limits for crystalline silica. In recent years the ACGIH Chemical Substance TLV Subcommittee has considered the role of particle size–selective TLVs (PSS-TLV) for other contaminants (1).

The objectives of the PSS-TLV is to identify the size fraction associated with the health effects of interest and to focus on the mass concentration within that size fraction in establishing a TLV. The potential hazard caused by chemical substances present in air as suspensions of particles or droplets (aerosols) depends on the particle size and mass concentration. This is important to worker health because the effects may depend on the level at which the particle deposits and on the association of specific occupational diseases/conditions with specific regions of the lung.

The PSS-TLVs are divided into three categories: (a) inhalable particulate mass (IPM-TLV) for those substances that are hazardous regardless of where they are deposited in the respiratory tract; (b) thoracic particulate mass (TPM-TLV) for the substances that have the greatest hazard when deposited in the airways and the gas exchange portions of the lungs; and (c) respirable particulate mass (RPM-TLV) for the substances that are hazardous when deposited in the gas exchange region. Each of these categories has a particle range based on the collection efficiency as a function of aerodynamic diameter. The particle size ranges for these size-selective criteria are IPMs less than 100 μm, TPMs less than 25 μm, and RPMs less than 10 μm.

These particle size fractions are considered as contributing to the health effect of a chemical contaminant based on the size most commonly associated with an industrial operation and the mass fraction of material contained within a specific size fraction. This concentration would then represent the TLV for that chemical. The use of the PSS methodology to determine exposure poses a new set of considerations for the practitioner. Since the size of the particle is inversely related to the energy required to produce it, the operation generating the particle is now as important as the contaminant itself in the evaluation of exposure and ultimately in health effects (2–4).

Some fibers, such as fibrous glass and asbestos, can also be classified as dusts. Fibers are defined as particles having a length-to-width ratio (aspect ratio) of at least 3 to 1. The main route of entry for dusts is by inhalation, although some studies on the effects of cutaneous exposure to fibrous glass have shown the potential to cause or increase the occurrence of dermatitis.

Fumes and Mists

A fume is a solid that has been vaporized and subsequently condenses. In the process of welding steel, for example, iron oxide fume is produced. Zinc oxide fume is produced when welding galvanized metal. Excessive exposure to zinc and other metals can cause metal fume fever, an acute illness with symptoms similar to those of influenza, which usually occur a few hours after initial exposure. A metallic taste in the mouth, dryness of nose and throat, weakness, fatigue muscular and joint pain, fever, chills, and nausea usually last less than 24 hours. A temporary immunity usually follows; however, when workers return to the job after a weekend or holiday, the symptoms may return.

A mist is a liquid that has been dispersed into the air as fine droplets. Cutting oils used in a machine shop become oil mists from the action of the metalworking machinery. Chromic acid mist can be generated during chrome-plating operations by the bursting of hydrogen gas bubbles. Fumes and mists enter the body by inhalation but also can have localized effects on the skin and mucous membranes.

Physical Agents

Some physical agents encountered in the workplace are noise, heat, cold, ionizing and nonionizing radiation, lasers, and vibration. Since the physical agents involve a field of energy, the whole body can be at risk. Ionizing radiation is found in nuclear facilities and many other industrial processes in small doses, especially for instrumentation purposes. Microwaves, a form of nonionizing radiation, are found in areas near radar telecommunication devices. Some physical agents mainly affect only a part of the body; for example, noise affects the ear and lasers the eye. Excessive vibration from pneumatic construction equipment can lead to "white finger" disease, now known as hand–arm vibration syndrome. Vibration, in addition to ergonomic factors, can lead to cumulative trauma disorders (CTDs) (1,5).

Biologic Agents

Relative newcomers to the industrial hygiene scene are the biologic agents, which include bacteria, viruses, and fungi. With the development of genetic engineering, resource recovery of municipal solid waste, and indoor air pollutants, more attention is being paid to this area of occupational health. The use of biologic agents in research laboratories and hospitals has led to the development of indicator organisms, which can provide a measure of exposure to biologic agents. Much more work has to be completed in this area to give physicians and industrial hygienists an understanding of the significance of exposure measurements, which at this time are undefined.

Air sampling can be conducted for many organisms, but the interpretation of results can be problematic. For example, in outbreaks of hypersensitivity pneumonitis in an office setting, culturing of the filters from the air-handling system may yield a growth of thermophilic actinomycetes. It may also be demonstrated that afflicted individuals showed an antibody response (serum precipitation) to the same organism. Although it may appear logical to infer that the air-handling system caused the disease, this approach overlooks the fact that it is not uncommon to culture the same organism from environments without the disease and for people to show antibody responses though they do not have or never had the disease. This caveat emerges: Just because an organism is present does not mean it is causing a health problem. This is even more so the case recently as the airborne fungi have also made their way into the health arena. The identification of certain species of fungi in the indoor environment has changed. Sampling methods continue to be improved in an attempt to evaluate the extent of exposure to biologic agents in the workplace.

MONITORING

Monitoring employee exposure to air contaminants is the most visible aspect of the industrial hygienist's job. After the sampling strategy is determined, monitoring is performed to assess the extent of exposure to an air contaminant. Personal or area samples are obtained for monitoring. In personal sampling, the sampling device or equipment, or both, is placed on the worker (Figs. 37.1 and 37.2) to ensure the most accurate exposure determination. For area sampling, the sampling apparatus is placed in the vicinity of the worker performing the job. Although more convenient, area monitoring often is less precise than personal monitoring. Methods for monitoring air contaminants are given below. For specific methods, the reader is referred to publications listed under Further Information.

Gases and Vapors

Organic gases and vapors can usually be collected with an adsorbing material, like activated charcoal or silica gel. The adsorbing material is contained in a small glass tube that is attached to a sampling pump,

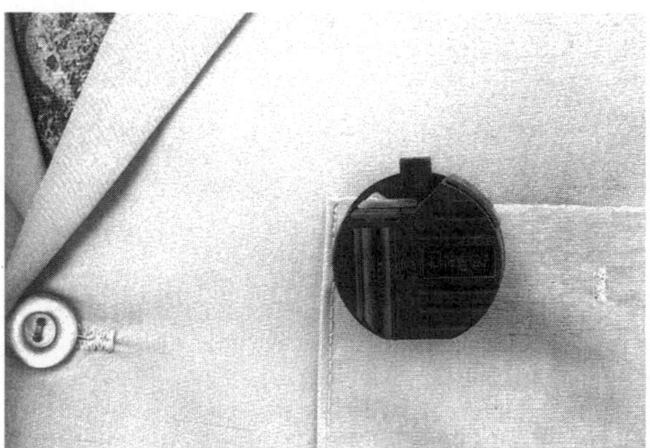

FIG. 37.1. A passive dosimeter air monitoring badge for formaldehyde. (Courtesy of Dräger Safety, Inc.)

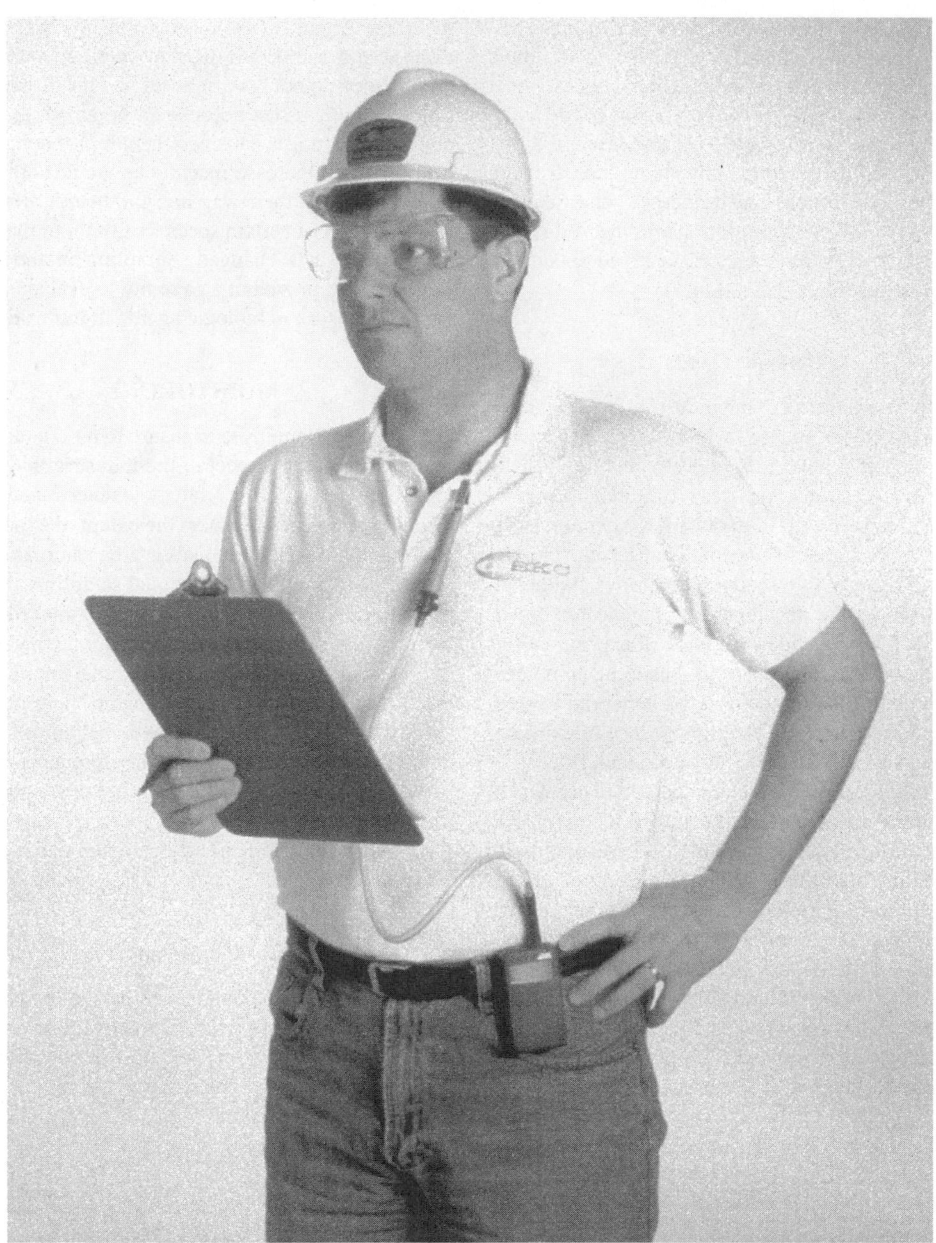

FIG. 37.2. A worker wearing an air sampling pump with a sorbent collection media to determine his exposure during the work shift. (Courtesy of SKC, Inc.)

which draws a known volume of air. Colorimetric tubes can also be used to determine the concentrations of contaminants in the work area. Designed similarly to the adsorbing tubes above, the solid material in the tube is chemically treated to cause a color reaction when the target substance is present. These types of sampling devices use a length of stain and the quantitation method for the target contaminant. Passive dosimeters that do not require an air-sampling pump are also used frequently. These devices consist of a collecting medium inside a badge. The air contaminant then diffuses from the air onto the col-

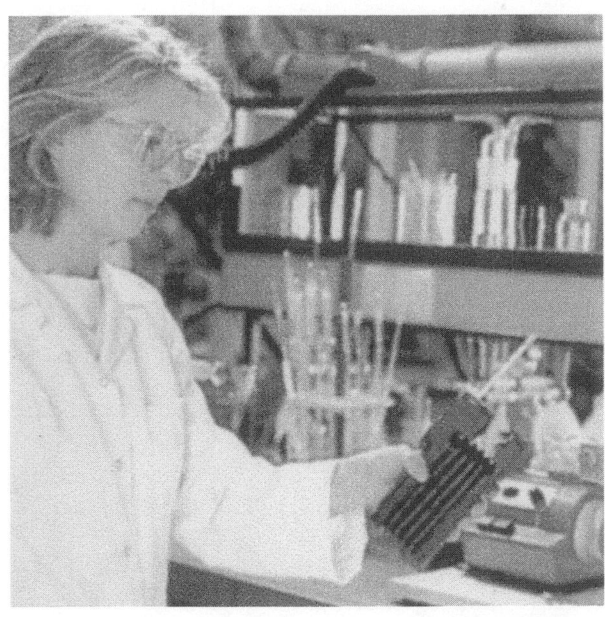

FIG. 37.3. Detector tubes that provide immediate air concentration indicated on a colorimetric scale. (Courtesy of Dräger Safety, Inc.)

lecting device. The concentration is determined based on the time the device was exposed to air and the amount of contaminant found on the collecting medium. The passive dosimeters can be either a colorimetric indicator or one that requires laboratory analysis. Inorganic substances can be collected in an impinger or bubbler whereby the contaminant is drawn into a liquid collecting medium using an air pump.

All of these methods, however, require the assistance of a qualified laboratory to analyze the sampling medium for the presence of the contaminant. Some methods that do not require laboratory analysis include detector tubes or direct-reading instruments that can give an immediate measure of the concentration of the air contaminant (Figs. 37.3 and 37.4). This ability is especially important to workers required to enter work spaces that are not adequately ventilated, such as confined spaces, to perform short-term tasks (Fig. 37.5). Gases and vapors are usually reported in parts per million (ppm) units, a volume per volume measurement.

Dusts

Dusts, including asbestos, coal, wood, and silica, can be monitored using a variety of instruments. The method used will depend on the type of dust, the size of the dust, the PEL or TLV, and the cost of the method. The most common method is to collect the dust on a preweighed filter medium using an air-sampling pump. The filter is then weighed after the sampling is completed and, along with the volume of air displaced during the sampling, the concentration of the contaminant can be determined. This method, also known as a gravimetric analysis, is used with nuisance-type dusts and dusts that do not require identification.

The type of dust may determine the sampling method. Asbestos, for example, can be sampled with the filter method mentioned above. The filter medium is not weighed, however, as it is for nuisance dusts, but undergoes a microscopic analysis to determine the fiber count, rather than weight.

The size of the dust may also determine the sampling method. If a total dust measurement is desired, the gravimetric analysis mentioned above can be used. This will collect both large dust particles and small dust particles based on the filter pore size. Respirable dusts (those of 10 μm or less in size) are monitored differently. In addition to an air-sampling pump, a cyclone is used to separate the respirable from the larger dusts. This method is used to monitor respirable dusts, such as silica, that affect the terminal parts of the lungs.

Cotton dust is sampled using a vertical elutriator, a sampling method specifically mentioned in the OSHA cotton dust standard. In this case the PEL or TLV may determine the particular sampling method used.

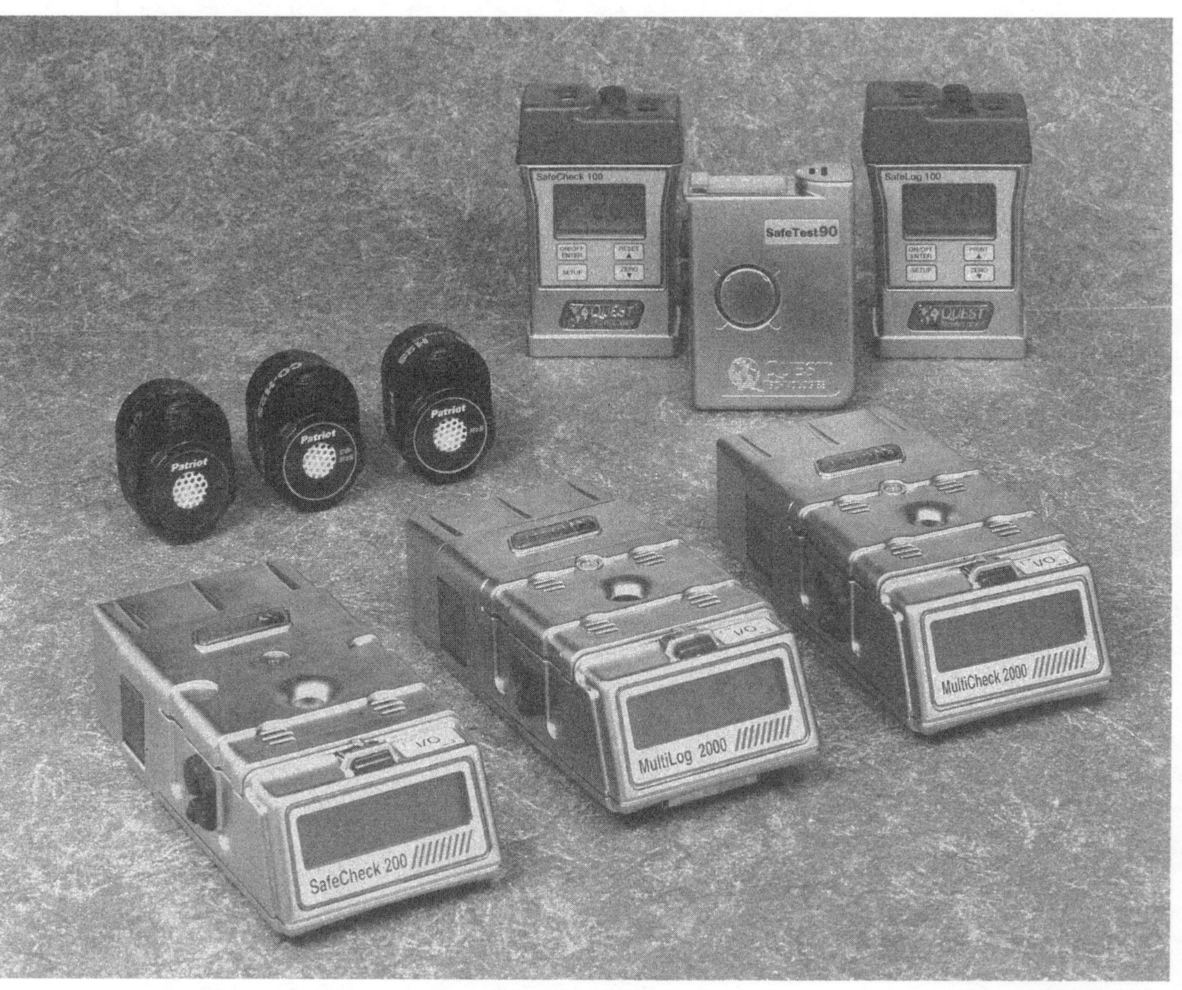

FIG. 37.4. Direct reading instruments for monitoring hazardous atmospheres and gases. (Courtesy of Quest Technologies.)

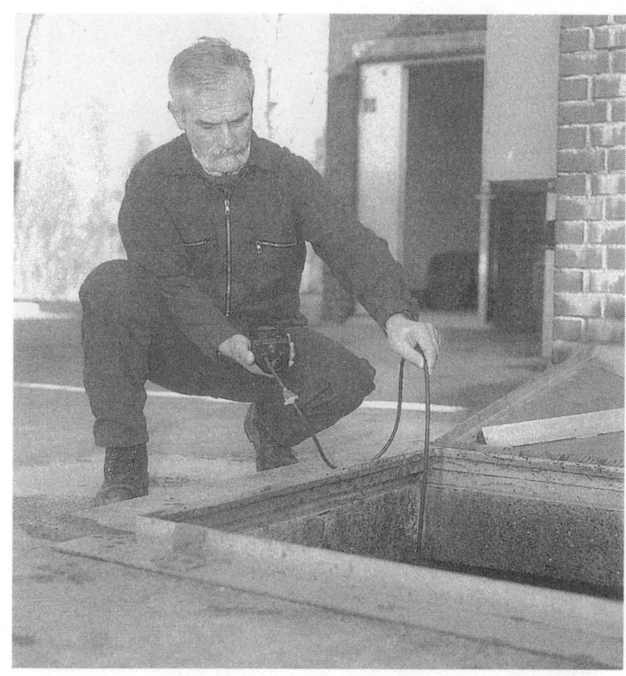

FIG. 37.5. Worker sampling a confined space with a direct reading instrument prior to entering the work area. (Courtesy of Dräger Safety, Inc.)

Cost is also a consideration for air sampling. New electronic instruments such as fibrous aerosol monitors used for monitoring asbestos and other fibrous materials can be expensive to purchase. Electronic instruments are also available to monitor total and respirable dusts. More sophisticated sampling analyses can also be expensive. Reliability and accuracy of results also come into consideration when evaluating the different methods. The ultimate choice of a sampling and analytic method, therefore, depends on consideration of all these various factors.

Fumes and Mists

Fumes and mists are collected on filters, like dusts, and analyzed in the laboratory. For example, a welder can be sampled for iron oxide fume through the use of a filter cassette, which is later analyzed by the chemist for the presence of iron.

Physical Agents

Physical agents such as noise, heat, and microwaves are usually monitored with electronic instruments that respond to the energy of the agent. Noise, for example, is monitored with a sound level meter or noise dosimeter. The sound level meter gives an immediate reading of the noise level; some instrument models are capable of integrating the noise dose over the exposure time (Fig. 37.6). Many of the sound level meters on the market currently are capable of assessing noise exposures under different conditions, and several have an electronic filter that collects sound level information by octave. This information can be essential to the industrial hygienist when control measures are considered and may also give the occupational medicine physician important information about the source of noise that can induce hearing loss. The noise dosimeter, another survey tool for the noisy work environment, accumulates the noise data over a period of time and reads out an average decibel level or a percent dose. [The reference used for the dose calculation is the PEL, i.e., 90 dBA (decibel measured on the A scale, slow response) for 8 hours' duration = 100% dose (see Chapter 26).]

Environmental temperature and humidity can also present a significant physical stress to workers in a variety of occupations. The industrial hygienist can measure the impact of these physical conditions as a heat stress index using other direct-reading electronic instruments.

Biologic Agents

Microorganisms can be sampled using a variety of methods, but commonly with a particle-sizing device.

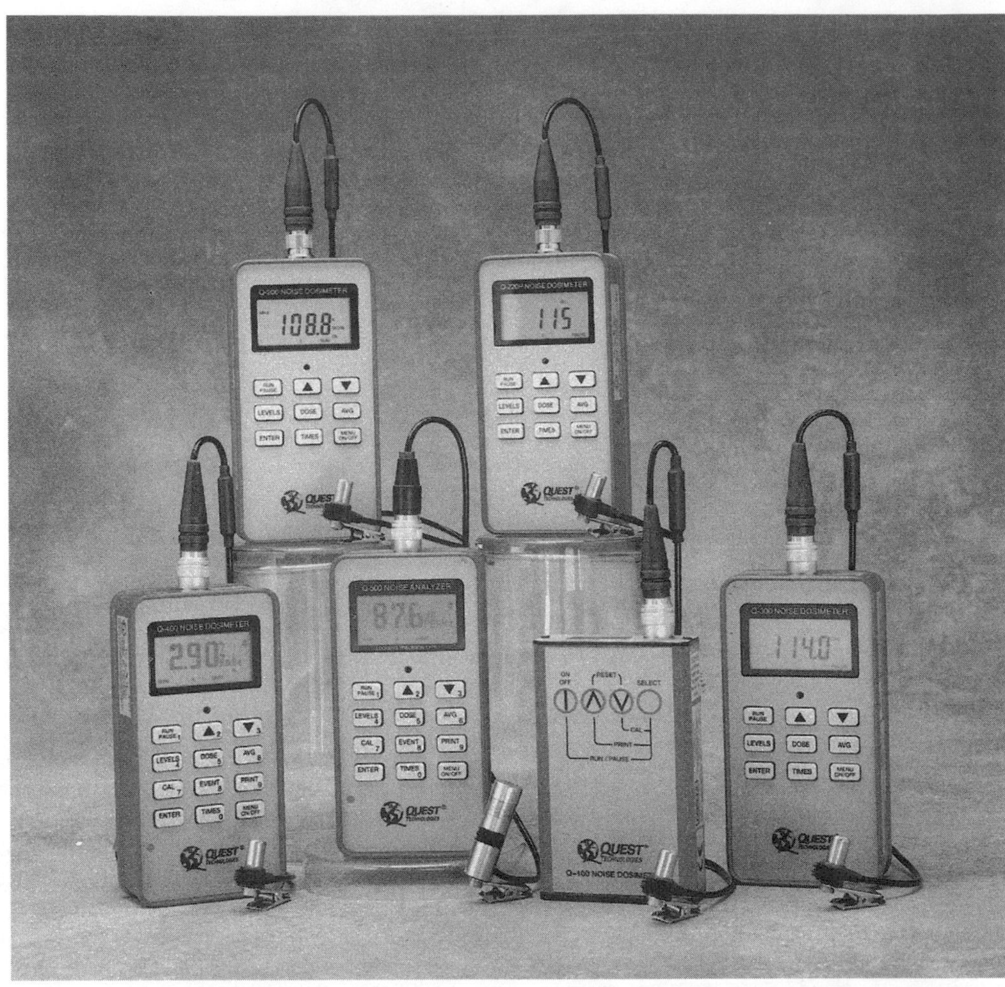

FIG. 37.6. Noise dosimeters and sound level meters used to evaluate a worker's exposure to noise. (Courtesy Quest Technologies.)

The various plates can then be incubated and counted to determine the airborne concentration. Typically most of the biologic agent (bioaerosol) sampling has been accomplished using a single-stage modification of the multistage samplers like the Anderson eight-stage cascade impactor. Since bioaerosol sampling was classically undertaken for bacteria or other infectious agents, the viable sample collected in the cascade-type impactor with agar plates was the most useful information for the practitioner. However, changes in the sampling methodology were indicated as the question in investigation became one of irritation and allergic-like reactions, and the need to assess the overall allergenic load became important. More recently, slit impactors like the Zefon Air-O-Cell (Fig. 37.7) have been extensively used in the nonviable sampling of bioaerosols. Another development in the viable sampling of biologic agents has been the specialized liquid impinger, which is designed to reduce the force and pressure normally encountered in conventional impingers (Fig 37.8). Sampling, however, is not usually recommended unless a source of a biologic agent is known to exist in the building or area.

However, when the decision to sample for bioaerosol contamination is made, several issues about the method of sampling and analysis must be assessed. Since there are currently no regulations covering the concentration of mold spores in a particular setting or an approved collection method, the decision to sample must be based on either identifying the source of contamination within a facility (i.e., home, office, school) or eliminating excessive mold

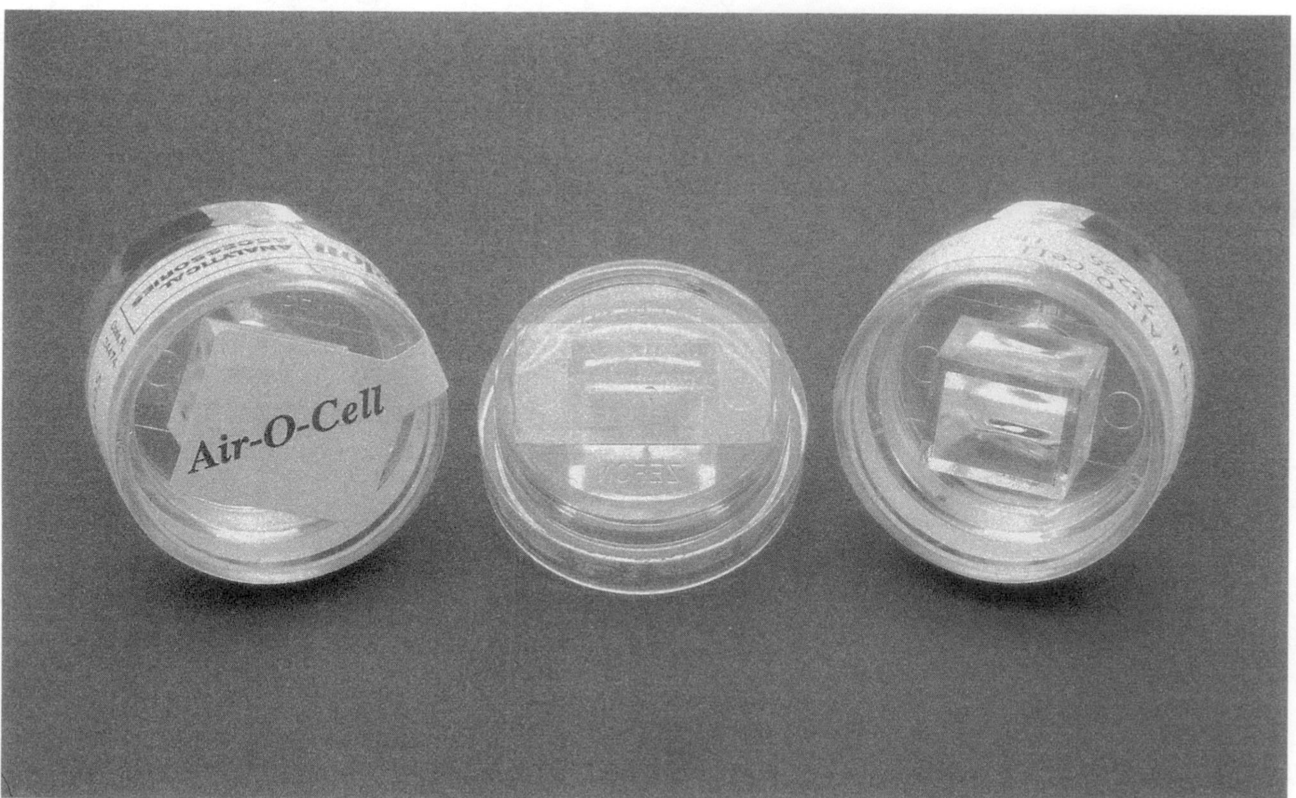

FIG. 37.7. Nonviable sampling Air-O-Cell cassettes used for particulate matter (fungal spore) collection. (Courtesy of Zefon, Inc.)

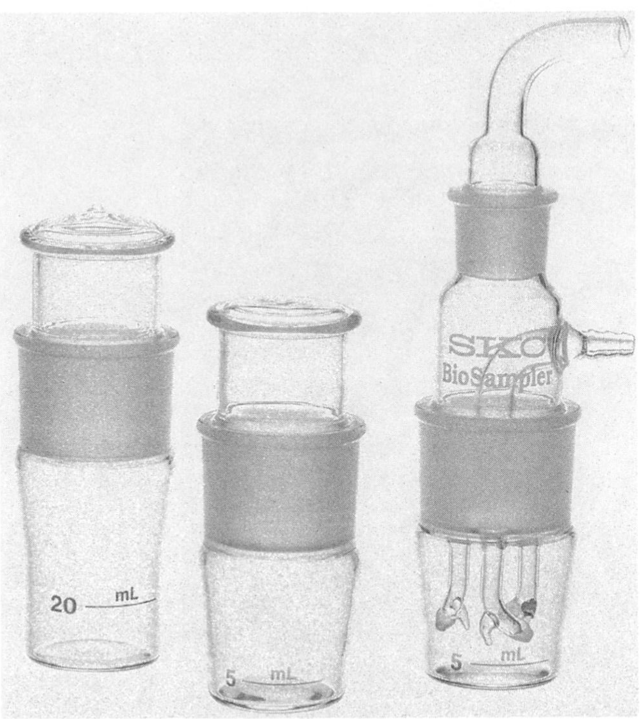

FIG. 37.8. Liquid sampler for viable sampling of bioaerosols. (Courtesy of SKC, Inc.)

exposures as a causative agent. Several states have adopted rules that address the presence of moisture or visible growth in a facility, but those typically only apply to public buildings, especially schools, or as a condition of property transfer or insurance.

Currently the Zefon Air-O-Cell (Fig. 37.7) is one of the predominant collection media utilized for mold sampling. When connected to an air pump with a fixed flow rate, a quantitative evaluation of spores can be derived. After microscopic examination, the results include an identification of the genus of mold spore present using morphologic characteristics and reported as spores per cubic meter of air. One of the limitations of this technique is that molds with similar spore morphologies, like *Aspergillus* spp. and *Penicillium* spp. cannot be exclusively identified. For this reason, viable sampling, the use of agar media plates, is still done on a case-by-case basis. Since the results from this method are reported as colony-forming units per cubic meter of air, the growth potential of the contamination can be ascertained.

Another common method for determining mold contamination is the surface sample. These samples are collected typically using either a swab method or a "tape-lift" method. Both samples are prepared for microscopic examination and spores identified in a similar fashion as the Air-O-Cell sample. The advantage of the swab sampling technique is that it could be converted to a viable sample if the swab contents were transferred to an agar plate in streak fashion. The development of a mold-sampling strategy is discussed in several texts (7,8).

OCCUPATIONAL EXPOSURE LIMITS

One of the most difficult questions asked of occupational health professionals is, What is the safe level of exposure to this chemical? To address the question definitively, all the current data and variations within exposures must be taken into account. To deal with the variability of exposures, the industrial hygiene professional relies on exposure guidelines to evaluate the significance of exposure levels to air contaminants. Workplace health professional should be familiar with as many of these guidelines as possible and should have them available for easy reference. The exposure limits suggested by the guidelines do not have the force of law in the United States but do offer the practitioner a wide variety of sources. Some of the available exposure guidelines are included here. Table 37.1 lists the voluntary exposure guidelines established by various sources, both in the United States

TABLE 37.1. *Recognized occupational exposure guidelines*

Guideline	Recommending organization
Threshold Limit Values (TLVs)	American Conference of Governmental Industrial Hygienists (ACGIH)
Biological Exposure Indices (BEIs)	ACGIH
Workplace Environment Exposure Limit (WEEL)	American Industrial Hygiene Association (AIHA)
Recommended Exposure Limits (RELs)	National Institute for Occupational Safety and Health (NIOSH)
Maximum Allowable Concentration (MAK)	Deutsche Forschungsgemeinschaft (Germany)
Occupational Exposure Limit (OEL)	Health and Safety Commission and Health Safety Executive (Britain)

and abroad. Table 37.2 lists the guidelines that have been established by the regulatory agencies in this country. Table 37.3, although not inclusive, lists some of the community-based exposure levels that are available for non–work-related exposure assessment. All levels refer to airborne exposures, except for the biologic exposure indices, which refer to safe biologic levels of the substance or its metabolite in body fluids or in expired air. Exposure guidelines can suggest to the occupational health professional how bad or good, in simplistic terms, a workplace or environmental exposure is. The TLVs developed by the ACGIH are updated annually and are meant to protect nearly all workers from adverse effects when they are repeatedly exposed to an agent. These values are the most comprehensive, have been in existence the longest, and are used by many regulatory authorities around the world. In the introduction to the TLVs, the TLV committee elaborates by stating that "because of wide variation in individual susceptibility, however, a small percentage of workers may experience discomfort from some substances at concentrations at or below the threshold limit; a smaller percentage may be affected by *aggravation* of a pre-existing condition or by development of an occupational illness" (1).

The TLV committee of the ACGIH points out that these levels are not to be used as a fine line between safe and dangerous concentrations. The committee also warns against the use of the guidelines as proof or disproof of an existing disease or physical condition. If a worker's exposure to an agent is below the level given in the guidelines, one cannot necessarily conclude that the exposure is safe for that person or that his or her symptoms are not related to the exposure. Similarly, overexposure to an agent does not necessarily mean that the agent is responsible for the noted symptoms. Other factors, especially potential confounders such as cigarette smoking, should be considered.

Although officially the TLVs are guidelines for good practices, they have assumed the power of law after OSHA adopted the 1968 TLVs as their PELs. The rationale for the TLV guidelines, which are based on industrial hygiene experience and experimental studies on animals and humans, can be found in the *Documentation of the Threshold Limit Values* published by the ACGIH.

The Biological Exposure Indices (BEIs), also published by the ACGIH, are warning levels of biologic response to a chemical or its metabolite (Tables 37.4 and 37.5). These values may be of use to a physician in determining a dose to a worker because other routes of entry besides inhalation may be involved (1). For example, blood lead analysis reflects the relative dose that the worker receives from all routes of exposure, including ingestion.

The use of biologic indices has been limited, however, because of the wide range in individual response to hazardous agents and the wide range in what is considered normal. In addition, sensitive analytic

TABLE 37.2. *Regulatory (occupational exposure) limits*

Regulatory limit	Regulatory agency
Permissible exposure limits (PELs)	Occupational Safety and Health Administration (OSHA)
New chemical exposure limit (NCEL)	U.S. Environmental Protection Agency (EPA)

TABLE 37.3. *Community-based exposure limits*

Exposure limit	Recommending body
Emergency Response Planning Guide (ERPG)	AIHA
Reference concentration (RC)	EPA

TABLE 37.4. *Airborne chemicals for which biologic exposure indices (BEIs) have been adopted*

Airborne chemical	Determinant
Acetone	Acetone in urine
Acetylcholinesterase inhibiting pesticides	Cholinesterase activity in red blood cells
Analine	Total *p*-aminophenol in urine
	Methemoglobin in blood
Arsenic, elemental and soluble inorganic compounds	Inorganic arsenic plus methylated metabolites in urine
Benzene	S-Phenylmercapturic acid in urine
	t,t-Muconic acid in urine
Cadmium and inorganic compounds	Cadmium in urine and blood
	Cadmium in blood
Carbon disulfide	2-Thiothiazolidine-4-carboxylic acid in urine
Carbon monoxide	Carboxyhemoglobin in blood
	Carbon monoxide in end-exhaled air
Chlorobenzene	Total 4-chlorocatechol in urine
	Total *p*-chlorophenol in urine
Chromium VI	Total chromium in urine
Cobalt	Cobalt in urine
	Cobolt in blood
N,N-Dimethylacetamide	*N*-Methylacetamide in urine
N,N-Dimethylformamide	*N*-Methylformamide in urine
	N-Acetyl-S-(*N*-methylcarbamoyl) cysteine in urine
2-Ethoxyethanol and 2-ethoxyethyl acetate	2-Ethoxyacetic acid in urine
Ethyl benzene	Mandelic acid in urine
	Ethyl benzene in end-exhaled air
Fluorides	Fluorides in urine
Furfural	Total furoic acid in urine
n-Hexane	2, 5-Hexanedione in urine
	n-Hexane in end-exhaled air
Lead	Lead in blood
Mercury	Total inorganic mercury in urine
	Total inorganic mercury in blood
Methanol	Methanol in urine
Methemoglobin inducers	Methemoblobin in blood
2-Methoxyethanol and 2-methoxyethyl acetate	2-Methoxyacetic acid in urine
Methyl chloroform	Methyl chloroform in end-exhaled air
	Trichloroacetic acid in urine
	Total trichloroethanol in urine
	Total trichloroethanol in blood
4,4′-Methylene bis (2-chloroaniline) (MBOCA)	Total MBOCA in urine
Methyl ethyl ketone (MEK)	MEK in urine
Methyl isobutyl ketone (MIBK)	MIBK in urine
Nitrobenzene	Total *p*-nitrophenol in urine
	Methemoglobin in blood
Parathion	Total *p*-nitrophenol in urine
	Cholinesterase activity in red cells
Pentachlorophenol (PCP)	Total PCP in urine
	Free PCP in plasma
Phenol	Total phenol in urine
Styrene	Mandelic acid in urine
	Phenylglyoxylic acid in urine
	Styrene in blood
Tetrachloroethylene	Perchloroethylene in end-exhaled air
	Perchloroethylene in blood
	Trichloroacetic acid in urine
Tetrahydrofuran	Tetrahydrofuran in urine
Toluene	*o*-Cresol in urine
	Hippuric acid in urine
	Toluene in blood
Trichloroethylene	Tricloroacetic acid in urine
	Free trichloroethanol in blood
	Trichloroethylene in blood
	Trichloroethylene in end-exhaled air

TABLE 37.5. *Airborne chemicals for which biologic exposure indices are proposed*

Airborne chemical	Determinant
Dichloromethane (methylene chloride)	Dichloromethane in urine
n-Hexane	2,5-Hexanedione (free) in urine
Methl *n*-butyl ketone	2,5-Hexanedione (free) in urine
Trichloroethylene	Trichloroacetic acid in urine
	Trichloroethanol (free) in blood
	Trichloroethylene in blood
	Trichloroethylene in end-exhaled air

methods specific for certain materials are lacking. The BEIs are particularly useful, however, in evaluating situations where skin absorption may occur, as indicated by the notation "skin" next to a substance's entry in the TLV book. The BEIs are usually based on epidemiologic and/or pharmacokinetic analysis of the metabolism of the agent in controlled human studies, The BEIs should be used only when relating to an 8-hour exposure (see the discussion of biologic monitoring under the heading "Lead" in Chapter 25).

The OSHA PELs are published in the Code of Federal Regulations (29 CFR 1910) for general industry. These limits were adopted in 1971 along with the other OSHA regulations. Most of the exposure limits are found in subpart Z of the regulations, where over 400 PELs are listed. In addition, there are permissible exposure limits in specific standards, such as lead (CFR 1910.1025.) These standards cover other aspects of lead exposure as well as the PEL.

In 1989, OSHA, through a generic rule-making procedure, updated the 1971 permissible exposure limits and added some PELs for substances not previously regulated in the air contaminants standard. This approach was a departure from OSHA's previous method of updating a PEL on an individual basis. At that time over 428 exposure limits were addressed.

On July 7, 1992, the United States Court of Appeals, Eleventh Circuit, issued a decision to vacate the air contaminants standard. Since OSHA did not appeal this decision to the Supreme Court, the decision stands. The decisions by both the court and OSHA have created a hodgepodge of PELs across the country. For the states covered by the federal OSHA program, the original PELs adopted when OSHA began are the standard to be complied with. However, states and territories with an OSHA-approved state plan had the opportunity to choose their regulatory limits. Some have reverted to the 1971 PELs, while others have kept the updated PELs or gone on to promulgate their own limits for selected contaminants. OSHA, nevertheless, believes the 1989 PELs are more protective and encourages employers to continue compliance efforts to meet those levels, particularly where engineering and work practice controls have already been implemented.

Most exposure limits are defined in 8-hour time-weighted averages. Other values refer to "ceiling" limits (2). A time-weighted average is usually based on an 8-hour work shift; however, some situations require appropriate adjustments for unusual work hours. The 8-hour time-weighted average is a method of calculating a full-shift average exposure by weighting short-term average concentrations by exposure time. For example, if an employee is exposed to carbon monoxide at 100 ppm for 4 hours and none for the remainder of the shift, the 8-hour time-weighted average would be 50 ppm. Ceiling values, which should never be exceeded, are usually assigned to strong irritants, cardiac sensitizers, and carcinogens. A short-term exposure limit (STEL) is another exposure limit used and is typically assigned to exposure times of 15 minutes or less.

Characteristically the work environment is dynamic and often workers are exposed to several chemicals simultaneously. When the chemicals have different toxicologic effects or target organs, the effects are not considered to be additive and are addressed as individual contaminants. However, if a worker is exposed to more than one chemical that acts on the same system, the combined additive effect of the agents must be considered. To evaluate this situation the exposure concentrations are entered into a mixture formula, and if the result exceeds 1, an overexposure situation exists. For example, if an employee is exposed to 800 ppm acetone (PEL of 1,000 ppm) and 130 ppm methylethyl ketone (PEL of 200 ppm), the calculation is made as follows:

$$\frac{C_1}{L_1} + \frac{C_2}{L_2} + \frac{C_3}{L_3} = E_m$$

where

E_m = the equivalent exposure for the mixture
C = the concentration of a particular contaminant
L = the exposure limit for that contaminant

$$\frac{800}{1000} + \frac{130}{200} = 1.45$$

As evidenced by the example, neither acetone nor methyl ethyl ketone alone was above regulated PELs, but their mixture suggests an overexposure. The Workplace Environmental Exposure Limits (WEELs) and National Institute for Occupational Safety and

Health (NIOSH) Recommended Exposure Limits (REL) are fewer in number but are also valuable guidelines to evaluate worker exposure. WEELs are published periodically in the *American Industrial Hygiene Association Journal.* NIOSH recommendations are found in the criteria documents and *Current Intelligence Bulletins.* Criteria documents are summaries of the scientific literature on a specific chemical, which also include recommended exposure guidelines. These documents also contain information on controlling the hazard, appropriate personal protective equipment, and the rationale for selecting the recommended guideline.

INDUSTRIAL HYGIENE SERVICES

If a patient's symptom or illness is suspected as being caused by the workplace environment, industrial hygiene data should be reviewed, if available. By comparing the level of exposures in the workplace to the various guidelines, the physician can form a preliminary opinion regarding the contribution of the workplace environment to a particular illness. For example, OSHA states that if an employee's airborne exposure to lead is maintained at 50 $\mu g/m^3$, the blood lead concentration should be approximately 40 µg/100 g whole blood. If hygiene data indicate that the employee's exposure at work is not high enough to produce the elevated blood levels observed, personal habits, such as eating or smoking at the workstation, or activities outside of work should be considered. The physician may learn that the individual was exposed to lead when stripping lead-based paint at home or while engaged in a hobby such as stained glass assembly. There are other substances to which OSHA requires an affirmative action by employers to institute medical surveillance and, depending on examination results, remove a worker from exposure. These can be found in the substance-specific regulations in 29 CFR 1910 and include as examples cadmium and noise.

Industrial hygiene data may be available from various sources for a particular workplace. Federal or state OSHA offices or the workers' compensation insurance carrier may have conducted an investigation of the facility and have industrial hygiene data that could prove helpful to the physician. A call to the employer or to the OSHA office will help in locating the survey if one has been done.

An industrial hygiene consultant or company industrial hygienist may also have done a survey of the workplace. This information would have to be obtained from the employer. NIOSH, a research arm of the federal government, also conducts industrial hygiene surveys, which can be requested by interested parties including employees, unions, and physicians. Although fewer in number, these reports are comprehensive and can prove useful to a physician.

If industrial hygiene data do not exist for a particular operation or plant, the physician can ask the local OSHA office to conduct an inspection based on suspected occupational health problems. This request can be initiated by writing or calling the local office. OSHA will investigate the physician's concern and report conclusions of the findings to the physician. This option should be kept in mind, since the physician may be the only person suspecting the workplace hazard and therefore the one who can then help correct the situation in the workplace for the patient and other workers. Another option is for the physician to discuss the concerns with the employer and have the employer request a consultation visit from the local OSHA consultants. This service is available from either OSHA directly or a state agency at no cost to the employer. The findings will not result in citation and the employer will be provided guidance and opportunity to remedy the hazards that are discovered during the consultation visit.

Often a physician may evaluate a patient who works for a company that does not have an industrial hygienist on staff. In this case, an industrial hygiene consultant can perform the needed services, which may range from a complete industrial hygiene survey to selective air sampling for certain substances such as carbon monoxide. A listing of industrial hygiene consultants can be found each year in the January/February issue of the *American Industrial Hygiene Association Journal.* Certified industrial hygienists (CIHs), as diplomats of the American Board of Industrial Hygiene, are industrial hygienists who by virtue of education in areas specified by the board and with at least 5 years of experience are eligible to take a comprehensive, rigorous 1-day examination on the practice of industrial hygiene. These individuals, after successful completion of the exam, are listed with the designation CIH after their names.

REFERENCES

1. Threshold limit values for chemical substances and physical agents and biological exposure indices for 2001. Cincinnati: American Conference of Governmental Industrial Hygienists.
2. Particle size-selective sampling in the workplace. Cincinnati: American Conference of Governmental Industrial Hygienists, 1985.
3. Particle size-selective sampling for particulate air contaminants. Cincinnati: American Conference of Governmental Industrial Hygienists, 1999.
4. Soderholm SC. Proposed international conventions for

particle size-selective sampling. *Ann Occup Hyg* 1989; 33:301–320.
5. McCunney RJ. Recognizing hand disorders due to vibrating tools. *J Musculoskel Med* 1992;9:91.
6. Miller G, Klonne D. Occupational exposure limits. In: DiNardi S, ed. *The occupational environment—its evaluation and control.* Fairfax, VA. *American Industrial Hygiene Association Press,* 1997:20–41.
7. Bioaerosols: assessment and control. Cincinnati: American Conference of Governmental Industrial Hygienists, 1999.
8. *Field guide for the determination of biological contaminants in environmental samples.* Fairfax: American Industrial Hygiene Association, 1996.

FURTHER INFORMATION

National Institute of Occupational Safety and Health (NIOSH/CDC), Department of Health and Human Services, 4676 Columbia Parkway, Cincinnati, OH 45226, 1-(800)-356-4674. *www.cdc.govniosh.*

Many educational materials related to the anticipation, recognition, evaluation, and control of workplace hazards are available from the two professional organizations for industrial hygienists. The American Conference of Governmental Industrial Hygienists (ACGIH) and the American Industrial Hygiene Association (AIHA) can also help in locating industrial hygienists, who may serve as consultants. A listing of industrial hygiene consultants is published annually in the January/February issue of the AIHA Journal.

ACGIH, 1330 Kemper Meadow Drive, Cincinnati, OH 45240-1634, *www.acgih.org.*

AIHA, 2700 Prosperity Avenue, Suite 250, Fairfax, VA 22031, *www.aiha.org.*

American Board of Industrial Hygiene (ABIH), 6015 W. St. Joseph, Suite 102, Lansing, MI 48917-3980, *www.abih.org.*

38

Workplace Safety

Myron C. Harrison

This chapter discusses the role physicians can play in workplace safety and in the prevention of work-related injury and illness. *Safety* is often defined as "an acceptable level of risk of injury or illness." "Acceptable" is a moving target. Workplace safety in the United States continually improved throughout the 20th century. The following examples are excerpted from a National Institute of Occupational Safety and Health (NIOSH) review of this progress (1).

In 1913, the Bureau of Labor Statistics documented approximately 23,000 industrial deaths among a workforce of 38 million in the U.S. Currently in the U.S. workforce of 130 million, there are approximately 5,000 industrial deaths annually. These rough numbers show a 95% decrease in incidence.

Similarly, data from the National Safety Council from 1933 through 1997 indicate that deaths from unintentional work-related injuries declined 90%, from 37 per 100,000 workers to 4 per 100,000.

The dramatic improvement in workplace safety, as measured by deaths, over the last 100 years is a testament to the efforts of workers, employers, labor organizations, government agencies, safety professionals, and health professionals. Nonetheless, there are tremendous opportunities for further improvement. According to the Bureau of Labor Statistics and NIOSH (2,3):

- Approximately 5.9 million nonfatal occupational injuries and illnesses occur yearly in private industry.
- Each year there are an estimated 3.6 million work-related injuries and illnesses treated in emergency departments, requiring the hospitalization of approximately 60,000 workers.
- Each day in the U.S. an average of 9,000 workers sustain a disabling injury (includes short-term disability).
- Each day 16 workers die from an injury in the workplace.
- Each day 137 workers die from work-related diseases.
- The annual direct and indirect costs of work-related injury and illness is $171 billion—equal to the annual costs of cancer.

Improvement in scientific knowledge and safety programs will contribute to continued progress. It is also important that physicians be more fully engaged in the prevention of work-related injury and illness. Traumatic injuries are decreasing and illnesses are becoming more prominent in the total burden of all work-related disease in the American workplace. Physicians have an active role in identifying the causes of work-related illness.

SAFETY PERSONNEL IN INDUSTRY

Almost all businesses have some type of designated safety position in their organization. In large manufacturing companies there are often safety departments with many practitioners. These jobs may be integrated with industrial hygiene, medical, toxicology, ergonomics, and environmental professionals into a single function. Smaller companies may have a single designated safety person, who may also have other roles. However the role is organized, the purpose of safety programs is to assist management in reducing the risk of work-related injury and illness. Specific responsibilities include advising management on ways to reduce injuries, illnesses, and accidents; coordinating interdepartmental activities, training, collection, and analysis of performance statistics; conducting research; and participating in health and safety committees.

The roots of the safety discipline are in industrial engineering and management. Safety personnel take the knowledge of health professionals and health scientists, and combine it with engineering knowledge and management skills to design programs that effect change in the workplace environment or worker behavior. Safety professionals come from many backgrounds, and most have experience in their company operations. Many of them are members of the American Society of Safety Engineers (ASSE), approximately 30,000 engineers who manage and consult on safety and health and environmental issues in industry, insurance, and government. Approximately 5,000 of those who practice safety are certified safety professionals (CSPs), a certification that is based on an examination.

Safety professionals are engaged in the prevention of accidents, incidents, and events that harm people, property, or the environment. They use qualitative and quantitative analysis of simple and complex products, systems, operations, and activities to identify hazards. They evaluate the hazards to identify what events can occur and the likelihood of occurrence, severity of results, risk (a multiple probability and severity), and cost. They identify what controls are appropriate and their cost and effectiveness.

Historically, risks in the workplace were associated with incidents such as falls or spills. But the focus of safety personnel and programs has gradually, and appropriately, extended to include work-related illnesses as well as injuries.

Industrial Hygiene Expertise

Another group of health professionals who are well educated in workplace safety skills are industrial hygienists. Their primary expertise is in assessing a work environment or job task in terms of all potential hazards (physical, chemical, or biologic), but many of them also design and administer safety programs in government, labor, industry, and academia. Most industrial hygienists are members of the American Industrial Hygiene Association (AIHA).

SAFETY PROGRAMS

Companies typically implement safety through written programs that define the activities necessary to address a specific hazard. These programs are often designed by safety personnel, but work best when they are "owned" and implemented by line management jointly with workers. Some examples:

- Emergency planning and preparedness
- Ergonomics
- Human factors and safe behavior
- Fire prevention
- Safe driving program
- Hazard communications
- Lockout/tag-out of hazards for purposes of equipment maintenance
- Medical and first aid programs
- Personal protective equipment
- Protection against slips, trips, and falls
- Tools and machine guarding
- Chemical safety
- Material handling
- Asbestos control
- Blood-borne pathogen control programs
- Electrical safety
- Office safety
- Injury or illness investigation

These programs are some of the building blocks of an overall safety and health management system, and they vary depending on the industry. Templates for these and other safety programs are easily found in books and on the Web (4–7). Each needs to be tailored to work within a specific organization.

Occupational Safety and Health Administration

Operating safely is a responsibility that is regulated in the U.S. by the Occupational Safety and Health Administration (OSHA) of the Department of Labor. The self-employed, family-operated agricultural businesses, and industries such as mining that are covered by other federal agencies are excepted. OSHA has promulgated a number of safety and health regulations and standards to protect employee health and safety. The agency is responsible for enforcing compliance with these regulations and standards. The specific regulations, standards, and guidance documents issued by OSHA are voluminous, and legal contests about the need for and interpretation of regulations are epic. Nonetheless, OSHA's mission can be boiled down to an important idea known as the "general duty clause," which simply states that employers have a general duty to keep their workplaces free from recognized hazards likely to cause death or serious physical harm.

In the furtherance of its mission, OSHA's regulations and standards generally require that employers do the following:

- Establish policies, procedures, and controls to ensure a safe workplace.
- Provide safety- and health-related information to employees.
- Provide training to employees.

- Provide employee access to appropriate exposure and medical records.
- Record and analyze injuries and illnesses.

In addition to these general responsibilities, OSHA has published hazard-specific regulations (e.g., standards for lead, asbestos, and benzene). These standards prescribe specific responsibilities for how an employer must manage each hazard. The programs also include rules for how a physician must examine and report findings for exposed workers. It is the responsibility of the employer to provide physicians who do these examinations with a copy of the applicable standard.

Some states have their own OSHA programs, such as CalOSHA in California. These state programs are required to be at least as stringent as the OSHA regulations and standards.

OSHA Voluntary Protection Programs (VPPs)

In the early 1980s, OSHA began to evaluate voluntary compliance programs as an alternative to a chronically understaffed inspection and enforcement approach. One result was the voluntary protection programs (VPPs), which are designed to recognize and promote effective safety and health management. In the VPP, management, labor, and OSHA establish a cooperative relationship at a workplace that has implemented a strong program.

The VPP concept recognizes that compliance enforcement alone can never fully achieve the objectives of the Occupational Safety and Health Act. Good safety management programs that go beyond OSHA standards can protect workers more effectively than compliance alone. VPP participants are facilities that have designed and implemented outstanding health and safety programs. The highest level participants (designated as "Star") meet all VPP requirements, and have demonstrated performance better than most others in their industry.

Voluntary Protection Programs Participants Association

A private nonprofit organization that assists companies in attaining and maintaining VPP status is the Voluntary Protection Programs Participants Association (VPPPA). It offers member companies networking with other VPP sites news and information on safety and health issues, and a representative voice with federal, state, and other governmental organizations. Working through VPPPA's mentoring program is an efficient way to jump-start a safety program.

National Institute of Occupational Safety and Health

The National Institute of Occupational Safety and Health (NIOSH) was created separately from OSHA for the express purpose of research. NIOSH is part of the Centers for Disease Control. In addition to occupational and health research, it is a resource for information on preventing workplace illness and injury and for training programs for occupational safety and health professionals.

The National Occupational Research Agenda

In 1996 the National Occupational Research Agenda (NORA) was developed by NIOSH with input from approximately 500 organizations and people nationwide. NORA was developed in recognition of the rapidly changing nature of the workplace and workforce and provides the framework for research to improve worker safety in the 21st century. NORA is a tool not only for NIOSH, but also for the entire occupational safety and health community. This process resulted in the following top 21 research priorities, which is notable for the emphasis on illnesses as opposed to injuries (8):

Disease and Injury

Allergic and irritant dermatitis
Asthma and chronic obstructive pulmonary disease
Fertility and pregnancy abnormalities
Hearing loss
Infectious diseases
Low back disorders
Musculoskeletal disorders of the upper extremities
Traumatic injuries

Work Environment and Workforce

Emerging technologies
Indoor environment
Mixed exposures
Organization of work
Special populations at risk

Research Tools and Approaches

Cancer research methods
Control technology and personal protective equipment

Exposure assessment methods
Health services research
Intervention effectiveness research
Risk assessment methods
Social and economic consequences of workplace illness and injury
Surveillance research methods

NIOSH's Health Hazard Evaluations

Few employers have the internal resources to investigate unexplained clusters of illness or exposures to new or previously unstudied hazards. Health hazard evaluations (HHEs) are investigations conducted by NIOSH epidemiologists and industrial hygienists in response to a written request to determine whether a substance normally found in the place of employment poses a risk to health. It's an option that a physician can suggest to management if there are unexplained patterns of disease that may be work related.

A typical HHE involves studying a specific operation or work area. The HHE may also evaluate other potentially hazardous working conditions, such as exposures to heat, noise, radiation, or musculoskeletal stresses. Based on the subject matter, NIOSH determines whether it is more appropriate for some other group to respond to the request. Sometimes these requests are referred to state-administered programs that are available to perform workplace hazard assessments.

THINKING ABOUT THE WORK-RELATEDNESS OF INJURY AND ILLNESS

Many physicians in private practice regularly diagnose and treat injuries or illnesses that are potentially related to a patient's work activities. Because most employers are required by OSHA to maintain a log of injuries and illnesses that are work related (as defined by OSHA criteria), physicians may be consulted on this issue.

It is important to understand that the determination of what belongs on the OSHA 300 log is a legal responsibility of company management. When asked about work-relatedness, it is very helpful to have knowledge of the job and the work environment. As the physician's judgment is particularly important to management's decision on work-relatedness, management is often willing to arrange for a job inspection. Inspections are often opportunities to become involved in company health and safety programs and to recommend appropriate preventive measures.

A physician's statement that an injury or illness is work related is a message to management that there is a health risk in the work environment that may need to be eliminated or controlled. Conversely, a statement that there is no discernible work-relatedness means that, in the judgment of the physician, management need not consider the workplace as a cause of the injury or illness. These statements on work-relatedness are important contributors to continuous improvement in the safety of the work environment.

Management's decision on work-relatedness for purposes of OSHA compliance may appropriately contradict a physician's statement on work-relatedness. Figure 38.1 illustrates the physician's role relative to "OSHA work-relatedness."

Understanding state regulations that define compensability for work-related injury or illness is another important responsibility in the practice of occupational medicine. But, like OSHA recordability, workers' compensation is not fully concordant with the fundamental issue of whether or not there is a remediable hazard in the workplace.

Other Questions that Physicians May Be Asked Relative to Recordability

Final rules on changes in OSHA's record-keeping regulation (29 CFR Part 1904) became effective on January 1, 2002. The new rules may bring about more congruence in the OSHA determination of work-relatedness and determinations for the purposes of managing risk. New provisions for recording musculoskeletal disorders and a new definition of standard threshold shifts for hearing loss will be delayed until January 1, 2003.

In addition to the issue of work-relatedness, there are other components of management's recordability decision that a physician may be asked to comment upon:

- Is the injury or illness a new case?
- Was a treatment medically necessary according to accepted clinical practices (includes restriction of work)?
- Was a prescription necessary according to accepted clinical practices?
- Did the medical care meet the new regulation's definition of first aid?

The complete OSHA revised rule for recording and reporting of occupational injuries and illnesses can be obtained at the OSHA Web site or regional OSHA offices (9).

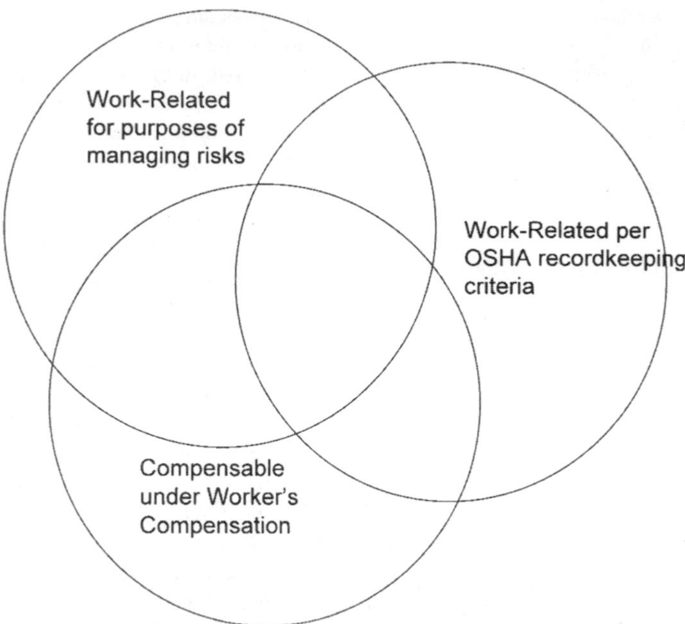

FIG. 38.1. Different determinations of work-relatedness.

Writing Medical Restrictions

An important occupational medicine activity is writing accurate statements to management about a patient's medical capabilities and limitations, whether or not the medical impairments are related to work. Requests to physicians for "medical restrictions" can emanate from many different employer needs, including the following:

Temporary Restrictions for Return to Work after Injury or Illness

One responsibility of a treating physician is to ensure that a patient does not engage in activities that could impede recovery or cause unnecessary pain. At the same time, physicians need to recognize that inappropriately restrictive limitations take away the employer's ability to accommodate duties that do not aggravate the medical problem. As an example, the restriction "no work" is unnecessarily restrictive for an employee who has a leg injury. An appropriate restriction is "no work that requires weight bearing."

If the injury or illness is work-related, OSHA recordability will be triggered if an employee loses a day of work or has significant restriction of duties because of a work-related injury or illness. Additionally, the total number of lost workdays because of a particular injury or illness is an important measurement. While these considerations are secondary to optimum medical treatment, unnecessary restrictions should be avoided.

Permanent Restrictions Regarding Ability to Work Safely

Misunderstanding about medical restrictions for permanent impairments or chronic disease is frequent. A physician needs to think carefully about two separate questions:

1. Does the applicant or employee have a medical condition that places him or her at increased risk of harm in the work environment?
2. Does the applicant or employee have an impairment that, in the specific job, creates increased risk to others or the environment?

In answering the first question, a physician should not restrict an employee against his or her wish to work unless the risk of harm is "high probability, severe and imminent" (10). Unless the above test is met, the choice, both ethically and legally, should be left to the individual. This creates a responsibility for the physician to adequately educate the individual regarding the risk.

It is widely recognized that employees at increased risk of a disease (work related or not) pose increased costs to employers in the form of health benefit costs, workers' compensation costs, and lost productivity. But, these alone are not legitimate considerations when determining medical fitness for work.

The second question is a different issue. Could the individual's medical condition pose a risk to others or the environment? Jobs that entail this potential (e.g., driving a school bus, operating a crane, or transporting environmentally hazardous material) are often termed "safety-sensitive" by employers. These jobs constitute a small percentage of all employment, but require ongoing medical screening for fitness. This screening may include testing for substance abuse. If an examiner diagnoses a medical condition that could result in sudden incapacitation or the chronic inability to exercise good judgment, it is appropriate to medically restrict the individual without his or her agreement.

The situation arises infrequently because individuals in safety sensitive jobs usually recognize the risk created by their impairment (substance abuse excluded). The appropriate medical restriction is simply "cannot work in safety-sensitive jobs." The challenge is to ensure that the physician, the patient, and the employer all agree on the correct definition of a safety-sensitive job. As an example, the presence of frequent, heavy lifting in a job, while it may create an increased risk of back injury, does not make a job safety-sensitive.

OCCUPATIONAL HEALTH AND SAFETY MANAGEMENT SYSTEMS

The hazard-specific safety programs that are implemented in many workplaces (see above) are important pieces of an overall system for managing safety. But writing and assembling them into a safety notebook does not, by itself, lead to a safe work environment. To achieve excellence in safety performance, an organization should implement an overall management system that pulls together health and safety activities and ensures continuous improvement. This is the approach that has been taken by many of the companies that lead their industries in safety.

A management system is written documentation of the steps necessary to accomplish defined objectives. Key elements of a management system are the following:

Objective—Clearly state the purpose of the system.

Scope—State the expectations and requirements of the system and its interfaces with other organizational systems.

Processes and procedures—Construct a flowchart of process steps that shows how the system works and gives detailed directions for accomplishing each step.

Responsible and accountable resources—Implement, administer, and execute a system of clear roles and responsibilities.

Verification and measurement—Verify that the system is being executed and set up measurements to assess performance against stated objectives.

Feedback mechanism—Facilitate continuous improvement by having management periodically review the results, and set up a process to ensure follow-up on the findings.

This general systems approach to achieving an objective is similar to quality initiatives in manufacturing and service industries. One commonly employed set of quality standards is those promoted by the International Organization for Standardization (ISO). The ISO 9000 series addresses quality in manufacturing. A similar approach is used in ISO's 14000 series, which address environmental management standards. Management systems do not need to follow the specific ISO approach to be effective, but they must incorporate all of the characteristics broadly described above (11).

There is no ISO standard for an occupational safety and health management system. The International Labor Organization recently published *Guidelines on Occupational Safety and Health Management Systems* (12). This publicly available document received input from many organizations in many countries, and is similar in approach to systems that have been developed in large manufacturing companies. It is a good starting point for learning more about these systems.

OSHA has shown increasing interest in occupational safety and health management systems as opposed to hazard-specific programs alone. Its current draft of a proposed safety and health program rule (29 CFR 1900.1) would require employers to establish a workplace safety and health program that implements many of the features listed above.

The Value of Errors

One important concept in the optimum implementation of a total quality management system is how an organization manages errors. The following excerpt describes a conceptual shift that must occur in order to effectively implement a quality management system. This example comes from the industry of patient care:

> To make health care safe we need to redesign our systems to make errors difficult to commit and create a culture in which the existence of risk is acknowledged and injury prevention is recognized as everyone's responsibility. A new understanding of accountability that moves beyond blaming individuals when they make mistakes must be established if progress is to be made (13).

A system that primarily identifies and punishes "bad guys" will not optimize safety in a work environment. Errors are the grist of an effective process to discover underlying system failures. Organizational denial sets a standard and becomes corrosive well beyond the sphere of safety. Sells (14) effectively describes a culture of organizational denial and its effects on management of health risks.

A related idea is the recognition and analysis of latent errors. Research into catastrophic airline accidents as well as industrial incidents such as the Chernobyl nuclear power and Bhopal plant accidents and the NASA's Challenger disaster has shown that accidents rarely result from a single error. Rather, accidents result from a combination of errors, including so-called latent errors. While a specific act may be the immediate cause of an accident, the root causes or vulnerabilities (the latent errors) were often present in the system for many years. This is particularly true in complex work endeavors (15).

One latent error in an organization can be the behavior of personnel in operations. Organizations that are high performers in terms of safety and health are able to identify behavioral patterns that increase risk. This is greatly facilitated by continued analysis of errors, near misses, difficulties, problems, behaviors, and attitudes.

Safety Culture

Petroleum companies work in some of the most hazardous conditions in the world and with some of the most hazardous materials used in industry. Most of them have made large investments to improve facilities and operational safety and health. They have also been among the leaders in the integration of safety and health management systems into their businesses. These investments have been accompanied by dramatic gains in safety performance.

Increasingly, these companies recognize that continued progress requires substantial gains in the area that is broadly known as human factors. Progress includes improving the design of man–machine interfaces, improving training, better management of variable work schedules, and better evaluation of capability and impairment. It also includes more attention to an organization's "safety culture"—the collective values and attitudes (usually unspoken) of the people in the organization influenced by factors such as management commitment, employee empowerment, and shared perceptions about safety and trust. It may be the most influential of all human factors in determining workplace safety and health.

Several petroleum companies, under the auspices of the International Association of Oil and Gas Producers (OGP), sponsored research at Leiden University (Netherlands) and University of Manchester (United Kingdom) to develop a diagnostic tool to determine a measure of a company's safety culture. The report of this research described five levels of safety culture as perceived by managers and safety professionals in the companies. The following descriptions are excerpted from this research (16):

1. *Pathologic:* "Many accidents are unavoidable—they are part of the job. Our safety record is good enough so that we do not get inspected frequently by the government. We rely on our legal staff for advice on safety requirements and related issues."
2. *Reactive:* "We measure the safety performance of our employees using indicators such as lost workday incident rate. We focus on results—a lack of incidents is evidence of satisfactory performance. We report incidents as required by legal and company requirements."
3. *Calculative:* "We monitor trends as well as the rates of injury and illness. We feel that accidents are preventable—root causes include hardware and procedures, but unsafe behaviors by workers are a primary cause. We have a lot of inspections and audits, which help to find any failures in our systems and processes. We assign accountability."
4. *Proactive:* "We investigate all incidents looking for system failures and human factors. When a hazardous situation is reported, we treat it as a potential incident. The workforce 'owns' many of the safety processes. Our audits and inspections are risk-based and reports focus on ways to improve our systems."
5. *Generative:* "Safety is how we do business. Since we have so few incidents, we don't focus on safety. It is part of the way we do our business. Despite our good sustained performance, we are concerned that the next accident is just around the corner. We use tools such as audits and haz-

ardous situation reporting to find better ways of improving our processes and systems for operating incident free."

Progress through these five stages demonstrates increasing integration of safety awareness and safe behaviors into the minute-to-minute operations of an organization. It also demonstrates increasing sophistication about the value of errors in the prevention of future serious incidents.

Understanding an organization's safety culture is an advantage to physicians who wish to play a preventive role in occupational injury and illness. Every unscheduled clinical encounter represents a system error, whether latent (behavior, perception, or attitude) or manifest (injury or illness). These encounters are opportunities not only to heal but also to consider, at least briefly, whether a change in the work environment or in worker behavior could prevent future harm.

REFERENCES

1. Improvements in workplace safety in the United States, 1900–1999. *MMWR* 1999;48:461–469.
2. Nonfatal occupational injuries and illnesses treated in hospital emergency departments in the United States, 1998. *MMWR* 2001;50:313–317.
3. NIOSH's strategic plan, 1997–2002. *www.cdc.govniosh/gpran1a.html.*
4. Occupational safety and health answers, Canadian Center for Occupational Health and Safety. *www.ccohs.-cao/shanswers.*
5. Wyman RJ. *Safety and the security professional, occupational safety and health strategies.* Butterworth Heinemann, 2000.
6. Safety info—an online library of safety programs, forms, references, and training materials at *www.safety-office2002.com.*
7. Zeimet DE, Ballard DN Jr. *Safety and health program for small businesses.* Des Plaines, IL: American Society of Safety Engineers, 1998.
8. NIOSH's National Occupational Research Agenda. *www.cdc.govnioshnorhmpg.html.*
9. Occupational Safety and Health Administration, injury and illness recordkeeping, *www.osha-slc.govrecord-keeping/index.html.*
10. Title I of the Americans with Disabilities Act, 29 CFR Part 1630.
11. Redinger CF, Levine SP, ed. *New frontiers in occupational health and safety: a management systems approach and the ISO model.* AIHA Publications, 1996.
12. International Labor Organization, Guidelines on occupational safety and health management systems, 2001. *www.ilo.org/public/english/support/publ/booksoh.*
13. Leape LL, et al. Promoting patient safety by preventing medical error. *JAMA* 1998;280:1444–1447.
14. Sells B. What asbestos taught me about managing risk. *Harvard Business Review* 1994(March-April);76–90.
15. Reason J. *Organizational accidents: the management of human and organizational factors in hazardous technologies.* Cambridge University Press, 1997.
16. Hudson P, Parker D. Profiling safety culture: the OGP interview study. Available from OGP at *www.ogp.org.-uk/index.html.*

39

Toxicology

Jonathan B. Borak and Richard C. Pleus

Toxicology is the scientific study of the mechanisms of action and effects of exposure caused by chemical agents in living organisms. The objectives of toxicology are to characterize the potential hazards of exposure to specific agents and to estimate the probability that such effects will follow anticipated types and levels of exposure. In particular, toxicology considers the effects of specific doses of specific agents under specific conditions of use and exposure. In that context, assessments of dose lead to characterizations of "toxicity," while considerations of the conditions of use and exposure produce assessments of "hazards."

To achieve those goals, toxicologists rely on specific types of information, including the identity and form of the agent; the conditions of exposure (e.g., route, level and duration of exposure); the pharmacokinetics of the agent (e.g., absorption, distribution, metabolism, and excretion); and its mechanisms of action. Some of the necessary information, such as the conditions of exposure, can be obtained by observation and reconstruction of exposure events. Other types of information, such as mechanisms of action and pharmacokinetics of particular agents, can often be found in the literature (e.g., standard reference books, scientific journals, and on the World Wide Web). However, there are numerous chemical agents for which only insufficient information is available. For those agents, toxicologists may need to derive their estimates and conclusions on extrapolations from the available, albeit limited information and analogies to better studied chemicals (e.g., comparative structure analysis).

Access to and understanding of toxicologic information are necessary for a wide array of decisions essential to the practice of occupational and environmental medicine. For clinicians evaluating patients' health complaints, knowledge about their chemical exposures is often critical. For occupational physicians developing work-site health and safety programs, toxicologic data are required to implement appropriate medical surveillance programs. Likewise, toxicologic information is central to setting occupational and environmental exposure limits, determining needs and choosing types of personal protective equipment for specific settings, evaluating the significance of environmental contamination, and prioritizing the remediation and cleanup of environmental hazards.

In general, there is a hierarchy of toxicologic information that underlies knowledge about specific agents and their risks to humans. This hierarchy is based on the species tested (human data are always more valuable for predicting human effects than comparable data from other species, and mammalian data are more valuable than data from lower species) and on the design of testing, with well-designed long-term studies generally providing more useful data than short-term studies. Such a hierarchy is reflected in standard testing protocols required for new chemical agents before they can be commercialized. For example, the United States Environmental Protection Agency (EPA) has published harmonized test guidelines for evaluating the health effects of pesticides and toxic substances. These guidelines include acute toxicity testing in animals (oral, dermal, inhalation, eye irritation, skin irritation, and skin sensitization), subchronic toxicity testing (rodents exposed for 28 and 90 days, oral and dermal), chronic toxicity and carcinogenicity testing in animals (at least two species exposed for at least 12 months), reproductive and fertility effects testing, developmental effects testing, and a variety of test protocols for mutagenicity, neurologic and behavioral toxicity, immunotoxicity, and skin penetration. The results of such testing are generally compiled and available, although usually in summary rather than in detail.

For predicting human health effects, animal and in vitro testing are of uncertain value. Although many chemicals cause similar effects in lab animals and humans, there are also others for which animal testing failed to predict human toxicity. One example is arsenic, a known human carcinogen for which there is essentially no animal model (some studies have reported increased cancer in hamsters after instillation into the lungs). A second example is thalidomide, a potent human teratogen with toxic activity not detected in standard rodent tests. There are also examples of toxic effects demonstrated in laboratory animals that have proven to be of no relevance to humans. Such effects have been related to genetic, metabolic, or structural peculiarities that predispose affected animals to toxicity. Examples of such species-specific toxicities include tubular nephritis and renal cancer in male rats exposed to certain solvents, effects related to the presence of a species- and gender-specific serum protein, α_{2u}-globulin; lung cancer in rats that suffer dust overload from a variety of particulates including titanium dioxide, carbon black and diesel exhaust, an effect related to anatomic peculiarities of the rat airway; and hepatomegaly and liver cancer in rodents exposed to peroxisome proliferators, a category of compounds that includes some halogenated solvents and some cholesterol- and triglyceride-lowering medications, e.g., the statins. Accordingly, toxicologic data derived solely from animal studies must be used with caution when predicting human risks.

The best evidence of human toxicity derives directly from observations of exposed humans, but there are practical and ethical limitations to such research. Clinical studies, in which humans are directly challenged by exposure are a requisite aspect of Food and Drug Administration (FDA) approval of new medications, but at the current time (early 2003) the EPA has severely limited its acceptance of such human data for ethical reasons. Accordingly, there may be significantly less use of direct human testing to evaluate industrial chemicals. Instead, human evidence of chemical toxicity will increasingly be obtained by epidemiologic assessments of exposed workers. As a result, the clinical observations of occupational physicians and the compiled results of workplace medical surveillance programs will play increasingly important roles in identifying and characterizing the human toxicity characteristics of chemical agents.

GENERAL PRINCIPLES

Toxicologic science rests on several basic principles that provide an important starting point to understanding the effects of toxic agents. The first law, formulated by the medieval physician and alchemist Paracelsus, states that the dose makes the poison: "What is there that is not poison? All things are poison...Solely the dose determines that a thing is not a poison." The full force of this principle remains paramount today. It is not sufficient to know that exposure occurred; to infer causation it is necessary to know the dose to which the receptor (e.g., the patient) was exposed.

The second law, attributed to the French surgeon Ambroise Paré (1510–1590), states that the effects of individual chemicals are specific, not general: "Poyson...kil by a certaine specifick antipathy contrary to our nature." This principle, that chemicals have specific rather than general effects, leads to the expectation that exposures to particular chemical agents will lead to characteristic and characterizable patterns of toxicity. In turn, this predicts the usefulness of well-conducted epidemiologic studies for understanding the human effects of chemical exposures.

The third law of toxicology states that humans are animals and that useful information about the possible human effects of chemical exposures can be gained by studying their effects in animals. It is this principle that underlies EPA's harmonized test guidelines and that allows risk assessors to extrapolate human risks from animal data. However, humans are not merely "giant rodents," and the toxicologic differences between men and mice can be enormous. For that reason, animal data are often necessary but rarely sufficient for determining the toxic hazards of chemical exposures in humans.

There are also other principles of importance to toxicologists, ones more frequently seen as relevant to concerns about causal inference. Consider, for example, the nine principles known as the Hill criteria. The first two Hill criteria, strength and consistency, indicate that one can feel most certain about toxicologic data that document large, rather than marginal, effects, especially when such findings have been replicated. The fourth Hill criterion, temporality, states that exposure must precede effect, while the fifth criterion, biologic gradient, states that chemical-induced effects are expected to follow a monotonic (i.e., unidirectional) dose-response curve. This fifth criterion can be seen as a corollary to the first law of toxicology ("Dose makes the poison"), while the third Hill criteria, specificity, echoes the second law of toxicology ("Chemicals cause specific, not general, effects").

These general principles provide starting points from which to interpret toxicologic data and understand toxicologic effects. Observations that conform to these principles provide more trustworthy evidence of true biologic effects, while those that diverge should be viewed with greater skepticism. Likewise, estimations and predictions that deviate from these principles require greater empirical proof before they can achieve general acceptance.

But it is not possible to understand toxicologic processes from general principles alone. Toxicologists must also rely on a variety of chemical-specific and situation-specific information in order to characterize, quantify, and predict toxicologic effects. Examples of such information include (a) identity, physical form, and properties of the agent; (b) exposure conditions (e.g., route and pattern of exposure); (c) dose and dose-response relationships; and (d) agent-specific pharmacokinetics (e.g., absorption, distribution, metabolism, and excretion).

IDENTITY, PHYSICAL FORM, AND PROPERTIES

The activity and potency of individual chemicals differ from one another, even when comparisons are drawn between chemicals that share molecular similarities. Knowledge that an agent belongs to a particular chemical family or category can often provide a useful basis for predicting the qualitative behaviors of the agent, and sophisticated computer-intensive studies, known as structure-activity relationship (SAR) analysis, have been used to screen families of chemicals to find those likely to have particular characteristics. However, quantitative toxicologic predictions usually require that the identity and characteristics of each specific chemical be known.

But knowledge of the chemical identify alone may be insufficient. Large differences in toxicity can result from differences in the physical form of an agent. One example is the differences in dispersion and availability of gases as compared to liquids. More volatile liquids, which are more prone to vaporize, pose greater inhalation hazards than do comparably potent but less volatile liquids. Likewise, because vaporization increases as temperature rises, the risks of inhalation exposure are greater in hot than cold climates. Another example involves particulate size; inhaled larger particles (e.g., >2.5 μm) tend to deposit in the upper airways, smaller particles (e.g., <1 μm) more readily penetrate deeply to the lower airways and alveoli, while very large particles (e.g., >10 μm) are mostly trapped in the nares and do not enter the airways. For such reasons, the EPA and other organizations have devoted substantial resources to determining the differential toxicity of exposure to ambient particulates of varying size. Likewise, occupational exposure limits increasingly differentiate between large and small particulate; the Occupational Safety and Health Administration (OSHA) distinguishes "total" from "respirable" particulates, and the American Conference of Governmental Industrial Hygienist's (ACGIH) draws the same distinction, but refers to its categories as "inhalable" vs. "respirable" particulates.

In addition, the physical array or electrical state of chemical molecules may influence toxicity. Amorphous silica (diatomaceous earth) is relatively harmless, but crystalline silica (e.g., quartz) is among the most important and well-recognized causes of toxic lung injury in human history. The valence state of an ion can make important toxicologic differences. Hexavalent chromium, for example, exhibits significantly greater toxicity than trivalent chromium, which is actually an essential trace element. Likewise, trivalent arsenic is more readily taken up by cells than is pentavalent arsenic and it is therefore four to ten times more potent on an equimolar basis; by contrast, metallic arsenic has so little bioavailability that it is essentially harmless.

EXPOSURE CONDITIONS

The first law of toxicology teaches that all things are poison under some exposure conditions, but not under others. Thus, it is necessary to characterize the situation and circumstances of exposure when evaluating or predicting the toxicity of specific agents. The critical importance of certain exposure variables, such as the route, duration, and level of exposure, is widely appreciated; they ultimately determine the exposure dose. Other variables, such as those related to ambient conditions (such as ambient temperature and humidity), can be less obvious but may explain significant toxicity differences between settings. For example, sulfuric acid mist formed during metal pickling operations is composed of airborne hygroscopic droplets. At high humidity, the acid droplets increase in size and have greater impact on upper airways, while at low humidity comparable levels of the acid mist (measured in units of mg/m^3) form smaller droplets that penetrate deeper into the lungs. As a result, workers exposed in humid climates suffer more severe upper respiratory irritation, while workers exposed to identical mist levels in dry climates experience fewer acute irritative symptoms, but suffer greater chronic lung damage.

An initial goal of toxicologic assessments is to evaluate and characterize the exposure and its setting. Concerns of primary importance include exposure route, exposure level and duration, and the patterns of exposure.

Routes of Exposure

The major routes of exposure to toxic chemicals include inhalation, ingestion, and dermal contact. Parenteral exposures can also be of concern, but mainly for exposure to medications and drugs, rather than industrial chemicals. For chemicals with predominant local effects (i.e., toxicity affecting the tissues directly contacted), routes of exposure predict the tissues harmed. Corrosives, for example, cause inflammation and necrosis of the tissues they contact, but generally little systemic toxicity. Accordingly, ingestion of corrosives causes mainly gastrointestinal injury, inhalation affects mainly the airways, and dermal contact leads to chemical skin burns.

In other cases, route of exposure determines rate and efficiency of systemic absorption. In general, uptake is most rapid and efficient after inhalation exposure, less so after ingestion, and least rapid and efficient after dermal contact. As a result, the rate of onset of systemic effects varies according to the exposure route. For example, inhalation of cyanide gas can induce almost immediate systemic effects and death, while similar effects are delayed for many minutes after ingestion and hours after skin exposure. Understanding such differences can help to explain the nature and onset of specific intoxications. Likewise, such concerns influence the design of biologic monitoring for exposed workers. The appropriate time for obtaining surveillance samples depends on whether dermal or inhalation exposures are more important. In creosote workers, for example, urinary biomarkers peak shortly after the work shift when inhalation is the major exposure route, but when dermal uptake predominates peak urine levels are found in the next morning's samples.

Finally, some agents have significantly greater toxicity by one exposure route than another. Chronic inhalation of mercury vapor can lead to renal and neurologic toxicities, and acute high-level mercury vapor inhalation can cause both pulmonary and systemic effects, but ingestion of elemental mercury at even extremely high doses is almost always without adverse effects.

Patterns of Exposure

Chemical exposures are often characterized according to their duration and frequency. Relatively short-term (e.g., hours or days), isolated exposures are referred to as acute, while exposures occurring over months or years are referred to as chronic. All other things being equal, chronic exposures can be expected to cause greater toxicity, particularly if the chemical accumulates following exposure (i.e., body burdens increase) or if resulting injuries accumulate over time (e.g., repair mechanisms are increasingly overwhelmed). But if exposure promotes accommodation or adaptation (e.g., induction of detoxification mechanisms), then toxicity may actually decline as exposures become more chronic.

A different concern involves the frequency and duration of exposure-free periods, a particular concern for workers assigned to unusual work schedules, e.g., longer than standard 8-hour shifts or more than 40 hours per week. Workers assigned to longer than standard shifts may have insufficient time to effectively eliminate absorbed doses before beginning their next shift. In that case, body burdens will rise over the course of a workweek, achieving levels that may be significantly greater than those of workers assigned to standard schedules. Such concerns are of particular relevance to chemicals with biologic half-lives between 2 and 100 hours. Chemicals with shorter half-lives can be eliminated over such short time periods that unusual work shifts are unlikely to lead to enhanced accumulation, while the accumulation of those with longer half-lives is unlikely to be affected by length of individual shifts, but would increase if workers are routinely assigned to workweeks of longer than 40 hours.

DOSE AND DOSE-RESPONSE RELATIONSHIPS

The toxic effects of chemical exposures are related directly to the quantities of the chemicals to which a person is exposed; exposure and dose are related, but they are not equivalent. The first law of toxicology states that at sufficiently high doses all things are poisons, while at sufficiently low doses nothing is poisonous: "Dose makes the poison." The Hill postulate on biologic gradients refines that concept: chemical-induced effects are expected to demonstrate monotonic dose-response relationships. In other words, one can expect that at some low exposure levels there will be essentially no toxicity, but as doses rise toxicity will increase (in severity, in frequency, or both). The toxicologic challenge is first to determine the proper measure of dose and then to characterize the dose-response relationship, the quantitative relationship between exposure and effect that provides the basis for predicting toxicity in light of known or expected dose.

A simplistic definition of dose is the quantity of a substance applied to an individual, i.e., the quantity inhaled, ingested, or contacting the skin. That simple definition, however, ignores a variety of toxicologically relevant concerns. For example, it is usually more important to know the quantity of chemical absorbed into the systemic circulation, rather than the quantity externally applied. Likewise, it is often more meaningful to know the quantity of the specific chemical metabolites formed in or transported to the toxicity-associated target organ. The aspect of toxicology that addresses such concerns is known as pharmacokinetics (discussed below).

Despite its limitations, this simplistic approach is routinely used for setting workplace exposure limits and predicting the toxic effects of ambient and workplace exposures. Calculation of the ingestion dose is the most straightforward; it is literally the quantity ingested, sometimes corrected for body size. That approach, however, ignores the variable absorption of different compounds from the alimentary tract, a process that is often dynamic. For example, ingested lead compounds are partially absorbed from the gut, but lead absorption is much enhanced by concomitant iron deficiency. Thus individuals of identical size and weight who ingest identical quantities of a lead compound would have identical external doses, but their internal doses might be very different if one was iron deficient and the other was not.

For inhalation exposures, dose is most simply calculated as the following product:

$$[\text{Air Concentration}] \times [\text{Exposure Duration}] \times [\text{Ventilation Rate}].$$

For example, suppose a worker breathing 20 L/min is exposed for 50 minutes to toluene at a concentration of 100 mg/m^3 (approximately 30 ppm). That worker's inhaled dose, 100 mg, can be calculated as follows:

$$\text{Inhaled Dose} = [100\ \text{mg/m}^3] \times [50\ \text{min}] \times [20\ \text{L/min}]$$

$$[50\ \text{min}] \times [20\ \text{L/min}] = [1{,}000\ \text{L}] = [1\ \text{m}^3]$$

$$\text{Inhaled Dose} = [100\ \text{mg/m}^3] \times [1\ \text{m}^3] = 100\ \text{mg}$$

This approach underscores that ventilation rate is a key determinant of inhalation dose, but it ignores the fact that absorption of inhaled compounds is generally variable and rarely complete. As ventilatory rates increase, the time allowed for uptake from each breath declines, thereby reducing uptake. Likewise, as inhaled chemicals accumulate, the concentration gradient that facilitates uptake is reduced and uptake therefore declines.

For dermal exposures, dose can be calculated as the following product:

$$[\text{Chemical Concentration}] \times [\text{Exposed Surface Area}] \times [\text{Duration of Exposure}].$$

This is the least precise of the simplistic dose calculations. There are wide differences in the rates and efficiencies of dermal uptake of various chemicals, depending on characteristics such as their water vs. fat solubility, and there are significant differences in uptake from the skin on different parts of the body. For example, the thin, moist skin of the axillae and groin permit much greater dermal uptake than does the drier, thicker skin on the palms and soles. In addition, the adequacy of postexposure skin cleansing is important, but often difficult to quantify.

These simplistic dose measurements are rarely better than first approximations of the biologically more relevant measure of the levels of the ultimate toxic agents found at specific subcellular sites where they disrupt physiologic functions. Unfortunately, it is difficult to achieve those more relevant measurements; for many chemicals, the ultimate toxic agents are not known with certainty and even when known, it may be technologically difficult to measure them at their sites of action. Accordingly, toxicologists must depend on estimated values for such measures of internal dose. The field of toxicology devoted to estimating such subcellular concentrations and describing their dynamic changes under physiologic conditions is pharmacokinetics (discussed below).

The dose-response relationship is typically depicted in graphical format (dose-response curve), where the dose is plotted on the abscissa (x-axis) and response is plotted on the ordinate (y-axis). For some purposes, relatively crude estimates of dose (e.g., simplistic measures of external dose) are sufficient, while others require sophisticated estimates of the concentrations of chemicals or their metabolites in target tissues and organs. Likewise, the response may be as simple as mortality rates or as complex as alterations in protein synthesis or gene transcription. As measurements of dose and response become more precise, there is greater likelihood that calculated dose-response relationships can predict toxicologic outcomes with high degrees of accuracy.

Most toxic chemicals cause multiple effects, some more harmful than others, and these effects may develop at different dose levels. For each, there may be different dose-response relationships. From the perspective of experimental toxicologists, such a multiplicity of dose-response curves is useful, providing insight into underlying biologic processes. For regulatory toxicologists, however, such multiplicity leads to conflict and dispute that arise often in setting workplace and ambient exposure limits. For example, chlorinated solvents at high doses may cause central nervous system (CNS) depression, cardiac dysrhythmias, and hepatitis, while lower doses cause only reversible effects, such as induction of hepatic enzyme systems and liver cell hypertrophy. If there is a different dose-response relationship for each effect, then there can be disputes about which one best serves as the basis for regulatory action. Such disputes turn on which effects are adverse and which adverse effect occurs at the lowest dose. Toxicologists often disagree on such issues.

Dose-response curves provide two apparently different types of information. First, they provide information about the activity of the agent on biologic systems. Second, they provide information about the susceptibility of populations to the agent's effects. In fact, however, these two information types are tightly related because activity levels of biologic systems are often distributed across populations in a manner similar to the distributions of susceptibility. As a first approximation, therefore, it is often possible to extrapolate dose-response curves derived from lab studies to general populations, and vice versa.

A key aspect of dose-response curves is their shape. For many agents, response varies as a normally distributed function of the dose. (This is most frequently the case when response is related to the logarithm of the dose, rather than the dose itself.) In such cases, the dose-response curve is sigmoid (i.e., S-shaped) when response is measured as cumulative response, and bell-shaped when response is measured as the percent responding at each dose. The often-justified assumption that dose-response curves have normal distributions makes toxicologic problem solving relatively easier because arithmetic calculations based on normal distributions are familiar and straightforward.

In other cases, dose-response curves are J-shaped or U-shaped; greater levels of toxicity are noted at very high and very low doses, with fewer toxic effects noted in between. This is most often found for chemicals that are essential to life, but cause toxicity when exposures are excessive. Examples include essential trace minerals, such as copper, selenium, and iron, and certain fat-soluble vitamins, such as vitamin A. For these agents, deficiency is associated with certain adverse effects, while overdose is associated with others. Such U-shaped dose-response curves are most obvious when the specific effects of deficiency and excess are not differentiated. Recent interest has focused on the theory of hormesis, which argues that many agents have paradoxical adverse effects at very low doses. This suggests that many agents may have U-shaped (or J-shaped) dose-response curves. The biologic basis for such low-dose hormetic effects has not been fully explained.

A second key aspect of dose-response curves is their slope, calculated as the rate that adverse effects increase as dose increases. This is particularly important for that range of the curve that corresponds to the levels of exposure likely to be encountered in the workplace or environment. For agents with steep dose-response curves (i.e., large slope factor), small increments of dose lead to large increments in response. Such agents have small margins of safety; there is only a relatively small difference between safe doses and harmful ones. By contrast, agents with shallow dose-response curves have large margins of safety. As a general rule, chemicals with steep dose-response curves require greater caution and controls than those that have shallow curves.

A third key aspect of dose-response curves is whether responses occur at all levels of dose, or only above some minimum level, the threshold. There are several reasons that any specific chemicals might cause no adverse effects below a threshold. For example, there might be limited amounts of detoxification capacity or limited amounts of reserve capacity for the function affected by the agent. In either case, adverse effects would be seen only when detoxification capacities have been overwhelmed or reserve capacity depleted. Cyanide is a toxin that demonstrates a detoxification-defined threshold. It is naturally detoxified by the actions of a mitochondrial enzyme, rhodanese; toxicity does not develop until the cyanide dose exceeds the capacity of rhodanese-mediated detoxification. Thus, the cyanide dose-response curve has a threshold defined by the intrinsic detoxification capacity of that enzyme. Carbon monoxide is a toxicant with a threshold defined by underlying reserve capacity. It binds to hemoglobin, thus preventing oxygen transport to the tissues. But most people have excess hemoglobin, far more than they need to transport sufficient oxygen, and therefore small doses of carbon monoxide cause no adverse effects; poisoning occurs only when the carbon monoxide dose is sufficient to substantially reduce oxygen transport.

PHARMACOKINETICS (ABSORPTION, DISTRIBUTION, METABOLISM, AND EXCRETION)

The simplistic dose measurements discussed above considered quantities of chemicals applied externally to exposed individuals. Such measures are rarely better than first approximations of the biologically more relevant measure, the levels of the ultimate toxic agents found at those specific subcellular sites where they disrupt physiologic functions. Unfortunately, it is usually difficult to achieve those more relevant measurements; for many chemicals, the ultimate toxic agents are not known with certainty, and even when they are known it may be technologically difficult to measure them at their sites of action. Accordingly, toxicologists must depend on estimated values for such measures of internal dose.

Pharmacokinetics is the field of toxicology devoted to estimating such subcellular concentrations. It is the study through measurement or modeling of the absorption, distribution, metabolism, and excretion of drugs or chemicals in a biologic system as a function of time. The National Research Council has called pharmacokinetics "the linkage between exposure and dose." It is sometimes referred to by the acronym ADME, reflecting its four principal components: absorption, distribution, metabolism, and excretion.

Absorption

Absorption is the transfer of chemicals from their sites of exposure into the systemic circulation. The rate and efficiency with which specific chemicals enter the body depend on their physical and chemical properties as well as the relevant routes of exposure. Most toxicants are absorbed passively by simple diffusion, but some undergo active uptake, a process of particular relevance to certain ingestion exposures. Accordingly, a useful approach to understanding differences in absorption begins with considerations of those factors that influence passive diffusion. The rates of diffusion of most materials across biologic membranes, and thus their rates of absorption, depend largely on two factors: lipid solubility and concentration gradients.

Lipid solubility is of major concern because body membranes are high in lipid content; lipid-soluble molecules cross those membranes much more rapidly and efficiently than do lipid-insoluble molecules. Nonionized and less polar molecules are generally more lipid soluble and therefore more likely to penetrate lipid membrane barriers than are water-soluble molecules. Thus the lipid solubility of chemicals is a useful predictor of molecules likely to be well absorbed.

Concentration gradients reflect the force that drives molecules across the biologic membranes. The greater the gradient, the greater the force and the more rapid the flow of molecules. Gradients reflect both the concentrations of administered chemicals as well as ways in which specific chemicals are stored, metabolized, and/or excreted. Chemicals that are readily stored in large quantities, for example, are likely to be more rapidly and efficiently absorbed because storage maintains concentration gradients that favor uptake. For similar reasons, there is greater uptake of chemicals that are rapidly and effectively metabolized or excreted.

The effects of lipid solubility and concentration gradients on efficiency of absorption differ according to the routes of exposure. Intact skin, for example, is an effective barrier to penetration because it consists of multiple layers, each with differing physical characteristics. The outer layer is the corneum stratum, a superficial membrane of keratinized cells that prevents foreign materials from contacting living cells and serves as the principal rate-limiting step for skin absorption. Lipid-soluble agents can penetrate the corneum stratum, but water-soluble chemicals penetrate slowly and incompletely. Hydration of the corneum stratum, as occurs with occlusive dressings and after continual use of work gloves, facilitates passage of water-soluble agents and subsequent dermal absorption. Once through the corneum stratum, water-soluble chemicals can more readily diffuse through the germinal layer of the epidermis, which consists of a porous, nonselective, aqueous medium. (Skin normally contains about 90 g of water per gram of dry tissue.)

Following inhalation, the amounts of chemicals absorbed across the lung depend on their physical form (e.g., solid vs. gas) and their solubility in blood and interstitial fluid. Solid particulates deposited in the lung can be absorbed, but they must first be solubilized, dissolving into interstitial and alveolar fluids, from which they are absorbed into the blood. Highly soluble gases are rapidly and efficiently absorbed across the alveolar membranes; relatively large amounts must be absorbed before the blood becomes saturated. The extent of saturation of blood is dependent on both the rate and efficiency of uptake from the lungs and the rate and efficiency of removal of the absorbed chemical from the blood. These latter issues of distribution and excretion are addressed below. For gases, especially those with appreciable lipid solubility, uptake rates are directly related to minute ventilatory volume and the concentration of gas in inspired air, and indirectly related to the level of saturation in blood.

Distribution

Systemic distribution of absorbed chemicals occurs through the bloodstream. For any individual chemical, distribution is regulated by its capacity to pass through the cell membranes, the specific affinity of various tissues for the chemical, and the volume of blood flow to the various organs. Most agents cross cellular membranes by passive diffusion. Small water-avid molecules (molecular weight less than 600) enter via aqueous channels in the cell membranes, while lipophilic molecules diffuse across lipid-rich areas of the membranes. As a general rule, the smaller the molecule and the greater its lipophilicity, the more rapidly it can pass the cell membrane. Some chemicals are actively transported into cells by mechanisms that require the input of cellular energy, such as when entry is opposite the concentration or ionic gradient or when the transport process is intended to select for some specific molecular structures over others.

After entering the bloodstream, chemicals distribute into the water compartments of the body; chemicals may remain in the plasma or move into the interstitial or intracellular fluid space. Many of the chemicals that remain within the plasma space do so because they bind with one or more plasma proteins, of which the most important is albumin. Once bound, the high molecular weight of the protein prevents passage of the substance outside the vascular space, thereby limiting further distribution. In addition to the water compartments, there are other sites of distribution within the body. Some chemicals bind to intra- or extracellular receptor sites, where they become relatively fixed in place, or they may enter storage tissues such as fat, liver, or bone where the chemical is sequestered. Lipophilic organic solvents, for example, are stored in adipose tissue; some metals, such as lead and aluminum, are stored in bone, while other metals, such as cadmium, are selectively bound to storage proteins (e.g., metallothionein) and sequestered in liver and kidney cells.

Binding to plasma proteins serves as a generally available chemical reservoir. Protein-bound molecules exist in equilibrium with unbound plasma molecules, and as unbound molecules are transported into cells and storage areas, or metabolized and excreted, bound molecules dissociate from binding sites and become biologically available. This process continues until levels of the chemical in extravascular fluid equilibrate with plasma levels of unbound chemical.

The distribution of absorbed chemicals is also influenced by cardiovascular factors such as rates and volumes of blood flow to various organs. When different species are compared, differential rates of blood flow to liver, kidney, or brain can explain observed differences in the distribution of specific agents across species. The uptake of a chemical into any specific organ is a factor of the chemical's lipid solubility, concentration gradients, the presence of active uptake mechanisms, and the rate and proportion of blood flow to the organ.

Some organs, particularly the CNS, have specialized barriers to distribution that protect them from potentially toxic exposures. There are three reasons that most toxicants do not enter the brain in appreciable quantities: the capillary endothelial cells of the CNS are tightly joined, leaving few or no pores between the cells; the capillaries of the CNS are largely surrounded by astrocytes, which provide an additional barrier to penetration; and the protein concentration in the interstitial fluid of the CNS is much lower than elsewhere in the body, which reduces movement of protein-bound chemicals into the CNS. Those agents that do enter the brain in significant amounts are generally lipid soluble, non–protein bound, nonionized, and of relatively small molecular size.

At the other extreme, fetuses can be more susceptible to toxicants than are the mothers. The placenta is a relatively ineffective barrier to many types of chemicals, and many workplace and environmental chemicals are readily transported from maternal to fetal circulation. Simple diffusion appears to be the mechanism by which most toxicants pass across the placenta, but some chemicals actually concentrate in the fetus. For example, carbon monoxide binds more tightly to fetal than adult hemoglobin, thus following carbon monoxide exposure in pregnant women fetal levels exceed those of the mothers. Fetuses are also more susceptible because the blood–brain barrier is not completely developed until after birth; thus some chemicals can more readily gain entrance into the fetal CNS. Fetal susceptibility to lead-induced neurotoxicity is an example. In addition, the placenta itself can accumulate chemicals and suffer toxic injury to harm the fetus. Cadmium is an example of a chemical that exerts fetotoxicity primarily by accumulation in and damage of placental tissues.

Metabolism

After systemic absorption, many chemicals are metabolically transformed by enzyme-mediated reactions occurring mainly in the liver and to a lesser extent in other metabolically active tissues such as the kidneys and lungs. The metabolic processes increase the water solubility of transformed compounds, which facilitates their excretion and elimination. Thus, it seems that such metabolic transformations serve an important detoxification role. However, not all transformations diminish the risks of toxicity. On the contrary, there are many examples in which specific enzymatic processes generate active metabolic intermediates that are more toxic than their parent compounds. Accordingly, biotransformation of absorbed chemicals can lead to detoxification, or activation and greater toxicity, or both.

The enzymatic reactions contributing to these chemical transformations are sometimes referred to as phase I and phase II reactions. There are a variety of phase I reactions, including oxidation, reduction, and hydrolysis, that generally increase the polarity of the metabolized molecule; as polarity increases, molecules become more water soluble and more readily excreted. The most important oxidative enzymes involved in such transformation reactions are the cytochrome P-450–containing monooxygenases located in the cellular endoplasmic reticulum. By means of a variety of specific reactions (e.g., hydroxylation, dealkylation, and epoxidation), the monooxygenases transform the underlying molecular structures, generally by introducing one or more oxygen atoms. Cytochrome P-450 enzyme systems are widely distributed and well preserved across species and they are found in a wide array of human tissues. However, there is increasing appreciation of genetic variability in the activities of some cytochrome enzymes, and such variations may explain observed differences in susceptibility to the toxic effects of certain families of chemicals.

Phase II reactions lead to conjugation of molecules to mainly acidic structures (e.g., sulfate, acetate, amino acids) and glutathione (a sulfur-containing tripeptide), rendering the molecules more water soluble and more readily excreted in urine and bile. Glutathione conjugation leads to formation of mercapturic acids, important urinary excretion products for common solvents such as benzene and trichloroethylene, and which also serve as biomarkers for biologic monitoring of workers exposed to those solvents.

Excretion

Toxic chemicals can be excreted in urine, bile, exhaled air, secretions from sweat glands and tears ducts, and breast milk. Urinary excretion is the most important route, especially for smaller molecules and those that are not protein bound. Large molecules preferentially undergo conjugation in the liver and excretion into the bile. For complex molecules, such as the metabolic products of phase II enzyme systems, urine excretion predominates when molecular weights are less than 250, while biliary excretion predominates for molecular weights greater than 350.

A variety of physiologic disturbances can alter the excretion of toxic materials. For many agents, urinary excretion is affected by urine pH and the sufficiency of blood flow to the kidneys. Diseases that alter normal function of renal tubules can increase or decrease urinary excretion of specific compounds, depending on whether those compounds are normally reabsorbed or secreted by the tubules. Conditions that compromise renal function (e.g., dehydration, hypovolemia, and hypotension) and numerous kidney diseases can decrease urinary excretion, thereby increasing the toxicity of compounds normally excreted in the urine.

Likewise, biliary excretion depends on the integrity of hepatobiliary tissues. Individuals with hepatic diseases are at increased risk of toxicity from chemicals that are transformed and excreted by the liver. In addition, some genetic syndromes reduce the normal capacity for hepatic uptake and biliary excretion. Similar reduced capacities are seen in premature and very young infants, thus rendering them at greater risk from some toxic insults. In contrast, certain drugs and chemicals, such as barbiturates, can induce hepatic metabolic activity, increase bile flow, and perhaps also increase blood flow to the liver, changes expected to enhance biliary excretion. Such agents have been used therapeutically to enhance excretion of toxic compounds in some affected individuals.

Exhaled air is also effective as a route of excretion for volatile chemicals, especially those existing in gas phase at body temperature. Elimination is by simple diffusion from the blood into the alveolar space. For such compounds, hyperventilation can increase excretion. For this reason, mechanical respiration and hyperventilation have been advocated as means to reduce body burdens in some forms of acute solvent poisoning.

Fat-soluble compounds, such as organic solvents and polycyclic aromatic hydrocarbons, concentrate in the fat-rich milieu of breast milk. For compounds such as polychlorinated biphenyls (PCBs), breast milk is the most important human route of excretion. For similar reasons, toxic reactions have been reported in the breast-fed infants of mothers exposed in the workplace to fat-soluble organic solvents (e.g., perchloroethylene).

Pharmacokinetic Models

To refine measures of dose and thereby make toxicologic predictions more precise, models can be constructed that link the various species- and chemical-specific data that result from studies of the absorption, distribution, metabolism, and excretion of chemicals and their metabolites. Such models, referred to as physiologically-based pharmacokinetic (PBPK) models, permit the solution of complex simultaneous equations describing ongoing processes within an exposed individual. These modeling techniques, generally simple in concept but enormously dependent on large computer systems, have been used to evaluate the simultaneous effects of multiple metabolic pathways, some leading to detoxification and elimination of the chemical while others produce the ultimate toxicant responsible for the compound's toxicity. The first explicit inclusion of a PBPK model in an OSHA regulation was the methylene chloride standard, which used such a model to calculate the permissible exposure limit. PBPK models have become a major aspect of regulatory toxicology, and it is common to find several modeling experts on most EPA regulatory panels.

TOXICITY TESTING

Substantial human toxicologic data are available for only a limited number of specific chemicals, most notably those that have been used historically for medical and therapeutic purposes. Because of ethical restrictions, it is often not possible to perform human testing, especially at doses anticipated to cause significant or irreversible toxic effects. The Helsinki Declaration of the World Medical Association prohibits experiments using healthy volunteers unless the potential benefits to participants outweighs the potential risks:

> Physicians should abstain from engaging in research projects involving human subjects unless they are confident that the risks involved have been adequately assessed and can be satisfactorily managed. Physicians should cease any investigation if the risks are found to outweigh the potential benefits. . . . Medical research involving human subjects should only be conducted if the importance of the objective outweighs the inherent risks and burdens to the subjects. This is especially important when the human subjects are healthy volunteers.

Consequently, most human toxicology data derive from controlled low-dose exposures, epidemiologic studies, and post hoc study of the victims of accidental high-dose exposures. Instead, the vast majority of quantitative toxicologic data derive from in vivo toxicity testing in nonhuman species, "test tube" testing of lower organisms (e.g., bacteria), and in vitro studies with cell cultures and subcellular materials.

Numerous types of tests can be conducted to provide toxicologic data that are otherwise unavailable from human studies (see the EPA's harmonized test guidelines, discussed at the beginning of this chapter).

Among the most forceful motivations for extensive toxicology testing are requirements of the federal Toxic Substances Control Act (TSCA), legislation adopted in 1976 and administered by the EPA. TSCA requires manufacturers to notify the EPA at least 90 days before the production of any new chemical substance and to submit data from a mandated array of tests as a component of premanufacturing notices intended to demonstrate that the substance poses no significant risks to public health or the environment. Based on a review of that data, the EPA may approve the production or new use, or limit the manufacture or distribution of the substance until additional test data are available. TSCA also requires the ongoing submission of new data as they are produced in further testing or as a result of clinical observations in exposed individuals.

Another potent stimulus to toxicologic testing has been the growing importance of quantitative risk assessment in setting exposure and cleanup standards. Most risk assessment guidelines require extra margins of safety to address gaps in the toxicologic database for individual chemicals. Thus, the risk assessment process tends to highlight data deficiencies and provides incentives, especially to the regulated community, to perform the testing necessary to provide the missing information.

A fundamental assumption underlying most animal testing is that the effects produced by the test compound are the same or similar to those observed or expected in humans. Unfortunately, this assumption can lead to dispute and uncertainty. Of particular concern is the increasing reliance on a limited number of genetically uniform strains of animals (in some cases actually genetically engineered strains), which have been selected in part because of their susceptibility to certain kinds of toxicologic effects. For example, the strain of mice used most often for cancer bioassays in the United States (B6C3F_1 mice) have high rates of spontaneous liver cancer; accordingly, the human relevance of increased rates of liver cancer in experimentally exposed mice has been challenged. Likewise, differences in the capacities of specific strains to metabolically activate or detoxify certain chemicals may render those strains of limited relevance to the risks in humans. Accordingly, the choice of species and strains can influence the results of testing and their meaningfulness as predictors of human disease.

Because occupational and environmental health professionals are often called upon to read and interpret toxicologic reports and data, it is important that they understand the purposes and differences of commonly used toxicologic tests.

Acute Toxicity Studies

Acute toxicity studies are performed by administering a test material to animals on one occasion and evaluating any resulting toxicity over the following hours, days, and even weeks. These studies can determine the median lethal dose for a chemical (LD_{50}). An LD_{50} is defined as the dose that would predictably kill one half of the animal population experimentally exposed. For inhalation studies, the LD_{50} or lethal concentration required to produce death in 50% of the animals, is determined. In addition to determining a material's lethality, these tests are used to evaluate a number of other toxic effects, including behavior, response to stimuli, reflexes, and effects on bodily functions and vital signs.

The results of acute toxicity testing provide basic information about a material's relative potential to cause acute or immediate toxic effects. This relative potential is often expressed in terms of toxicity ratings of classes. One example of a well-known classification system is given in Table 39.1. Discovery that a material has a "6" or "supertoxic" rating using this classification system would help the clinician quickly appreciate the highly toxic nature of the material and its potential to severely injure or kill an individual at extremely low doses. Such classification systems are only qualitative, but they serve a practical and useful purpose as first approximations of the likely toxicologic hazards posed by individual chemicals and the levels of precautions needed for their use.

Dermal Irritation and Sensitization

The ability of a chemical to irritate the skin is usually determined in rabbits. The fur on the back of the rabbit is removed with clippers, and the chemical is applied to the skin under a covered patch for a period of usually 3 days. The degree of skin irritation is scored for erythema and eschar formation, edema formation, and corrosive action. These dermal observations are repeated at various intervals after the covered patch is removed. Increasing attention has focused on finding skin irritancy testing methods that do not require the use of whole animals.

Cutaneous sensitization is usually evaluated in guinea pigs. Through initial skin testing and testing with subsequent challenge doses, both irritant and challenge scores can be determined. A comparison of these scores is then used to determine the material's ability to sensitize.

Eye Irritation

Most compounds that are generally available for human use are tested for irritant effects following topical application of the agents to the eyes of experimental animals, often referred to as the Draize test. Rabbits are the preferred species for testing. The procedure involves applying material in liquid or solid form to the lower conjunctival sac of one eye in each of at least six animals. The eyes are then examined periodically following exposure (e.g., at 1, 2, and 3 days) and scored according to the severity of irritation noted. The irritation score for a particular material gives useful information regarding the material's po-

TABLE 39.1. *Example of a numerical toxicity rating system*

	Probable oral lethal dose (human)	
Toxicity rating of class	Dose	For 70-kg person (150 lb)
6—supertoxic	Less than 5 mg/kg	A taste (less than 7 drops)
5—extremely toxic	5–50 mg/kg	Between 7 drops and 1 tsp
4—very toxic	50–500 mg/kg	Between 1 tsp and 1 oz
3—moderately toxic	0.5–5 g/kg	Between 1 oz and 1 pt (or 1 lb)
2—slightly toxic	5–15 g/kg	Between 1 pt and 1 qt
1—practically nontoxic	Above 15 g/kg	More than 1 qt (2.2 lb)

From Gosselin R, et al. *Clinical toxicology of commercial products,* 5th ed. Baltimore: Williams & Wilkins, 1984:1–2.

TABLE 39.2. *Examples of threshold-based toxicity guideline values by exposure scenario*

Term	Acronym	Defined	Agency	Reference[a]
For emergency response	*Developed to assist emergency response personnel in planning for catastrophic chemical releases to the community, and are short-term community exposure limits applicable to most members of the general public*			
Emergency response planning guideline	ERPG	An estimate of a concentration range below which it is believed nearly all individuals could be exposed for up to an hour without observing adverse effects. Three levels of ERPGs have been developed for different health effect end points. ERPG-1, ERPG-2, and ERPG-3[b] values have been established for over 90 chemicals.	American Industrial Hygiene Association's (AIHA)	AIHA, 2002
Acute exposure guideline levels	AEGL	Three-tiered exposure guidelines for emergency chemical releases spanning exposure durations of 10 minutes to 8 hours. Modeled after the ERPGs, and motivated by requirements of the Clean Air Act, AEGLs are developed by an international committee representing U.S. federal and state agencies, European agencies, industry, and others including ACOEM. Peer-reviewed and published by National Academy of Sciences.	Lead Agency: U.S. Environmental Protection Agency (EPA)	NRC, 2001
For occupational exposures	*Developed to protect healthy adult workers from the effects of chronic exposures over their working lifetimes.*			
Threshold limit value time-weighted average	TLV-TWA	A time-weighted average concentration for a conventional 8-hour workday and a 40-hour workweek, to which it is believed that nearly all workers may be repeatedly exposed, day after day, without adverse effect. (NIOSH and OSHA have developed similar toxicity guideline values.[c])	American Conference of Governmental Industrial Hygienists (ACGIH)	ACGIH, 2000, 2001
Threshold limit value short-term exposure limits (STELs) and ceiling (C)	TLV-STEL	A 15-minute TWA exposure which should not be exceeded at any time during a workday even if the 8-hour TWA is with the TLV-TWA.	ACGIH	ACGIH, 2000, 2001
	TLV-C	A concentration that should not be exceeded during any part of the working exposure.		
Immediately dangerous to life and health	IDLH	A condition that poses a threat of exposure to airborne contaminants when that exposure is likely to cause death or immediate or delayed permanent adverse health effects or prevent escape from such an environment. IDLH concentrations are established at levels that ensure that a worker can escape from a given contaminated environment in the event of failure of the respiratory protection equipment.	National Institute for Occupational Safety and Health (NIOSH)	NIOSH, 1999
For nonoccupational exposures	*Estimates of a daily chemical exposure to the human population that is likely to be without an appreciable risk of deleterious effects during a lifetime. These values generally consider sensitive subpopulations, whereas worker guideline values do not.*			
Reference dose	RfD	An estimate (with uncertainty spanning perhaps an order of magnitude) of a daily oral exposure to the human population (including sensitive subgroups) that is likely to be without an appreciable risk of deleterious effects during a lifetime.	U.S. EPA	EPA, 2002
Reference concentration	RfC	An estimate (with uncertainty spanning perhaps an order of magnitude) of a continuous inhalation exposure to the human population (including sensitive subgroups) that is likely to be without an appreciable risk of deleterious effects during a lifetime.		
Minimal risk level	MRL	An estimate of the daily human exposure to a hazardous substance that is likely to be without appreciable risk of adverse noncancer health effects over a specified duration of exposure.	Agency for Toxic Substances and Disease Registry (ATSDR)	ATSDR, 2000

[a]For full reference, see Further Information section.

[b]ERPG-1 is the maximum airborne concentration below which it is believed that nearly all individuals could be exposed for up to 1 hour without experiencing other than mild transient adverse health effects or perceiving a clearly defined objectionable odor. The ERPG-2 is the maximum airborne concentration below which it is believed that nearly all individuals could be exposed for up to 1 hour without experiencing or developing irreversible or other serious health effects or symptoms that could impair an individual's ability to take protective action. The ERPG-3 is the maximum airborne concentration below which it is believed that nearly all individuals could be exposed for up to 1 hour without experiencing or developing life-threatening health effects.

[c]OSHA has developed permissible exposure limits (PELs) and NIOSH has developed recommended exposure limits (RELs) toxicity guideline values for the workplace (OSHA, 1999; NIOSH, 1999). OSHA has established values for PEL-TWAs, short-term exposure limits (PEL-ST), and ceiling exposure limits (PEL-C) for over 160 chemicals. NIOSH has established values for REL-TWAs, short-term exposure limits (REL-ST), and ceiling exposure limits (REL-C) for over 650 chemicals. The values and definitions of PEL and REL are not equal to each other or to ACGIH values and definitions (for example, the REL-TWA considers a 10-hour workday). The references for these toxicity guideline values are presented in the Further Information section.

ACOEM, American College of Occupational and Environmental Medicine; OSHA, Occupational Safety and Health Administration.

tential to irritate human eyes on contact. Increasing attention has focused on finding eye irritancy testing methods that do not require the use of whole animals.

Subchronic Exposure

The objective of subchronic exposure studies is to evaluate and characterize the potential toxicity of a compound when administered to experimental animals on a daily basis over a period of 3 to 4 months. The subchronic study is usually performed in two animal species, using the same route of exposure that is expected in humans. Observations on the test animals include mortality, body weight changes, diet consumption, hematology, and clinical chemistry measurements. At the end of the experiment, the gross and microscopic condition of the animals and selected organs and tissues are evaluated and recorded. One of the objectives of the subchronic study is to attempt to demonstrate some form of toxic effect, at least in the high-dose group of experimental animals. Use of short-term acute toxicity studies prior to the subchronic test is helpful in planning an appropriate subchronic dose regimen. Subchronic studies also aim at determining the exposure level at which there is no adverse effect or adverse effects are not observable.

With appropriate modifications, the basic subchronic test can be used to evaluate mutagenesis, teratogenesis, and effects on reproductive capacity. Except for carcinogenesis and some forms of cytotoxicity, the subchronic test usually reveals most forms of toxicity to adult animals. These findings form a reasonable basis to predict the material's potential toxicity to humans when exposed through the same route of exposure.

Chronic Exposure/Cancer Bioassays

Chronic toxicity studies, used to evaluate a chemical's cumulative toxicity, often allow simultaneous consideration of cancer and noncancer end points. Standard protocols in most countries include testing of both a rat and a mouse strain; specific strains may vary across studies. U.S. studies most often use Fischer rats and $B6C3F_1$ mice, but European studies generally use other rodent strains, and larger mammals, including cats, dogs, guinea pigs, rabbits, and even primates, have sometimes been used. Differences between studies can sometimes be explained by the choice of test species and strain.

A commonly employed testing protocol includes 50 male and 50 female animals for each of three exposure levels plus gender-specific control groups, with rats exposed for 24 to 30 months and mice exposed for 18 to 24 months. The high-dose group is usually administered a level known to cause mild toxicity (maximum tolerated dose, MTD) determined in prior subchronic studies. The test chemical can be administered orally (diet or gavage) or by inhalation; dermal exposure is less common. At the termination of the study, animals are sacrificed and all animals, including those that die during the study, are subjected to gross and microscopic pathologic examinations and all pathologic changes are noted.

The bioassay is designed to assess whether test chemicals produce carcinogenic effects, which are often defined as any of the following changes:

1. The development of types of neoplasms not seen in controls.
2. An increased incidence of the types of neoplasms occurring in controls.
3. The occurrence of neoplasms earlier than in controls.
4. An increased multiplicity of neoplasms in an individual animal.

As a first approximation, it is assumed that chemicals capable of causing cancer in animals can also cause cancer in humans. There is sufficient evidence that all human carcinogens (with the possible exception of arsenic) are also animal carcinogens; for at least 19 of those carcinogens, humans and animals demonstrate the same target organs. But the converse may not always be true. There are numerous animal carcinogens for which there is little or no evidence of human carcinogenicity. It is uncertain whether such disparities reflect intrinsic species-specific differences of susceptibility. An alternative explanation is that they are due to the relatively low potency of the carcinogens coupled with the small numbers of exposed humans, resulting in an unperceived increase in disease.

As a general rule, animal studies provide valuable insights into the potential of chemicals to cause chronic injury and cancer in humans, but animal findings alone are insufficient to determine the human carcinogenicity of a chemical.

In Vitro Assays

In vitro assays provide a rapid and relatively inexpensive means of characterizing certain toxic effects, especially mutagenicity and DNA reactivity. Mutagenesis is the ability of chemicals to cause changes in the genetic material in the nucleus of cells in ways that can be transmitted during cell division. In vitro assays include bacterial mutagenicity tests, and the use of normal or genetically altered animal or human cells. Collectively, these assays provide data on gene mutations (e.g., base pair substitutions, frameshift mutations, etc.), chromosomal aberrations, primary DNA damage, and morphologic transformation. Since mutations are thought to be an important mechanism for the initiation of cancer, mutagenic tests are often required as a component of screening for potential carcinogens.

The most widely utilized bacterial test system for identifying mutagenic activity is the *Salmonella typhimurium* microsomal test (Ames assay) that detects gene mutation affecting the ability of *Salmonella* to synthesize histidine, an essential amino acid. Bacteria lacking the ability to synthesize histidine are exposed to the suspect mutagen and then grown in a culture medium lacking histidine. If the test chemical is mutagenic, some bacteria "back-mutate," thereby regaining the ability to synthesize histidine, and will survive in the histidine-free medium. Comparison of such chemically induced mutations rates and the rate of spontaneous back-mutations permits an estimate of the mutagenic potential and potency of the test chemical.

The mouse lymphoma (L5178Y), the Chinese hamster ovary (CHO), and the V70 hamster fibroblast cell lines are commonly used for mutation testing in mammalian cells. These assays detect forward-mutations that confer resistance to toxic chemicals. The end points for these assays are most commonly the genes controlling hypoxanthine-guanine phosphoribosyltransferase (*hprt* gene) and thymidine kinase (*tk* gene). As with the Ames assay, the potency of chemicals is characterized by comparing the mutation rates among treated and untreated cells.

Other assays are often used to indirectly detect mutations or damage at the chromosome, rather than gene level. These tests include the presence of sister chromatid exchange (SCE), which reflects the breakage and repair of sister chromosomes, the micronucleus assay, which reflects breakage and loss of large pieces of individual chromosomes or nondisjunction during mitosis, and karyotype analysis, which evaluates the number and gross configuration of the chromosomes.

ADVICE TO CLINICIANS

Understanding toxicologic principles and testing methods can assist the physician in evaluating patients with symptoms or illness suspected to be the result of toxic exposures. In evaluating such patients, a detailed and comprehensive exposure history, both occupational and otherwise, is of primary importance. Likewise, a comprehensive and thoughtful clinical evaluation is required. It is generally important to distinguish between subjective symptoms and objective physical pathology; diseases and pathologies may cause symptoms and complaints, but such symptoms and complaints do not define the pathology, although they may raise suspicions in the minds of competent clinicians. Numerous occupational medicine diseases were first detected by perceptive clinicians evaluating common, but unexplained, symptoms in exposed workers. Ultimately, such diseases were defined by the discovery of specific objective pathologies in those patients.

Knowing what exposures a patient may have encountered, the magnitude of these exposures, and the period of time during which exposures occurred provides critical data necessary for a physician to evaluate the role and responsibility of exposures for a particular illness. Beyond workplace exposures and concerns about diet, smoking and use of drugs and alcohol, patients should be asked about their home location and type, sources of drinking water (in communities where well water is used), hobbies and nonoccupational activities, and contact with others potentially exposed to chemicals.

Frequently, information concerning workplace exposures can be obtained through consultation with medical and industrial hygiene professionals at the patient's place of employment. The OSHA Hazard Communication Standard requires that information regarding the materials used or handled be made available to the employee. In addition, the OSHA Access to Employee Medical and Exposure Records regulation provides for employee access to applicable exposure records. Most employers can provide Material Safety and Data Sheets (MSDSs), which are useful to identify the exposures of individual workers. (The appendix to this chapter outlines information required by OSHA to be included on the MSDS of regulated chemicals.) For environmental exposures, it is often necessary to obtain exposure records from multiple sources, including local sources of drinking water, regional or state air pollution monitoring programs, and EPA chemical release inventories.

Once a list of suspect chemicals has been established, evaluating whether any chemical is likely to have been medically significant requires detailed knowledge of the specific agents in question. These situations can be approached in either of two directions. Most often, the evaluation begins with the patient evaluation, leading to a detailed characterization of the patient's illness, particularly the organs affected and the nature of physiologic disturbances. There is often a list of chemicals that are well recognized as able to cause such effects, and the clinician should look to determine whether the patient has had such exposures. In addition, systematic literature reviews usually reveal longer list of agents of known or suspected association with diagnosed conditions. These should also become suspects and the patient's history should be searched to determine whether there has been exposure to any of those additional agents.

A history of historical exposures to agents associated with the patient's conditions raises the possibility of causal associations, but such information alone is not sufficient to actually attribute causation. For that purpose, knowledge of the exposure dose and exposure duration is critical; without quantitative dose-related data, it is not possible to evaluate the probability that any given exposure has led to a specific disease. As stressed earlier, the first law of toxicology states, "Dose makes the poison." The exception to this important rule is for situations in which rapid intervention and treatment are necessary. In such cases, actions based solely on clinical suspicion are often justified, situations of special relevance to acute poisonings for which early administration of antidotes and other therapies may be lifesaving. In those cases, reasonable possibility is often sufficient justification for intervention, even when evidence is not sufficient to conclude causation with any degree of certainty.

FURTHER INFORMATION

AIHA: *The AIHA 2002 emergency response planning guidelines and workplace environmental exposure level guides handbook.* Fairfax, VA: American Industrial Hygiene Association, 2002.

A quick reference guide providing emergency response planning guideline (ERPG) and workplace environmental exposure level (WEEL) limits. Each includes background information and user guidance.

ACGIH: *Documentation of the threshold limit values (TLVs) and biological exposure indices (BEIs) with Appendices,* 6th ed. Cincinnati: American Conference of Governmental Industrial Hygienists, Inc., 2000.

ACGIH: *2001 TLVs and BEIs. Threshold limit values for chemical substances and physical agents.* Cincinnati: American Conference of Governmental Industrial Hygienists, 2001.

ACGIH, 2000 is a three-volume set presenting literature reviews and justification for the occupational exposure limits established by ACGIH for a wide array of specific chemicals substances and physical agents.

ACGIH, 2001 is a pocket guide providing the exposure limits and other key information contained in the three-volume set, but in abbreviated tabular form.

ATSDR, 2000. *Minimal risk levels (MRLs) for hazardous substances.* Available online at *www.atsdr.cdc.govmrls.html.*

MRLs, intended to serve as screening levels, are used by Agency for Toxic Substances and Disease Registry (ATSDR) health assessors and other responders to identify contaminants and potential health effects of possible concern at hazardous waste sites.

Ellenhorn MJ, ed. *Ellenhorn's medical toxicology: diagnosis and treatment of human poisoning,* 2nd ed. Baltimore: Williams & Wilkins, 1997.

This reference book provides an extensive discussion of individual intoxications, with emphasis on acute poisonings, their diagnosis, and treatment. This is an excellent and widely used text in emergency departments and poison control centers.

EPA: Integrated Risk Information System. Washington, DC: Environmental Protection Agency, 2003. http://www.epa.gov/IRIS/.

Greenberg MI, Hamilton RJ, Phillips SD, eds. *Occupational, industrial, and environmental toxicology.* St. Louis: Mosby, 1997.

This comprehensive reference book is unique in its approach, which organizes its discussion of toxicology almost entirely in terms of the types of work and workplaces, rather than the categories of chemicals and agents.

Hayes AW, ed. *Principles and methods of toxicology,* 4th ed. Philadelphia: Taylor & Francis, 2001.

This massive textbook and reference contains detailed discussions of the principles of toxicology and methods of toxicology testing. Systematic and highly detailed, this book is not aimed at clinicians and provides only very limited clinical information.

Klaassen CD, ed. *Casarett and Doull's toxicology: the basic science of poisons,* 6th ed. New York: McGraw-Hill, 2001.

This is a standard textbook covering the basic principles of toxicology, especially strong in its discussions of the metabolic and mechanistic processes that underlie toxic injuries. Systematic and highly detailed, this book is not aimed at clinicians and provides only very limited clinical information.

Liverman CT, Ingalls CE, Fulco CE, et al., eds. *Toxicology and environmental health information resources: the role of the National Library of Medicine.* Washington, DC: National Academy Press, 1997.

This is a concise overview of the toxicology and environmental health resources offered by the National Library of Medicine (NLM), including description of key databases overviews of similar resources external to the NLM.

NRC (National Research Council). *Standing operating procedures for developing acute exposure guideline levels for hazardous chemicals.* Washington, DC: National Academy Press, 2001.

NRC (National Research Council). *Acute exposure guideline levels for selected airborne chemicals, vol. 1.* Washington, DC: National Academy Press, 2000.

The first of these two books describes the detailed methodology being used to develop acute exposure guideline limits as mandated by the Clean Air Act, and subsequently adopted by all federal and numerous international agencies. The second illustrates the in-depth literature reviews and toxicologic reasoning that underlies the exposure limits thus established.

NIOSH: *Registry for toxic effects of chemical substances. Department of Health & Social Services, Public Health Service, Centers for Disease Control and Prevention.* NIOSH, 2000. Accessed on DIALOG (Knight-Ridder Information, Inc.).

RTECS is a comprehensive database of basic toxicity information on more than 100,000 chemical substances used in industrial, commercial, and household situations. Reports of toxic effects and data on skin/eye irritation, mutation, reproductive consequences, and tumorigenicity are included.

NIOSH: *NIOSH pocket guide to chemical hazards.* U.S. Department of Health and Human Services Centers for Disease Control and Prevention. NIOSH publication No. 99-115, April 1999.

This guide provides key information and data in abbreviated tabular form for more than 600 toxic chemicals found in the workplaces, including OSHA permissible exposure limits and NIOSH recommended exposure limits, chemical and physical properties, and abbreviated toxicity summaries.

National Library of Medicine. *Hazardous Substances Data Bank.* National Library of Medicine Toxicology Data Network, 2000. Available at *http://toxnet.nlm.nih.govcgi-binsishtmlgen?HSDB.*

The Hazardous Substances Data Bank (HSDB), which contains more than 4,500 entries, focuses on the toxicology of potentially hazardous chemicals. It is enhanced with information on human exposure, industrial hygiene, emergency handling procedures, environmental fate, regulatory requirements, and related areas.

Sullivan JB, Krieger GR, eds. *Clinical environmental health and toxic exposures,* 2nd ed. Philadelphia: Lippincott Williams & Wilkins, 2001.

A comprehensive reference that discussion the toxicology of a wide array of industrial activities and a large inventory of industrial chemicals including limited discussions of clinical management of exposure victims.

Verma DK. Adjustment for occupational exposure limits for unusual work schedules. *Am Ind Hyg Assoc J* 2000;61: 367–374.

This review discusses four approaches to using toxicologic information to adjust occupational exposure limits to protect workers assigned to unusual work schedules.

Wexler P, Hakkinen PJ, Kennedy G, et al., eds. *Information resources in toxicology,* 3rd ed. New York: Academic Press, 2000.

This is a very useful overview of worldwide resources pertaining to toxicology. Includes substantial subject bibliographies, guides to literature, databases, and standard toxicology texts.

APPENDIX: MATERIAL SAFETY DATA SHEETS

The 1970 Occupational Safety and Health Act requires employers to provide employees with safe working conditions. One means, as stated in the OSHA Hazard Communication Final Rule (29 CFR 1910.1200), requires the following information to be included on Material Safety Data Sheets for hazardous chemicals covered by the regulation:

I. The identity used on the label, and
   A. If the hazardous chemical is a single substance, its chemical and common name(s);
   B. If the hazardous chemical is a mixture that has been tested as a whole to determine its hazards, the chemical and common name(s) of the ingredients that contribute to these known hazards, and the common name(s) of the mixture itself; or
   C. If the hazardous chemical is a mixture that has not been tested as a whole;
      1. The chemical and common name(s) of all ingredients that have been determined to be health hazards and comprise 1% or more of the composition; except that chemicals identified as carcinogens are to be listed if the concentrations are 0.1% or more; and
      2. The chemical and common name(s) of all ingredients that have been determined to present a physical hazard when present in the mixture;
      3. Physical and chemical characteristics of the hazardous chemical (such as vapor pressure, flash point);
      4. The physical hazards of the hazardous chemical, including the potential for fire, explosion, and reactivity;
      5. The health hazards of the hazardous chemical, including signs and symptoms of exposure and any medical conditions that are generally recognized as being aggravated by exposure to the chemical;
      6. The primary route(s) of entry;
      7. The OSHA permissible exposure limit, ACGIH threshold limit value, and any other exposure limit used or recommended by the chemical manufacturer, importer, or employer preparing the Material Safety Data Sheet, where available;
      8. Whether the hazardous chemical is listed in the National Toxicology Program (NTP) Annual Report on Carcinogens (latest edition), or has been found to be a potential carcinogen in the International Agency for Research on Cancer (IARC) Monographs (latest editions), or by OSHA;
      9. Any generally applicable precautions for safe handling and use that are known to the chemical manufacturer, importer, or employer preparing the Material Safety Data Sheet, including appropriate hy-

gienic practices, protective measures during repair and maintenance of contaminated equipment, and procedures for cleanup of spills and leaks;

10. Any generally applicable control measures that are known to the chemical manufacturer, importer, or employer preparing the Material Safety Data Sheet, such as appropriate engineering controls, work practices, or personal protective equipment;
11. Emergency and first-aid procedures;
12. The date of preparation of the Material Safety Data Sheet or the last change to it; and
13. The name, address, and telephone number of the chemical manufacturer, importer, employer, or other responsible party preparing or distributing the Material Safety Data Sheet, who can provide additional information on the hazardous chemical and appropriate emergency procedures, if necessary.

40

Epidemiology and Biostatistics

Joseph K. McLaughlin and Loren Lipworth

Epidemiology is the study of the distribution and determinants of disease in human populations (1). Its approach is population based, as compared to a clinical or individual perspective. This chapter introduces some basic epidemiologic and biostatistic concepts as they apply to etiologic investigations in occupational medicine and provides a framework for the evaluation of epidemiologic evidence in determining causality. The fundamental goal of an epidemiologic investigation is to obtain valid and reasonably precise estimates of an exposure–disease association in occupational groups. Case reports and other forms of anecdotal data in the clinical literature may alert an investigator to potential health risks, but cannot provide evidence of an association. For example, hypotheses linking organic trivalent arsenic compounds to skin cancer (2) and vinyl chloride to angiosarcoma of the liver (3) have been derived, to a considerable extent, from astute clinical observations. However, it was epidemiologic studies that provided a systematic method for identifying, verifying, and quantifying such health risks.

STRENGTHS AND LIMITATIONS OF EPIDEMIOLOGY

Much of the success of epidemiology in enhancing our understanding of the causes of disease is due to the fact that the risk of cancer, heart disease, stroke, and other chronic diseases is measured directly in human populations (4). With the epidemiologic method, there is no need to rely on questionable extrapolations across species to estimate the impact of an exposure in humans. Instead, it is possible in epidemiology to examine the consequences of environmental, occupational, or endogenous exposures in the manner in which they actually occur in humans, not the artificial manner in which laboratory studies of animals are done (5). The issues of dose, route of exposure, concomitant exposures, and host factors are also directly assessed (6). Thus, an agent can be considered etiologically related to disease when an alteration in the frequency or intensity of exposure to this agent is followed by a change in the frequency of occurrence of one or more types of disease. In fact, it was through epidemiologic studies that the serious health risks associated with tobacco, ionizing radiation, asbestos, and a number of other occupational exposures were identified (7).

Although epidemiology may be the only direct way to evaluate harmful or potentially harmful exposures in humans, the method has several shortcomings (1,4,6,7). Low-level risks are difficult to detect without very large expensive studies, and these weak associations (10% to 50% increases in risk) are now becoming more common in epidemiology as we may have already uncovered most of the easy-to-identify common causes of serious diseases such as cigarette smoking and lung cancer and saturated fats and cardiovascular disease. Very small observed increases in disease rates for exposed compared with unexposed groups in epidemiologic studies are more likely to be accounted for by bias (systematic error), confounding (distortion of the exposure–disease association by an extraneous variable), or chance occurrence. It should be added, however, that it is also difficult to demonstrate effects in experimental studies of laboratory animals at low exposure levels; hence, very high doses are typically given to animals in carcinogenicity studies. The long latency (time from exposure to disease) of most chronic diseases is another obstacle in epidemiologic research. Latency periods of 5 to 50 years between initial exposure and actual cancer occurrence, for example, make the identification of a cancer-causing agent quite difficult and make the timely epidemiologic evaluation of agents newly introduced into the environment or workplace virtually impossible. Furthermore, in occupational settings, individuals often encounter many concomitant exposures, the effects of which are difficult to disentangle, although this does allow for the detection of synergistic effects of exposures such as cigarette smoking and alcohol intake on oral, laryngeal, and esophageal cancer, and cigarette smoking and asbestos on lung cancer. Sometimes epidemiologists must use surrogate measures such as job title or place of employment instead of direct information on exposures, thus allowing the opportunity for misclassification (information bias). Another major limitation of the epidemiologic approach is the inability to adjust for the effects of unknown confounders, which, unlike known confounders that can be controlled through statistical methods, distort risk estimates.

OBSERVATIONAL VERSUS EXPERIMENTAL STUDIES

Conclusive evidence regarding disease causation in humans can, in theory, come only from double-blind randomized trials. Randomization produces, on average, equal distribution of both known and unknown confounding factors in the study and control groups, and double-blind designs minimize the potential for several types of bias. However, epidemiologic studies cannot achieve the experimental control of randomized trials. From an ethical point of view, researchers could not randomly assign humans to two groups, one to receive 300 rad of ionizing radiation (an established carcinogen) and one to serve as a control group to assess the short- and long-term effects of radiation. An exception may occur when there is evidence that a particular factor may actually prevent disease, but even under these conditions, trials aiming at disease prevention in humans are impractical or extremely complex. For instance, in clinical trials of cancer treatment, the outcome under investigation (death, metastasis, or recurrence) is a relatively frequent event, and the corresponding study size is manageable. In contrast, among healthy individuals, the frequency of occurrence of any particular cancer is low, so that the corresponding study size must be large with a very long follow-up period.

In the absence of strong human experimental evidence (which is invariably the situation in most cause-and-effect controversies), disease causation in humans can best be assessed through well-conducted observational or nonexperimental studies, in which the issues of bias and confounding are evaluated on a study-by-study basis. Some populations provide an opportunity to conduct "natural experiments," such as workers exposed to a particular agent during the course of their work or an ethnic or religious group with unique dietary habits. The most effective observational studies in epidemiology are the so-called analytic investigations, which are designed to explore whether an association between a particular agent or characteristic and a particular type of disease actually exists, at the individual level, and to quantify the magnitude of the association after eliminating, as far as possible, all recognizable confounding and bias. The two most common types of analytic study designs in occupational epidemiology are the cohort and case-control studies.

TYPES OF OBSERVATIONAL STUDIES IN EPIDEMIOLOGY

Cohort Studies

The most common type of study in occupational epidemiology is the cohort study, which is also known as a follow-up, longitudinal, or prospective study. The cohort study identifies populations of individuals exposed or not exposed to a particular factor and follows them forward in time until a sufficient number of cases of disease have developed. The frequency of occurrence of the disease (or diseases) under investigation in the two (or more, if several exposure categories or levels can be ascertained) groups is calculated and compared. The well-known cohort studies of cigarette smokers are examples of this type of study.

The prospective or classic type of cohort study relies on the collection of current exposure information and identifies new cases of disease as they occur in the future. However, this type of study takes a long time to complete and analyze, since the investigators usually have to wait many years before acquiring enough cases of disease (or deaths if disease outcome is measured by mortality). Thus, a variant of the prospective cohort study has been developed, the retrospective cohort study, in which preexisting records are used to characterize the past exposure status of the study subjects, and disease occurrence or, more typically, mortality is determined up to the present or a particular date in the recent past. This is the typical type of cohort design found in most occupational studies, since the need to wait for a long follow-up period is eliminated, as it is already inherent in the design.

All analytic epidemiologic studies involve some type of sampling, although often the sampling process is not clearly defined. The source population that is sampled over the study period is often called the study base or base population, while the subjects who are actually investigated comprise the study group or study population (1). In the absence of randomization, the issue of study base, or source population, is of paramount importance in determining whether the comparison group in an observational study is appropriate. The comparison group in a cohort study should represent the same study base or source population as the exposed or study group. Ideally, therefore, the nonexposed group should be an internal comparison group sampled from the study cohort. For instance, in an occupational study, exposed and unexposed workers in the same cohort are likely to have undergone the same employment selection process and may be similar with respect to several lifestyle factors such as smoking and alcohol consumption. An external comparison group from a similar occupation or industry may also meet some of the criteria for selection and comparability of lifestyle factors. Often, however, general population incidence or mortality rates (specific for age, sex, race, geographic area, and calendar time) are used in place of an internal comparison group in order to estimate an expected number of new cases (or deaths), which is compared with the corresponding number observed in the exposed cohort. Since disease rates vary by geographic area, it is often more appropriate to use state or regional rates (if available and statistically stable) rather than the national disease experience for comparison. For instance, if the exposed cohort is from an area with unusually high or low background disease rates and the national disease experience is used as a comparison, a misleading result could be reported. The validity of the use of general population rates depends on the accurate recording of exposed person-time, as well as on the use of similar and adequate criteria for diagnosis of cases or attribution of deaths in the exposed and the general population.

Sometimes, if one of the comparison groups (e.g., general population) has a deficiency, it may be useful to have more than one comparison group. If the results are consistent across the two comparison groups, the findings are strengthened; however, if the results are not consistent, the interpretation of the findings can be quite difficult (8).

When using general population rates in occupational epidemiology, as opposed to internal comparison groups, there is strong potential for bias due to the "healthy worker effect," because both sick and well, and employed and unemployed, individuals comprise the comparison group. Employed people, as a result of preplacement physical examinations and other selection factors, are generally healthier than unemployed people and have lower mortality rates for most major diseases (9). The healthy worker effect, however, is usually not as pronounced for cancer as it is for respiratory and heart diseases.

Advantages and Disadvantages

The primary methodologic advantage of the cohort design (both prospective and retrospective) is that information on exposure is recorded before the development of the disease under study. Thus, the investigator knows that exposure to the suspected risk factor preceded the onset of the disease, eliminating recall bias (differential recall between ill and healthy individuals), to which case-control studies are potentially vulnerable (10). Also, a cohort study traces in a more natural way the time sequence of causal phenomena and provides a fuller picture of the health effects of the hypothesized disease-causing agent relative to a case-control study. Thus, a particular exposure that may cause more than one disease can be better studied in a cohort study compared with a case-control study, which usually investigates only one disease.

For the prospective cohort design, however, the time between exposure and occurrence of disease is often long, thereby increasing the cost and difficulty of maintaining and following the cohort, particularly in a mobile society such as the United States, as well as the length of time before data can be meaningfully analyzed. Therefore, it is not an efficient way to study rare diseases. However, with this design, predisease information can be collected, along with repeated measures of the study exposure over the course of the investigation. Increased information on the early stages of the natural history of the disease and advances in the precision of exposure measures over time make this design important in etiology research (11).

In the retrospective cohort study design, both exposure and disease have already taken place, and therefore this design has advantages over the prospective cohort approach for diseases with long latency. For these reasons, the retrospective cohort design is commonly used in occupational studies. However, while retrospective cohort studies are usually faster and less expensive than prospective cohort studies, it is often difficult to find reasonably complete records to adequately characterize the cohort and its exposure experience, and there is usually little if any ability to control for potential confounders such as cigarette smoking, alcohol consumption, and other lifestyle factors, which are normally collected at the start of a prospective cohort study. Since most of these studies are of occupational groups with unusually high exposures to a particular agent, an attributable risk estimate cannot be meaningfully interpreted, as the exposure level is not representative of the general population (11).

Relatively rare diseases such as cancer are difficult to study using either cohort approach, as even for the more common cancers such as lung or breast cancer, unless the relative risk associated with the exposure is very large, it is unlikely that there will be enough cases to provide adequate information on the effects of the exposure. A cohort study can be advantageous if the exposure of interest is rare in the general population and responsible for only a small proportion of a particular disease, but common among a particular group of workers.

Confounding is just as common in cohort as in case-control studies, and in retrospective cohort investigations typically this problem cannot be addressed as there is usually little if any information on confounding factors such as cigarette smoking. In prospective cohort studies, in contrast, confounding can often be taken into consideration provided information on potential confounding factors is collected at baseline enrollment. Cohort studies allow estimation of the risk of disease among unexposed and exposed individuals, providing direct measures of the relative risk (or of several relative risks according to the level or category of exposure) and absolute risks.

Case-control Studies

Because of the logistical and cost disadvantages of the cohort design, case-control studies have predominated in cancer and other areas of epidemiology. While cohort studies follow individuals from exposure to disease development, case-control studies ascertain previous exposure experience among a group of subjects who have been recently diagnosed with the disease under study (cases) and a group of subjects free of the disease (controls) sampled from the source population (study base) from which the cases were ascertained (12). Information on past exposures and lifestyle habits and other confounders is obtained by use of a self- or interviewer-administered questionnaire. The proportion of cases with a particular exposure is compared with that of the controls to determine whether there is an association between the exposure and the disease.

In some occupational investigations, a case-control study within a cohort (sometimes called a nested case-control study) is initiated. This study is usually begun after the completion of a retrospective cohort study and is identical to the case-control study described above except that the study base is the occupational cohort under study. This methodologic maneuver is usually done when an increased risk is observed in the cohort for a particular cancer or other disease, more specific exposure information is desired, and detailed personnel records are available for the cohort. Employment records of individuals with that disease are examined to obtain occupational titles along with any available information about specific exposures, and these are compared with similar data obtained from the records of a sample of fellow workers without the disease. This comparison may help isolate a particular exposure or occupational process that may be responsible for the increased disease risk in the cohort and also provide an opportunity to assess confounding by lifestyle factors, such as smoking, through interviews with workers or their next of kin. Nested case-control studies can also reduce costs, since it is much less expensive to interview or examine in detail only the records of individuals with the disease of interest and a sample of controls than to interview or examine the records of all the individuals in the cohort, which often includes thousands of subjects.

The primary challenge in case-control studies is the selection of cases and controls from the same study base or source population, uninfluenced by their exposure status (12). Without this, valid comparisons between groups cannot be made. Cases may be identified from population-based disease registry files or from all clinics serving a well-defined geographic area, and these should be compared with controls selected from the same general populations from which those cases were drawn. Cases may also be identified from hospital or physician records, and the controls should be chosen from among patients treated for other conditions in those same hospitals or physicians' offices or, in certain circumstances, different hospitals near the residence of the case. Under such circumstances, the comparability of the two groups can be ensured only if the catchment area for the different hospitals and clinics is the same for cases and controls, and patients residing outside the catchment area are excluded. Moreover, hospital controls with conditions associated directly or indirectly with the exposure of interest should be excluded since their exposure patterns do not represent the exposure distribution in the source population for the cases. For instance, hospital controls with conditions requiring extensive pain relief should be excluded in studies of analgesic use and chronic renal or liver failure, and overrepresentation of poor and less educated controls in such studies could introduce a selection bias since patterns of analgesic use vary substantially by demographic characteristics (13). Only an appropriately stratified analysis controlling for the selection factors (that is, race, gender, socioeconomic status) will eliminate the associated selection bias for all other variables, including analgesic use.

In general, a selection bias will be introduced when controls are selected through a process that is associated with the exposure under consideration, and controlling for the suspected selection factors in the analysis of the data may reduce (but not necessarily eliminate) this problem, depending on whether the selection factors can be correctly identified and accurately measured (1). It is possible to undertake analytic procedures to increase confidence in the comparability of the case and control series. This can be done by (a) comparing cases and controls with respect to the frequency of reporting of exposures or characteristics unlikely to be relevant to the etiology of the study disease; or (b) examining a group of patients not expected to share the etiologic background of the true cases, although they went through the same study procedures as the cases. In the case-control approach, as in the cohort approach, a second control group can be used to address any shortcomings of the first, but an inconsistent result across control groups makes interpretation difficult (10). The nested case-control approach ideally reflects the study base principle, since the controls are chosen from within the cohort (the source population of the cases).

Advantages and Disadvantages

Although there is more criticism of case-control than cohort study designs, they do have distinct advantages in the assessment of disease risk (12). Case-control studies are more suitable for the study of rare diseases and diseases with long latency periods than the cohort designs. Moreover, they are often statistically more powerful, since large numbers of cases of a particular disease can be ascertained from the general population and enrolled in relatively short periods of time, although the frequency of exposure to the suspected agent may not be high in the general population. For risk evaluation, a much larger number of exposure variables can be examined using the case-control design, and such studies can be relatively inexpensive and quick compared with prospective cohort studies. Moreover, by obtaining information on past exposures through questionnaires, case-control studies are able to adjust for potential confounding factors such as cigarette smoking and to obtain lifetime occupational histories, making them useful in identifying occupational determinants of disease (9,14).

Because exposure information is collected after the onset of disease, information bias concerning exposure to suspected agent(s) is more common in case-control investigations, since the existence of a serious disease such as cancer can influence recollection and reporting (recall bias) and can affect certain biochemical and immunologic variables. This type of bias usually is assumed to be in the direction of overreporting by cases compared with controls, thus creating a spurious association between an exposure and the disease under study. Although this is a potential bias, there are few documented occurrences (10). The use of controls with an illness such as hospital controls may help reduce the potential for recall bias, since they, too, have recently experienced a disease.

The relative risk cannot be directly calculated in a case-control study; however, the odds ratio provides a very good approximation of the relative risk if the disease under study is uncommon in the population, as is every cancer type. Thus, while cohort studies allow estimation of the risk for disease among unexposed and exposed individuals, direct estimation of the actual risk associated with a particular exposure is not possible using the case-control approach unless ancillary information on underlying rates of the disease is available.

Cohort studies are usually considered the design of choice if the exposure is rare in the general population, but a case-control study is appropriate if a rare exposure accounts for a large proportion of the cases. Adenocarcinoma of the vagina in young women with *in utero* exposure to diethylstilbestrol would be an example of the identification of a rare causal exposure using the case-control design.

Cross-sectional Studies

In a cross-sectional study, also called a survey or prevalence study, individuals are selected regardless of exposure or disease status. Cross-sectional surveys usually rely on random or probability sampling procedures to select subjects. This allows for the examination of the prevalence of a particular disease in a representative sample of the population, and analyses are conducted by various combinations of age, sex, and other variables and the presence or absence of disease, data that are all obtained at the same time, usually by interview. However, many cross-sectional occupational studies do not employ random sampling in the selection of study subjects.

Advantages and Disadvantages

A cross-sectional study or prevalence survey has no methodologic advantage over the cohort or case-control designs. Cross-sectional studies are useful for hypothesis generation and health services planning if random sampling is employed. If the information is not gathered using a random sampling procedure, estimates of the prevalence of a disease or of an association between a factor and a disease are of little value, since they are not representative of a study base or source population and are subject to numerous biases.

Since exposure and disease status are usually measured at the same time in a cross-sectional study, there is no way to ascertain the time sequence, that is, whether the agent or exposure preceded the disease or whether individuals with particular medical conditions selected certain jobs or volunteered for the study. Diseases of short duration (either because of cure or death) are not good candidates for this study design; conversely, long-duration diseases are usually overrepresented in cross-sectional studies. In occupational settings, this type of study is likely to include information only on currently employed individuals, thereby missing retired employees and persons who may have quit due to ill health that may be related to the exposure under study (14).

BIOSTATISTICAL ASPECTS OF EPIDEMIOLOGIC INVESTIGATIONS

Measures of Association

We now describe some basic statistical measures of risk commonly used in occupational epidemiology and the approaches used to evaluate their variability. The essence of all the techniques is a comparison of the observed number of disease cases with the expected number of disease cases, that is, the number that would be expected if the exposure neither increased nor decreased the risk of disease. If the measure of association (commonly referred to as the relative risk) equals 1.0, then the exposure has no effect on disease occurrence. If the relative risk is greater than 1.0, then there is a positive association between exposure and disease, and if the relative risk is less than 1.0 then there is an inverse association. Thus, a relative risk of 10 indicates that individuals exposed to the agent under study have 10 times the risk of developing the disease as compared with those not exposed to the agent.

The 2 × 2 Table

The simplest statistical technique, the 2 × 2 table, is useful when occupationally exposed and unexposed individuals are followed for equal amounts of time for disease occurrence. The basic measure of association derived from the 2 × 2 table is the relative risk. It is the ratio of the proportions of individuals developing the disease among the exposed compared with the unexposed. For example, if 58 of 150 exposed individuals show abnormal pulmonary function while 27 of 200 unexposed individuals show abnormal pulmonary function, the relative risk associated with exposure is (58/150)/(27/200) = 2.9. This is interpreted to mean that exposed individuals are at nearly three times the risk of abnormal lung function compared with unexposed individuals.

In occupational studies, however, the duration of follow-up among subjects is usually variable, and this must be accounted for in the analysis. For example, if the exposed group were followed for a longer time, more cases of disease would be expected in this group, even if the exposure had no effect on disease. The most commonly used measure of association that accounts for variable follow-up is the incidence rate ratio (often also referred to as the relative risk), which is the ratio of the incidence rate of disease among the exposed to the incidence rate of disease among the nonexposed (1). The incidence rate for each exposure group is calculated by dividing the observed number of cases of disease by the total person-years of follow-up in that group. For example, suppose 350 person-years are observed in an occupationally exposed group, producing 30 events, while 776 person-years are observed in an unexposed group, producing 40 events. The ratio of disease incidence rates is (30/350)/(40/776) = 1.7. This is interpreted to mean that the incidence in the exposed group is approximately 70% higher than in the unexposed.

As indicated above, the relate risk (or incidence rate ratio) can be directly calculated from a cohort study since the two incidence rates are available. In a case-control study, the relative risk cannot be directly calculated but can be estimated by the odds ratio if the disease under study is uncommon in the population.

Standardized Mortality Ratio

The calculation of a relative risk or incidence rate ratio relies on the use of an internal control group; that is, data are collected from an occupational group in which some are exposed to a potentially hazardous substance and some are not. Unfortunately, such an internal control group is not always available, and in these situations, we must rely on external comparisons. The observed number of disease cases in an exposed cohort is compared with the expected number using a set of known, standard disease rates. The estimate of the relative risk is called the standardized mortality ratio (SMR) (9,11,14) and is the ratio of the observed number of events (O) to the number expected if the exposure had no effect (E). The expected number of events is computed by applying standard rates to the study cohort. The study cohort is usually stratified by age, sex, year of birth, and race. To obtain the expected number, the observed number of person-years in each age-sex-year-race stratum are multiplied by the standard disease rate for that stratum. The expected number from each stratum is then summed to obtain the total expected number of events.

For example, suppose a retrospective cohort study is conducted to examine cancer risk in an occupational group exposed to high airborne concentrations of a potential carcinogen. The expected number of cancer deaths is computed from the sum of the product of the number of observed person-years in each category of age, calendar period, race, and sex, and the corresponding mortality rate in the community. If 47 observed deaths from malignant neoplasms occurred, and 39.4 were expected, the SMR would be 47/39.4 = 1.2. This can be interpreted to mean that the occupationally exposed group has a 20% higher risk of cancer death compared with the reference population.

Assessing Chance Variation

The role of statistics in occupational epidemiology is to detect patterns (exposure-disease associations) in the data and to determine if these patterns (associations) could be accounted for by chance. The goal of the statistical analysis is to obtain a valid comparison of disease risk in an occupationally exposed group and in a comparable unexposed group. This comparison should be supplemented with an evaluation of the likelihood that the observed differences in disease rates are artifacts due to chance or represent a real exposure effect. The role of chance is evaluated in epidemiologic studies through significance testing and calculation of confidence intervals. If a risk estimate is statistically significant at a specified level, chance can be ruled out as a likely explanation of the observed exposure-disease association. This, however, does not rule out bias or confounding as candidate explanations in nonexperimental research.

Chance variation refers to the natural variation in the occurrence of health outcomes observed among similarly exposed individuals. Two statistical tools for assessing the role of chance are the *p* value and the confidence interval. The *p* value is the probability of observing, by chance alone, a difference in disease occurrence between the exposed and unexposed as large as or larger than what was actually observed, assuming the null hypothesis, that is, that the exposure has no effect on disease occurrence and that differences in disease rates are due solely to chance. The smaller the *p* value, the less consistent are the data with the null hypothesis. For example, a *p* value of .005 means that the probability of obtaining by chance alone an exposure effect as large as or more extreme than what was observed is only 1 in 200. Based on this result, one can conclude either that a rare "chance event" has occurred or, more likely, chance can be ruled out as an explanation for the study results.

P values smaller than .05, an arbitrarily chosen threshold value often referred to as the alpha or nominal level, are generally referred to as "statistically significant," although they are frequently overemphasized and are of limited use in the interpretation of epidemiologic data. A *p* value of .05 does not completely rule out chance as an explanation for the results; rather, it means that chance could explain the observed risk estimate only one out of 20 times. The *p* value gives no indication of the observed magnitude of the effect of the exposure. Small differences from very large studies may be statistically significant, because of the influence of sample size on measures of statistical significance, although they may be too small to be of practical or scientific significance. Therefore, it is important to present a quantitative estimate of the effect of exposure (relative risk), along with a measure of the uncertainty of the estimate (the standard error), often presented as a confidence interval.

The confidence interval provides a range of values containing the true relative risk with a desired degree of confidence, usually 95%. The "true" relative risk is the risk that would be observed based on an infinite amount of data, that is, if sampling variability could be eliminated. A 95% confidence interval that includes 1.0 (e.g., 0.8–2.4) implies that a value of 1.0 for the relative risk, and thus the null hypothesis of no exposure effect, is consistent with the data. If 1.0 is not included in the interval (e.g.,

1.2–2.4), the null hypothesis is rejected and chance is ruled out as a likely explanation. Inspection of a confidence interval is a rapid method of evaluating statistical significance; however, the actual p value cannot be immediately deduced from a confidence interval. The p value and the confidence interval complement each other, and both are sometimes reported.

Sample Size and Power

A fundamental issue in planning a study is the number of subjects needed to assess the potential exposure-disease relationship. The calculation of sample size begins with the specification of a fixed, low probability of inferring that the exposure is associated with the disease when in fact it is not (called the type I error). Typically this is set at 5% (alpha or nominal level). Ideally, there should be enough subjects to avoid stating that there is no association between the exposure and the disease when in fact there is (type II error). The power of a study is the probability of observing an association of a given magnitude between an exposure and a disease when in fact it exists. The larger the sample size, the greater the power to detect a specified difference in risk; conversely, the smaller the sample size, the lower the power to detect a difference in risk. Also, for a fixed sample size, the smaller the magnitude of an actual association, the lower the power of a given study to detect it. Rare or very common exposures also require very large studies.

Certain study designs tend to produce greater power when testing or evaluating a hypothesis. For example, if the disease is rare, greater power is generally available in a small- to moderate-sized case-control study than in a large cohort study. In contrast, if the exposure is rare, it may be advantageous to follow a group exposed to the rare agent using a cohort design. Unfortunately, issues of sample size and power are usually constrained by practical concerns about time, cost, and the availability of appropriate study subjects.

Multiple Hypothesis Testing

A serious problem that warrants special consideration is the issue of multiple hypothesis testing in epidemiology. Epidemiologic studies often involve the collection of large amounts of data regarding numerous potential risk factors and health outcomes. Interviews and questionnaires often include items of secondary importance for various reasons. For example, a researcher might simply want to be comprehensive and to consider as many factors as possible, or a researcher might want to obscure the real purpose of the questionnaire to minimize reporting bias by asking about an assortment of other exposures or risk factors. In any event, once the data are collected, it is standard epidemiologic practice to analyze all the variables, to compute risk estimates, and to assess statistical significance.

If a large number of risk factors are tested for statistical significance, there is a high probability of declaring at least one risk factor significant, even if there is no real association between the disease and any of the risk factors. Several solutions have been proposed for dealing with the problem (15). A classic solution is to require a smaller alpha level (p value) when testing each risk factor. For example, if one wants at most a .05 probability of finding any of N risk factors significant when actually none of the risk factors is associated with the disease, one may test each risk factor at the .05/N nominal level. The approach is often referred to as the Bonferroni method for adjusting for multiple comparisons (16,17). However, there are some intuitive difficulties with this approach. The approach treats all factors as if they are equally important and equally likely to affect disease risk. If N is large, one would require a very small p value before declaring any risk factor significant. Suppose, for example, that it was considered likely that smoking was an important risk factor for a particular disease (based on previous research) and a sufficiently large number of secondary risk factors (e.g., 25) were also being evaluated. In this case a Bonferroni-type approach might lead us to declare the effect of smoking not statistically significant for any p value less than .05 but greater than .002 (.05/25). Moreover, the different associations in a study are typically of interest on a one-at-a-time basis, often to different investigators with different interests. In such situations, procedures adjusting for multiple comparisons are inappropriate and would produce improperly imprecise single intervals (15). Finally, one should never substitute statistical significance testing for scientific judgment.

INTERPRETATION OF EPIDEMIOLOGIC DATA

Because of the absence of randomization of exposure among study subjects in epidemiologic study designs, it is paramount that, in addition to ruling out chance, the role of bias and confounding in individual studies be evaluated before a reported exposure-disease association can be assessed for causality.

Chance

The role of chance is evaluated in epidemiologic studies by the use of significance testing and confidence limits. If a risk estimate is statistically significant at a specified level (e.g., .05) or if the confidence interval excludes 1.0, we can assume that chance is an unlikely explanation for our results. It does not completely exclude chance as an explanation; rather, it simply means that chance could explain the risk estimate we observe only 1 of 20 times.

Bias

Bias, or systematic error, generally results from flaws inherent in nonexperimental study designs or in data collection and generally cannot be corrected at the data analysis stage. Selection bias involves systematic differences in the study exposure between those selected and not selected for inclusion in the study. Examples may include enrolling only currently employed workers in a cohort study or ignoring the exposure experience of the deceased cases in a case-control study or having a high loss to follow-up among the exposed but not the unexposed in a cohort study. Information bias involves systematic differences in measuring the exposure of interest between the compared groups, and includes recall and interviewer bias (18). Detection bias is another problem in occupational studies where the exposed workers often have better medical care and follow-up than the general population to which they are compared in typical SMR studies.

Confounding

Confounding refers to the effect of an extraneous variable, related independently to both exposure and disease, that may partially or completely account for an apparent association between a study exposure and disease (18). For example, in a case-control study of a blue-collar occupation and bladder cancer or a case-control study of alcohol consumption and heart disease, cigarette smoking would be an obvious confounding variable, since it is related to blue-collar employment and bladder cancer and also to alcohol consumption and heart disease. Only when potential confounding variables have been identified and measured can confounding be evaluated in the analysis phase of the study by stratification of the study subjects according to the suspected confounding variables. In this manner, the effect of the study exposure on disease risk among those in different categories of the confounding variable (for example, smokers and nonsmokers) can be estimated. Confounding can also work in the other direction (negative confounding) to mask an association between an exposure and disease.

EVALUATION OF CAUSALITY

If bias, confounding, and chance can be confidently excluded as likely explanations for the exposure-disease association under study, then an investigator is obligated to assess whether the observed association may be causal in nature. Much has been written about the meaning and philosophic implications of causality, but here we focus mostly on practical ways to assess the likelihood of a causal association in epidemiology. The likelihood of causality can be assessed using the following set of criteria or principles developed by epidemiologists during the heated debate of the late 1950s and early 1960s over the association of cigarette smoking and lung cancer (19,20).

Strength of the Association

In general, the higher the magnitude of the risk estimate, the stronger the evidence that the observed exposure effect is real and the less likely the finding may be accounted for by bias, uncontrolled confounding, or chance. A relative risk of 4.5 is considerably more persuasive than a relative risk of 1.25, since the latter represent only a 25% increase in risk. The use of this criterion has become increasingly difficult as small elevations in risk, usually between 20% and 50%, have become more common in epidemiology. The alternative explanations of bias, confounding, and chance are more plausible when the excess risk is low.

Dose-response Effect

If the risk of the disease increases with increasing exposure, a causal interpretation of the association is more plausible. This is sometimes referred to as the biologic gradient principle. The failure to demonstrate a dose-response effect does not necessarily rule out a causal interpretation, however, as a threshold effect or a saturation effect may be possible (18). These latter effects are uncommon in reality but often invoked in argument.

Time Sequence

The exposure or risk factor must precede the development of the disease in order for it to have caused the disease. There appears to be no exception to this principle. In studying chronic diseases with long latency periods, however, the temporal sequence is often difficult to establish. To a great extent this difficulty depends on the particular study design employed; cohort designs, for example, ensure the proper temporal sequence.

Consistency

The plausibility of a causal association is increased greatly if similar results are reported in other epidemiologic studies conducted among different populations using various study designs, because it is unlikely that bias or confounding would explain the results of each of these studies. Consistency observed in studies of a particular design (e.g., case-control studies) may reflect the same flaw (e.g., the same source of information bias), and thus replication using different designs is important. In epidemiology, more than in other fields of biomedical research, it is the collective evidence that is critically important, rather than the results of a particular study.

Biologic Plausibility and Coherence

Does the exposure-disease association make biologic sense given what is known about the natural history of the disease and the nature of the exposure? Is the association consistent with experimental evidence? (For example, if a threshold or saturation effect is observed, are there experimental data to suggest a mechanism for such an effect?) Is there a suitable or relevant animal model? Do other types of descriptive evidence support the association, such as secular trends of the exposure and the disease? Unfortunately, for many diseases little is known about their etiologies or natural histories, so the information necessary to judge biologic plausibility or coherence is often limited.

The first three principles can be applied internally to an individual study and used to assess the findings. The last two principles refer to results outside a particular study and relate more to external issues of coherence and consistency. All of the criteria or principles should be viewed as guidelines. Except, perhaps, for time sequence, none is required for a causal interpretation.

In the end, a causal interpretation in epidemiology rests on sound scientific judgment, a commodity often in short supply.

REFERENCES

1. MacMahon B, Trichopoulos D. *Epidemiology: principles and methods,* 2nd ed. Boston: Little, Brown, 1996.
2. International Agency for Research on Cancer. IARC monographs on the evaluation of the carcinogenic risk of chemicals to humans. 23. Some metals and metallic compounds. Lyon: IARC, 1980.
3. McLaughlin JK, Lipworth L. A critical review of the epidemiologic literature on health effects of occupational exposure to vinyl chloride. *J Epidemiol Biostat* 1999;4:253–275.
4. Hoover RN. Detection of environmental cancer hazards: epidemiologic methods. *J Med Soc NJ* 1978;75:746.
5. Ames BN, Gold LS. Too many rodent carcinogens: mitogenesis increases mutagenesis. *Science* 1990;249:970.
6. Fraumeni JF Jr, Hoover RN. Current views of epidemiologic methods. *Fed Reg* 1985(March 14);Part II:58–64.
7. Doll R, Peto R. *The causes of cancer.* New York: Oxford University Press, 1981.
8. Wacholder S, et al. Selection of controls in case-control studies. II. Types of controls. *Am J Epidemiol* 1992;135: 1029.
9. Monson RR. *Occupational epidemiology,* 2nd ed. Boca Raton, FL: CRC, 1990.
10. Wacholder S, et al. Selection of controls in case-control studies. III. Design option. *Am J Epidemiol* 1992;135: 1042.
11. Breslow NE, Day NE. *Statistical methods in cancer research, vol 2. The design and analysis of cohort studies.* Lyon, France: International Agency for Research on Cancer, 1987.
12. Wacholder S, et al. Selection of controls in case-control studies. I. Principles. *Am J Epidemiol* 1992;135:1019.
13. Eggen AE. The Tromso study: frequency and predicting factors of analgesic drug use in a free-living population (12–56 years). *J Clin Epidemiol* 1993;46:1297.
14. Chekoway H, Pearce N, Crawford-Brown DJ. *Research methods in occupational epidemiology.* New York: Oxford University Press, 1989.
15. Rothman KJ, Greenland S. *Modern epidemiology,* 2nd ed. Philadelphia: Lippincott-Raven, 1998.
16. Cupples LA, et al. Multiple testing of hypotheses in comparing two groups. *Ann Intern Med* 1984;100:122.
17. Mantel N. Assessing laboratory evidence for neoplastic activity. *Biometrics* 1980;36:381.
18. Kleinbaum DG, Kupper LL, Morgenstern H. *Epidemiologic research: principles and quantitative methods.* Belmont, CA: Lifetime Learning, 1982.
19. Hill AB. The environment and disease: association or causation? *Proc R Soc Med* 1965;58:295.
20. U.S. Department of Health, Education and Welfare. *Smoking and health: report of the Advisory Committee to the Surgeon General.* Public Health Service publication No. 1103. Washington, DC: U.S. Government Printing Office, 1964.

FURTHER INFORMATION

Alderson M. *Occupational cancer.* London: Butterworth, 1986.

Anderson S, et al. *Statistical methods for comparative studies: techniques for bias reduction.* New York: John Wiley & Sons, 1980.

Armitage P. *Statistical methods in medical research.* New York: John Wiley & Sons, 1971.

Breslow NE, Day NE. *Statistical methods in cancer research, vol 1: The analysis of case-control studies.* Lyon, France: International Agency for Research on Cancer, 1980; Vol. II: *Design and analysis of cohort studies.* Lyon, France: International Agency for Research on Cancer, 1987.

Chekoway H, Pearce N, Crawford-Brown DJ. *Research methods in occupational epidemiology.* New York: Oxford University Press, 1989.

Cochran WG. *Planning and analysis of observational studies.* New York: John Wiley & Sons, 1981.

Fleiss JL. *Statistical methods for rates and proportion,* 2nd ed. New York: John Wiley & Sons, 1981.

Fletcher RH, Fletcher SW, Wagner EH. *Clinical epidemiology: the essentials,* 3rd ed. Philadelphia: Lippincott-Raven, 1996.

Gordis L. *Epidemiology,* 2nd ed. Philadelphia: WB Saunders, 2000.

Kahn HA, Sempos CT. *Statistical methods in epidemiology.* New York: Oxford University Press, 1989.

Kleinbaum DG, Kupper LL, Morgenstern H. *Epidemiologic research: principles and quantitative methods.* Belmont, CA: Lifetime Learning, 1982.

Last JM. *A dictionary of epidemiology,* 4th ed. New York: Oxford University Press, 2001.

MacMahon B, Trichopoulos D. *Epidemiology: principles and methods,* 2nd ed. Boston: Little, Brown, 1996.

Miettinen OS. *Theoretical epidemiology: principles of occurrence research in medicine.* New York: John Wiley & Sons, 1985.

Monson RR. *Occupational epidemiology,* 2nd ed. Boca Raton, FL: CRC, 1990.

Rosner B. *Fundamentals of biostatistics.* Boston: Duxbury, 1982.

Rothman KJ, Greenland S. *Modern epidemiology,* 2nd ed. Philadelphia: Lippincott-Raven, 1998.

Sackett DL, Haynes RB, Guyatt GH, et al. *Clinical epidemiology: a basic science for clinical medicine,* 2nd ed. Boston: Little, Brown, 1991.

Schlesselman JJ. *Case-control studies: design, conduct, analysis.* New York: Oxford University Press, 1982.

Siemiatycki J. *Risk factors for cancer in the workplace.* Boca Raton, FL: CRC, 1991.

41

Occupational Medical Surveillance

Philip Harber, Craig Conlon, and Robert J. McCunney

Occupational health surveillance includes the systematic collection, analysis, and dissemination of data on groups of workers and workplaces for the prevention of illness and injury. Surveillance may include health surveillance, hazard surveillance, or both. Surveillance activity may be active or passive. Active surveillance depends on collecting data specifically for the purpose of the surveillance program (e.g., blood lead level tests), whereas passive surveillance utilizes information collected for other purposes (e.g., death certificates). One form of surveillance—screening—is designed to detect early signs of work-related illness. A well-run program can aid in the early recognition of a relationship between exposure to a hazard and disease, in the assurance of the safety of new substances, and as an indicator of the effectiveness of existing control measures. Medical practitioners should always aggressively look to take full advantage of any surveillance program for additional benefits, such as wellness and health counseling.

The primary purpose of medical surveillance is to prevent disease, rather than to diagnose and treat existing disease. Therefore, methods of interpreting results must be focused on this purpose. Surveillance testing is often, but not always, designed to be of benefit to the specific worker tested. However, in some situations, the testing is performed for the benefit of a group rather the specific workers tested. Medical surveillance should be linked with environmental surveillance, rather than being used in isolation. The utility is determined by the adequacy of interpretation of the results and the actions based on them to prevent disease.

This chapter describes the series of steps necessary for implementing a successful occupational medical surveillance program. The steps are summarized in Table 41.1. Elements of specific programs are included as examples for several of the steps; in addition, examples illustrate application of specific surveillance modalities.

TABLE 41.1. *Steps for medical surveillance program implentation*

Needs assessment
Selection of programmatic goals and target population
Choice of testing modalities
Collection of data
Interpretation of data to benefit the individual
Intervention based on results
Interpretation of data for the benefit of groups of workers
Communication of results
Program evaluation

STEP 1: NEEDS ASSESSMENT

The first stage of medical surveillance is needs assessment. Physicians who provide clinical services to workers and industry are often confronted with questions such as, Do certain workers need special tests? In many instances, medical surveillance is unlikely to be of benefit, whereas in others it can be of significant value.

In most cases, considerable judgment is required before a program can be designed and implemented. In Table 41.2, an approach to evaluating the need for medical surveillance is outlined. Every setting calls for the physician to have an understanding of the work process, job duties, and potential exposures to hazardous substances and working conditions.

A surveillance program should be designed to consider all of the perspectives of all the stakeholders in-

TABLE 41.2. *Needs assessment*

Review process and potential for exposure
- Industrial hygiene survey
- Work-site visit

Review toxicity of materials
- Basic toxicology
- Available texts and databases
- Available guidelines
  - Occupational Safety and Health Administration (OSHA) guidelines
  - National Institute for Occupational Safety and Health (NIOSH) criteria documents
  - American Conference of Governmental Industrial Hygienists (ACGIH)
- Medical literature
  - Human studies
    - Epidemiologic investigation
    - Clinical case series and reports
  - Animal studies

Does potential toxicity of material or job process require medical surveillance?

Do ergonomic or other job stressors require medical surveillance?

volved. These include workers, worker representatives (e.g., unions), former workers, employers, line supervisors, regulatory agencies, insurers, and clinicians.

The Work Site

A plant visit is often necessary to design an effective program. During the plant visit, questions can be raised regarding previous problems and current concerns. Why is attention now being paid to medical surveillance? Has a new report appeared? Has a new Occupational Safety and Health Administration (OSHA) standard been introduced? Is there a change in the process? Has a new material or process been introduced? Is there a legitimate health risk? Did an injury occur? An understanding of these matters at the work site can assist the physician in making a decision as to whether a program is needed, and, if so, what it is intended to accomplish.

The physician should ascertain whether an industrial hygiene audit has been conducted. Industrial hygienists from OSHA, the workers' compensation carrier, the plant, a consulting firm, or a corporate office often perform periodic evaluations of working conditions that often include air sampling and evaluation of other routes of potential exposure such as ingestion and skin contact. It may be necessary to request a reevaluation, however, if substantial changes have occurred in the work process.

Hazard Identification and Risk Assessment

The need for and nature of surveillance activity is determined by a risk assessment. This includes determination of the potential hazards, the seriousness of the health consequences, and identification of the population at risk. In addition to assessing the risk posed by chemical exposure, risk assessment should also consider ergonomic hazards and risk associated with the quality of the work environment. Speaking with line management and the affected workers is critical for gaining an understanding of the work environment.

Next, the toxicity of the materials should be reviewed. Guidelines are available from the American Conference of Governmental Industrial Hygienists (ACGIH) and from criteria documents prepared by the National Institute for Occupational Safety and Health (NIOSH). For some substances, an OSHA standard dictates the type of medical surveillance program required for certain work situations.

Review generally requires consultative help from a physician board certified in occupational medicine. Results of human studies, especially epidemiologic investigations, and clinical case series can also be of assistance in formulating an opinion as to the need for medical surveillance. A decision regarding the need for and type of medical surveillance program can now be made. Since few situations conform to recommended guidelines, consideration should also be given to the potential for emergencies, results of animal studies, and public relations issues.

STEP 2: SELECTING PROGRAMMATIC GOALS AND TARGET POPULATION

The next stage is deciding about programmatic goals. Table 41.3 lists general reasons for instituting medical surveillance programs. The target population must be carefully defined to be consistent with the goals chosen. For example, if the goal is to detect current exposures, then current workers represent the optimal target group. However, if the goal is to detect cancers, which generally have a long latency period (time from exposure to onset of disease), then focusing only on those currently employed is usually inappropriate; that is, those who have retired are often at higher risk because of their longer latency. OSHA regulations typically do not

TABLE 41.3. *Purposes of medical surveillance programs*

For benefit of Individual workers
Screening for disease
Risk factor identification
Assessment of environmental exposures of the individual worker
Identifying overexposures
Fitness for duty
Preplacement testing
Worker selection
Job accommodation
Detection of nonoccupational disease
Health promotion
Baseline for future reference
Substance abuse detection
For benefit of groups of workers
Detection of new hazards
Identification of sites of exposure to known hazards
Assuring safety of current practices
Assessing absence patterns
Projecting health care resource needs
Planning of preventive programs

address screening former rather than current employees.

Screening for Occupational Disease

Screening is the search for a previously unrecognized disease at a stage at which intervention can slow, halt, or reverse the progression of the disorder. An effective screening program should identify disease at an early stage, before it would otherwise become evident based on symptoms.

Screening has been very effective in improving treatment and survivability of nonoccupational ailments such as hypertension and cervical and breast cancers. In fact, certain occupational disorders such as noise-induced hearing loss, bladder cancer, and some of the pneumoconioses lend themselves well to the principles of screening. In contrast, screening efforts for certain malignancies such as lung cancer have generally proved to be futile and at best only advance the point of diagnosis without improving outcome. In the latter setting, this advancement of the point of diagnosis is known from an epidemiologic perspective as "lead-time effect."

Screening is considered a secondary preventive measure in the control of occupational illness, since the primary control measure is to reduce the hazardous exposure. Screening is based on a number of principles, including the following:

1. The screening test must be selective and geared to the population at risk.
2. The disease should be identified in its latent stage, not when symptoms appear.
3. Adequate follow-up study is necessary.
4. The screening test should be both valid and reliable.
5. Benefits outweigh the costs and, where feasible, tests are noninvasive.
6. Treatment should be both available and effective at a stage when the disease is detectable.
7. The program should represent an optimal use of resources.

Regulatory Requirements

Surveillance activities are often mandated by specific regulations. In particular, many OSHA standards require that surveillance activities be conducted. In addition to OSHA, testing may be mandated by other federal agencies. Requirements may vary from state to state, but if a state regulation is based on a federal OSHA regulation, it must at least meet the federal standards. Surveillance activities include medical testing and recording of information. Requirements for testing are generally based on exposure levels. For example, if exposure to airborne lead or noise exceeds the "action level," testing is mandatory. In comparison to the United States, several other countries, such as Germany, require more testing (1).

Table 41.4 lists several common types of surveillance examinations that are used in the screening for occupational diseases. Surveillance examinations may be mandatory as defined by OSHA or other federal agencies. However, some surveillance examinations are well accepted in the occupational medicine community, but federal standards have not been promulgated. OSHA standards should be carefully reviewed when designing occupational surveillance activities.

OSHA Standards and Other Regulatory Agencies

Example of OSHA Mandated Surveillance Programs: The OSHA Asbestos Standard

The OSHA asbestos standard mandates a medical surveillance program for all employees who are or will be exposed to airborne concentrations of fibers of asbestos at or above the time-weighted average (TWA) and/or excursion limit. The employee's exposure to airborne asbestos is not to exceed 0.1 fiber per cubic centimeter of air as an 8-hour TWA. The excursion limit refers to an airborne concentration of 1.0 fiber per cubic centimeter of air over 30 minutes.

TABLE 41.4. *Regulatory mandated screening*

Standard/agency	Agent	Target (organ)	Tests/actions	Frequency
Asbestos/OSHA	Asbestos	Lung, colon	CXR, PFT, OB	Annual
Benzene/OSHA	Benzene	Blood, CNS	CBC, PFT	Annual (PFT q 3 years)
Beryllium/DOE	Beryllium	Lung, skin	BeLPT, PFT, CXR	
Blood-borne pathogens/OSHA	Viral pathogens	Immune system, blood	Hep B vaccination; monitor exposure	Initial and prn
Cadmium/OSHA	Cadmium	Kidney, bone	PFT, CXR Urine: Cr, Cd, β-2 Mg Blood: Cd, Cr	6–12 months
Cotton dust/OSHA	Cotton dust	Lung	History, examination, PFT	6–24 months
Formaldehyde/ OSHA	Formaldehyde	Upper and lower respiratory tract	History, examination, PFT	Annual
Hazard communication	Chemicals	Not specific	Training and information	Initial assignment
HAZWOPER/ OSHA	Hazardous waste and emergency response	Blood, lungs, kidney, liver, CNS, CV	CBC, CXR, EKG, chem panel, optional TMST	Annual
Hearing conservation/ OSHA	Noise	Hearing	Audiogram	Annual
Lead/OSHA	Lead	Blood, kidney, bone, CNS, fertility	Blood lead and ZPP	6 months
Methylene chloride	Methylene chloride	Skin, CNS, CV, blood, liver	Optional: EKG, LFTs, carboxyHgb, Hct, cholesterol	Annually
Respiratory protection/OSHA	Respirators	Lung, cardiovascular	History w/ optional exam, PFT	12–36 months
Proposed tuberculosis/ OSHA	Tuberculosis	Lung	PPD, CXR	6–12 months

The table includes several common types of surveillance examinations that are used in the screening for occupational diseases. Surveillance examinations may be mandatory as defined by OSHA or other federal agencies. However, some surveillance examinations are well accepted in the occupational medicine community, but federal standards have not been promulgated.

β-2 Mg, beta-2-microglobulins; BeLPT, beryllium lymphocyte proliferation test; CBC, complete blood count; Cd, cadmium; Cr, creatinine; CXR, chest x-ray; EKG, electrocardiogram; Hep B, hepatitis B vaccination; Hct, hematocrit; Hgb, hemoglobin; LFTs, liver enzyme blood tests; OB, stool test for occult blood; PFT, pulmonary function test; PPD, tuberculin skin test; TMST, treadmill stress test; ZPP, zinc protoporhyrin.

From *http://www.osha.gov/comp-links.html; http://tis.eh.doe.gov/be/berule.pdf* for the DOE, Federal Register, Part III, 10 CFR, Part 850, Chronic Beryllium Disease Prevention Program; final rule.

These limits should not take into consideration whether the employee is wearing personal protection, such as a respirator.

If the employee could be exposed at or above the TWA or excursion limit, then the employee is placed under medical surveillance. Before the employee is assigned to such a position a preplacement examination is provided by the employer and at the employer's expense. The examination would include at a minimum:

A medical and work history

A complete physical examination of all systems with emphasis on the respiratory system, the cardiovascular system, and digestive system

Completion of the standardized respiratory disease questionnaire available from OSHA

Posterior-anterior chest x-ray with interpretation and classification per OSHA

Pulmonary function tests including forced vital capacity (FVC) and forced expiratory volume in 1 second (FEV_1)

Any additional tests deemed appropriate by the examining physician

Periodic examinations are done annually with the same components as listed above except the chest x-ray, which is performed is performed every 5 years until the employee has reached more than 35 years of age and it has been more than 10 years since the initial asbestos exposure. Then the chest x-ray is done every 2 years until the worker is 45 years old, and annually thereafter.

The asbestos standard requires an examination of employees when they are terminated from the company unless their last examination has occurred within the last year. The physician must provide a written opinion to the employer after each examination. This opinion must include whether the employee

has any detected medical conditions that would place the employee at an increased risk of material health impairment from exposure to asbestos;

has any recommended limitations on duties or on the use of personal protective equipment such as clothing or respirators;

has been informed by the physician of the results of the medical examination and of any medical conditions resulting from asbestos exposure that require further explanation or treatment;

has been informed by the physician of the increased risk of lung cancer attributable to the combined effect of smoking and asbestos exposure.

Screening for Nonoccupational Disease

Often, screening is conducted in the work site for nonoccupational disorders (general medical screening). Occupational physicians have long played a role in evaluating the presence of unrecognized illness in an asymptomatic person. Now many preventive medicine and screening programs have become part of health promotion activities.

Unfortunately, consensus is lacking on the type and content of a periodic medical evaluation that physicians should offer the asymptomatic person. Guidelines, however, have been proposed. The effectiveness of various ancillary procedures has also been critically reviewed. Not surprisingly, few of the ancillary procedures commonly used in medical practice today meet all criteria of screening (see Chapter 19 for a discussion of periodic medical examinations).

Screening programs often encounter difficulties involved in evaluating people with abnormal tests. Screening programs must include a plan for appropriate follow-up of those with positive results. False-positive tests occur when the screening test is positive but the individual does not have the disease. False-positive results are inherent in most laboratory reference limits, simply because of the manner by which those limits are established. In general, 1 of every 20 healthy people has an abnormal test result without evidence of illness.

Surveillance to Detect Exposure Rather than Disease

Medical surveillance is not limited to screening (from which the participant generally benefits). In some settings, medical surveillance is designed to detect exposure rather than disease. For example, biologic monitoring (discussed later) measures concentrations of chemical agents or their metabolites in biologic specimens. This type of testing may be useful for determining if exposure is occurring even at levels that do not imply the presence of disease.

Baseline for Future Reference

Another purpose of medical surveillance is to serve as a baseline for future evaluation. A previous electrocardiogram is often useful when interpreting a current one. Similar considerations apply to many other tests. Change over time is often more important than the actual value itself. For example, a worker whose FEV_1 declines from 119% of predicted to 81% of predicted over 1 year warrants review even though both results are within normal limits.

Raw data, rather than interpretive conclusions alone (e.g., normal/not normal), should be kept on file for future reference. Documentation of the technique employed is essential to ensure that future testing is performed by comparable methods.

Special considerations apply in tests subject to a "learning effect." Spirometry results, in particular, are subject to this problem because the test is effort dependent and people often perform better on the second test since they have learned how to improve their performance.

Example of Baseline Testing: Surveillance for Noise-induced Hearing Loss

Occupational noise exposure is common and can lead to noise-induced hearing loss. Detection of any progressive decline in auditory acuity is useful both for the individual affected and as an indicator of adequate workplace protection. Audiometric testing measures hearing thresholds at specific frequencies (pure tone frequencies). The results of testing at any time must be compared to the employee's baseline audiogram to determine whether there has been a change in auditory acuity (i.e., a threshold shift). A temporary threshold shift is a reversible difference, frequently resolving after several days away from heavy noise exposure. Conversely, a standard or permanent threshold shift is an irreversible change in auditory acuity in comparison to previous results. OSHA standards define a standard threshold shift as a change in hearing threshold relative to the baseline audiogram of an average of 10 dB or more at 2,000, 3,000, and 4,000 Hz in either ear (2).

For occupational health audiometric surveillance, change in threshold, rather than the absolute auditory threshold itself, is of most importance. Deviation from perfect hearing is common even without occupational noise exposure; it is an inevitable consequence of aging (presbycusis). Therefore, baseline testing is particularly important in determining whether there has been a change over time.

Risk Factor Identification

Medical surveillance programs are also used to detect precursors of disease or factors associated with a greater than average likelihood of developing disease. Unlike true screening, persons with positive results do not have specific, well-defined diseases but rather a greater than average risk of developing disease without appropriate intervention. Here the interpretation is often more difficult than for screening, and the importance of carefully counseling the employee about the significance of the findings is paramount. For example, one genetic variant type is associated with a markedly increased likelihood of developing chronic beryllium disease among exposed workers (3–5). Significant ethical questions are raised if such a test is proposed in order to exclude otherwise healthy workers from jobs with potential exposure. Practical and ethical issues of genetic testing are discussed in Chapter 35.

STEP 3: CHOOSING TESTING MODALITIES

After establishing the need for medical surveillance and selecting general goals, the best tools must be selected. This section briefly reviews the major techniques. Physicians should avoid the temptation to recommend tests in a reflex-like fashion. Exposure to potentially hazardous substances does not necessarily indicate the need for special tests. Decisions should be based not only on the relative toxicity of the substance but also on the extent of control measures, sampling results, work practices, and usefulness of the tests themselves. Lay personnel who have responsibilities for health and safety in the work site may have unrealistic expectations about the value of medical monitoring. In particular, they must be apprised that medical surveillance is not a substitute for primary control measures.

Unnecessary tests may lead to difficulties in assessing false-positive results and may also cause alarm among healthy workers and needlessly increase health care costs. For example, many blood tests for metals and solvents can be obtained, but the interpretation of the results is clinically unclear and problematic.

Questionnaires

Questionnaires are simple, inexpensive tools that for many disorders serve as a reasonably sensitive way to obtain an overview of a potential problem, which can provide the basis for further investigation. Questionnaires are often used in conjunction with other techniques.

Surveillance questionnaires require as much attention to technical detail as do other testing methods. The questionnaire should be designed and pilot tested considering the specific exposures of concern (e.g., chemicals or ergonomic hazards in the workplace). Generic health questionnaires generally are ineffective for occupational health surveillance. In addition, the questionnaire must be designed for the target population. The wording of the questionnaire should match the educational levels of those completing it, and the language should be appropriate.

The most appropriate method of questionnaire administration for the specific situation should be selected. Often, carefully designed questionnaires may be self-administered. But interviewer-administered questionnaires are necessary when information is complex or the population is not literate. Sometimes, the worker completes the questionnaire and then reviews it in person with an occupational physician or nurse.

When questionnaire data are used for aggregate analysis (combining results from many workers for statistical analysis), it is critically important that systematic bias be avoided. Staff members who are administering questionnaires must be carefully trained to avoid influencing worker responses.

Several standard questionnaires are available. For respiratory disease, the American Thoracic Society questionnaire is widely used (6). OSHA mandates that a specific questionnaire be employed for respirator medical surveillance (7).

Questionnaires are also particularly valuable in ergonomic surveillance. A variety of questionnaires have been developed to allow workers to rate their perceived ergonomic stress (i.e., exposure) as well as to report symptoms.

Physical Examination

A physical examination is a time-honored method for detecting signs of illness. Although its effectiveness in screening settings is limited, some signs of illness may be uncovered. A physical examination also offers people the personally perceived benefit of being examined. Although this value can be overlooked, people generally appreciate the opportunity of discussing their health concerns with a qualified provider in an appropriate setting. In fact, effective physician counseling in these settings can help to motivate people to control health risks. A physical examination is relatively inexpensive. Its effectiveness increases if directed primarily toward the target organ. In many diseases, however, physical signs are a late finding.

Chest Radiography

Chest radiography gained favor as a screening device in the early detection of tuberculosis. The method continues to find application in screening for nonmalignant lung disorders such as silicosis, asbestosis, and chronic beryllium disease. Annual chest radiographic examination, especially in young workers, may be unnecessary in routine monitoring programs. For most occupational hazards, adequate information can be obtained if chest films are administered less frequently and programs include an annual review of symptoms and pulmonary function (8). The method is discussed in more detail later in this chapter.

Effective chest radiography depends on quality control regarding technical factors such as contrast and penetration. The radiologist's usual interpretation should be supplemented by a standardized coding system to ensure comparability among physicians performing the interpretation, to permit aggregate data analysis, and to allow comparison with past and future results. The International Labor Organization (ILO) has developed a system for coding chest radiographs (the ILO System). Under this system, posteroanterior (PA) films are interpreted in a standardized fashion. The shape and number (profusion) of opacities consistent with pneumoconiosis are described with a series of letters and numbers by comparing the patient's radiograph with a set of reference films supplied by the ILO. The presence of pleural disease and other abnormalities is coded in the standardized manner. Epidemiologic studies and comparisons over time are facilitated, since a 12-point scale rather than a long verbal description describes the number of opacities. Where important decisions are based on interpretation of radiographic surveillance, each radiograph may be interpreted by several readers according to the ILO system; those readers who tend to overinterpret or underinterpret thus may be identified.

Radiologists, chest physicians, occupational medicine specialists, and others may be certified as B readers by NIOSH if they successfully complete a course and pass a standardized and exacting test. Lists of B readers in each geographic area can be obtained from NIOSH.

The occupational implications of abnormal chest radiographs must be considered carefully. According to the ILO system, a positive report indicates findings "consistent with" pneumoconiosis but does not indicate that such disease actually is present. The radiographic findings must be integrated with exposure information and other clinical findings to achieve an accurate diagnosis. Even though interpretation by B readers using the ILO system is useful, inconsistency may occur (9–13). The ILO system was designed for epidemiologic purposes and not for establishing clinical diagnoses in individuals.

Radiography is a relatively sensitive method for detecting early pneumoconiotic changes. Workers who have abnormal radiographs and yet have no physiologic impairment raise difficult questions about job placement. For example, should a coal miner with early radiographic abnormality be precluded from any coal mining work (i.e., considered disabled for such work) even if pulmonary function is completely normal? The current consensus is that removal would be advisable to prevent the abnormality from possibly developing into progressive massive fibrosis (PMF) with attendant morbidity. Early pulmonary fibrotic changes viewed radiographically in asbestos-exposed workers raise similar questions; optimally, the worker without physiologic impairment can continue working if the work environment or work practices can be successfully modified to prevent any further asbestos exposure.

Pulmonary Function Testing

Pulmonary function testing is an integral component of most screening programs designed to detect nonmalignant occupational lung disorders. This procedure should be conducted in accordance with standard guidelines (14,15). Pulmonary function testing can be a sensitive screening device for some occupational lung disorders. Cigarette smoking and nonoccupational medical conditions, especially asthma and chronic obstructive lung disease, can affect results.

Properly performed and interpreted, spirometry is simple, economical, and reliable (16–19). Guidelines for spirometry testing have been published by both the American College of Occupational and Environmental Medicine (15) and the American Thoracic Society (14). Results depend in part on the manner in which the technician encourages the patient to perform the test. Calibration errors can also produce inaccurate spirometry. The person supervising the testing must be trained in principles of spirometry. Although such training is required only by selected OSHA standards (e.g., cotton dust), persons administering spirometry tests ideally should complete a course approved by NIOSH. The spirometer should be checked daily for accuracy, including the newer automated spirometers, which may lead to complacency because of ease of operation.

Since a variety of parameters may be derived from spirometry, the physician must decide in advance which factors are of significance. The FEV_1, FVC, and their ratio (FEV_1/FVC) are collected. In addition, the average rate over the midportion of the forced expiratory flow ($FEF_{25-75\%}$) is commonly obtained. In general, the FEV_1, the FVC, and the FEV_1/FVC ratio are most important. An appropriate reference group should be chosen to compare each subject's value with the predicted value. Normal ranges are calculated through the use of gender-specific regression equations that employ age and height as the major variables. Adjustment of predicted values for race may be advisable, since blacks average 10% to 15% lower predicted values at the same age and height. If the automated spirometer prints predicted values as well as observed values, the interpreter must know the source of prediction equations and whether race adjustment has been accomplished.

Longitudinal testing is potentially valuable. After age 25, FEV_1 and FVC decline with age; acceleration of the annual decline (whether due to nonoccupational cause such as smoking or an occupational cause) indicates significant risk of developing respiratory disability in the future. However, precise measurement of annual decline is difficult because the magnitude of the change is comparable to the variability of measurement (20). Estimates of rate of decline in individuals must be based on at least three measurements over a several-year period. Thus, although declines of FEV_1 of greater than 35 mL per year may further warrant medical evaluation, imprecision of estimating the annual decline rate requires caution in interpretation.

When spirometry data will be used for longitudinal comparisons, special attention to detail is necessary (21,22). Small changes over time, particularly in a large group of workers, might be significant. Unfortunately, small differences in technique (e.g., effort urged by the technician, differences in equipment, control groups, or time of day of the test) may similarly affect results. Attention to adjustment of the spirometer for barometric pressure and ambient temperature is needed.

To ensure repeatability, the original tracing rather than only the numeric summary should be kept on file. When workers are tested at several sites (e.g., different plants), a group of individuals should be tested at all sites to ensure comparability. For multisite surveillance programs, physicians who interpret tests are advised to do so according to a common algorithm.

Biologic Monitoring

Biologic monitoring (23,24) may serve three purposes: (a) as a measure of workplace exposure, (b) as a measure of early effect of exposure on the individual, and (c) as an indicator of personal susceptibility. Biologic monitoring relies on measurements made in biologic specimens (e.g., blood, urine, exhaled air). They may be analyzed for the quantity of an environmental chemical or one of its metabolites to provide an estimate of the worker's chemical exposure. Mere detection of a chemical, however, does not imply the presence of a disease or of toxicity. Other forms of biologic monitoring include measuring direct effects on red cell enzymes, protein-losing nephropathies (e.g., β_2-microglobulin in cadmium toxicity), or cholinesterase levels.

Biologic monitoring can be helpful when evaluating a hazardous exposure that a person may have experienced. For example, if people who live in a basement apartment are concerned about the presence of solvents thought to contain xylene, measurement of urinary levels of methyl-hippuric acid (a metabolic product of xylene) can indicate that exposure to xylene has occurred. Unfortunately, it is uncommon for a specific blood or urinary level of a hazardous material to be associated with particular adverse health effects. Certain substances such as inorganic lead, however, are notable exceptions.

Biologic monitoring data are used to assess exposure to a hazard rather than to make a clinical diagnosis. Therefore, interpretation mandates careful attention to the timing of the specimen acquisition. Was it obtained in a worst-case situation, reflecting the highest possible exposure of the individual? Alternatively, was the specimen obtained during average work, which may not reflect peak exposures? Finally, was the specimen obtained when the person was not working or exposed, thus not reflecting actual exposure for materials that are cleared rapidly?

The biologic half-life of the agent determines whether it is detectable following exposure. Measurement of substances with long half-lives (such as the blood lead level) reflects longer-term exposure, but rapidly disappearing agents (e.g., carbon monoxide) reflect the period immediately preceding acquisition of the sample. Timing of sample acquisition is most critical for substances that have a short half-life. Thus, obtaining a blood lead specimen after a 24-hour absence from work might be appropriate, whereas obtaining a carbon monoxide analysis of exhaled air after such a time lapse would be invalid.

Biologic monitoring accounts for factors that affect total exposure, including breathing capacity, work effort, and underlying medical conditions. Such factors may not be adequately reflected in routine air measurements conducted in an industrial hygiene audit.

Biologic monitoring offers other advantages:

1. It measures the parameter most directly related to potential health effects. Results can aid in formulating a more refined estimate of risk of illness secondary to exposure.
2. Nonoccupational exposures and individual variability are assessed.
3. Multiple exposures and other routes of exposure, such as dermal and ingestion, can be evaluated.

Biologic monitoring, however, has limitations:

1. Effectiveness is dependent on adequate toxicologic data. (For most substances used in commerce today, adequate toxicologic data do not exist.)
2. Test results can be affected by other factors such as alcohol and pregnancy. (At the same blood lead levels, women have higher levels of zinc protoporphyrin than men.) Dietary deficiencies can lead to enhanced toxicity of a variety of hazardous substances. Cigarette smoking can also interfere with monitoring results. Workers who smoke cigarettes, for example, may have levels of cadmium higher than their nonsmoking counterparts (25).
3. For some substances, relatively short biologic half-lives affect the monitoring. In monitoring for dimethylformamide, a solvent used in the production of adhesives, 24-hour urinary samples near the time of last exposure can indicate the level of exposure a worker has experienced. Beyond 48 hours from the time of last exposure, the major metabolite, *N*-methylformamide (NMF) is not detectable (26).
4. Monitoring is ineffective for surface-acting agents such as sulfur dioxide and ammonia.

Example: Biologic Monitoring for Exposure to Metals

Occupational exposure to metals is common and can lead to adverse effects. Surveillance programs targeting workers exposed to the heavy metals (lead, mercury, and arsenic) have been effective at decreasing the morbidity associated with such exposures.

Lead

Inhalation or ingestion can result in inorganic lead accumulation. Metal smelting operations (e.g., during primary metal refining or during secondary smelting to recover lead from existing materials such as storage batteries) can produce significant exposures. Lead incorporated into paints can be ingested (especially by children) or may be inhaled if the surface is subjected to heat, sanding, or grinding. Nervous system effects are the main consequences of lead exposure. In children, lead encephalopathy (including apathy, coma, and seizure) may be seen, while adults tend to have peripheral nervous system effects (e.g., wrist drop and abnormalities of nerve conduction). More subtle effects on central nervous system functioning, particularly in children, are receiving considerable attention. Lead inhibits hemoglobin synthesis and therefore can produce anemia. Lead also produces renal disease; acute lead nephropathy is characterized by proximal tubular damage, while more chronic exposure can produce progressive renal fibrosis and renal failure. Hypertension may be related. Gastrointestinal symptoms (e.g., abdominal pain and constipation) also occur. Lead rarely can produce joint pain and also precipitate gout. Lead has adverse reproductive effects as well. Persons with lead exposure who have any of these health problems require both careful medical evaluation and assessment of the work environment to evaluate exposure.

Workers with significant potential exposure to lead must be placed in a medical surveillance program. The OSHA standard is very explicit about criteria for inclusion. Decisions regarding the need for medical surveillance depend on a number of factors, including the toxicity of the agent, working conditions, and level and degree of exposure. Blood lead level determination is useful as a reflection of exposure. Zinc protoporphyrin (ZPP) levels are much more nonspecific (affected by many causes of interference with heme synthesis). ZPP testing may be of some utility in reflecting long-term exposure and is performed because the requirement has not been deleted from the OSHA lead standard. Blood lead measurements should be performed by competent laboratories certified by the Centers for Disease Control and Prevention (CDC). In general, these measurements should be made every 6 months.

Detection of blood lead levels (BLLs) above 40 μg/100 mL in itself does not prove that clinical toxic effects are present but does indicate that significant overexposure has occurred. Although diagnosis of clinical toxicity is an individual matter, OSHA mandates certain implications of BLL surveillance: It requires that workers with BLL greater than 60 μg/100 mL on one test or whose 6-month average BLL is greater than 50 μg/100 mL be removed from exposure until the lead concentration returns to legally acceptable levels (40 μg/100 mL); during such periods of removal, the mandated medical removal protection requires that employers continue workers' pay at the usual rate. Conversely, the OSHA criterion value of 40 does not ensure adequate workplace control of exposure. Minor physiologic effects occur at levels well below 40, and a pattern of results of those of the community population indicate a lack of workplace control. For example, the state of California requires that laboratories report all values >25.

Interpretation of biologic monitoring data should be based on knowledge of the kinetics of disposition. Blood lead concentrations are indicative of recent and acute exposures, while urine measurements provide an integrated measure of more chronic exposure. However, elevated BLL may persist after cessation of exposure because of a high body burden of lead due to prior chronic overexposure. ZPP and hematocrit levels may be affected by lead exposure, but the results may be difficult to interpret in the presence of chronic disorders (e.g., iron deficiency anemia and increased serum bilirubin).

Mercury

Mercury exposure occurs in many industrial processes. Chloralkali cells used for producing chlorine can lead to exposure, as can use of mercury in instrument production, dental offices, laboratories, and the paper pulp industry. After inhalation, ingestion, or uptake from the skin, mercury is widely distributed in the body and accumulates in the brain. Chronic exposure to inorganic mercury can produce tremors, a psychoaffective disorder known as erethism (a personality change with withdrawal, anxiety, irritability), gingivitis, and renal disorders. In contrast to inorganic mercury exposure, organic mercury leads to cerebellar findings, which are more prominent than the psychological effects.

As with many other parameters of biologic monitoring, there is only a loose association between clinical toxicity and measurement of blood and urine mercury. Nevertheless, blood and urinary levels of mercury do reflect exposure, and therefore mercury-exposed workers should have such urine testing periodically. Hair levels, if specimens are obtained properly and analyzed carefully, may have utility in a small number of cases as a reflection of long-term or distant exposures. However, this method is highly subject to contamination and is often inaccurate.

Arsenic

Arsenic exposure is often a consequence of smelting of other metals, since arsenic is a common contaminant of ores of lead, copper, and zinc. It also is used in the chemical and pesticide industries. Chronic exposure produces dermatologic effects, including hyperkeratosis, eczematous dermatitis, increased pigmentation, and an increased risk of lung cancer. Hepatic toxicity and sensory neuropathy may occur from industrial arsenic exposures.

For surveillance purposes, urinary arsenic provides the best indicator of exposure. Arsenic has a short blood half-life, and therefore blood levels rarely are useful except as an indicator of very recent exposure. Surveillance programs also may include periodic liver function testing and examination of the skin in arsenic-exposed workers.

Ingestion of ocean fish or shellfish can lead to brief but rather high urinary arsenic concentrations. Therefore, a careful dietary history is important in any worker found to have an increased urinary arsenic level. In the evaluation of an increased concentration of urinary arsenic, it is advisable to recommend abstinence from seafood for a short period of time. Sputum cytology, despite being part of the recommended surveillance for the OSHA arsenic standard, is not routinely considered an effective screening device.

Surveillance of Medical and Workers Compensation Reports

Medical surveillance also may be based on systematic review of routine medical reports and workers' compensation files. Recognition of patterns of illness associated with particular work sites or work processes can be particularly helpful in identifying opportunities for preventive intervention.

Certain health events should trigger concern about possible occupational etiologies. These are considered *sentinel health events–occupational* (27). For example, new onset of asthma in the health care industry or nonviral hepatitis in the chemical industry warrant investigation. Furthermore, clusters of similar events should raise concerns. However, many clusters are simply chance events, particularly if the health effect is relatively common (e.g., lung and breast cancer) (28,29).

Evaluation of sentinel health events and of case clusters is fundamentally anecdotal. However, systematic, preplanned surveillance of reported health events may be particularly effective when there is an a priori suspicion of significant exposures. In such instances, the surveillance program directors should design a method to ensure collection of reports of health events. In so doing, particular care is necessary to avoid violating confidentiality.

Example of Records-based Surveillance: Ergonomics Surveillance

One method of detection of ergonomic problems relies on the reports of work-related musculoskeletal disorders. For such purposes, the surveillance program should systematically collect reports of diagnoses of work-related problems by workers' personal health care providers and by employer-related providers.

Cumulative trauma disorders (CTDs) are increasingly recognized. Medical surveillance programs are essential for their detection and prevention (30). As an adjunct to work site biomechanical analyses, worker-based clinical assessment can yield considerable useful information.

Review of absence records, productivity data, and reports of clinical diagnoses may also be useful for ergonomic medical surveillance. On a research basis, several surveillance programs have been instituted in areas at high risk of cumulative injury, even including clinical examination. Unfortunately, reliance on clinical signs is inappropriate. Even classic findings such as in Phalen's test actually have limited sensitivity and specificity.

When ergonomic surveillance is performed, it is important to note that the case definition differs significantly from the usual clinical case definition. The epidemiologic (or surveillance) definition is not meant to be specifically interpreted as the presence of a clinical diagnosis; similarly, one should not wait until the establishment of firm clinical diagnoses to be concerned.

Health care provider reports have been proposed by OSHA as the basis for determining that a sufficient hazard exists to require implementing a workplace program (e.g., reports of clinical diagnoses are used as a surrogate "exposure measure"). Therefore, it is critical that such diagnoses and attributions of causation be accurate. Optimally, the health care provider should be well trained in musculoskeletal disorders and also understand workplaces. Currently, there is considerable controversy about the minimal qualification of clinical providers who can serve as the trigger to require instituting specific programs.

Cancer Risk Screening

In the occupational setting, a number of techniques have been attempted to screen for cancer. Assuming that the development of environmentally related cancer proceeds in an orderly sequence, screening efforts theoretically may be focused at several points.

One technique is *assessment of exposure* to carcinogens. Persons with greater exposure have greater risk. Monitoring techniques include the assessment of mutagens in body fluids. Detection of urinary mutagens is the only assay that has shown some reliability in many groups of workers. The measurement of adducts created by binding of carcinogens or their metabolites to body chemicals (such as DNA or hemoglobin) can provide a measure of exposure. (See Chapter 35 for a more detailed discussion.)

Oncogene activation determination, although not currently useful, holds considerable promise. Activation of certain genes such as *ras* is believed to occur early in the malignant transformation process. Activation of such oncogenes may be determined by the detection of the protein products that are coded by the genes. For example, certain carcinogens (e.g., polycyclic aromatic hydrocarbons) activate the *ras* genes; these genes produce a protein known as p2l. Testing for p2l in serum may be useful for early lung cancer detection (31).

Cytogenetic monitoring is the study of numerical and structural chromosomal aberrations, which may occur naturally or secondary to exposure to environmental agents. As an attempt to assess damage to the gross structure of chromosomes, cytogenetic monitoring has been used to determine increases in chromosomal abnormalities among groups exposed to carcinogens. To date, however, these results have proved to be of little value in the evaluation of individual risk of developing malignancy secondary to a toxic exposure (see Chapter 23).

Cell surface antigens may change in the development of malignancy. Hence, immunologic studies of exfoliated cells such as those in sputum may permit earlier detection of lung cancers than traditional cytologic methods.

Cytologic morphology of malignant cells theoretically might be of benefit for tumors in locations that allow facile collection of shed cells (e.g., sputum, urine, or cervical cytology). Unfortunately, although routine cytopathology can detect cancers before development of symptoms, treatment options for some cancer sites may not always lead to improved survival.

Clinical testing methods have also been utilized. These aim at detecting malignancies at a stage that is more advanced than the stage addressed by the aforementioned methods. Radiographic screening for lung cancers in high-risk groups is controversial. Recently, the possible application of a relatively expensive technique—spiral chest computed axial tomography—has been suggested as a possible screening modality for lung cancer (32–34). If this proves effective, it may become useful for very high risk exposed workers. Other clinical techniques have included colonoscopy or cystoscopy for gastrointestinal and uroepithelial malignancies.

STEP 4: COLLECTION OF DATA

Actual collection of data should be conducted in a carefully planned manner. Testing may be conducted by the medical department of the employer, by a contract health provider selected by the employer, by a union selected contract provider, or by the personal physicians of the individual workers. In some instances, testing can be done at the work site based on on-site facilities or by the use of mobile testing vans. In other settings, workers travel to the testing location (e.g., clinicians' offices).

Administration of the test itself is only one part of medical surveillance testing. In many instances, the clinician performing the test is competent to manage all aspects, whereas in others, specialists in occupational health are necessary.

The meaning of surveillance data depends on its source and type. Some surveillance data must automatically generate an investigation to find preventable factors (e.g., report of a fatality or of a highly work-specific disease). Other surveillance-based diagnoses are important only when they occur in excess or in time-space clusters (e.g., common cancers). Elevated rates of common diseases (e.g., hepatitis) or common symptoms (e.g., cough, back pain) warrant follow-up study. It is important to interpret data in the context of the following:

1. Specific occupational diagnoses (e.g., confirmed toluene diisocyanate [TDI] asthma)
2. Diagnoses often associated with work (e.g., nonviral hepatitis)
3. Nonspecific clinical diagnoses (e.g., bronchitis)
4. Indicators of symptoms rather than disease (e.g., hand-wrist pain, cough)
5. Exposure indicators (e.g., blood lead level)
6. Possible physiologic effect (e.g., spirometry)
7. Nonspecific genotoxic or genetic findings (e.g., cytogenetics)
8. Markers of personal risk (e.g., atopic history in animal handlers)
9. Indications of possible early disease (e.g., β_2-microglobulin or *N*-acetylglucosaminidase in the urine of cadmium workers)

STEP 5: INTERPRETATION OF DATA TO BENEFIT THE INDIVIDUAL

To benefit the individual worker, several questions should be asked. For screening: Is a disease present? For risk factor identification: Is a significant precursor of a disease present, and is there an appropriate intervention to reduce the risk of disease developing? For work practices and environmental exposure assessment: Is this particular worker more highly exposed to an environmental agent (chemical or physical) than are co-workers?

A clear plan should be established for interpreting the results and presenting the findings to management and workers that avoids creation of either false anxiety or assurance. In general, ideal screening programs have high sensitivity (test is positive in a high percentage of persons with disease). The price paid for this high sensitivity is often low specificity (i.e., some workers with positive screening tests are free of disease). The predictive value of a test is of considerable interest because this represents the percentage of persons with a positive test who actually have the disease. For example, bilateral pleural thickening has an approximately 80% predictive value of being associated with previous exposure to asbestos. In reviewing these findings on a routine chest radiograph, the physician can counsel the patient accordingly, especially if other causes such as pleurisy, obesity, and rib fractures have been considered (35).

The opposite problem must also be avoided—false assurance. The worker (and health care provider as well) must understand that a negative test result may not prove the absence of disease. The predictive value of a negative test (e.g., if the test result is normal, what is the probability that the individual is truly free of disease?) is the relevant question in interpreting normal results. This figure depends on the sensitivity of the test and the prevalence of the disease.

Example: Nonspecific Testing (such as Liver Function Testing)

A perplexing situation often arises when minor abnormalities may be normal variants or may be due to nonoccupational factors. Because many industrial materials, particularly at high dose, can cause liver function abnormalities, liver function testing frequently is included in surveillance testing (36,37). Unfortunately, many otherwise normal persons have slightly elevated concentrations of liver enzymes without disease. Furthermore, many nonoccupational factors such as obesity, alcohol use, and infections can cause minor liver enzyme elevations. Thus, interpreting liver function data from a surveillance program requires careful thought and planning. If relatively minor abnormalities are detected, one must consider an occupational cause rather than ascribing the abnormalities to drinking. A careful examination with attention to occupational as well as nonoccupational factors is necessary. The physician should carefully and discreetly ask about hazardous exposures, even materials that the worker may be reticent to discuss (e.g., "Is work performed using unauthorized materials or in unauthorized manners?"). If there is any question about occupational hazards being contributing factors, a work-site visit, discussion with production supervisors, and industrial hygiene consultation may be needed. Minor functional abnormalities may allow intervention to prevent significant occupational disease, and an active approach is therefore needed in the occupational setting.

STEP 6: INTERVENTION BASED ON RESULTS

The intensity of intervention for risk factors must be chosen based on the gravity of the disease and the ability of the intervention to be effective. If an abnormality is found, a decision must be made about whether it was caused or aggravated by work conditions. Although the epidemiologic (group perspective) approach can help assess whether work conditions are contributing to disease in the population of workers, evaluating the individual case may be more problematic. For example, is a liver function abnormality a consequence of solvent exposure, nonoccupational disease (e.g., chronic active hepatitis), or lifestyle (e.g., alcohol use)? Implications for workers' compensation and employer liability should be addressed. In addition, reporting of certain diagnoses may be mandatory. The role of the director of the surveillance program in such determination of causality needs to be clearly defined in advance. Often, this physician may be more knowledgeable than the patient's personal physician or the specialist in understanding occupational toxicology and should therefore provide appropriate assistance in such decisions. The physician's ethical responsibility to the worker in this situation must be the foremost consideration, and a physician (no matter in whose employ) must never withhold any information for fear of adverse effects on the employer.

Several approaches to ensuring follow-up may be employed. Workers found to have abnormalities may be referred to their personal physicians. A clear policy consistent with local, state, and federal laws should be stated regarding which costs will be borne by the employer and which are the responsibility of the individual worker or the worker's health insurer. In addition, the surveillance program director should establish a plan for referral of people who do not have a personal physician. Optimally, the physician to whom the patient is referred should prepare a report to the referring physician (surveillance program director) regarding the test results, nature of the diagnosis, treatment, and related information.

STEP 7: INTERPRETATION OF AGGREGATE DATA FOR THE BENEFIT OF GROUPS OF WORKERS

Analysis of aggregate data may reveal information that is useful for preventing occupational disease. Analysis of aggregate data requires epidemiologic skills. If the clinician performing the testing has not had formal training, it is often worthwhile to consult a board certified specialist in occupational medicine or an epidemiologist. Formal statistical analysis of data requires time, staff, and skills often not available in the clinical setting. Improvements in microcomputer equipment, however, are making data interpretation more efficient. Occupational health systems can provide information related to white blood cell counts at certain areas of a plant, for example.

There are several ways by which analysis of medical surveillance data can provide beneficial information to groups of workers, rather than just the person tested:

1. Index case investigation: In some instances, detection of a single case can alert the clinician to a preventable risk for a group of workers. For example, PPD conversions or one case of TDI asthma (if confirmed) may indicate that exposures need control.
2. Case clusters: The occurrence of several cases in close spatial-temporal relationship warrants investigation, even if the illness is not specific for occupational causation. Case clusters can occur by chance, and proper investigation, not panic, should be employed.
3. Temporal or geographic trends: Even if individual results are "normal," aggregate data analysis may show a significant pattern. For example, an increase in average blood lead level over 1 to 2 years in a battery-manufacturing plant may mean that work practices or process controls need reassessment. Similarly, if urinary mercury levels in one area of a thermometer plant are higher than in other areas, investigation is needed.
4. Association with exposure status: The clinical and laboratory results should be linked to exposure data. Where process descriptions or industrial hygiene sampling data are available, these should be linked with the medical data. This process requires joint planning of data collection and interpretation.

Health surveillance data can be used to detect new hazards through the review of rates of disease and abnormalities in groups of workers. If the rate of abnormality in an exposed group is higher than that of an unexposed group, an industrial hazard should be suspected. The reference (unexposed) group must be comparable to the exposed group, except for the exposure under consideration. For example, lung cancer rates or frequency of spirometric abnormality should not be compared between a plant employing many heavy smokers and one that has essentially a nonsmoking population.

Relatively small changes in a variable may be more important in an aggregate analysis than when evaluating one person. For example, a 100-mL difference from predicted FEV_1 would hardly prompt a diagnosis of lung disease in an individual. But if a population of exposed workers averages 100 mL less compared to an unexposed population, an occupational hazard could be present.

Aggregate analysis can identify new sites of known hazards. For example, although hazards of asbestos are well known, detection of pleural plaques on surveillance chest radiographs can lead to identifying processes not otherwise known to involve asbestos exposure or to contamination of raw materials (e.g., vermiculite ore) with tremolite asbestos fibers. Similarly, although ergonomic factors associated with low back pain are well known, a geographic or temporal clustering of back injuries should prompt the clinician to suspect a particular area of the plant as having poor equipment design or work practices. Aggregate analysis of surveillance data can document the safety of materials and processes; in the absence of such data analysis, doubts may persist.

The ability to perform aggregate analysis depends on integration of various types of data. Personnel characteristics (e.g., job history) and industrial hygiene data (e.g., levels of exposures), in addition to the clinical information, can be entered into computer programs for data analysis. However, confidentiality needs to be guarded in accordance with ethical and legal standards. When providing contractual service for a small employer without a corporate health department, the physician should urge aggregate as well as individual analysis of medical monitoring results.

Medical surveillance analysis ideally includes observation of absence patterns that may represent an occupational hazard. Some ergonomic hazards have been detected in this manner (38,39), and chemical exposure hazards may be pinpointed as well.

Identification of Overexposures and Disease Patterns

Physicians should encourage discussion during medical surveillance examinations because an employee may feel more comfortable reporting concerns about work to a health professional than to a line supervisor. Furthermore, because of the physician's role as health advocate, workers often feel more comfortable in addressing concerns in a clinical setting (40,41).

Medical surveillance may also detect patterns of illness. Sentinel health events–occupational (SHE-O) are medical diagnoses that are frequently associated with occupational causation (27). When they occur, they should be investigated. Workers' compensation claims, although not necessarily accurate, may provide clues to show that a pattern of illness is developing; this has been successfully applied to skin disease surveillance (42,43). Sentinel physicians, community-based clinicians who report disease of possible occupational origin, have been used for community-wide surveillance in the SENSOR program (44,45), but this method is less applicable for the company-based than for public health agency–based programs.

STEP 8: COMMUNICATION OF RESULTS

Information about surveillance data may be directed to several different targets: the worker, the management, worker representatives (e.g., unions), insurers, and government.

The worker must be given surveillance testing results in a timely manner and in an understandable fashion (46). Workers should be given a summary of their information, and access to the complete data must be assured. If values out of the "reference range" are noted, their significance should be explained in a clear and understandable manner. Interpretation (not just test values themselves) should be provided by a clinician (e.g., plant physician) whom the workers trust and who is accessible for additional discussion if needed. As a practical matter, it is often difficult to succinctly interpret data in an easily understandable manner. A BLL of 35, while below the level at which OSHA mandates action, indicates exposure that should be limited.

The communication to the worker therefore should avoid implying the diagnosis of toxicity, but also should avoid giving the impression that everything is fine if it is below the OSHA standard of 40. Similarly, small-airway abnormality (isolated abnormality of the $FEF_{25-75\%}$) is unlikely to produce symptoms, but should not be ignored because it may be a harbinger of early abnormality (e.g., "Your breathing test showed normal FEV_1 and FVC, but one test, the $FEF_{25-75\%}$, was not in the normal range. This is not a major problem now, but it may be an indicator of an early problem. You should see Dr. X if you would like to discuss this.") It is important to avoid overemphasizing the importance of a borderline deviation in a test for which significance is uncertain.

Implications of certain test results must be reported to management. For example, detection of a medical condition that makes work unsafe for the individual, the public, or co-workers cannot be ignored. However, management is not generally entitled to the specific medical information, only the clinician's opinion about its implications. Therefore, physicians who perform testing must be prepared for this awkward situation.

Worker representatives (e.g., unions) also have limited access to medical data. Particularly if confidential data are involved, extreme caution is needed. Ethical considerations as well as the OSHA regulations should be considered.

Interpretations must clearly indicate the difference between group analysis and abnormalities in individuals. A smaller deviation from normality may be of greater concern in a group than in an individual. The results should not be construed to indicate the presence of "disease" in the traditional sense. Often, it is useful to indicate both the magnitude of the effect found and the estimated likelihood (considering all factors) that it is due to occupational exposure.

In reporting the interpretations, the clinician must be sensitive to the concerns of workers. Many may fear loss of jobs if any abnormality is found, whereas in other situations the workplace psychosocial environment might encourage inappropriate compensation claims that are not specifically occupational in origin.

Under certain circumstances, results must be reported to governmental agencies. For example, if a specific occupational disease is diagnosed based on surveillance, it is mandatory to record it on the OSHA 300 log (see Chapter 3). Similarly, patterns of abnormalities, even if not absolutely proven, often must be reported to the Environmental Protection Agency and other agencies.

Many workers have personal physicians, some of whom may have very limited knowledge of the testing performed. Therefore, interpretation often must be done for both the worker and the worker's physician.

STEP 9: PROGRAM EVALUATION

Occupational health surveillance involves much more than simply performing tests. The program should be evaluated on a periodic basis. Many of the criteria proposed by the CDC for evaluating public health surveillance systems are directly applicable to occupational health surveillance (47). Evaluation should include at least consideration of the presence of sufficient quality resources (48,49), and optimally the evaluation should consider the actual program outcomes. Table 41.5 summarizes questions for assessing program structure.

In addition to structural analysis, audit of performance is advisable. Quality control must be considered. Are the results accurate and precise? For chemical tests, samples may be split and submitted to different laboratories. Known reference standards may be submitted in a blind fashion to the laboratory. For physiologic tests, such as spirometry, quality control can be assessed by reviewing hardcopies of tracings or directly assessing the laboratory's quality assurance procedures. Often, the medical surveillance program clinician should personally conduct (or arrange for a consultant to conduct) a quality assurance audit of facilities used. In addition, the appropriateness of the target populations should be as-

TABLE 41.5. *Program evaluation questions*

Stakeholder involvement:
- Are all of the appropriate stakeholders involved?
- Does the program meet the needs from all perspectives?

Program goals:
- Is there a specific, well-defined health effect or exposure for which the program operates?
- Is the population to be tested carefully defined to include those at greatest risk and not extend resources on those with minimal risk?

Regulatory and legal concerns:
- Is there a specific OSHA standard regulating the program?
- Is confidentiality appropriately protected?
- Do providers of service have appropriate licensees and certifications?
- Are results reported and recorded as required?

Testing quality:
- Is there a quality assurance program to assure that tests are accurate?
- Do staff have appropriate training and certifications (e.g., NIOSH spirometry course certificate, B reader certification, formal audiometry training certificate)?
- Is equipment up-to-date and well maintained?
- Do the physicians and others performing testing understand the nature of the workplace exposures?
- Does the testing facility understand requirements of OSHA?

Communication:
- Are test results of individual workers provided to them?
- Are employers provided only the information to which they have true need and legal access?
- Is a qualified clinician available to explain the implications test results to individual workers?
- Is there a clear, written policy about who has access to the data (e.g., union representatives)?
- Are the purposes of the program adequately explained to individual workers in an appropriate language and level?
- Are results of clinical testing appropriately provided to the personal physicians of workers?

Integration with exposure assessment?
- Are exposure data concomitantly collected?
- Are exposure data for the individual worker available to help the clinician interpret the test results?
- Is a database available that links exposure and clinical test results?
- Does the surveillance program director have sufficient training to interpret exposure data? If not, is an appropriate consultant available?

Follow-up:
- Is a plan for follow-up of individuals with positive screening results in place?
- Is there appropriate feedback so that workplace changes can be made based on the results of the surveillance program?

Record keeping:
- Are records maintained for future reference?
- Are there provisions for custodial responsibility for records, radiographs, raw data (e.g., audiometry and spirometry graphs)?

Aggregate analysis:
- Are the tests conducted with sufficient consistency to allow comparability from different test sites?
- Are the data for individual workers aggregated into a large database for future analysis?
- Is there sufficient capability to do simple statistical analyses?

sessed. Of workers at risk, what percentage actually underwent medical surveillance? Conversely, how much testing, and so forth, was wasted on workers without specific risk factors warranting the testing? The effectiveness of the surveillance program can be gauged by determining if it was successful in leading to interventions that could decrease disease or injury rates. Often, surveillance programs include significant screening components, in which subsequently more detailed evaluations determine if disease is truly present. The sensitivity and specificity of the surveillance/screening testing can therefore be evaluated. This process requires that the true situation be ascertained. Finally, the cost of the program must be considered in interpreting its value.

Actual outcomes should also be addressed if possible. These include measures of the acceptability of the entire program to all involved. The cost of the program should also be considered. Costs include the direct cost of testing, the cost of program management, the impact of additional testing generated by false positives, lost work time while going for testing, and the nonmonetary costs of anxiety induced by the program. Several measures should be considered: (a) the sensitivity of the testing (proportion of individuals with the disease who are detected as positive); (b) the predictive value of a positive result (if the test is positive, how likely is it that there actually is a problem); and (c) the predictive value of a negative result, which is particularly important in occupational health surveillance. Testing is performed not only to detect positive individuals but also to evaluate the efficacy of workplace controls. Employers should not be falsely assured unless negative results of surveillance testing can be considered accurate.

REFERENCES

1. Straif K, Silverstein M. Comparison of U.S. Occupational Safety and Health Administration standards and German Berufsgenossenschaften Guidelines for Preventive Occupational Health Examinations. *Am J Ind Med* 1997;31(4):373–380.
2. *http://www.osha.govOshStd_data1910_0095.html.*
3. Newman LS. To Be2+ or not to Be2+: immunogenetics and occupational exposure. *Science* 1993;262(5131):197–198.
4. Saltini C, et al. Immunogenetic basis of environmental lung disease: lessons from the berylliosis model. *Eur Respir J* 1998;12(6):1463–1475.
5. Rossman MD, et al. Human leukocyte antigen class II amino acid epitopes: susceptibility and progression markers for beryllium hypersensitivity. *Am J Respir Crit Care Med* 2002;165(6):788–794.
6. Ferris BG. Epidemiology standardization project (American Thoracic Society). *Am Rev Respir Dis* 1978; 118(6 pt 2):1–120.
7. Pappas GP, et al. Medical clearance for respirator use: sensitivity and specificity of a questionnaire. *Am J Ind Med* 1999;35(4):395–400.
8. Kreiss K. Approaches to assessing pulmonary dysfunction and susceptibility in workers. *J Occup Med* 1986; 28(8):664–669.
9. Wagner GR, et al. The NIOSH B reader certification program: an update report. *J Occup Med* 1992;34(9): 879–884.
10. Meyer JD, et al. Prevalence of small lung opacities in populations unexposed to dusts: a literature analysis. *Chest* 1997;111(2):404–410.
11. Ducatman AM, Yang WN, Forman SA. "B-readers" and asbestos medical surveillance. *J Occup Med* 1988;30 (8):644–647.
12. Welch LS, et al. Variability in the classification of radiographs using the 1980 International Labor Organization Classification for Pneumoconioses. *Chest* 1998; 114(6):1740–1748.
13. Balmes JR. To B-read or not to B-read. *J Occup Med* 1992;34(9):885–886.
14. American-Thoracic-Society. Standardization of spirometry, 1994 update. *Am J Respir Crit Care Med* 1994;152 (3):1107–1136.
15. Townsend MC. ACOEM position statement: spirometry in the occupational setting. American College of Occupational and Environmental Medicine. *J Occup Environ Med* 2000;42(3):228–245.
16. Enright PL, et al. Spirometry reference values for women and men 65 to 85 years of age: cardiovascular health study. *Am Rev Respir Dis* 1993;147(1):125–133.
17. Enright PL. Surveillance for lung disease: quality assurance using computers and a team approach. *Occup Med* 1992;7(2):209–225.
18. Harber P, Discher D. Occupational respiratory function testing—an algorithmic approach. *Occup Med* 1997;12 (3):485–512.
19. Harber P, Lockey JE. Pulmonary function testing in pulmonary prevention. *Occup Med* 1991;6(1):69–79.
20. Schouten JP, Tager IB. Interpretation of longitudinal studies: an overview. *Am J Respir Crit Care Med* 1996; 154(6 Pt 2):S278–S284.
21. Enright PL, et al. Spirometry in the Lung Health Study: II. Determinants of short-term intraindividual variability. *Am J Respir Crit Care Med* 1995;151(2 Pt 1): 406–411.
22. Enright PL, et al. Spirometry in the Lung Health Study. 1. Methods and quality control. *Am Rev Respir Dis* 1991;143(6):1215–1223.
23. Derosa CT, et al. The Agency for Toxic Substances and Disease Registry's role in development and application of biomarkers in public health practice. *Toxicol Ind Health* 1993;9(6):979–994.
24. Biological markers in environmental health research. Committee on Biological Markers of the National Research Council. *Environ Health Perspect* 1987;74:3–9.
25. Zielhuis RL, et al. Smoking habits and levels of lead and cadmium in blood in urban women. *Int Arch Occup Environ Health* 1977;39(1):53–58.
26. Krivanek ND, McLaughlin M, Fayweather WE. Monomethylformamide levels in human urine after repetitive exposure to dimethylformamide vapor. *J Occup Med* 1978;20(3):179–182.
27. Mullan RJ, Murthy LI. Occupational sentinel health events: an up-dated list for physician recognition and public health surveillance. *Am J Ind Med*1991;19(6): 775–799.
28. Fleming LE, Ducatman AM, Shalat SL. Disease clusters: a central and ongoing role in occupational health. *J Occup Med* 1991;33(7):818–825.
29. Fleming LE, Ducatman AM, Shalat SL. Disease clusters in occupational medicine: a protocol for their investigation in the workplace. *Am J Ind Med* 1992;22(1):33–47.
30. Silverstein BA, et al. Work-related musculoskeletal disorders: comparison of data sources for surveillance. *Am J Ind Med* 1997;31(5):600–608.
31. Brandt-Rauf PW. Oncogene proteins as biomarkers in the molecular epidemiology of occupational carcinogenesis: the example of the ras oncogene-encoded p21 protein. *Int Arch Occup Environ Health* 1991;63(1):1–8.
32. Patz EF Jr, Black WC, Goodman PC. CT screening for lung cancer: not ready for routine practice. *Radiology* 2001;221(3):587–591; discussion 598–599.
33. Jett JR. Spiral computed tomography screening for lung cancer is ready for prime time. *Am J Respir Crit Care Med* 2001;163(4):812; discussion 814–815.
34. van Klaveren RJ, et al. Lung cancer screening by low-dose spiral computed tomography. *Eur Respir J* 2001; 18(5):857–866.
35. Albelda SM, et al. Pleural thickening: its significance and relationship to asbestos dust exposure. *Am Rev Respir Dis* 1982;126(4):621–624.
36. Herip DS. Recommendations for the investigation of abnormal hepatic function in asymptomatic workers. *Am J Ind Med* 1992;21(3):331–339.
37. Hodgson MJ, Goodman-Klein BM, van Thiel DH. Evaluating the liver in hazardous waste workers. *Occup Med* 1990;5(1):67–78.
38. Park RM, et al. Use of medical insurance claims for surveillance of occupational disease: an analysis of cumulative trauma in the auto industry. *J Occup Med* 1992;34 (7):731–737.
39. Park RM. Medical insurance claims and surveillance for occupational disease: analysis of respiratory, cardiac, and cancer outcomes in auto industry tool grinding operations. *J Occup Environ Med* 2001;43(4):335–346.
40. Welch L. The role of occupational health clinics in surveillance of occupational disease. *Am J Public Health* 1989;79[suppl]:58–60.

41. Herbert R, et al. The Union Health Center: a working model of clinical care linked to preventive occupational health services. *Am J Ind Med* 1997;31(3):263–273.
42. O'Malley M, et al. Surveillance of occupational skin disease using the Supplementary Data System. *Am J Ind Med* 1988;13(2):291–299.
43. Mathias CG, et al. Surveillance of occupational skin diseases: a method utilizing workers' compensation claims. *Am J Ind Med* 1990;17(3):363–370.
44. Jajosky RA, et al. Surveillance of work-related asthma in selected U.S. states using surveillance guidelines for state health departments—California, Massachusetts, Michigan, and New Jersey, 1993–1995. *MMWR CDC Surveill Summ* 1999;48(3):1–20.
45. Matte TD, Baker EL, Honchar PA. The selection and definition of targeted work-related conditions for surveillance under SENSOR. *Am J Public Health* 1989;79 [suppl]:21–25.
46. Schulte PA, Singal M. Interpretation and communication of the results of medical field investigations. *J Occup Med* 1989;31(7):589–594.
47. CDC. Updated guidelines for evaluating surveillance systems: recommendations from the guidelines working group. *MMWR* 2001;50(RR-13):1–30.
48. Harber P, Hsu P. Program optimization: a semi-quantitative approach. *Occup Med* 1991;6(1):145–151.
49. Harber P. Pulmonary prevention: programmatic characterization. *Occup Med* 1991;6(1):133–143.

42

Risk Assessment in the Workplace

John Whysner and Kenneth H. Chase

The workplace and the environment have always contained risks. Traditionally, accidents have been, and continue to be, the most important risks that must be assessed. However, the vast number of chemicals now used in the workplace and found in the environment have increased the complexity of assessing risk. In the past, certain jobs have been considered more hazardous than others based on risks that are clearly visible; however, the risks associated with exposures to chemicals are often hidden. The possibility of exposure may be hard to detect, and the effects of some chemicals may not develop until years or decades after exposure.

The practicing physician will be increasingly called on to provide guidance to individuals exposed to a variety of occupational and environmental hazards (1). But how can the physician estimate the degree of risk that confronts a patient, and how can this risk be made understandable in a lay person's terms? One possibility is to use the tool of risk assessment, which is a quantitative approach to this problem that has been developed extensively over the past three decades.

This chapter describes a general approach to this problem, and provides a case illustration of a hypothetical situation in which sufficient information is available to make a reasonable risk calculation. Unfortunately, such information is often unavailable, or the time required for risk assessment calculations is prohibitive. However, by understanding the elements of the risk calculation, those parameters that increase or decrease risk can be appreciated. Such calculations are similar to those used by government agencies to determine regulatory limits for chemicals in the workplace or environment. Regulatory bodies, such as the U.S. Environmental Protection Agency (EPA) have numerous risk assessment documents available. For additional information on this subject, see refs. 2–4.

CLINICAL APPROACH TO EVALUATING RISK

The example given here is a hypothetical one involving a worker who has discovered that he has been exposed to compound X, by the dermal route, at his workplace. He has no clinical symptoms or abnormal laboratory findings, but he wants to know whether he can get cancer as a result of the exposure. Often the hypothetical risk is small, and in the occupational setting many jobs involve some risk. The approach to this patient should include the following three steps:

1. Risk assessment of current and past exposure based on actual dose, if available.
2. Modification of risk factors in the workplace through counseling, personal protective equipment, and engineering controls.
3. Reassessment of risks to provide the worker with input for determining acceptability of the risk.

A review of the available information on compound X shows that it is a known human carcinogen based on human epidemiology data. In this case the human data do not supply good dose-response information. However, on the basis of rodent studies, the cancer oral slope factor is listed as 1×10^{-1} per mg/kg-day^{-1}. This means that for a daily exposure over a lifetime exposure (actually a 30-year exposure) of 1 mg per kilogram body weight, the total lifetime risk would be 0.1 or 10%. Such information is typically available from a regulatory agency such as the EPA and may be found in the on-line database at *www.epa.gov/iris/index.html.* In this case, only an oral slope factor is given by EPA, but this can usually be used as an approximation of the slope factor for dermal exposure.

A call to the company where the employee is working reveals that the average surface concentration of compound X in his work area was measured by standard swipe tests and found to be 70 μg/100 cm^2. His job put him in the contaminated area for only one fourth of his working days. It is assumed that the work practices were constant over his work lifetime, which was 30 years. The man was not a smoker, and opportunities for oral exposure or inhalation exposures appear to have been minimal. Repeated measurements of air concentration (in this case) were negligible.

For dermal absorption, a simplifying upper limit assumption can be made that one half of the surface area of the hands and arms was in equilibrium with the contaminated surface area. This would provide a health protective upper limit of exposure estimate. Studies have shown that dermal absorption of compound X is about 10%. As can be seen from Fig. 42.1, the lifetime average daily dose (LADD), calculated based on the foregoing assumptions, is 0.1 μg/kg-day or 1/10,000 of a milligram. By multiplying the oral slope factor by the LADD, the hypothetical additional cancer risk for a lifetime for the worker would be 1/100,000. If the worker continues at the same job with the same exposure, each additional year will add an additional hypothetical cancer risk of approximately 1/3,000,000. (The 1/100,000 risk is accumulated over 30 years; one thirtieth of 1/100,000 is 1/3,000,000 per year.)

It is recognized that physicians usually have neither the information nor the time to perform such a calculation. Also, there are numerous uncertainties in the assumptions involved in risk assessment. Consequently, this risk assessment represents, at best, a rough estimate, which may greatly overestimate risk. The correlation of 0.1 μg/kg-day with an excess cancer risk is an upper limit of risk, and some would argue that the human risk is 100 or 1,000 times less or may even be zero at these low levels. This is because

Dermal Daily Dose Calculation:

$$\frac{70\ \mu g}{100\ cm^2} \times 1500\ cm^2 \times \frac{0.25\ day}{day} \times \frac{0.1\ \mu g\ absorbed/day}{\mu g\ exposed} = \frac{26\ \mu g}{day}$$

Lifetime Average Daily Dose (LADD) calculation:

$$\frac{26\ \mu g/day \times 240\ working\ days/year \times 30\ years}{25{,}550\ days/lifetime \times 70\ kg} = 0.1\ \mu g/kg\text{-}day$$

Where:

$\frac{70\ \mu g}{100\ cm^2}$ = measured environmental surface level

1500 cm^2 = one-half of the surface area of the arms

0.25 day/day = fraction of day exposed

$\frac{0.1\ \mu g\ absorbed/day}{\mu g\ exposed}$ = absorption efficiency of 10%

FIG. 42.1. Calculation of cancer risk for a worker exposed to compound X.

high-dose animal cancer studies are used with linear-at-low-dose extrapolation methods. This extrapolation method may not be appropriate for certain types of carcinogens as is discussed below (see Dose-Response Relationships).

RISK COMMUNICATION AND HAZARD REDUCTION

Putting all of these uncertainties aside, how can an excess cancer risk of 1/3,000,000/year be explained to the patient? By referring to Table 42.1, the physician can explain that the risk of cancer from this exposure is about the same as the risk of dying in an earthquake if one lives in California or in a flood, but greater than being struck by lightning. By further comparison, the risk is about 1/10,000 that of smoking one pack of cigarettes per day.

Is this an acceptable risk? This is a complex issue. Government regulatory agencies have used 1/10,000 to 1/1,000,000 excess lifetime cancer risk as benchmarks for policy decisions. But such guidelines are for involuntary risks. For voluntarily risks, as may be the case for those associated with certain occupational exposures, acceptability must be evaluated by the patient.

The next step is to consider ways to reduce the current hazard. Table 42.2 presents a number of factors that contribute to a risk. The patient can be counseled on the importance of personal hygiene and the use of protective equipment to reduce exposure. Steps such as approaching management, unions, or the shop foreman can also be considered to attempt reduction of exposure. For example, if the area of skin exposed could be reduced to one fifth by the use of protective clothing, and if surface contamination can be reduced to one fourth, then the resulting incremental risk will be one twentieth of the 1/3,000,000/year risk previously determined, or 1/60 million/year. From Table 42.1, this is one sixth that of being struck by lightning and less than 1/300 of the risk of dying in a flood. Finally, the physician should attempt to discover whether the patient is exposed to other hazards in the workplace. Typically, there are multiple chemicals in the workplace, some of which may be of greater hazard than the chemical of concern to the worker.

TABLE 42.1. *Risks*

Situation	Deaths/person/ year (odds)
Motorcycling	1 in 50
Smoking (20 cigarettes/day)	1 in 200
Influenza	1 in 5,000
Auto driving (U.K.)	1 in 5,900
Leukemia	1 in 12,500
Drinking (1 bottle wine/day)	1 in 13,300
Struck by auto	1 in 20,000
Taking contraceptive pills	1 in 50,000
Floods	1 in 455,000
Earthquake (California)	1 in 588,000
Lightning (U.K.)	1 in 10 million
Release from nuclear reactor at site boundary	1 in 10 million

From (5).

Note: Some problems arise with the conversion of lifetime to yearly risks for hazards, such as carcinogens, that are cumulative. For the purpose of this table, this difficulty has been ignored, since both are approximations.

TABLE 42.2. *Exposure factors that proportionally increase the calculated risk of cancer, assuming a linear-at-low-dose relationship*

For all routes
Years of exposure
Hours of exposure per day
Concentration of toxic substance[a]
For dermal exposure
Surface area of skin exposed[a]
Length of time substance remains on skin[b]
For oral exposure
Mouthing episodes from contaminated hands, cigarettes, food, etc.[b]

[a]Reduced by personal protective equipment and work practices.

[b]Reduced by hygiene.

RISK ASSESSMENT METHODS AND TERMINOLOGY

Risk assessment is a statistical procedure employed by various regulatory agencies in an attempt to define an acceptable level of risk for exposure to a hazardous substance. Risk assessment uses available scientific evidence from human (epidemiology) and animal studies to develop models to predict toxicity of the various substances at low levels of exposure. Limitations inherent in this process include the reliability of the data, the accuracy of extrapolating results from animals to humans, and the legitimacy of assuming a linear relationship between low doses of a substance and the adverse health effect, which is the cancer slope factor as was used in the worker risk calculation present earlier in this chapter. Now, U.S. governmental agencies, such as the EPA, recognize the possible presence of a threshold dose for carcinogens, below which exposure to a substance is not a health risk, as will be discussed (6).

Hazard Identification

Hazard identification relies on the results of well-designed human or animal studies for the purposes of risk assessment. Human epidemiology studies of workers exposed to a chemical may provide evidence of carcinogenicity. If a number of such studies have shown statistically significant increases in a cancer end point, and the studies are consistent, then a carcinogenic effect is suggested. If the increased rate of cancer is substantial and the studies have taken place in different settings so that confounding factors or bias are unlikely to produce the results, then the chemical may be deemed a known human carcinogen. It should be noted, however, that such a designation is confined to a particular cancer end point, and although some chemicals may cause more than one type of cancer, this is not necessarily the case. For example, many of the known human carcinogens cause only lung cancer associated with inhalation exposure.

For most chemicals, more information is available from tests in experimental animals (usually mice and rats) than from epidemiology studies. For regulatory purposes, sufficient evidence of carcinogenicity in either humans or in experimental animals begins the risk assessment process. Although positive studies in experimental animals do not prove that a chemical can cause cancer in humans, the health protective principle used by regulatory agencies requires that the chemical be treated *as if* it has the potential to cause cancer in humans.

The use of animal tests to determine this potential to cause cancer in humans is problematic. Several cancer mechanisms have now been found whereby the positive findings in rodents do not apply to humans (7). Of course, this is not a problem for known human carcinogens, which are designated International Agency for Research on Cancer (IARC) group 1, EPA group A, National Toxicology Program (NTP) group K, and American Conference of Governmental Industrial Hygienists (ACGIH) group A1. However, for lesser designations that are based on animal tests, the risk assessment process may concern risks that are not applicable to humans.

Dose-response Relationships

For most carcinogenic effects, no threshold dose is assumed to exist by U.S. government agencies, as shown in Fig. 42.2 (curve B). Only at zero dose is there assumed to be no effect. This is the assumption

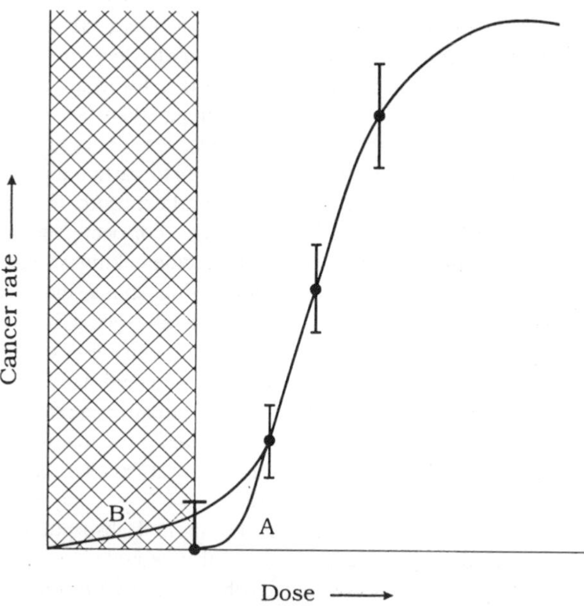

FIG. 42.2. Alternative dose-response curves for carcinogenicity. In curve A, the data points are fitted to the curve with threshold. In curve B, the data points are fitted to the curve without threshold (linear model). The shaded area indicates the "no observed effect level" (NOEL).

used in the determination of a cancer slope factor as used earlier in this chapter. The "linear-at-low-dose" model predicts that the line can be extrapolated to smaller and smaller dose with declining risk of cancer. Various regulatory agencies have usually determined the range of 1/10,000 to 1/10,000,000 as an acceptable lifetime risk due to a chemical. The dosage associated with this risk is called a "virtually safe dose" (VSD).

The "no-threshold" theory of carcinogenesis is based on the premise that only one molecule of a carcinogen needs to interact with DNA to initiate cancer development. This theory, however, has been the subject of considerable scientific challenge by authors who claim that large numbers of chemical molecules are required for a measurable response (8). Presumably, the metabolic system can successfully detoxify small amounts of carcinogens. Additionally, chemical carcinogens act through different mechanisms. Many chemicals that act by a non–DNA-reactive mechanism exert their effects by enhancing the development of tumors rather than by creating neoplastic cells (9).

The classic sigmoidal dose-response curve for most toxic effect appears in Fig. 42.2 (curve A) and exhibits a threshold at low doses below which the effect does not occur. For example, a very small dose of a chlorinated hydrocarbon will not produce chloracne; a minimal amount of exposure is required to alter the metabolism of the skin to produce these changes. The hatched area in the diagram is called a "no observed effect level" (NOEL). For regulatory purposes, limits on exposure are usually set at a fraction of the NOEL, usually 1/10 to 1/1,000. This adjusted dosage is called a reference dose (RfD) or an acceptable daily intake (ADI). The RfD is set well below the NOEL because the NOEL is usually based on animal studies rather than human epidemiology studies, and uncertainties exist in extrapolation from animals to sensitive humans. This approach is used by U.S. Government agencies for noncarcinogenic effects and by other governments for many carcinogenic effects as well (2). The EPA has now also considered using such an approach that they term the margin of exposure (MOE) (6). In this case, the MOE is the dose (actually, the 95% lower statistical confidence limit of the dose) associated with a 10% cancer incidence divided by the determined environmental exposure. In other words, a risk is not calculated, but this ratio gives an estimate of how different an exposure is from the exposure that could hypothetically cause a significant increase in cancer.

Calculation of Exposure

The assessment of risk requires an estimate of the person's exposure. For this estimate, a measurement of the concentration of the chemical in the worker's environment is preferred. Depending on the exposure scenario, such a measurement may be the concentration of a substance in air, on a surface, or in a solid matrix such as soil.

To perform relevant measurements and estimate an exposure, it is first necessary to assess the routes and conditions by which a worker may be exposed. Such exposure scenarios are usually specific to an absorption route, which may be oral, dermal, or inhalation. Inhalation estimates are the easiest to perform; by knowing the airborne level, one can calculate the exposure, as shown in Fig. 42.3. The air concentration is usually measured in milligrams or micrograms per cubic meter (mg/m^3 or $\mu g/m^3$). For the respiratory route, it is often assumed that there is total absorption of the inspired toxic vapors, although this is not the case for most substances. For an adult, air is inhaled at a rate of 1 m^3/hour at rest and 2 m^3/hour for moderately vigorous activity. An exposure estimate (dose) can be calculated by simply taking the product of the measured concentration and the air volume inhaled over a specified time interval.

Dermal and oral absorption are more complicated to model. Dermal exposure is probably the most difficult to estimate, as evidenced by the sample calculation for the hypothetical worker in Fig. 42.1. The skin surface levels are assumed equal to the levels on environmental surfaces. The efficiency of absorption is usually less than unity, and can be 10% or less for exposures to particulate or soil bound chemicals.

For oral exposure, the amount of ingestion must be estimated. For occupational exposures, there may be acute accidental ingestions that can be quantified. For chronic ingestions, the scenarios are more complex and generally occur by hand-to-mouth activities or "mouthing episodes" of smoking, eating, nail biting, or other personal habits. Soil ingestion directly from soil or from airborne soil particles has been estimated to average 25 mg/day for adults (10). The calculation of daily oral exposure is performed as shown in Fig. 42.3.

For dermal absorption, a method has been developed that provides an upper limit of exposure. This method was used in the example given at the beginning of the chapter. In this method, the assumption is made that part of the skin is in contact with the concentration equal to the surface concentration of the toxic substance in the environment for a period of

```
Inhalation:

Daily exposure  =  air level  X   1-2m³   X  hours
                                  hour        day

Oral (Soil):

Daily exposure  =  soil level  X  25 mg soil/day  X  % absorption

Dermal (Surfaces):

Daily exposure  =  surface level  X  1500 cm²  X

                     fraction of day exposed  X  % absorption

(The simplifying assumption of concentration equivalence between
of one-half the area of the arms and environment surface levels
will generally lead to an overestimation of exposure.)

All Routes:

Lifetime Average Daily Dose  =

     Daily exposure X days exposure/year  X  years exposure
                25,550 days/lifetime  X  70 kg
```

FIG. 42.3. Formulas for calculating daily exposure by route. See text for explanation of terms.

time. This assumption may be further refined by wipe samples utilizing an appropriate solvent. Then, the equation for dermal exposure can be expressed as shown in Fig. 42.3. In this case, the absorption efficiency for a 24-hour contact must be known. Usually animal studies are performed to determine this factor. The surface area exposed may include the hands only, the hands and forearms, or other exposed areas of the body.

The use of personal protective equipment will modify any of the above calculations. In fact, such calculations can be utilized to estimate the benefits of such protection. The presumed efficiency of air filtration devices or barrier clothing, which reduce exposures, can be included in these calculations.

PRINCIPLES OF RISK ASSESSMENT

Risk assessment is a quantitative approach to the risk of exposure from toxic chemicals, although it uses qualitative information for hazard identification. Usually it is not possible to perform all of these calculations on an individual patient. Such calculations are time-consuming and are usually performed on groups or an occasional patient involved in litigation. However, an understanding of the risk factors can be useful in reducing hazards and in explaining risk to the patient. Three principles of risk assessment worth noting are the following:

1. For carcinogens, lowering the exposure can usually decrease the upper limit risk of cancer to a level comparable to insignificant risks (Table 42.1).
2. For most toxic effects and arguably for some carcinogens, keeping exposure below a certain level reduces the effect to zero.
3. Cancer risk is based on lifetime dose, which is determined by multiple factors (see Table 42.2). Reduction in these factors will reduce the risk of cancer proportionately.

For clinical purposes, it is important to realize that risk estimates are based on a number of statistical assumptions that may not be directly pertinent to the individual patient. Also, for animal carcinogens, risk assessment does not tell us the site or type of cancer that could be produced in humans, and we do not know if any cancer risk will be present. For those chemicals that are human carcinogens, the risk of a particular exposure will be dependent on both the target organ dose and the genetic susceptibility of the individual.

REFERENCES

1. Bunn WB. Right-to-Know laws and evaluation of toxicologic data. *Ann Intern Med* 1985;103:947.
2. Whysner JA, Williams GM. International cancer risk assessment: the impact of biologic mechanisms. *Regul Toxicol Pharmacol* 1992;15:41–50.
3. National Research Council. *Risk assessment in the federal government: managing the process.* Washington, DC: National Academy Press, 1983.
4. Office of Science and Technology Policy. Chemical carcinogens: notice of review of the science and its associated principles. *Fed Reg* 1984;49(100):21594.
5. Dinman BD. Occupational health and the reality of risk: an eternal dilemma of tragic choices. *J Occup Med* 1980;22:153.
6. U.S. Environmental Protection Agency. Proposed guideline for carcinogen risk assessment. *Fed Reg* 1996; 61:17960–18011.
7. International Agency for Research on Cancer. Consensus Report. In: Species differences in thyroid, kidney, and urinary bladder carcinogenesis. Capen CC, Dybing E, Rice JM, et al., eds. IARC scientific publication No. 147. Lyon: IARC, 1999:1–14.
8. Cohen SM, Ellwein LB. Cell proliferation in carcinogenesis. *Science* 1990;249:1007–1011.
9. International Expert Panel on Carcinogen Risk Assessment. The use of mechanistic data in the risk assessments of ten chemicals: an introduction to the chemical-specific reviews. *Pharmacol Ther* 1996;71:1–5.
10. LaGoy PK. Estimated soil ingestion rates for use in risk assessment. *Risk Analysis* 1987;7(3):355–359.

FURTHER READING

Faustman EM, Omenn GS. Risk assessment. In: Klaassen CD, ed. *Toxicology: the basic science of poisons,* 6th ed. New York: McGraw-Hill, 2001:83–104.

National Research Council. *Improving risk communication.* Washington, DC: National Academy Press, 1989.

Slovic P. Perception of risk. *Science* 1987;280.

U.S. Environmental Protection Agency. *Risk assessment guidance for Superfund,* vol 1. Human Health Evaluation Manual. Part A. EPA/540/1-89/002, 1989.

43

Ergonomics

Stacy R. Rose, Erin K. Walline, J. Steven Moore, and Jonathan B. Borak

Ergonomics is a broad field that covers issues such as biomechanics, work physiology, anthropometry, and man–machine interfaces. In terms of occupational medicine, ergonomics is most recognized as a discipline related to musculoskeletal disorders. Low-back pain among workers has been recognized and studied for decades. In the 1980s, upper extremity disorders, especially carpal tunnel syndrome, became a major concern for employers, employees, insurance providers, and health care providers. Unfortunately, scientific knowledge about these disorders and their causes is often limited, published in a great variety of journals, and often follows the development of beliefs. This chapter discusses low back pain and upper extremity pain as they relate to work. Knowledge in this field continues to evolve and it is therefore necessary to periodically reexamine one's theories and beliefs about ergonomics and related disorders.

The word *ergonomics* implies something favorable, e.g., an ergonomically designed workstation is good. It is the lack of ergonomic considerations that increases risk of discomfort or injury. As a result, there is no really such thing as an *ergonomic disorder,* because an ergonomically designed job would not cause such a disorder.

A deficiency in ergonomic design or work organization may lead to the presence of risk factors, such as for low back pain. Overexposure to these risk factors may contribute to workers (and others) developing low back pain. In ergonomics, risk factors are external sources of stress to the worker, and are often called *stressors*. The effect of such stressors on the body is called *strain*. For example, the strength requirements of a job reflect a stressor, while the forces on the musculoskeletal system represent strain. When the magnitude of this strain exceeds the biomechanical tolerance of the musculoskeletal system, overexertion injury is likely. By contrast, if the magnitude of strain were not excessive, but the temporal pattern of its application stimulated degenerative or adaptive responses in specific components of the musculoskeletal system, then the more likely outcome would be a nontraumatic illness.

This chapter discusses ergonomics from the perspective of physicians who may need to apply ergonomics-related knowledge and skills in the course of managing workers with musculoskeletal disorders, performing plant walkthroughs, or serving as a member of an ergonomics team. Upper extremity disorders and low back pain are emphasized. The areas of ergonomics that correspond to this clinical context are called *occupational biomechanics* and *work physiology,* which, like industrial hygiene, are disciplines that emphasize assessment of exposure (stress), not assessment of disease resulting from strain. The ergonomist can characterize the biomechanical and physiologic stresses of a job by using a variety of tools to estimate exposure. Under ideal conditions, this estimate of exposure can be translated into internal stresses on the body (essentially a measure of dose). A dose-response curve can then be formulated to predict the risk of developing consequent disorders. The response aspect of such dose-response curves can be measured in terms of occurrence of musculoskeletal conditions, injuries and illness recorded in the Occupational Safety and Health Administration (OSHA) 200 log, or by means of a symptom survey.

In the practice of occupational medicine, activities such as determination of work-relatedness and management of the return to work often entail consideration of ergonomic exposure data. Because musculoskeletal disorders are common conditions among adults that are not always due to employment, it is important to differentiate work-related from non–work-related disorders. For this purpose, work-related exposure assessments are critical. The exposure assessment defines whether a hazardous condition is present or absent; it is not about making medical diagnoses. For example, in assessing a person's ability to return to work, the physician should compare the patient's physical capabilities with the physical demands of the job, the latter determined in part by means of exposure assessment.

One contemporary research objective of ergonomics is to develop exposure assessment tools that are (a) consistent with or derived from relevant physiologic, biomechanical, and epidemiologic principles (content validity); (b) able to discriminate between adverse and nonadverse exposures (predictive validity); and (c) applicable to a variety of circumstances of exposure (external validity/generalizability). There are a variety of checklists available to help assess whether circumstances reported to be associated with increased occurrence of upper extremity and/or low back conditions are present. While these may be effective in identifying risk factors, they are insufficient for hazard assessment and determination of work-relatedness because they do not consider whether magnitude, duration, or frequency of exposure to the risk factor was sufficient to cause or contribute to the development of specific conditions. Other tools attempt more thorough description of the physical demands of a job by assessment of the magnitude and temporal pattern of one or more stressors, but many of these tools lack published data on reliability (e.g., interrater agreement) and predictive validity (accurate hazard classification). Therefore, practitioners are cautioned to apply and interpret the results of an exposure assessment carefully.

This chapter discusses the principles and overview tools available for assessing exposure to the upper extremities and back, and acquaints practitioners with the fundamentals of occupational biomechanics so that they will be able to understand the ergonomics-related exposure for certain types of musculoskeletal disorders, and develop a fundamental approach for the recognition and estimation of these risk factors, such as when conducting a walkthrough survey or viewing a videotape.

PROXIMAL UPPER EXTREMITY DISORDERS

The upper extremity can be conveniently divided into two anatomic regions: the proximal upper extremity (shoulder girdle and upper arm) and the distal upper extremity. The proximal and distal upper extremity differ in terms of their anatomy and their disorders. The muscles of interest in the proximal upper extremity do not extend below the elbow. Excluding the neck (particularly the trapezius muscle), the most common proximal upper extremity disorders involve the glenohumeral joint, especially the rotator cuff. The supraspinatus tendon is the primary site of pathology for most rotator cuff disorders.

Epidemiology of Proximal Upper Extremity Disorders

The epidemiologic literature for proximal upper extremity disorders related to work is limited. Some studies lack anatomic or clinical specificity (e.g., neck disorders are often combined with shoulder disorders). Other studies present nonspecific exposure assessments (e.g., forcefulness or repetitiveness measured according to distal, not proximal upper extremity activity). When the National Institute for Occupational Safety and Health (NIOSH) evaluated this literature for evidence that generic risk factors were associated with shoulder disorders, it concluded that there was evidence of a positive association for repeated or sustained shoulder posture above 60 degrees' flexion or abduction, limited evidence of a positive association for highly repetitive work, and insufficient evidence of an association for force and vibration (1).

Theories of Pathogenesis for Rotator Cuff Disorders

Multiple plausible theories have been proposed for the pathogenesis of rotator cuff disorders. For the purposes of this chapter, we assume that a single pathologic process leads to supraspinatus tendon tears and calcification. Mechanisms leading to acute-onset disorders of the rotator cuff complex (e.g., strains, falls, dislocations) are excluded from consideration. It is likely that pathogenesis includes a variety of separate factors (e.g., prior trauma, congenital or acquired deformity, normal anatomic variations, and both work and nonwork activities), although a detailed consideration of their interactions is beyond the scope of this chapter. Ultimately, it is likely that compromised or inadequate repair of damaged collagen fibers within the avascular zone of the tendon is a factor in all cases.

Impaired Healing

The presence of a watershed or avascular zone in the supraspinatus tendon has been described and demonstrated by several investigators (2–4). It is believed that the avascular zone compromises the ability of the tenocytes within this portion of the tendon to repair damage to collagen fibers or their matrix. This impaired ability to repair the tendon implies that degenerative changes within this portion of the tendon will accumulate over time; therefore, the degree and progression of tendon degeneration increase with increasing exposure to potential sources of injury and/or with age. Potential sources of injury to the tendon's collagen fibers or matrix may be ischemic, mechanical (impingement), or physiologic (contractile load).

Ischemia

It has also been proposed that the function and viability of the tenocytes within the supraspinatus tendon are compromised because of ischemia in the avascular zone; thus they are unable to maintain the normal structure of the tendon over a lifetime. This lack of maintenance manifests itself as degenerative changes within the substance of the tendon. The positive correlation between the prevalence of supraspinatus tendon degeneration and tears with age is consistent with this theory. It is not clear that task variables related to work are necessary in this pathogenetic model; however, Rathbun and Macnab (4) postulated that shoulder adduction with neutral rotation would subject this avascular portion of the tendon to pressure from the humeral head, thus "wringing out" the blood from this already avascular area. If this were true, the duration of shoulder adduction would probably be more important than the number of shoulder adductions.

Impingement

Neer (5) estimated that 95% of rotator cuff tears were the end result of impingement. Neer (6) proposed that the subacromial bursa and supraspinatus tendon were mechanically impinged on the underside of the anterior aspect of the acromion process or coracoacromial ligament as the shoulder approached 80 degrees' abduction or flexion when internally or externally rotated. Below 80 degrees' flexion or abduction, the greater tuberosity of the humerus is generally not in immediate contact with the acromion process or the coracoacromial ligament. Beyond this degree of elevation, the humeral head is displaced down and away from the acromion and the ligament, thus relieving these structures of this contact stress. This contact stress is postulated to cause mechanical stress and disruption of collagen fibers within the tendon. This mechanism of collagen disruption may be combined with the phenomenon of impaired healing in the avascular zone. The critical link between this proposed model of supraspinatus tendon disease and biomechanical task variables is passage of the shoulder through the 80 degrees' abduction or flexion arc. Since this biomechanical stress occurs in only a limited portion of these arcs, it is anticipated that the number of times the shoulder performs this task (per unit time) is more relevant than the duration of time the shoulder is in this position. Anatomic variations in the size and shape of the acromion as well as hypertrophy of tissues related to the coracoacromial arch are also important factors (7,8).

Static Tensile Loading

Using electromyography, several investigators have demonstrated that the supraspinatus muscle is activated throughout most of the shoulder's range of motion, and they have postulated that the level of tension in the supraspinatus muscle during arm elevation was sufficiently high to increase the intramuscular pressure and hereby compromise intramuscular blood flow (9,10). Intramuscular pressures of 20 mm Hg may be sufficient to prevent perfusion of the muscle and its associated tendons (11). If perfusion is sufficiently reduced, tenocytes or other tendon components may suffer ischemic injury. Experimental data suggest that work involving overhead arm movements may cause intramuscular pressures capable of reducing intramuscular perfusion. Lifting combined with arm elevation (shoulder load) also contributes to the magnitude of supraspinatus muscle activation. From a temporal perspective, this proposed model is more related to the duration of the intramuscular pressure rather than to its frequency.

Exposure Assessment for the Proximal Upper Extremity

There are currently no exposure assessment tools with demonstrated ability to identify those jobs that are not associated with increased risk of proximal upper extremity disorders. Some tools combine exposure scoring for the proximal and distal upper extremity, such as Rapid Upper Limb Assessment (RULA) (12), Rapid Entire Body Assessment (REBA) (13), and appendix B of the Washington State ergonomics standard (14). But combining proximal and distal upper extremity risk factors into one composite score reduces these tools' specificity. In addition, these tools lack evidence of their predictive validity. Given their limitations and lack of scientific validation, we do not recommend that practitioners use them as the basis for predicting the presence or absence of upper extremity musculoskeletal hazards.

DISTAL UPPER EXTREMITY DISORDERS

The distal upper extremity is defined as the elbow, forearm, wrist, and hand. Disorders of the distal upper extremity may occur in the muscle-tendon units or peripheral nerves (15). Each muscle-tendon unit is a composite of tissues that begins with a proximal aponeurotic tendon inserted into bone, a proximal myotendinous junction, muscle, a distal myotendinous junction, a distal cord-like tendon, and, for some units, a tendon sheath. Each of these components manifests unique clinical disorders.

Epidemiology of Distal Upper Extremity Disorders

Several published studies have described the spectrum of distal upper extremity disorders associated with specific manufacturing jobs and tasks (Table 43.1) (16,17). These disorders can be grouped into two major categories: disorders of the muscle-tendon unit (e.g., tendon entrapment, peritendinitis, epicondylitis) and disorders of the nervous system (e.g., carpal tunnel syndrome, cervical spondylosis). Such studies demonstrate that muscle-tendon disorders are much more common in manufacturing operations than is carpal tunnel syndrome. Moreover, even when carpal tunnel syndrome is believed to be causally associated with specific work activities, it is almost always accompanied by other muscle-tendon unit disorders in the same individual or among other workers performing the same task. It is useful to compare the circumstances of a particular case to this epidemiologic context when determining the work-relatedness of carpal tunnel syndrome.

Studies of office workers have revealed similar findings. Hales et al. (18) noted that tendon and muscle were the most commonly affected tissues among cases with "potential work-related upper extremity musculoskeletal disorders," and that such conditions were approximately six times more prevalent than conditions related to possible nerve entrapment. Gerr et al. (19) reported that the majority of distal upper extremity disorders detected in their longitudinal study were tendon related. At baseline, they noted 40 cases with tendon-related disorders compared to three cases with carpal tunnel syndrome. The most common distal upper extremity condition was de Quervain's tenosynovitis. During follow-up, the authors found 199 new tendon-related distal upper extremity disorders compared to three new nerve entrapment disorders. A causal relationship between computer work and carpal tunnel syndrome was cast into further doubt by Stevens et al. (20), who found that their subjects with documented carpal tunnel syndrome did not differ from comparison groups in terms of average hours of keyboard, typewriter, or mouse use per day or years.

Reviews have been published that summarize and evaluate evidence that generic risk factors are associated with distal upper extremity disorders (1,21). For example, NIOSH evaluated the epidemiologic literature describing the relationship of selected combinations of repetition, force, posture, and vibration to carpal tunnel syndrome and hand/wrist tendinitis (1), and concluded that there was insufficient evidence of a causal relationship for posture; evidence of a causal relationship for repetition, force, and vibration; and

TABLE 43.1. *Number and type of disorders reported in previous studies of work-related distal upper extremity musculoskeletal disorders*

Study	Total disorders (no.)	Muscle-tendon disorders[a] (%)	Carpal tunnel syndrome (%)
Hymovich and Lindholm (1966)	62	100	0
Ferguson (1971)	62	95	5
Kuorinka and Koskinen (1979)	17	100	0
Luopajarvi et al. (1979)	89	95	5
Armstrong and Langholf (1982)	78	87	13
Armstrong et al. (1982)	32	93	7
Viikari-Juntura (1983)	6	80	20
Silverstein (1985)	43	52	48
Moore and Garg (1993)	104	83	21

[a]Disorders of the muscle-tendon unit include some specific conditions, such as stenosing tenosynovitis, epicondylitis, peritendinitis, etc., and may include nonspecific conditions, such as hand-wrist pain.

Adapted from Moore JS, Garg A. The spectrum of upper extremity disorders associated with hazardous work tasks. In: Kumar S, ed. *Advances in industrial ergonomics and safety IV.* London: Taylor & Francis, 1992:723–730.

strong evidence for some combinations of these risk factors. For hand/wrist tendinitis, NIOSH reported evidence of a causal association with repetition, force, and posture, and strong evidence for some combinations of these risk factors (e.g., repetition and force). Such reviews may contribute to determining *if* an exposure attribute is a risk factor for a particular health outcome but, as noted by NIOSH, they may not define *when* increased risk is present (1). In addition, there may be concerns about the external validity of such association (e.g., whether the reported associations can be generalized to populations, jobs, facilities, or industries other than those of the original studies).

Theories of Pathogenesis for Distal Upper Extremity Disorders

Models of pathogenesis are important in investigating and understanding the link(s) between exposure and disease development. When ergonomists or health care providers see a patient who is experiencing pain or discomfort characteristic of one of these disorders, they may consider interventions based on the unique relationships between patterns of hand usage and the specific disorder (i.e., by reducing exposure dose). Interventions that mainly modify generic risk factors not linked to the person's condition may not be effective.

Theories have recently been proposed to explain the pathogenesis of four specific distal upper extremity neuromusculoskeletal disorders (22). Using biomechanical and physiologic principles along with clinical observations and experimental studies, pathogenic pathways were proposed leading from the "initial state" (defined as normal anatomy and function) to the "final state" (defined as the established pathology). For each disorder, the proposed model identified a critical biomechanical or physiologic attribute considered as the best characterization of "dose." In addition, two temporal patterns of exposure (duration versus repetition) were used to characterize "dosage." The contributions of long-term exposure versus novel, unaccustomed work were viewed as potentially relevant effect modifiers, but they were not incorporated into the models.

Tendon Entrapment of the Dorsal Wrist Compartments

The first of the four disorders was tendon entrapment of the dorsal wrist compartments, usually diagnosed as stenosing tenosynovitis. These entrapment syndromes usually manifest clinically as pain localized to the affected compartment, with increased pain with firm palpation or loading (stretching or contraction) of the tendons that pass through the compartment. Swelling and reduced range of motion secondary to pain may also be present; thickening of the extensor retinaculum is the characteristic pathology. The most common of these disorders is de Quervain's tenosynovitis, tendon entrapment at the first dorsal wrist compartment.

The model proposed for such tendon entrapment emphasizes compressive force applied to the extensor retinaculum when loaded tendons that pass through those compartments change direction. It is not currently known whether duration or repetition is the critical temporal factor.

Lateral Epicondylitis

The second disorder, lateral epicondylitis, is commonly known as "tennis elbow." Clinically, it usually manifests as pain localized to the lateral side of the elbow and proximal forearm that increases with firm palpation or loading (stretching or contraction) of the affected muscle-tendon units (usually the extensor carpi radialis brevis). The characteristic pathology of this condition is collagen degeneration and disorganized repair within the tendon.

Two models were proposed for lateral epicondylitis. One emphasized the role of eccentric exertions of the extensor carpi radialis brevis leading to microscopic tears within its tendon. The other emphasized contact pressure on the underside of the extensor carpi radialis brevis tendon from the radial head occurring with certain arm positions. It is not currently known whether duration or repetition is the critical temporal factor.

Peritendinitis

Peritendinitis, the third disorder, is widely recognized in countries outside the United States. It manifests clinically as an acute inflammatory condition with pain, redness, swelling, tenderness, and dysfunction of the affected muscle-tendon units. It most typically occurs on the extensor side of the distal half of the forearm (extensor carpi radialis longus and brevis, abductor pollicis longus, and extensor pollicis brevis). The pathogenic model for peritendinitis focuses on localized muscle fatigue.

Carpal Tunnel Syndrome

Carpal tunnel syndrome, the fourth disorder, is defined as symptomatic compression of the median nerve at the wrist. Clinically, it most often manifests as numbness or tingling (paresthesia) in the fingers innervated by the median nerve (thumb, index, middle, and part of the ring). Symptoms characteristically occur during sleep or with static grasp. The diagnosis is best supported by electrodiagnostic studies because physical findings are generally unreliable (23).

Seven plausible pathogenic models were presented for carpal tunnel syndrome. The key factors for the seven models were thickening of the flexor tenosynovium; digital flexor tendon–median nerve traction; flexor tendon hypertrophy; contact pressure on the median nerve from the flexor tendons; lumbrical muscle retraction into the carpal tunnel; hypertrophy of the transverse carpal ligament; and intraneural ischemia from nonneutral wrist posture or flexor tendon tension. Except for the ischemia model (which requires that ischemia be prolonged), it is not known whether duration or repetition is the critical temporal factor.

Exposure Assessment for Distal Upper Extremity

Several methods have been proposed as means to assess exposure and thereby identify distal upper extremity musculoskeletal hazards, and this area of study remains uncertain. Several of those specific methods are described below.

Generic Risk Factors

Since the 1980s, identification of generic risk factors has been advocated as exposure and risk assessment for the distal upper extremity (24–33). The risk factors most often listed include repetitiveness, forcefulness, pinch grasp, awkward posture, localized mechanical compression, vibration, gloves, and cold temperature. By and large, the construct validities of the generic risk factors are based on clinical and epidemiologic data (24–31). In general, practitioners who use this generic risk factor approach to distal upper extremity risk assessment make their determinations based on the presence of one or more risk factors (24–34). If risk factors are present, the job is assumed to expose workers to increased risks of distal upper extremity conditions, while if those risk factors are absent, then the job is seen as without such risks. But a recently published study demonstrated that most of the individual risk factors, as well as most combinations of risk factors, had essentially no predictive validity for the identification of workers with and without a history of distal upper extremity morbidity (35). Likewise, the method has poor concordance with models of pathogenesis for the various distal upper extremity disorders.

Threshold Limit Value for Hand Activity Level

According to the American Conference of Governmental Industrial Hygienists (ACGIH), the purpose of its threshold limit value (TLV) for hand activity level (HAL) is to specify combinations of hand activity and peak force for hand, wrist, and forearm to which it is believed nearly all workers may be repeatedly exposed without adverse health effects (36). Based on epidemiologic, psychophysical, and biomechanical studies, the TLV for HAL is intended for "mono-task" jobs performed four or more hours per day. In a mono-task job, similar sets of motions or exertions are performed repeatedly, such as work on an assembly line or use of a keyboard.

As shown in Fig. 43.1, the TLV for HAL has two components—average HAL and peak hand force. HAL can be determined by trained observers using a 0 to 10 rating scale. Verbal anchors on the scale provide guidelines such as "0 = hand idle most of the

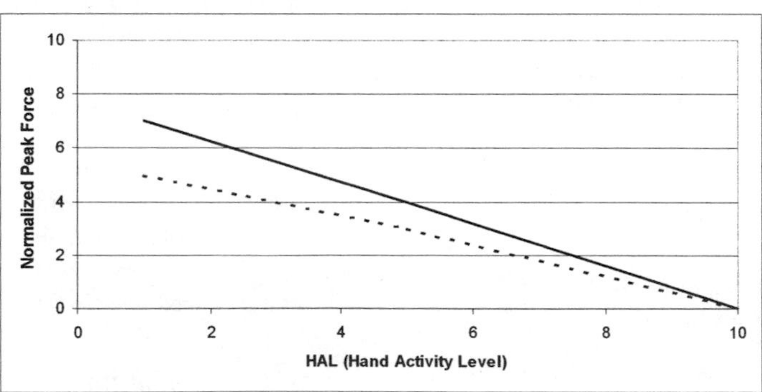

FIG. 43.1. The TLV for HAL. (Adapted from American Conference of Governmental Industrial Hygienists. Ergonomics: Notice of intent to establish–Hand Activity Level. In: *Threshold limit values for chemical substances and physical agents and biological exposure indices* [ACGIH], 2000.)

time; no regular exertions" and "10 = rapid, steady motion/difficulty keeping up or continuous exertion." The HAL can also be calculated from a table using measurements of the frequency of exertions and the work/recovery ratio. Peak hand force can be determined using ratings by a trained observer or ratings by workers using a Borg scale, or measured using instrumentation (e.g., strain gauges or electromyography). Peak hand force is normalized to a 0 to 10 scale that corresponds to 0% to 100% of the applicable population reference strength. The TLV documentation outlines the scientific basis for the recommended limits and explains the calculation of normalized peak force.

According to the TLV documentation, the significantly elevated prevalence of musculoskeletal disorders is associated with exposures exceeding the TLV (36). Appropriate control measures should be utilized so that the force for a given level of hand activity is below the TLV. Since it is not possible to specify a TLV that protects all workers in all situations without profoundly affecting work rates, an action limit is defined to indicate when general controls, including surveillance, are recommended (36).

The reliability of the HAL scale is good (37). But the reliability of the methods used to assess peak force and of the TLV as a whole has not been reported, nor has the predictive validity of the TLV for HAL. The TLV for HAL has poor concordance with the models of pathogenesis for distal upper extremity disorders.

The Strain Index

The Strain Index (SI) is based on a theory that the exertional demands of a job determine the magnitude of risk for developing distal upper extremity disorders among workers performing hand-intensive work (38). It relies on measurements and/or estimation of six task variables that describe the exertional demands (physical stress) of a job: (a) intensity of exertion (how much); (b) duration of exertion (how long within the job cycle); (c) exertions per minute (how frequent); (d) hand/wrist posture (how bent); (e) speed of work (how fast); and (f) duration per day (how long). There are three primary variables that describe the magnitude (intensity), duration, and frequency of hand exertions (tensile loads) per task cycle. When combined with hand/wrist posture, they account for compressive loads that arise when loaded tendons change direction at particular anatomic sites (e.g., the extensor retinaculum). Speed of work accounts for reduced recovery efficiency when exertions are highly dynamic. Duration of task per day integrates these stresses across varying durations of task performance. Biomechanical, physiologic, and epidemiologic principles link this description of exposure (external physical stress) to dose and dosage (internal physical strain).

As an example, consider a task that involves 12 exertions per minute (one every 5 seconds) where the duration of each exertion is 4 seconds (80% of each task cycle). The intensity of exertion is estimated as "somewhat hard" and the wrist posture is "fair" (nonneutral) when this exertion is performed. The speed of work is fair (nominal pace) and duration per day for this task is 8 hours. Table 43.2 demonstrates the procedure for calculating the SI score based on this exposure data. Task variable rating values and multiplier values are determined from tables provided on an SI worksheet. Several individuals and organizations have developed software that facilitates job analysis from digitized video as well as SI calculators or spreadsheets.

Interpretation of the SI score is the last step. Data suggest that an SI score of 5.0 best discriminates between jobs with and without a history of workers developing distal upper extremity disorders (39–41). In the example, the SI score of 13.5 indicates that the job is "hazardous."

In the 1995 SI paper, the SI scores (and score ranges) for jobs in a pork processing plant were compared to indicators of distal upper extremity morbidity, including the dichotomous morbidity classifications ("positive" and "negative") as well as incidence rates (38). Examination of the data suggested that a criterion SI score of 5.0 provided good discrimination between positive and negative jobs. Logistic modeling of these data supported that impression. The SI score that corresponded to a 0.5 probability for the job being a positive job was 4.7. As this criterion value was based on a relatively small number of data,

TABLE 43.2. *An example demonstrating the calculation of a Strain Index score*

	Intensity of exertion	Duration of exertion	Efforts per minute	Hand/wrist posture	Speed of work	Duration per day
Exposure data	Somewhat hard	80%	12	Fair	Fair	4–8 hours
Ratings	2	4	3	3	3	4
Multipliers	3.0	2.0	1.5	1.5	1.0	1.0

SI score = 3.0 × 2.0 × 1.5 × 1.5 × 1.0 × 1.0 = 13.5

it was recommended that users interpret SI scores in the 3 to 7 range cautiously. The predictive validity of the SI has been successfully established in other food processing and manufacturing industries (39–41).

The SI has some limitations, such as the concern that three of the six task variables (intensity, posture, and speed of work) are estimated rather than measured. Several theoretical approaches to calculating a composite SI score in the context of multiple-task analysis (job rotation and complex tasks) are being evaluated. A mathematical formulation for the SI has been developed that links it to the models of pathogenesis for specific distal upper extremity disorders discussed previously.

Summary

We have reviewed the epidemiology and assessment of exposure for risk of proximal and distal upper extremity disorders. Since knowledge in this area is evolving, the astute occupational physician should be aware of the settings in which upper extremity disorders occur because the settings provide clues to understanding associations between the reported disorders and work. Several methods for distal upper extremity exposure assessment have been presented. The generic risk factor method suffers from poor predictive validity. The TLV for HAL is limited by its lack of predictive validity and generalizability. The SI is the recommended method for assessing exposure to the distal upper extremity. There are currently no valid or reliable methods available for the proximal upper extremity.

ERGONOMIC CONSIDERATIONS OF LOW BACK PAIN

We now discuss the ergonomics of low back pain in terms of its epidemiologic context, physiologic and biomechanical models, and a psychophysical model. There in only a 5% to 10% likelihood of identifying a specific cause for a given patient's low back pain, although a definite structural diagnosis can be reached in up to 50% of cases (42,43).

Epidemiologic Context

Several comprehensive reviews of the epidemiology of low back pain have been published (44,45). Low back pain is the second most common cause for physician visits and the most common cause for decreased work capacity among people aged 25 to 44 years. Approximately 10% to 17% of adults have one or more episodes of back pain each year, and each year about 2% of all employees have a compensable back injury. These injuries are associated with approximately 29 days lost per 100 workers per year. Each year, they cause 21% of all workplace injuries and illnesses and 33% of workers' compensation payments and medical costs. Overexertion is considered the most common cause, associated with 25% of all reported injuries. Sixty-seven percent of overexertion injury claims involve lifting, while 20% involve pulling or pushing. Individuals who suffer low back pain as a result of overexertion and who have significant time loss from work have an especially poor prognosis for returning to their original jobs.

The precise cause for most forms of low back pain is unclear, although one likely source is muscle strain—acute failures at the myotendinous junctions (46,47). Such failures are believed associated with extremely high tensile loads in the muscle-tendon units, generally associated with forceful eccentric actions of a muscle, e.g., the muscles are contracted to near-maximal tension and simultaneously stretched or twisted. A second major cause is degenerative diseases of the spine (45). Current models for low back pain emphasize the stimulation of nociceptors scattered throughout various anatomic structures, such as the facet joint capsule and posterior longitudinal ligament. Degenerative changes are typically classified according to two locations—discs and facets. There is a general belief that disc degeneration plays a central role in the etiology of most episodes of low back pain, but disc degeneration per se is not necessarily symptomatic. As disc degeneration progresses, a permanent loss of disc height may elicit secondary changes in other structures, including the facet joints and ends of the vertebral bodies, which may stimulate nociceptors and cause pain. For any given patient, the underlying pathophysiology of low back pain is generally unclear.

Low Back Pain Exposure Assessment Tools

Biomechanical Models for Estimating Low Back Pain Risk Factors

The biomechanical basis for low back pain has been reviewed (48). The majority of studies examined the biomechanical characteristics of lumbar motion segments in cadavers (Fig. 43.2). A lumbar motion segment is two vertebral bodies and the intervening disc, with or without intact posterior elements. These lumbar motion segments may be susceptible to compression, tension (or distraction), shear, and torsion. As the levels of disc compression force increase, a level is reached that causes permanent deformation of the motion segment, mainly manifested as fracture of the cartilaginous endplate. During healing, the cartilaginous surface is probably replaced by fibrous scar and, as a result, there is less efficient fluid transfer between the vertebral body and the disc. Thus, discs lose hydration characteristics and their ability to maintain disc integrity. This may lead to a gradual but permanent loss of disc height. It is unlikely that a single cartilaginous end-plate fracture would lead to end-stage disc degeneration, but repeated exposure to high disc compression forces may lead to multiple cartilaginous end-plate fractures and sclerosis of significant portions of the end plate. Accordingly, disc degeneration is better characterized as a *disease process* related to repeated episodes of high disc compression forces and that requires significant time to develop. The maximum compressive strength of lumbar motion segments has been investigated, but there is a wide range in the compressive strength of individual vertebral segments (49).

In a few studies, investigators were able to directly measure intradiscal pressure among volunteers assuming various postures and during certain activities (48). Such studies form the basis for biomechanical models of disc compression. Once validated, these models allow estimation of disc compression forces for a variety of other postures and activities. Chaffin and Park (50) demonstrated that the incidence of low back pain correlated with predicted disc compression forces at the L5-S1 disc

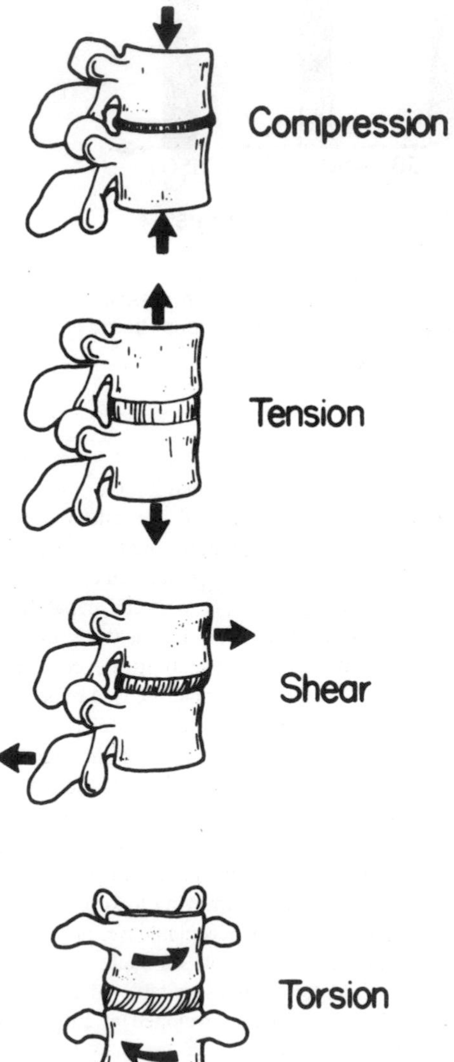

FIG. 43.2. A lumbar motion segment. Compression, shear, and torsion are the three primary forces that affect the lumbar spine. (From Pope MH, Andersson GBJ, Frymoyer JW, et al. *Occupational low back pain: assessment, treatment, and prevention.* St. Louis: Mosby-Year Book, 1991.)

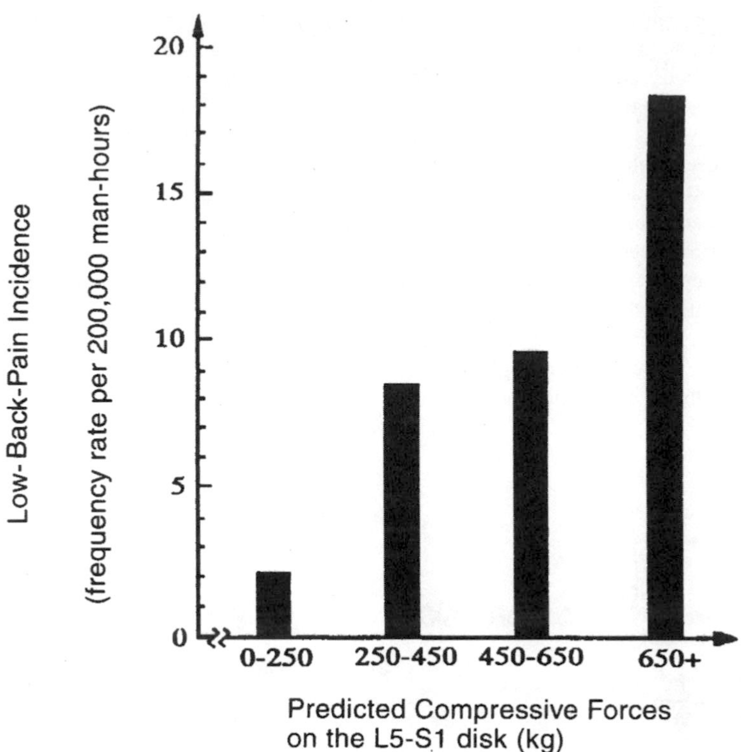

FIG. 43.3. Relationship between incidence rate of low back pain and disc compression. (From Chaffin DB, Park KS. A longitudinal study of low back pain as associated with occupational lifting factors. *Am Ind Hyg Assoc J* 1973;34:513.)

(Fig. 43.3). This has provided validation for estimations of risk for low back injury based on disc compression, and NIOSH has adopted a disc compression criterion ("action limit") indicating that disc compressive forces should not exceed 770 lb (350 kg) (51,52). It should be noted, however, that a variety of other models of low back pain have been developed. Figure 43.4 is a printout from a three-dimensional biomechanical model (53).

Psychophysical Criteria for Low Back Pain

For many people, overexertion is considered a significant contributor to low back pain. One aspect of overexertion reflects an individual's strength; it is useful to compare the strength required by a job task versus the worker's maximal strength. If job demands greatly exceed the worker's capabilities, the worker would be considered incapable of performing the task, and is at risk of overexertion injury if the job is attempted. There is epidemiologic evidence that strength demands, expressed as a ratio of job requirements to maximum strength, predict increased risks of injury (Fig. 43.5) (50). In particular, when strength requirements exceeded a worker's capabilities, the risk of musculoskeletal injury was three times greater than when the worker's capabilities exceeded the job demands. These studies have focused on strength required for isometric exercises.

Another measure of strength is *maximum acceptable weight*. An individual is directed to lift a box of standardized size to a given height with a specified frequency over the course of about 45 to 60 minutes. During the trial, the subject can adjust the weight of the box by adding or removing load so as to derive a weight, the maximum acceptable weight, that the subject would find acceptable for such work over an 8-hour day. A comprehensive table of maximum acceptable weights was developed at Liberty Mutual (54), but its purpose was to assist in developing design criteria for jobs, rather than as a toll for assessing the work capacity of individuals.

Whenever the strength requirements of a job exceed the maximum acceptable weights for the worker, the worker is presumed to be at increased risk for overexertion injury. Such use of the maximum acceptable weight tables has not undergone adequate validation, although Snook and associates (55) estimated that up to one third of compensable low back pain incidents may have been related to performing exertions that exceeded the maximum acceptable weight of 75% of females.

Physiologic Model for Estimating Risk for Low Back Pain

The physiologic model, often called the energy expenditure model, reflects the aerobic demands of a task (56). Jobs with significant aerobic demands are believed to lead to whole-body fatigue, and as a result they increase risks for overexertion injury, loss of dexterity, and falling (57). An example of a job involving high-energy expenditure is carrying large numbers of heavy boxes from a moving van to a second-story apartment. The weight of the boxes could be less than 10 lb and thus pose minimal stresses in terms of disc compression and strength, but the carrying combined with walking and climbing would pose significant aerobic demand.

Because it is possible to perform exercise solely with the upper extremities, there is a different threshold for whole-body fatigue when performing solely upper extremity work (57). For job design and analysis, NIOSH recommends two energy expenditure criteria (52). When activities require repeated bending and lifting of the torso, the maximum energy expenditure should be less than 3.12 kcal per minute; when performing primarily arm work, the maximum energy expenditure should be less than 2.18 kcal per minute.

Estimation of energy expenditures can be made by incorporating laboratory estimates for varying component tasks, which are then summed by means of a model that aggregates energy expenditure for the entire task (56). Component tasks may include lifting, walking, carrying, lowering, etc. By entering the weight of the object, the distance and speed of the carrying or walking, as well as the origin and destination heights of lifting and lowering tasks, the energy expenditure of the job can be estimated with reasonable accuracy. In addition, the major components of the task that contribute to the energy expenditure can also be identified so that intervention can be targeted as appropriate.

The NIOSH Guide for Manual Lifting

Prior to 1981, exposure assessment of manual handling tasks involved the estimation of *disc forces and static strength demands* based on the two-dimensional model, estimation of *strength demands* in comparison to maximum acceptable weights using the Liberty Mutual tables, and estimation of the *energy expenditure demands* of the job using either standardized tables or the energy expenditure model. Given the complexity of these job analysis techniques, a simplified method seemed necessary for wider implementation. To that end, NIOSH convened a committee of experts to develop guidelines, the 1981 NIOSH Lifting Guide (51). That NIOSH guide was widely accepted and highly successful. The guide was quantitative, simple and easy to use, effective, and greatly increased awareness regarding the ergonomic assessment and management of low back pain in the workplace. It also led to formal recognition that prevention must include both engineering controls and administrative controls. Unfortunately, the NIOSH guide did not meet all needs. It was limited to two-handed sagittal plane lifting and it could not contribute to the analysis of activities involving asymmetric lifting. In addition, the 1981 guide did not consider the effects of compromised couplings (e.g., box handles) or the duration of lifting, especially when the lifting was performed intermittently throughout the day. To address those issues, NIOSH undertook efforts leading to the 1991 Revised NIOSH Lifting Guide (52).

In the Revised NIOSH Lifting Guide, the action limit (AL) and the maximum permissible limit (MPL) terminology have been replaced by a single limit called the recommended weight limit (RWL). The criteria for the RWL are (a) a compressive force less than 770 lb; (b) greater than 75% capable females and 99% capable males in terms of strength; (c) energy expenditure less than 3.12 kcal per minute near the floor or less than 2.18 kcal per minute above bench height; and (d) a nominal risk of low back pain based on epidemiologic data.

Both NIOSH lifting guides were based on the principle that there is an acceptable weight limit for a standard lifting location. The weight corresponding to that standard lifting location is the *load constant*. In the Revised NIOSH Lifting Guide, the *load constant* is 51 lb. That load constant is then multiplied by a series of factors, each between 0 and 1, that discount the load constant. Six such factors (or multipliers) are described in the revised NIOSH guide: the horizontal multiplier (HM), the vertical multiplier (VM), the

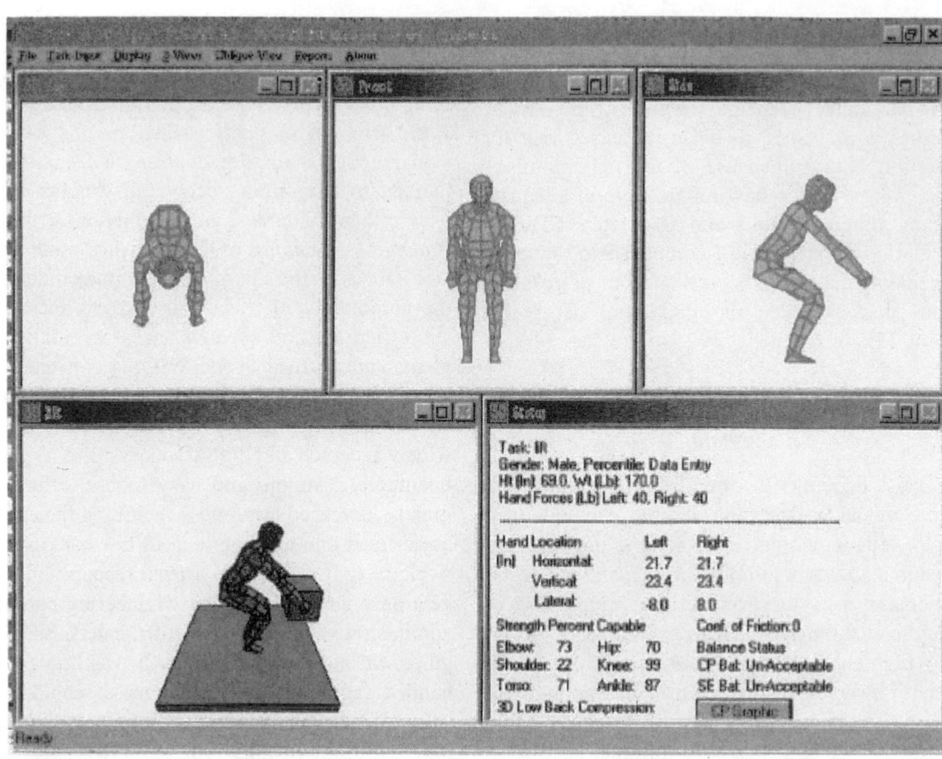
Task: lift
Gender: Male, Percentile: Data Entry
Ht (In): 69.0, Wt (Lb): 170.0
Hand Forces (Lb) Left: 40, Right: 40
Hand Location Left Right
(In) Horizontal: 21.7 21.7
Vertical: 23.4 23.4
Lateral: -8.0 8.0
Strength Percent Capable
Coef. of Friction: 0
Elbow: 73 Hip: 70
Shoulder: 22 Knee: 99
Torso: 71 Ankle: 87
Balance Status
CP Bal: Un-Acceptable
SE Bal: Un-Acceptable
3D Low Back Compression:
Ready

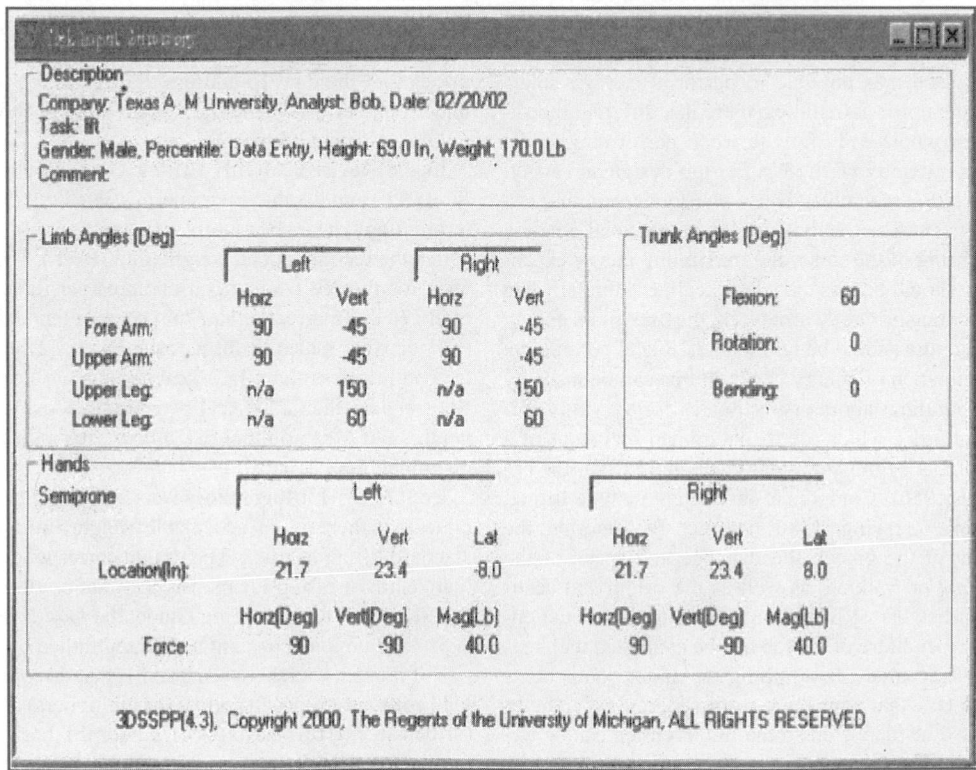
Description
Company: Texas A_M University, Analyst: Bob, Date: 02/20/02
Task: lift
Gender: Male, Percentile: Data Entry, Height: 69.0 In, Weight: 170.0 Lb
Comment:
Limb Angles (Deg)
Left Right
Horz Vert Horz Vert
Fore Arm: 90 -45 90 -45
Upper Arm: 90 -45 90 -45
Upper Leg: n/a 150 n/a 150
Lower Leg: n/a 60 n/a 60
Trunk Angles (Deg)
Flexion: 60
Rotation: 0
Bending: 0
Hands
Semiprone
Left Right
Horz Vert Lat Horz Vert Lat
Location(In): 21.7 23.4 -8.0 21.7 23.4 8.0
Horz(Deg) Vert(Deg) Mag(Lb) Horz(Deg) Vert(Deg) Mag(Lb)
Force: 90 -90 40.0 90 -90 40.0
3DSSPP(4.3), Copyright 2000, The Regents of the University of Michigan, ALL RIGHTS RESERVED

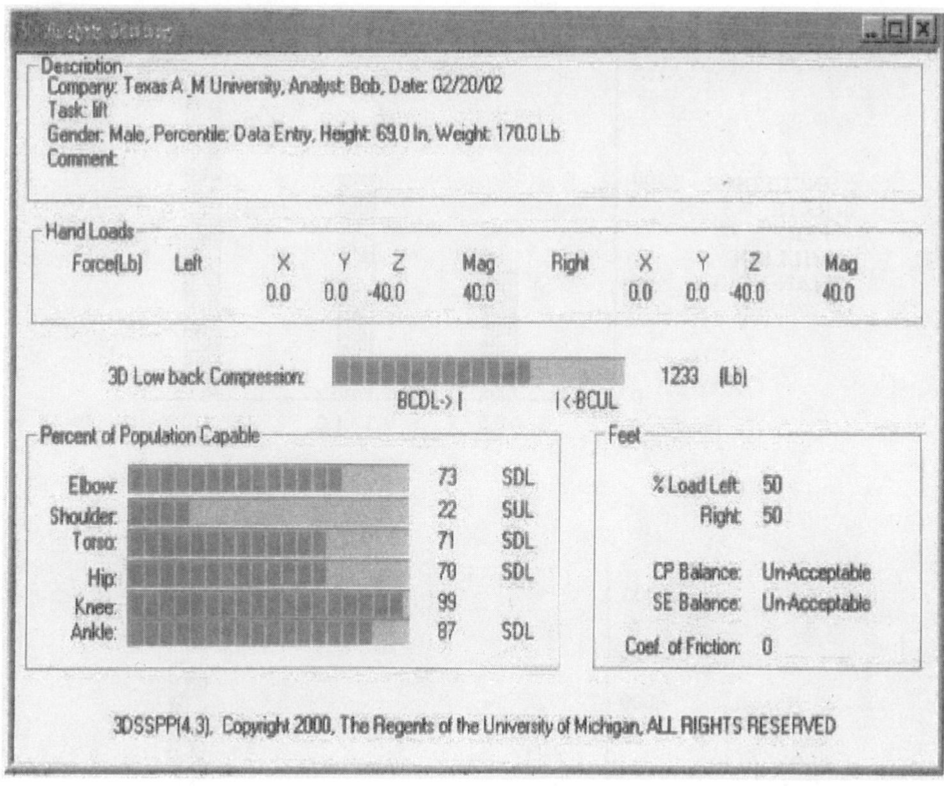

FIG. 43.4. Printout from the University of Michigan's 3-dimensional static strength prediction model (3DSSPP) sample output screen *(top)*, task input summary *(bottom)*, and analysis summary *(above)* for a 40-lb box lift.

distance multiplier (DM), the frequency multiplier (FM), the asymmetry multiplier (AM), and the coupling multiplier (CM). The RWL is determined by the following equation:

$$RWL = Load\ Constant \times HM \times VM \times DM \times FM \times AM \times CM$$

As shown in Fig. 43.6, the *horizontal distance* is the distance from the midpoint between the ankles to the midpoint between the hands. In general, the horizontal multiplier is associated with the greatest degree of penalty as it deviates from the ideal location. The *vertical distance* is defined by the vertical location of the hands above the floor at the origin of the lift. If the hands are at separate heights, their vertical heights are averaged. The *vertical travel distance* is the distance between the origin and destination at the lift. Asymmetry is defined by the *asymmetric angle,* which is the angle that the asymmetry line makes from the midsagittal plane, measured in degrees. The *asymmetry line* is the line joining the midpoint between the angles with the midpoint of the hands as projected on the floor. As a result, the asymmetry angle does not necessarily measure torsional twisting, but is more of a reflection of the hands relative to the feet. Couplings were classified as good, fair, and poor according to a variety of criteria including the length and height of the object, the types of handles available, whether the objects were asymmetric, sagging, or unstable, and whether gloves were required. The *frequency multiplier* refers to the number of lifts per minute, measured over an interval of 5 minutes. An additional set of considerations is based on the total time during the day that lifting occurs.

The Revised NIOSH Lifting Guide is a tool to estimate the demands of a job rather than an individual performing a particular job.

Postural Stresses

There is a fourth risk factor for low back pain not previously addressed, *static postural stresses,* which refer to prolonged awkward postures, such as

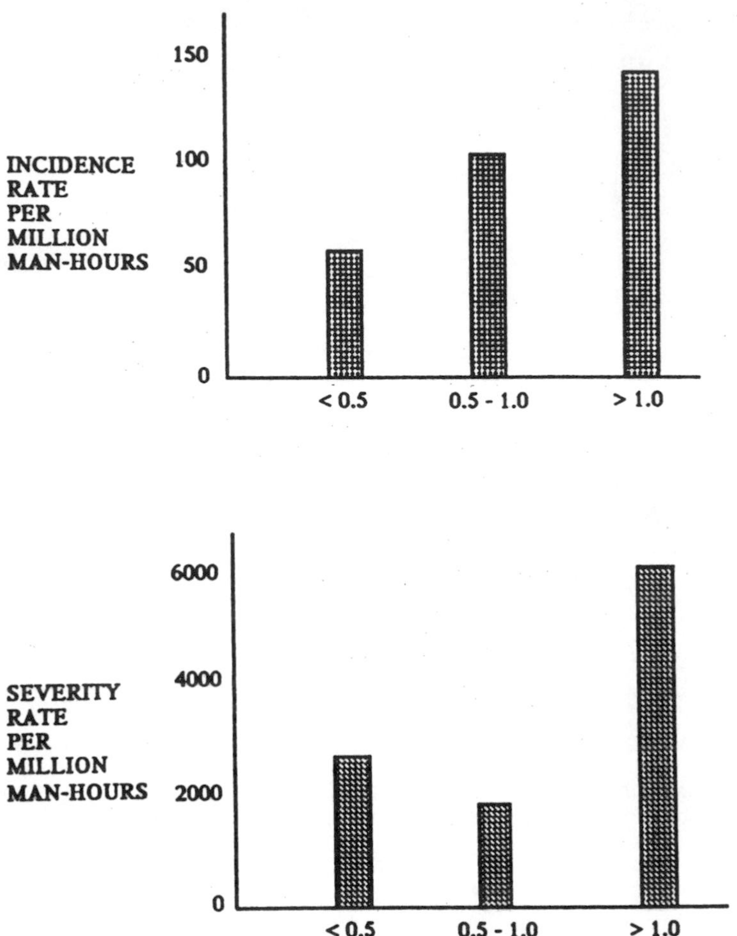

FIG. 43.5. The incidence and severity rates for musculoskeletal injuries with increasing strength demands. The job strength rating is a ratio of the required strength divided by the worker's maximum strength. (From Chaffin DB, Park KS. A longitudinal study of low back pain as associated with occupational lifting factors. *Am Ind Hyg Assoc J* 1973;34:513.)

bending over for several minutes to perform a task that is at or below knee height. Such postures are associated with static muscular work leading to localized muscle fatigue of the support structures of the spine.

Summary

A variety of methods are available to estimate the physical demands of jobs in terms of their effects (or potential effects) on the lumbar spine and associated structures. Disc compression forces may be estimated with a three-dimensional model (53). Strength demands may be assessed in terms of static strength with a two- or three-dimensional model and in terms of maximum acceptable weight using the Liberty Mutual tables (53,54). The energy expenditure model or standardized tables may be used to estimate the aerobic demands of tasks (56). In addition, it is possible to integrate all three of these components to derive a more simple model that is reflected in the 1991 Revised NIOSH Lifting Guide (52).

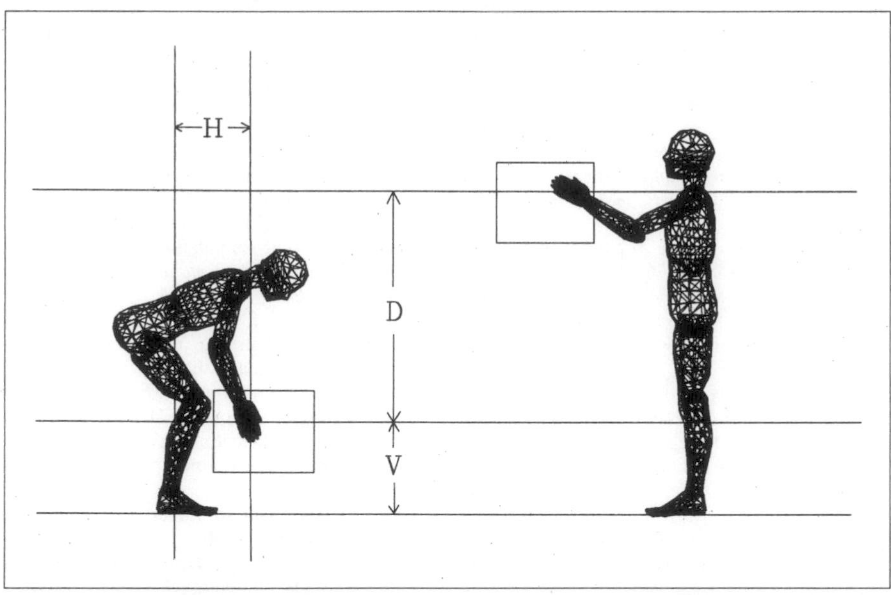

FIG. 43.6. Definition of distances used in the NIOSH Guide for Manual Lifting. In general, these distances are measured at the origin of the lift. *H* is the average distance between the malleoli and the center of the hands. The vertical distance, *V,* is average distance from the floor to the center of the hands. The vertical travel distance, *D,* is the difference in vertical height between the origin and the destination.

ERGONOMICS AND OSHA

OSHA proposed a final rule for an ergonomics program standard on November 14, 2000 (58). The standard became effective on January 16, 2001, but it was rescinded by the U.S. Senate on March 6, 2001. The purpose of the standard was to protect general industry workers from exposures to risk factors that significantly increased their risk for musculoskeletal disorders (MSDs) of the upper extremities, back, and lower extremities. The standard relied on an "action trigger" intended to identify jobs with risk factors of sufficient magnitude, duration, or intensity to warrant employer examination. When a worker experienced and reported musculoskeletal symptoms, the employer was required to determine the severity of the condition in terms of days away from work, restricted work activity, medical treatment required beyond first aid, or persistence of symptoms for more than 7 days. If any of these criteria were met, the condition was called an "MSD incident." Once that determination was made, the employer was to determine whether the employee's job had risk factors that met the level of the standard's action trigger. If an employee reported an MSD incident and the job met the standard's action trigger, the employer was required to establish an ergonomics program for that job. The ergonomics program was required to contain the following six elements: hazard information and reporting, management leadership and employee participation, job hazard analysis and control, training, MSD management, and program evaluation. Subsequently, OSHA decided to pursue industry-specific ergonomics guidelines rather than mandated regulatory programs.

REFERENCES

1. Bernard BP, ed. *Musculoskeletal disorders and workplace factors.* NIOSH publication No. 97-141. Cincinnati: Department of Health and Human Services, 1997.
2. Moseley HF, Goldie I. The arterial pattern of the rotator cuff of the shoulder. *J Bone Joint Surg* 1963;48B: 780–789.
3. Rothman RH, Parke WW. The vascular anatomy of the rotator cuff. *Clin Orthop* 1965;41:176–188.
4. Rathbun JB, Macnab I. The microvascular pattern of the rotator cuff. *J Bone Joint Surg* 1970;52B:540–553.
5. Neer CS. Impingement lesions. *Clin Orthop* 1983;173: 70–77.
6. Neer CS. Anterior acromioplasty for the chronic impingement syndrome in the shoulder. *J Bone Joint Surg* 1972;54A:41–50.

7. Bigliani LU, Ticker JB, Flatow EL, et al. The relationship of acromial architecture to rotator cuff disease. *Clin Sports Med* 1991;10:823–828.
8. Fu FH, Harner CD, Klein AH. Shoulder impingement syndrome: a critical review. *Clin Orthop* 1991;269: 162–173.
9. Jarvholm U, Palmerud G, Herberts P, et al. Intramuscular pressure and electromyography in the supraspinatus muscle at shoulder abduction. *Clin Orthop Rel Res* 1989;245:102–109.
10. Herberts P, Kadefors R. A study of painful shoulder in welders. *Acta Orthop Scand* 1976;44:381–387.
11. Edwards RHT, Hill DK, McDonell M. Myothermal and intramuscular pressure measurements during isometric contractions of the human quadriceps muscle. *J Physiol* 1972;224:58–59.
12. McAtamney L, Corlett EN. RULA: a survey method for the investigation of work-related upper limb disorders. *Appl Ergonomics* 1993;24:91.
13. McAtamney L, Hignett S. Technical note: Rapid Entire Body Assessment (REBA). *Appl Ergonomics* 2000;31: 201.
14. Washington State Department of Labor and Industries. Appendix B: criteria for analyzing and reducing WMSD hazards for employers who choose the Specific Performance Approach. WAC 296-62-05174. May 2000. Web site: *www.lni.wa.govwisha.*
15. Moore JS. Function, structure, and responses of components of the muscle-tendon unit. *Occup Med State of the Art Rev* 1992;7(4):713–740.
16. Moore JS, Garg A. The spectrum of upper extremity disorders associated with hazardous work tasks. In: Kumar S, ed. *Advances in industrial ergonomics and safety, IV*. London: Taylor & Francis, 1992:723–730.
17. Moore JS. Carpal tunnel syndrome. *Occup Med State of the Art Rev* 1992;7(4):741–763.
18. Hales T, Sauter S, Petersen M, et al. NIOSH Health Hazard Evaluation Report: U.S West Communications, Phoenix, AZ, Minneapolis, MN, and Denver, CO. NIOSH report No. 89-299-2230. Cincinnati: DHHS, 1992.
19. Gerr F, Marcus M, Ensor C, et al. A prospective study of computer users: I. Study design and incidence of musculoskeletal symptoms and disorders. *Am J Ind Med* 2002;41:221–235.
20. Stevens JC, Witt JC, Smith BE, et al. The frequency of carpal tunnel syndrome in computer users at a medical facility. *Neurology* 2001;56:1568–1570.
21. Kuorinka I, Forcier L, eds. *Work-related musculoskeletal disorders (WMSDs): a reference book for prevention.* Bristol, PA: Taylor & Francis, 1995.
22. Moore JS. Biomechanical models for the pathogenesis of specific distal upper extremity disorders. *Am J Ind Med* 2002;41:353–369.
23. Rempel D, Evanoff B, Amadio PC, et al. Consensus criteria for the classification of carpal tunnel syndrome in epidemiologic studies. *Am J Public Health* 1998;88(1): 1447–1451.
24. Armstrong TJ. *An ergonomics guide to carpal tunnel syndrome.* Cincinnati: American Industrial Hygiene Association, 1983.
25. Silverstein BA, Fine LJ, Armstrong TJ. Carpal tunnel syndrome: causes and a prevention strategy. *Semin Occup Med* 1986;1:213–221.
26. Armstrong TJ, Radwin RG, Hansen DW, et al. Repetitive trauma disorders: job evaluation and design. *Human Factors* 1986;28:325–336.
27. Silverstein BA, Fine LJ, Armstrong TJ. Occupational factors and carpal tunnel syndrome. *Am J Ind Med* 1987;11:343–356.
28. Armstrong TJ, Fine LJ, Goldstein SA, et al. Ergonomic considerations in hand and wrist tendinitis. *J Hand Surg* 1987;12(A)[2 pt 2]:830–837.
29. Armstrong TJ, Lifshitz Y. Evaluation and design of jobs for control of cumulative trauma disorders. In: *Ergonomic interventions to prevent musculoskeletal disorders in industry.* Chelsea, UK: Lewis, 1987:73–85.
30. Keyserling WM, Armstrong TJ, Punnett L. Ergonomic job analysis: a structured approach for identifying risk factors associated with overexertion injuries and disorders. *Appl Occup Environ Hyg* 1991;6(5):353–363.
31. Keyserling WM, Stetson DS, Silverstein BA, et al. A checklist for evaluating ergonomics risk factors associated with upper extremity disorders. *Ergonomics* 1993; 36:807–831.
32. U.S. Department of Labor, Occupational Safety and Health Administration. *Ergonomics Program Management Guidelines for Meatpacking Plants.* OSHA report No. 3123. Washington, DC: OSHA, 1990.
33. Cohen AL, Gjessing CC, Fine LJ, et al. *Elements of ergonomics programs: a primer based on workplace evaluations on musculoskeletal disorders.* NIOSH publication No. 97-117. Cincinnati: U.S. Department of Health and Human Services, Public Health Service, Centers for Disease Control and Prevention, National Institute for Occupational Safety and Health, 1997.
34. Department of Labor (Occupational Safety and Health Administration): 29 CFR 1910 Ergonomics Program; Proposed Rule. *Fed Reg* 1999 (November 23);64(225): 65768–66078.
35. Moore JS, Rucker NP, Knox K. Validity of generic risk factors and the strain index for predicting nontraumatic distal upper extremity morbidity. *AIHA J* 2001;62:229.
36. American Conference of Governmental Industrial Hygienists. Ergonomics: hand activity level. In: *Documentation of the threshold limit value for hand activity level.* Cincinnati: ACGIH, 2000.
37. Latko WA, Armstrong TJ, Foulke JA, et al. Development and validation of an observational method for assessing repetition in hand tasks. *AIHA J* 1997;58(4):278–285.
38. Moore JS, Garg A. The Strain Index: a proposed method to analyze jobs for risk of distal upper extremity disorders. *AIHA J* 1995;56:443–456.
39. Knox K, Moore JS. Predictive validity of the strain index in turkey processing. *J Occup Environ Med* 2001; 43:451–462.
40. Rucker NP, Moore JS. Predictive validity of the strain index in manufacturing. *Appl Occup Environ Hyg* 2002; 17:63–73.
41. Moore JS, Garg A. Participatory ergonomics in red meat packing plant. Part 2: Case studies. *Am Ind Hyg Assoc J* 1997;58:498–508.
42. Frymoyer JW, Pope MH, Constanza MC, et al. Epidemiologic studies of low back pain. *Spine* 1980;5(5): 419–423.
43. Pope MH, Wilder DG, Stokes IAF, et al. Biomechanical testing as an aid to decision making in low back pain patients. *Spine* 1979;4:135–140.

44. Andersson GBJ. The epidemiology of spinal disorders. In: Frymoyer JW, ed. *The adult spine: principles and practice*. New York: Raven Press, 1990:107–146.
45. Garg A, Moore JS. Epidemiology of low back pain in industry. *Occup Med: State of the Art Rev* 1992;7(4): 593–608.
46. McCully KK, Faulkner JA. Injury to skeletal muscle fibers of mice following lengthening contractions. *J Appl Physiol* 1985;59(1):119–126.
47. Nikolau PK, MacDonald BL, Glisson RR, et al. Biomechanical and histological evaluation of muscle after controlled strain injury. *Am J Sports Med* 1987;15(1): 9–14.
48. Garg A. Occupational biomechanics and low back pain. *Occup Med: State of the Art Reviews* 1992;7(4):609–628.
49. Jäger M. Biomechanisches Modell des menschen zur Analyze und Beurteilung der Belastung der Wirbelsaule beider Handhabung von Lastten [PhD thesis]. Dortmund, Germany: Universitat Dortmund, 1987.
50. Chaffin DB, Park KS. A longitudinal study of low back pain as associated with occupational lifting factors. *AIHA J* 1973;34:513-525.
51. National Institute for Occupational Safety and Health. *A work practices guide for manual lifting*. Cincinnati: DHHS (NIOSH), 1981.
52. Waters TR, Putz-Anderson V, Garg A, et al. Revised NIOSH equation for the design and evaluation of lifting tasks. *Ergonomics* 1993;36(7):749–776.
53. University of Michigan. 3-Dimensional Static Strength Program. Ann Arbor, MI: Center for Ergonomics, 1989.
54. Snook SH, Ciriello VM. The design of manual handling tasks: revised tables of maximum acceptable weights and forces. *Ergonomics* 1991;34(9):1197–1213.
55. Snook SH, Campanelli RA, Hart JW. A study of three preventive approaches to low-back injury. *J Occup Med* 1978;20:478–481.
56. Garg A, Chaffin DB, Herrin GD. Prediction of metabolic rates for manual materials handling jobs. *Am Ind Hyg Assoc J* 1978;39:661–674.
57. Garg A, Rodgers SF, Yates JW. The physiological basis for manual lifting. In: Kumar S, ed. *Advances in industrial ergonomics and safety IV*. London: Taylor & Francis, 1992:867–874.
58. U.S. Department of Labor (Occupational Safety and Health Administration). Ergonomics Program; Final Rule. *Fed Reg* 2000(November 14);65:68261–68870.

FURTHER INFORMATION

Moore JS, Garg A, eds. Ergonomics: low back pain, carpal tunnel syndrome, and upper extremity disorders in the workplace. In: *Occupational medicine: state of the art reviews,* vol 7, no. 4. Philadelphia: Hanley & Belfus, 1992.

This book is a compilation of review articles dealing with a variety of topics related to the lower back and upper extremity. Aside from topics discussed in this chapter, there are reviews of electrodiagnostic medicine, clinical management of low back pain, and the role of dynamic variables in ergonomics.

Kasdan ML, ed. *Occupational hand and upper extremity injuries and diseases.* Philadelphia: Hanley & Belfus, 1991.

This book offers a comprehensive overview of issues particularly pertinent to the treatment of a broad spectrum of upper extremity disorders, including traumatic and nontraumatic injuries.

Rodgers SH, ed. *Ergonomic design for people at work,* vols 1, 2. New York: Van Nostrand Reinhold Company, 1986.

These two volumes are classics in the field of ergonomics. Rodgers and the Human Factors Section of Eastman Kodak provide an easy-to-read yet scientifically rigorous treatise on almost all of the major topics in ergonomics.

Pope MH, Andersson GBJ, Frymoyer JW, et al. *Occupational low back pain: assessment, treatment, and prevention.* St. Louis: Mosby Year Book, 1991.

This book is a useful summary of contemporary concepts related to low back pain—especially issues related to pathogenesis, epidemiology, patient care, prevention, and legal aspects.

Frymoyer JW, ed. *The adult spine: principles and practice.* New York: Raven Press, 1991.

This two-volume book (>2,000 pages) is the most comprehensive summary of knowledge related to the adult spine. It includes sections addressing the cervical spine, the lumbar spine, and the sacrum and coccyx.

44

Medical Center Occupational Health

Marilyn V. Howarth and Mark Russi

The 10 million health care workers in the United States constitute 8% of the total U.S. workforce (1). Health care workers include all employees working in medical centers despite differences in job responsibilities that alter their individual risks. Workers directly involved in patient care include nurses, physicians, dentists, podiatrists, nursing assistants, physician assistants, and therapists, among others. Others do not provide direct patient care but perform functions that are essential to the operations and support of medical center activities, such as security, dietary, laboratory, pharmacy, maintenance, housekeeping, and administrative.

Large medical centers often have great diversity in their employees' jobs and in the complexity of their organizational structures. Employees who work in food service, security, housekeeping, maintenance, pharmacy, and direct patient care may be employed directly or work as independent contractors. The employer is responsible for providing a safe and healthy workplace, and, under the workers' compensation system, providing care for work-related illness and injury. The out-sourcing of employees to independent contractors may influence medical care of work-related injuries of out-sourced employees.

The structure of the medical center environment shapes both the scope of occupational health services needed and the risks of health care workers. When medical centers perform teaching and research, occupational exposures often broaden to include animals and concentrated microbiologic laboratory specimens. Zoonoses, animal allergies, and potential exposures to a broader range of laboratory chemicals become important to consider.

Community factors may also affect the spectrum of illness found in the patient population, impacting employee exposure and risk. State and federal regulations for testing those at risk for tuberculosis vary based on prevalence of illness in the patient population. Knowing the seroprevalence of human immunodeficiency virus (HIV) in a particular patient population is useful in counseling a health care worker after a percutaneous blood exposure. Awareness of current local health issues is important in the provision of medical center occupational health.

Providers of occupational medicine services in the medical center environment have confronted new challenges presented by for-profit market forces. Such forces may change the organization of and expectation for services in medical centers. Financial pressures may require changes in service not driven by science or institutional needs. Providing occupational medicine services in this climate requires continual reevaluation of priorities to maximally meet the needs of employees and medical center budgets.

MEDICAL CENTER OCCUPATIONAL HEALTH SERVICES

Occupational health services in the medical center should provide direct patient services to employees and consultation services geared toward risk management, exposure reduction, and compliance with regulatory requirements. Most health care organizations consider accreditation by the Joint Commission on Accreditation of Health Care Organizations (JCAHO) to be essential. The standards employed by the JCAHO cover nearly all facets of medical center operations (2). The National Institute for Occupational Safety and Health

(NIOSH), a branch of the Centers for Disease Control and Prevention (CDC), makes recommendations related to worker safety and health. The Occupational Safety and Health Administration (OSHA) regulates medical center exposures through a broad range of workplace standards. In addition, many state health agencies have regulations regarding immunizations and confidentiality.

Occupational health often serves as a liaison between administration and employee to protect both parties in legal and ethical matters. The preservation of employee confidentiality as prescribed by state and federal regulation is a responsibility of occupational health providers. Often occupational health takes a leading role in the development and implementation of medical center policies. Policies addressing human resources issues, infection control, and safety should clearly delineate the role of occupational health services.

Injuries and illness may be reduced or prevented by active and passive surveillance. Identifying hazards experienced by health care workers is an integral part of an overall risk reduction strategy in medical centers. Industrial hygienists and other safety professionals frequently work in close partnership with occupational health providers in determining the need and extent of surveillance for exposures in the medical center. The establishment of a multidisciplinary safety committee provides ongoing evaluation of health and safety activities in the medical center, and occupational health providers often direct such committees.

Similarly, assessment of individual susceptibility before beginning a job allows for enhanced counseling about risk and job accommodation when necessary. Preplacement evaluations are performed to evaluate whether health care workers have communicable diseases that might place patients at risk. In addition, screening is carried out for preexisting conditions that would likely be exacerbated on the job (e.g., latex allergy, serious ongoing musculoskeletal injury, animal allergy, asthma). Preventing an employee from beginning a job based on a medical condition is a rare circumstance. Part of the preplacement evaluation is the identification of qualified individuals with disabilities as defined by the Americans with Disabilities Act. Qualified individuals may require accommodation to perform essential job functions.

Assessing immunity for communicable disease is another important part of preplacement evaluation. Measles, mumps, rubella, hepatitis B, and chickenpox are infections that can be acquired on the job and for which effective immunizations are available. Encouraging or requiring immunization of health care workers when immunity is not present serves to protect vulnerable patient populations and the potentially exposed health care worker. OSHA's blood-borne pathogens standard requires that employers offer hepatitis B vaccine at no charge to employees at risk (3). Similarly, OSHA requires postvaccination for hepatitis B titers for at-risk employees.

Health care workers exposed to hazards on the job may require medical surveillance. Medical surveillance should be performed on a periodic basis, whenever there is a change in process and/or personnel, and on leaving the job. Medical surveillance in medical centers may be appropriate for employees exposed to TB, noise, waste anesthetic gases, chemotherapeutic agents, ethylene oxide, latex, lasers, radiation, heavy metals in radiation mold manufacture, plastics and solvents in rehabilitation appliance fabrication, and all respirator users. Findings on exposure assessment, performed by an industrial hygiene professional, should dictate whether or to what extent medical surveillance is required based on OSHA standards (4).

Workers' compensation laws require the provision of medical care for workers injured on the job, although the specific provisions vary widely state to state. Occupational health services provide care for medical center employees and sometimes employees of other employers. Occupational health can be instrumental in the reduction of lost work time, by negotiating modified duty when appropriate and expediting access to appropriate medical services. Occupational health can be helpful in disability management and return to work issues for non–work-related disability.

OCCUPATIONAL INJURY AND ILLNESS AMONG HEALTH CARE WORKERS

Beginning in the 1970s, OSHA focused its efforts on workplaces well known for risk of death and catastrophic injury. Over the last three decades, epidemiologic data has repeatedly shown that health care workers are at risk for a variety of injury and illness on the job (5). Table 44.1 presents a partial list of occupational hazards by location in the hospital workplace. These hazards can be classified as physical, chemical, and biologic.

TABLE 44.1. *Occupational hazards by location in the hospital*[a]

Location	Hazard
Central supply	Ethylene oxide Infection Broken equipment (cuts) Soaps, detergents Steam Flammable gases Lifting Noise Asbestos insulation Mercury
Dialysis units	Infection Formaldehyde
Dental service	Mercury Ethylene oxide Anesthetic gases Ionizing radiation Infection
Food service	Wet floors Sharp equipment Noise Soaps, detergents Disinfectants Ammonia Chlorine Solvents Drain cleaners Oven cleaners Caustic solutions Pesticides Microwave ovens Steam lines Ovens Heat Electrical hazards Lifting
Housekeeping	Soaps, detergents Cleaners Solvents Disinfectants Glutaraldehyde Infection Needle punctures Wastes (chemical, radioactive, infectious) Electrical hazards Lifting Climbing Slips, falls
Laboratory	Infectious diseases Toxic chemicals Benzene Ethylene oxide Formaldehyde Solvents Flammable and explosive agents Carcinogens Teratogens Mutagens Cryogenic hazards Wastes (chemical, radioactive, infectious) Radiation
Laundry	Wet floors Lifting Noise Heat Burns Infection Needle punctures Detergents, soaps Bleaches Solvents Wastes (chemical and radioactive)
Maintenance and engineering	Electrical hazards Tools, machinery Noise Welding fumes Asbestos Flammable liquids Solvents Mercury Pesticides Cleaners Ammonia Carbon monoxide Ethylene oxide Freons Paints, adhesive Water treatment chemicals Sewage Heat stress Cold stress (refrigeration units) Falls Lifting Climbing Strains and sprains
Nuclear medicine	Radionuclides Infection X-irradiation
Office areas and data processing	Video display terminals Air quality Ergonomic/body mechanics Chemicals Ozone
Operating rooms	Anesthetics Antiseptics Methyl methacrylate Compressed gases Sterilizing gases Infection Electrical Sharp instruments Lifting
Pathology	Infectious diseases Formaldehyde Glutaraldehyde Flammable substances Freons Solvents Phenols

TABLE 44.1. *Continued*

Location	Hazard
Patient care	Lifting
	Pushing, pulling
	Slips, falls
	Standing for long periods
	Infectious diseases
	Needle punctures
	Toxic substances
	Chemotherapeutic agents
	Radiation
	Radioactive patients
	Electrical hazards
Pharmacy	Pharmaceuticals
	Antineoplastic agents
	Mercury
	Slips, falls
Print shops	Inks
	Solvents
	Noise
	Fire
Radiology	Radiation
	Infectious diseases
	Lifting
	Pushing, pulling

[a]Although this list is not exhaustive, it demonstrates the variety of hazards that can exist in a hospital environment. Stress is reported by hospital workers in all job categories and is not listed separately by location.

Adapted from National Institute for Occupational Safety and Health. Guidelines for protecting the safety and health of health care workers. Department of Health and Human Services. NIOSH publication No. 88–119, 1988.

PHYSICAL HAZARDS IN THE MEDICAL CENTER ENVIRONMENT

Musculoskeletal Injury

The Bureau of Labor Statistics (BLS) in 1996 reported the incidence of nonfatal injury in health services as 8.5 per 100 full-time workers (6). This rate is quite high considering that the occupations of manufacturing and construction, traditionally considered hazardous, range from 9.2 to 10.1 per 100 full-time workers. The types of injuries seen in the medical center setting has been reported to be distributed as follows: regional low back pain 50%, hand/wrist disorders 16.5%, lower extremity disorders 16.2%, rotator cuff 7%, neck 4.8%, trunk 4%, and elbow 1.5% (7).

Comparing the rates of injury in hospitals and nursing/personal care facilities (10 per 100 full-time workers and 16.2 per 100 full-time workers, respectively) points to several important risk factors for injury. The number of nonambulatory patients in nursing and personal care facilities is greater than in hospitals. Acute back-related disorders, in particular of the low back, occur with high frequency during patient transfers. It has been suggested that the high rate of low back disorders among health care workers may be due to the mismatch in size between patient and health care worker. Large nonambulatory patients moved by relatively small or average-sized health care workers represents a common scenario. Other risk factors relevant to all lifting include heavy weight lifted, long horizontal distance between the lumbosacral spine and hands when lifting patients from beds and chairs, and increased frequency of lifting.

A number of personal risk factors for back disorders have also been identified. They include increasing age, female gender, obesity, tobacco use, prior back injury, hypertension, systemic arthritis, job dissatisfaction, psychosocial stressors, and poor physical fitness (8).

Ergonomics is the study of fitting the task to the worker to reduce the likelihood of injury. Assessing the task-related and personal risk factors for injury is the first step in maximizing the ergonomics of a task. Proper ergonomics can reduce both the incidence of acute injury as well as the incidence of disorders due to repeated or cumulative trauma. Ergonomists are trained professionals with knowledge of the engineering, equipment, and musculoskeletal biomechanics necessary to match job task to worker. In medical centers, maximizing ergonomics can prevent injury when applied to patient transfers, keyboarding, material handling, and housekeeping activities. Ergonomics programs can be implemented to reduce injuries in jobs with high injury rates or can be implemented proactively to prevent these injuries. Proactive programs may incorporate a zero lifting policy, for example, which prohibits nearly all lifting of any consequence (9).

Other examples of ergonomic intervention in hospitals include the proper maintenance and lubrication of the wheels on carts used by employees in dietary and patient transport; the use of a spring-loaded platform to raise the bottom of laundry carts for employees working in the laundry; training to push carts rather than pull them; and decreasing the size of the laundry bags (7).

Repetitive trauma is also a hazard in medical centers. The BLS reported hospitals as the third-ranking industry in number of nonfatal illness cases of disorders associated with repeated trauma (10). Despite the high number of cases, risk factors for repeated trauma disorders remain a subject of debate. The number of keystrokes at computer workstations performed per day has been quantified in the effort to identify a predictor for the development of hand and wrist disorders including carpal tunnel syndrome. However, no clear correlation has been found between the number of keystrokes and the development of these conditions. Improving the ergonomics of a computer workstation may increase the comfort and decrease the symptoms in those already symptomatic from hand, wrist, and other musculoskeletal symptoms. The properly designed, ergonomically correct workstation includes an adjustable chair, an adjustable back rest, adjustable keyboard height, adjustable page holder, properly located monitor, and padded wrist rest. Administrative control of rest breaks is also important. A comprehensively designed ergonomics program has been shown to be effective in reducing the incidence of upper extremity work-related musculoskeletal disorders in a university medical center setting (11). OSHA has stimulated much discussion on this topic with proposed ergonomic standards that have been published for comment, accepted, and rescinded (12).

Noise

Occupational noise exposure occurs in several locations within the medical center setting. Excessive noise exposure may be found in the central supply area, operating room, food service, laundry, engineering, facilities maintenance, and print shops. Noise overexposure has a cumulative and permanent negative effect on the hair cells of the cochlea of the inner ear. Engineering controls to reduce noise production and hearing protection to reduce exposure remain the most important strategies to prevent permanent hearing loss.

OSHA has set 90 dB as the time-weighted average (TWA) for an 8-hour workday and a maximum allowable exposure level of 115 dB for a short-term exposure. NIOSH has recommended an exposure limit of 85 dB as an 8-hour TWA (13). Noise levels in operating rooms have been measured at 118 dB when powered bone-cutting tools are in use (14). Occupational hearing loss has been documented in operating room personnel (15).

Noise exposure elevates heart rate and blood pressure, increases psychologic stress, and impairs concentration and focus (16). All areas within a medical center that may approach the OSHA limits for noise should be monitored for noise. Chronic overexposure to noise should be avoided by the use of engineering controls and personal protective equipment when necessary. When hearing conservation programs are necessary, they should be initiated and managed through occupational health services (17).

Heat

Kitchen facilities, the boiler room, and the laundry are the most common areas for heat overexposure in a medical center. Excessive heat exposure can cause health effects including dermatitis, syncope, heat cramps, heat exhaustion, and heat stroke. Medications that enhance heat stress include sympathetic blocking agents, anticholinergics, antidepressants, antihistamines, calcium channel blockers, cocaine, diuretics, and ethanol, among others. Engineering controls such as physically insulating sources of heat and enhancing ventilation provide the best strategy in medical centers to avoid heat stress. Providing water and allowing frequent breaks to those whose jobs require working in heat-exposed areas can also be helpful (18).

Lasers

Lasers (light amplification by stimulated emission of radiation) are used in hospital operating rooms, as well as in a number of outpatient settings. Laser types used include argon, carbon dioxide, dye, excimer, and neodymium:yttrium-aluminum-garnet (Nd:YAG). Most lasers used in surgical procedures are class 4, which means that eye or skin exposure by direct beam is extremely dangerous, and that eye exposure by specular or diffuse reflection is hazardous.

Damage to the cornea, lens, or retina may lead in some cases to permanent visual field loss or blindness. Wavelengths less than 315 nm and greater than 1,400 nm are absorbed primarily by the cornea and may cause a corneal burn. Those from 315 nm to 400 nm are absorbed by the lens and may induce cataracts with chronic exposure. Wavelengths from 400 nm to 1,400 nm are transmitted to the retina, where they may cause irreparable tissue burns (19). Wavelengths less than 400 nm cause primarily photochemical injury to the skin, while those between 400 nm and 1,400 nm are more likely to result in thermal burns.

Lasers also generate a smoke plume containing potentially infectious organisms or toxic byproducts of tissue combustion. Cellular residues and viruses, including human papilloma virus, have been detected in such aerosols. Studies have also demonstrated that pyrolysis products from laser-induced tissue vaporization may have mutagenic activity, as demonstrated by sister chromatid exchange and micronuclei assays (20,21).

Operating suites where lasers are used are designed to prevent scatter of laser light. Such suites must also be kept well lit in order to minimize pupillary diameter. Eye protection designed to protect against the wavelengths of light produced by a specific laser type is imperative, as is skin protection. Local exhaust ventilation effectively reduces plume exposure.

The American National Standards Institute (ANSI) has published recommendations for safe practice around lasers, and for the medical evaluation and monitoring of personnel who routinely use class 3b and class 4 lasers. The recommendations call for evaluation of visual acuity and macular vision prior to job assignment, following a laser accident, and at the close of employment. Funduscopic examination or further testing as determined by the examiner should be carried out if an abnormality is detected on the screening exam (22).

Ionizing Radiation

Health care workers represent the largest group of individuals occupationally exposed to radiation, most at levels well below the permissible yearly exposure limit of 50 millisievert (mSv) (5 rem). The average dose among health care workers has been reported to be 0.7 mSv/year, and less than 0.05% of exposed health care workers exceeded 50 mSv/year (23). Exposure of health care workers to radiation is regulated by OSHA; performance of radiation machinery is regulated by the Center for Radiologic devices of the Food and Drug Administration (FDA); use of certain radioactive isotopes is regulated by the Nuclear Regulatory Commission (NRC). Radiation exposure may occur to individuals involved with diagnostic imaging procedures, radiation oncology treatments, or administration of radioactive isotopes.

In diagnostic imaging, fluoroscopic procedures such as cardiac catheterization, vascular procedures, and certain interventional radiologic procedures have the potential for the highest individual exposures. When workers are required to stand adjacent to a patient receiving x-rays, bodily protection with aprons containing 0.5 mm of lead is required. Substantial radiation doses may also occur to the hands of technicians who repeatedly stabilize body parts, such as the cervical spine of a trauma patient, and 0.5-mm-lead–containing gloves should be used under such circumstances (23). For imaging procedures that do not require staff to stand adjacent to the patient during x-ray use, most exposure to health care workers occurs through scatter of x-rays from the patient. A shielded barrier containing 1/16-inch lead or more provides adequate protection for staff.

Sources of exposure during radiation oncology treatment include external beams from linear accelerators, gamma knives, or cobalt-60 therapy machines, and loading of radioactive sources for brachytherapy. External beam machines are housed within thick concrete walls to reduce outside scatter, and gamma knife procedures are performed in similar settings (19). Workers who come into direct contact with radioactive sources, such as in the implantation of radioactive seeds for brachytherapy, should utilize bodily protection, such as lead-containing aprons, neck protectors, and gloves. Certain patients in whom seeds have been implanted may need to be hospitalized in radiation-shielded rooms to minimize exposure to others.

Patients who have undergone nuclear imaging procedures generally present minimal risk to those around them due to the low levels of radiation used in such imaging. Staff who administer radioactive isotopes must see that shielding is utilized for vials and syringes, and should don protection while handling isotopes. Certain patients who receive therapeutic doses of isotopes, such as iodine 125 or iodine 131, may require hospitalization immediately following treatment to minimize exposure to family or others.

Violence

Bureau of Labor Statistics data confirm that health care and social service workers have a high incidence of assault injuries (25). Other studies describe a very high incidence of verbal threat and other aggressive behaviors toward health care workers that may not result in physical injury (26,27). The perpetrator of violent incidents toward health care workers may be patients, their families, their visitors, or co-workers.

The long-term consequences of ongoing threats of violence and altercations that do not result in physical harm have not been well studied. However, such incidents may contribute to job stress. Severe physical and emotional consequences of violence on the job have been well documented (26,27).

Factors implicated in the increased rate of violence in medical centers include deinstitutionalization of the mentally disabled, inadequate staffing, increase in weapons taken into the medical center, presence of money and drugs, and ease of entry. Several areas of the medical center are clear robbery targets due to the perceived availability of money and drugs (e.g., pharmacy, emergency departments). Trauma centers and tertiary care facilities that treat high acuity and critically ill patients often have frustrated family members and visitors. Victims of intended homicide who are being treated in the medical center may still be at risk for violence from the perpetrator, thereby placing staff caring for them at risk as well. Low staffing levels may increase the risk of health care workers by increasing the length of time that they work alone. Lack of training in recognizing and managing escalating hostility and aggressive behavior may also contribute to risk (28).

The OSHA guidelines recommend the following components for successful prevention of violence in the medical center environment: (a) management commitment and employee involvement, (b) work-site analysis, and (c) safety and health training (29). A written program encompassing a wide variety of strategies is essential for broad participation and support. The written program includes a clear statement of zero tolerance for violence in the workplace and establishes and encourages prompt reporting of all incidents of violence in the workplace, regardless of the presence or absence of physical injury. The written program establishes employee–management groups to identify strategies to reduce the risk of violence. Key participants in this effort are security personnel and other safety personnel with appropriate training (30).

Work Stress

Work stress has been associated with occupational injury and the length of recovery from injury (31). Work stressors fall into three categories: job/task demands, organizational factors, and physical conditions (32). Work stress can be exacerbated by factors in one or all of these categories and by a variety of personal non–work-related situations. Cost containment can lead to staff reduction and longer shifts. The increased acuity of hospitalized patients adds to the work demands of the staff who care for them. Patients and their family members often direct their anger and frustration at staff. Recent concerns regarding infection with agents of bioterrorism are surely adding to the stress, although no published reports are yet available quantifying the magnitude of these effects.

As the workers' compensation provider for the medical center, occupational medicine providers are well positioned to perform surveillance on rates of department-specific illness and injury. Clusters of back injury or complaints of indoor air quality may represent a symptom of a particularly stressful working environment. Intervention, often with the support of human resources, to identify and reduce local stressors is beneficial (33).

When employee assistance programs (EAPs), providing confidential individual counseling, are available, occupational medicine providers can take a very proactive role in utilizing them. The data for EAP utilization for medical center employees is higher than for employees in nonmedical fields (34). However, it is still modest at best. Encouraging employees to use EAP services for a full range of challenging life circumstances (e.g., eldercare, adolescent child counseling, personal chronic medical illness, chronic pain, bereavement, substance abuse) may reduce stress in and out of work.

Shift Work

Shift work for health care workers provides continuous 24-hour attention to hospitalized patients. Health care workers participate in shift work in a variety of ways. They may work on rotating shifts, moving between day, afternoon, and night shift, or they may work on one of these shifts continuously. The effects of shift work are to disrupt normal circadian physiologic rhythms leading to a changed sleep–wake cycle in addition to social disruptions with family and friends (35). The acute effects of shift work begin with disturbed sleep and lead to daytime sleepiness and decreased mental focus and performance. Rotating shift workers have a reduction in sleep stage 2 and rapid eye movement (REM) sleep. Studies have shown an increased use of sick leave and, in general, decreased health status among shift workers when compared with day workers (36). Shift workers who do not successfully adjust to shift work develop a syndrome of chronic fatigue, sleep disturbance, depression, mood disturbance, and personality changes. There is also an increase in the incidence of cardiovascular diseases and gastrointestinal disorders including peptic ulcer disease among shift workers (37). Epilepsy can be stimulated with sleep deprivation.

Despite the need for shift work, there are strategies to reduce its ill effects. The natural sleep–wake cycle is approximately 25 hours. Therefore, work schedules that rotate clockwise, in other words, day to evening to night to day, should be preferred over day to night to evening to day. In addition, it is preferable to have a slowly rotating schedule rather than weekly changes in rotating shift work (38,39). Both the direction of shift change and the speed of rotation remain subjects of controversy.

CHEMICAL HAZARDS

Anesthetic Gases

Health care personnel working in operating rooms, labor and delivery areas, postanesthesia recovery units, and certain ambulatory settings are at risk for exposure to anesthetic gases. Exposure may occur to nitrous oxide alone, or in combination with halogenated agents such as fluroxene, methoxyflurane, enflurane, halothane, isoflurane, desflurane, or sevoflurane. Scavenging devices are capable of reducing exposures to below 25 ppm for nitrous oxide and below 0.5 ppm for halogenated agents. Nitrous oxide levels as high as 300 ppm in hospital operating rooms and 1,000 ppm in dental operatories using scavenging equipment have been documented (40). Personnel working in postanesthesia care units may also be highly exposed to anesthetic gases due to exhalation by surgical patients of absorbed agents. Specific concern has been raised regarding exposures to desflurane and sevoflurane, due to the higher concentrations at which these two anesthetic agents are typically administered (41). During inhaled induction with a rebreathing bag or a circle circuit system, sevoflurane concentrations as high as 20 ppm have been demonstrated, with nitrous oxide concentrations of approximately 100 ppm (42).

Approximately 20 epidemiologic studies have evaluated an association between anesthetic gas exposure and adverse reproductive outcomes. The data suggest an elevated spontaneous abortion rate among highly exposed women. A study of dental assistants concluded that the relative risk of spontaneous abortion was elevated among women who worked with nitrous oxide for 3 hours or longer per week in offices not using scavenging equipment (43).

Female dental assistants with at least 5 hours of exposure per week to unscavenged nitrous oxide were only 41% as likely as unexposed women to conceive during each menstrual cycle [95% confidence interval (CI) 23–74%, $p < .003$], adjusted for age, race, smoking habits, and reproductive/gynecologic history (44). Among those exposed to scavenged nitrous oxide, there was no relationship between the number of hours of exposure and fertility. Similarly, questionnaire-based data regarding congenital anomalies collected prior to widespread use of gas scavenging systems noted increased rates of congenital anomalies among more highly exposed workers (45–47).

A large American Dental Association survey revealed no statistically significant increases in cancer risk among exposed men or women with the exception of highly exposed female chairside assistants, who had higher rates of cervical cancer (48). A study of Ontario hospital personnel revealed no elevation in cancer risk among exposed individuals (47). A large survey of U.S. operating room personnel was suggestive of increased leukemia and lymphoma risk among female study participants. There was no increased cancer risk among exposed men (45). A survey of cancer mortality among physicians revealed no increase among anesthesiologists (49).

There is no OSHA standard for waste anesthetic gases in general or for specific agents in use today. The NIOSH recommended exposure limit (REL) is 25 ppm TWA (over the time of exposure). The REL for halogenated anesthetics is a ceiling level of 2 ppm. The American Conference of Governmental Industrial Hygienists (ACGIH) threshold limit values (TLVs) are 50 ppm for nitrous oxide and halothane, and 75 ppm for enflurane. ACGIH has not set TLVs for other halogenated anesthetic gases.

Reduction of exposures is best accomplished through a multidisciplinary effort including regular maintenance and inspections of anesthesia delivery equipment and scavenging systems, maintenance of room ventilation rates, provision of training to staff members, and regular (at least every 3 months) measurement of nitrous oxide levels. In most situations, control of nitrous oxide to a TWA concentration of 25 ppm during anesthetic administration will result in levels of approximately 0.5 ppm of the halogenated agent (50).

Hazardous Drugs

The principal hazardous drugs of concern in medical centers are antineoplastic agents. Exposure to antineoplastic drugs may occur in a wide range of occupations. Pharmacists may be exposed if drugs are mixed outside of a biologic safety cabinet, if inadequate personal protective equipment is used, or if a spill occurs. Personnel who transport medications are also at risk for exposure from spills. Oncology nurses and other nursing and medical personnel who administer medications are at risk if medication vials are opened at the bedside, if trapped air is emptied from a syringe, if skin contact with drug or a patient's urine occurs, or if soiled linens from a patient administered hazardous drugs are improperly disposed. Housekeeping and maintenance personnel who clean linens and patient rooms similarly have potential for exposure to excreta containing hazardous medication or hazardous medication metabolites. A recent survey of cancer treatment centers in the U.S. and Canada found surface contamination with antineoplastic agents in 75% of pharmacy preparation areas and in 65% of oncology drug administration areas (51).

Human epidemiologic studies over the past 15 years have evaluated risk of spontaneous abortion infertility, ectopic pregnancy, stillbirth, low birth weight or preterm delivery, and congenital anomalies. Data for many studies were gathered prior to widespread implementation of safety precautions designed to minimize exposures among pharmacy and nursing personnel.

Spontaneous abortions have been reported among exposed personnel in hospital environments where adequate exposure controls were absent (52–56). Infertility was examined in a questionnaire-based case-control study of staff participating in National Cancer Institute clinical trials. Subjects reporting infertility were 1.5 times as likely as controls to have been exposed to chemotherapeutic drugs prior to onset of infertility (95% CI 1.1–2.0) (57). Some studies have shown elevated rates of congenital anomalies among hospital personnel with poorly controlled exposure to antineoplastic agents (58,59).

Several antineoplastic agents are listed as known carcinogens by the International Agency for Research on Cancer (IARC) (60–62). Elevated risk of secondary tumors, particularly leukemias and lymphomas, in chemotherapy recipients is also well documented. Among health care workers with occupational exposures to antineoplastic drugs, however, there are almost no data regarding increased risk of malignancy (53).

Adverse health effects have also been reported among health care workers exposed to hazardous drugs other than antineoplastic agents. Upper respiratory symptoms, bronchospasm, and pulmonary function abnormalities have been observed in personnel administering aerosolized pentamidine (63,64). Pulmonary function abnormalities have also been reported in healthy adult volunteers exposed to aerosolized ribavirin (65,66).

There is no OSHA standard specific to hazardous drugs, though OSHA developed practice guidelines for personnel handling cytotoxic medications in 1986 and updated them in 1995 (67). The guidelines recommend a written hazardous drug safety and health plan to address operating procedures; use of vertical flow biologic safety cabinets (class II type B or class III) for preparation of drug solutions; and use of personal protective equipment including gloves, gowns, and eye and face protection. They also specify practices around handling, administration, and disposal of drugs, and outline guidelines pertaining to patient care and management of linen and other reusable items. Waste disposal, spill cleanup procedures, medical surveillance, hazard communication, training, and record keeping are also addressed.

Glutaraldehyde

Glutaraldehyde (1,5-pentenedial) is an effective microbiocide used for cold sterilization of endoscopes and bronchoscopes, histologic tissue fixation, and in the development of radiographs. Glutaraldehyde's antimicrobial activity stems from its ability to react with amino groups and crosslink proteins on cell surfaces. Glutaraldehyde is generally used as a 2% aqueous solution. Because it is more effective in an alkaline environment, sodium bicarbonate is added to achieve a pH of 7.5 to 8.0.

Technical personnel assigned to the cleaning and disinfection of endoscopes and bronchoscopes are commonly exposed, but nurses and physicians working within endoscopy or bronchoscopy suites may also have significant contact if fumes are not adequately ventilated or scopes are not adequately rinsed. Radiology and histology technicians have potential air or skin contact. Other hospital personnel may be exposed during glutaraldehyde spills (68).

Glutaraldehyde is a skin, eye, and respiratory tract irritant. Skin contact causes irritation, pruritus, and erythema. Eye contact may result in conjunctival swelling and erythema, and contact with high concentrations may result in corneal injury. Upper respiratory tract exposure may cause nasal irritation, throat irritation, and cough. Epistaxis has been reported rarely (69).

Health care workers are also at risk for developing glutaraldehyde allergic conditions. Allergic contact dermatitis has been frequently reported and does not always abate following cessation of exposure (70). An association between glutaraldehyde exposure and occupational asthma is well established (71–73). Cases may occur at exposure levels below currently applicable guidelines. While the pathophysiology of glutaraldehyde-induced asthma is uncertain, immunoglobulin E (IgE) antibodies specifically directed at glutaraldehyde-modified albumin have been detected in glutaraldehyde-exposed individuals with occupational asthma (74).

Although glutaraldehyde has mutagenic properties, human studies do not implicate it as a carcinogen, teratogen, or cause of spontaneous abortion.

There is no OSHA standard applicable to glutaraldehyde. The NIOSH REL is a ceiling level of 0.2 ppm, and the ACGIH TLV is a ceiling level of 0.05 ppm.

A detailed set of recommendations for the safe handling of glutaraldehyde in health care facilities has been developed by the Association for the Advancement of Medical Instrumentation (AAMI) in conjunction with ANSI. The recommendations address engineering and work practice controls, training of staff, and personal protective equipment. Local exhaust ventilation, routed either to a filtering system or an outside duct, is generally necessary to maintain air levels below recommended limits. Eye protection, impervious gowns, and nitrile or butyl rubber gloves are recommended to prevent skin or mucous membrane contact. Due to the potential hazard of eye contact, eyewash stations should be readily accessible to any personnel with potential for glutaraldehyde contact. Monitoring of workplace levels should take place after initiating use of glutaraldehyde; whenever a major change in protocol, work practices, or ventilation occurs; and on some regular basis based on volume of use and work practices (68).

Formaldehyde

Formaldehyde is usually found as an aqueous solution ("formalin") containing 30% to 50% formaldehyde and 5% to 15% methanol. Exposure occurs among workers in anatomy, pathology, and histology laboratories, where formalin is used as a tissue fixative. Individuals who use formaldehyde to sterilize dialysis equipment and other medical devices may also be exposed. Elevated breathing zone exposures have been commonly reported. One study of an anatomy laboratory reported TWA exposures up to 2.94 ppm, nearly four times the current OSHA permissible exposure limit (PEL), and a second reported peak exposures approaching 5 ppm (75,76). Dissection tables that contain local exhaust ventilation systems are capable of reducing formaldehyde in gross anatomy laboratories to as low as 0.03 to 0.09 ppm (77,78).

Inhaled formaldehyde is primarily absorbed by the upper respiratory tract. Exposures <10 ppm may cause intense irritation of mucous membranes. High exposure levels may cause tracheobronchitis, chemical pneumonitis, and pulmonary edema. Among asthmatics, bronchospasm and airway inflammation may occur at levels as low as 0.3 ppm. Allergic reactions to formaldehyde are common, and skin contact or inhalation can result in urticaria, allergic contact dermatitis, or occupational asthma.

There is limited evidence of formaldehyde's carcinogenicity in humans, but sufficient evidence in experimental animals (79,80). The human cancer risks have been evaluated in more than 50 epidemiologic studies and three meta-analyses (81–83). Different abnormalities were found in two broadly defined groups: professionals (e.g., embalmers, anatomists, and pathologists) and industrial workers (e.g., workers making formaldehyde resins, plywood, particleboard, and apparel). Formaldehyde-exposed professionals had excess leukemia (11 of 13 studies show relative risks of 1.1 to 3.1), brain cancer (six of nine studies show relative risks of 1.2 to 3.3), and colon cancer (six of nine studies show relative risks of 1.1 to 2.3).

The OSHA PEL for formaldehyde is 0.75 ppm as an 8-hour TWA. The NIOSH REL is 0.016 ppm as a 10-hour TWA and 0.1 ppm as a 15-minute ceiling. The ACGIH TLV is 0.3 ppm as a ceiling. OSHA requires that a baseline medical examination be offered to workers prior to first assignment to an area where formaldehyde levels are expected to be >0.5 ppm. An annual symptom questionnaires and periodic medical examination are required by OSHA to be offered to workers exposed to formaldehyde levels >0.5 ppm as an 8-hour TWA, and to those exposed to formaldehyde levels >2 ppm on a 15-minute TWA.

Ethylene Oxide

Ethylene oxide exists at room temperature and standard pressure as a colorless gas. Because it is used as a cold sterilizing agent for medical supplies, exposures are of concern to those involved in surgical sterilizing, as well as to those who manufacture or package medical supplies and medical devices sterilized with ethylene oxide. Contact has been described in health care workers exposed to ethylene oxide off the gassing from recently sterilized medical devices. Nurses and hospital central supply workers may experience episodic exposures to high levels of ethylene oxide if closed sterilization equipment malfunctions or if an accidental release occurs (84–86). Levels greater than 200 ppm have been described during such accidents.

The most important exposure route for ethylene oxide is inhalation, but contact with high concentrations of its vapor and splash exposures to liquid ethylene oxide can cause burns of the skin and eyes and also initiate allergic reactions.

Bronchitis, asthma, pulmonary edema, and reactive airway dysfunction syndrome (RADS) have been associated with high-level occupational exposures (87). However, there are few reports of severe inhalation exposure in humans. Ethylene oxide–related occupational asthma has been reported in a chronically exposed worker with IgE against ethylene oxide–albumin complexes (88). Sensitization can occur after skin and inhalation exposure, resulting in contact dermatitis, urticaria, periorbital edema, and allergic rhinitis.

Central nervous system (CNS) effects reported after acute or subacute inhalation exposure to ethylene oxide include drowsiness, incoordination, headache, nausea and vomiting, seizures, aseptic meningitis, and coma. An association has been reported between chronic workplace exposures and progressive cognitive impairment, although these reports have been challenged (89–92). Peripheral nervous system effects following high-dose exposure include delayed-onset toxic axonopathy and wallerian degeneration.

Ethylene oxide exposure can cause a variety of genotoxic effects after acute or chronic exposure (93,94). Exposure of nurses to ethylene oxide has been associated with increased risks of spontaneous abortion (95). Ethylene oxide has been judged "carcinogenic to humans" by IARC and "known to be a human carcinogen" by the National Toxicology Program (96,97). Epidemiologic studies of exposed workers have yielded inconsistent results.

The OSHA PEL for ethylene oxide is 1 ppm as an 8-hour TWA and 5 ppm as a 15-minute excursion limit. The NIOSH REL is 0.1 ppm as a 10-hour TWA and 5 ppm as a 15-minute ceiling. The ACGIH TLV is 1 ppm as a ceiling. OSHA requires that a baseline medical examination be offered to workers prior to first assignment to an area where ethylene oxide levels are expected to be >0.5 ppm as an 8-hour TWA. Annual medical surveillance, including a detailed work and medical history, physical examination, complete blood count, and pregnancy or fertility testing, if requested, must be offered to workers exposed to levels >0.5 ppm as an 8-hour TWA for 30 or more days per year.

Elemental Mercury

Health care workers may sustain exposures to elemental mercury in several settings. Dentists and dental technicians may contact mercury as a component of dental amalgam. In hospitals and other clinical settings, mercury may spill from broken thermometers or manometers. Mercury has also been used to fill balloons, which serve as propulsive weights for bouginage dilators, Cantor tubes, and Miller-Abbott tubes.

The most important exposure route for elemental mercury is inhalation; about 80% of an inhaled dose is retained. The amount absorbed across the skin is estimated to be about 1% of that absorbed from the lungs. Only about 0.01% of an ingested dose is absorbed from the gastrointestinal (GI) tract (98).

Dental amalgams have contained as much as 50% elemental mercury (99). When amalgam is mixed at the patient's side immediately before use, mercury vaporizes into the room air and may also adhere to hands and clothing or spill onto surfaces. Potentially harmful exposures in dental offices have been documented in the past, and elevated mercury levels in urine and tissues have confirmed exposure among dental workers (100–102). Current exposure levels are better controlled due to improvements in ventilation and use of prepackaged alloys.

The principal effects of elemental mercury exposure involve the nervous system, but generally do not occur at urine mercury levels less than 100 μg/g creatinine. Neurologic effects include motor disorders (e.g., tremor and incoordination); intellectual dysfunction (e.g., memory loss, decreased verbal IQ); psychologic abnormalities (e.g., decreased libido, irritability, depression); and peripheral sensorimotor neuropathy of both large myelinated and small nerve fibers (103). Subclinical changes (e.g., subtle tremor, slowed nerve conduction, decreased verbal intelligence, decreased memory) have been demonstrated with urine levels of 35 to 50 μg/g creatinine, but such effects are usually reversed following removal from exposure (104–106).

Under conditions of heavy exposure, renal glomerular effects due to mercury-induced immunologic mechanisms may occur (107). Tubular defects may lead to low-molecular-weight (LMW) proteinuria (e.g., β_2-microglobulin, retinol binding protein). LMW proteinuria, and increased urine levels of renal enzymes such as *N*-acetylglucosaminidase (NAG) have also been reported (108,109).

The OSHA PEL for elemental mercury is a ceiling limit of 0.1 mg/m^3. The NIOSH REL is 0.50 mg/m^3 as a 10-hour TWA. The ACGIH TLV is 0.025 mg/m^3 as an 8-hour TWA. Adequate spill management procedures in settings where mercury is used is an important method to minimize exposures to health care workers. In dental offices, proper training of personnel in preparation of amalgams and disposal of waste, use of precapsulated alloys, provision of adequate room ventilation, and avoidance of skin contact contribute to decreased workplace exposures.

ALLERGIES IN THE MEDICAL CENTER ENVIRONMENT

Allergies of Animal Workers

Medical research is an important activity for many large medical centers, and the use of a variety of laboratory animals is quite common. Employees who work with animals have an increased risk of developing allergies to antigens found in hair, dander, urine, serum, and saliva. Atopy, prior history of exposure to laboratory animals, as well as animals in the home are risk factors for the development of laboratory animal allergy. The extent of exposure to laboratory animals on the job remains the most important risk factor

(110). Laboratory animal allergy is an immediate type I hypersensitivity reaction mediated through IgE antibody, which can occur via inhalation or direct skin contact. Symptoms most typical of early allergy are rhinoconjunctivitis (80% prevalence), and rashes and urticaria (40% prevalence) (111). Much more serious reactions of bronchospasm and asthma including anaphylaxis occur (112).

Employees who will work with animals should have a preplacement screening evaluation (113). History of allergy to domestic pets, laboratory animals, atopy, and asthma, as well as family history of allergy, asthma, or atopic conditions should be addressed. In the event that the screening process identifies potential risk factors, specific testing (IgE) to allergens relevant for the work scenario should be considered. Employees who are identified on preplacement as having bronchospasm or asthma related to exposure to laboratory animals may be qualified individuals under the Americans with Disabilities Act (114). Continued exposure to laboratory animal allergens may exacerbate their asthma and place them at risk for life-threatening anaphylactic reactions.

Reducing allergen exposure is important in reducing the primary sensitization to allergens as well as the expression of symptoms in previously sensitized employees. Controls to reduce exposure include the use of hairless animals for experimentation, the use of laminar flow cage racks, and the establishment of ventilation systems that are equipped with high-efficiency particulate air (HEPA) filters to eliminate the allergens prior to air exhaust from the rooms. In addition, dust-free bedding and the use of biologic safety cabinets for manipulation of materials contaminated with animal secretions are useful.

The greatest exposure to employees is associated with tasks of direct animal handling, cage cleaning, and feeding (110). Generally, researchers themselves have a lower risk of sensitization due to their intermittent animal exposure. Administrative controls that may be useful to reduce exposure are the appropriate use of washing and showering facilities, and the use of employer-provided clothes that are left at work and laundered by an appropriate facility.

Personal protective equipment may be effective in primary prevention of laboratory animal allergy. The use of gloves, gowns, respirators, goggles, shoe coverings, and hair coverings reduces the allergen transport out of the animal facility and reduces the total allergen accessible to the respiratory tract and mucous membranes of the employee. Rarely are respirators useful to decrease or eliminate symptoms once an animal worker has been sensitized. Whenever respiratory protection is considered, the OSHA respiratory protection standard describes in detail the appropriate and necessary components of a comprehensive program.

Medical surveillance should be performed on a regular basis for employees who are at greatest risk of exposure (e.g., workers performing tasks involving the direct handling of animal materials, cage cleaning, and feeding). Medical surveillance could be accomplished using a questionnaire method (113). In the event that symptoms of early laboratory animal allergy are detected, reducing exposure should be the first method of intervention. In the early stages, improving personal protective equipment use should also be tried. Failure of exposure reduction may necessitate medical removal of the employee from animal exposure to avoid the real risk of worsening symptoms.

Latex Allergy

In the wake of Universal Precautions and the blood-borne pathogens standard, health care workers began using greatly increased quantities of latex gloves (115,116). An unintended consequence was enhanced exposure to a wide range of potent allergenic latex-associated proteins. There has ensued an epidemic of latex allergy among health care workers that has led to enormous morbidity and cost.

Latex is an elastic and durable material, which accounts for its continued widespread use in barrier protection for health care workers. As a naturally occurring material extracted from the commercial rubber tree, its sap is a complex mixture of protein, lipid, and phospholipid. The raw sap is often processed with ammonia or sodium sulfate and vulcanized with sulfur. Accelerants such as thirams, carbamates, and mercapto compounds are used to decrease production time. These additives may play a role in glove reaction (117). Latex contains more than 200 proteins, and at least 60 have been shown to be allergenic.

Corn starch powder is added to gloves to enhance the ease of removal from the mold and donning of the gloves. The powder has been shown to adhere to protein and contribute to its wide environmental distribution. In addition, it allows for respiratory exposure to bystanders who may not themselves have skin contact with latex protein (118). The mechanism of corn starch's role in the development of latex sensitization requires further investigation. However, corn starch powder has been shown to be an irritant to the skin and may enhance the likelihood of latex protein entry into skin (119).

Irritant contact dermatitis is the most common reaction to latex gloves. This is not an allergic reaction to latex protein, but rather an irritation of the skin caused by the rubbing of glove material and sweating. Allergic contact dermatitis is characterized by a prominent cutaneous inflammatory response. The onset of symptoms may be several hours to days, but generally the peak reaction occurs 1 to 2 days after exposure. This is a delayed type IV hypersensitivity reaction. The accelerators and antioxidants associated with latex, not latex protein itself, cause allergic contact dermatitis. True latex allergy is an immediate type I hypersensitivity reaction, mediated by IgE antibodies previously formed to latex proteins (120). Prevalence of allergy to latex among occupationally exposed persons has been found to be 8% to 17% (121). Anaphylaxis to latex proteins has occurred during dental and medical examinations and surgery as well as during the donning of gloves and in the presence of others donning latex gloves (122).

Preplacement evaluations, done for all health care workers, should include a latex allergy questionnaire (123). Most latex-allergic health care workers can be accommodated in the medical workplace depending on their area of specialty and their level of reaction. Those who have type 1 latex allergy with bronchospasm or hives caused by airborne exposure should have no direct contact with latex and work only in latex-safe environments. Those with symptoms of urticaria, rhinitis, conjunctivitis, and dermatitis occurring only on direct contact of latex with the skin or mucous membranes can be offered a less pervasive workplace accommodation. Accommodation would include the following in most cases: wearing only latex-free gloves, wearing gloves whenever touching a latex-containing material, and reducing latex aeroallergen in the work environment by having co-workers wear only latex-free gloves.

Employees with type I latex allergies may be considered qualified individuals under the Americans with Disabilities Act, though this question has not been fully tested in the courts. The identification of latex allergy early in its natural history provides an opportunity for the intervention and prevention of the progression of symptoms. The careful selection of gloves that are appropriate to the task promotes primary prevention of latex allergy and reduction of symptoms in employees already sensitized to latex. OSHA requires that the selection of personal protective equipment be based on the understanding of the nature of the exposure from which the worker is to be protected. Therefore, selecting latex-free gloves for health care workers who do not have blood and body fluid exposure should eliminate latex sensitization on the job in that group. Appropriate and adequately protective latex-free gloves are also available for health care workers with blood and body fluid exposure (124,125).

The FDA has an approved method for the quantification of protein on latex (American Society for Testing and Materials, ASTM D5712-95, modified Lowry test method) and it has labeling requirements for medical examination gloves. Labels on gloves can indicate that the glove has been found to be below the limit of quantification of 50 μg of protein per gram of glove. The FDA also has labeling requirements for medical devices that come into direct contact with patients (126).

Latex allergy may affect up to 17% of health care workers, depending on the extent of exposure and the presence of underlying medical conditions. Work with accommodation requires exposure assessment and exposure reduction to latex on the job. Health care institutions should establish multidisciplinary latex allergy task forces to coordinate and successfully manage latex issues in hospitals (127). Glove selection should include consideration of selecting powder-free low-protein latex gloves whenever latex gloves must be used. For some health care settings, becoming latex safe is financially advantageous (128).

BIOLOGIC HAZARDS

Infection Control and Immunization of Health Care Workers

An effective infection control program is essential to minimize the spread of infectious disease within the medical center setting. Patients are at risk from infectious health care workers just as health care workers may be at risk for transmission of infection from patients. An effective infection control program includes the prompt assessment of patients and health care workers for signs or symptoms of infectious disease and proper containment or personal protective equipment use. Medical center facility design has been shown to directly affect the spread of infection. Primary design and renovation of medical centers should include consideration of modern techniques of engineering control (e.g., ventilation, selection of finishes for surfaces, flooring, privacy curtains, disposable versus reusable medical equipment) (129,130).

There are a variety of immunizations that health care workers can obtain to minimize the spread of infectious diseases. The Advisory Committee on Immunization Practice (ACIP) strongly recommends the following vaccines for health care workers who have not already received them or who cannot document natural immunity: hepatitis B, influenza, measles, mumps, rubella, varicella, and tetanus (131).

On preplacement exam, a health care worker's immunity to infectious agents can be assessed and immunizations updated as needed. Other pathogens commonly found in the hospital setting, for which no vaccines are currently available, are enteric pathogens, *Staphylococcus aureus,* cytomegalovirus (CMV), cryptosporidium, scabies, and herpes simplex. Hepatitis A is a vaccine-preventable illness to which health care workers can be exposed. The ACIP does not currently recommend hepatitis A vaccine for health care workers.

Infection by varicella, CMV, and rubella can present teratogenic risk for pregnant medical center employees. Immunization for varicella and rubella prior to pregnancy reduces this risk. ACIP had recommended that women refrain from becoming pregnant for 3 months after receiving live vaccines (e.g., rubeola, mumps, and rubella). Recent recommendations by the ACIP have shortened the waiting period for rubella to 28 days, after no cases of congenital rubella syndrome were reported among 680 live births born to women inadvertently immunized for rubella early in pregnancy (132).

Occupational health services play an important role in the restriction of health care workers exposed to or infected with diseases that are infectious. State and local regulations may also restrict the work of health care workers with infectious diseases. In general, it is prudent for medical centers to develop policies and guidelines for health care workers with infectious diseases. Table 44.2 lists work restrictions for health care workers with infectious diseases (133). Distribution of these guidelines to supervisory staff assists in case ascertainment and active surveillance. Health care workers with known infectious disease or a suspected infectious disease should seek guidance from occupational health services as to the need for restrictions on the job.

Tuberculosis

The incidence of tuberculosis (TB) in the U.S. has decreased over the last few years. In 1998, 6.79 cases of TB were reported per 100,000 U.S. population compared with 12.25 in 1980 (134). The risk to health care workers had increased substantially in the 1980s, complicated by the emergence of multidrug-resistant TB and the need to hospitalize patients not responding to traditional outpatient antibiotics. Despite the recent decreasing incidence in the population, individual health care workers may remain at high risk without careful adherence to engineering and administrative controls. Health care workers performing bronchoscopies, intubations, respiratory care, and administration of aerosolized medications may be at particularly high risk considering the close proximity of their work to potentially infectious patients undergoing procedures that induce cough (135).

Identifying high-risk procedures, establishing prevention strategies to reduce exposure, and identifying potentially infectious patients before they expose health care workers in large numbers are important strategies to prevent transmission. Tuberculosis is more prevalent among those infected with HIV, the homeless, prison inmates, persons from countries with high rates of TB, residents of long-term-care facilities, and intravenous drug users. Use of epidemiologic indicators in addition to signs and symptoms of disease is a good strategy to increase early identification of TB in patients. Medical surveillance of health care workers through the use of purified protein derivative (PPD) testing and symptom questionnaires may lead to the early detection of exposure and infection.

Tuberculosis Exposure Control Program

The CDC issued guidelines in 1990 and 1994 recommending that health care facilities at risk for TB transmission develop and implement programs preventing occupational exposure to TB (135). The guidelines include recommendations for administrative, engineering, and work practice controls and personal protective equipment. Departments of infection control have often taken responsibility for the development and implementation of TB exposure control programs. Coordination of and communication between a variety of departments in the health care institution is essential (e.g., nursing, occupational health, respiratory care, reception, facilities, purchasing).

Administrative controls are a key element in primary prevention of infection. Establishing a screening method to be employed by clinical and nonclinical staff can help in early identification and isolation of potentially infectious patients. The process for isolation of potentially infectious patients must be easy and quick for staff to implement. Once the patient is isolated, administrative and work practice controls continue to be important. They include limiting patient access to staff and visitors who are wearing appropriate respiratory protection, using signs to inform

TABLE 44.2. *Work restrictions for health care workers with infectious diseases or exposures to infectious diseases*

Condition necessitating relief from all patient contact:
Infectious conjunctivitis (until the discharge ceases)
Acute diarrhea with symptoms* (e.g., fever, abdominal cramps, bloody stools)
Until symptoms resolve and infection with *Salmonella* is ruled out
Or if caused by *Salmonella,* consult with local and state health authorities regarding the need for negative stool cultures
Diphtheria (until antimicrobial therapy completed and two cultures obtained ≥24 hours apart are negative)
Hepatitis A* (until 7 days after onset of jaundice)
Herpes simplex infection on the hands (herpetic whitlow) (until lesions heal)
Active measles infection (until 7 days after the rash appears)
Postexposure to measles (susceptible personnel should remain out of the workplace from days 5 to 21 after exposure, and/or 4 days after rash appears)
Meningococcal infection (until 24 hours after start of effective therapy)
Active mumps (until 9 days after onset of parotitis)
Postexposure to mumps (susceptible personnel should remain out of the workplace from days 12 to 26 after exposure, and/or 9 days after onset of parotitis)
Pediculosis (until treated and observed to be free of adult and immature lice)
Active pertussis (from beginning of catarrhal stage through the 3rd week after onset of paroxysms or until 5 days after start of the effective therapy)
Active rubella (until 5 days after rash appears)
Postexposure to rubella (susceptible personnel should remain out of the workplace from days 7 to 21 after exposure and/or 5 days after rash appears)
Scabies (until treated and cleared by medical evaluation)
Staphylococcus aureus infection of skin (until lesions have resolved)
Group A streptococcal infection* (until 24 hours after starting adequate therapy)
Active tuberculosis (until proven noninfectious)
Active varicella (chicken pox) (until all lesions dry and crust)
Postexposure to varicella (chicken pox or shingles) (susceptible personnel should remain out of the workplace from days 10 to 21) (28th day if varicella zoster immunoglobulin given)
Generalized varicella zoster or localized zoster in an immunosuppressed person (shingles) (until all lesions dry and crust)

Diseases necessitating partial work restrictions:
Acute febrile viral respiratory infection (during community outbreaks of influenza and respiratory syncytial virus considering excluding symptomatic personnel from caring for high-risk patients)
Diarrhea caused by enteroviral infection (restrict from care of infants, neonates, and immunocompromised until symptoms resolve)
Hepatitis B "e" antigen positive in personnel performing exposure-prone procedures (personnel should be excluded from invasive procedures until recommendations from an expert review panel are made based on the specific job tasks and their risk for exposing patients)
Orofacial herpes simplex (personnel should not take care of high-risk patients until lesions heal)
Human immunodeficiency virus (personnel should be excluded from invasive procedures until recommendations from an expert review panel are made based on the specific job tasks and their risk for exposing patients)
Staphylococcus aureus respiratory infections (personnel should not take care of high-risk patients until acute symptoms resolve)
Localized varicella zoster (personnel should keep lesions covered and should not take care of high-risk patients until lesions dry and crust)

Conditions necessitating no work restriction:
Cytomegalovirus infection
Mild diarrhea lasting less than 24 hours without other symptoms
Hepatitis B—acute or chronic antigenemia (should follow standard precautions)
Hepatitis C—no recommendations for work restriction at this time.
Genital herpes simplex
Postexposure pertussis (asymptomatic personnel) prophylaxis recommended
Purified protein derivative (PPD) converter

*Food handlers should also remain out of work with these infections.

staff who might enter the patient's room about the respiratory hazard, and restricting the performance of diagnostic and therapeutic procedures that would lead to respiratory droplet formation to the patient's room.

Engineering controls, in general, reduce hazards or control them to minimize the opportunity for exposure. The isolation of potentially infectious patients in negative pressure respiratory isolation rooms can be an effective engineering control for TB (129). The degree of effectiveness can be enhanced by keeping doors and windows closed, ensuring that rooms that can function as both negative pressure infectious isolation and positive pressure protective isolation are set properly, and performing in-use testing such as smoke-trail visualization to document effectiveness.

Laboratory health care workers may also be exposed when clinical specimens are manipulated in a manner that would generate respirable aerosols. Engineering controls in mycobacteriology laboratories include the use of class I or II biologic safety cabinets. Routine maintenance and effectiveness testing are essential and well described in CDC documents (136).

Personal protective equipment is considered the last line of defense when administrative, engineering, and work practice controls do not offer adequate protection to the employee. Appropriate respirators should be used by everyone entering the isolation room of a patient with known or suspected TB, while transporting the patient, and while performing procedures with high risk of aerosol production on these patients. The OSHA respirator standard outlines the principles of respirator selection and use (137). It requires that the employer institute a respiratory protection program whenever respirators are in use. NIOSH published *TB Respiratory Protection Program in Health Care Facilities: Administrator's Guide* in 1999 (138). This document outlines the required elements of the respiratory protection program for TB and offers appendices including names and addresses of respirator manufacturers, respirator-fit testing procedures, and checklists useful for the evaluation of the overall program.

Medical surveillance for tuberculosis for health care workers is required (135). The frequency of employee evaluations is based on the risk assessment performed as part of the respiratory protection program. TB skin testing should be performed as part of preplacement evaluations. The two-step method offers the opportunity to better detect latent infection in new employees by taking advantage of the booster effect.

OSHA has not finalized a standard on TB, despite publishing a proposed standard in 1997 (139). OSHA has used the CDC guidelines in issuing compliance directives. Hospitals have not traditionally been a major focus of OSHA site visits and compliance evaluations. However, OSHA has issued citations to hospitals based on the compliance directives on TB. The JCAHO has adopted the OSHA compliance directives and used them in the process of auditing hospitals. Since hospitals are audited regularly by JCAHO for accreditation, it is expected that hospitals would be implementing measures to comply with the OSHA directives.

Blood-borne Pathogens

Prevention

A broad range of blood-borne infections can be transmitted to health care workers via needle sticks; splashes onto mucous membranes of the mouth, eyes, and nose; or exposures to abraded skin. While an exact tally of such exposures is not at hand, due in part to the practical challenges of active surveillance, it has been estimated that well over 500,000 needle sticks occur annually in the U.S., of which at least 5,000 involve HIV-contaminated blood (140). Despite the hazard, a number of studies document substantial underreporting of blood and body fluid exposures among health care workers. In the operating room setting, it is estimated that in as many as 15% of all procedures at least one person at the surgical table sustains a needle stick, and blood contact may occur in as many as 50% of all surgical procedures (141,142). A study comparing incident reports of blood exposures with the actual frequency of such exposures observed at the operating table demonstrated that only approximately 2% to 11% were reported (143). Studies of percutaneous exposures with hollow-bore needles have also demonstrated significant differences between the frequency of needle sticks reported and that estimated through retrospective questionnaires. Since early prophylactic therapy is now indicated for exposures to HIV-infected blood or body fluids, underreporting may place health care workers at unnecessary risk of infection.

A number of guidelines and regulations have been designed to reduce blood-borne exposures among health care workers. Universal Precautions, developed by the CDC in 1987, were incorporated into the OSHA blood-borne pathogens standard of 1991, along with a requirement for annual training, exposure reduction plans, engineering controls, and provision of hepatitis B vaccine to potentially exposed health care workers. In 1995, Standard Precautions were introduced, combining Universal Precautions with body substance isolation, to establish a single set of procedures for patient care and handling of blood and potentially infectious body fluids. Standard Precautions include use of barrier protections, such as gloves, gowns, and facial protection, where exposures to blood or body fluids may occur. They also include basic elements of infection control, such as handwashing and proper sharps disposal. Fundamental to the concept of Standard Precautions is the assumption that all blood and body fluids, except sweat, are potentially infectious, regardless of the infectious status of the patient.

Substantial evidence has accumulated that needlestick injuries can be reduced through educational programs and replacement of standard instruments with safer devices. Significant reductions in injury rates have been demonstrated for phlebotomy devices with engineered safety features and for needleless intravenous delivery systems (144–147). Reductions in the rates of percutaneous injury among operating room staff following implementation of blunt needles for certain procedures have also been documented (148–150). Several studies show the value of educational programs addressing needle safety (151–153). Based on the potential for safer devices to reduce blood-borne pathogen exposures among health care workers, the OSHA blood-borne pathogens standard was amended in 2001 to require that employers document consideration and implementation of appropriate commercially available and effective safer medical devices designed to eliminate or minimize occupational exposure. Employers are also required to maintain a sharps injury log containing information regarding the type and brand of device involved in an exposure incident, and an explanation of how and where the incident occurred (154).

Although a broad range of infections can be transmitted percutaneously or mucocutaneously, the blood-borne pathogens of greatest significance for health care workers are HIV, hepatitis B virus (HBV), and hepatitis C virus (HCV).

HIV

Of the 453,462 AIDS cases reported to the CDC through December 31, 2000, for whom occupational information was known, 23,047 were employed in health care. The group included 5,026 nurses, 5,105 health aides, 3,014 technicians, 1,730 physicians, 1,032 therapists, 479 dental workers, 440 paramedics, and 114 surgeons. At the time of this writing, the CDC is aware of 57 health care workers in the U.S. documented to have become HIV-positive following occupational exposure: 24 nurses, 19 laboratory workers, six physicians, two surgical technicians, one dialysis technician, one respiratory therapist, one health aide, one morgue technician, and two housekeeper/maintenance workers. Another 138 cases of HIV infection have occurred among health care workers who did not report other risk factors for infection, but for whom seroconversion after exposure was not documented. Among U.S. health care workers infected on the job, the majority—48—suffered percutaneous exposure. Five became infected following mucocutaneous exposure, two following both cutaneous and mucocutaneous exposure, and two from an unknown exposure route (155). Nearly all transmissions have been due to exposures to HIV-infected blood.

Based on a combined study of 6,202 health care workers percutaneously exposed to HIV, of whom 20 seroconverted, a 0.3% risk of HIV infection following needle-stick exposures is commonly quoted. Characteristics that may be associated with higher risk of seroconversion include deep injury, visible contamination of the device with blood, needle placement directly into an artery or vein, and exposure to an individual with elevated viral titers (156). Risk of seroconversion following mucous membrane exposure has been estimated at 0.09%, based on one seroconversion in six studies (157). The risk of seroconversion following isolated skin exposure has not been quantified, but is likely to be of extremely low magnitude.

When percutaneous or mucocutaneous exposures to HIV-contaminated blood or body fluids occur, current U.S. Public Health Service recommendations call for prophylactic treatment of exposed individuals with antiretroviral medications (158). Several lines of evidence support use of prophylaxis. A case-control study assessed risk factors for seroconversion in 33 health care workers who became HIV positive following blood-borne occupational exposure to HIV (159,160). Compared to a control group that did not seroconvert, cases were significantly less likely to have used antiretroviral prophylactic medication (zidovudine) when adjusted for other HIV transmission risk factors. A study of HIV-positive pregnant women demonstrated that administration of zidovudine during pregnancy markedly lowered transmission of HIV to the fetus (7.6% transmission in treatment group, 22.6% transmission in placebo group, $p < .001$). Viral load testing at a later date revealed that a relatively small proportion of the difference could be attributed to reduction in maternal viral load, suggesting that zidovudine may have acted prophylactically in the fetus (161). Subsequent studies utilizing alternate dosing regimens or other antiretrovirals have yielded similar results. Animal studies have shown mixed results, but demonstrate decreased drug efficacy if treatment is not begun until 48 or 72 hours following exposure, or if animals are treated for only 3 or 10 days (162).

Despite convincing evidence that prophylaxis can prevent HIV infection, it clearly is not always effective. Several seroconversions have occurred despite prophylaxis with one or more antiretroviral medications, likely due to viral resistance, late initiation of therapy, inadequate length of therapy, or an overwhelming inoculum of virus. Clinicians prescribing combination antiretroviral therapy to exposed health care workers should consider probable patterns of viral resistance based on knowledge of source patient medication history (163).

Physicians who treat health care workers exposed to HIV-infected blood or body fluids should put into place mechanisms to begin prophylaxis as soon as possible following exposure, to ascertain source patient infectious status, and to monitor side effect and serologic results in the exposed. Drug toxicities also should be monitored closely in health care workers receiving prophylaxis. A broad range of side effects has been reported; one individual suffered fulminant hepatic failure requiring liver transplant following prophylactic treatment with a nevirapine-containing regimen. Mechanisms should also be put into place to provide prophylactic medications to health care workers working in HIV-endemic areas of the world where such medications may not be readily available (166).

Hepatitis B

The estimated number of new hepatitis B infections among health care workers declined from 17,000 (386 per 100,000) in 1983 to 400 (9.1 per 100,000) in 1995. Although new infections among health care workers have fallen sharply in recent years due to widespread implementation of Standard Precautions and hepatitis B vaccine, prevalence figures among surgeons of from 13% to 18% attest to the high risk of hepatitis B transmission in the past (167). Not surprisingly, hepatitis B prevalence rates are higher among physicians with frequent blood contact than among those who rarely performed invasive procedures.

Risk of HBV infection following exposure is dependent on exposure characteristics, body fluid to which the health care worker is exposed, and whether or not the source patient has e-antigenemia. Percutaneous exposure to HBV-infected blood is associated with a risk of 1% to 6% if the source patient is e-antigen negative, but 22% to 31% if the source patient is e-antigen positive (158). Viral titers may vary considerably, and may be as high as 1 billion virions per milliliter of blood or serous fluid. Titers are generally several orders of magnitude lower in saliva, semen, and vaginal secretions. In contrast to HIV and HCV, HBV is resistant to drying, ambient temperatures, simple detergents, and alcohol, and may survive on environmental surfaces for up to 1 week (168). Hence, contaminated sharp objects may pose a threat to health care workers for several days following the last contact with a source patient.

The incubation period of the virus ranges from 7 to 23 weeks, and less than half of individuals who become infected with hepatitis B manifest acute symptoms. Fulminant hepatitis may develop in approximately 1% of patients. Chronic infection develops in approximately 5% of patients. In individuals whose infections do not become chronic, hepatitis B surface antibody develops as surface antigen levels fall. It has been estimated that cirrhosis develops in approximately 20% to 35% of individuals with chronic hepatitis B, and that 20% of those with cirrhosis will develop hepatocellular carcinoma (169).

The single most effective step to prevent hepatitis B infection among health care workers is vaccination. Despite an OSHA requirement that employers provide vaccine free of charge to health care workers, a surprising number of workers remain at risk. A 1992 survey conducted at 150 hospitals revealed that slightly more than half of eligible employees had completed the vaccine series (170). A more recent survey of more than 100 hospitals revealed that approximately two thirds of employees had completed the vaccine series (171).

Administration of hepatitis B vaccine, which contains recombinantly produced surface antigen, generates immunity in greater than 90% of individuals who receive three vaccine doses. Immunity lasts for at least 12 years following immunization, even if surface antibody titers fall or become undetectable; there is currently no recommendation for periodic booster doses. Individuals who do not produce surface antibody following vaccination should have the three vaccine series repeated. Those who do not mount a surface antibody response to the vaccine following repetition of the series should be counseled regarding their susceptibility to hepatitis B and should receive hepatitis B immune globulin and possibly additional vaccine if exposed percutaneously or mucocutaneously to hepatitis B–contaminated blood or body fluids. Hepatitis B immune globulin, which should be administered as soon as possible, but which may be effective when administered as late as 7 days following exposure, is approximately 75% effective in preventing HBV infection in those without vaccine-induced protection (172).

Hepatitis C

An estimated 1.8% of the U.S. population is infected with hepatitis C virus (173). Primary risk factors for the disease in the general population are intravenous drug abuse and receipt of contaminated blood transfusions. Among health care workers, several surveys show hepatitis C prevalence to be approximately equivalent to that of the general population. Needle-stick exposures are independently associated with increased risk.

Following percutaneous exposure to infected blood, risk of hepatitis C seroconversion among exposed health care workers ranges from 0% to 10%, with an average risk of 1.8% (174,175). Infection following mucocutaneous exposure appears to be less common, though several case reports document its occurrence. HCV viral titers are low compared to HBV, and virus is generally not detected in urine, feces, or vaginal fluids.

The incubation period for hepatitis C varies from 2 to 24 weeks, and averages 6 to 7 weeks (168). Antibodies to HCV may be detected within 5 to 6 weeks of infection, and may persist regardless of whether virus is actively replicating. The vast majority of those who become infected with hepatitis C have no acute symptoms, and chronic hepatitis develops in approximately 85%.

There is no known neutralizing antibody to HCV, and no vaccine is available. Administration of immune globulin has not been shown to be effective and is not recommended following exposure. Several studies have demonstrated the efficacy of interferon-α-2b as an effective treatment of chronic hepatitis C, and treatment early in the course of chronic disease may be associated with higher cure rates (176–178). To date, treatment efficacy has been demonstrated in individuals with liver enzyme elevations, but it is not known whether there is an advantage to treating prior to any liver enzyme elevation, or whether treating acute illness begets a more favorable prognosis than treating early chronic disease (168). One report has demonstrated high cure rates when interferon-α-2b was begun during acute disease at an average of 89 days following infection (179). However, the study population's early clinical hepatitis C course was atypical in that all subjects had liver function test abnormalities.

Health care workers exposed percutaneously or mucocutaneously to hepatitis C–infected blood or body fluids should have hepatitis C antibody checked at baseline, and at 6, 12, and 24 weeks. Individuals who seroconvert should undergo polymerase chain reaction (PCR) testing to detect viral replication, and should be referred to a liver specialist for consideration of early treatment with interferon and ribavirin.

Infected Health Care Workers

Since the onset of the AIDS epidemic, there have been two instances in which health care workers transmitted HIV to patients. The first was a well-publicized case in which a Florida dentist transmitted HIV to six patients in his practice (180–182). More recently, a French orthopedic surgeon who likely became infected on the job in 1983 transmitted HIV to a patient on whom he performed a 10-hour surgical procedure in 1992 (183). Of 982 other patients who underwent procedures with the same surgeon, serologic testing revealed no other transmissions (184). Numerous serologic surveys of patients treated by other HIV-positive health care workers, including dentists, surgeons, obstetricians, and other physicians, have revealed no other transmissions of HIV from health care workers to patients. In contrast, more than 350 patients have become infected with hepatitis B following procedures by hepatitis B–infected health care workers (185,186). Transmissions have taken place during dental procedures prior to widespread use of examining gloves, and during vaginal hysterectomies, major pelvic surgeries, and cardiac surgeries, and nearly all transmissions were linked to hepatitis B e-antigen–positive health care providers. Clusters in which hepatitis C was transmitted from health care providers to patients have been recently reported (187,188). The CDC has estimated that the risk for transmission of HIV or hepatitis B lies between 1/42,000 and 1/420,000 (189).

On July 12, 1991, the CDC issued guidelines addressing HIV and hepatitis B infection of health care workers, particularly among those who performed certain exposure-prone procedures (190). The guidelines stated that infected health care workers who adhere to Universal Precautions and who do not perform invasive procedures pose no risk for transmitting HIV or hepatitis B to patients, but that those who perform certain exposure-prone procedures pose a small risk for transmitting hepatitis B or HIV. Exposure-prone procedures were characterized as those in which a needle tip was digitally palpated in a body cavity, or those in which a health care worker's fingers and a needle or other sharp instrument or object are simultaneously present in a poorly visualized or highly confined anatomic site. Initial efforts to develop standard lists of procedures meeting these criteria were abandoned shortly after the guidelines were issued.

The guidelines stated further that health care workers performing exposure-prone procedures should know their HIV antibody status, and if nonimmune to hepatitis B, their hepatitis B surface antigen and hepatitis B e-antigen status. Health care workers infected with HIV or hepatitis B (and e-antigen positive) were further instructed not to perform exposure-prone procedures unless they had sought counsel from an expert review panel and been advised under what circumstances, if any, they might continue to perform these procedures. Such circumstances would include notifying prospective patients of the health care worker's seropositivity before they underwent exposure-prone invasive procedures. Mandatory testing of health care workers for HIV antibody, hepatitis B surface antigen, or hepatitis B e-antigen was not recommended.

Several court decisions have rejected health care workers' discrimination claims regarding forced alterations of medical practice (191). In contrast, a number of professional organizations have affirmed the ability of most physicians to continue to perform invasive procedures. Decisions regarding a health care worker's continued ability to perform invasive procedures should take into account the surgeon's adherence to appropriate precautions and nature of the specific invasive procedures performed. The higher frequency of transmission from hepatitis B e-antigen–positive surgeons, compared to the very low chance of transmission from HIV-positive or hepatitis C–positive surgeons, should also be considered. While the accumulated evidence provides very little support for restricting surgical privileges among HIV-positive or hepatitis C–positive surgeons, greater hazards may exist among hepatitis B–infected surgeons with e-antigenemia. Suppression of hepatitis B viral replication with antiviral medications may influence transmission potential, and could play a role in future decision making for such cases.

CONCLUSION

Occupational medicine professionals practicing in the medical center face a unique and diverse spectrum of challenges. The size, location, and scope of services offered by the medical center affect the occupational exposures experienced by medical center employees. A thorough risk assessment will help clinicians design appropriate preplacement and medical surveillance programs. Maintaining an awareness of emerging infectious diseases in the local community and using the information to identify illness in health care workers at an early stage will help to avoid outbreaks among staff. Active surveillance of injury among medical center staff identifies clusters and sentinel events that are opportunities for future prevention. A comprehensive program of prevention strategies, appropriate treatment, and consultation in occupational medicine is of value to the medical center and the community. Reduction of workers' compensation costs and costs due to lost time and productivity are measurable outcomes, but represent only a part of the overall value of the service.

The Medical Center Occupational Health Section of the American College of Occupational and Environmental Medicine supports and continually updates the Guidelines for Employee Health Services in Health Care Facilities. This is an on-line guidance document found at *http://www.occenvmed.net*. Medical professionals may find this site useful for the information that it contains and also for the many links that it offers to other relevant sites.

ADDITIONAL SOURCES OF INFORMATION

Occupational and Environmental Medicine Resources: *http://www.occenvmed.net.*

Centers for Disease Control and Prevention: *http://www.cdc.gov.*

National Institute of Occupational Safety and Health: *http://www.cdc.gov/niosh/.*

Occupational Safety and Health Administration: *http://www.osha.gov/.*

REFERENCES

1. NIOSH. *Worker Health Chartbook, 2000.* Publication No. 2000-127. Cincinnati: U.S. Department of Health and Human Services, Public Health Service, Centers for Disease Control, National Institute for Occupational Safety and Health, 2000.
2. Joint Commission on Accreditation of Health Care Organizations. *Comprehensive accreditation manual for hospitals (CAMH).* Oakbrook Terrace, IL: JCAHO, 1999.
3. OSHA. Bloodborne pathogens. 29 CFR 1910.1030.
4. OSHA. *Framework for a comprehensive health and safety program in the hospital environment.* Washington, DC: U.S. Government Printing Office, U.S. Department of Labor, Occupational Safety and Health Administration, 1993.
5. NIOSH. *Guidelines for protecting the safety and health of health care workers.* Publication No. 88-119. Department of Health and Human Services, National Institute for Occupational Safety and Health, 1988.
6. U.S. Department of Labor, Bureau of Labor Statistics. Safety and Health Statistics 1996. Available at *http://stats.bls.gov/news.release.*
7. Hegman KT, Garg A. Ergonomic issues in medical centers. In: McCunney RJ, ed. *Medical center occupational health and safety.* Philadelphia: Lippincott Williams & Wilkins, 1999:231–245.
8. Bernacki EJ, Schaefer JA. Human factors and ergonomics programming in the health care industry. In: Orford R, ed. *Clinics in occupational and environmental medicine: occupational health in the health care industry.* Philadelphia: WB Saunders, 2001;1(2): 261–277.
9. Garg A. *Prevention of injuries to health care workers: a manual for implementing zero lifting policy.* Milwaukee: University of Wisconsin-Milwaukee, 1998.
10. U.S. Department of Labor, Bureau of Labor Statistics. Safety and Health Statistics 2000. Available at *http://stats.bls.gov/news.release.*

11. Bernacki EJ, Guidera JA, Shaefer JA, et al. An ergonomics program designed to reduce the incidence of upper extremity work related musculoskeletal disorders. *J Occup Environ Med* 1999;41(12):1032–1041.
12. Office of the Federal Register, National Archives and Records Administration. 29 CFR 1910.900, OSHA Ergonomics Program Standard (as amended). 2000(November 14);65(220).
13. NIOSH: *Occupational noise exposure: criteria for a recommended standard 1998.* NIOSH publication No. 98-126. Cincinnati: U.S. Department of Health and Human Services, Public Health Service, Centers for Disease Control, 1998.
14. Ray CD, Levinson R. Noise pollution in the operating room: a hazard to surgeons, personnel, and patients. *J Spinal Disord* 1992;5:485–488.
15. Willett KM. Noise-induced hearing loss in orthopedic staff. *J Bone Joint Surg* 1991;73B:113–115.
16. Belli S, Sani L, Scarfiiccia G, et al. Arterial hypertension and noise: a cross-sectional study. *Am J Ind Med* 1984;6:59–65.
17. OSHA. Occupational exposure to noise. 29 CFR 1910. 95.
18. NIOSH. *Criteria for recommended standard: occupational exposure to hot environments.* Cincinnati: U.S. Department of Health and Human Services, Public Health Service, Centers for Disease Control, National Institute for Occupational Safety and Health, 1986.
19. Vetter RJ, Classic KL. Ionizing radiation and laser safety. In: Chase KH, Orford RR, eds. *Clinics in occupational and environmental medicine. Occupational health in the healthcare industry.* Philadelphia: WB Saunders, 2001;1:409–422.
20. Stocker B, Meier T, Fliedner TM, et al. Laser pyrolysis products: sampling procedures, cytotoxic and genotoxic effects. *Mutat Res* 1998;412:145–154.
21. Plappert UG, Stocker B, Helbig R, et al. Laser pyrolysis products—genotoxic, clastogenic, and mutagenic effects of the particulate aerosol fractions. *Mutat Res* 1999;441:29–41.
22. American National Standards Institute. American National Standard for the safe use of lasers in health care facilities. ANSI Z136.3. New York: ANSI, 1996.
23. Hendee WR, Edwards FM. Trends in radiation protection of medical workers. *Health Physics* 1990;58: 251–257.
24. Singer CM, Baraff LJ, Benedict SH, et al. Exposure of emergency medicine personnel to ionizing radiation during cervical spine radiography. *Ann Emerg Med* 1989;18:822–825.
25. Department of Labor, Bureau of Labor Statistics. *Survey of occupational injuries and illnesses, 1995. Summary 97-7.* Washington, DC: U.S. Government Printing Office, May 1997.
26. Caldwell ME. Incidence of PTSD among staff victims of patient violence. *Hosp Community Psychiatry* 1992; 43(6):838–839.
27. Hales T. Occupational injuries due to violence. *J Occup Med* 1988;30(6):483–487.
28. Simonowitz JA. Healthcare workers and workplace violence. *Occup Med* 1996;11:277–291.
29. OSHA. Guidelines for preventing workplace violence for health care and social service workers. OSHA 3148. Washington, DC: U.S. Department of Labor, Occupational Safety and Health Administration, 1998.
30. Warshaw LJ, Messite J. Workplace violence: preventive and interventive strategies. *J Occup Environ Med* 1996;38(10):993–1006.
31. Bigos SJ, Battie MC, Spengler DM, et al. A prospective study of work perceptions and psycho-social factors affecting the report of back injury. *Spine* 1991; 16:1–6.
32. Hurrell JJ, Murphy LR. Psychological job stress. In: Rom WN, ed. *Environmental and occupational medicine,* 3rd ed. Philadelphia: Lippincott-Raven, 1998: 905–914.
33. Sauter S, Murphy LR, Hurrell JJ. Prevention of work-related psychological disorders: a national strategy proposed by the National Institute for Occupational Safety and Health. *Am Psychol* 1990;45:1146–1158.
34. Blum TC, Martin JK, Roman PM. EAP prevalence, components and utilization. *J Employ Assist Res* 1992;1(1):209–229.
35. Colligan MJ, Rosa RR. Shift work effects on social and family life. *Occup Med* 1990;5:315–322.
36. Naitoh P, Kelly TL, Englund C. Health effects of sleep deprivation. *Occup Med* 1990;5:209–238.
37. Knuttson A, Akerstedt T, Jonsson BG. Prevalence of risk factors for coronary artery disease among day and shift workers. *Scand J Work Environ Health* 1988;14: 317–321.
38. Knauth P. Speed and direction of shift rotation. *J Sleep Res* 1995;4[suppl 2]:41–46.
39. Kecklund G, Akerstedt T. Effects of timing of shifts on sleepiness and sleep duration. *J Sleep Res* 1995;4 [suppl 2]:47–50.
40. Dames BL, McGlothlin JD. Controlling exposures to nitrous oxide during anesthetic administration. Publication No. 94-100. Cincinnati: National Institute for Occupational Safety and Health, 1994.
41. Westphal K, Byhahn C, Strouhal U, et al. Exposure of recovery room personnel to inhalation anesthetics. *Anaesthes Reanim* 1998;23:157–160.
42. Hoerauf KH, Wallner T, Akca O, et al. Exposure to sevoflurane and nitrous oxide during four different methods of anesthetic induction. *Anesth Analg* 1999; 88(4):925–929.
43. Rowland AS, Baird DD, Shore DL, et al. Nitrous oxide and spontaneous abortion in female dental assistants. *Am J Epidemiol* 1995;141:531–538.
44. Rowland AS, Baird DD, Weinberg CR, et al. Reduced fertility among women employed as dental assistants exposed to high levels of nitrous oxide. *N Engl J Med* 1992;327:993–997.
45. Ad Hoc Committee on the Effect of Trace Anesthetics on the Health of Operating Room Personnel, American Society of Anesthesiologists. Occupational disease among operating room personnel. *Anesthesology* 1974;41:321–340.
46. Cohen EN, Gift HC, Brown BW, et al. Occupational disease in dentistry and chronic exposure to trace anesthetic gases. *J Am Dent Assoc* 1980;101:21–31.
47. Guirguis S, Pelmear P, Roy M, et al. Health effects associated with exposure to anesthetic gases in Ontario hospital personnel. *Br J Ind Med* 1990;47:490–497.
48. Cohen EN, Gift HC, Brown BW, et al. Occupational disease in dentistry and chronic exposure to trace anesthetic gases. *J Am Dent Assoc* 1980;101:21–31.
49. Doll R, Peto R. Mortality among doctors in different occupations. *Br Med J* 1977;I:1433–1436.

50. McMartin HL, Rose VE, Smith DL, et al. NIOSH criteria for a recommended standard: occupational exposure to waste anesthetic gases and vapors. NIOSH publication No. 77-140. Washington, DC: Department of Health, Education, and Welfare, 1977.
51. Connor TH, Anderson RW, Sessink PJ, et al. Surface contamination with antineoplastic agents in six cancer treatment centers in Canada and the United States. *Am J Health Syst Pharm* 1999;56:1427–1432.
52. Hemminki K, Kyyroenen P, Lindbohm M-L. Spontaneous abortions and malformations in the offspring of nurses exposed to anaesthetic gases, cytostatic drugs, and other potential hazards in hospitals, based on registered information of outcome. *J Epidemiol Community Health* 1985;39:141–147.
53. Skov T, Maarup B, Olsen J, et al. Leukaemia and reproductive outcome among nurses handling antineoplastic drugs. *Br J Ind Med* 1992;49:855–861.
54. Selevan SG, Lindbohm M-L, Hornung RW, et al. A study of occupational exposure to antineoplastic drugs and fetal loss in nurses. *N Engl J Med* 1985;313: 1173–1178.
55. Stuecker I, Caillard J-F, Collin R, et al. Risk of spontaneous abortion among nurses handling antineoplastic drugs. *Scand J Work Environ Health* 1990;16: 102–107.
56. Valanis B, Vollmer WM, Steele P. Occupational exposure to antineoplastic agents: self-reported miscarriages and stillbirths among nurses and pharmacists. *J Occup Environ Med* 1999;41:632–638.
57. Valanis B, Vollmer W, Labuhn K, et al. Occupational exposure to antineoplastic agents and self-reported infertility among nurses and pharmacists. *J Occup Environ Med* 1997;39:574–580.
58. Hemminki K, Kyyroenen P, Lindbohm M-L. Spontaneous abortions and malformations in the offspring of nurses exposed to anaesthetic gases, cytostatic drugs, and other potential hazards in hospitals, based on registered information of outcome. *J Epidemiol Community Health* 1985;39:141–147.
59. McDonald AD, McDonald JC, Armstrong B, et al. Congenital defects and work in pregnancy. *Br J Ind Med* 1988;45:581–588.
60. International Agency for Research on Cancer. *IARC monographs on the evaluation of the carcinogenic risk of chemicals to humans: some antineoplastic and immunosuppressive agents,* vol 26. Lyon, France: IARC, 1981.
61. International Agency for Research on Cancer. *IARC monographs on the evaluation of the carcinogenic risk of chemicals to humans: overall evaluations of carcinogenicity,* an updating of IARC monographs vols 1 to 42[suppl 7]. Lyon, France: IARC, 1987.
62. International Agency for Research on Cancer. *IARC monographs on the evaluation of the carcinogenic risk of chemicals to humans: pharmaceutical drugs,* vol 50. Lyon, France: IARC, 1990.
63. Balmes JR, Estacio PL, Quinlan P, et al. Respiratory effects of occupational exposure to aerosolized pentamidine. *J Occup Environ Med* 1995;37:145–150.
64. Gude JK. Selective delivery of pentamidine to the lung by aerosol. *Am Rev Respir Dis* 1989;139:106.
65. California Department of Health Services Occupational Health Surveillance and Evaluation Program. *Health care worker exposure to ribavirin aerosol:* field investigation Fl-86-009. Berkeley: California Department of Health Services, 1986.
66. Connor JD, Hintz M, Van Dyke R. Ribavirin pharmacokinetics in children and adults during therapeutic trials. In: Smith RA, Knight V, Smith JAD, eds. *Clinical applications of ribavirin.* Orlando: Academic Press, 1984.
67. U.S. Department of Labor, Occupational Safety and Health Administration. OSHA instruction CPL 2-2.20B CH-4, Directorate of Technical Support, April 14, 1995.
68. ANSI/AAMI. Safe use and handling of glutaraldehyde-based products in health care facilities. ANSI/AAMI ST58, 1996.
69. Wiggins P, McCurdy SA, Zeidenberg W. Epidstaxis due to glutaraldehyde exposure. *J Occup Med* 1989; 31:854–856.
70. Nethercott JR, Holness DL, Page E. Occupational contact dermatitis due to glutaraldehyde in healthcare workers. *Contact Dermatitis* 1988;18:193–196.
71. Chan-Yeung M, McMurren T, Catonio-Begley F, et al. Occupational asthma in a technologist exposed to glutaraldehyde. *J Allergy Clin Immunol* 1993;91: 974–978.
72. DiStefano F, Siriruttanapruk S, McCoach J, et al. Glutaraldehyde: an occupational hazard in the hospital setting. *Allergy* 1999;54:1105–1109.
73. Gannon PJ, Bright P, Campbell M, et al. Occupational asthma due to glutaraldehyde and formaldehyde in endoscopy and x-ray departments. *Thorax* 1995;50: 156–159.
74. Curran AD, Burge PS, Wiley K. Clinical and immunologic evaluation of workers exposed to glutaraldehyde. *Allergy* 1996;51:826–832.
75. Akbar-Khanzadeh F, Vaquerano MU, Akbar-Khanzadeh M, et al. Formaldehyde exposure, acute pulmonary response, and exposure control options in a gross anatomy laboratory. *Am J Ind Med* 1994;26:61–75.
76. Uba G, Pachorek D, Bernstein J, et al. Prospective study of respiratory effects of formaldehyde among healthy and asthmatic medical students. *Am J Ind Med* 1989;15:91–101.
77. Coleman R. Reducing the levels of formaldehyde exposure in gross anatomy laboratories. *Anat Rec* 1995; 243:531–533.
78. Martin WD, Nemitz JW, Hendley A, et al. Three years of experience with a dissection table ventilation system. *Clin Anat* 1995;8:297–302.
79. International Agency for Research on Cancer. Wood dust and formaldehyde. *IARC Monogr Eval Carcinog Risks Hum* 1995;62.
80. National Toxicology Program. *Ninth report on carcinogens: 2000 summary.* Research Triangle Park, NC: U.S. Department of Health and Human Services, 2000.
81. Collins JJ, Acquavella JF, Esmen NA. An updated meta-analysis of formaldehyde exposure and upper respiratory tract cancers. *J Occup Environ Med* 1997; 39:639–651.
82. Blair A, Saracci R, Stewart PA, et al. Epidemiologic evidence on the relationship between formaldehyde exposure and cancer. *Scand J Work Environ Health* 1990;16:381–393.
83. Partanen T. Formaldehyde exposure and respiratory cancer—a meta-analysis of the epidemiologic evidence. *Scand J Work Environ Health* 1993;19:8–15.

84. Sobaszek A, Hache JC, Frimat P, et al. Working conditions and health effects of ethylene oxide exposure at hospital sterilization sites. *J Occup Environ Med* 1999; 41:492–499.
85. Wesolowski W, Sitarek K. Occupational exposure to ethylene oxide of hospital staff. *Int J Occup Med Environ Health* 1999;12:59–65.
86. Zey JN, Mortimer VD, Elliott LJ. Ethylene oxide exposures to hospital sterilization workers from poor ventilation design. *Appl Occup Environ Hyg* 1994;9: 633–641.
87. Deschamps D, Rosenberg N, Soler P, et al. Persistent asthma after accidental exposure to ethylene oxide. *Br J Ind Med* 1992;49:523–525.
88. Dechamp C, Dubost R, Forissier MF, et al. Airway hyperreactivity to ethylene oxide with positive RAST (radio allergo sorbent test). *Clin Exp Allergy* 1990;20: 74.
89. Crystal HA, Schaumburg HH, Grober E, et al. Cognitive impairment and sensory loss associated with chronic low-level ethylene oxide exposure. *Neurology* 1988;38:567–569.
90. Estrin WJ, Bowler RM, Lash A, et al. Neurotoxicological evaluation of hospital sterilizer workers exposed to ethylene oxide. *Clin Toxicol* 1990;28:1–20.
91. Klees JE, Lash A, Bowler RM, et al. Neuropsychologic "impairment" in a cohort of hospital workers chronically exposed to ethylene oxide. *Clin Toxicol* 1990;28:21–28.
92. Dretchen KL, Balter NJ, Schwartz SL, et al. Cognitive dysfunction in a patient with long-term occupational exposure to ethylene oxide. *J Occup Med* 1992;34: 1106–1113.
93. Fuchs J, Wullenweber U, Hengstler JG, et al. Genotoxic risk for humans due to work place exposure to ethylene oxide: remarkable individual differences in susceptibility. *Arch Toxicol* 1994;68:343–348.
94. Major J, Jakab MG, Tompa A. Genotoxicological investigation of hospital nurses occupationally exposed to ethylene-oxide: I. Chromosome aberrations, sister-chromatid exchanges, cell cycle kinetics, and UV-induced DNA synthesis in peripheral blood lymphocytes. *Environ Mol Mutagen* 1996;27:84–92.
95. Hemminki K, Mutanen P, Saloniemi I, et al. Spontaneous abortions in hospital staff engaged in sterilizing instruments with chemical agents. *Br Med J* 1982;20: 1461–1463.
96. International Agency for Research on Cancer: Some industrial chemicals. Ethylene oxide. *IARC Monogr Eval Carcinog Risks Hum* 1994;60:73–159.
97. National Toxicology Program. *Ninth report on carcinogens: 2000 summary.* Research Triangle Park, NC: U.S. Department of Health and Human Services, 2000.
98. Russi M, Borak J. Chemical hazards of health care workers. In: Orford RR, ed. *Clinics in occupational and environmental medicine. Occupational health in the healthcare industry.* Philadelphia: WB Saunders, May 2001.
99. Kelman GR. Urinary mercury excretion in dental personnel. *Br J Ind Med* 1978;35:262–265.
100. Buchwald H. Exposure to dental workers to mercury. *Am Ind Hyg Assoc J* 1972;33:492–502.
101. Kelman GR. Urinary mercury excretion in dental personnel. *Br J Ind Med* 1978;35:262–265.
102. Joselow MM, Goldwater LJ, Alvarez A, et al. Absorption and excretion of mercury in man. XV. Occupational exposure among dentists. *Arch Environ Health* 1968;17:39–43.
103. Kishi R, Doi R, Fukuchi Y, et al. Residual neurobehavioural effects associated with chronic exposure to mercury vapour. *Occup Environ Med* 1994;51:35–41.
104. Chang YC, Yeh CY, Wang JD. Subclinical neurotoxicity of mercury vapor revealed by a multimodality evoked potential of chloralkali workers. *Am J Ind Med* 1995;27:271–279.
105. Langworth S, Almqvist O, Soderman E, et al. Effects of occupational exposure to mercury vapour on the central nervous system. *Br J Ind Med* 1992;49: 545–555.
106. Liang Y-X, Sun R-K, Sun Y, et al. Psychological effects of low exposure to mercury vapor: application of a computer-administered neurobehavioral evaluation system. *Environ Res* 1993;60:320–327.
107. Tubbs RR, Gephardt GN, McMahon JT, et al. Membranous glomerulonephritis associated with industrial mercury exposure. *Am J Clin Pathol* 1982;77:409–413.
108. Cardenas A, Roels H, Bernard AM, et al. Markers of early renal changes induced by industrial pollutants. I. Application to workers exposed to mercury vapour. *Br J Ind Med* 1993;50:17–27.
109. Langworth S, Elinder CG, Sundquist KG, et al. Renal and immunological effects of occupational exposure to inorganic mercury. *Br J Ind Med* 1992;49:394–401.
110. Hollander A, Heederick D, Doeks G. Respiratory allergy to rats: exposure-response relationship in laboratory animal workers. *Am J Respir Crit Care Med* 1997; 155:562–567.
111. Hunskaar S, Fosse RT. Allergy to laboratory mice and rats: a review of the pathophysiology, epidemiology, and clinical aspects. *Lab Anim* 1990;24:358–374.
112. Platts-Mills TA, Longbottom J, Edwards J, et al. Occupational asthma and rhinitis related to laboratory rats: serum IgG and IgE antibodies to the rat urinary allergen. *J Allergy Clin Immunol* 1987;79:505–515.
113. Phipatanakul W, Wood RA. Allergens of animal and biological systems. In: Fleming DO, Hunt D, eds. *Biological safety: principles and practice,* 3rd ed. Washington, DC: ASM Press, 2000.
114. Americans with Disabilities Act, 1990, 42 U.S.C. 12101 *et seq*.
115. Centers for Disease Control and Prevention. Guidelines for prevention of transmission of human immunodeficiency virus and hepatitis B virus to health-care and public safety workers. *MMWR* 1989;38:3–31.
116. Occupational Safety and Health Administration. Occupational exposure to bloodborne pathogens. 29 CFR 1910.1030. *Fed Reg* 1991;56:64175–64182.
117. Conde-Salazar L, del-Rio E, Guimaraens D. Type IV allergy to rubber additives: a 10-year study of 686 cases. *J Am Acad Dermatol* 1993;29:76–180.
118. Allmers H, Brehler R, Chen Z, et al. Reduction of latex aeroallergens and latex-specific IgE antibodies in sensitized workers after removal of powdered natural rubber latex gloves in a hospital. *J Allergy Clin Immunol* 1998;102(5):841–846.
119. Brehler R, Voss W, Mueller S. Glove powder effects skin roughness, one parameter of skin irritation. *Contact Dermatitis* 1998;39(5):227–230.
120. Occupational Safety and Health Administration. Technical information bulletin: potential for allergy to natural rubber latex gloves and other natural latex products. Washington, DC: OSHA, 1999.

121. Liss GM, Sussman GL, et al. Latex allergy: epidemiological study of 1351 hospital workers. *Occup Environ Med* 1997;54(5):335–342.
122. National Institute for Occupational Safety and Health. *NIOSH alert: preventing allergic reactions to latex in the workplace.* NIOSH Publication No. 97–135. Washington, DC: Department of Health and Human Services, 1997.
123. Sussman G, Gold M. *Guidelines for the management of latex allergies and safe latex use in healthcare facilities.* Ottawa: CHA Press, 1996.
124. Nelson JR, Roming TA, Bennett JK. A whole-glove method for the evaluation of surgical gloves as barriers to viruses. *Am J Contact Dermatitis* 1999;10(4): 183–189.
125. Hamann CP, Nelson JR. Permeability of latex and thermoplastic elastomer gloves to the bacteriophage phi X174. *Am J Infect Control* 1993;21(6):289–296.
126. Food and Drug Administration. *Natural rubber-containing medical devices: user labeling.* 21 CFR Part 801 [Docket No.96N-0119], 1997.
127. Hunt LW, Boone-Orke JL. A medical-center-wide, multidisciplinary approach to the problem of natural rubber latex allergy. *J Occup Environ Med* 1996;38(8): 765–770.
128. Phillips VL, Goodrich MA, Sullivan TJ. Healthcare worker disability due to latex allergy and asthma: a cost analysis. *Am J Public Health* 1999;89(7): 1024–1028.
129. Noskin GA, Peterson LR. Engineering infection control through facility design. *Emerg Infect Dis* 2001 (March-April);7(2).
130. Livornese LL, Dias S, Samuel C, et al. Hospital-acquired infection with vancomycin-resistant *Enterococcus faecium* transmitted by electronic thermometers. *Ann Intern Med* 1992;117:112–116.
131. Centers for Disease Control and Prevention. Immunization of health care workers: Recommendations of the Advisory Committee on Immunization Practices (ACIP) and the Hospital Infection Control Practices Advisory Committee (HICPAC). *MMWR* 1997;46 (RR-18):1–44.
132. Reef SE, Frey TK, Abernathy E, et al. The changing epidemiology of rubella in the 1990s: on the verge of elimination and new challenges for control and prevention. *JAMA (in press).*
133. Bolyard EA, Tablan OC, Williams WW, et al. Guideline for infection control in health care personnel, 1998. *Am J Infect Control* 1998;26(3):289–354.
134. MacKay AP, Fingerhut LA, Duran CR. *Health, United States, 2000.* DHHS publication No. 00-1232. Hyattsville, MD: National Center for Health Statistics, U.S. Department of Health and Human Services, 2000.
135. Centers for Disease Control and Prevention (CDC). Guidelines for preventing the transmission of mycobacterium tuberculosis in health care facilities. *MMWR* 1994;43(RR-13).
136. Centers for Disease Control, National Institutes of Health. *Biosafety in microbiological laboratories,* 3rd ed. Atlanta: CDC and NIH, 1993.
137. OSHA. Respiratory Protection. 29 CFR 1910.134 (a) (2).
138. DHHS (CDC). *TB Respiratory Protection Program in Health Care Facilities: Administrator's Guide.* DHHS NIOSH publication No. 99-143. Atlanta: DHHS, September 1999.
139. Occupational Health and Safety Administration. Proposed standard for occupational exposure to tuberculosis. *Fed Reg* 1997;62:54159.
140. Bell DM. Occupational risk of human immunodeficiency virus infection in healthcare workers: an overview. *Am J Med* 1997;102[suppl 5B]:9–14.
141. Centers for Disease Control and Prevention. Evaluation of blunt suture needles in preventing percutaneous injuries among health-care workers during gynecologic surgical procedures—New York City, March 1993–June 1994. *MMWR* 1997;46:25–29.
142. Quebbeman EJ, Telford GL, Hubbard S, et al. Risk of blood contamination and injury to operating room personnel. *Ann Surg* 1991;214:614–620.
143. Lynch P, White MC. Perioperative blood contact and exposures: a comparison of incident reports and focused studies. *Am J Infect Control* 1993;21:357–363.
144. Centers for Disease Control and Prevention. Evaluation of safety devices for preventing percutaneous injuries among health-care workers during phlebotomy procedures. Minneapolis–St. Paul, New York City, and San Francisco, 1993–1995. *MMWR* 1997;46:21–29.
145. Mendelson MH, Short LJ, Schechter CB, et al. Study of a needleless intermittent intravenous-access system for peripheral infusions: analysis of staff, patient, and institutional outcomes. *Infect Control Hosp Epidemiol* 1998;19:401–406.
146. Gartner K. Impact of a needleless intravenous system in a university hospital. *Am J Infect Control* 1992;20: 75–79.
147. L'Ecuyer P, Schwab E, Iademarco E, et al. Randomized prospective study of the impact of three needleless intravenous systems on needlestick injury rates. *Infect Control Hosp Epidemiol* 1996;17:803–808.
148. Centers for Disease Control and Prevention. Evaluation of blunt suture needles in preventing percutaneous injuries among healthcare workers during gynecologic surgical procedures—New York City, March 1993–June 1994. *MMWR* 46:25–29.
149. Hartley JE, Ahmed S, Milkins R, et al. Randomized trial of blunt-tipped versus cutting needles to reduce glove puncture during mass closure of the abdomen. *Br J Surg* 1996;83:1156–1157.
150. Mingoli A, Sapienza P, Sgarzini G, et al. Influence of blunt needles on surgical glove perforation and safety for the surgeon. *Am J Surg* 1996;172:512–517.
151. Haiduven D, DeMaio T, Stevens D. A five-year study of needle stick injuries: significant reduction associated with communication, education, and convenient placement of sharps containers. *Infect Control Hosp Epidemiol* 1992;13:265–271.
152. White M, Lynch P. Blood contacts in the operating room after hospital-specific data analysis and action. *Am J Infect Control* 1997;25:209–214.
153. Gerberding J. Procedure-specific infection control for preventing intraoperative blood exposures. *Am J Infect Control* 1993;21:364–367.
154. *Fed Reg* 2001(January 18);66(12):5317–5325.
155. Department of Health and Human Services. Centers for Disease Control and Prevention. Surveillance of Health Care Workers with HIV/AIDS. Available at: *http:www.cdc.govhivpubsfactshcwsurv.htm.*
156. Cardo DM, Culver DH, Ciesielski CA, et al. A case-control study of HIV seroconversion in health care workers after percutaneous exposure. *N Engl J Med* 1997;337:1485–1490.

157. Bell DM. Occupational risk of human immunodeficiency virus infection in healthcare workers: an overview. *Am J Med* 1997;102[suppl 5B]:9–14.
158. Centers for Disease Control and Prevention. Updated U.S. Public Health Service guidelines for the management of occupational exposures to HBV, HCV, and HIV and recommendations for postexposure prophylaxis. *MMWR* 2001;50(RR-11):1–42.
159. Centers for Disease Control and Prevention. Case-control study of HIV seroconversion in health-care workers after percutaneous exposure to HIV-infected blood—France, United Kingdom, and United States, January 1988–August 1994. *MMWR* 1995;44: 929–933.
160. Cardo DM, Culver DH, Ciesielski CA, et al. A case-control study of HIV seroconversion in health care workers after percutaneous exposure. *N Engl J Med* 1997;337:1485–1490.
161. Balsley J. Efficacy of zidovudine in preventing HIV transmission from mother to infant. *Am J Med* 1997; 102(5B):45–46.
162. Van Rompay KKA, Otsyula MG, Marthas ML, et al. Immediate zidovudine treatment protects simian immunodeficiency virus-infected newborn macaques against rapid onset of AIDS. *Antimicrob Agents Chemother* 1995;39:125–131.
163. Beltrami EM, Cheingsong R, Respess R, et al. Antiretroviral drug resistance in HIV-infected source patients for occupational exposures to healthcare workers [Abstract P-S2-70]. In: *Program and abstracts of the 4th Decennial International Conference on Nosocomial and Healthcare-Associated Infections.* Atlanta: CDC, 2000:128.
164. Russi M, Buitrago M, Goulet J, et al. Antiretroviral prophylaxis of health care workers at two urban medical centers. *J Occup Environ Med* 2000;42: 1092–1100.
165. Centers for Disease Control and Prevention. Serious adverse events attributed to nevirapine regimens for postexposure prophylaxis after HIV exposures–worldwide, 1997–2000. *MMWR* 2001;49(51–52):1153–1156.
166. Russi M, Hajdun M, Barry M. A program to provide antiretroviral prophylaxis to health care personnel working overseas. *JAMA* 2000;283(10):1292–1293.
167. West DJ. The risk of hepatitis B infection among health professionals in the United States: a review. *Am J Med Sci* 1984;287:26–33.
168. Beltrami EM, Williams IT, Shapiro CN, et al. Risk and management of blood-borne infections in health care workers. *Clin Microbiol Rev* 2000;13:385–407.
169. Hoofnagle JH. The clinical spectrum and course of chronic hepatitis B. Program of the Workshop on Management of Hepatitis B. Bethesda, MD: 2000:12–14.
170. Agerton TB, Mahoney FJ, Polish LB, et al. Impact of the bloodborne pathogens standard on vaccination of healthcare workers with hepatitis B vaccine. *Infect Control Hosp Epidemiol* 1995;16:287–291.
171. Mahoney FJ, Steward K, Hu H, et al. Progress toward elimination of hepatitis B virus transmission among health care workers in the United States. *Arch Intern Med* 1997;157:2601–2605.
172. Grady GF, Lee VA, Prince AM, et al. Hepatitis B immune globulin for accidental exposures among medical personnel: final report of a multicenter controlled trial. *J Infect Dis* 1978;138:625–638.
173. Alter MJ, Druszon-Moran D, Nainan DV, et al. The prevalence of hepatitis C virus infection in the United States, 1988 through 1994. *N Engl J Med* 1999;341: 556–562.
174. Centers for Disease Control and Prevention. Recommendations for follow-up of health-care workers after occupational exposure to hepatitis C virus. *MMWR* 1998;47:603–606.
175. Mitsui TK, Iwano K, Masuko C, et al. Hepatitis C virus infection in medical personnel after needlestick accident. *Hepatology* 1992;16:1109–1114.
176. Vogel W, Graziadei I, Umlauft F, et al. High-dose interferon-alpha2b treatment prevents chronicity in acute hepatitis C: a pilot study. *Dig Dis Sci* 1996;41 [suppl 12]:81S–85S.
177. Camma C, Almasio P, Craxi A. Interferon as treatment for acute hepatitis C: a meta-analysis. *Dig Dis Sci* 1996;41:1248–1255.
178. Noguchi S, Sata M, Suzuki H, et al. Early therapy with interferon for acute hepatitis C acquired through a needlestick. *Clin Infect Dis* 1997;24:992–994.
179. Jaeckel E, Cornberg M, Wedemeyer, et al. Treatment of acute hepatitis C with interferon alfa-2b. *N Engl J Med* 2001;345:1452–1457.
180. Centers for Disease Control. Possible transmission of human immunodeficiency virus to a patient during an invasive dental procedure. *MMWR* 1990;39:489–493.
181. Centers for Disease Control. Update: transmission of HIV infection during an invasive dental procedure—Florida. *MMWR* 1991;40:21–33.
182. Centers for Disease Control and Prevention. Update: investigations of persons treated by HIV-infected health-care workers—United States. *MMWR* 1993;42: 329–331, 337.
183. National Public Health Network of France. Roseau National de Sante Publique. HIV transmission from an orthopedic surgeon to a patient. Press Release, 1997.
184. Lot F, Seguier J-C, Fegueux S, et al. Probable transmission of HIV from an orthopedic surgeon to a patient in France. *Ann Intern Med* 1999;130:1–6.
185. Henderson DK. SHEA Position Paper: Management of healthcare workers infected with hepatitis B virus, hepatitis C virus, human immunodeficiency virus, or other bloodborne pathogens. *Infect Control Hosp Epidemiol* 1997;18:349–362.
186. Harpaz R, Von Seidlein L, Averhoff FM. Transmission of hepatitis B virus to multiple patients from a surgeon without evidence of inadequate infection control. *N Engl J Med* 1996;334:549–554.
187. Ross RS, Viazov S, Gross T, et al. Transmission of hepatitis C virus from a patient to an anesthesiology assistant to five patients. *N Engl J Med* 2000;343:1851–1854.
188. Esteban JI, Gomez J, Martell M. Transmission of hepatitis C virus by a cardiac surgeon. *N Engl J Med* 1996;334:555–560.
189. Bell DM, Shapiro CN, Gooch BF. Preventing HIV transmission to patients during invasive procedures. *J Public Health Dent* 1993;53:170–173.
190. Centers for Disease Control and Prevention. Recommendations for preventing transmission of human immunodeficiency virus and hepatitis B virus to patients during exposure-prone invasive procedures. *MMWR* 1991;40:1–8.
191. Burris S. Human immunodeficiency virus-infected health care workers. *Arch Fam Med* 1996;5:102–106.

45

Fitness for Duty in the Transportation Industry

Natalie P. Hartenbaum

While employees in the transportation industry suffer types of injuries that are similar to those of other workers, most of their interactions with occupational health professionals are for medical fitness evaluations. Unlike many careers where the concern is the potential of injury to the examinee, for transportation workers the assessment must include a determination of whether the worker presents a risk to co-workers or the general public. Many of the jobs considered "safety-sensitive" in transportation have some degree of federally mandated medical standards. These range from the very clearly defined aviation standards, to those for railroad engineers, which essentially only require adequate hearing, vision, and color vision. Transportation industry workers include not only truck drivers, airline pilots, flight attendants, locomotive engineers, and conductors, but also workers in support roles whose jobs may have similar public safety ramifications.

Fitness evaluations in most employment setting are subject to the Americans with Disabilities Act (ADA); however, where regulated standards exist, these are not overridden by the ADA (1). Suits have been filed on behalf of employees denied employment based on federal medical standards and have been decided for and against the employer in the lower courts. In one decision, the Supreme Court upheld a company's right to have standards that are more stringent than the federal requirements, provided they are not based on a disability that significantly impairs the individual from performing activities of daily living (2). This case concerned vision requirements. In the majority of cases, ensuring public safety is given key consideration.

HIGHWAY—FEDERAL MOTOR CARRIER SAFETY ADMINISTRATION

One of the most common medical examinations in many occupational medicine practices is the commercial driver medical fitness examination, more commonly known as the Department of Transportation (DOT) exam. (This should not be the preferred term because DOT also encompasses railroad, aviation, pipeline, transit, maritime, and other areas of transportation.) Responsibility for the Federal Motor Carrier Safety Regulations, which includes the medical standards, had been under the authority of the Federal Highway Administration until 1999 (3). At that time a new agency of DOT, the Federal Motor Carrier Safety Administration (FMCSA), was created to oversee highway safety issues. This agency reports directly to the secretary of DOT.

This examination may seem quick, easy, and of little significance; however, there have been several high-profile motor vehicle accidents in which medical factors were found to be at least in part responsible. A study by the Association for the Advancement of Automotive Medicine (AAAM) (4) demonstrated deficiencies in the proper performance of this regulated examination. Even in cases where the medical examiners were aware that their work was being reviewed, the paperwork was not completed properly, or medical qualification decisions were not based on federal standards, available guidelines, or recommendations. Unfortunately, even when guidelines are available, many examiners are unaware of them or are unsure how and when they should be applied. Other studies have also demonstrated that examiners are unaware of local regulations or other medical requirements for drivers (5).

To determine whether an individual is able to safely perform a job, one of the first considerations must be identifying the key tasks. In addition to driving, there are many other tasks that may be impacted by the driver's medical condition:

- Entering and exiting the cab, which may be 5 feet off the ground;

- Loading and unloading freight;
- Working with load securement devices.

Drivers who are physically unable to tie down their load could find material flying off the back of their vehicle, resulting in accidents or fatalities to other drivers and passengers. Drivers physically unable to inspect their equipment may be driving an unsafe vehicle.

Other work conditions or stressors that may cause an acute deterioration of the driver's underlying medical status include hazardous material, adverse weather conditions, long absences from home, tight or irregular work schedules, noise, and vibration.

Some accident investigations have concluded that accidents have resulted from a driver's being improperly certified under the FMCSA regulations (6). An increasing number of suits are being filed where the driver's medical condition is alleged to be the case of an accident resulting in injury or fatality. There is controversy over the degree to which medical conditions affect an individual's ability to drive safely and how to identify those at higher risk. Commercial driver medical examiners must base their determination on the driver's status at the time of the examination, but it is difficult to determine whether the condition may deteriorate during the certification period. The examiner's best recourse in this circumstance is to certify for less than a full 24-month period. A frustration of many examiners is the inability to place restrictions on the driver, other than requiring use of a hearing aid or corrective lenses and in very specific circumstances a skill performance evaluation certificate or exemption. Once a medical certificate is given, the driver may use it for any commercial carrier willing to accept it.

The degree of acceptable risk in a commercial driver has not been defined in the United States. The Canadian Cardiovascular Society defined acceptable risk in patients with cardiovascular disease as a 20% annual risk of sudden incapacitation in a driver of a private vehicle, and a 1% annual risk in a driver of a commercial vehicle (7).

One significant area of confusion is which drivers require the commercial driver medical fitness examination. Under federal regulations the definition of a commercial vehicle for the purposes of the commercial driver's license (CDL) and drug and alcohol testing is different from that for indicating which drivers require the examination only. The examination is required if the driver operates a vehicle in interstate commerce

- with a gross vehicle or gross combination weight, or gross vehicle weight rating or gross combination weight rating, of greater than 10,001 pounds; or
- that is designed to transport 15 or more passengers, including the driver; or
- that is used to transport hazardous material of a quantity requiring placarding.

A CDL and testing for controlled substances are not required unless the driver is operating a vehicle

- with a gross vehicle weight or gross vehicle weight rating of greater than 26,001 pounds;
- that is designed to transport 16 or more passengers, including the driver; or
- that, regardless of size, is used to transport hazardous materials requiring placarding under the Hazardous Materials Regulations.

A proposed rule published in the *Federal Register* (8) sought comments on requiring medical evaluation for drivers operating vehicles designed to carry, for direct compensation, between 9 and 15 passengers a distance of greater than 75 miles. If adopted, these drivers would have to meet the medical qualification standards but would not require CDLs or drug or alcohol testing.

Most states have adopted the federal medical standards for intrastate (within the same state) commercial driving, although states may have different criteria for requiring medical certification. Many states have mechanisms in place to permit drivers who were operating intrastate prior to adoption of the federal standards to continue to do so. Many states also grant waivers or exemptions under specific circumstances. This chapter addresses only the medical regulations for drivers involved in interstate commerce.

Drivers are required to be examined if they do not have a current medical certificate or have not been medically certified within the past 24 months. In addition, they are also required to be examined if their physical or mental condition affects their ability to operate a vehicle safely. Carriers are responsible for ensuring that a driver is reexamined if there is any health concern.

Federal regulations state that the commercial driver examination can be performed by any "licensed, certified, and/or registered health care professionals permitted by their state's laws and regulations" to perform the examination. This includes doctors of medicine or osteopathy and, depending on the state, may also include physician assistants, advanced practice nurses, or doctors of chiropractic.

There are 13 requirements that a commercial driver must meet to be medically certified (Fig. 45.1). These intentionally leave a great deal of discretion to the individual examiner in deciding whether the potential risk of a medical condition causing sudden incapacita-

§391.41 Physical qualifications for drivers

a) A person shall not drive a commercial motor vehicle unless he/she is physically qualified to do so and, except as provided in 391.67, has on his/her person the original, or a photographic copy, of a medical examiner's certificate that he/she is physically qualified to drive a commercial motor vehicle.

(b) A person is physically qualified to drive a commercial motor vehicle if that person --

(b)(1) Has no loss of a foot, a leg, a hand, or an arm, or has been granted a skill performance evaluation certificate pursuant to 391.49;

(b)(2) Has no impairment of: (b)(2)(i) A hand or finger which interferes with prehension or power grasping; or

(b)(2)(ii) An arm, foot, or leg which interferes with the ability to perform normal tasks associated with operating a commercial motor vehicle; or any other significant limb defect or limitation which interferes with the ability to perform normal tasks associated with operating a commercial motor vehicle; or has been granted a skill performance evaluation certificate pursuant to 391.49.

(b)(3) Has no established medical history or clinical diagnosis of diabetes mellitus currently requiring insulin for control;

(b)(4) Has no current clinical diagnosis of myocardial infarction, angina pectoris, coronary insufficiency, thrombosis, or any other cardiovascular disease of a variety known to be accompanied by syncope, dyspnea, collapse, or congestive cardiac failure;

(b)(5) Has no established medical history or clinical diagnosis of a respiratory dysfunction likely to interfere with his/her ability to control and drive a commercial motor vehicle safely;

(b)(6) Has no current clinical diagnosis of high blood pressure likely to interfere with his/her ability to operate a commercial motor vehicle safely;

(b)(7) Has no established medical history or clinical diagnosis of rheumatic, arthritic, orthopedic, muscular, neuromuscular, or vascular disease which interferes with his/her ability to control and operate a commercial motor vehicle safely;

(b)(8) Has no established medical history or clinical diagnosis of epilepsy or any other condition which is likely to cause loss of consciousness or any loss of ability to control a commercial motor vehicle;

(b)(9) Has no mental, nervous, organic, or functional disease or psychiatric disorder likely to interfere with his/her ability to drive a commercial motor vehicle safely;

(b)(10) Has distant visual acuity of at least 20/40 (Snellen) in each eye without corrective lenses or visual acuity separately corrected to 20/40 (Snellen) or better with corrective lenses, distant binocular acuity of at least 20/40 (Snellen) in both eyes with or without corrective lenses, field of vision of at least 70° in the horizontal meridian in each eye, and the ability to recognize the colors of traffic signals and devices showing standard red, green, and amber;(b)(11) First perceives a forced whispered voice in the better ear at not less than 5 feet with or without the use of a hearing aid or, if tested by use of an audiometric device, does not have an average hearing loss in the better ear greater than 40 decibels at 500 Hz, 1,000 Hz, and 2,000 Hz with or without a hearing aid when the audiometric device is calibrated to American National Standard (formerly ASA Standard) Z24.5 1951;

(b)(12)(i) Does not use a controlled substance identified in 21 CFR 1308.11 Schedule I, an amphetamine, a narcotic, or any other habit-forming drug.(b)(12)(ii) Exception. A driver may use such a substance or drug, if the substance or drug is prescribed by a licensed medical practitioner who:

(b)(12)(ii)(A) Is familiar with the driver's medical history and assigned duties; and

(b)(12)(ii)(B) Has advised the driver that the prescribed substance or drug will not adversely affect the driver's ability to safely operate a commercial motor vehicle; and:

(b)(13) Has no current clinical diagnosis of alcoholism.

FIG. 45.1. Federal motor carrier safety regulations—physical qualifications for drivers. 49 CFR 391.41.

tion is acceptable or not. Unfortunately, the wide variance of knowledge, training, and understanding of the mental, emotional, and physical requirements of commercial driver tasks may lead to different determinations on the same driver's examination by different examiners. In 1977, the Federal Highway Administration (FHWA) issued medical advisory criteria to serve as guidelines for examiners and to further clarify factors in determining driver fitness. The most recent version was issued in October 2000 as a part of the new Medical Examination Report. Additional information is contained in the *Federal Register* of April 7, 1997 in the form of regulatory guidance, responses to specific questions addressed to the agency. Also, the FHA has sponsored several conferences in an effort to offer examiners more specific recommendations for several medical diagnoses. These conference reports contain recommendations by specialists concerning pulmonary (9), cardiac (10), neurologic (11), and psychiatric (12) disorders and can be found on the Internet at *www.fmcsa.dot.gov/rulesregs/medreports.htm.* Other resources are also available to examiners, such as the DOT medical examination: A Guide to Commercial Driver Medical Certification (Hartenbaum NP, ed., 2nd edition. Beverly, MA: OEM Press, 2000), and the Commercial Driver Medical Examiner (CDME) Review, published by the American College of Occupational and Environmental Medicine, Arlington Heights, IL.

Physical Requirements for Commercial Drivers

This section provides an overview of the regulations, and examples of the issues to consider. In many cases, the examiner will be unable to make a determination of the driver's medical status, including compliance and complications from an existing disease, during the office visit. As advised in the regulations, additional information from either treating physicians or specialists may be necessary to make a fully appropriate qualification determination.

The four areas where the standards leave no discretion to the examiner are vision, hearing, insulin-requiring diabetes, and epilepsy.

Vision

The driver must have central visual acuity of at least 20/40 in each eye and in both, with or without corrective lenses. The use of monovision contact lenses is not acceptable. Normal color vision is not required, but the driver must be able to identify the colors of traffic signals—red, green, and amber. Vision can be tested with a Snellen chart or any of the automated or standardized vision testing machines or simple identification of the color by colored lights or objects. The driver must also have a horizontal field of vision of at least 70 degrees in the horizontal plane. There are a number of drivers who had been in the FHA vision waiver program, which terminated in 1994 due to court action. These drivers are permitted to continue commercial driving in interstate commerce. Since 1998, a number of drivers have been granted exemptions from the vision requirement. Additional information can be obtained from the FMCSA.

Hearing

A forced whisper at 5 feet can be used to screen for significant hearing deficits. The examiner should whisper three to five words or phrases not all containing sibilants ("s" sounds) while the driver covers first one ear and then the other. If the driver is unable to pass this screening test, an audiometric test should be performed. Unlike the Occupation Safety and Health Administration (OSHA) standards, the hearing range of interest is 500, 1,000, and 2,000 Hz, the frequencies responsible for speech recognition. The driver should be considered qualified only if the average (add the three values on one side, then divide by three, then do same on the opposite side) hearing loss is not greater than 40 dB in the better ear, with or without a hearing aid.

Diabetes

Under the current regulations, drivers cannot be medically qualified if they are taking insulin for control of their diabetes. A driver who is not using insulin but whose glucose is not well controlled and most likely should be on insulin should also not be qualified. When evaluating diabetic drivers, it is important to assess not only their glycemic control but also whether there has been any effect of the disease on the nervous system, heart, or kidneys. Many of the older oral hypoglycemic agents can cause hypoglycemia, and this has been shown to decrease the ability to drive safely. In addition, drivers who are aware of their low blood sugar but do not take appropriate action (13,14), and drivers who are prone to hypoglycemia but have hypoglycemic unawareness, either because of their disease or medications such as beta blockers, present a danger. Whether there have been episodes of hypoglycemia should also be reviewed. Drivers who had been in the diabetes waiver program may continue to be qualified upon meeting certain criteria. New exemptions are currently not being issued for insulin-taking diabetics.

Epilepsy

A medical examiner should not issue a medical certificate to a driver with a seizure disorder or other medical condition that is likely to cause loss of consciousness or the ability to operate the vehicle. In those cases where a nonepileptic seizure or other loss of consciousness of unknown etiology occurred, the medical examiner may consider certification if antiseizure medication is not required. The advisory criteria recommend a 6-month waiting period prior to qualification and a complete neurologic evaluation that indicates a low likelihood of recurrence. If a drug reaction or metabolic condition was determined to be the cause of the seizure, the driver should be fully recovered without residual deficits prior to certification. The neurology conference recommended that after a single seizure episode that required medication, drivers should not be medically qualified until they have been seizure free and off medication for 5 years. With an established history of seizure disorder, a 10-year seizure- and medication-free period was recommended. Drivers currently requiring medication for their seizures should not be qualified.

Other Medical Issues

The nine other regulations address the other medical issues and provide discretion to the examiner. It is important to carefully evaluate each patient using all available information. Final qualification determination should not be made until the examiner reviews all the necessary information. The motor carrier has the responsibility to ensure that only medically qualified drivers operate commercial vehicles and that the examiner has the necessary information on the driver's task and the regulatory requirements. The actual medical decision is the responsibility of the medical examiner. If the driver has a medical condition that appears stable at the time of the examination but may deteriorate over the following 2 years, the examiner may certify the driver for less than a 2-year period. The following are examples of some of the more common medical conditions and guidance from the FMCSA- or FHWA-sponsored conference.

Loss of Arm, Foot, or Leg or Impairment of Hand, Finger, Arm, Foot, or Leg or Other Limb Defect

Drivers who are able to safely operate a commercial vehicle despite their limb impairment may be eligible for exemption from this requirement through a Skill Performance Evaluation (SPE) certificate (formerly referred to as a limb or orthopedic waiver). The medical examiner should evaluate all other medical conditions and if the driver is otherwise qualified, indicate that a SPE certificate is required on the medical certificate. The driver, either individually or with the carrier, is then required to obtain this certificate by applying through their state's office of the FMCSA. In addition to an assessment by an orthopedist or physiatrist, a road test is also required. A complete description of the program can be found in the Code of Federal Regulations or in the *Federal Register* (15).

Cardiac Disease

This area was covered in depth by one of the FHWA-sponsored conferences. While the report is more than 10 years old, more recent reviews of the literature and recommendation by specialists in other countries have similar recommendations (16–18). Cardiac disorders such as arrhythmias, either primary or as a result of myocardial ischemia, or valve dysfunction, which may cause emboli or congestive failure, may result in sudden incapacitation. These conditions might require the driver to be medically disqualified. It is important to assess not only the current status of the disease but also its natural history, the likelihood of progression, and the potential effects of medications.

Drivers who have had myocardial infarctions or other ischemic events should have a normal resting electrocardiogram (ECG) and stress test prior to resuming vocational driving. Their medications should be reviewed to ensure that there are no side effects that may be impairing. The cardiac conference participants recommended return to work after a waiting period and follow-up as presented in Fig. 45.2.

When evaluating drivers with valvular disease, care should be taken to identify coexistent coronary artery disease and to determine the risk of arrhythmias. The current status of the valvular dysfunction should be noted as well as any progression of the disease and the natural history. Participants in the cardiac conference recommended against qualifying those drivers taking Coumadin, but participants in the pulmonary conference recommended that drivers on anticoagulants could be qualified under certain conditions. Recent guidance from the FHWA details recommendations on the use of Coumadin in commercial drivers (Fig. 45.3).

Arrhythmias are the most likely cardiac disorder to cause sudden incapacity. The American Heart Associ-

	Return to Work	Follow up
Myocardial Infarction	3 month wait—EST negative	Stress test 1 year then 2 years until age 55, then annually
CABG	3 month wait—EST negative	EST every 2 years first 6–10 years then annually
PTCA	3 week wait—EST negative	EST at 3-6 months then annually

FIG. 45.2. Recommended return-to-work wait after cardiac event. (Adapted from U.S. Department of Transportation, Federal Highway Administration, Office of Motor Carriers. Conference on cardiac disorders and commercial drivers. Publication No. FHWA-MC-88-040, 1987.)

ation (AHA) and North American Society of Pacing and Electrophysiology (NASPE) addressed several specific arrhythmias in a review (19). The cardiac conference report suggested disqualification for those drivers with ventricular fibrillation, ventricular tachycardia, type II second-degree (A-V) block, and third-degree blocks. Qualification of drivers with pacemakers was controversial and would require individual assessment. The AHA and NASPE considered whether the individual was pacemaker dependent, that is, if the pacemaker malfunctioned, would the individual be unable to continue to function. In general, implantable cardiac defibrillators are not thought to be compatible with commercial driving (16–18,20).

Pulmonary and Allergic Disease

Aside from the effects of the disease itself, one of the major concerns in this category is the adverse effect of the medications used in treatment. Some antihistamines have been found to be as impairing as alcohol (21,22), and many of the antitussives contain sedating narcotics. Sleep apnea is becoming more recognized as a cause of motor vehicle accidents and the revised Medical Examination Report for Commercial Driver Fitness Determination (23), which must be used by November 6, 2001, requires questioning a driver about symptoms. In addition, screening tests such as the Berlin Questionnaire (24) and the Epworth Sleepiness Scale (25) can be used for screening. Drivers with sleep apnea should not be qualified under the regulations unless the sleep apnea is well controlled and monitored. Periodic demonstration of compliance and effectiveness of treatment should be reviewed. Cough syncope may cause sudden incapacitation and should be disqualifying.

Borderline pulmonary function may be sufficient under normal driving conditions, but it is important to remember that commercial drivers must also drive in adverse weather conditions. In addition, they must load and unload their vehicles and perform other maintenance activities. Any of these activities may increase the respiratory demand, potentially beyond the individual's reserve. The pulmonary conference participants recommended using pulmonary function testing to further evaluate drivers with borderline pulmonary status. Further evaluation with arterial blood gases was recommended if the forced expiratory volume in 1 second (FEV_1) was less than 65% predicted or the forced vital capacity (FVC) was less than 60% of predicted. If the partial pressure of oxygen is less than 65 mm Hg or the partial pressure of carbon dioxide is greater than 65 mm Hg, then the driver should not be considered qualified for commercial operations.

Hypertension

Guidance for qualification determination in drivers with hypertension had been issued in the advisory criteria. A much simpler format was included with the new Medical Report Form. It was advised that drivers with blood pressures of >180 systolic or >104 diastolic should not be medically qualified. Drivers whose blood pressure is less than 160/90 and on no medications could be qualified for the full 2-year period provided there are no other medical concerns. Details for drivers with blood pressure in between these values can be found in Fig. 45.4. A recent addition to the advisory criteria included in the Medical Examination Report addressed those drivers whose blood pressure was in the range considered acceptable by the FMCSA but on medication. The advisory criteria suggested that individuals with a clinical diagnosis of hypertension and on medication should be subject to more frequent evaluation, suggesting 1 year if the blood pressure was in the mild to moderate range at the time of diagnosis. As part of the evaluation of the driver with hypertension, attention should be paid to the presence of end-organ damage (cardiac,

Part 391 of the Federal Motor Carrier Safety Regulations has been designed to protect both the health and safety of the driver and the general public. As drivers age and as the indications for anticoagulation with coumadin increase. It is important to review the effect of coumadin on the commercial driver's health and risk to the general public from commercial drivers on coumadin. Based on reviews of the medical literature, regulations from other regulatory agencies, and the policies of other countries, the following recommendations have been reached.

1. Coumadin is a medical treatment which can improve the health and safety of the driver and should not, by its use, medically disqualify the commercial driver. The emphasis should be on the underlying medical condition(s) which require treatment and the general health of the driver.

2. The medical examiner responsible for making the qualification determination should confer with other doctors who have treated the driver.

3. The International Normalized Ratio (INR) is now the best available methods to monitor the anticoagulant effect of coumadin. It also allows results from different laboratories to be compared. This method is strongly recommended for monitoring the effect of coumadin.

4. A driver on coumadin should be educated about the potential interaction of coumadin with other medications and diet, the increase risk of bleeding with trauma and the need for regular monitoring of coumadin's effect.

5. The medical certification of commercial drivers on coumadin and over age 65 should receive careful consideration because of the increased sensitivity to coumadin and the risk for significant bleeding.

6. The medical certification of commercial drivers with cerebrovascular disease and who are on coumadin is not recommended because of the increased risk of intracranial hemorrhage with sudden loss of consciousness.

7. An individual should not be medically certified during the first 3 months on coumadin because the major risk from side-effects of coumadin occur within these first months on treatment.

8. An individual should have a physical examination every year under section 391.43, instead of every 2 years, because of the need to monitor closely both the effect of coumadin and the underlying medical condition(s).

Revised: April 1996
US Department of Transportation
Federal Highway Administration

FIG. 45.3. Federal Highway Administration regulations for the commercial driver on Coumadin.

On initial exam		Within 3 months		Certify
If 161-180 and/or 91-104, Qualify 3 months only.	→	If $\leq$ 160 and/or 90, Qualify for 1 yr. Document Rx & control the 3rd month	→	Annually if acceptable BP is maintained
If > 180 and/or 104, not qualified until reduced to < 181/105. Then qualify for 3 months only.	→	If $\leq$ 160 and/or 90, qualify for 6 mos. Document Rx & control the 3rd month	→	Biannually

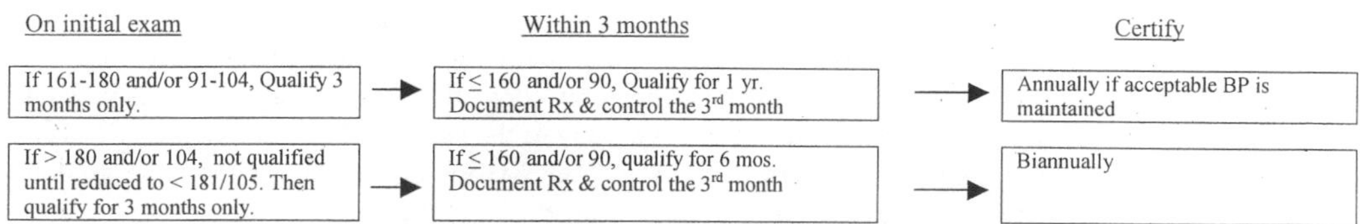

FIG. 45.4. Guidelines for blood pressure evaluation.

renal, and ophthalmic) and any potential side effects of pharmacologic treatment.

Arthritic, Rheumatic, Orthopedic, Muscular, Neuromuscular or Vascular Diseases

Various medical conditions can produce sudden or progressive difficulty in operating motor vehicles. A complete neurologic and musculoskeletal examination should be performed on any individual in whom a more focused examination or medical history suggests abnormalities. This assessment should address range of motion, strength, and coordination. Factors in determining whether the driver meets the medical qualifications include the medical condition, its severity, the degree of limitation, the course of the disease since diagnosis, and whether progressive or sudden limitations might occur. If the disease is stable and progression is slow, a shorter duration of certification may be appropriate.

Psychiatric Disorders

Drivers with psychiatric disorders may have impaired judgment, attention, or reasoning due to either the disorder or the medication used for treatment. The driver must have adequate ability to maintain alertness and to react quickly and appropriately to various adverse situations, including traffic, hazardous road conditions, and environmental factors. If there are periods of instability such as occurs with schizophrenia or other psychoses, disqualification may be appropriate. In addition to evaluating the effectiveness or side effects of medications, compliance with treatment regimens should be ensured.

Drug Use or Alcoholism

Testing for controlled substances is no longer a part of the medical examination. The examiner is still instructed to evaluate whether the driver has a current clinical diagnosis of alcoholism or uses a schedule I substance or other habit-forming drugs, and if so, the driver should not be qualified. The examiner may make this determination by taking a history, or may suspect a problem based on the medical examination. Prior to qualifying such a driver, the examiner should obtain clearance from a substance abuse professional. The advisory criteria suggest that there may be situations where a driver is using a controlled substance or other habit-forming drug under the direction of a licensed health care practitioner. Prior to the examiner's considering the driver to be medically qualified, he should ensure that the medication is used in the dose and manner prescribed. The prescribing practitioner should be aware of the driver's responsibilities and safety issues, and should state, preferably in writing, whether the medication will interfere with the driver's ability to safely operate the commercial vehicle and perform required tasks. The advisory criteria state that drivers on methadone, even under a health care professional's supervision, should not be qualified to operate commercial vehicles in interstate commerce.

Many other medications, such as antihistamines, may interfere with the driver's ability. The examiner is instructed to review the driver's medications, both prescription and over the counter, and how they might affect driving. The examiner is also to instruct the driver to read warning labels on all medications. Drivers should be advised to avoid medications while driving unless they are certain that there are no side effects. For those medications with a high likelihood of sedation, discussion with the treating provider to consider an alternate treatment would be indicated.

MARITIME—COAST GUARD

The Coast Guard has medical standards for employees who hold certain merchant marine licenses. The standards that are specified in Title 46, Code of Federal Regulations parts 10, 12, and 14, require that the individual be physically fit. There are specific requirements only for visual acuity and color vision. The Coast Guard issues period Navigation and Vessel Inspection Circulars (NVICs). The most recent addressing mariner fitness was issued in February 1998 (NVIC 2-98) and it provides guidelines for the medical examiner who is evaluating an individual for this type of work. Drug and alcohol testing is required for certain positions.

The examination must be reported on a specific form and the original provided to the examinee. Aside from NVIC 2-98, the *Marine Safety Manual* (volume 4, chapter 3) provides guidelines for the examiner. Licensed medical doctors (MD or DO), licensed physician assistants, or licensed nurse practitioners may perform the examination. There is no requirement for training. The form is presented to the Coast Guard Marine Safety Office for processing and review. If additional information is needed or a problem of potential qualification error is identified, the issue may be referred to the Regional Examination Center or possibly to the National Maritime Center in Washington, D.C. Mariners who do not meet the guidelines may be eligible for a waiver.

In determining whether the individual is fit to be qualified under Coast Guard requirements, it is necessary to understand the work environment and job tasks. Living and work spaces are often cramped, and environmental factors such as storms may make the work even more hazardous. With no ready resource for additional personnel, mariners should be able to function in emergency situations requiring fire fighting or launching life rafts or boats. Much of the work requires heavy physical labor.

Employees in the maritime industry not only must be fit to perform their jobs, but also should not have any medical conditions that may require sudden or frequent evaluation and treatment. These individuals may

Potentially Disqualifying Conditions – Coast Guard – Adapted from NVIC 2-98, US Coast Guard
Mariners may apply for waiver

Vision –
- Not correctable to 20/40 in each eye, or unable to recognize color coded indicator lights, diagrams, piping systems, valves and wiring (Deck officer) or
- Not correctable to 20/50 in each eye or unable to distinguish colors red, green, blue or yellow (Engineer Officer)

Hearing – checked at 500Hz, 1000 Hz, 2000 Hz, and 3000 Hz and averaged
- Original deck and engineer officer license - Averaged unaided hearing threshold of 70dB or less, each ear and less than 90% speech discrimination.
- Renewal or raise of grade – average unaided hearing threshold of less than 70 dB or less than 80% functional speech discrimination
- Deck officers may use hearing aids (threshold must be 40dB or less in ear), Engineer officers may not use hearing aids

Speech – severe speech impediment

Cardiac
- History of multiple myocardial infarctions
- New York Heart Association class II, III or IV
- Heart irregularity
- Hypertension –original license greater than 150/90, renewal or raise in grade 160/100 if under age 50, 175/100 if over age 50 or on medication

Pulmonary –
- Lung disease including chronic or active asthma
- Tuberculosis or other active pulmonary disease

Gastrointestinal
- Chronic/recurrent pancreatitis
- Esophageal varices – one episode of GI bleeding in past 6 months or 2 episodes in past 2 years

Genitourinary
- Chronic renal failure

Orthopedic
- Amputation, arthritis or deformity resulting in impairment

Endocrinologic
- Insulin dependent diabetes or poorly controlled non-insulin dependent diabetes. Documentation must be provided that diabetes is not affecting eyesight
- Addison's disease, Cushing's syndrome- adrenal dysfunction, hyperaldosteronism
- Obesity sufficient to impair normal activity or prevent rapid response in emergency situation

Hematologic/ Oncologic
- Hemophilia
- Leukemia
- Malignancies – Untreatable, recurrent or currently undergoing treatment

Neurologic
- Any convulsive disorder resulting in altered state of consciousness, regardless of control by medication
- Condition which limits balance (Parkinson's, Meniere's)
- Chronic organic/traumatic brain syndrome
- Neurosylphilis
- Narcolepsy
- Senility
- Somnambulism

Psychiatric
- Primary Psychosis
- Any condition requiring use of psychotropic medication
- Mental retardation
- Drug addiction
- Current or chronic alcohol abuse/ alcohol dependence/ alcoholism

Allergies
- Any sever allergy, which could cause sudden incapacitation, or be life-threatening

Infectious disease
- Amy communicable disease which could present hazard to crewmembers or passengers

Medications
- Anticoagulants

Systemic corticosteroids
Psychotropic medications
Medication causing impairing side effects
HIV
- Requires review

Miscellaneous
Any other condition which may cause deterioration of performance or sudden incapacitation or compromise shipboard safety.

FIG. 45.5. Potentially disqualifying conditions—Coast Guard. Mariners may apply for waiver. (Adapted from NVIC 2-98, U.S. Coast Guard.)

be away from home for months at a time and access to medical care may be unavailable or suboptimal.

In addition to being physically fit, the codified physical requirements for an original license as master, mate, pilot, or operators are as follows:

1. Vision correctable to at least 20/40 in each eye and uncorrected vision of at least 20/200 in each eye.
2. Color vision must be satisfactory and tested with one of the following: pseudoisochromatic plates (Dvorine, 2nd edition; AOC; revised edition or AOC-HRR [American Optical Company/Hardy-Rand-Ritter] Ishihara 16-, 24-, or 38-plate editions); Eldridge Green Color Perception Lantern; Farnsworth Lantern; Keystone Orthoscope; Keystone Telebinocular; School of Aviation Medicine Color Threshold Tester; Titmus Optical Vision Tester; or the Williams Lantern.

For an original license as an engineer, radio officer, offshore, installation manager, barge supervisor, or ballast control operator, applicants must have correctable vision of at least 20/50 in each eye and uncorrected vision of at least 20/200 in each eye. They must be able distinguish the colors red, green, blue, and yellow.

There are several potentially disqualifying medical conditions listed in NVIC 2-98 (Fig. 45.5). In general, for these conditions, unless the examiner is convinced that the condition is stable and not a potential threat, the examiner should indicate on the designated form "needs further evaluation" or "not competent." Mariners can apply for a waiver if the examiner does not find them qualified. Additional requirements for a waiver can be found in the *Marine Safety Manual* or NVIC 2-98.

RAILROAD—FEDERAL RAILROAD ADMINISTRATION (FRA)

Many jobs in the rail industry involve moderate to heavy work. Others, such as train dispatchers, may have fewer physical demands, but the tasks may require a great deal of concentration. Drug testing is required for all railroad employees covered by the Hours of Service Regulations (49 CFR 28) including conductors, engineers, signalmen, and many others. In addition, many employees also fall under the FMCSA authority for either drug testing or physical requirements. Only railroad engineers are covered with specific federal medical standards. Federal medical requirements for locomotive engineers are significantly less detailed than those for either pilots or commercial drivers, requiring only an evaluation of distant visual acuity, color vision, and hearing every 3 years; some states require more frequent evaluation. Although the color vision requirement is that the engineer be able to identify the colors of the signals, both the FRA and the National Transportation Safety Board (NTSB) (26) recognize that more accurate color vision is necessary. Yarn or simple color identification tests are not adequate in screening for color vision defects in these employees. Ishihara pseudoisochromatic plates or similar tests should be used as a minimal screening tool. If the engineer is unable to pass the screening color vision test, additional evaluation should be considered (27).

Many railroads also require an evaluation for other medical conditions that might cause sudden impairment. Engineers with medical conditions such as seizures, heart disease, sleep apnea, or insulin-requiring diabetes mellitus should receive careful evaluation. Similar to the commercial drivers, engineers may not have normal work, rest, and mealtime schedules. The FRA also requires that railroads ensure that employees in safety sensitive positions not use medications, whether prescription or over the counter, that may interfere with safety (28).

AVIATION—FEDERAL AVIATION ADMINISTRATION (FAA)

The FAA has a significant organizational structure governing the medical certification of pilots. Pilot medical examinations must be performed by designated aviation medical examiners (AMEs). These are physicians (MD or DO) who are selected for AME designation based on their professional credentials, aviation experience, and continuing training. AMEs are required to forward all examinations for FAA review through the Internet-based Airman Medical Certification System (AMCS).

AMEs are authorized to grant airman medical certificates unless any of 15 specifically disqualifying medical conditions are found. The AME may defer issuance of the airman medical certificate to the FAA if clinically appropriate. Nine regional flight surgeon offices and the Civil Aeromedical Institute (CAMI) Aeromedical Certification Division and Aeromedical Education Division provide support and guidance for the AME. In addition, CAMI supports and conducts ongoing research and training in human factors and the effect on safety in aviation. Pilots may appeal a disqualification decision through the Aeromedical Certification Division and the federal air surgeon.

There are three classes of airmen medical certificate:

Class 1 medical certificates are required for pilots or airline transport pilots (ATPs). These have the most stringent medical requirements. The class 1 certificate is valid through the end of the examination month and 6 months for ATP duties, 1 year for other commercial activities, and 2 or 3 years for private pilot duties.

Class 2 medical certificates are for commercial, non-airline workers such as crop dusters, charter pilots, and corporate pilots. A class 2 certificate is valid through the end of the examination month plus 1 year for commercial activities and 2 or 3 years for private pilot use.

Class 3 medical certificates are for private pilot activities only. These have the least restrictive medical requirements and are valid through the end of the examination month plus 3 years for those under age 40 and 2 years for those over age 40.

There are specific standards for vision, hearing, and blood pressure. In general, the physical requirements are designed to minimize the risk of an adverse medical event potentially causing injury to the pilot, the passengers, or individuals on the ground. The medical requirements for each class of medical certificate can be found in Part 67 of the Federal Aviation Regulations (14 CFR 67). Details are not covered here as only a designated AME may perform the examination. Specific questions can be directed to the Aeromedical Certification Division at (405) 954-4821, the Aeromedical Education Division at (405) 954-4803, or one of the regional flight surgeon offices.

There are approximately 20,000 air traffic control specialists (ATCSs) employed by the FAA. They work in en route centers, terminal radar centers, airports, and flight service stations. ATCSs must meet the medical standards contained in FAA order 3920.3A, the Air Traffic Control Specialist Health Program, and can be examined only by senior AMEs who have been designated by the FAA to examine air traffic controllers.

The military or local municipalities may also employ air traffic controllers.

TRANSIT—FEDERAL TRANSIT ADMINISTRATION (FTA)

The FTA regulates public transportation. Bus operators generally fall under the medical requirements of the FMCSA, as they require a commercial driver's license. The FRA regulates engineers of regional rail lines. Subway and trolley operators are not covered by federal medical standards, although companies may have specific job requirements.

OTHER CONCERNS

Jobs in the transportation industry share several common features regarding hazards. The Department of Labor Report of Workplace Injuries and Illnesses in 1999 reported that within the service-producing sector the highest incidence rate was found in transportation (7.3 cases per 100 full-time workers) (29). The highest rate was found in air transportation (13.3 per 100 full-time workers) (Fig. 45.6). Highway crashes were the cause of the highest number of fatal on-the-job injuries, 898 fatalities in 1999, with just over two fifths of those being truck drivers, the highest number over an 8-year period (30).

Transport of goods and passengers occurs 24 hours a day, 7 days a week. While a tired production line worker may make errors or be injured, a tired pilot, bus driver, truck driver, or railroad engineer may cause widespread catastrophe. Hours of service regulations in the transportation field attempt to ensure that workers get sufficient sleep. But studies have shown that commercial drivers, despite mandated off-duty time, often do not get sufficient sleep (31). Operator fatigue has been identified as a problem only partially addressed by methods currently in place according to the NTSB (32). Ongoing efforts are underway to identify optimal methods to avoid fatigue and maintain service (33). Rosekind et al. (34) identified six major areas for a complete program to address worker fatigue in 24-hour operations: (a) education and training, (b) hours of service, (c) scheduling practices, (d) countermeasures, (e) design and technology, and (f) research.

Much of the freight and maintenance work must be performed in various weather conditions, ranging from extreme heat to extreme cold. Employees involved in passenger transport may be asked to assist with passengers' belongings. They also must deal at times with difficult and demanding passengers, as for example flight attendants must deal with passenger air rage. They also must be prepared to assist passengers in emergencies, such as illness or accidents, and stress either may result from the emergency or may be involved in its cause.

Another concern in the transportation industry, as in all work settings, is musculoskeletal disorders. Loading or unloading freight and carrying or repairing equipment can result in injury if not performed carefully or appropriately. Truck drivers have been thought to be at increased risk of back and neck com-

	Total Cases	Lost Workday Cases		Cases without lost workdays
		Total[1]	With days away from work[2]	
Transportation	7.3	4.4	3.1	2.8
Railroad transportation	3.6	2.8	2.4	8
Local and interurban passenger transit	9.1	4.7	3.5	4.4
Trucking and warehousing	8.7	5.1	3.6	3.6
Water transportation	8.0	4.4	3.8	3.6
Transportation by air	13.3	9.4	6.6	3.9
Transportation services	3.8	2.2	1.3	1.6

[1] Total cases includes days away from work, on restricted duty or both.
[2] Days away from work includes days away from work with or without restricted duty.

FIG. 45.6. Incidence rates (per 100 full-time workers) of nonfatal occupational injuries and illness by transportation type—1999. (Adapted from U.S. Department of Labor, Bureau of Labor Statistics. *Workplace injuries and illness in 1999.* Publication No. USDL 00-357, 2000. Washington, DC: Department of Labor.)

plaints due to vibration and frequent lifting (35). Newer designed cabs may reduce the risk of musculoskeletal disorders.

Diesel fuel is used in both rail (36) and the trucking industry (37), and is believed to be the cause of an increased risk of lung cancer in those exposed. In the event of a spill or accident, workers also may be exposed to whatever hazardous material they are transporting.

Some studies have found an increased risk of cancer among pilots and flight attendants (38). Cosmic radiation has been suggested as a cause, but the amount of exposure and relationship are controversial.

For the occupational health care professional who evaluates workers in safety-sensitive positions in the transportation industry, it is important to remember that their medical status affects not just them but also their co-workers and the general public. For many positions, workers who can do some but not all of their job may be able to be accommodated. If an individual is unable to meet mandated federal medical standards, the only option an employer may have is to find an alternate position if one is available. Both the medical examiner and employer are responsible to ensure not only that the individual is able to perform his job, but also that he can do so without unacceptable risk to others.

REFERENCES

1. Equal Employment Opportunity Commission. *Americans with Disabilities Act Technical Assistance Manual.* Washington, DC: EEOC, 1992.
2. *Sutton v. United Air Lines, Inc.,* 119 S. Ct. 2139, 144 L. Ed. 2d 450, 9 A.D. Cases (U.S. 06/22/1999) U.S. Supreme Court (no. 97-1943, June 22, 1999, vol 1).
3. Department of Transportation, Office of the Secretary. Organization and delegation of powers and duties; redelegation to the director, Office of Motor Carrier Safety. Final rule. *Fed Reg* 1999(October 9);64: 38356–38357.
4. Association for the Advancement of Automotive Medicine. Prototype state medical review program. DTFH 61-90-C-00098, 1995.
5. King D, Benbow SJ, Barrett JA. The law and medical fitness to drive—a study of doctor's knowledge. *Postgrad Med J* 1992;68:624–628.
6. National Transportation Safety Board. Fatigue, alcohol, other drugs and medical factors in fatal-to-driver heavy truck crashes. Washington, DC: PB90-917992, NTSB/ SS-90/01, 1990.

7. Brennan FJ, et al. Assessment of the cardiac patient for fitness to drive: 1996 update. *Can J Cardiol* 1996;12 (11):1164–1170.
8. U.S. Department of Transportation, Federal Motor Carrier Safety Administration. Safety requirements for operators of small passenger-carrying commercial motor vehicles used in interstate commerce; notice of proposed rulemaking (NPRM); request for comments; 49 CFR parts 385, 390 and 398; published: 01/11/2001; 66 FR 2767-2780.
9. U.S. Department of Transportation, Federal Highway Administration, Office of Motor Carriers. Conference on respiratory/pulmonary disorders and commercial drivers. Publication No. FHWA-MC-91-004. Washington, DC: DOT, 1991.
10. U.S. Department of Transportation, Federal Highway Administration, Office of Motor Carriers. Conference on cardiac disorders and commercial drivers. Publication No. FHWA-MC-88-040. Washington, DC: DOT, 1987.
11. U.S. Department of Transportation. Federal Highway Administration. Conference on neurological disorders and commercial drivers. Publication No. FHWA-MC-88-042. Washington, DC: Office of Motor Carriers, 1988.
12. U.S. Department of Transportation. Federal Highway Administration. Conference on psychiatric disorders and commercial drivers. Publication No. FHWA-MC-91-006. Washington, DC: Office of Motor Carriers, 1991.
13. Cox DJ, Gonder-Frederick LA, Kovatchev BP, et al. Progressive hypoglycemia's impact on driving simulation performance: occurrence, awareness, and correction. *Diabetes Care* 2000;23:163–170.
14. Laberge-Nadeau C, Dionne G, Ekoe J, et al. Impact of diabetes on crash risk of truck-permit holders and commercial drivers. *Diabetes Care* 2000;25(5):612–617.
15. U.S. Department of Transportation, Federal Motor Carrier Safety Administration. Final rule; technical amendment. *Fed Reg* 2000(May 1);65:25285–25290.
16. Canadian Medical Association. *Determining medical fitness to drive: a guide for physicians,* 6th ed. 2000. Available and updated on the Internet: *www.cma.ca.*
17. Driver and Vehicle Licensing Agency. For medical practitioners: at a glance guide to the current medical standards of fitness to drive. Swansea, 1999. Available and updated on the Internet: *http://www.dvla.gov.ukat_a_glanceaag_intro.htm.*
18. Australasian Faculty of Occupational Medicine for the National Road Transport Commission. Medical examination of commercial vehicle drivers. April 1997. Available and updated on the Internet: *www.nrtc.gov.au.*
19. Epstein AE, et al. Personal and public safety issues related to arrhythmias that may affect consciousness: implications for regulation and physician recommendations. *Circulation* 1996;94:1147–1166.
20. Petch MC. Driving and heart disease. *Eur Heart J* 1998; 19:1165–1177.
21. Reidel WJ, Schoenmakers EAJM, O'Hanlon JF. Sedation and performance impairment with antihistamines. In: Kalinger MA, ed. *Management of allergy in the 1990s.* Toronto: Hans Huber, 1989:38–49.
22. Kay GG. The effects of antihistamines on cognition and performance. *J Allergy Clin Immunol* 2000;105(6 pt 2) [suppl]:S622–S627.
23. Department of Transportation, Federal Motor Carrier Safety Administration. Physical Qualification of Drivers; medical examinations; certificates. Final rule. *Fed Reg* 2000(October 5);65(194):59363–59379.
24. Netzer NC, Stoohs RA, Netzer CM, et al. Using the Berlin Questionnaire to identify patients at risk for the sleep apnea syndrome. *Ann Intern Med* 1999;131(7): 485–491.
25. Krieger J. Clinical approach to excessive daytime sleepiness. *Sleep* 2000;23[suppl 4]:S95–S98.
26. National Transportation Safety Board. Railroad accident report on near head-on collision and derailment of two New Jersey Transit commuter trains near Secaucus, New Jersey, February 9, 1996. RAR-97-01.
27. U.S. Department of Transportation, Federal Railroad Administration. Final rule, qualification and certification of locomotive engineers. *Fed Reg* 1999;64: 60966–60997.
28. U.S. Department of Transportation, Federal Railroad Administration. Safe use of prescription and over-the counter drugs. *Fed Reg* 1998(December 24);63(247): 71334.
29. U.S. Department of Labor, Bureau of Labor Statistics. Workplace injuries and illness in 1999. Publication No. USDL 00-357. Washington, DC: Department of Labor, 2000.
30. U.S. Department of Labor, Bureau of Labor Statistics. National Census of Fatal Occupational Injuries, 1999. Publication No. USDL 00-236. Washington, DC: Department of Labor, 2000.
31. Mitler MM, Miller JC, et al. The sleep of long-haul drivers. *N Engl J Med* 1997;337:755–761.
32. National Transportation Safety Board. Safety report: evaluation of U.S. Department of Transportation efforts in the 1990s to address operator fatigue. NTSB/SR 99-01. Washington, DC: NTSB, May 1999.
33. National Transportation Safety Board and NASA Ames Research Center. Fatigue symposium proceedings, November 1–2, 1995, Washington, DC.
34. Rosekind MR, Gander PH, Gregory KB, et al. Managing fatigue in operational settings II: an integrated approach. *J Behav Med* 1996;21:166–170.
35. Magnusso ML, Pope MH, Wilder DG, et al. Are occupational drivers an increased risk for developing musculoskeletal disorders? *Spine* 1996;21:710–717.
36. Larkin EK, Smith TJ, Stayner L, et al. Diesel exhaust exposure and lung cancer: adjustment for the effect of smoking in a retrospective cohort study. *Am J Ind Med* 2000;38:399–409.
37. Steenland K, Deddens J, Stayner I. Diesel exhaust and lung cancer in the trucking industry: exposure–response analyses and risk assessment. *Am J Ind Med* 1998;34: 220–228.
38. Ballard T, Lagorio S, De Angelis G, et al. Cancer incidence and mortality among flight personnel: a meta-analysis. *Aviat Space Environ Med* 2000;71(3):216–224.

46

The Construction Industry: Its Occupational Health and Safety Experience and Needs

Jean Spencer Felton

> For we must admit that the workers in certain arts and crafts sometimes derive from them grave injuries, so that where they hoped for a subsistence that would prolong their lives and feed their families, they are too often repaid with the most dangerous diseases and finally, uttering curses on the profession to which they had devoted themselves, they resent their post among the living.
>
> Bernardino Ramazzini, 1700 A.D.

Human creation of shelters as protection against the elements dates back to the late Stone Age. The construction of permanent dwellings began around 10,000 B.C., when agriculture replaced hunting and gathering as a way of life and means of survival (1). Since the agricultural revolution, the development of new technologies has seen the introduction of new building materials such as bricks, bronze, iron, granite, and steel as well as architectural changes that have altered the mode of assembly of these materials. The development of roads, an adaptation of animal paths, dates to 4000 B.C., and with the coming of the Bronze Age and the availability of metal tools, stone paving became much more attainable (1). The demand for such arteries increased with the appearance of wheeled vehicles around 2000 B.C. (1). The Industrial Revolution in Great Britain brought with it the incorporation of glass and iron in structures.

Whereas the early buildings were assembled by carpenters working with wood, other craftsmen came on the scene in the Middle Ages to erect the cathedrals. Some 101 different building personnel were involved, such as porters, stonecutters, sculptors, masons, plasterers, and roofers, among others (2).

Injuries and occupational illnesses have always been concomitants of construction. While lead poisoning had been identified in England in 1776, Thomas Cadwalader described the West Indian gripes and lead poisoning, such observations being published by Benjamin Franklin (3). With Percival Pott's description of scrotal cancer among young chimney sweeps (4), early proscriptive legislation appeared as the Act for the Better Regulation of Chimney Sweepers and Their Apprentices in 1788 (5), specifying protection of a single craft. In the United States in 1789, merchant seamen were the first craft group selected for medical care through what was to become the Public Health Service (6).

During the 18th and 19th centuries, little appeared in the literature concerning occupational injuries, for "the injured slave represented the loss of valuable property—the loss of a white employee represented only the loss of 'another Irishman'" (6). Child labor was rampant, and John Spargo (7) observed, "It is a sorry but indisputable fact that where children are employed, the most unhealthful work is generally given them." The enactment in 1910 of the child labor laws did much to prevent job-associated injuries.

The passage of the early workers' compensation laws marked a move from the then-current principle of needing to prove employer liability, to the principle of no-fault compensation in connection with work-associated injuries. Immediately thereafter, big corporations experienced great decreases in the numbers of disabling injuries (6). Scott Nearing (8), America's eminent sociologist, pointed to the essence of construction industry injuries as far back as 1914 when he wrote that as long as it was cheaper to have accidents than to provide safety devices and exercise ordinary care, injuries may be expected.

Even with the passage of the Occupational Safety and Health Act of 1970, there has been persistent opposition by industry to new occupational safety legislation (9), and Congress has overturned the Occupational Safety and Health Administration's (OSHA) ergonomics standard. And, finally, have we progressed from the view of a major contractor a quarter-century ago who considered 15 or 20 fatalities a year to be a reasonable cost of doing business (10)?

CONSTRUCTION ACTIVITY—THE NATURE OF THE INDUSTRY

The construction industry, because of the admixture of trades, the frequent change of work sites, the variability in duration of employment, and the variety of tasks—maintenance, repair, and creation—differs vastly from other historic organizational undertakings. The workforce in the U.S. is undergoing constant change in its diversity as a result of increasing immigration to this country and the high reproductive rate of those newly arrived.

The construction sector, as defined in the North American Industry Classification System, "comprises establishments primarily engaged in the construction of buildings and other structures, heavy construction (except buildings), additions, alterations, reconstruction, installation, and maintenance and repair." Included also are "those establishments engaged in blasting, test drilling, landfill, leveling, earthmoving, excavating, land drainage, and other land preparation" (11). The activities composing the industry are defined on the basis of their unique production processing, and, similar to other industries, are distinguished by such processes and by the use of specialized human resources and "physical capital" (11). While construction activities are usually administered or managed at a relatively fixed place of business, the actual work, as indicated earlier, is performed at one or more project sites. The establishments involved in these various kinds of construction operate as general contractors, design builders, engineer construction contractors, joint-venture contractors, and turnkey construction contractors. Construction management firms are included.

Special trade contractors embrace such crafts as plumbing, painting, and electrical work, and work for builders and general contractors is conducted under subcontract or directly for project owners. Those organizations engaged in demolishing buildings, dismantling machinery, excavating, boring, foundation drilling, and grading for buildings are included.

The subsector of building, developing, and general contracting constitutes land subdivision and development, and residential and nonresidential building construction. Heavy construction incorporates highway, bridge, and tunnel construction; water, sewer, and pipeline construction; and power—and communication—transmission line construction. The third subsector subsumes plumbing, heating, air conditioning; painting and wall covering; electrical wiring, masonry, stone, drywall, insulation, and tile installation; carpentry; floor laying; roofing, siding, and sheet-metal work; concrete work; water-well drilling; structural steel erection; glazing; excavation; demolition; and machinery installation (12).

Construction is one of the economy's largest industries, and while general contractors may specialize in one type of construction, for example residential building, they assume full responsibility for the complete job, except for a few highly specific tasks. Although such contractors may do a portion of the work with their own crews, they frequently subcontract most of the work to special trade contractors (13).

Construction put in place during January 2001 was estimated at a seasonally adjusted annual rate of $830.5 billion, representing a 3% increase over that of January 2000 (14). Private residential construction was seen to total $263.3 billion, while nonresidential building construction reached $237.9 billion. Public construction was estimated at $188.9 billion (14).

In 1988, there were 5,098,000 jobs in construction, increasing to 5,985,000 in 1998, and projected to reach 6,535,000 in 2008, representing over 4% of all jobs in the U.S. (15). Since October 2000, employment in construction increased, on average, by 37,000 per month, while in the prior 12 months the average monthly increase was only 23,000 (16).

Employment in construction was at a cyclical trough in 1992 of 4.5 million, and then increased 39.6% to 6.3 million in 1999. Employment in the economy as a whole grew 18.8%. In 1999, the construction workweek averaged 39.0 hours, with weekly earnings at $668.07. The hourly earnings of workers in construction reached $17.13, in contrast to $13.24 for all workers. Despite these individual gains, there were 792 mass layoffs in 1999's construction industry, involving 106,686 initial claims for unemployment insurance benefits (17). The injuries and work fatalities sustained are discussed later.

The construction industry itself is optimistic about future growth. Despite a slowdown in the economy, the Associated Builders and Contractors (ABC) forecast a 10th year of growth and expansion. There will be a continuing construction boom in the southeastern U.S., while highway development will remain strong nationwide. The key to the growth lies with the skilled crafts worker. Some 250,000 new workers are needed yearly just to fill the demand resulting from attrition and retirement (18).

In 1998 the Center to Protect Workers' Rights (CPWR), the research and development unit of the Building and Construction Trade Department of the AFL-CIO, published *The Construction Chart Book* (19). While some of its information may be out of date, the book and its graphs give insights into this burgeoning and needed industry (19). Although newer, advanced technologies are changing radically the types of skills required in much of construction, skilled craftspersons will remain essential to the industry. Joint labor–management apprenticeships and training programs will continue to maintain the skilled workforce needed.

A breakdown of 1992 data reveals the distribution end of the goals of the construction dollar: materials, 30.1%; subcontracting, 25.9%; wages, 22.3%; benefits, 5.6%; services, 1.7%; rentals, 1.6%; power and fuel, 1.6%; other, 11.2%. The varying size of construction establishments is as follows: one to nine employees, 519,300 establishments; 10 to 99 employees, 110,000 establishments; 100 to 499 employees, 4,600 establishments; and 500 or more employees, 200 establishments. Thus, most construction companies are small (1.4 million employees in establishments of one to nine workers), and, as will be seen later, this factor may account for the human injury toll encountered in these undertakings (19).

Nearly 2 million companies were under sole proprietorship in 1994, but it was the approximately 200 corporations that produced the largest income in 1994 of nearly $370 million (19). Women owned 10.0% of all construction companies in 1992, compared to a 34.1% ownership overall in industry. Blacks owned 2.4% of building companies, in contrast to 3.6% of all industry. Hispanics were higher in construction ownership at 5.3%, with but 4.5% ownership of all industries (19).

The occupational distribution showed managers, carpenters, laborers, and some others comprising 52% of the personnel involved, while 21 other trades made up the remainder of construction participants (19).

Union membership in 1996 was higher at 21% in construction than the 16% affiliation in all other industries (19). Such membership, as shown by selected occupation, placed ironworkers highest at 57%. Some 40% of electrical workers and 37% of sheet-metal workers followed (19).

Age considerations are of interest, for construction workers as a group are slightly younger that those of other industries. The average age in 1996 was 37.0 years, in contrast to 38.0 years of wage-and-salary workers in all industries. Employees in racial minorities, as a percentage of all workers in a particular industry in 1996, were at the 10% level, with Hispanic employees at 12% in construction. The number grew from 8.9% in 1985 to the 812,000 men and women encountered 11 years later. Hispanic workers who were unionized earned a greater hourly wage (19).

Of all growing groups in this industry, women have outpaced most others and receive higher wages in construction than in all industries. In 1996, there were 813,000 women so employed, representing 10% of the total workforce. Union pay was higher for women members than for those not in organized labor (19). Most of the women (53%) were in administrative support, with another 29% in management, leaving 19% actually involved in the manual trades.

While many are working longer today in all jobs, construction personnel averaged 39.7 hours per week. Certain crafts, in greater demand, put in more overtime, but, in keeping with a belief common to all occupations, "overtime for several weeks worsens productivity and increases costs per unit of production," an observation resulting from studies both by the Business Roundtable and the National Electrical Contractors Association (19).

Those workers in construction having a high school diploma or higher education were at the 68.7% level with those in all industries at 87.2% (19).

Although apprentice programs are the best route to learning a trade, most learn the details of their craft through on-the-job training, by working under the supervision of experienced workers (20).

BASELINE FOR CONSTRUCTION SAFETY

In keeping with federal legislation, the construction industry comprises the construction, alteration, and/or repair of structures, in addition to painting and decorating, and "no contractor or subcontractor...shall require any laborer or mechanic employed in the performance of the contract to work in surroundings or under working conditions which are unsanitary, hazardous, or dangerous to his health or safety" (21).

STATISTICS ON CONSTRUCTION SAFETY

Despite the above precautionary federal note, workers in construction face special hazards, as evidenced by the significant number of work-related illnesses, injuries, and fatalities recorded each year. While sources of information vary in their content, recent data show over 8.5 million persons employed in construction, with 90.6% of them being male (22).

Injuries sustained on the job, in contradistinction to illnesses, are more readily categorized because their occurrence as to place and time is much more obvious. The designation of an illness as occupational in etiology is less exact because such illnesses may take years to manifest themselves and may be influenced in their development by such adverse lifestyle factors as smoking, or such nonoccupational factors as age, family history, or exposure to nonavocational noise (23).

Innumerable epidemiologic studies have been conducted of the morbidity and mortality associated with work in the industry, shedding light on the type of injury and the cause, and the gender, age, ethnicity, union membership, and trade of the individuals sustaining the injuries. In addition, the influence of drug and alcohol usage, the temporary or permanent status of the employees, socioeconomic status, the element of injury repetition, and the state or country in which the injuries took place are other variables that have been studied.

Note that the term "accident" is not used now, as the designation "unintentional injury" is preferred (24). A study of sufficient depth usually discloses a fault in the worker's behavior, in the work process, in the manufacturing system, or in the equipment that can account for the injurious effect on the employee. A contemporary definition of "accident" includes the absence of intention, thus being supportive of the preferred term: "An undesirable or unfortunate happening that occurs unintentionally and usually results in injury, damage, or loss" (25).

It must be emphasized that the many reviews of construction-related injuries involve different cohorts of workers; different points in time, as there is the usual delay in analysis; different sources of data collection and reporting; and occasionally, different definitions of the terminology utilized. While the standard statistical base in the U.S. is that of the Bureau of Labor Statistics (BLS) of the Department of Labor, other sources may vary in the elements utilized in epidemiologic approach, rendering comparisons not always feasible.

Overall Injuries

Injuries and illnesses accounted for 1,833,380 days away from work nationwide in 1997. Construction laborers, carpenters, welders, and cutters were among the ten occupations with the highest injury-related absences, accounting for 111,000 lost days (22). The construction industry in the period 1980–1995 had a rate of 15.3 fatal occupational injuries per 100,000 workers, or 18.3% of the nearly 94,000 deaths recorded in that period (27). Nonfatal injuries in private industry in 1997 with and without lost workdays showed construction at 47% of all injuries or a total of 486,000, almost evenly divided between injuries involving lost workdays and those not involving lost workdays (25).

All industries demonstrated an increase in the percentage of nonfatal occupational injury cases, with lost workdays involving restricted work activity (limited duty) only between 1992 and 1997 (29). Construction was the lowest of eight industrial divisions at 18% of such injured workers, bespeaking the fact that restricted work in that industry may not be feasible.

Fatalities

In 1999, fatal work injuries numbered 6,023, essentially the same as those job-related deaths in 1998 (30). The construction industry experienced the greatest number of fatalities of any industry, accounting for one fifth of the total, or 1,190 deaths. Of these losses, 709 were of special trades contractors, 280 were in heavy construction exclusive of building, and 183 general building contractors were injured fatally at work. Of 717 on-the-job falls that resulted in death, half occurred in construction, such as falls from a roof, ladder, or scaffolds (30).

These data include those deaths occurring in 1999 that resulted from traumatic occupational injuries, such injuries being defined as follows:

> Any intentional or unintentional wound or damage to the body resulting from acute exposure to energy, such as heat, electricity, or kinetic energy from a crash or from the absence of such essentials as heat or oxygen caused by a specific event, incident, or series of events within a single workday or shift. Included are open wounds, intracranial and internal injuries, heatstroke, hypothermia, asphyxiations, acute poisonings resulting from short-term exposures limited to the worker's shift, suicides and homicides, and work injuries listed as underlying or contributory causes of death (30).

It is to be noted that work-related fatal illnesses are not included in this particular BLS census because the delay in the development of symptoms or the latency of linking illnesses to work "make identification of a universe problematic" (30). However, in a separate compilation, some 529 fatalities are credited to "exposure to harmful substances or environments." There were 278 electrocutions and 106 deaths resulting from "exposure to caustic, noxious, or allergenic substances or environments." Some numbers were reported by specific occupation for the construction trades. Of 633 fatalities where the occupation and event or exposure was known in 1999 data, 542 were among tradesmen other than supervisors. Carpenters and electricians and their apprentices accounted for 208 of these job-related deaths (31).

The essence of these figures lies in the fact that the construction industry accounted for 20% of the fatalities, three times its 6% share of total employment.

Nonfatal Injuries

Databases vary based on the reporting sources and the particular selection of the industries included for compilation. For examples, the BLS figures exclude the self-employed, farms with fewer than 11 employees, private households, federal government agencies, and, for national estimates, employees in state and local government agencies (32). Such omissions may minimize some of the totals of injuries actually sustained by comparable craftsmen working at other sites.

In this tabulation of nonfatal occupational injuries and illnesses for 1999, the average annual employment for the construction industry was given as 6,337,300; special trade contractors numbered 4,024,100; general building contractors totaled 1,453,300; and those workers engaged in heavy construction other than building totaled 860,000.

For the year, there were 493,000 cases of injury. Resulting from these injuries were 190,600 workers who lost work time. An additional 252,900 injuries were sustained, but no time was lost from the job. If illnesses were added to the total number of injuries, the figures rose to 501,400, of which 243,800 workers lost 193,800 days of work. The greatest percentage of injuries was experienced by the special trade contractors at 63.5%.

The incidence rate of nonfatal injuries, or the number of injuries per 100 full-time workers, was 8.4 for construction, second only to durable goods manufacture at 8.8. By size of establishment, the rate was highest among construction workers in establishments of 50 to 249 employees at 10.5 (32).

The illnesses encountered among construction workers in 1999 are as follows:

Total cases	8,400
Skin disorders	1,700
Dust diseases of the lungs	100
Respiratory conditions due to toxic agents	600
Poisonings	200
Disorders due to physical agents	600
Disorders associated with repeated trauma	3,100
All others	2,000

Over the years, since 1996, the incidence rate of nonfatal occupational injuries and illnesses declined from 9.9 to 8.6, with lost-time cases decreasing from 3.7 to 3.3, and cases without lost workdays decreasing from 5.4 to 4.4 (32).

Characteristics of Injuries

Details of lost work time injuries and illnesses are available for 1999 (33). Of the ten occupations with the greatest number of lost-time injuries and illnesses, construction laborers and carpenters ranked fourth and seventh with 46,500 and 35,000, respectively, out of a total of 1,702,500.

Of 582,300 musculoskeletal disorders, the construction industry experienced 48,800, with a median of 10 days away from work. In that industrial division, construction laborers sustained 11,000 such injuries, with a median or 7 days lost from work.

Sprain and strain led the injuries and illnesses in every major industry division, while the trunk, including the back, was the body part most affected by disabling work incidents in all industries except finance, insurance, and real estate (32). With the same exceptions, overexertion while maneuvering objects and coming in contact with objects and equipment led all other disabling events or exposures. Among construction workers, heating, air conditioning, and refrigeration mechanics had the highest median days away from work (each with 10 days) along with public transportation attendants (33).

Worker characteristics are of interest in reviewing construction experience. Of 193,800 nonfatal injuries and illnesses, men accounted for 188,600, and women 4,600. Workers of ages 35 to 44 years had 59,200 injuries, whereas those of ages 25 to 34 years numbered 58,200 injuries. When race or ethnic origin was reported (162,300 cases), the following percentages of the injuries and illnesses were noted:

White, non-Hispanic	74.8%
Black, non-Hispanic	5.9%
Hispanic	17.7%
Asian or Pacific Islander	0.008%
American Indian or Alaskan Native	0.0067%

Most of the lost-time injuries were encountered among the following construction crafts:

- Construction laborers
- Carpenters
- Electricians
- Plumbers and pipefitters
- Helpers

The 193,800 lost-time injuries in the construction industry were classified as follows:

Sprains, strains	72,400
Cuts, lacerations	19,700
Fractures	19,100
Bruises, contusions	13,900
Multiple injuries	8,500
Heat burns	2,400
Chemical burns	1,900
Amputations	1,400
Carpal tunnel syndrome	1,200
Tendonitis	800

The numbers shown in the breakdowns do not always approach the total results because of "the inability to obtain detailed information about all cases in the sample, mistakes in recording or coding the data, and definitional difficulties"; thus, nonsampling errors occur (33).

While the numbers of injuries shown are presented with some inexactitude, they still depict great losses in wages and productivity, high health care costs, and personal hurt. Factors that influence the numbers shown are the level of economic activity, working conditions and practices, worker experience and training, and the number of hours worked (33).

As indicated earlier, some conditions such as long-term latent illnesses caused by exposure to carcinogens, are often difficult to tie to the workplace and are not fully recognized or reported, and thus are believed to be underrepresented. The great majority of the reported new illnesses, e.g., contact dermatitis or carpal tunnel syndrome, are most readily identified with work activity (33).

While other details concerning the injuries sustained in construction could be dissected from the BLS data, one can see that a problem exists. Because of the idiosyncratic means of conducting most of the industrial processes, where workers, workplace, work authority, and work demands shift with such great frequency, programs that emphasize occupational safety and health are difficult to conduct.

International Scene

Even though the rate of occupational injuries and illnesses in construction in the U.S. has decreased from 14.6 cases per 100 full-time workers in 1998 to 8.6 in 1999, the problem exists universally. U.S. Surgeon General David Satcher (35) observed that the overall issue of injuries is still a neglected area in national, and particularly international, health policies. Injuries represent a primary cause of death, posing an enormous public health burden worldwide. Satcher concludes, "The global community can increase its collective investment in safety and injury prevention. This investment opportunity is simply too compelling to ignore, with enormous potential gains for all people."

Concern has been expressed internationally. Construction in Spain has accounted for nearly 250 fatalities a year (36). In Kuwait, construction is the most hazardous industry, accounting for 34% of all disabling injuries and 42% of all fatalities in 1996 (37). For the most recent reporting period in Great Britain—April 1 through September 30, 2000—the construction industry sustained 62 fatalities, including employees, the self-employed, and even four members of the public (38). Of 87 reported deaths following work events, 50% were falls that occurred in Israel's construction industry (39). The characteristics of construction injuries in Korea showed that fatalities occurred more often in older workers; falls from a height were the most common accidents; fractures led the injuries by type; fatalities resulted most often from head, face, and neck trauma; and most of the injuries "occurred from...temporary construction or fabric[ation]" (40).

Construction workers have been studied in Japan with concerns involving back pain and shoulder stiffness (41,42), asbestos-related malignancies, and injury fatalities (43). In Finland, asbestos exposure and resulting radiographic abnormalities were surveyed (44), as were construction site injuries (45). Italian construction workers were investigated in connection with injuries and fatalities (46,47) and the development of asbestosis and mesothelioma in connection with the application of asbestos products (48,49).

New construction in China accounted for 55% of the fatalities (50), and its workers had an average annual mortality rate of 57.5 per 100,000 such workers, with falls the leading cause of death at 46.4% (51). Similar studies have emanated from Ireland (52), Taiwan (53), Canada (45,55), South Africa (56), Australia (57), Germany (58), and Great Britain (5,60), among others.

Given this universality of concern, have other efforts been made to define the elements causative of, and associated with, this human trauma and these lives lost?

PERTINENT RESEARCH INTO RELATED FACTORS

Many epidemiologic studies have been conducted in an effort to identify characteristics of the injured, the work practices involved, the external negating influences or risk factors, and the idiosyncrasies of construction when compared with other industrial divisions.

Experience by State

Whereas national data are gathered by the U.S. Department of Labor, injury epidemiology has been conducted in some of the states. In North Carolina, for the years 1977 to 1991, the construction industry was among the largest contributors to unintentional work fatalities, logging some 16.8% of over 2,500 deaths. Decentralized and rural industries were the most hazardous (61). In a more recent review of nearly 4,000 deaths occurring between 1988 and 1994, a major cause of work-related motor vehicle incidents included back-overs on construction sites and injuries to drivers caused by shifting loads while transporting construction materials. High in frequency also were injuries associated with erecting, moving, and disassembling scaffolds and working on scaffolds. Electrocutions occurred most often among craftsmen who were neither electricians nor linemen (62).

In West Virginia, there were 182 fall injuries in 1991, most of the events occurring among young white males working as craftsmen or laborers on nonunion jobs. The counties with rates exceeding the state rate were located around or near major industrial areas. One third of the injured claimants had been employed in these occupations 2 years or less, 26% being employed 6 months or less. Fall protection devices were not in common usage (63). In a later period, 1996 to 1999, there were 163 work-related fatalities (23 in construction), 93% of whom were male, with a mean age of 42 years and 80% being West Virginia residents (64).

Similar state studies incriminating the construction industry have been conducted in Alaska (65), Washington (66), Massachusetts (67), and Iowa and Illinois (68).

Why some jurisdictions convert collected data to publications in the medical literature is probably dependent on many factors. Academicians in public and occupational health believe that information concerning injuries and fatalities should be made known to other investigators similarly troubled by the harm accruing from work. As great numbers of construction personnel are affected by the risks of work, attention should be directed to both the lay and professional readerships concerning these employment mishaps. Primarily, though, it is hoped that such studies will aid in developing better preventive measures and help in planning further research priorities. From such state-based publications in national media should develop a greater awareness of the hazards of building and the means needed to reverse the trend of trauma associated with a burgeoning industry.

Factor of Age

As construction continues to increase nationwide to meet both human and industrial needs, questions arise as to the safety of certain workers. Despite the mass layoffs in the last decades of the 20th century, many employees are working at older ages, and many young workers disdain a college education in favor of immediate financial gain.

In the Netherlands, as an example, an increase in the morbidity and disability rates is expected owing to the aging of the workforce. Advancing age brings new health problems in addition to exacerbating previously existing disorders, particularly musculoskeletal disturbances among construction workers. One function of an occupational health service (OHS) would be to maintain or improve the health of such seniors (69).

In the U.S., the Centers for Disease Control and Prevention found that the construction industry had one of the highest workplace fatality rates for older workers (aged 65 and older) when compared with younger employees in the industry, aged 16 to 64. Older men were at a higher risk for fatalities caused by machines, and older women for fatal falls and homicide. Such elevated rates require special preventive action (70).

Attention has been given the injuries sustained by adolescents in New Zealand, as studied by University of North Carolina researchers. Data obtained form an emergency department covered occupational injuries among youths aged 15 through 19 years. The injury rate was 13.8 per 200,000 hours worked (100 full-time equivalents) during a 4-year period. The rate for males was 206 injuries, and for females, 5.8 injuries. The hands, eyes, and lower extremities were the prominent sites of trauma, with lacerations, sprains/strains, and foreign bodies the leading types of injury. The rate was highest for 16- and 17-year-olds, decreasing for workers of ages 18 and 19. The rates of injuries in the construction sector were the highest of all occupational groups at 27 injuries per

200,000 hours (71). The focus of OHS efforts is clearly directed.

Adolescents were similarly reviewed in the state of Washington, covering the period 1988 to 1991. Again, construction displayed one of the highest rates of 21.1 injuries per 100 workers. When adjusted for hours worked, the rate for 16- and 17-year-olds was 19.4 per 100 full-time equivalents in contrast to adults at 10.6 per full-time equivalents. Of nearly 18,000 workers' compensation claims from 11- to 17-year-olds, there were three fatalities, 22 amputations, and almost 500 fractures. The 16- and 17-years-olds sustained 89% of all the injuries (72). A British study summarized the issue well: "Our findings indicate that it is time to look at the occupational health of children as a major concern" (73).

Fatalities

The severest construction injuries lead to the death of workers, with the attendant effects on survivors, both the families of those killed and fellow workers, particularly those associates who were witness to the injury. Other elements of concern are the disruption of work and productivity losses; the costs of medical care, workers' compensation, employee replacement, potential liability suits, and rectification of effects on fellow workers, including psychotherapy if indicated; possible prolonged downtime at the construction site; and property damage or loss, potential police costs, and administrative expenses. The unintentional injury costs in the U.S. in 1999 reached nearly $469 billion overall (74).

An early OSHA study analyzed nearly 3,500 construction fatalities for the period 1985 to 1989 (75). The primary findings showed deaths from the following causes:

Fall from elevation	33%
Struck by an object	22%
Caught in between	18%
Shock (electrical)	17%
Other	10%

OSHA conducts about 700 fatality investigations annually. Little difference is noted in the days of occurrence, the age of the workers lost, or in the union or nonunion status of the work site, the last paralleling the numbers in such association. Firm size and percentage of fatalities were in a direct match, and the causes of fatalities were similar in both federal OSHA states and state-plan states. The four major causes of death, as noted above, did not vary significantly over the 5-year period. Roofs and scaffolds were the primary locations of fatalities due to falls from elevation, 40% of these falls involving elevations greater than 30 feet; 25% were from distances of 11 to 20 feet; and 25% were from distances of 21 to 30 feet (75).

"Struck by" fatalities involved trucks, cranes, graders, or scrapers, many of the deaths being caused by poor rigging of the loads being moved or poor storage of materials. Seventy-nine percent of trenching fatalities occurred in trenches under depths of 15 feet, 38% taking place in trenches less than 10 feet deep. Electric shock losses involved, in 74% of the fatalities, voltages in excess of 480 V, and 65% of the losses involved contact with overhead power lines. Of the latter, 53% were related to construction equipment (75).

Fatalities and Type of Work

While there has been some improvement over the years, there is still considerable concern. Secretary of Labor Alexis Herman stated, following the release of 1999 data that showed a total of nearly 1,500 fatal work injuries overall, that the report "shows that we must do more to prevent workplace fatalities in the construction industry, just as we have reduced homicides in the workplace" (76). Because of the industry's accounting for 20% of all workplace deaths, the highest for any industry, preventive action is indicated.

In an effort to understand the causation of these deaths, several epidemiologic studies have focused on the type of work. Particular attention has been directed to deaths by electrocution, "fatal incidents involving workers who contacted energized electrical conductors or equipment," such equipment ranging from contact with a broken light bulb to an energized overhead power line (77–79). Construction workers were four times more likely to be electrocuted at work than were workers in all industries combined, 80% being associate with wiring, appliances, and transmission lines (78). Those craftsmen most at risk were male, young, and nonwhite, and worked as electricians, structural metal workers, and laborers (78). In addition, the painting and roofing trades had greater proportions of electrical death (79).

Falls from elevations are potentially fatal in all industries and are seen in a myriad of work settings, from a stock clerk retrieving goods from a shelf or changing a light bulb while using a 4-foot ladder, to an ironworker connecting steel columns or bolts 200 feet in the air (80). From 1980 through 1994, falls were, overall, the fourth leading cause of death at the workplace, being experienced from ladder use (fixed or portable), from scaffolds used in all varieties of construction activity, from roof and floor openings and edges, and from poles, towers, bridges, tanks, and platforms (80).

Fall protection has been well outline by the National Institute for Occupational Safety and Health (NIOSH) (81). In need of clarification, among other statistical findings, is the reason for the highest fatalities rates being observed within subregions of the southern states in the United States (82).

Forklift operation caused over 1,000 deaths from 1980 through 1994, resulting in nearly 28,000 years of productive life lost. Most common were overturns, striking of pedestrians, and crushing of workers. Construction caused 16% of the total fatalities. Most deaths could have been prevented through the use of restraining belts or traffic control (83). NIOSH has suggested the needed precautionary measures (84).

In the period 1980 to 1992, there were 2,144 work-related motor vehicle fatalities in the U.S. construction industry, the rate not diminishing over the years as with falls, electrocutions, and machinery-contact fatalities (85). Construction accounted for 25% of all pedestrian deaths, but 6% were flaggers or surveyors. Half of the 34 pedestrian deaths among women involved flaggers, while only 3% of male deaths were seen in flaggers. It was concluded that modes of prevention should become a research priority in construction.

Machinery-related fatalities in construction were fourth in number between 1980 and 1992, resulting in 1,900 deaths. Involved primarily were workers in three divisions: precision production, craft, and repair; transportation and material moving; and handlers, equipment cleaners, helpers, and laborers (86). The machinery involved mostly included cranes, excavating equipment, and tractors. Prevention programs were indicated not only for operators but also for those persons working on foot around machines (86).

The role of socioeconomic status in construction injuries has not been addressed specifically, but research into injury mortality overall has shown that it "is an important structural factor that influences injury" (87). While workplace injury data do consider race or ethnic origin, level of occupation, age, and gender, the social factors viewed as determinants of premature morbidity, death, and disability outcomes have not been applied to injury studies. Socioeconomic status has been suggested as an important risk factor for injury mortality (87), and such research is indeed indicated. However, in a review of work-related injuries in an inner-city population in Philadelphia, it was concluded that poor and minority workers were at risk for a broad range of occupational injuries, many in construction. Such injuries could result in a considerable amount of lost time with serious medical and economic consequences (88).

Types of Injuries and Illness

Injuries

The injuries sustained in construction do not differ clinically from those sustained in other industrial divisions, although certain body traumas are more prevalent. Injuries resulting from work in vessels or with tools under air pressure have been identified (89). Nail-gun injuries to the hand are relatively unique to the construction industry in both the U.S. (90,91) and England (92). The industry was noted in Washington State as the highest in the number of claims for work-related musculoskeletal disorders of the neck, back, and upper extremity (93). Shoulder tendonitis was prominent among Swedish construction workers (94), and nasal malignancies have been seen in woodworkers (95), the condition being either an illness or injury as individually perceived. Hand-transmitted vibration was common in construction workers using hammer drills, hand-held portable grinders, and jigsaws (96).

Occupational Illness

A common assumption is that construction workers are physically injured with regularity, but probably do not contact job-generated illnesses. Much evidence to the contrary points to the presence of a broad variety of both acute disorders and those with long periods of latency.

The pairing of diseases and jobs has been done for the construction trades, in which some 12 craft groups have been shown to have exposure to toxic materials potentially productive of occupational illnesses (97), exclusive of cancer and skin irritation.

Two examples are given:

Job Title	Hazardous Job Task (Associated Disease)
Insulator	Installed installation before 1975 (asbestosis)
	Remove insulation installed before 1975 (asbestosis)
	Work with glue solvents (acute solvent syndrome)
	Use *n*-hexane as glue solvent (peripheral neuropathy after prolonged high exposure)

Use epoxy in isocyanate sealants, adhesives, or foams [allergic contact dermatitis (ACD), occupational asthma (OA)]

Sheet metal worker
- Installed insulation before 1975 (asbestosis)
- Remove insulation installed before 1975 (asbestosis)
- Machine metal (ACD, OA, hypersensitivity pneumonitis)
- Machine lead (lead poisoning)
- Degrease metal (acute solvent syndrome)
- Solder or braze (ACD, OA)
- Braze using cadmium-based solder (cadmium poisoning)
- Forge metal (carbon monoxide poisoning)
- Weld (lead poisoning, ACD, OA, cadmium poisoning, metal fume fever, carbon monoxide poisoning, acute inhalation injury from NO_2, ozone and phosgene, siderosis, manganese poisoning, polymer fume fever)

Similar matchings are made for roofers; brick, block and stone masons; concrete or terrazzo workers; carpenters; construction, industrial, or maintenance painters; electricians/repairers of transformers, electrical, or electronic equipment; plumbers, pipe fitters, or steamfitters; welders, cutters, or burners; heating and air condition installers; and dry wall tapers and plasterers (97).

An attorney firm in California has made available on the Internet a list of chemicals commonly found in construction and industrial settings, stating, "They should never be used without protective clothing and breathing protection. . . . To easily learn how dangerous the...chemicals are, [one should] ask your local dump operator how to legally dispose of them" (98). The chemicals used in construction include the following:

- Benzene
- Polyvinyl chloride
- Trichloroethylene
- Perchloroethylene
- Polychlorinated biphenyls
- Methyl ethylketone
- Chlorinated hydrocarbons: dioxins and furans
- Fiberglass

Most of the evidence of human toxicity is given in the descriptions of the chemicals.

Outstanding over the years in occupational medicine (OM) has been the exposure to lead and the resulting lead poisoning. As recently as 1992, NIOSH sought assistance in the prevention of such intoxication specifically in workers engaged in maintenance, repainting, or demolition of bridges or other steel structures coated with lead-containing paints. The operations involved in the production of extremely high concentrations of lead dust and fumes included abrasive blasting, sanding, burning, cutting, or welding (99). Symptoms of such toxicity may be mild and go undetected for a while, may be acute, or may lead to fatality.

Lead poisoning in bridge demolition workers has been described by NIOSH (100,101), and in an effort to control such intoxication, several public agencies initiated the Connecticut Road Industry Surveillance Project (CRISP) to incorporate protective measures into contracts in addition to the use of regulatory measures (101,102). While action proved effective in that state, other jurisdictions still had workers with elevated blood lead levels. The lead in construction standard promulgated by OSHA in mid-1993 was effective in lowering the hazardous levels (103). The action was necessary in light of this nation's deteriorating infrastructure (103,104). Despite the positive effects of CRISP and application of the OSHA standard, lead poisoning persists in construction (105–109).

The striking history of workers' exposure to asbestos has been well documented, a tale highly illustrative of the industrial denial of the hazards associated with this universally applied insulating material (110). While its use has been restricted in keeping with federal regulation (111), there are four classes of construction activity involving contact with this material (112):

- Class I: removal of thermal system insulations.
- Class II: removal of other types of asbestos-containing materials such as flooring or roofing.
- Class III: repair and maintenance operations where asbestos-containing materials are disturbed
- Class IV: custodial activities involving cleanup of asbestos-containing waste and debris.

Medical examinations of asbestos workers are mandated, and the examining physician must be apprised of the current standards, the worker's job description, and the information to be given the examinee.

The progressive form of diffuse pulmonary fibrosis was observed early, and subsequently the excess risk of lung cancer and mesothelioma was noted among asbestos workers (113). There is a small association between exposure to asbestos and some gastrointestinal cancer (114), and contact with asbestos waste still can produce pleural mesothelioma (115). Asbestos-related disease persists in Ireland (116) and in Australian construction workers (117), and Australia "has one of the highest national incidences of mesothelioma in the world and the rate is still rising" (118).

Other illnesses stemming directly from construction work have been observed. Pulmonary diseases such as silicosis, frequently complicated by tuberculosis and cancer, have been noted (119). It is impossible to determine with any accuracy which exposed workers will develop a lung disorder and which, with an equivalent exposure, will not. But in view of OM's being subsumed under preventive medicine, the awareness of workers' respiratory environment is mandatory in forestalling the onset of frank disease. Also, construction workers face some of the highest respirable crystalline silica dust concentrations (masonry, heavy construction, painting, shipbuilding and repair, and bridge, tunnel and elevated highway construction) (120,121).

Construction boilermakers have manifested pulmonary symptoms and lower lung function (122), while construction workers have developed respiratory tract malignancies, pulmonary and pleural fibrosis, airway diseases, inhalation injuries, and respiratory infection (123). Lung cancer has been associated with construction in Canada (124), China (125), Argentina (126), and Uruguay (127).

Dermatoses have been described among construction workers (128,129), as have the prolonged exposures to sources of vibration (130). Long work periods with environmental heat led to increased inhalation of particulates (manganese, nickel, and chromium), especially among boilermakers, pipefitters, and welder-fitters (131), and in the highway construction industry (132). Hearing loss is common in this industry, warranting frequent audiometric testing (133–135). Among recent reviews have been meta-analyses of epidemiologic studies of workers exposed to asphalt. Such contact produced irritation of the eyes, nose, and throat, and also of the lower respiratory tract. Whether such work contacts produce chronic respiratory disorders like bronchitis or lung cancer remains to be determined (136).

Lastly, tremors have been detected in crafts workers exposed to aluminum (137).

From a larger view, partly because of the transfer abroad of hazardous work processes from industrialized countries, there is substantial exposure to asbestos in developing countries. The prevention of resulting malignancies can only result from political and economic changes (138).

The difficulties with the identification of work-related illness include the mobility of the construction craftsman from job to job, the late appearance of symptoms specific to particular toxic exposure, the lack of knowledge of the poisonous content of building materials on the part of both the contract employer and the worker, and the constant pressure toward completion of the project. Until physicians in general practice, to whom many construction workers go, become sensitized to the effects of common work contactants, occupational diseases may go unrecognized for years.

Related Factors

The federal Healthy People 2010 report states in the section on occupational safety and health that "little is known about factors such as gender, genetic susceptibility, culture, and literacy that may increase the risk for occupational disease and injury." Specialists agreed that "many high-risk populations have been underserved by the occupational safety and health community, resulting in important unanswered questions about the profile of hazards these workers face, the number of cases of work-related injuries and illnesses, the mechanisms of these injuries and illnesses, and the optimal approach to preventing them" (139).

However, some efforts have been made to identify relationships of factors in the construction scene. Hispanic workers in the industry have been reviewed and in one study it was concluded that minority status was a predictor of trade and that the resulting affiliating trade was a predictor of injury risk. It was suggested that increasing union membership among such workers would be helpful (140).

While many of the research efforts in the construction industry involved union members as study subjects (141,142), none pointed up any contrast in injury or illness as determined by unionization of the craft or particular members. Currently, in an investigation jointly sponsored by the CPWR and Duke University, the medical care received through union programs and workers' compensation is being studied (143).

COMORBIDITY AND MORTALITY PATTERNS

An area clouded by a lack of definition is the presence of coexisting disease and causes of death among construction workers. Are the symptoms or disorders of certain bodily organ systems immediately related to the occupational exposure(s), or would they have appeared irrespective of the trade or vocation? Roofers demonstrated significantly increased proportionate mortality rates (PMRs) for lung, bladder, esophageal, laryngeal, and other cancers, in addition to pneumoconiosis and other nonmalignant respiratory diseases (144). Carpenters had an elevated PMR for pulmonary cancer and mesothelioma, and gastric, bone, and breast cancer (141). Both worker groups had, in addition, elevated PMRs for injuries. Operating engineers, responsible for the operation of heavy earth-moving equipment used in the construction of building, bridges, roads, and other facilities, had significantly elevated mortality for lung and bone malignancies, in addition to leukemia and aleukemia (145).

Construction workers in North Carolina displayed elevated PMRs for malignancies of the buccal cavity, pharynx, and lung "possibly related to work" (146). A death-certificate study project covered cause-of-death data for 1,713,413 black and white men and women, considering, in addition, occupational and industry categories. Occupations in construction with the highest PMRs for selected causes of deaths, other than injuries, were as follows (147):

- Malignant neoplasm of trachea, bronchus, and lung—insulation workers (white males)
- Malignant neoplasm of brain and nervous system—electrical and electronic engineers (white males)
- Malignant neoplasm of esophagus—painters, construction workers (black males)
- Alcohol-associated disorders—painters, construction workers (black males)
- Ischemic heart disease other than acute myocardial infarction—crane and tower operators (black males)
- Pneumonia and influenza—helpers, construction trades (black males)
- Suicide—painters (white females)

A similar review of occupation and industry codes on death certificates for causes other than injuries, showed the following for elevated PMRs (148):

- Cancer and several other chronic diseases—white male construction workers
- Cancer, mental disorders, alcohol-related disease, digestive diseases, poisonings, homicides—males younger than age 65 years
- Similar causes, but to a lesser degree—black men and white women in construction
- Cancer of the connective tissue and suicide—white women
- Bone cancer and melanoma—brick masons
- Gastric cancer—roofers and brick masons
- Renal and bone cancer—concrete/terrazzo finishers
- Nasal cancer—plumbers
- Pulmonary tuberculosis—laborers
- Scrotal cancer and aplastic anemia—electricians
- Acute myeloid leukemia—boilermakers
- Rectal cancer and multiple sclerosis—electrical power installers
- Lung cancer—structural metal workers

There are unquestionably lifestyle factors involved in the etiology of many of these disorders, which makes work-relatedness extremely difficult to establish. Further, many claims of job origin of one or another of these illnesses are filed late, thus placing environmental and clinical findings in different time frames. There may be familial or genetic factors to cloud the etiologic understanding, and the clinical evidence may be manifested years after the employee in question left a specific point of contact, a challenge to the limited record retention system encountered in construction. Lastly, many of the laborers may be in the U.S. illegally, further rendering an investigation difficult or even unwanted. The relationship of work exposures to disease development has been explored among foreign workers also (149–151), with the same conclusions of a "small but significant role [of occupation]" (149), or that "occupational exposures seem to contribute" (150).

Additional factors concerning all-case mortality include, as intimated earlier, alcohol consumption (62,146,152,153), aging (69), preexisting disease (154), all anthropometric measurements (weight, height, body mass index, lean body mass) in construction workers with prostatic cancer (155), and smoking (156,157), among others.

There is an aftermath to construction injuries. Acute musculoskeletal injuries frequently result in chronic symptoms, changes that not only affect the quality of life but also require job accommodations (158). The increase in use of temporary workers introduces stresses not associated with most permanent employment. Such status can limit the reporting of injuries and hence the needed care and increased fear of future trauma because of the added vulnerability (159). Lifestyle factors can lead to prolonged unemployment among construction workers, worsening the associated stress and the effects of previous injuries; the factors include age greater than 40 years, poor subjective health, smoking, frequent and heavy use of alcohol, low job satisfaction, and single marital status (160).

Construction workers have had a high suicide rate, relating possibly to "sociodemographic differences, self-selection for occupation, ease of access to lethal agents, or job stress" (161). It is difficult to do follow-up of injuries or illnesses sustained on the job because of turnover in the construction industry, which relates to the strongest predictor of job change, i.e., extrinsic satisfaction, and somewhat less so to satisfaction with a supervisor (162). Finally, a factor that can relate to the underlying psychopathology or stress on the job or elsewhere is the matter of injury repetition; in the past such workers were labeled "accident-prone." Early addressing of the individual's job behavior is indicated (162).

PSYCHOSOCIOLOGY ON THE CONSTRUCTION CULTURE

The construction industry differs vastly from other manufacturing enterprises and businesses. Most corporate work is conducted at a fixed location, with a cadre of workers employed for long periods of time, and with a single employer, fixed hours of employment, and usually a company safety-and-health culture targeted toward the well-being of employees. In contrast, construction workplaces are mobile, with the various craft members moving from job to job, having to adapt to new work sites and to different building contractors whose attitudes toward safety may vary widely. Work sites are usually multiemployer, which thwarts a uniform approach to training, and with anywhere from 10 to 50 subcontractors on site, each may inadvertently create hazards for the others (164). Furthermore, about 82% of employers have fewer than ten employees, and the workers buy their own tools, which may differ greatly in their design from brand to brand. All of the tasks are distinctly challenging ergonomically, running the gamut from heavy overhead applications to procedures conducted at floor level. If the work is recompensed on a piecework basis, workers invariably speed up the rate at which they perform work tasks, making injuries more likely (164).

Workers in construction "could be inadequately informed because conditions in the...industry work against establishing and maintaining occupational health and safety program," since many are self-employed or employed in small companies. If employed by larger companies, they are usually assigned to a particular job/work site only for limited periods (165). These realities are obstacles to educating construction workers about desirable work practices that help prevent occupational injuries and illnesses. In addition, attempts to educate a mobile workforce can be costly, and experience has shown that there is a lack of interest among construction workers, exacerbated somehow by their fear of the loss of their job and livelihood (166). Apprehension among workers is common when ergonomic changes that would improve productivity are suggested, because from the worker's perspective such changes could lead to job loss if the work can be completed by fewer crafts people (164).

In the construction work arena, there is a tendency for workers to feel that it is not "masculine" to follow prescribed safety measures and that exposure to risk is an unavoidable reality of life in construction ("it goes with the territory"), and that an appearance of fearlessness must be maintained (167). This attitude has been well expressed by Dr. Eleanor Fendler, who manages formula development of protective skin products. She aptly characterizes this worker group: "It's sissy to complain about your hands. It's macho to have these rough, tough hands, even if they do hurt. It's considered part of the job" (168).

Another risk factor that thwarts safety indoctrination is the influx of illegal immigrants who are willing to work under hazardous conditions at low wages (169) and are reluctant to voice complaints for fear of detection of their illegal status and possible deportation. Self-employment also negatively impacts efforts at health and safety maintenance, as the self-employed often have longer hours of exposure, the economic and time pressures faced by those paid according to their output are greater, and the self-employed often have inadequate access to treatment (170,171).

Compounding the risk for construction workers is the hierarchy among them, often manifested by bullying or "mobbing" of those lower in the pecking order by crafts workers whose hourly wage is higher. Such behavioral pressures can lead to distraction and inattention on the part of abused workers, putting them at greater risk for injuries on the job.

A study of nearly 8,000 construction laborers was conducted to determine whether substance abuse was associated with an increased risk of work-related injuries. For the 422 workers with a diagnosis of substance abuse, the rate of time-loss injuries per 100 workers was 15.1, compared with 10.9 for all workers in the cohort. For those in the 25- to 34-year-old age group, the rate for substance abuse was 23.6, compared with 12.2 for nonusers (172).

Another psychosocial problem in the construction world is the hostile reception often given women workers, which puts them at even greater risk than that associated with the primary safety and health hazards encountered by workers in general. Specific difficulties women have faced as manifestations of a hostile workplace include restricted access to sanitary toilets, ill-fitting protective clothing and equipment, and inadequate on-the-job training. These injustices, which are amenable to remediation, have unquestionably had an adverse effect on women's ability to work safely (173). Incidents of gender harassment occur, even in this presumably enlightened age, and 41% of subjects in a NIOSH study stated that they had been mistreated because they were female. Women workers in construction had the second highest rate of sexual harassment complaints per 100,000 women in the workforce, second only to female miners (173). Most will not speak up because they fear losing their jobs or being subject to further acts of discrimination as retaliation (174).

Women in the construction industry have demonstrated an increased PMR for all diseases related to asbestos exposure (175), and the average fatality rate of 1.80 per 100,000 workers for female construction workers was higher than the rate for women in any other industry (176). Black women younger than 65 years of age at death had a significantly elevated PMR for traumatic fatalities (177). More women are entering the industry (178), and are manifesting, overall, a greater risk of carpal tunnel syndrome, burns, sprains, and fractures than males (179).

Personal attitudes toward safety measures are influenced by cost factors. For example, there are cases of worker deaths in trenches whose walls were not shored up. Some operators omit shoring in order to lower costs, hoping that the job will be finished before the soil caves in. Some operators would sooner pay the OSHA fine, since such flouting of the laws, even if the offending operator is caught, is less expensive than the cost incurred by properly shoring up the trench walls (180).

Another risk that often distinguishes the milieu of construction work is the temporary employment of adolescents to supplement the regular workforce during the summertime. Even though the Fair Labor Standards Act (FLSA) prohibits assigning them to tasks or tools that account for a great number of injuries, such assignments are often given to these inexperienced employees, putting them at a disproportionate risk for injury. While vacation employment is commonplace in nonhazardous industries, construction work may injure or even kill the unguided, inexperienced, or overutilized teenager (181).

Ringen et al. (182) provide an excellent summary of the work idiosyncrasies in the construction industry:

- Injuries frequently develop incrementally.
- Chronic work-related illnesses are unrecognized and underreported.
- The medical profession fails to recognize occupational illness.
- As a worker's location on site may change regularly in relation to other workers, the potential exposure as a bystander to such hazards also changes.
- Ambient conditions (ventilation and temperature) can change markedly.
- Weather dictates the employment of many outdoor workers.
- Workers leave because of the uncertainty of employment and the hazards involved, thus leaving a workforce of inexperienced, temporary, and transient tradespersons.
- The work, in the main, is characterized by high turnover and small operations.
- Stress is increased by frequent relocations, long commutes, a lack of health insurance, and an occupation-forced inability to have long-term individual health care provider.
- The many moves of the workers, the inconsistency in health care, and the odd employment sites "limit [both] the clinician's or the researcher's ability to trace the individual's work history or exposure to hazards."

Pairing these job factors with the high-risk factors for musculoskeletal disorders (MSDs)—rapid work pace, monotonous work, low job satisfaction, little decision-making power, and high levels of work stress—substantiates the findings that men who work as construction laborers, carpenters, and industrial truck or tractor equipment operators are at the highest risk for MSDs (183). Thus there is a need for an ergonomics standard.

Contaminant Spread

Construction workers are highly likely to bring contaminating materials into their homes via labor-soiled clothing, inadequate end-of-the-workday cleansing, and by means of vehicular transport. In a 1981 to 1983 survey, it was estimated that about 48,000 families with children under 6 years of age had members who were occupationally exposed to lead, supporting the position that these children should be targeted for blood lead screening (184). In a British review, the hypothesis was tested that, among excesses of childhood leukemia associated with extreme population mixing, the incidence was higher for those children of fathers whose work involved contact with many individuals (particularly children), as was noted in certain childhood infections. The excess in the high category related to the father's occupation in the construction industry (185).

Lead is often transported home. NIOSH found that the hands of lead-exposed workers were seven times more contaminated with lead compared with worker controls. Automobiles driven by such workers were significantly higher in surface lead contamination, the highest level being on the armrests. The study suggested that construction workers' occupational exposures, together with poor hygiene practices, were the primary causes of lead contamination. Preventive measures must be taken (186).

Lead carried home in this fashion results in paraoccupational or "take-home" exposure to workers' families. Oddly, the lead contamination inside some 27 automobiles sampled was not associated with personal exposure to airborne lead in the work environment. The workers considered highly exposed to lead, such as blasters, regularly changed out of work clothing and showered before getting into their cars. It was other workers who were only minimally exposed to lead who did not follow these hygienic practices and thus carried home the material. Some 20 automobiles sampled demonstrated the presence of lead, primarily on the driver's side floor, armrests, and steering wheels (187). All crafts persons at lead-abatement sites must practice personal cleaning at workday's end before going home. Details concerning personal hygiene practice are provided by NIOSH (188,189).

Home contamination has been addressed by the Workers' Family Protection Act, passed by Congress in 1992 (190). A report to Congress cited the effects of 13 different classes of substances that could be taken into the home by contaminated workers (190). A reverse of this path of spoiliation is seen when craftspersons experience adverse health effects from working on facilities containing contaminated building materials. In one report, workers were rendered ill following renovation of a building where water incursion allowed fungal growth. While the matching of contactants to symptoms was not complete, personal protective equipment was advised for similar future undertakings (191).

The transport and installation of fungus-contaminated gypsum wallboard in a new seven-story, 170-room hotel required the removal of the building material and replacement by more acceptable board as the indoor concentrations were 50 times higher than outdoor levels. Occupancy permission by local building officials was not granted until replacement was effected (192).

Regulatory Canopy

With so much research, so many publications, and federal and state regulation of construction, why are occupational injuries and illnesses still sustained in the industry at an unacceptable rate? In an effort to address this issue, the federal government has attempted multiple modes of intervention.

The formalized regulations legislated by Congress and promulgated by OSHA are numerous and sufficiently detailed to cover every work procedure in construction (193). A summarized, abbreviated version of the regulations has been published as a pocket booklet "to aid employers, supervisors, and safety and health personnel in their efforts toward achieving compliance with OSHA standards in the workplace" (194). The directorate of construction has been created to serve as OSHA's source for standards and regulations (195), and one of its four divisions is the Division of Construction Services, whose mission is "to enhance safety awareness and reduce construction accidents" (196).

Under the provisions of the Contract Work Hours and Safety Standards Act (Construction Safety Act), the Advisory Committee on Construction and Safety and Health (ACCSH) was established. It comprises 15 members representing employers, employees, state safety and health agencies, and the public, plus one member, usually designated by NIOSH, to advise OSHA's assistant secretary regarding the establishment of construction standards and policy matters affecting federally financed or assisted construction (197).

A relatively recent (1998) activity of ACCSH was the formation of a work group to comment on revisions of the *Field Instructional Reference Manual* (FIRM) concerning multiemployer work sites. A proposed draft of revisions (June 10, 1999) has been circulated for comment (198). ACCSH has prepared a draft of another document on preventing musculoskeletal disorders in construction workers (September 1, 1999) (199). Every ergonomic challenge in construction is covered, and checklists are presented so that work sites can be evaluated. In addition, outreach training programs on construction safety and health have been authorized for certain workers in the trades to enable them to teach courses on construction safety and health.

Corrective Action

With the knowledge that in a single year (1999) 17 workers were fatally injured each day, of whom 20% were in construction (30), it is clear that corrective intervention is indicated. As previously described, all the regulatory mechanisms are in place, and guidelines for safe and healthful work have had wide distribution to employers, unions, and individual workers, both through governmental publications and the Internet. However, as discussed, compliance is subject to the cost-cutting and other unfortunate business expediencies commonly practiced by both contractors and crafts personnel.

Quality educational programs emphasizing work without injury or disease are sorely needed, but delivering them directly to the innumerable individuals composing the multiemployer workforce, at the incalculable number of construction sites, challenges the capabilities of all the official agencies combined. Compulsory training should instead be directed toward the contractors so that they can communicate the crucial safety messages to their workers, possibly under the auspices and supervision of national labor and management organizations (200). Large companies with international building responsibilities are not the problem. It is the fragmentation of the industry, with its thousands of contractors ranging "from `mom and pop' operators with nothing but a pickup truck and a magnetic sign" to huge international corporations that makes a universal program of rectification so difficult (201).

It is imperative that contractors be trained so that they, in turn, can train their field supervisors, who, through daily tailgate conferences, can pass on to their work crews the principles and procedures for working without bodily injury or loss of life (202). Training must be site specific, particularly for new workers, so that safety and health hazards unique to that particular job can be emphasized (200,203). Educational media can be utilized, including CDs, posters, pocket cards, booklets, and Internet resources, as well as items in Spanish, if needed.

Educational Content

The following vital topics should be covered in the process of educating workers:

- Hazards inherent in manual maneuvers that can result in musculoskeletal injuries.
- Toxic chemicals present in work materials (204,207) in areas of previous contamination [such as those that may be encountered during repair of moldy buildings (208), bridge repair (102), demolition of old structures (209), or during the admixture of other work substances], which may cause excessive exposure via additive effects.
- Observance of all precautions required by legal mandate.
- Procedures to be followed in the event of injury, toxic spill, evacuation, and emergency response as well as availability of definitive health care, including pertinent equipment on site (210–212).
- Precautions to be taken if construction work involves entry into confined spaces (203).
- Craft-specific practices to be utilized, including the use of equipment of new design (or new to the workers). Manufacturers' representatives may assist in the indoctrination.
- Distribution and explanation of appropriate Material Safety Data Sheets (MSDSs).
- Avoidance of work at times of high personal stress and sources of personal counseling to help resolve the causative problem(s) (217).
- Recognition of the diversification of the construction workforce and the behavioral precautions required to maintain equity among workers, regardless of racial, religion, sexual orientation, or national origin (218,219).
- Importance of reporting all injuries so that appropriate care can be initiated and complications avoided (220).
- Need to utilize all indicated and appropriate personal protective equipment (PPE) and to determine that such PPE is correctly fitted and adequately maintained, or replaced as needed (216,221).
- Familiarization with potential reproductive health hazards and their effects, as determined by potential work contact with such substances and the gender of the worker (222).
- Education of lead-exposed construction workers about their children's potential risk for excessive lead exposure (223).

RESOURCES FOR SAFETY TRAINING AND COMMUNICATION

A single training program is not adequate, since working conditions change as a structure evolves, requiring new materials, new heights, and the addition of different crafts personnel. Periodic refresher classes must be given at intervals to be determined by the extent of labor turnover, the addition of more updated equipment, and the stage of completion of a building project.

It must be assumed that the building corporation, through its safety professionals, is familiar with the hazards unique to a particular construction project. Such a body of knowledge is mandatory for the institution of any training program. While contractors and their supervisors should undertake the training of construction personnel, other avenues of education can also be effective. A variety of educational resources have been utilized in communicating the precepts of on-the-job safety and its concomitant preservation of worker health.

On-site Classrooms

An example of the provision of high-quality, cost-effective, professional training is a company (Construction Safety and Health, Austin, TX) that offers sessions at construction job sites. By means of mobile classrooms that are modified airport-bus vehicles seating 14 people, the travel time of workers is reduced and the building site and structure are immediately at hand to serve as visual aids in the learning process, making training more reality-based (224).

Trade Unions

Working through a specific labor organization allows tailoring of the safety message to the unique hazards and exposures of a particular trade so that educational material can be sharply focused and tailored to that trade (225).

Organizational Alliances

Through triangular "robust collegial relationships among small-scale builders, the inspectorate [OSHA] and the industry association," knowledge of construction health and safety needs can be increased, relevant material can be included in written contracts, and injuries can be reduced in number (226).

Full-time Safety Director

In a large construction company, a full-time safety director or specialist can be effective in training workers prior to the onset of building, particularly since the educational content can be designed to emphasize the resolution of ergonomic problems inherent in the project (227).

OSHA Training Courses

OSHA standards stipulate a requirement for worker training: "The employer shall instruct each employee in the recognition and avoidance of unsafe conditions and the regulations applicable to his work environment to control or eliminate any hazards or other exposure to illness or injury" (228). The employer or a representative can acquire training skills and teaching content via the courses offered by OSHA.

Partnership between Federal Agency and Industry Association

Because of the hazards inherent in highway work zones—"segment[s] of the roadway marked to indicate that construction, maintenance, or utility work is being performed"—the American Road and Transportation Builders Association joined with the Federal Highway Administration to create the National Work Zone Safety Information Clearinghouse. The objective was to provide information and referrals to government agencies, public and private organizations, and the general public concerning the safe the effective operation of traffic work zones. The rationale for such a partnership organization in the road and transportation building sector is seen in a single year's 700 roadway fatalities, 24,000 injuries due to vehicular crashes, and 52,000 property-damage-only crashes that occur in traffic work zones. The clearinghouse offers links to multiple training sources relating to work-zone safety (229,230). Similar partnerships in other sectors of the construction industry would undoubtedly be beneficial.

OSHA Consultation

Training can be enhanced through utilization of consultant visits by OSHA health and safety specialists. Among other functions, on-site consultants will "offer training and education for you [the employer] and your employees at your workplace and, in some cases, away from the site" (231). Comparable consultative assistance in training is offered by some states (232).

Academia

Universities, through their schools of public health or medicine, offer programs in occupational health, and program instructors can be called upon to assist in training.

Publications

An example of a succinct publication that can be used for training purposes in an employer handout titled *Construction Safety Pocket Guide,* published by Genuine Publishing, Amsterdam, New York. It is comprehensive and includes topics such as "Things to Know Before Starting Work," "Protecting Your Body," "Working with Equipment," and "Working Safely with Others." The appendices cover MSDSs, construction material hazards, and a glossary of terms and acronyms. The messages are clear and practical; the handbook is "aimed at the men and women who do the hammering, digging, and climbing [on construction sites]" (233).

Mode of Communication

A 1995 article in *Synergist* alerted industrial hygienists (IHs) that "effective communication and interpersonal skills are becoming increasingly important for health and safety professionals" (234). While the authors deemed gaining the cooperation of construction workers a difficult task, they stressed that by observing the following cardinal rules for communicating with this group, barriers to communication could be surmounted to effectively transmit important safety and health information:

- Know the industry.
- Talk the talk of the construction world in order to establish credibility.
- Assure management that work will not be interrupted (more applicable to the IH).
- Be familiar with the different duties of workers.
- Do not use acronyms; they are puzzling to many people.
- Never talk down to workers or use technical terms with which they are unfamiliar.
- Treat workers as peers and view them as partners in accomplishing a healthier workplace.
- Never return shabby treatment.
- Practice what is preached: Wear a hard hat where indicated in order to retain credibility.
- Do not rely too heavily on written materials; not all workers can read.
- Seek assistance from a worker or workers during the presentation; it will enhance communication.

Review of Injuries

In the event of an injury, particularly a serious one, fellow workers are usually emotionally shaken, for either they were witness to the event or have thoughts of "But for the grace of God...." It is imperative that a review of the circumstances leading to the trauma be promptly undertaken with the crew. The usual causes of injury, where applicable, should be sought. Was an unsafe work method or process used? Were the customary work procedures followed? Did the injured worker use substitute equipment or materials? Was the worker distracted while engaged in work? Was there any dissatisfaction, expressed or latent, among the workers? Were the work movements speeded up in order to meet new production goals? Had the injured worker been upset because of personal problems? Were there conflicts with supervisors?

Following the review and inquiry into the circumstances surrounding the injury, a demonstration of the proper procedures for the particular operation should be performed, observing all safety or health precautions, so that differences in technique can be identified and repetition of the unplanned injury avoided in the future. If illustrative material is available, it should be used to emphasize the physical or emotional causative factors that may have been involved in the injury or loss of the worker. Both the review and inquiry and the demonstration of proper procedure for the work task should be performed as quickly as possible after the injury incident, while all memories are fresh.

Risk Behavior

Although most physical and ergonomic causes of injury can be identified through adequate investigation and study, the identification of psychosocial etiologies is more elusive. Recently, certain psychosocial elements or deficits in the lifestyle of construction workers have been explored in an attempt to explain the many injuries and illnesses among this group. It has been found that in the construction trades there is a need for preventive measures directed toward alcoholism, respiratory tuberculosis among laborers and drywall workers, and accidental drug or alcohol poisoning among painters and drywall workers (235).

A 1998 study revealed a positive dose–response relationship between smoking and the rate of early retirement due to permanent disability in the construction industry (236). This finding bespeaks not only the premature and avoidable loss of skilled personnel, but also an undue burden for society (236). A Chinese review found that a large proportion of workers who were injured in construction were smokers and beer drinkers (237). While it was not demonstrated that smoking was the immediate cause of the sustained trauma, it was thought to have exerted an indirect effect by reducing workers' concentration, in addition to presenting a real risk of fire. Smokers, the investigators believed, risk their own health by smoking and also have a general tendency toward risky behavior at work.

Last, as described in 1991 by Bigos and co-workers (238), and emphasized more recently by Marks (239), job satisfaction may be the only significant predictive factor for lost-time injuries due to low back disorders. This points up the necessity for occupational health professionals to systematically address all the causative factors that may be associated with back injuries in the construction industry, including lifestyle and psychosocial factors.

Over the years, many occupational health practitioners have sought behavioral etiologies for accidental injuries (most often successfully), but it is only in recent times that the concept of behavior-based safety (BBS) has been established. Events that led to the development of the BBS paradigm are the following: (a) academic psychologists began research on behavioral techniques for injury prevention; (b) Proctor & Gamble used BBS principles to manage safety throughout the corporation; and (c) in 1979, an organization was founded by a psychologist and a physician who pioneered the application of BBS principles in the industrial setting (240).

The goals of BBS are the identification and definition of site-specific critical behaviors by means of peer-to-peer behavioral observation and feedback. The objective is the conversion of at-risk behaviors (causative behaviors) to safe behaviors. For example, the goals of one BBS program were (a) zero injuries; (b) zero nuclear or radiologic incidents; (c) zero fire impairments for more that 30 days; and (d) zero joint company/union safety committee concerns for more that 30 days. All of the accepted elements of first-rate safety programs are included, plus emphasis on management's involvement, toolbox or tailgate meetings, communication to all levels of personnel, brown-bag meetings between senior-level managers and floor-level employees, and multiple modes of training (241). While "accident proneness" is a bygone concept, there are always behavior-based reasons that repetition of injury occurs, and BBS may aid in their identification. Currently, there is still controversy over the appropriateness and usefulness of the BBS concept, and negative views have been expressed even by OSHA's chief. There is great reluctance to blame workers' behavior for injuries; the prevailing feeling seems to be that employers have not provided safe workplaces (242). Time will probably bring acceptance, in part, of both positions.

Miscellany

Other problems, many alluded to earlier, beset workers in the construction industry. Compared with white-collar workers, construction workers had, upon baseline examination, a higher rate of hearing deficits, signs of obstructive lung diseases, increased body mass index, and musculoskeletal abnormalities in a study conducted by Arndt and colleagues (243).

In another study (244), construction workers who died between 1984 and 1986 and who were younger than 65 years of age (and most likely still employed immediately prior to death) had significantly increased PMRs for cancer, asbestos-related disease, mental disorders, alcohol-related disease, and digestive diseases as well as falls, poisonings, work-related trauma, and homicides.

Young persons are employed in the building trades both here and abroad (245). During the years 1992 to 1997, there were 53 fatalities in the construction industry among workers under 18 years of age (246). These could have been avoided; young workers can be employed safely, provided there is compliance with all laws and regulations (247).

Workers in some specific occupations in the construction industry are at greater risk, and these are currently receiving attention. One such occupation is flag persons (flaggers)—individuals who are responsible for safely coordinating vehicular traffic through road work sites. To lower the rate of injuries and fatalities among flaggers, a change in training standards and better traffic barricading are necessary (248). In addition, garments should be used that will provide the maximum conspicuity for the wearer utilizing high visibility and reflective materials. ANSI/ISEA 107-1999 is a voluntary consensus standard applicable to all workers in need of increased visibility (249).

Regardless of occupational rank or occupation, any construction worker is at extreme risk around cranes because of the lack of delineation of the danger area's boundaries (250). Work assignments such as those described require special preventive measures, and the employees so engaged should be involved in the design of the intervention mode, the determination of its use, and its field testing and evaluation (164).

WRITTEN PROGRAMS FOR INJURY PREVENTION

Every employer must have a written program concerning the prevention of job-related illnesses and injuries and ensure that it is given to all employees. In certain states, a written program is mandatory. The program must be operation-specific and cover all work processes involved in a construction project. In addition, provisions for prompt injury review should be included in the program, especially for fatal injuries.

An excellent example of such a publication is the *NAHBOSHA Jobsite Safety Handbook,* a joint project of OSHA and the National Association of Home Builders (251). It covers the following topics:

- Orientation and training
- Personal protective equipment
- Housekeeping and access around site
- Stairs and ladders
- Scaffolds and other work platforms
- General
- Planking
- Scaffold guardrails
- Fall protection
- Floor and wall openings
- Alternatives
- Work on roofs
- Excavations and trenching
- Foundations
- Tools and equipment
- Vehicles and mobile equipment
- Electrical
- Fire prevention

In addition, locations of all OSHA offices are provided.

While the brochure is intended for workers constructing homes, variations in content can be provided for different kinds of construction projects.

There are other publications to assist an employer in the preparation of a written safety management program, for example, Tompkins's (252) *How to Write a Company Safety Manual* and Washington Industrial Safety and Health Act Services' (253) *How to Write an Accident Prevention Report.*

The purposes of a written safety program and the general content, as outlined by the State of Washington, are:

- To identify and eliminate hazards in the workplace.
- To orient new employees as to what they need to know to work safely.
- To provide ongoing training to improve the skill and competence of employees in safety issues.
- To involve workers in maintaining a safe workplace.
- To plan for emergencies that might occur.

The need for a program is substantiated by the federal government. OSHA states, "Employers and contractors are advised and encouraged to institute and maintain...a program that provides adequate systemic policies, procedures, and practices to protect their employees from, and allow them to recognize, job-related safety and health hazards" (194).

If a particularly serious injury requires investigation, a detailed outline is available via the Internet that provides coverage of all aspects of an inquiry into the causation and details of an unintentional work-related trauma (254).

Comments

It is important that, whenever possible, occupational health professionals (OHPs) assist construction companies, particularly contractors and subcontractors, in developing safety and health programs regardless of the professional's practice venue. Employers may obtain access to OHP consultation through a private consultant's office, a group clinic, an academic center, a hospital or medical center, an armed services establishment, an occupational health facility chain, or a health maintenance organization (HMO). The assistance of an OHP is crucial in overcoming the current resistance to construction safety measures occasioned primarily by fear of additional costs. Life is too precious to be weighed against fiscal issues and cost savings. Safety and health programs are less costly than the cost incurred when there is a fatality, although it is difficult to convince the "bottom-liners" of this reality.

Another element has entered into consideration of work-related morbidity and mortality. In some instances, job-related deaths have been ruled murder. For example, in a precedent-setting case in Cook County, Illinois, after 8 years of legal maneuvering, three managers were eventually sentenced to up to 3 years in jail for manslaughter (255). As pointed out in a review of the subject, in 1988 the Department of Justice ruled that "employers whose workers are killed or injured on the job can be prosecuted for murder, manslaughter, or assault under state law and cannot seek refuge under Federal laws or workplace safety" (255). An accompanying editorial stated, "No matter what nuances of social history, . . . homicide prosecutions cannot possibly be a major instrument for securing workplace safety. . . . Reliance on such prosecution in lieu of safety standards and practice is a sign of weakness, not strength, in the institutions of public health" (256). The jury is still out, however.

That there is currency in the concern over the morbidity and fatalities associated with the construction industry is seen in the recent issue of the OSHA standard that improves the safety of workers erecting steel buildings (257). As described, the standard will require "certification of proper curing of concrete in footings and in piers for steel columns, pre-planning of key erection activities, additional crane safety, safe and secure walking surfaces, procedures to minimize the collapse of lacing loads on steel joists, and adequate worker training" (258,259). A new Cable Safe system is available for workers at heights (260).

OSHA continues to offer courses pertinent to the construction industry (261), partnerships with contractors continue (262,263), ergonomics projects specific to construction have been undertaken (264), training in construction safety is available via the Internet (265,266), and drug testing continues to show a decline in work injury rates (267,268).

The National Safety Council, in its method of data collection, has estimated that in 1998, 1,230 deaths occurred in the construction industry among its 8.14 million workers, who constitute 61% of the country's total workforce (269). This is a 16% increase over the industry's fatalities in the previous year (269). The annual increase in fatalities for all industries was only 2%.

The Occupational Safety and Health Act of 1970 was created "to assure so far as possible every working man and woman in the nation safe and healthful working conditions and to preserve our human resources" and, further, "to stimulate employers and employees to institute new and to perfect existing programs" (270).

Have these ideal goals been realized as we read "Do Construction Workers Fall Through the Cracks?" or "Only a fundamental change in the attitude of Americans and their government toward the day-to-day exposure to the risk affecting the health, safety, and lives of workers makes possible the aggressive pursuit [of OSHA's objectives]" (271).

A recent newspaper headline screamed, "Builders in Demand—Construction Industry Seeking Skilled Workers." Skilled workers are needed because there is "a reluctance of young people to do physical labor to get their hands dirty" (272). It is hoped that the older workers who will be seeking jobs will benefit from this millennium's efforts to preserve the lives of construction workers through the prevention of unintentional illness or injury and fatality. This will aid in reaching the 2010 target goal of 10.2 deaths per 1,000 workers, which will be a significant improvement over the 1998 baseline of 14.6 deaths per 1,000 (273).

The employment projections to the year 2008 see an increase in women in the labor force to 48%, Asians to 6%, and Hispanics to 13%. The black labor pool will grow by 20%, twice as fast as the 10% growth rate for whites (274). All the more are there indications for greater safety and health measures in construction as many trainees come into new work settings. In a contemporary summary of construction safety, it was concluded that the "industry faces worker shortages that, combined with continued growth, place increased pressure on companies to aggressively pursue safety" (275). The key points of the review are as follows (275):

- A good reputation and a strong safety program equal more business.
- The cost associated with an injured employee far outweighs the cost of an OSHA fine.
- Companies that practice safety retain their employees.
- Make safety a commitment and either hire or designate a safety director.
- Train and retain employees.
- Communicate to all employees, especially those who understand little or no English.

Much work in both health and safety at the construction workplace remains. The dedicated occupational health professional can aid construction personnel in having a "safe working life and a retirement free from long-term consequences of occupational disease and injury" (276). May the effort begin.

REFERENCES

1. *The history of building construction.* Encyclopedia Britannica CD, 2001.
2. Dickerson OB. Cathedral workers during the Middle Ages. *J Occup Med* 1967;9:605–610.
3. Felton JS. Man, medicine, and work in America: a historical series. IV Thomas Cadwalader, M.D., physician, Philadelphian and philanthropist. *J Occup Med* 1969;11:374–380.
4. Hunter D. *The diseases of occupation,* 6th ed. London: Hodder and Stoughton, 1978:791.
5. Thomas MW. *The early factory legislation.* London: Thames Bank Publishing, 1948:11.
6. Howard JM. The history of occupational injuries in the United States (1776–1976). *J Trauma* 1977;17: 411–418.
7. Spargo J. *The bitter cry of children.* New York: Macmillan, 1906:175.
8. Nearing S. *Social adjustment.* New York: Macmillan, 1914:239.
9. Szasz A. Industrial resistance to occupational safety and health legislation: 1971–1981. *Social Problems* 1984;32:104–116.
10. Constructing a safer workplace. *Environ Health News* (University of Washington) 2000:1–3.
11. Executive Office of the President, Office of Management and Budget. *North American Industry Classification System, United States 1997.* Washington, DC: U.S. Government Printing Office, 1997:89.
12. *Ibid,* pp. 89–104.
13. Career Guide to Industries. Construction. Bureau of Labor Statistics, U.S. Department of Labor, *http://stats.bls.gov/oco/cg/cgs003.htm.*
14. Highlights from the value of construction put in place,

press release, March 1, 2001: *http://www.census.gov/pub/const/c30_curr.html.*
15. Employment Projections. Bureau of Labor Statistics, U.S. Department of Labor: *http://stats.bls.gov/news.release/ecopro.t01.htm.*
16. Abraham KG. Commissioner's statement on the employment situation, March 9, 2001: *http://www.bls.gov/new.release/pdf/jec.pdf.*
17. Industry at a glance. Construction. Bureau of Labor Statistics, U.S. Department of Labor: *http://stats.bls.gov/1ag.construction.htm.*
18. Continued growth seen for construction industry. *Safety and Health* 2001;163:24–25.
19. *The construction chart book—the U.S. construction industry and its workers,* 2nd ed. The Center to Protect Workers Rights, April 1998: *http://www.cpwr.com/Cover.html.*
20. Construction Trade Occupations. Carpenters: *http://stats.bls.gov/oco/ocos202.htm.*
21. Occupational Safety and Health Administration. Occupational Safety and Health Standards for the Construction Industry. General Safety and Health Provisions. 29 CFR, part 1920.20(a)(I).
22. *Worker Health Chartbook, 2000.* Washington, DC: U.S. Department of Health and Human Services, Public Health Service, Centers of Disease Control and Prevention, National Institute for Occupational Safety and Health, September 2000:7.
23. *Ibid,* p. 12.
24. Mortality patterns—United States, 1997. *MMWR* 1999;48:664–668.
25. *Random House Webster's College Dictionary,* 2nd ed. New York: Random House, 1997:8.
26. Ref. 22, supra, p. 22.
27. *Ibid,* p.34.
28. *Ibid,* p.95.
29. *Ibid,* p.96.
30. *National census of fatal occupational injuries, 1999.* Washington, DC: United States Department of Labor, Bureau of Labor Statistics, August 17, 2000.
31. 1999 Census of Fatal Occupational Injuries data: *http://stats.bls.gov/oshcfo:1.htm.*
32. *Workplace injuries and illnesses in 1999.* Washington, DC: United States Department of Labor, Bureau of Labor Statistics, December 12, 2000.
33. *Lost-worktime injuries and illnesses: characteristics and resulting time away from work, 1999.* Washington, DC: United States Department of Labor, Bureau of Labor Statistics, March 28, 2001.
34. Current labor statistics—injury and illness data. *Monthly Labor Rev* 2001;124:94.
35. Satcher D. Injury: an overlooked global health concern. *JAMA* 2000;284:950.
36. Spain gets tough on construction safety. *Safety and Health* 2001;163:21,23.
37. Kartam NA, Bouz RG. Fatalities and injuries in the Kuwaiti construction industry. *Accid Anal Prev* 1998;38:805–814.
38. Fatal injuries in the construction industry notified to HSE [Health and Safety Executive] and local authorities: *http://www.hse.gov.uk/press/e00214.htm.*
39. Koton S, Ifrah R, Lerman Y, et al. Workers' health in Israel. *Public Health Rev* 1998;2:189–203.
40. Jeong BY. Occupational deaths and injuries in the construction industry. *Appl Ergon* 1998;29:355–360.
41. Shirai Y, Miyamoto M, Genbun Y, et al. Combination of low back pain and previous low back pain and should stiffness in construction employees. *Nippon Ika Daigaku Zasshi* 1998;65:307–311.
42. Kuwashima A, Aizawa Y, Nakamura K, et al. National survey on accidental low back pain in workplace. *Ind Health* 1997;35:187–193.
43. Sun J, Sibata E, Hisanaga N, et al. A cohort mortality study of construction workers. *Am J Ind Med* 1997;32:35–41.
44. Koskinen K, Zitting A, Tossavainen A, et al. Radiographic abnormalities among Finnish construction, shipyard, and asbestos industry workers. *Scand J Work Environ Health* 1998;24:109–117.
45. Salminen ST. Epidemiological analysis of serious occupational accidents in southern Finland. *Scand J Soc Med* 1994;22:225–227.
46. Pianosi G, Zocchetti C. Work-related accidents in unions in Lombardy. *Med Lav* 1995;86:332–340.
47. Pianosi G. Fatal occupational accidents in Lombardy. *Med Lav* 1995;86:534–541.
48. Germani D, Belli S, Bruno C, et al. Cohort mortality study of women compensated for asbestosis in Italy. *Am J Ind Med* 1999;36:129–134.
49. Ascoli V, Scalzo CC, Facciolo F, et al. Malignant mesothelioma in Rome, Italy 1988–1995: a retrospective study of 79 patients. *Tumori* 1996;82:526–532.
50. Xia ZL, Courtney TK, Sorock BS, et al. Fatal occupational injuries in a new development area in the People's Republic of China. *J Occup Environ Med* 2000;42:917–922.
51. Xia ZL, Sorock GS, Zhu J, et al. Fatal occupational injuries in the construction industry of a new development area in East China, 1991 to 1997. *Am Ind Hyg Assoc J* 2000;61:733–737.
52. Brenner H, Ahern W. Sickness absence and early retirement on health grounds in the construction industry in Ireland. *Occup Environ Med* 2000;57:615–620.
53. Wu TN, Liu SH, Hsu CC, et al. Epidemiologic study of occupational injuries among foreign and native workers in Taiwan. *Am J Ind Med* 1997;31:623–630.
54. McVittie DJ. Fatalities and serious injuries. *Occup Med* 1995;10:285–293.
55. Guidotti TL. Occupational injuries in Alberta: responding to recent trends. *Occup Med* 1995;45:81–88.
56. Lerer LB, Myers JE. Application of two secondary documentary sources to identify the underreporting of fatal occupational injuries in Cape Town, South Africa. *Am J Ind Med* 1994;26:521–527.
57. State of the work environment: construction industry, Western Australia 1994/95: *http://www1.safetyline.wa.gov.au/pagebin/injrstat0024.htm.*
58. Rothenbacher D, Brenner H, Arndt V, et al. Disorders of the back and spine in construction workers: prevalence and prognostic value for disability. *Spine* 1997;22:1481–1486.
59. HSE campaigns to improve standards in construction industry. *Soc Occup Med Newsletter* 2001;(83):40–41.
60. Dong W, Vaughan P, Sullivan K, et al. Mortality study of construction workers in the UK. *Int J Epidemiol* 1995;24:750–757.
61. Loomis DP, Richardson DB, Wolf SH, et al. Fatal occupational injuries in a southern state. *Am J Epidemiol* 1997;145:1089–1099.
62. Lipscomb HJ, Dement JM, Rodriguez-Acosta R.

Deaths from external causes of injury among construction workers in North Carolina, 1988–1994. *Appl Occup Environ Hyg* 2000;15:569–580.

63. Cattledge GH, Schneiderman A, Stanevich R, et al. Nonfatal occupational fall injuries in the West Virginia construction industry. *Accid Anal Prev* 1996;28: 655–663.
64. Helmcamp JC, Lundstrom WJ. Work-related deaths in West Virginia from July 1996 through June 1999: surveillance, investigation, and prevention. *J Occup Envir Med* 2000;42:156–162.
65. Husberg BJ, Conway GA, Moore MA, et al. Surveillance for nonfatal work-related injuries in Alaska, 1991–1995. *Am J Ind Med* 1998;34:493–498.
66. Silverstein B, Welp E, Nelson K, et al. Claims incidence of work-related disorders of the upper extremities: Washington state, 1987 through 1995. *Am J Public Health* 1998;88:1827–1833.
67. Overview of fatal injuries at work in 1995: *http:www.state.ma.usdphohspcfo:02-htm.*
68. Reynolds SJ. Prevalence of elevated blood leads and exposure to lead in construction trades in Iowa and Illinois. *Am J Ind Med* 1999;36:307–316.
69. de Zwart BC, Frings-Dresen MH, van Duivenbooden JC. Senior workers in the Dutch construction industry: a search for age-related work and health issues. *Exp Aging Res* 1999;25:385–391.
70. Kisner SM, Pratt SG. Occupational fatalities among older workers in the United States: 1980–1991. *J Occup Environ Med* 1997;39:715–721.
71. Dufort VM, Kotch JB, Marshall SW, et al. Occupational injuries among adolescents in Dunedin, New Zealand, 1990–1993. *Ann Emerg Med* 1997;30: 266–273.
72. Miller ME, Kaufman JD. Occupational injuries among adolescents in Washington state, 1988–1991. *Am J Ind Med* 1998;34:121–132.
73. White L, O'Donnell C. Working children and accidents: understanding the risks. *Child Care Health Dev* 2001;27:23–34.
74. Numbers speak volumes: unintentional-injury costs, United States, 1999. *Safety and Health* 2000;162: 78–79.
75. *Analysis of construction fatalities—the OSHA data base 1985–1989.* Washington, DC: U.S. Department of Labor, Occupational Safety and Health Administration, November, 1990.
76. Job-related deaths decline in 1999. *Safety and Health* 2000;162:20.
77. *Worker deaths by electrocution—a summary of NIOSH surveillance and investigative findings.* Washington, DC: U.S. Department of Health and Human Services, Public Health Service, Centers for Disease Control and Prevention, National Institute for Occupational Safety and Health, May, 1998.
78. Ore T, Casini V. Electrical fatalities among U.S. construction workers. *J Occup Environ Med* 1996;38: 587–592.
79. Janicek CA. Occupational fatalities caused by contact with overhead power lines in the construction industry. *J Occup Envir Med* 1997;39:328–332.
80. *Worker deaths by falls—a summary of surveillance findings and investigative case reports.* Washington, DC: U.S. Department of Health and Human Services, Public Health Service, Centers for Disease Control and Prevention, National Institute for Occupational Safety and Health, November, 2000.
81. *NIOSH alert: request for assistance in preventing worker injuries and deaths caused by falls from suspension scaffolds.* Washington, DC: U.S. Department of Health and Human Services, Public Health Service, Center for Disease Control and Prevention, National Institute for Occupational Safety and Health, September, 1990.
82. Cattledge GH, Hendricks S, Stanevich R. Fatal occupational falls in the U.S. construction industry, 1980–1989. *Accid Anal Prev* 1996;28:647–654.
83. Collins JW, Landen DD, Kisner SM, et al. Fatal occupational injuries associated with forklifts, United States, 198–1994. *Am J Ind Med* 1999;36:504–512. See also Collins JW, Smith GS, Baker SB, et al. A case-control study of forklift and other powered industrial vehicle incidents. *Am J Ind Med* 1999;36: 522–531.
84. *NIOSH alert: preventing injuries and deaths of workers who operate or work near forklifts.* Washington, DC: U.S. Department of Health and Human Services, Public Health Service, Centers for Disease Control and Prevention, National Institute for Occupational Safety and Health, December, 1999.
85. Ore T, Fosbroke DE. Motor vehicle fatalities in the United States construction industry. *Accid Anal Prev* 1997;29:613–626.
86. Pratt SG, Kisner SM, Moore PH. Machinery-related fatalities in the construction industry. *Am J Ind Med* 1997;32:42–58. See also Suruda A, Liu D, Egger M, et al. Fatal injuries in the United States construction industry involving cranes 1984–1994. *J Occup Environ Med* 1999;41:1052–1058.
87. Cubbin C, Le Clere FB, Smith GS. Socioeconomic status and the occurrence of fatal and nonfatal injury in the United States. *Am J Public Health* 2000;90:70–77.
88. Frumkin H, Williamson M, Magid D, et al. Occupational injuries in a poor inner-city population. *J Occup Environ Med* 1995;37:1374–1382.
89. Welch LS, Weeks J, Hunting KL. Fatal and non-fatal injuries from vessels under air pressure in construction. *J Occup Environ Med* 1999;41:100–103.
90. Hoffman DB, Jebson PJ, Steyers CM. Nail gun injuries of the hand. *Am Fam Physician* 1997;56:1643–1646.
91. Beaver AC, Cheatham ML. Life-threatening nail gun injuries. *Am Surg* 1999;65:1113–1116.
92. Kenny N, O'Donaghue D, Haines J. Nail gun injuries. *J Trauma* 1993;35:943–945.
93. Washington Department of Labor and Industries. Work-related musculoskeletal disorders of the neck, back, and upper extremity in Washington State, 1990–1998: *http://www.cdc.gov/niosh/elcosh/docs/d0300/d000376/d000376.html.*
94. Stenlund B, Goldie J, Hagberg M, et al. Shoulder tendonitis and its relation to heavy manual work and exposure to vibration. *Scand J Work Environ Health* 1993;19:43–49.
95. Comba P, Belli S. Etiological epidemiology of tumors of the nasal cavities and the paranasal sinuses. *Ann Ist Super Sanita* 1992;28:121–132.
96. Palmer KT, Griffin MJ, Bendall H, et al. Prevalence and pattern of occupational exposure to hand transmitted vibration in Great Britain: findings from a national survey. *Occup Environ Med* 2000;57:218–228.

97. Diseases and jobs: *http://www.haz-map.com/jobtasks.htm.*
98. Alexander R. Toxic exposures in the construction industry: *http://consumerlawpage.com/article/construction-toxics.shtml.*
99. *NIOSH alert: request for assistance in preventing lead poisoning in construction workers.* Washington DC: U.S. Department of Health and Human Services, Public Health Service, Centers for Disease Control and Prevention, National Institute for Occupational Safety and Health, April, 1992.
100. Lead poisoning in bridge demolition workers—Georgia 1992. *MMWR* 1993;42:388–390.
101. Lead toxicity among bridge workers, 1994. *MMWR* 1995;44:913–920.
102. Controlling lead toxicity in bridge workers—Connecticut, 1991–1994. *MMWR* 1995;44:76–79.
103. Levin SM, Goldberg M, Doucette JT. The effect of the OSHA lead exposure in construction standard on blood lead level among iron workers employed in bridge rehabilitation. *Am J Ind Med* 1997;31:303–309.
104. Reynolds SJ, Fuortes LJ, Garrels RL, et al. Lead poisoning among construction workers renovating a previously deleaded bridge. *Am J Ind Med* 1997;31: 319–323.
105. Osorio AM, Melius J. Lead poisoning in construction. *Occup Med* 1995;10:353–361.
106. Goldberg M, Levin SM, Doucette JT, et al. A task-based approach to assessing lead exposure among iron workers engaged in bridge rehabilitation. *Am J Ind Med* 1997;31:310–318.
107. Hipkins KL, Materna BL, Kosnett MJ, et al. Medical surveillance of the lead exposed worker: current guidelines. *AAOHN J* 1998;46:330–339.
108. Goldberg M, Clark WL, Levin SM, et al. An assessment of lead controls for torch cutting and rivet removal on steel structures. *Appl Occup Environ Hyg* 2000;15:445–452.
109. Vork KL, Hammond SK, Sparer J, et al. Prevention of lead poisoning in construction workers: a new public health approach. *Am J Ind Med* 2001;39:243–253.
110. Castleman BI. *Asbestos: medical and legal aspects,* 4th ed. Englewood Cliffs, NJ: Aspen Law & Business, 1996.
111. Occupational Exposure to Asbestos, CFR 1926.1101, 1994 and subsequent dates, 1995–1998.
112. *Asbestos standard for the construction industry (rev.).* OSHA 3096. Washington, DC: U.S. Department of Labor, Occupational Health and Safety Administration, 1995:2.
113. Seaton A. Asbestos: past, present, and future. *Schweiz Med Wochenschr* 1995;125:453–457.
114. Kang SK, Burnett CA, Freund E, et al. Gastrointestinal cancer mortality of workers in occupations with high asbestos exposure. *Am J Ind Med* 1997;31: 713–718.
115. Szeszenia-Dabroska N, Wilczynska U, Szymczak W, et al. Environmental exposure to asbestos in asbestos cement workers: a case of additional exposure from indiscriminate use of industrial wastes. *Int J Occup Med Environ Health* 1998;11:171–177.
116. O'Reilly D, Reid J, Middleton R, et al. Asbestos related mortality in Northern Ireland: 1985–1994. *J Public Health Med* 1999;21:95–101.
117. Yeung P, Rogers A, Johnson A. Distribution of mesothelioma cases in different occupational groups and industries in Australia, 1979–1995. *Appl Occup Environ Hyg* 1999;14:759–767.
118. Yeung P, Rogers A. An occupation-industry matrix analysis of mesothelioma cases in Australia 1980–1985. *Appl Occup Environ Hyg* 2001;16:40–44.
119. Pearce N, Matos E, Boffetta P, et al. Occupational exposures to carcinogens in developing countries. *Ann Acad Med Singapore* 1994;23:684–689.
120. U.S. Department of Health and Human Services. *Tracking healthy people 2010.* Washington, DC: U.S. Government Printing Office, 2000:20–26.
121. Anderson JT, Hunting KL, Welch LS. Injury and employment patterns among Hispanic construction workers. *J Occup Environ Med* 2000;42:176–186.
122. Hessel PA, Melenka LS, Michaelchuk D, et al. Lung health among boilermakers in Edmonton, Alberta. *Am J Ind Med* 1998;34:381–386.
123. Sullivan PA, Bang KM, Hearl FJ, et al. Respiratory disease risks in the construction industry. *Occup Med* 1995;10:313–334.
124. Finkelstein MM. Occupational associations with lung cancer in two Ontario cities. *Am J Ind Med* 1995;27: 127–136.
125. Wang QS, Boffetta P, Parkin DM, et al. Occupational risk factors for lung cancer in Tianjin, China. *Am J Ind Med* 1995;28:353–362.
126. Pezzotto SM, Poletto L. Occupation and histopathology of lung cancer: a case-control study in Rosario, Argentina. *Am J Ind Med* 1999;36:437–443.
127. De Stefani E, Kogevinas M, Boffetta P, et al. Occupation and risk of lung cancer in Uruguay. *Scand J Work Environ Health* 1996;22:346–352.
128. Mattison P. Dermatitis on construction sites. *Occup Health Lond* 1993;45:122, 124.
129. Goh CL. Common industrial processes and occupational irritants and allergens—an update. *Ann Acad Med Singapore* 1994;23:690–698.
130. Beaumont D, Noeuveglise M, Vibert ML. Screening of vibration-induced disorders in the building industry using digital tactilometry. *Cent Eur J Public Health* 1995;3[suppl]:103–106.
131. Rappaport SM, Weaver M, Taylor D, et al. Application of mixed models to assess exposures monitored by construction works during hot processes. *Ann Occup Hyg* 1999;43:457–469.
132. Blute NA, Woskie SR, Greenspan CA. Exposure characterization for highway construction. Part I: Cut and cover and tunnel finish stages. *Appl Occup Environ Hyg* 1999;14:632–641.
133. Reilly MJ, Rosenman KD, Kalinowski DJ. Occupational noise-induced hearing loss surveillance in Michigan. *J Occup Environ Med* 1998;40:667–674.
134. Neitzel R, Seixas NS, Camp J, et al. An assessment of occupational noise exposures in four construction trades. *Am Ind Hyg Assoc J* 1999;60:807–817.
135. Hessel PA. Hearing loss among construction workers in Edmonton, Alberta. *J Occup Environ Med* 2000; 42:57–63.
136. *Health effects of occupational exposure to asphalt.* Washington, DC: U.S. Department of Health and Human Services, Public Health Service, Centers for Disease Control and Prevention, National Institute for Occupational Safety and Health, December, 2000.
137. Bast-Pettersen R, Skaug V, Ellingsen D, et al. Neu-

robehavioral performance in aluminum welders. *Am J Ind Med* 2000;37:184–192.

138. Partanen T, Jaakkola J, Tossavainen A. Silica, silicosis, and cancer in Finland. *Scand J Work Environ Health* 1995;21[suppl 2]:84–86.
139. Linch KD, Miller WE, Althouse RB, et al. Surveillance of respirable crystalline silica dust using OSHA compliance data (1979–1995). *Am J Ind Med* 1998;34: 547–558.
140. Freeman CS, Grossmann EA. Silica exposures in workplaces in the United States between 1980 and 1992. *Scand J Work Environ Health* 1995;21[suppl 2]: 47–49.
141. Robinson CF, Petersen M, Sieber WK, et al. Mortality of Carpenter's Union members employed in the U.S. construction or wood products industries. *Am J Ind Med* 1996;30:674–694.
142. Stern FB, Sweeney MH, Ward E. Proportionate mortality among unionized construction ironworkers. *Am J Ind Med* 1997;331:176–187.
143. Welcome to the Center to Protect Workers' Rights: *http:www.cpwr.com.*
144. Stern FB, Ruder AM, Chen G. Proportionate mortality among unionized roofers and waterproofers. *Am J Ind Med* 2000;37:478–492.
145. Stern F, Haring-Sweeney M. Proportionate mortality among unionized construction operating engineers. *Am J Ind Med* 1997;32:51–65.
146. Wang E, Dement JM, Lipscomb H. Mortality among North Carolina construction workers, 1988–1994. *Appl Occup Environ Hyg* 1999;14:45–58.
147. Burnett C, Maurer J, Rosenberg HM, et al. *Mortality by occupation, industry, and cause of death: 24 reporting states, 1984–1988.* Washington, DC: U.S. Department of Health and Human Services, Public Health Service, Center for Disease Control and Prevention, National Institute for Occupational Safety and Health, June, 1997:5–7.
148. Robinson C, Stern F, Halperin W, et al. Assessment of mortality in the construction industry in the United States, 1984–1986. *Am J Ind Med* 1995;28:49–70.
149. Chow WH, McLaughlin JK, Malker HS, et al. Occupation and stomach cancer in a cohort of Swedish men. *Am J Ind Med* 1994;26:511–520.
150. Porru S, Aulenti J, Donato F, et al. Bladder cancer and occupation: a case-control study in northern Italy. *Occup Environ Med* 1996;53:6–10.
151. Markovic-Denic L, Janhovic S, Marinkovic J, et al. Brick mortar exposure and chronic lymphocytic leukemia. *Neoplasma* 1995;42:79–81.
152. Brenner H, Arndt V, Rothenbacher D, et al. The association between alcohol consumption and all-cause mortality in a cohort of male employees in the German construction industry. *Int J Epidemiol* 1997;26:85–91.
153. Maier H, Tisch M, Dietz A, et al. Construction workers as an extreme risk group for head and neck cancer? *HNO* 1999;47:730–736.
154. Brenner H, Arndt V, Rothenbacher D, et al. Body weight, pre-existing disease, and all-cause mortality in a cohort of male employees in the German construction industry. *J Clin Epidemiol* 1997;50:1099–1106.
155. Andersson SO, Wolk A, Bergstrom R, et al. Body size and prostate cancer: a 20-year follow-up study among 135,006 Swedish construction workers. *J Natl Cancer Inst* 1997;89:385–389.
156. Bolinder G, Alfredsson L, Englund A, et al. Smokeless tobacco use and increased cardiovascular mortality among Swedish construction workers. *Am J Public Health* 1994;84:399–404.
157. Rothenbacher D, Arndt V, Fraisse E, et al. Early retirement due to permanent disability in relation to smoking in workers of the construction industry. *J Occup Environ Med* 1998;40:63–68.
158. Welch LS, Hunting KL, Nessel-Stephens L. Chronic symptoms in construction workers treated for musculoskeletal injuries. *Am J Ind Med* 1999;36:532–540.
159. Morris JA. Injury experience of temporary workers in a manufacturing center. *AAOHN J* 1999;47:470–478.
160. Liira J, Leino-Arjas P. Predictors and consequences of unemployment in construction and forest work during a 5-year follow-up. *Scand J Work Environ Health* 1999;25:42–49.
161. Liu T, Waterbor JW. Comparison of suicide rates among industrial groups. *Am J Ind Med* 1994;25: 197–203.
162. Schnake M, Dumler MP. predictors of propensity to turnover in the construction industry. *Psychol Rep* 2000;86:1000–1002.
163. Brown B. Solving the problem of repeat injuries. *Occup Haz* 1999;61:50,54.
164. Schneider S. Implement ergonomic interventions in construction. *Appl Occup Environ Hyg* 1995;10: 822–824.
165. Behrens VJ, Brackbill RM. Worker awareness of exposure: industries and occupations with law awareness. *Am J Ind Med* 1993;22:695–701.
166. Gyi DE, Haslam RA, Giff AGF. Case studies of occupational health management in the engineering construction industry. *Occup Med* 1998;48:263–271.
167. Dedobbeleer N, German P. Safety practices in construction industry. *Occup Med* 1987;29:863–868.
168. Nash IL. Skin care: staring from scratch. *Occup Haz* 2000;62:53–55.
169. Marsicans L. Getting lost in the rubble—is industrial hygiene receiving the attention it deserves in the construction health and safety arena? *Synergist* 1995;6: 18–19.
170. James C. Occupational injuries amongst building workers in Queensland. *Saf Australia* 1993;M.V. 8–11, abstracted in *J Occup Health Saf Aust NZ* 1993;9:112.
171. Mayhew C, Gibson G. Self-employed builders: factors which influence the probability of work-related injury and illness. *J Occup Health Saf Aust NZ* 1996;12:61–67.
172. Pollack ES, Franklin GM, Gulton-Kehoe D, et al. Risk of job-related injury among construction laborers with a diagnosis of substance abuse. *J Occup Environ Med* 1998;40:573–577.
173. *Women in the construction workplace: providing equitable safety and health protection.* Washington, DC: U.S. Department of Labor, Occupational Safety and Health Administration, June 1999. Available at *http:// www.osha-slc.gov/doc/accsh/haswicformal.html.*
174. Women in construction need improved workplace culture, safety, and health. *Synergist* 1998;9:25.
175. Germani D, Belli S, Bruno C, et al. Cohort mortality study of women compensated for asbestosis in Italy. *Am J Ind Med* 1999;36:129–134.
176. Ore T. Women in the U.S. construction industry: an analysis of fatal occupational injury experience, 1980 to 1992. *Am J Ind Med* 1998;33:256–262.

177. Robinson CF, Burnett CA. Mortality patterns of U.S. female construction workers by race, 1979–1990. *J Occup Med* 1994;36:1228–1233.
178. Welch LS, Goldenhar LM, Hunting KL. Women in construction: occupational health and working conditions *J Am Med Womens Assoc* 2000;55:89–92.
179. Islam SS, Velilla AM, Doyle EJ, et al. Gender differences in work-related injury/illness: analysis of workers compensation claims. *Am J Ind Med* 2001;39: 84–91.
180. Suruda A, Smith G, Baker SP. Deaths from trench cave-in in the construction industry. *J Occup Med* 1988;30:552–555.
181. Herman AM. A message from the secretary of labor. Washington, DC: U.S. Department of Labor: *http://www.dol.gov/*. See also: NIOSH warns: employment may be hazardous for adolescent workers: *http://www.cdc.gov/niosh/95-115.html.*
182. Ringen K, Englund A, Welch L, et al. Why construction is different. *Occup Med* 1995;10:255–259.
183. Scientists confirm MSDS can be attributed to specific jobs. *Occup Haz* 2001;63:24–25.
184. Roscoe RJ, Gittleman JL, Deddens JA, et al. Blood lead levels among children of lead-exposed workers: a meta-analysis. *Am J Ind Med* 1999;36:475–481.
185. Kinlen LS. High-contact paternal occupations, infection and childhood leukemia: five studies of unusual population-mixing of adults. *Br J Cancer* 1997;76: 1539–1545.
186. Piacitelli GM, Whelan EA, Sieber WK, et al. Elevated lead contamination in homes of construction workers. *Am Ind Hyg Assoc J* 1997;58:447–454.
187. Piacitelli GM, Whelan EA, Ewers LM, et al. Lead contamination in automobiles of lead-exposed bridge-workers. *Appl Occup Environ Hyg* 1993;10:849–855.
188. Preventing lead poisoning in construction workers. NIOSH alert, April 1992: *http://www.cdc.gov/niosh/91-116.html.*
189. NIOSH update: children of construction workers at increased risk for lead poisoning: *http://www.cdc.gov/niosh/leadpois.html.*
190. Report to Congress on Workers' Home Contamination Study Conducted Under the Workers' Family Protection Act (29 U.S.C. 671A): *http://www.cdc.gov/niosh/contamin.html.*
191. Weber A, Page E. Renovation of contaminated building materials at a facility serving pediatric cancer outpatients. *Appl Occup Environ Hyg* 2001;16:2–31.
192. Ellringer PJ, Boone K, Hendrickson S. building materials used in construction can affect indoor fungal levels greatly. *Am Ind Hyg Assoc J* 2000;61:895–899.
193. Occupational Safety and Health Standards for the Construction Industry, 29 CFR, part 1926.
194. *Construction Industry Digest*. OHA 2202, 1998 (revised). Washington, DC: U.S. Department of Labor, Occupational Safety and Health Administration, 1998.
195. Directorate of Construction (OSHA): *http://www.osha-slc.gov.*
196. Division of Construction Services (OSHA): *http://www.oshaslc,gov.*
197. Advisory Committee on Construction Safety and Health (ACCSH): *http://www.osha-slc.gov.*
198. Advisory Committee on Construction Safety and Health (ACCSH) Multi-Employer Citation Policy Work Group: *http://www.osha-slc.gov.*
199. Advisory Committee on Construction Safety and Health. Preventing musculoskeletal disorders in construction workers (draft): *http://www.osha-slc.gov.*
200. Ringen K. National conference on ergonomics, safety, and health in construction. *Appl Occup Environ Hyg* 1994;9:239–241.
201. Salwen P. Commitment, communication: keys to worker safety in construction. *Occup Health Saf* 1989;58:34,36–37.
202. OSHA Outreach Training Program: *http://www.osha-slc.gov/training.*
203. Culver C. Build a safer construction site. *Safety and Health* 1993;147:74–76.
204. Fairfax F. Construction health exposures. *Appl Occup Environ Hyg* 1994;9:168–170.
205. Linch KD, Cocalis JC. An emerging issue: silicosis prevention in construction *Appl Occup Environ Hyg* 1994;9:539–542.
206. Moran JB. Mortality among construction laborers: new dimensions. *Appl Occup Environ Hyg* 1994;9: 764–768.
207. Maclean J, Malaby F. Multiple solvent exposure on a construction site. *Appl Occup Environ Hyg* 1995;10: 17–18.
208. Rautiala S, Reponen T, Hyvarinen A, et al. Exposure to airborne microbes during the repair of moldy buildings. *Am Ind Hyg Assoc J* 1996;57:279–284.
209. OSHA Instruction TED 1.15, Sec. IV construction operations, Chap. 1: Demolition, September 22, 1995.
210. *NIOSH alert: request for assistance in preventing silicosis and deaths in construction workers.* DHHS (NIOSH) Pub. No. 96-1112. Washington, DC: U.S. Department of Health and Human Services, Public Health Service, Centers for Disease Control and Prevention, National Institute for Occupational Safety and Health, May, 1996.
211. OSHA Instruction CPL2-2.53. Guidelines for first aid training programs, January 7, 1991.
212. OSHA directive STD 1-82-29 CFR, part 1910.151(6), medical services and first aid; 29 CFR, part 1926.50 and 51. medical service and first aid, March 8, 1982.
213. Derocher RJ. Confined spaces—does construction need its own standard? *Safety and Health* 2000;161: 51–55.
214. Bushkin SE, Paulozzi LN. Fatal injuries in the construction industry in Washington State. *Am J Ind Med* 1987;11:453–460.
215. Goldenhar LM, Sweeney MH. Tradeswomen's perspectives on occupational health and safety: a qualitative investigation. *Am J Ind Med* 1996;29:516–520.
216. National Institute for Occupational Safety and Health and Chicago Women in Trades. *Providing safety and health protection for a diverse construction workforce: issues and ideas.* DHHS (NIOSH) publication No. 99-140. Cincinnati: NIOSH, 1999.
217. Heberle KD. *Construction safety manual.* New York: McGraw-Hill, 1998.
218. Anderson JTL, Hunting KL, Welch LS. Injury and employment patterns among Hispanic construction workers. *J Occup Environ Med* 2000;42:176–186.
219. Latinos' safety and health risks. *Safety and Health* 2000;161:12–13.
220. Brown B. Do you really want it reported? *Synergist* 2000;11:28–29.
221. Personal Protective Equipment (rev), OSHA 3088.

Washington, DC: U.S. Department of Labor, Occupational Safety and Health Administration, 1998. See also OSHA regulations (29 CFR). Criteria for personal protective equipment (part 1926.95).
222. Greaves WW. Reproductive hazards. In: McCunney RJ, ed. *A practical approach to environmental medicine,* 2nd ed. Boston: Little, Brown, 1994:447–464.
223. Whelan EA, Piacitelli GM, Gerwel B, et al. Elevated blood levels in children of construction workers. *Am J Public Health* 1997;87:1352–1355.
224. Freestone AE. Training travels in Texas—classroom on wheels facilitates learning. *Safety and Health* 2000; 161:30–32.
225. Lusk SL, Kerr MJ, Kauffman SA. Use of hearing protection and perceptions of noise exposure and hearing loss among construction workers. *Am Ind Hyg Assoc J* 1998;59:466–470.
226. Mayhew C, Ferris R. The impact of the legislative requirement for the completion of workplace health and safety plans on small-scale Queensland builders. *J Occup Health Saf Aust NZ* 1998;14:357–362.
227. Dessoff AL. Seek simple solutions for ergonomics problems in construction. *Safety and Health* 1996;153: 62–65.
228. OSHA Regulations (29 CFR). Safety training and education (part 1926.21).
229. Work Zone Safety Information Clearinghouse: *http://wzsafety.tamu.edu*.
230. Busick J. The quest for workzone safety. *Occup Haz* 1999;61:155–156,158,160.
231. *Consultation services to the employer*. OSHA 3047 (revised). Washington, DC: U.S. Department of Labor, Occupational Safety and Health Administration, 1997:7.
232. *On-site consultation*. South San Francisco: CAL/OSHA Consultation Services, [n.d]. p. 10.
233. *Construction safety pocket guide: http://www.genium.com/training/cspg.shtwl*.
234. Communication skills imperative in construction health and safety. *Synergist* 1995;6:10.
235. Wang E, Dement JM, Lipscomb H. Mortality among North Carolina construction workers, 1988–1991. *Appl Occup Environ Hyg* 1998;40:63–68.
236. Rothenbacher D, Arndt V, Fraisse E, et al. Early retirement due to permanent disability in relation to smoking in workers of the construction industry. *J Occup Environ Med* 1998;40:63–68.
237. Nong JW. Occupational injuries among construction workers in Hong Kong. *Occup Med (Lond)* 1994;44: 247–252.
238. Bigos SJ, Battie MC, Spengler GM, et al. A prospective study of work perceptions and psychological factors affecting the report of back injuries. *Spine* 1991; 16:1–6.
239. Marks N. An evaluation of a multifaceted back care program for the construction industry. *Appl Occup Environ Hyg* 1997;12:642–647.
240. Sharing Solutions (program announcement). The Behavior-Based Safety Leadership Conference, Dallas, Texas, March 11–12, 1998.
241. Findley M. Management needs behavior-based safety initiatives too. *Safety and Health* 2000;161:44–48.
242. Behavior-based safety—is it the Holy Grail of the workplace? *Safety and Health* 2000;161:35–42.
243. Arndt V, Rothenbacher D, Brenner H, et al. Older workers in the construction industry: results of routine health examination and a five-year follow-up. *Occup Environ Med* 1996;53:686–691.
244. Robinson C, Stern F, Halperin W, et al. Assessment of mortality in the construction industry in the United States, 1984–1986. *Am J Ind Med* 1995;28:49–70.
245. Fassa AG, Facchini LA, Dall'Agnol MM, et al. Child labor and health: problems and perspectives. *Int J Occup Environ Health* 2000;6:55–62.
246. Windau J, Sygnatur E, Toscano G. Profile of work injuries incurred by young workers. *Mo Labor Rev* 1999; 122:3–10.
247. *Facts for employers—super jobs for teens*. Berkeley: Labor Occupational Health Program, University of California, 1998.
248. Baron J, Stroe TL, Francescutti LH. The construction flagperson: a target for injury. *Occup Med (Lond)* 1998;48:199–202.
249. Bradley JC. Workplace solutions [Solutions for workers who need enhanced visibility]. *Safety and Health* 2001;136:66. See also Nighswonger T. Do your workers need high-visibility apparel? *Occup Haz* 2001;63: 45–46, 48.
250. California Fatality Assessment and Control (FACE) Program. Construction Superintendent Dies when Crushed by Falling Crane Boom in California. California FACE report No. 96CA003, October 2, 1996; see also Suruda A, Liu D, Egger M, et al. Fatal injuries in the United States construction industry involving cranes, 1984–1994. *J Occup Environ Med* 1999;41:1052–1058.
251. *NAHBOSHA jobsite safety handbook*. Washington, DC: NAHB and OSHA, [n.d.].
252. Tompkins NC. *How to write a company safety manual,* 2nd ed. Boston: Standard Publishing, 1998. See also Goldsmith PE. Turning action into words: the art of the safety manual. *Synergist* 2001;12:13.
253. Washington Industrial Safety and Health Act (WISHA) Services. *How to write an accident prevention program*. Olympia, WA: Department of Labor and Industries, WISHA Services, February 2, 1996.
254. Menesini M, Rice J. Investigating accidents: *http://www.cdc.gov/niosh/elcosh/docs/d0200/d000290/d000290.html*.
255. Rosner D. When does a worker's death become murder? *Am J Public Health* 2000;90:535–540.
256. Edgar H. Homicide prosecutions and progress toward workplace safety. *Am J Public Health* 2000;90: 533–534.
257. Steel erection (part 1926) (safety protection for ironworkers) 1218-AA65, final rule. *Fed Reg* 2000(November 30);65(231).
258. Karr A. OSHA unveils three standards in final Clinton days. *Safety and Health* 2001;163:16.
259. OSHA National News Release, USDL:01-24, Jan. 17, 2001. OSHA issues new steel erection standard.
260. New safety system bids to cut construction industry fatalities—and boost speed of working: *http:www.shu.ac.ukcgi-binnews*.
261. OSHA Training Institute Schedule. *Job Saf Health Q* 2001;12:17–21.
262. OSHA Trade News Release, OSHA partners with contractors, February 14, 2000.
263. Associated General Contractors of America News Release, January 9, 2001. Injuries, illnesses, and fatalities to be reduced in industry partnership: *http://www.incongress.com*.
264. de Jong AM, Schaefer WF, Vink P. Evaluation of par-

ticipative projects in the construction industry: an analysis of the effectiveness of the results in practice: *http://www.cdc.gov/niosh/elcosh*.
265. Workplace diversity training on line: *http:trainingonline.com*.
266. Safety management training course: *http://www.agc.org/safety_info/safety_management.asp*.
267. Krispin K. The new face of drug testing. *Safety and Health* 2001;163:44–46, 48.
268. Myers L. Construction company drug testing reduces work injuries, study finds: *http:www.news.cornell.eduChronicles6.29.00drug-testing.html*.
269. Hoskin A. Safety and health report. *Safety and Health* 1999;159:88–90.
270. Occupational Safety and Health Act of 1970. Public Law 91-596, December 29, 1970.
271. Do construction workers fall through the cracks? *Safety and Health* 1997;155–159.
272. Bayer R. Whither occupational health and safety? (Editor's note). *Am J Public Health* 2000;90:532.
273. Builders in demand—construction industry seeking skilled workers. *Press Democrat* April 16, 2000;J1.
274. BLS Releases New 1998–2008 Employment Projections: *http://stats.bls.gov/news.release/ecopro.nr0.htm*.
275. Rospond KM. Construction safety at a crossroads. *Safety and Health* 2001;163:54–56, 58.
276. National health plan includes job safety goals. *Occup Haz* 2000;62:28.

47

Health Risk Communication

Victor S. Roth, David H. Garabrant, and Craig F. Turet

Clear and understandable communication to employees of the potential health risks from work-related exposures and the proper training of these employees in the safe performance of their job tasks go hand in hand.

BASIS OF HEALTH RISK COMMUNICATION

There are several reasons for the promulgation by employers to their employees of information regarding potential health and safety threats posed by the workplace. Primary among those reasons is the training mandated by the Occupational Safety and Health Administration (OSHA) standards. Additionally, employers realize that properly trained workers increase workplace efficiency, decrease injury and illness, decrease workers' compensation costs, and decrease litigation.

Health Risk Communication and Mandatory/Nonmandatory OSHA Training

The health and safety training regulations contained in OSHA standards include not only mandatory but also nonmandatory training. Numerous OSHA standards explicitly require the employer to train employees in the safety and health aspects of their jobs. Other OSHA standards make it the employer's responsibility to limit certain job assignments to employees who are "proficient," ("meeting a stated level of achievement") (1) and/or "competent" ("possessing the skills, knowledge, experience, and judgment to perform assigned tasks or activities satisfactorily as determined by the employer") (1) in the performance of specific job tasks. Risk reduction is typically handled through proper training, signage, and personal protective equipment (2).

Health Risk Communication and the Hazard Communication Standard

In November 1983, OSHA promulgated the Hazard Communication Standard (HazCom), a regulation covering a broad range of chemical hazards. This standard contains specific provisions regarding the evaluation of health hazards, labeling of containers, use of chemical information sheets known as Material Safety Data Sheets (MSDSs), and training of employees. The HazCom standard originally applied only to chemical manufacturers, importers, and distributors, but was later expanded to cover many additional employers. Presently, all companies and employers that handle any hazardous substance in any form are required to comply with the standard (3).

HazCom, commonly known as the "worker right to know" law, mandates that workers receive training and information on all the potentially hazardous chemicals with which they work. It is a performance-based standard because it specifies what employers must do but not how they must do it. The basic components of the standard are as follows (4):

1. Manufacturers must produce a MSDS for all hazardous chemicals that they produce and sell.
2. MSDSs must be shipped to all downstream users of the hazardous chemicals.
3. In all workplaces in which hazardous chemicals are present, the employer is responsible for the following:
    a. Labeling all hazardous chemicals in the workplace
    b. A written hazardous chemicals program that is accessible to employees who ask for it
    c. A system for managing MSDSs with worker access to them
    d. A training program for all employees who may experience an exposure to a potentially hazardous chemical
4. The training program must include information on the following:
    a. Location and identity of hazardous chemicals
    b. Physical hazards
    c. Health effects (acute and long-term)
    d. Proper work practices and personal protection

e. First aid
f. Emergency response (including fire, leak, and spill)
g. Workers' rights under HazCom
h. Labeling systems
i. MSDS systems

HazCom and its components were revised in 1987 to include health care institutions. The purpose of this inclusion was to "enable hospital managers to learn more about the types of hazardous materials used in the health care setting and allow hospital employees to work with these materials in a more safe manner" (5). On February 15, 1989, OSHA announced that the 1987 HazCom revision was effective immediately, preempting individual states' hazardous substances regulations. According to the revised standard, manufacturers must determine whether chemicals they produce are hazardous; a pharmacy compounding a drug mixture may even be considered a manufacturer according to the standard (6).

Some employers believe that compliance with the HazCom means only obtaining and filing appropriate MSDSs. In reality, the employer should also arrange for the worker to have access to this information through training and MSDS retrieval. HazCom is a proactive standard, and is explicit about employers' responsibility to train workers, not just to respond to requests for information when workers ask for it.

Health Risk Communication and the Blood-borne Pathogen Standard

Physician and other health care worker interest in OSHA regulations increased with the publication of the Bloodborne Pathogens Standard (7). The Bloodborne Pathogens Standard is the first standard promulgated by OSHA that addresses a biologic hazard in the workplace. This standard applies to all workers with occupational exposure to blood or other potentially infectious materials. The goal of the standard is to reduce the occupational risk of morbidity and mortality associated with diseases such as hepatitis B and human immunodeficiency virus (HIV) (8). To achieve compliance, the employer must determine and document exposure. Also, a written exposure control plan must be available that stipulates the use of appropriate methods of compliance such as engineering controls, work practice controls, and use of personal protective equipment (9). The Bloodborne Pathogens Standard includes requirements for employee hazard communication and training as well as management of regulated waste, contaminated laundry, and proper housekeeping procedures. OSHA recognizes the benefits of prophylactic hepatitis B vaccine and therefore requires that the vaccine be available at no charge to employees at risk, that is, those with occupational exposure to blood or other potentially infectious materials.

The main points that relate to employee training that are contained in the OSHA Bloodborne Pathogens Standard (1910.1030) include (a) epidemiology and symptoms of bloodborne diseases; (b) modes of transmission of bloodborne pathogens; (c) methods of recognizing tasks that involve exposure to blood or other potentially infectious materials; (d) methods to prevent exposure including personal protective equipment; (e) information on appropriate action following an exposure incident; and (f) information on the hepatitis B vaccine.

On November 6, 2000, Congress passed the Needlestick Safety and Prevention Act, directing OSHA to revise its bloodborne pathogens standard to describe in greater detail its requirement for employers to identify and make use of effective and safer medical devices. That revision was published on January 18, 2001, and became effective April 18, 2001.

Specifically, the revised OSHA Bloodborne Pathogens Standard obligates employers to consider safer needle devices when they conduct their annual review of their exposure control plan. Safer sharps are considered appropriate engineering controls, the best strategy for worker protection. There is increased employee/employer communication in the revision, as it obligates the employer to involve frontline employees in selecting safer devices, anticipating that this will help ensure that workers who are using the equipment have the opportunity for input into purchasing decisions. The revision also mandates a new needlestick log, as this organized information for all such injuries will help both employees and employers track all needlesticks to help identify problem areas or operations. The updated standard also includes the following provisions, designed to maintain the privacy of employees who have experienced needlesticks (10):

- Employers must review their exposure control plans annually to reflect changes in technology that will help eliminate or reduce exposure to bloodborne pathogens. That review must include documentation of the employer's consideration and implementation of appropriate commercially available and effective safer devices.
- Employers must solicit input from nonmanagerial health care workers regarding the identification, evaluation, and selection of effective engineering controls, including safer medical devices. Examples of employees include those in different departments of the facility (e.g., geriatric, pediatric, nuclear medicine, etc.).

- Employers with 11 or more employees who are required to keep records by current record-keeping standards must maintain a sharps injury log. The log must be maintained in a way to ensure employee privacy and will contain, at minimum, the following information:
- Type and brand of device involved in the incident, if known;
- Location of the incident; and
- Description of the incident.

The federal government is ensuring that this revision is communicated to those workers who are most affected, that is, those in health care. OSHA's attempt to communicate the revisions added to the Bloodborne Pathogens Standard and OSHA's education effort to that effect include a collection of written materials designed to explain specific aspects of the revised standard and "outreach period." The written materials are also available on OSHA's Web site, *www.osha.gov*.

During the outreach period, in which communication, education, and awareness of the revisions to the Bloodborne Pathogens Standard was a priority, OSHA enforced the new provisions of the standard that required employers to maintain a sharps injury log and involve nonmanagerial employees in selecting safer medical devices on July 17, 2001 (11).

The Bloodborne Pathogens Standard is further detailed in Chapters 31 and 44.

Health Risk Communication and Material Safety Data Sheets (MSDSs)

Material Safety Data Sheets, directly related to an OSHA standard (HazCom), are a foundation of a successful safety and health program. MSDSs are available from the workplace in which the chemical is being used, from the manufacturer of the chemical, and, in most cases, on the Internet. In most cases, a worker brought in for medical evaluation following a chemical exposure will be accompanied by the appropriate MSDSs.

MSDSs provide information that can be used during employee training and chemical exposure incidents and give vital information to medical professionals caring for the affected employee. They inform employees of the health hazards of chemicals with which they are working and let them know what situations have the potential to produce explosion or decomposition hazards. The purpose of these sheets is to communicate critical facts about working safely with the hazardous material.

The MSDSs provide workers with enough information about a specific chemical substance to understand (a) potential acute and chronic health effects; (b) recommended personal protective equipment; (c) proper work practices; (d) first-aid treatment following exposure; (e) spill, leak, and fire precautions and appropriate responses; and (f) other additional information that may be necessary to work safely with the potentially hazardous substance (4).

MSDSs vary with respect to thoroughness and the extent to which chemicals are specified on the sheet. Thus, the physician treating a patient with an exposure identified on the MSDS should realize that the information contained in the document might be incomplete. Some chemicals may not be listed at all, and the broad class of materials to which they belong may identify others. In some cases, it is necessary to contact the manufacturer listed on the MSDS to obtain additional information.

An example of MSDS variability is highlighted in a study that analyzed reproductive health hazard descriptions on almost 700 MSDSs for lead- or ethylene glycol ether–containing products submitted by Massachusetts companies to the Department of Environmental Protection under provisions of the Massachusetts Right-to-Know Law (12). More than 60% of the MSDSs made no mention of potential effects of these chemicals on the human reproductive system. Those that did mention these adverse effects were much more likely to address fetal development risks and omit any male reproductive effects. MSDSs from larger companies (employing 100 or more workers) mentioned reproductive system effects more frequently than MSDSs from smaller companies. A significant proportion (53%) of the MSDSs prepared after promulgation of the OSHA HazCom still contained no information on reproductive risks.

The specific chemical identity of a hazardous substance may be withheld from the MSDS if it is determined that the information regarding this chemical is a trade secret (information used in one's business that gives that employer an opportunity to obtain an advantage over competitors who do not know how to use the chemical in this way). However, the MSDS must contain information concerning the *properties* and *effects* of the hazardous chemical and also must indicate that the specific chemical is being withheld as a trade secret. If a treating physician or nurse determines that a medical emergency exists that requires additional information about the specific chemical, the manufacturer, importer, or employer shall immediately disclose the specific chemical identity of a trade secret chemical to that physician or nurse. In nonemergency situations, health professionals must request information about trade secret chemicals in writing, detailing the need for such information. The health professional may be required to sign a confidentiality agreement, stating that information disclosed will not be used for any purpose other than for the health needs asserted.

MSDSs must be readily accessible to employees when they are in their work areas during their shifts. Some employers keep the MSDSs in a binder in a central location. Others computerize the information and provide access to employees through computer terminals either saved on the on-site computer hard drive, on a floppy disc or CD-ROM, or on the company's Internet or Intranet Web site specific to that location.

With chemicals becoming more abundant in the workplace, and with new and more complex chemicals being developed, the MSDS is a valuable tool for the occupational physician in conducting occupational medicine evaluations for surveillance purposes and in evaluating exposure-related symptoms. It is therefore important that the physician advise potentially exposed workers and their employers that all pertinent MSDSs should accompany the employee when he or she is evaluated for chemical exposure.

Health Risk Communication and the Emergency Planning and Community Right-to-Know Act

Concern over the safety of manufacturing, transporting, using, and disposing of extremely hazardous chemicals is worldwide. Tragic incidents such as occurred at Bhopal, India, and Love Canal, New York, amplify this concern.

In the United States, there is an increased awareness and concern about process incidents involving hazardous materials. This fear permeates down to the local level in communities where explosive or toxic chemicals are manufactured or regularly used on site. Population growth resulted in large residential areas and institutional buildings being built near pre-existing chemical plants and chemical storage tanks. Occupational physicians are regularly asked to see patients who request evaluation due to their fear of potential or actual adverse physiologic effects to themselves or other family members from living in the vicinity of such work sites.

Passage of the Emergency Planning and Community Right-to-Know Act of 1986, also known as the Superfund Amendments and Reauthorization Act Title III, has broadened the need to convey information about the health effects of chemicals from the workplace to the general community (13). MSDSs constitute the primary source of health effects information about hazardous chemicals under Title III, although MSDSs were originally intended to be used in the occupational setting. This act mandates that every facility using, storing, or manufacturing hazardous chemicals reveal to the public its inventory of such chemicals and notify public officials and appropriate health personal every time a hazardous chemical is released. These facilities must also cooperate fully with physicians who treat the victims of hazardous chemical exposure.

Health Risk Communication and Process Safety Management of Highly Hazardous Chemicals

Recognizing the tragic events that can result from the accidental release of hazardous chemicals led OSHA to issue in 1992 the regulation known as the Process Safety Management of Highly Hazardous Chemicals. The main points related to training are as follows:

Initial training: Employees presently involved in operating a process, and employees about to become involved in operating newly assigned processes, shall be trained in an overview of the process and procedure. The training shall include safety and health hazards emergency operations including shutdown, and safe work practices applicable to the employee's job task.

Refresher training: Refresher training shall be provided at least every 3 years, and more often if necessary, to employees involved in an operating process to ensure that the employees understand and adhere to the current and proper operating procedure of the process.

Documentation of training: The employer shall prepare a record that contains the identity of each employee who undergoes training, the date of such training, and the means used to verify the employee's understanding of the training. Posttraining exams are not mandatory. In most cases, the employee's attendance at the training session(s) assumes retention by the employee of the material presented.

Health Risk Communication and OSHA Posters

In August 2000, OSHA introduced a new workplace poster for informing workers of their rights to a safe workplace (14). The posters are free and may also be downloaded from the OSHA Web site.

"Making sure workers are safe on the job is a top priority of the Department of Labor, and OSHA's new poster is another way we do that," Secretary of Labor Alexis M. Herman said. "Redesigned as part of President Clinton's and Vice President Gore's plain language initiative, it gives workers and employers information they need to make sure their workplace is a safe workplace."

Employers are not obligated to replace the posters they already have, but they are required to post an

OSHA notice of employee rights in a prominent location. The new poster tells workers in plain language that they have the right to a safe workplace, how they may file a complaint, report an emergency, or seek OSHA advice, and that they have a right to confidentiality.

The poster must be displayed in a conspicuous place where employees and applicants for employment can see it. Title 29 Code of Federal Regulations, 1903.2(a)(3), states that reproductions or facsimiles of the poster shall be at least 8½ by 14 inches with 10-point type.

Health Risk Communication and OSHA Partnerships

The OSHA Strategic Partnership Program for Worker Safety and Health (OSPP), adopted on November 13, 1998, is an expansion and formalization of OSHA's substantial experience with voluntary programs. In a partnership, OSHA enters into an extended, voluntary, cooperative relationship with groups of employers, employees, and employee representatives (sometimes including other stakeholders, and sometimes involving only one employer) in order to encourage, assist, and recognize their efforts to eliminate serious hazards and achieve a high level of worker safety and health.

There are two types of partnerships available with OSHA:

Comprehensive: Each participating employer is committed to implement in a timely manner an effective workplace safety and health program. The hallmarks of an effective program are management leadership and employee involvement, hazard analysis, hazard prevention and control, safety and health training, evaluation, and compliance with applicable OSHA requirements.

Limited: The employer may choose to require that the partners establish comprehensive work-site safety and health programs. However, the employer may alternatively choose to focus on eliminating a prevalent hazard in a particular industry or on solving some other problem.

Partnerships have the potential to transform the relationship between OSHA and an employer or even an entire industry. Partners recognize that working together to solve workplace safety and health problems is to everyone's advantage and is much less costly than paying penalties for violations and rising workers' compensation premiums.

A partnership benefits workers by reducing risk of injury, illness, or death on the job; increasing practical safety and health knowledge and skills; affording the opportunity to work cooperatively with OSHA and the employer; enhancing employee morale and quality of work life.

A partnership benefits employers by involving stakeholders in the process of identifying and solving problems relating to workplace safety and health; providing employers with an opportunity to learn how to systematically manage safety and health at their work sites; reducing workers' compensation insurance premiums and costs of injuries and illnesses; increasing productivity, enhancing employee morale, reducing absenteeism; improving the company's relationship with OSHA; and providing opportunities to help other businesses, the employer's industry, and the community through outreach activities.

Partnerships benefit OSHA through the opportunity to work cooperatively to improve worker protection; establishing alternatives to traditional enforcement activity; enabling OSHA to increase its emphasis on serious hazards; providing a means to gather data and track reductions in injuries and illnesses and other indices of worker safety and health; offering opportunities to leverage the agency's limited resources; and producing models of effective, voluntary, and cooperative compliance.

Health Risk Communication and Employee Involvement in OSHA Work-site Consultations

Employees now play a larger role in OSHA work-site consultation visits. The on-site consultation programs funded by OSHA and managed by state agencies provide expert advice from trained consultants to assist employers in identifying workplace hazards and in establishing safety and health programs (15).

OSHA claims that since it is the employees who often have firsthand knowledge of hazards in the workplace, the workers' participation in the visit and their suggestions for correcting problems helps to ensure the effectiveness of the consultation in improving workplace conditions.

The OSHA consultation is free, but employers who request OSHA's help agree, in advance, to correct all serious hazards identified by the consultant. OSHA gives top priority for these consultations to hazardous industries with fewer than 250 employees on site or no more than 500 employees nationwide.

The new rule allows authorized employees the right to accompany the OSHA consultant during the physical inspection of the workplace. Authorized employee representatives are also permitted to participate in opening and closing conferences with the OSHA consultant (either separately or jointly with the employer). In cases where there is no authorized representative, or where such a representative cannot be determined, the OSHA consultant should speak to a reasonable number of employees about workplace safety and health.

Under the revised rule, employers must post a list of the serious hazards identified by the consultant and the dates for completing the corrective action for these problems. This list must be posted in a prominent place, easily observed by all affected employees for 3 days or until the hazards are corrected, whichever is later. A copy of the posted list will also be given to the authorized employee representative who participated in the consultation. The rule does allow for electronic posting of the hazards list, if the employer demonstrates that electronic posting is as effective as hardcopy posting.

The rule also offers special recognition through the Safety and Health Achievement Recognition Program (SHARP) for employers who complete a consultation visit and meet specific requirements (correcting all hazards and demonstrating that all the elements of a safety and health program are in place). SHARP participants receive a 1-year exemption from scheduled OSHA inspections.

The final rule, Consultation Agreement: Changes to Consultation Procedures, 29 CFR Part 1908, was published in the October 26, 2000 *Federal Register* and was effective on December 26, 2000.

Health Risk Communication and Effective Presentations

As part of the Construction Safety and Health Outreach Program, the OSHA Office of Training and Education, released the document, "Presenting Effective Presentations with Visual Aids" in May 1996 (16). This information is available on the OSHA Web site.

According to the document, OSHA is concerned that training information presented be understood by the employee; otherwise the training will not be effective. Therefore, employers must include training material that is appropriate in content and vocabulary to the educational, literacy, and language background of employees. This will ensure that all employees, regardless of their cultural or education background, will receive adequate training on how to eliminate or minimize their occupational exposure.

Training sessions should be designed so that sufficient time is allocated not only to present the information but also to allow for questions and review of materials as needed. The trainer needs to provide an environment in which participants feel sufficiently comfortable in order to ask questions and make comments. Asking questions and discussing aspects of a training program can clarify information and reinforce important learning objectives.

Health Risk Communication and Concerns with Health and Safety Training

It is well established that health and safety training and communication decrease mortality and morbidity in the workplace. In a study of blood lead levels and exposure to lead in construction workers (17), completed questionnaires contained, among other items, the participants' information on personal protective equipment and training. The authors concluded that the trend toward lower blood lead levels in those performing lead abatement provided evidence that employee training, implementation of engineering controls, and proper use of personal protective equipment are effective in controlling lead poisoning.

In many cases, even with proper worker training, it is management that is responsible for communicating health risk of exposure to the worker. The use of engineering and work practice controls to protect workers from lead-containing dusts and fumes generated during rehabilitation of steel structures is mandated by the OSHA Lead in Construction Standard (1993). A study compared lead exposures at one site without controls to exposures at sites utilizing two lead exposure controls [(a) paint removal prior to oxy-acetylene torch cutting of steel and (b) encapsulation of rivets prior to their removal to reduce lead exposure] (18). The results indicated that, for torch cutting, exposures at the control site were not significantly different from those at an uncontrolled site. The results for rivet busting also showed no significant differences at the control site compared to the uncontrolled site. One of the conclusions reached by the authors was that this was a management problem arising from a lack of coordination among different contractors and from a failure to provide day-to-day guidance and assessment of the control.

Of additional concern, even when properly trained workers use personal protective equipment such as respirators, is whether or not these devices actually protect the worker, to the degree expected, from the harmful effects and, therefore, the risks of potential exposure. Again, using lead as an example, a recent study of negative pressure and powered air purifying respirators came to the conclusion that this may not be the case (19). The negative pressure half-mask respirators showed a mean effective protection factor of 6.5 and a mean corrected effective protection factor of 4.6, while the assigned protection factor for these respirators was 10. For the powered air purifying half-mask respirators, the means for effective protection factor and corrected effective protection factor were 18.2 and 11.9, respectively, while the assigned protection factor for these respirators was 50. The uncorrected and corrected within-mask lead concentrations for both types of respirators exceeded the OSHA permissible exposure limit (PEL) for lead from 19% up to 58%.

Silicosis is another example in which proper training of workers about limiting the level of a specific (silica) exposure, even to levels below the current OSHA standard, could prevent future disease. A recent study cites the risk of silicosis [International Labor Organization (ILO) category 1/1 or more] following a lifetime of exposure at the current OSHA standard of 0.1 mg/m^3 as at least 5% to 10%, and the lung cancer risk at this level is likely to be increased by 30% or more. Available data suggest that 30 years' exposure at 0.1 mg/m^3 might lead to a lifetime silicosis risk of about 25%, whereas reduction of the exposure to 0.05 mg/m^3 might reduce the risk to less than 5%. Lowering silica exposures to the National Institute of Occupational Safety and Health (NIOSH) recommended limit of 0.05 mg/m^3, which is half the current OSHA standard, may result in substantial health benefits (20).

Employers and employees should not feel complacent about the training and knowledge they have had to date, even if this training and communication is in full compliance with OSHA rules and standards. Training and communication is a continuous, ongoing, and evolving process that never ends.

EVALUATING THE ADEQUACY OF WARNINGS AND HAZARD COMMUNICATIONS

Warnings should be supplements to, not substitutes for, programs that focus on designing out and guarding against hazards. The warning process requires both communication from a source and information processing by the recipient. To be effective, the warning must be consistent with the recipients' attitudes and beliefs, must be comprehensible to the recipients at their level of technical competence, and must be capable of influencing their behavior (21). In evaluating whether a warning is needed, the following principles should be considered:

- A significant hazard exists.
- The people exposed to the hazard are not likely to know of the hazard, its consequences, or safe behavior.
- The hazard is not obvious.
- People need to be reminded at the proper time to ensure awareness of the hazard and of safe behavior.

The ultimate measure of the effectiveness of a warning is behavioral compliance. Common reasons that warnings fail to produce safe behavior include insufficient salience of the message, lack of understanding, attitudes and beliefs that are discordant with the warning, and insufficient motivation to follow the recommended behavior. While much of the expertise needed to evaluate the adequacy of warnings comes from the areas of cognitive psychology, human factors, and communications science, the content of warnings regarding health risks also falls squarely in the domain of occupational and environmental physicians and toxicologists who understand mechanisms of toxicity, clinical toxicity in humans, and long-term risks to humans at various levels of exposure. Individuals who design and run hazard communication programs often include assessments of the effectiveness of the communications either through empiric tests of user responses, posttraining exams, comparisons of programs across other products or devices that present similar hazards, or by determining the extent to which the warning complies with standards. Occupational physicians often play a critical role in developing and in evaluating hazard communications and warnings because of their specialized knowledge and their experience in communicating information to laymen regarding health risks. Their involvement in the evaluation of warnings with respect to the adequacy and accuracy of health hazard information is also critical.

The adequacy of a warning or other communication requires consideration of (a) the dangerousness of the agent, (b) the form of the warning, (c) the responsibility of the manufacturer to provide warnings, and (d) the likelihood that those who foreseeably will use the product will adequately understand the risks and actions they must take.

Necessary Skills for Risk Communication

The effectiveness of warnings and risk communications depends on the credibility of the source. When physicians participate in risk communications, they have greatest credibility when their expertise is relevant to the warning issues and when they are held to be trustworthy. Because apparent conflicts of interest may affect how their trustworthiness is perceived, physicians must consider whether they appear to be independent of outside influence and whether their message will be perceived as legitimate. An effective communication program should rely on individuals who are perceived as credible by the audience. Likability also influences the effectiveness of communications, and attributes such as physical appearance, personal warmth, sensitivity, and intelligence affect the success of the communication.

The effectiveness of warnings is also dependent on the content and the channel through which they are communicated. The warning must stand out amidst the clutter of noise and visual stimuli in order to be noticed, and must be clear and unambiguous. One of the greatest challenges in risk communications is understanding the recipients' attitudes and beliefs that will influence their response to and interaction with a hazardous situation or a warning. The recipients must have expectations about the adverse consequences of exposure and must be motivated to avoid exposure in order for warnings to be effective. Risk communicators should consider the audience's perception of the magnitude of the hazard, the costs of compliance to the recipient, the perceived effectiveness of the precautionary action, and the audience's competence (reading ability, language skills, educational background).

Legal Implications of Health Risk Communications

Health risk communication also can be a critical issue in litigation that is based upon claimed personal injury or product liability. A health risk communication that is inaccurate, incomplete, ambiguous, or missing completely can leave one vulnerable to a "failure to warn" claim, whereas a clearly worded warning can help shield against such claims.

In this age of litigation, an injured person often looks exhaustively for someone to hold accountable for the sustained injury, for compensation. If the injury resulted from the use of a product (i.e., industrial equipment, chemical product), the injured person may claim that the product was defective, and, therefore, that the product manufacturer must be held liable. Under most states' products liability laws and judicial decisions, a person injured by a "defective" product may file suit and prevail not only against the manufacturer of the product, but also against those who provided the injurious components or ingredients within the product, those who distributed or supplied the product, and those who provided (or failed to provide) instructions as to how the product should be used safely.

Although not typically thought of as a "defect," a product may be characterized as "defective" if it lacks an appropriate, clearly worded warning or set of instructions as to how the product can be used safely.[1]

Warnings or instructions typically are required whenever there is a hidden danger associated with use of the product, or where the product will be dangerous if used without certain precautions. Warnings generally are not required where the danger or potential danger is generally known or obvious. Thus, an effective, complete warning must include whatever information and guidance is necessary to make the use of that product safe. At a minimum, a warning/instruction should, therefore, adequately inform the user of (a) what the intended use(s) of the product is; (b) what risks may exist if the product is used for its intended purpose(s); (c) what steps should be taken so as to reduce or eliminate those risks; and (d) what steps should be taken if the risks become a reality, and the anticipated injury occurs.

As a general proposition, a warning must be communicated to the foreseeable users of the product, whether or not the foreseeable users are the one(s) who purchased the product in the first instance. Thus, depending upon the particular circumstances, it may not be sufficient for a warning to be given exclusively to an employer, if it is clearly foreseeable that employees will be the ultimate users of the product.[2]

An adequate warning must address foreseeable uses of the product-not necessarily every use that the product could ever be put to, but at least the uses of the product that can reasonably be anticipated. With respect to a chemical product, that may include cautions not only as to the chemical product itself, but further as to foreseeable mixtures of the chemical product with other substances. Given the realities of litigation, it is advisable to err on the side of over-inclusiveness, rather than under-inclusiveness, while being mindful that a warning that becomes too long, detailed and complex may thereby become unintelligible and ineffective.

---

[1]Under the product liability laws of most states, a product can be "defective" due to (a) a manufacturing defect; (b) a design defect; (c) and/or a lack of warnings or instructions as to how the product might be used safely.

[2]There are some narrow exceptions to that general rule which can vary from jurisdiction to jurisdiction. For example, a manufacturer of prescription medication may have a duty to warn the prescribing physician about known risks, but it may be the prescribing physician's responsibility to instruct or warn his/her patient as to the safe use of the medication.

An important distinction exists between a "failure to warn" claim that is asserted based on strict liability and one that is based upon negligence principles. Under strict liability, the central issue is whether the product is defective because it lacked an adequate warning as to a danger that was knowable, thereby making it unfit, unsuitable or unsafe for its intended purpose. The degree of care taken, and the actual knowledge possessed by the person or entity that manufactured or supplied the product, generally is not relevant. Thus, if a chemical product is sold without a warning that dermal contact can cause a skin rash, and if it is scientifically determinable that the chemical product can, in fact, cause skin rash, then the product may well be defective when sold due to this lack of warning. A person who develops a rash following dermal contact with the product may assert a strict liability failure to warn claim against the manufacturer, and the manufacturers' lack of knowledge will not be an effective defense.

Under negligence principles, however, the focus is upon the reasonableness of the defendant's conduct in failing to warn. Thus, if the manufacturer knew or reasonably should have known that its product could cause a rash, or knew that it should test the safety of its product before selling it but chose not to do so, then the defendant-manufacturer might well be found to have been negligent in failing to warn its customer.[3]

SUMMARY OF HEALTH RISK COMMUNICATION

Over the years, there have been many advances in health risk communication, including from OSHA to employer, from OSHA to employee, from employer to employee and from employee back to the employer and OSHA. Increase in communication and knowledge will only serve to benefit all concerned. As communication and training increase knowledge of health risks involved in occupational tasks and exposures, one can assume that the work force will be healthier, safer, and live longer. The employer will benefit with healthier and safer employees who have decreased absences from the workplace due to job related illness or injury.

[3]Many jurisdictions today hold that there is no longer a doctrinal distinction between failure to warn claims asserted under strict liability versus negligence theories, since both ultimately require a showing that the manufacturer/supplier knew or should have known of the particular danger.

REFERENCES

1. *Training curriculum guidelines—Non-mandatory—1926.65 App E* in OSHA Regulations (Standards–29 CFR).
2. Steinmann J. Analysis methods for new work cell standards: risk analysis and risk reduction help in dealing with the revised Robot Standard. *Occupational Health and Safety* 1998;67(12):24–27.
3. O'Neill BM, et al. Right-to-know laws: a guide to maintaining compliance. *Occupational Health and Safety* 1988;57(6):28–49.
4. Sattler B. Rights and realities: a critical review of the accessibility of information on hazardous chemicals. *Occup Med State of the Art Rev* 1992;7:189.
5. Fluke C. What is "right to know"? Reviewing the Hazard Communication Standard. *J Healthcare Material Manage* 1989;7(2):87–89.
6. Myers CE. Pharmacy implications of the revised OSHA Hazard Communication Standard. *Am J Hosp Pharm* 1989;46(5):990–991.
7. Zuber TJ, Geddie JE. Occupational Safety and Health Administration regulations for the physician's office. *J Fam Pract* 1993;36(5):540–550.
8. Barlow R, Handelman E. OSHA's final bloodborne pathogens standard. Part II. *AAOHN J* 1992;40(12): 562–567.
9. Barlow R, Handelman E. OSHA's final bloodborne pathogens standard. Part I. *AAOHN J* 1993;41(1):8–15.
10. OSHA National News Release, USDL, Office of Public Affairs. Needlestick requirements take effect April 18. April 12, 2001.
11. OSHA National News Release, USDL: 01-140. Prevention is the best medicine. OSHA announces outreach effort on needlestick prevention. May 9, 2001.
12. Paul M, Kurtz S. Analysis of reproductive health hazard information on material safety data sheets for lead and the ethylene glycol ethers. *Am J Ind Med* 1994;25(3):403–415.
13. Hadden SG. Providing citizens with information about health effects of hazardous chemicals. *J Occup Med* 1989;31(6):528–534.
14. OSHA National News Release, USDL, Office of Public Affairs. OSHA introduces new "plain language" workplace poster. August 9, 2000.
15. OSHA Trade News Release USDL, Office of Public Affairs. OSHA expands employee involvement in safety and health consultation visits. October 26, 2000.
16. OSHA USDL Office of Training and Education Construction Safety and Health Outreach Program. Presenting effective presentations with visual aids. May 1996.
17. Reynolds SJ, Seem R, Fourtes LJ, et al. Prevalence of elevated blood leads and exposure to lead in construction trades in Iowa and Illinois. *Am J Ind Med* 1999;36(2): 307–316.
18. Goldberg M, Clark NL, Levin SM, et al. An assessment of lead controls for torch cutting and rivet removal on steel structures. *Appl Occup Environ Hyg* 2000;15(5):445–452.
19. Spear TM, DuMond J, Lloyd C, et al. An effective protection factor study of respirators used by primary lead smelter workers. *Appl Occup Environ Hyg* 2000;15(2): 235–244.
20. Finkelstein MM. Silica, silicosis, and lung cancer: a risk assessment. *Am J Ind Med* 2000;38(1):8–18.
21. Wogalter MS, Dejoy DM, Laughery KR. *Warnings and risk communications*. Philadelphia: Taylor & Francis, 1999:1–23, 85–122, 189–219.

48
Reproductive Hazards

William W. Greaves and Kevin Soden

The question, "Doctor, if I work with substance X, will it hurt my baby?," presents a physician with an often difficult task. The physician's response not only must incorporate the scientific literature on substance X and data on the work exposure, but also must be sensitive to the fears and concerns of the patient. Even the manner used to inform the patient of the facts must be measured so misinterpretation or an irrational fear is not created. The answer to the patient's question should be designed to provide accurate information in proper perspective with the risks of everyday living and in a manner understandable to the patient.

Employee concerns about reproduction become important for pregnant women and women in the childbearing period, as well as for men. The circumstances of their concerns may be varied. Maybe a relative, or even the patient, has been unable to conceive, or has experienced a fetal loss during pregnancy or the birth of a malformed child. All are bitter disappointments and produce tremendous personal stress. Perhaps a chemical substance or video display terminals recently received media attention, and now the patient is concerned because it is used in his or her workplace or workstation. Determining the exact cause of the concern is important. Factual information alone will not alleviate the individual's concern if the root cause of that concern is not addressed. One cannot address emotional fears with only facts; the basis of the concern must be considered.

A 1991 Supreme Court decision (1) does not allow employers to keep pregnant or fertile women from working in jobs that may injure a fetus and cause an adverse reproductive outcome. Rather, employees decide as individuals whether they will perform potentially hazardous jobs after receiving information on potential risks. This presents a singular conundrum for the employer and the occupational physician in the event that the employee does not choose to avoid a specific exposure that scientific evidence links with an adverse reproductive outcome. Under section 5a(1), the general duty clause of the Occupational Safety and Health Act of 1970, an employer may be cited for failing to provide working conditions free from recognized hazards that are likely to cause serious harm. Although with few exceptions employers cannot be held liable for recovery beyond workers' compensation, an injured child of an employee is apparently not bound by this limitation. At this time a prudent course of action for an employer is an approach based on the scientific literature, including both an employee educational and monitoring program for adverse reproductive outcomes and a policy to link employee removal from specific work activities to specific work performance.

This chapter discusses issues that help the occupational physician respond to the woman or man concerned about reproductive hazards. The response should consider four areas:

1. The scientific literature on the substance(s) in question
2. The true and potential levels of exposure
3. The control measures used to assure safety
4. The specific concerns of the individual

These four areas are covered in later sections that describe the potential interferences with the normal reproductive process, the evaluation of a suspected problem, and guidelines useful for the practicing physician.

CASE EXAMPLES

Case 1

A 28-year-old married woman has been your patient for several years. You know her medical history well. She has been employed in the data processing department of a large company for the past 6 years. Her husband has seen you for periodic maintenance visits only. He has worked for a local foundry since his military service in Vietnam. The woman is visibly anxious and relates marital trouble as well as financial difficulties. She tells you that she and her husband have been trying to start a family for 3 years; she asks you if their work has made them sterile. What do you tell her?

Case 2

Over the past 5 years, you have been employed part-time as the medical director of a company. Initially, you were asked to provide preplacement and periodic examinations for the employees in addition to acute care both in-plant and at your office when necessary. Lately, the company has been asking you to address several policy decisions. You are now asked if the company should be concerned about potential hazards of substances used at a small chemical plant. Reproductive hazards are mentioned during the discussion. How do you respond?

Discussion

These two case examples of a concerned individual and a concerned company illustrate scenarios faced by physicians who practice occupational medicine. Both address the issue of reproductive hazards in the workplace and both present a challenging task.

REPRODUCTIVE TOXICOLOGY

An understanding of normal reproduction is a necessary foundation for the recognition of adverse effects to the reproductive processes of men and women. With this understanding of the normal or usual outcome, the actions of toxins or stressors can be more fully appreciated.

Male

Sexual differentiation begins about 7 weeks after conception and is completed by the fourth month in the male. Follicle-stimulating hormone (FSH) acts on the Sertoli cells in the testes to produce the release of a second hormone from the hypothalamic-pituitary axis, luteinizing hormone (LH). LH stimulates the testicular Leydig cells to produce testosterone. Although males and females have identical FSH and LH, it is the hormonal effects on sex-specific target cells that produce sexual differentiation.

In adult men, the high rate of cell division during the 70 to 80 days of spermatogenesis makes this process susceptible to adverse influences. Spermatogonia undergo mitosis into spermatocytes; spermatids are produced by further cell division through meiosis and mature into the characteristic head and tail shape of sperm. Normal sperm production is about 20 to 350 million per day, with human ejaculate containing from 50 to 150 million per milliliter. Less than 20 million sperm per milliliter is considered to be clinical infertility (2). Fertility criteria have been defined as greater than 40% motile sperm, greater than 20 million sperm per milliliter of semen (normal sperm count is approximately 40–60 million/mL), and greater than 70% normal morphology (3).

Female

The entire complement of ova is present at birth, and their number gradually decreases with age. Only about 400 mature ova are released during ovulation in a lifetime. The release of specific factors from the hypothalamus and hormones from the pituitary produces the development of the ovarian follicle. The follicle expels the mature ovum at the peak of the estrogen and luteinizing hormone levels, approximately 14 days after the beginning of menses. Fertilization and early development occur during the ensuing few days and are followed by implantation onto the wall of the uterus.

The embryonic stage of development progresses from about the third through eighth weeks of pregnancy and includes organogenesis. Organ growth occurs during the ninth through 40th weeks of fetal development. Adverse reproductive outcome can occur after harmful exposure during any of these stages, although the period of organogenesis is considered to be especially susceptible (Table 48.1).

TABLE 48.1. *Stages of embryonic development and adverse outcome to toxic agents*

Month	Stage	Adverse outcome
0	Conception and implantation	Embryonic death
1	Embryonic organogenesis	Birth defects
3	Fetal	Developmental deficits, metabolic dysfunction, cancer
9	Birth	
	Neonatal	Functional deficits

Adapted from Radike M. Reproductive toxicology. In: Williams PL, Burson JL, eds. *Industrial toxicology, safety and health applications in the workplace.* New York: Van Nostrand Reinhold, 1985:353.

INTERFERENCE WITH THE REPRODUCTIVE PROCESS

The potential interferences with the reproductive process are several. A healthy baby is the normal outcome if a healthy sperm fertilizes a healthy ovum that passes unimpeded through the fallopian tubes, implants in the uterus, develops normal organs, and grows to term. Interference with this basic process can occur with a change in libido or in the following steps, each with an example of an interfering exposure:

1. The production of sperm: Chromosomal or gene changes (nonlethal or lethal) can occur; fewer numbers may be produced (e.g., ionizing radiation).
2. The production of ova: Changes in hormonal patterns may interfere with ovulation (e.g., estrogen deficiency).
3. The fertilized ovum may not pass through the fallopian tube to the uterus (e.g., scar tissue from pelvic inflammatory disease). Effects on normal muscular, ciliary, and secretory activity may occur.
4. The fertilized ovum may not implant in the uterus. The endometrial lining may be altered, or the fertilized ovum may be damaged in the cleavage and blastocyst stages. This effect usually is lethal and produces an abortion recognized only as an abnormal menstrual period in humans but is the equivalent to resorptions in rats and mice and occasionally in rabbits (e.g., infectious diseases).
5. The embryo may be affected as its tissues differentiate or its organs develop. Congenital malformations, or structural aberrations, can occur during organogenesis, from days 21 to 56 of gestation (e.g., rubella infection, thalidomide administration) (4).
6. The fetus may not grow normally, resulting in spontaneous abortions, stillbirths, or premature births. A disease or toxic state in the mother can affect the fetus (e.g., diabetes mellitus), and the risk of spontaneous abortion increases with maternal age and history of prior spontaneous abortions (5). Postnatal growth and development may likewise be altered, the effect possibly not manifested until several years after birth (e.g., ethyl alcohol). In practice, of course, it is difficult to detect a pregnancy, even with good symptoms of morning sickness, until several weeks after conception. Because the woman is in fact pregnant but unaware of it, protection of the fetus at this stage can be a difficult task.

TERATOGENS

An agent or factor that causes physical birth defects or malformations in the developing embryo is termed a *teratogen.* A teratogen is a substance that produces birth defects or congenital malformations without producing toxicity in the mother. The effects of a teratogen are dose related: a high dose is embryolethal, a moderate dose produces a defect, and a low dose may produce no effect. If a birth defect results from maternal toxicity, the defect may be caused by the toxic effects on the mother rather than a direct manifestation of the substance itself. The type of defect or malformation also depends on the day(s) during the period of organogenesis that exposure to the teratogen occurred.

The following are the general principles of teratology (6):

1. Susceptibility to teratogenesis depends on the genotype of the conceptus and the manner in which the genotype interacts with environmental factors.
2. Susceptibility to teratogenic agents varies with the developing stage of the fetus at the time of exposure.
3. Teratogenic agents act through specific mechanisms on developing cells and tissues, thus initiating abnormal embryogenesis.
4. The final manifestations of abnormal development are malformation, growth retardation, functional disorder, or death.
5. The access of adverse environmental influences to developing tissues depends on the nature of the influences (agents).
6. Manifestations of abnormal development increase from no effect to the totally lethal level as the dosage increases.

About 10% to 20% of normal conceptions (where the sperm has fertilized the ovum and pregnancy is recognized) fail to reach full growth and delivery. Similarly, 30% to 40% of spontaneous abortions have a chromosomal anomaly (7). This relatively high level of "normal" spontaneous abortions needs to be recognized in evaluating rates of adverse reproductive outcome.

Congenital anomalies, or birth defects, have been reported in about 3% of all newborn children (Table 48.2); anomalies in another 3% of live births become manifest during postnatal or later development (8). Two thirds of all congenital anomalies or malformations have no known cause, while drugs and chemicals are implicated in 3% (Table 48.3).

TABLE 48.2. *Frequency of selected reproductive end points*

Event	Frequency per 100	Unit
Azoospermia	1	Men
Birthweight[a] <2,500 g	7	Live births
Failure to conceive after 1 year of unprotected intercourse	10–15	Couples
Spontaneous abortion 8–28 weeks of gestation	10–20	Pregnancies or women
Chromosomal anomaly among spontaneously aborted conceptions 8–28 weeks	30–40	Spontaneous abortions
Chromosomal anomalies among amniocentesis specimens to unselected women over 35 years	2	Amniocentesis specimens
Stillbirth	2–4	Stillbirths + live births
Birth defects	2–3	Live births
Chromosomal anomalies	0.2	Live births
Neural tube defects	0.01–1.00	Live births + stillbirths
Severe mental retardation	0.4	Children to age 15 years

[a]More usefully analyzed as a continuous variable.

Adapted from Bloom AD, ed. *Guidelines for studies of human populations exposed to mutagenic and reproductive hazards.* White Plains, NY: March of Dimes Birth Defects Foundation, 1981:47.

TABLE 48.3. *Causes of congenital anomalies*

Cause	Percent
Maternal metabolic imbalance	1–2
Infections	2–3
Chromosomal aberrations	3–5
Drugs and environmental agents	
Radiation	1
Drugs and chemicals	3
Known genetic transmission (autosomal dominant, autosomal recessive, sex-linked recessive)	20
Combinations and interactions	
Unknown	
Unknown factors	69–73

From American Medical Association Council on Scientific Affairs.

Effect of toxic chemicals on the reproductive system. *JAMA* 1985;253:3431.

HUMAN DATA

The medical literature provides the primary source of information to the physician confronted with a reproductive outcome issue. Like any epidemiologic literature, the literature on reproductive outcomes must be assessed for its scientific merit as well as for what it has to say on the subject. Textbooks, such as those listed in the References and Further Information at the end of this chapter, detail aspects of study design and interpretation that should be considered in a critical review. Major points to consider include the following (9):

1. Exposure levels: Frequently, good industrial hygiene data are not available and proper grouping of potentially exposed employee populations by time of exposure cannot be performed. Because reproductive effects are dose dependent, lack of exposure data may become a major limitation of an otherwise good study.
2. Selection of controls: Important variables that can also affect reproductive outcome include age, parity, nutritional and socioeconomic status, and smoking and alcohol habits.
3. Background incidence of events: Relatively common events of everyday living, such as infertility, menstrual disorders, and spontaneous abortions, require a large sample size and a large total number of cases to detect an increased incidence of the condition in the population under study. Rare events, such as a specific congenital malformation, require a smaller total number of cases to detect an effect, but rare events also require a larger population at risk to obtain that smaller number of cases.
4. Reliability of ascertainment: Once an abnormal outcome has occurred, determining the nature of the disorder becomes of paramount importance in the search for a cause. Early abortion, frequently recognized as a late heavy menses or a change in libido, is subject to self-assessment, which may confound the outcome evaluation.
5. Multiple exposures: When multiple exposures may be exerting effects, the points noted above may severely limit the inferences that can be made regarding a specific compound. In such a case, a valid assessment may still be made of the production process or work activity that involves the multiple exposures.
6. Interpretation of findings: Answering such questions as whether sufficient data are available to reach a final decision, whether a hazard exists, and what kind of action needs to be taken can be challenging tasks. Potentially confounding factors (Table 48.4), comparability of cases and con-

TABLE 48.4. *Potentially confounding factors for a number of adverse reproductive effects*

Adverse reproductive effect	Potentially confounding factors
Impaired spermatogenesis	Surgical procedures such as vasectomy; diseases and illnesses such as varicocele, fever, mumps, and diabetes; organophosphates; certain therapeutic drugs
Reduced fertility	Contraceptive use, male lead exposure
Spontaneous abortion	Maternal age, cigarette smoking, alcohol consumption, history of spontaneous abortions, male welding[a] (stainless steel), ethylene glycol ethers[b]
Low birth weight	Race, cigarette smoking, parity, maternal nutrition
Birth defects	
Down syndrome	Maternal age
Neural tube defects	Ethnic factors

[a]Adapted from Hjollund NH, Bonde JP, Jensen TK, et al. Male-medicated spontaneous abortion among spouses of stainless steel welders. *Scand J Work Environ Health* 2000;26(3):187–192.

[b]Adapted from Correa A, Gray RH, Cohen R, et al. Ethylene glycol ethers and risks of spontaneous abortion and subfertility. *Am J Epidemiol* 1996;143(7):707–717.

trols, and the other points noted above must be evaluated.

Epidemiologic data provide the information necessary to take action on a potential reproductive hazard. For the practicing physician, these data come from two primary sources: the medical literature and monitoring programs on a plant- or company-wide basis.

A first step in assessing the role of the workplace in affecting reproductive experience is to apply simple and straightforward techniques to monitor reproductive experience. Monitoring can ensure the safety of the workplace, focus industrial hygiene and safety efforts, and assist in employee health promotion. Monitoring allows reproductive outcome to be viewed dispassionately. If attention is focused on reproductive hazards at the time an unfortunate event has occurred, it is extremely difficult to obtain unbiased data.

A useful approach to reproductive surveillance or monitoring has two major steps:

I. Establish objectives
   A. Assess outcome for normality during pregnancy, delivery, or postnatal development
   B. If not normal, determine type of abnormality (Table 48.5)
II. Explore etiology
   A. Past and family history
   B. Lifestyle and substance use

TABLE 48.5. *Reproductive end points for which population estimates are available*

End point	Population survey[a]
Infertility of male and female origin	NSFG, PYS
Conception delay	NSFG, PYS
Birth rate	NSFG, NNS, NFMS, PYS
Pregnancy complications	NSFG, NNS, NFMS, PYS
Gestation at delivery (prematurity, postmaturity)	NSFG, NNS, NFMS
Early fetal loss (<28 weeks' gestation)	NSFG, NNS, NFMS, PYS
Late fetal loss (≥28 weeks' gestation)	NSFG, NNS, NFMS, PYS
Sex ratio	NSFG, NNS, PYS
Birth weight	NSFG, NNS
Apgar score	NNS
Congenital defect	NNS
Infant morbidity and mortality	NSFG, NNS
Childhood morbidity and mortality	NNS, NFMS, PYS

[a]These surveys also contain data on the following related topics: onset of menses, fertility expectations, birth spacing, contraceptive use, sterilization, care-seeking for infertility, prenatal care, spontaneous and induced abortions, maternal smoking and alcohol consumption, chronic diseases, and venereal infections in pregnancy.

NSFG, 1982 National Survey of Family Growth; NNS, 1980 National Natality Survey; NFMS, 1980 National Fetal Mortality Survey; PYS, Parnes Youth Survey.

From U.S. Congress, Office of Technology Assessment. *Reproductive health hazards in the workplace.* OTA-BA-266. Washington, DC: U.S. Government Printing Office, 1985:165.

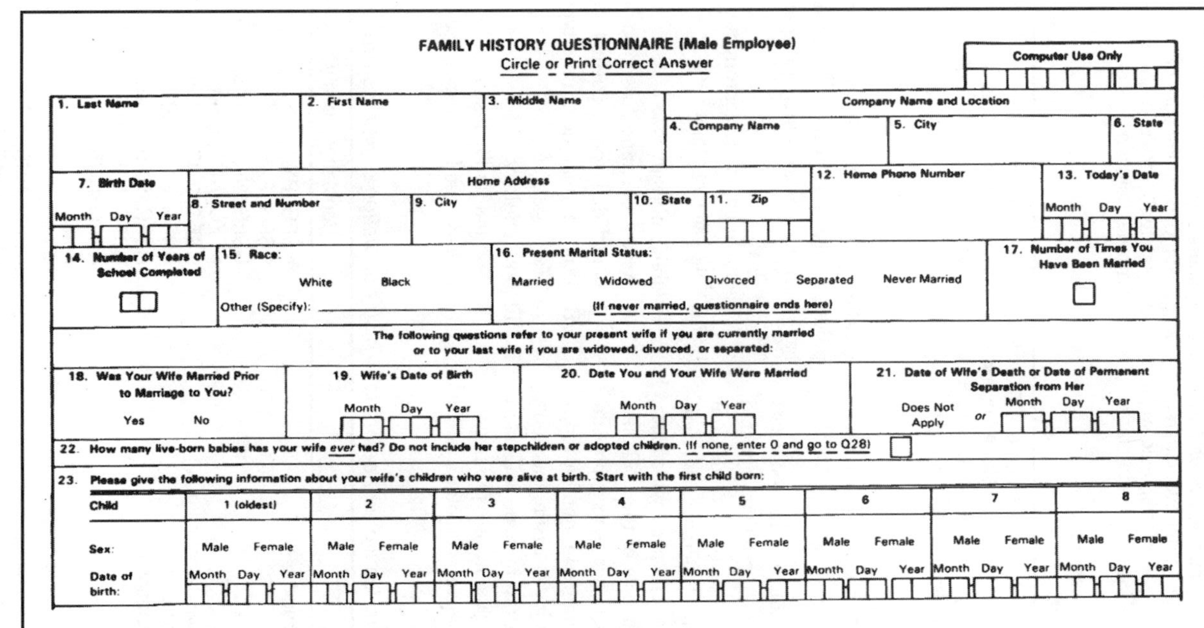

FAMILY HISTORY QUESTIONNAIRE (Male Employee)
Circle or Print Correct Answer

Computer Use Only

1. Last Name | 2. First Name | 3. Middle Name | Company Name and Location: 4. Company Name | 5. City | 6. State

7. Birth Date: Month Day Year

Home Address: 8. Street and Number | 9. City | 10. State | 11. Zip

12. Home Phone Number

13. Today's Date: Month Day Year

14. Number of Years of School Completed

15. Race: White Black Other (Specify): ____

16. Present Marital Status: Married Widowed Divorced Separated Never Married
(If never married, questionnaire ends here)

17. Number of Times You Have Been Married

The following questions refer to your present wife if you are currently married or to your last wife if you are widowed, divorced, or separated:

18. Was Your Wife Married Prior to Marriage to You? Yes No

19. Wife's Date of Birth: Month Day Year

20. Date You and Your Wife Were Married: Month Day Year

21. Date of Wife's Death or Date of Permanent Separation from Her: Does Not Apply or Month Day Year

22. How many live-born babies has your wife *ever* had? Do not include her stepchildren or adopted children. (If none, enter 0 and go to Q28)

23. Please give the following information about your wife's children who were alive at birth. Start with the first child born:

Child	1 (oldest)	2	3	4	5	6	7	8
Sex:	Male Female	Male Female	Male Female	Male Female	Male Female	Male Female	Male Female	Male Female
Date of birth:	Month Day Year	Month Day Year	Month Day Year	Month Day Year	Month Day Year	Month Day Year	Month Day Year	Month Day Year

FIG. 48.1. Reproductive history questionnaire. (From Levine RJ, Blunden PB. Family history questionnaire, CIIT:FSA.1 3-83. Chemical Industry Institute of Toxicology, P.O. Box 12137, Research Triangle Park, NC 27709.)

24. **How many of your wife's children who were alive at birth had an abnormality or defect? *All* abnormalities or defects should be included even if you do not think they are relevant or if they were not discovered at birth.** (If none, enter 0 and go to Q26) ☐

25. **Please give the following information about your wife's children with an abnormality or defect:**

Sex:	Male Female	Male Female	Male Female	Male Female
Date of birth:	Month Day Year	Month Day Year	Month Day Year	Month Day Year
Abnormality or defect (describe):				
How many months pregnant was your wife at his/her birth?	Months Pregnant: ☐	Months Pregnant: ☐	Months Pregnant: ☐	Months Pregnant: ☐

26. **How many of your wife's children who were born alive are no longer living?** (If none, enter 0 and go to Q28) ☐

27. **Please give the following information about your wife's children who are no longer living:**

Sex:	Male Female	Male Female	Male Female	Male Female
Date of birth:	Month Day Year	Month Day Year	Month Day Year	Month Day Year
Date of death:	Month Day Year	Month Day Year	Month Day Year	Month Day Year
Cause of death (describe):				
How many months pregnant was your wife at his/her birth?	Months Pregnant: ☐	Months Pregnant: ☐	Months Pregnant: ☐	Months Pregnant: ☐

28. **How many miscarriages or stillborn children has your wife *ever* had?** (If none, enter 0 and go to Q30) ☐

FIG. 48.1. *(Continued)*

29. Please give the following information about your wife's miscarriages or stillborn children:

Miscarriage or Stillbirth	First	Second	Third	Fourth	Fifth	Sixth
Date of miscarriage or stillbirth:	Month Day Year	Month Day Year	Month Day Year	Month Day Year	Month Day Year	Month Day Year
How many months pregnant was your wife at the time?	Months Pregnant:	Months Pregnant:	Months Pregnant:	Months Pregnant:	Months Pregnant:	Months Pregnant:

30. How many pregnancies has your wife *ever* had that were terminated by medical or surgical means and did not result in a live birth, such as an ectopic pregnancy, tubal pregnancy, therapeutic or induced abortion? (If none, enter 0 and go to Q32)

31. Please give the following information about such pregnancies terminated by medical or surgical means:

Date pregnancy ended:	Month Day Year	Month Day Year	Month Day Year	Month Day Year	Month Day Year	Month Day Year
How many months pregnant was your wife at the time?	Months Pregnant:	Months Pregnant:	Months Pregnant:	Months Pregnant:	Months Pregnant:	Months Pregnant:

32. Have you or your wife had any operation which keeps you from having children, such as a vasectomy, hysterectomy, or tubal ligation? Yes No (If no, go to Q34)

33. Please enter the date of the appropriate operation you or your wife had which keeps you from having children:

Operation	Vasectomy	Hysterectomy	Tubal Ligation (Tubes Tied)	Other (Please Specify):
Date of operation:	Month Day Year	Month Day Year	Month Day Year	Month Day Year

34. Are you and your wife presently doing anything to prevent a pregnancy? Yes No *or* Does Not Apply (widowed, divorced, separated, sterilized)

FIG. 48.1. *(Continued)*

C. Nonoccupational influences
   1. Diseases
   2. Injuries
   3. Hobbies
D. On-the-job substance exposure

The essential objective of monitoring is to answer one principal question: Is there an unusually high incidence of an abnormality? This question is answered by assessing reproductive outcome and comparing the results to what normally would be expected. If the concern deals with the ability to reproduce, the ability to reproduce itself must be assessed. If the concern deals with an outcome such as birth defects, this outcome must be assessed. Then, if an abnormality is detected, the specific type of abnormality is determined and the reason it happened is explored.

Determining the precise abnormality may require extensive study of the individuals involved, including both parents and the fetus or newborn. The occupational physician will usually obtain the services of other medical specialists for the clinical evaluation of these individuals. The usual incidence of adverse reproductive outcomes by type of abnormality can be compared to that from various population-monitoring surveys (Table 48.5). Whether an abnormal incidence is present among a specific group of workers and/or their spouses can then be determined.

Assessing etiologic factors that may result in abnormalities of the reproductive process requires consideration of several items. Both past medical history and family history are extremely important, as are lifestyle and substance use. The prior reproductive experience of both the employee and the spouse, as well as that of blood relatives, must be investigated. Smoking and alcohol use and medications taken before or during a pregnancy are as important to assess as substances an individual may encounter on the job.

Virtually all the data required to monitor reproduction adequately are historical. Other than the laboratory tests that may be needed to specify the type of abnormality that occurred on the occasion that a pregnancy outcome is abnormal and the data needed to indicate on-the-job substance exposure, everything else is obtainable by history or questionnaire.

Most questionnaires contain a great deal of information that is not needed and may omit the information required. A good history form should be clear, nonbiased, codable, and time specific from both a preemployment and postemployment standpoint. Basic questionnaires developed for men and women by the Chemical Industry Institute of Toxicology focus on the most recent marriage of the employee and can be expanded to include all partners (Fig. 48.1). The institute has more elaborate questionnaires, but these require a trained interviewer for their administration.

Once baseline information has been obtained, periodic updates ensure data reliability and timeliness in the event a problem is detected. Data are ideally analyzed by job type or department, and if a pattern emerges, special studies can be conducted. Adverse reproductive outcomes occur at a relatively predictable rate, just as causes of death or illness occur at a relatively predictable rate in a population. If an unusual amount of an adverse outcome is encountered in a specific group of employees, vigorous investigation is required. If the rate of occurrence in a company or plant is consistent with the usual experience, however, and no discernible differences occur among employees with different work experiences, assurance can be given that the work environment is not the source of an adverse health outcome. If a true hazard is uncovered, steps must be taken to abate it. A monitoring system can then serve to demonstrate the effectiveness of the abatement efforts.

ANIMAL DATA

In many cases, results on human populations are unavailable; consequently, animal studies need to be reviewed. Animal data can suggest estimates of possible human effects, although extrapolation to human experience is problematic. Ideally, human data from epidemiologic studies on reproductive experience should be reviewed to form a reliable assessment.

Items of importance to reproductive studies on test animals include the following:

1. Species: Studies on humans, nonhuman primates, and nonprimates may show marked variations in the rate of biotransformation. For example, the amount of phenylacetic acid excreted in the urine after conjugation to glutamine is almost 100% in humans, 30% to 90% in nonhuman primates, and none in nonprimates (10).
2. Dose-response: Measurable responses increase as the dosage frequency, duration, and intensity increase. Accurate dosage data are necessary to correlate dosage levels to the adverse outcome responses. For example, the concentration of a substance in parts per million (ppm) in a test animal's drinking water or feed may be known, but because the amount of water or feed the animal actually consumed may not be known, the total dose ingested is unknown. Higher doses in water or feed produce maternal toxicity and subsequent decreased maternal intake, which alters the dose delivered to the embryo or fetus. This altered

TABLE 48.6. *Agents associated with adverse female reproductive capacity or developmental effects in human and animal studies*[a]

Agent	Human outcomes	Strength of association in humans	Animal outcomes	Strength of association in animals
Anesthetic gases[b]	Reduced fertility, spontaneous abortion	1,3	Birth defects	1,3
Arsenic	Spontaneous abortion, low birth weight	1	Birth defects, fetal loss	2
Benzo(a)pyrene	None	NA[c]	Birth defects	1
Cadmium	None	NA	Fetal loss, birth defects	2
Carbon disulfide	Menstrual disorders, spontaneous abortion	1	Birth defects	1
Carbon monoxide	Low birth weight, fetal death (high doses)	1	Birth defects, neonatal mortality	2
Chlordecone	None	NA	Fetal loss	2,3
Chloroform	None	NA	Fetal loss	1
Chloroprene	None	NA	Birth defects	2,3
Ethylene glycol ethers	Spontaneous abortion	1	Birth defects	2
Ethylene oxide	Spontaneous abortion	1	Fetal loss	1
Formamides	None	NA	Fetal loss, birth defects	2
Inorganic mercury[b]	Menstrual disorders, spontaneous abortion	1	Fetal loss, birth defects	1
Lead[b]	Spontaneous abortion, prematurity, neurologic dysfunction in child	2	Birth defects, fetal loss	2
Organic mercury	CNS malformation, cerebral palsy	2	Birth defects, fetal loss	2
Physical stress	Prematurity	2	None	NA
Polybrominated biphenyls (PBBs)	None	NA	Fetal loss	2
Polychlorinated biphenyls (PCBs)	Neonatal PCB syndrome (low birth weight, hyperpigmentation, eye abnormalities)	2	Low birth weight, fetal loss	2
Radiation, ionizing	Menstrual disorders, CNS defects, skeletal and eye anomalies, mental retardation, childhood cancer	2	Fetal loss, birth defects	2
Selenium	Spontaneous abortion	3	Low birth weight, birth defects	2
Tellurium	None	NA	Birth defects	2
2,4-Dichlorophenoxyacetic acid (2,4-D)	Skeletal defects	4	Birth defects	1
2,4,5-Trichlorophenoxyacetic acid (2,4,5-T)	Skeletal defects	4	Birth defects	1
Video display terminals	Spontaneous abortion	4	Birth defects	1
Vinyl chloride[b]	CNS defects	1	Birth defects	1,4
Xylene	Menstrual disorders, fetal loss	1	Fetal loss, birth defects	1

[a]Major studies of the reproductive health effects of exposure to dioxin are currently in progress.
[b]May have male-mediated effects.
[c]Not applicable because no adverse outcomes were observed.
Key: 1, limited positive data; 2, strong positive data; 3, limited negative data; 4, strong negative data.
CNS, central nervous system.
Adapted from *Reproductive and developmental hazards, case studies in environmental medicine.* Atlanta: Agency for Toxic Substances and Disease Registry, 1993.

dose cannot be accurately correlated to a response. A useful maximal dosage end point to determine whether the substance has an effect on the embryo or fetus is the dosage just below that which produces maternal toxicity.

3. Route of administration: The skin or dermal exposure LD_{50} (the lethal dose for 50% of the test animals in the experiment) of many substances is about ten times that for ingestion, and ingestion itself is about ten times that for intravenous exposure. Occupational exposures occur frequently through the lung or inhalation route. Inhalation is a more efficient route of exposure than all others except intravenous.
4. Period of the reproductive process during which the animal is exposed to the substance: The first day of gestation may be referred to as day 0 or day 1, which introduces 1 day of error, a factor that becomes important during extrapolation of animal effects to humans. For example, a heart defect in animals is often assumed to produce a heart defect in humans when exposure occurs during the appropriate period of heart organogenesis.
5. Summary of effects: Adverse effects are generally described, along with a test of statistical significance. Often little consideration is given to biologic significance.

Outcome effects noted in animal studies include anatomic, biochemical, and functional changes. External appearance, gross pathologic weight, and gross volume of reproductive organs (e.g., ovary, testes, prostate) and the pituitary and adrenal glands are noted. Microscopy of these tissues is performed, and the numbers per milliliter and gross microscopic appearance of sperm can be determined. Biochemically, the synthesis and total content of nucleic acids and the activities of various enzymes contained within reproductive organs have been investigated. Circulating levels of hormones such as FSH and LH can be noted. Abnormalities of these parameters may suggest interference with the reproductive process, but their actual impact is uncertain in most cases.

Effects of reproductive outcome can be identified through single-generation and multigeneration studies. The Food and Drug Administration (FDA) protocol established in 1966 for single-generation studies is widely used to assess new drugs. Segment 1 studies (fertility studies) are characterized by >treatment occurring before mating; theoretically, they can be used as a summary outcome assessment of all stages of reproduction. Segment 2 studies (teratology studies) have treatment occurring during organogenesis. Segment 3 studies test the effect on parturition and the postnatal period.

Multigeneration studies frequently follow the FDA protocol for food additives. Time-consuming and expensive to complete, these studies begin by treating males and/or females, then by mating to produce two litters, F1a and F1b. The F1a litter is killed and examined, while some animals in the F1b litter are mated to form the second-generation litters, F2a and F2b. The F2a is examined; the F2b is mated to produce the third-generation litters, F3a and F3b, which are both examined for abnormalities. Both single-generation and multigeneration studies use rats or mice as the usual test animal at several exposure levels of the test compound. The lowest level produces neither adverse reproductive effects nor parental toxicity. The highest level produces maternal toxicity. In pregnant rats, the maximum tolerated dosage is defined as the exposure producing 10% maternal deaths. The usual indicator for maternal toxicity is a less than expected weight gain during pregnancy. The no-effect level of a compound (in a given species by a given route of exposure under laboratory conditions) is the highest dosage level, or exposure, producing neither maternal toxicity nor adverse reproductive outcome. For the great majority of compounds, adverse reproductive outcomes tend to occur very close to the adult toxic dose (Table 48.6).

CLINICAL ASPECTS

Some physicians respond to the woman who asks, "Will compound X hurt my baby?" by writing "No chemical use allowed" on a slip that is returned to the place of employment. Unfortunately, this blanket response may needlessly heighten the patient's charged emotions and create volatile workplace situations and employee relations problems. This "reflex-type" response overlooks the myriad of chemicals present in the home environment, in addition to neglecting a critical review of available information. Guidelines and methods for setting policy (11,12) and for determining if an individual may work in a job have been proposed (Fig. 48.2).

The algorithm of Fig. 48.2 provides a step-by-step process for assessing the work capability of the pregnant employee. This algorithm refers to four major categories of medical management outcome for the pregnant worker: (a) she may continue working; (b) she may continue working, but job modification is desirable; (c) she may continue working only with job modification; and (d) she may not work.

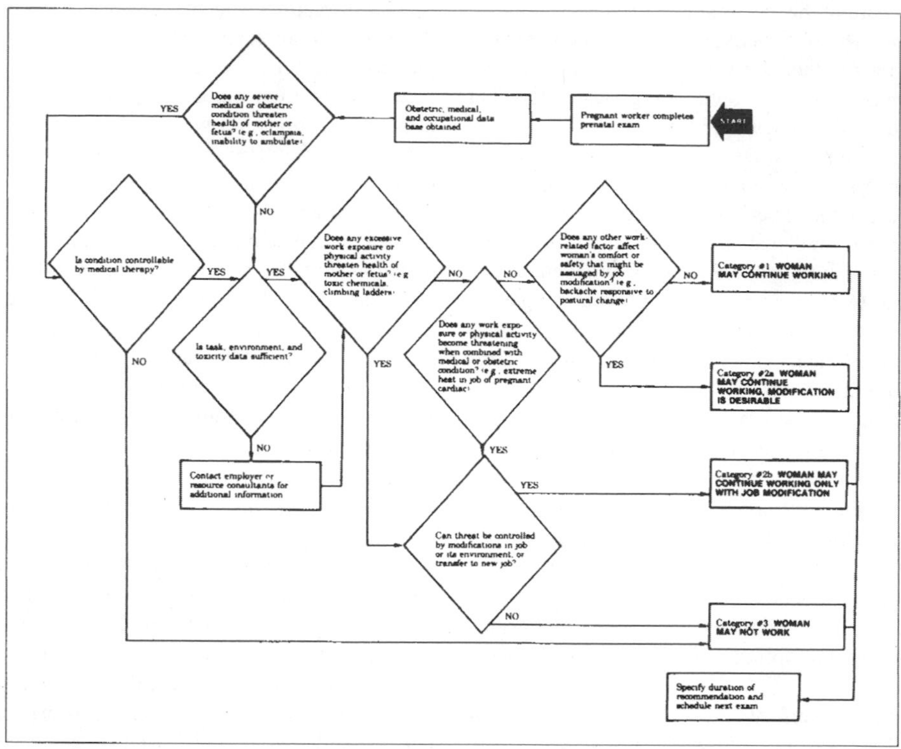

FIG. 48.2. Algorithm for medical management of the pregnant worker. (From U.S. Department of Health and Human Services. *Guidelines on pregnancy and work.* NIOSH publication No. 78-118, 1977:14.)

These categories are dependent to an extent on exposure limits. The published Occupational Safety and Health Administration (OSHA) standards and the American Conference of Governmental Industrial Hygienists (ACGIH) recommended threshold limit values (TLVs) can be used as starting points for exposure limit guidelines. When reviewing toxicologic and epidemiologic studies, a search for no-effect levels, the highest dose level at which a toxic effect is not observed, is of value. When neither published standards nor apparently safe levels in animals are available, caution is suggested. If available, a no-effect level can be reduced by a safety factor of 10, 100, 1,000, or more to set an acceptable exposure level in humans.

One set of guidelines (13) suggesting caution concerning potential exposure utilizes the following three terms: *Avoid:* It is suggested that no exposure should occur. This term is used where there are no data on a no-effect level. *Minimize:* It is suggested that exposure should be kept at the lowest feasible level. This term is used in those instances where a no-effect level is apparently present in animals, but such a level in humans has not been reported. *Limit:* The exercise of caution in degree of exposure or frequency of exposure is suggested. This term is used for those substances for which human studies indicate a level of nonhazardous exposure. One should then keep exposure below the level at which hazardous effects have been noted. The guidelines refer only to the workplace, where exposure may be expected to occur throughout the workday and over a period of time, not to an occasional or infrequent exposure to minimal amounts of substances intended for consumer use.

Another decision faced by the physician concerns the length of time into a pregnancy that an employee may continue to work without harming herself or her child. For the uncomplicated situation, the guidelines for continuation of various job tasks during pregnancy listed in Table 48.7 are very useful. These guidelines are generally recognized and have been produced by the American Medical Association's Council on Scientific Affairs (14). Algorithms to investigate and manage the infertile couple have been

TABLE 48.7. *Guidelines for working at various job tasks during pregnancy*

Job task	Week of gestation
Secretarial and light clerical	40
Professional and managerial	40
Sitting with light tasks	
Prolonged (more than 4 hours)	40
Intermittent	40
Standing	
Prolonged (more than 4 hours)	24
Intermittent	
More than 30 minutes per hour	32
Less than 30 minutes per hour	40
Stooping and bending below knee level	
Repetitive (more than 10 times per hour)	20
Intermittent	
Two to twenty times per hour	28
Less than two times per hour	40
Climbing	
Vertical ladders and poles	
Repetitive (four or more times per 8-hour shift)	20
Intermittent (less than four times per 8-hour shift)	28
Stairs	
Repetitive (four or more times per 8-hour shift)	28
Intermittent (less than four times per 8-hour shift)	40
Lifting	
Repetitive	
Less than 25 lb	40
25 to 50 lb	24
More than 50 lb	20
Intermittent	
Less than 25 lb	40
25 to 50 lb	40
More than 50 lb	30

From American Medical Association Council on Scientific Affairs. Effect of pregnancy on work performance. *JAMA* 1984;251:1995.

proposed (15), and a general audience publication on workplace hazards and female reproductive health has been produced by the National Institute of Occupational Safety and Health (NIOSH) (16).

A final issue requires elaboration. How does a physician determine work-relatedness of an adverse reproductive outcome? Occupational physicians are frequently called on to ascertain whether a disease or injury is related to the patient's work. The legal implications of the decision require a greater degree of certainty than do usual treatment situations; the cause must be established to a reasonable degree of medical certainty. Physicians can better respond to the demands of this situation if they understand how an examination for impairment, disability, or work-relatedness of a condition differs from an examination for treatment.

In an examination for treatment, the physician's primary responsibility is the patient's welfare; in contrast, in an examination for impairment, the physician also has increased responsibility to society. This different responsibility in the examination for impairment requires total objectivity and a legal requirement of truth that may at times conflict with the patient's interest. A great deal of miscommunication between the physician and patient can occur if these different roles are not understood. Determining the goal of the examination before seeing the patient assists the physician in structuring the evaluation.

Three steps may be used to determine the cause of a medical condition such as an adverse reproductive outcome and whether the cause is work related when sufficient evidence is available. First, a review of the historical, physical, and laboratory data must meet the necessary criteria to establish a diagnosis. Sometimes medical conditions unrelated to work can be aggravated by occupational factors. In such cases, a review of the natural history of the preexisting condition is conducted to determine whether it has been altered adversely by exposure.

Second, a search of the medical literature can reveal whether there is any evidence that the substance or situation in question is capable of producing the established medical condition. The epidemiologic literature defines the circumstances of exposure under which the condition can result. A well-established diagnosis based on objective criteria will allow a meaningful literature search; going to the literature without an established diagnosis, with only disparate symptoms and signs, rarely provides useful information.

Third, if the diagnosis and initial literature search suggest an occupational reason for the adverse reproductive outcome, then a workplace evaluation is conducted. The physician can either visit the workplace or obtain necessary data from the workplace. The medical, safety, industrial hygiene, or personnel department at the workplace may be able to give exposure information. If this information is not available, an industrial hygienist from a consulting firm, insurance carrier, or the state or local government can perform the necessary testing. With these data, the physician must then determine if exposure to the specific substance at the recorded level matches the circumstances of exposure sufficient to produce the patient's condition, as defined by the scientific literature.

CASE EXAMPLE UPDATES

Case 1

The 28-year-old woman had asked you if her work or her husband's work has made them sterile. What do you tell her?

A first question to be addressed is whether she or her husband is in fact sterile. Establishing the diagnosis with an infertility clinical examination by an appropriate consultant produces two alternatives for the practitioner: (a) The patient and her husband may not be sterile. Address the patient's concerns and fears regarding workplace exposures by providing in an understandable manner factual information about the risks of everyday living. The latest information on the risks associated with video display terminals in an office, dioxin from Agent Orange in Vietnam, lead and other heavy metals in a foundry, and stress from marital and financial difficulties in one's personal life can be addressed. (b) The patient or her husband probably is sterile. Perform a complete investigation into the specific cause by determining the circumstances of exposure with data from the medical literature and the workplace.

Case 2

As company medical director, you were asked about potential hazards of substances used at a chemical plant. How do you respond?

The company has a responsibility to protect its employees from hazardous workplace exposures. An overall corporate policy on health and safety can address this issue. The policy would cover legal requirements and medical standards. Medical standards can include a monitoring program to provide unbiased data to ensure the safety of the workplace or to address a hazard at the earliest moment. For this case, do a complete exposure inventory within the specific departmental unit of concern, or the entire company, and compare this to a scientific literature review of the substances in the inventory to determine the level of evidence linking those substances with any specific potential adverse reproductive outcome. Then, monitor the reproductive outcomes of the employees, with particular attention to the specific outcomes or end points identified by linking the exposure inventory and the scientific literature.

REFERENCES

1. *International Union v. Johnson Controls,* 111 US 1196 (1991). http://supct.law.cornell.edu/supct/html/89-1215.ZO.html.
2. Radike M. Reproductive toxicology. In: Williams PL, Burson JL, eds. *Industrial toxicology, safety and health applications in the workplace.* New York: Van Nostrand Reinhold, 1985:345.
3. McLeod J, Ving W. Male fertility potential in terms of semen quality: a review of the past, a study of the present. *Fertil Steril* 1979;31:103.
4. Manson JM, Wise LD. Teratogens. In: Amdur MO, Doull J, Klaassen CD, eds. *Casarett and Doull's toxicology: the basic science of poisons,* 4th ed. New York: Pergamon, 1991:235.
5. Kline JK. Maternal occupation: effects on spontaneous abortions and malformations. In: Stein ZA, Hatch MC, eds. Reproductive problems in the workplace. *Occup Med State of the Art Rev.* Philadelphia: Hanley & Belfus, 1986:381–403.
6. American Medical Association Council on Scientific Affairs. Effects of toxic chemicals on the reproductive system. *JAMA* 1985;253:3431.
7. Bloom AD, ed. *Guidelines for studies of human populations exposed to mutagenic and reproductive hazards.* White Plains, NY: March of Dimes Birth Defects Foundation, 1981:47.
8. Kalter H, Warkany J. Congenital malformations: etiologic factors and their role in prevention. *N Engl J Med* 1983;308:424.
9. Barlow SM, Sullivan FM. *Reproductive hazards of industrial chemicals: an evaluation of animal and human data.* London: Academic, 1982:23–27.
10. O'Flaherty EJ. Absorption, distribution, and elimination of toxic agents. In: Williams PL, Burson JL, eds. *Industrial toxicology, safety and health applications in the workplace.* New York: Van Nostrand Reinhold, 1985: 47–48.
11. Bond MB. Role of corporate policy in the control of reproductive hazards of the workplace. *J Occup Med* 1986;28:193.
12. Logan DC. Reproduction and the workplace: an industry perspective. In: Stein ZA, Hatch MC, eds. Reproductive problems in the workplace. *Occup Med State of the Art Rev.* Philadelphia: Hanley & Belfus, 1986: 473–481.
13. Greaves WW. *Teratogenicity and fetotoxicity assessments.* Milwaukee: Ergotopology, 1983.
14. American Medical Association Council on Scientific Affairs. Effect of pregnancy on work performance. *JAMA* 1984;251:1995.
15. Royal College of Obstetricians and Gynecologist. *The initial investigation and management of the infertile couple.* London: RCOG Press, October 1998.
16. National Institute of Occupational Safety and Health. The effects of workplace hazards on female reproductive health. DHHS (NIOSH) publication No. 99-104 *(www.cdc.govniosh,99-104pd.html).*

FURTHER INFORMATION

American Medical Association Council on Scientific Affairs. Effects of physical forces on the reproductive cycle. *JAMA* 1984;251:247.

A referenced summary of known hazardous physical forces. Little support for adverse reproductive outcomes due to physical forces was reported. Hazards are known for atmospheric pressure (over 12,000 ft above sea level), hyperthermia (greater than 40°C), and ionizing radiation (depends on dose and duration).

CDC leading work-related diseases and injuries—United States: disorders of reproduction. *MMWR* 1985;34:537.

A hypothesis-generating summary of possible causes of adverse reproductive outcome estimates.

Christian MS, et al. *Assessment of reproductive and teratogenic hazards. Vol 3. Advances in modern environmental toxicology.* Princeton: Princeton Scientific Publishers, 1983.

A discussion of historical incidents, specific environmental exposures, and systems for rapid detection of potential hazards, and a description of toxicity and screening texts.

Freedman A. *Industry response to health risk.* Report No. 811. New York: Conference Board, 1981.

An extensive compilation of interviews and data from corporate executives and health staff on corporate response to public health needs. It is synthesized and written well, presenting practical points for the practice of occupational medicine.

Gabbe SG, Turner LP. Reproductive hazards of the American lifestyle: work during pregnancy. *Am J Obstet Gynecol* 1997;176(4):826–832.

A literature review (40 references) on the impact of work on pregnancy and suggestions to practitioners.

Grasso P, Parazzini F, Chatenoud L, et al. Exposure to video display terminals and risk of spontaneous abortion. *Am J Ind Med* 1997;32(4):403–407.

No association emerged between VDT exposure and spontaneous abortion, the estimated odds ration being 1.0% [95% confidence interval (CI): 0.8–1.2].

Kline J, Stein Z, Susser M. *Conception to birth: epidemiology of prenatal development. Vol 14: Monographs in epidemiology and biostatistics.* New York: Oxford University Press, 1989.

An extensively referenced and critical review of prenatal development. The text presents a synthesis and evaluation of current knowledge.

Levine RJ, et al. A method for monitoring the fertility of workers: I. Method and pilot studies. *J Occup Med* 1980; 22:781.

Surveillance for adverse reproductive outcome using an excellent questionnaire is reported. This directs more intensive investigation if an abnormality is detected.

Lewis RJ. *Reproductively active chemicals: a reference guide.* New York: Van Nostrand Reinhold, 1991.

This reference work details experimental data on about 3,000 chemicals and includes a Chemical Abstract Service number cross-index and a synonym cross-index.

Mattison DR, ed. *Reproductive toxicology.* New York: Alan R. Liss, 1983.

A collection of papers addressing reproductive biology and toxicology, including male, female, prenatal, perinatal, and postnatal. The section on reproductive toxicology surveillance presents useful methods and data sources.

McMartin KI, Chu M, Kopecky E, et al. Pregnancy outcome following maternal organic solvent exposure: a meta-analysis of epidemiologic studies. *Am J Ind Med* 1998; 34(3):288–292.

This metaanalysis suggested an increase in major malformations following maternal organic solvent exposure, however, the findings are tempered by the limitations of the metaanalysis methodology.

Office of Technology Assessment Task Force. *Reproductive hazards in the workplace.* Philadelphia: Lippincott-Raven, 1988.

Extensive introduction to the full range of issues and literature on the subject.

Paul M, ed. *Occupational and environmental reproductive hazards: a guide for clinicians.* Baltimore: Williams & Wilkins, 1993.

A comprehensive text covering a broad range of issues and questions arising from clinical practice.

Robert E. Intrauterine effects of electromagnetic fields (low frequency, mid-frequency RF, and microwave): review of epidemiologic studies. *Teratology* 1999;59(4):292–298.

Review stating there is no convincing evidence that electromagnetic fields in occupation or daily life do harm to the human reproductive process.

Rowland AS, Baird DD, Shore DL, et al. Ethylene oxide exposure may increase the risk of spontaneous abortion, pre-term birth, and post-term birth. *Epidemiology* 1996;7(4):363–368.

Among exposed women, the age-adjusted relative risk of spontaneous abortion was 2.5 (95% CI = 1.0–6.31), for preterm birth 2.7 (95% CI = 0.8–8.8), and for postterm birth 2.1 (95% CI = 0.7–5.9). The estimated relative risk of any of these adverse outcomes among exposed women was 2.5 (95% CI = 1.0–6.1) after adjusting for age, nitrous oxide, and number of mercury amalgams prepared.

Schardein JL. *Chemically induced birth defects.* New York: Marcel Dekker, 1985.

A useful reference regarding acknowledged chemical hazards that may interfere with reproductive outcome.

Schnorr TM, Grajewski BA, Hornung RW. Video display terminal and the risk of spontaneous abortion. *N Engl J Med* 1991;324:727.

A study of 18- to 33-year-old telephone operators in eight southeastern states found no significant differences in spontaneous abortion in women who did or did not work with video display terminals.

Stein ZA, Hatch MC. Reproductive problems in the workplace. *Occup Med State of the Art Rev.* Philadelphia: Hanley & Belfus, July–December 1986.

A review of the background and issues regarding occupational reproductive hazards.

Sweet AY, Brown EG, eds. *Fetal and neonatal effects of maternal disease.* St. Louis: Mosby-Year Book, 1991.

A detailed discussion of effects from a wide variety of infectious diseases and organ system disorders.

49

Environmental Health

Tee L. Guidotti and Weimin Song

Environmental affairs are a natural extension of the role of the occupational physician. Environmental affairs involving health are often managed by occupational physicians in large employer organizations, such as corporations, but not government regulatory agencies, because they are governed by different regulations. Because of the content of toxicology and epidemiology in their training, occupational physicians are already equipped with considerable knowledge that can be applied to environmental health problems.

TABLE 49.1. *Specialty areas in environmental health*

Air quality management (monitoring and control of air pollution)
Consumer safety
Control technology (engineering and control technology)
Emergency preparedness (disaster management)
Environmental medicine
Environmentally related chronic disease epidemiology
Food protection (toxicology and microbiology)
Genetics (including epidemiologic studies and studies of genotoxicity)
Housing conservation and rehabilitation
Institutional environmental health (sanitation in schools, health facilities, prisons, etc.)
Noise control
Radiation health physics
Recreational health and safety (control of injuries and health problems associated with sports and recreation)
Risk assessment
Solid waste management
Toxic substances management (including hazardous waste control)
Toxicology (study of health effects, handling by the body, and pertinent factors of the host influencing the response to toxic agents)
Traffic safety
Vector control
Water supply and treatment
Water quality management (including wastewater treatment)

Environmental health issues must be thought of differently from issues in occupational medicine. Occupational health issues most often affect small populations of healthy adults under circumstances of greater exposure of limited duration occurring in a small area. Environmental health issues concern the general population, including the very young, the very old, the ill, and other vulnerable populations under circumstances of less exposure over longer periods in a larger area. Furthermore, environmental exposures may often be multiple, continuous in nature, and penetrating through several routes of entry.

Table 49.1 lists the numerous specialty areas that have developed within the broad field of environmental health sciences that are concerned with particular aspects of the natural and manmade cycles.

This chapter provides an overview of water quality, solid waste, hazardous waste, and global ecologic issues. It combines the points of view on environmental health from a developed society (the United States and Canada) with those from a developing nation (China), as represented by the two authors. Throughout, we use examples from each to illustrate basic principles. Issues of air pollution in the indoor environment and air quality are covered in Chapters 53 and 59, respectively.

WATER QUALITY

Water is critical for maintaining life and many physical and biochemical processes. Usually, daily intake of 2 to 3 L of water is necessary for an adult to sustain physiologic function. Water resources must be accessible and of suitable quality to protect human health. All water resources are part of the hydrologic cycle in which water flows from the oceans to the atmosphere; falls from the atmosphere as rain onto the ocean, land, or fresh water, including lakes, rivers, and underground; and then returns to the oceans as runoff or to the atmosphere by evaporation. Underground water is usually cleaner than surface water because it has been effectively filtered. Natural filtering systems composed of soil and rocks cleanse the water, trapping disease-causing microorganisms and particulates containing toxic elements. However, once polluted, groundwater is much more difficult to decontaminate than surface water.

Water Resources Management

On a global scale, there is no shortage of total water resources. However, the problem is water's availability in the right place at the right time in the right form. Unfortunately, 99% of the earth's water is unavailable or unsuitable for beneficial human use because of its salinity or form and location (ice caps and glaciers). Today, world per capita use of water is 710 m^3/year, and it is estimated that total human use of water is 6,000 km^3/year (1). Because of waste and pollution of water resources, the secure fresh water available for human use is not sufficient. Water resources are often polluted by human activities such as domestic sewage as well as industrial and agricultural waste. In general, protection of water resources from pollution is urgent and important for sustainable development.

Water resources management involves three fundamental issues: (a) assurance of a secure and reliable supply of water, (b) treatment of drinking water to assure safety from microbiologic and chemical hazards and to ensure acceptability by the public, and (c) handling and treatment of wastewater so that it can be safely discharged and will not come into contact with drinking water supplies. Critical deficits in water supply, water treatment, and sewage treatment infrastructure both increase the risk of exposure to agents of infectious and parasitic disease and to a growing volume of industrial chemicals, heavy metals, and, in rural areas, algal toxins. The coordination between environmental and public health objectives is important to manage water resources. The technologies of water distribution and treatment, as well as wastewater treatment and discharge, are increasingly complex and the cost of maintenance is very high.

Purification of drinking water can be accomplished in many different ways such as coagulation, flocculation, settling, filtration, and chlorination. Filtration and chlorination are used on a large scale. These techniques, especially chlorination, have drastically reduced the incidence of water-borne diseases to present negligible levels, except for incidents where there is a break in the system, resulting in downstream contamination. Although there are adverse health effects from the by-products of chlorination, it is by far the cheapest and most effective method of disinfection. The reason for this is that the chlorine continues to act downstream, providing a margin of safety all the way to the tap. Alternative technologies, such as ozonation, irradiation, or ultraviolet treatment, do not disinfect water beyond the point of treatment.

Conventional methods of wastewater management include disposal and treatment of household wastewater by way of septic tank disposal systems in rural areas and centralized water treatment plants that collect wastewater in cities from sewer systems. The septic tank is designed to separate solids from liquid, digest and store organic matter through a period of retention, and allow the clarified liquid to discharge into the seepage bed. Through a piping system, the treated sewage can then seep into the surrounding soil. In soil, the wastewater can be further treated by the process of natural oxidation and filtration.

The conventional treatment for wastewater in a centralized water treatment plant is categorized as primary, secondary, and tertiary. In primary treatment, the sewage is held in settling tanks and the particles are allowed to sediment. Organic material is digested by bacterial action and the sludge that forms is eventually dried and disposed of separately. Secondary treatment allows further bacterial degradation of the wastewater organics by bacteria in an oxygen-rich environment. In this process biochemical oxygen demand (BOD) is greatly reduced. Tertiary treatment involves chemical purification of the remaining bacteria and organics before the effluent is released, usually into a river or ocean. Occasionally, raw sewage is still released without treatment, especially when primary treatment facilities are out of order or a flood has overloaded the sewer lines. For this reason, flood channels and sewer lines are not built to interconnect, as they once were.

Microbiologic Hazards

Water is a vehicle for the distribution of microorganisms, whether in surface or ground water. Even rain and snow contain microorganisms. Most significant waterborne pathogens come from sewage contamination of drinking water.

Waterborne diseases can be divided into two types, according to mode of transmission. One is caused by drinking water polluted with pathogenic bacterial agents such as *Salmonella, Shigella, Vibrio cholerae,* and *Yersinia enterocolitica,* or parasites such as *Cryptosporidium parvum* and *Giardia lamblia*. Most common and widespread health risks are associated with drinking water contamination by human and animal excreta, particularly feces. In these circumstances, case occurrence is closely related to consumption of contaminated water. Once measures of purification and disinfection are taken, the outbreak ceases. The second type of waterborne disease occurs when the individual is infected by contacting the polluted water with skin and/or mucous membranes. For example, schistosomiasis, also known as bilharzia, is a serious disease, most common in the Middle and Far East, spread by contact with a free-swimming larva (cercaria) that enters the body through the skin and matures into a blood fluke.

Within limits, a flowing body of water is a self-purifying medium insofar as bacteria and viruses are concerned. A river or stream can dilute, oxidize, and remove pathogens as long as its capacity is not exceeded and sufficient time elapses before water is withdrawn downstream. The principal causes of waterborne diseases are the following: (a) polluted water is provided for drinking without proper purification and disinfection; (b) the treated, secure water is re-polluted by pathogens in the process of transportation or storage; and (c) the water supply is inadequate, forcing people to use unsafe water sources.

In the U.S., the first two causes accounted for 89% of all outbreaks of waterborne diseases during the period of 1971 to 1985 (2). By far the most important waterborne illness in the U.S. is diarrhea. The type and degree of pathogen entry into water depends on the nature of the contamination and the health of the population from which the sewage in wastewater originates. Runoff from a feedlot for cattle, for example, poses much less of a threat to human health than leakage from a sewer line. In the U.S., outbreaks of waterborne disease are usually limited to enteritis associated with any of a number of viruses or, less commonly, giardiasis. Typhoid and cholera are exceedingly rare in the U.S. and usually are imported cases rather than outbreaks associated with water-related disease.

In China from 1979 to 1985, 212 of such episodes of centralized water supply contamination occurred in which 69% were from polluted water sources, 25% were from pollution of the water supply network, and 3% from a polluted water storage pool (3). Dysentery and diarrhea are ranked among the main avoidable causes of death in children in China. In 1995, the mortality rate for children under the age of 5 in China was 275.2 per 100,000, ranking fourth among all deaths (4). The number of children living in rural areas was 14 times the number living in urban areas.

Fecal coliform bacteria are an important class of microbial water pollutant from human and animal feces. Because fecal coliforms exist in human and animal intestines and excreta and the survival time of coliforms in water is similar to that of most pathogenic bacteria, it is used as an index for water pollution by feces and indicates the possible presence of pathogens.

Chemical Contamination

With increased industrialization and the widespread use of chemicals in industry, agriculture, and life activities, accompanied by generation of enormous volumes of industrial and domestic waste, public concern has grown regarding the importance of protecting drinking water from contamination with chemical agents. These concerns reflect the broader problem of chemical risk management and control measures. Chemical contamination of drinking water mainly comes from two sources: (a) contamination of both ground and surface water sources by chemicals, solvents, pesticides, metals, and the like; and (b) the process of drinking water treatment creating by-products of chlorination.

Sources of water pollution can be divided into point source and non-point sources. Point sources include such facilities as municipal sewage and industrial plants that generate waste. Non-point origins include such diffuse sources as runoff and seepage from agricultural and urban areas, mining, livestock grazing, and construction sites.

Leakage of potentially toxic substances into groundwater has occurred in many communities as a result of leakage from supposedly secure disposal sites. For example, groundwater in California's Silicon Valley and wells near Tucson, Arizona, have been contaminated with trichloroethylene (TCE), an industrial degreasing agent. Gasoline leakage from underground tanks has been a common problem, compounded recently by the leakage and rapid distribution of methyl tertiary butyl ether (MTBE), a gasoline additive that may be an animal carcinogen (5).

Contamination of surface or groundwater by waste dumped illegally is likely to occur more frequently as the cost of legal waste disposal increases. Evidence of links to organized crime have been found in some parts of the world.

The process of chlorination can produce a small amount of by-products by reaction of chloride with organic substances existing in untreated water. One or more kinds of trihalomethanes (THMs) including chloroform, bromodichloromethane, dibromochloromethane, and bromoform can be detected in virtually every chlorinated water supply. Chloroform and chlorophenols formed during the chlorination of drinking water have been shown to be animal carcinogens and are listed by the International Agency for Research on Cancer (IARC) as possible human carcinogens (group 2B). A number of epidemiologic studies have shown a positive association between the ingestion of chlorinated drinking water and mortality rates from cancer, particularly bladder cancer (6), although the degree of evidence for this association is considered inadequate by IARC (7). Guidelines for drinking water quality suggest an excess lifetime cancer risk of 10^{-5} or less associated with this source of chlorinated compounds (8). The generation of by-products can be reduced by optimizing the treatment process. Removal of organic substances prior to disinfection will reduce the formation of potentially harmful by-products.

Eutrophication refers to algae blooms in lakes or reservoirs polluted by phosphorus and nitrogen. Blooms of cyanobacteria (often called blue algae) are a common kind of eutrophication. These bacteria are capable of producing cyanobacterial toxins. The major route of human exposure to cyanobacterial toxins is the consumption of drinking water. A minor form of exposure occurs with recreational activities in lakes and rivers. Blue-green algae have been known for over 100 years to produce a distasteful odor and human poisoning in lakes, ponds, and dugouts. Aquatic animals that live in eutrophic freshwater ecosystems may be killed by microcystins (one of the cyanobacterial toxins), but in many cases the toxicity is sublethal, so that the animals can survive long enough to accumulate the toxins and transfer them along the food chain. In recent years, the concern over cyanobacterial toxins has focused on the adverse health effects related to cancer. An epidemiologic survey in Haimen City in China found a close relationship between the incidence of primary liver cancer and the use of drinking water from ponds and ditches with a microcystin concentration range from 0.058 to 0.460 g/L (9). Cyanobacterial blooms tend to occur repeatedly in the same water supply. Therefore, some human populations are at risk of repeated ingestion of cyanobacterial toxins. However, available data are not sufficient to allow a quantitative assessment of human exposure.

SOLID AND MUNICIPAL WASTE DISPOSAL

The amount of waste produced by human society is increasing. Commercial and domestic solid waste is a great practical problem for many local governments. Industrial wastes are usually much smaller in volume but are more likely to contain hazardous materials, such as toxic chemicals, flammable liquids, and asbestos.

Waste disposal is necessary for a modern society. Disposal of solid waste is primarily an urban problem. With the growth of industry, population, and size of an urban area, the amount of solid waste increases progressively. The U.S. per capita figure for garbage production has topped 4 lb per person per day, and that amount is rising at roughly 5% per year (10). The basic considerations for solid waste disposal are to minimize its hazard, reduce its quantity, and reuse the recyclable resources to the extent possible. Of particular importance is the development of new methods for waste disposal that will not endanger the public health, create a nuisance, or create an environmental time bomb. For example, waste placed in landfills may cause further problems from the production of methane gas or migration of noxious liquids from the sites to contaminate the surrounding areas. Disposal sites are also capable of producing a significant air pollution problem.

The composition of solid waste is very complex. Generally, solid waste is made up of five components, listed in Table 49.2. The terms used to describe these various components are universally agreed upon by solid waste technologists. The garbage component tends to provide the nutrients and breeding grounds for flies and rats, whereas the rubbish and debris provide the housing. Buried solid waste can create ground and surface water pollution.

In recent decades, production and use of plastic have increased dramatically. During the period from 1990 to 1995 the average world rate of increase in plastic utilization was 8.9% (11). The world production of plastic is now about 100 million tons per year. A lot of this ends up as waste, discarded into surrounding environments. For example, in Shanghai, wrapping plastic waste accounts for 7% of all municipal solid waste. Because plastic is hard to degrade or decompose in a general environment and its half-life

TABLE 49.2. *Typical composition of domestic and commercial solid waste*

Component	Characteristics	Origins
Garbage	Putrid; attracts rodents and flies; suitable for hogs and animal feed recovery	Food wastes at all levels of handling
Rubbish and debris	Nonputrid; organic and inorganic; combustible and noncombustible	Packaging; grass, shrub and tree clippings; leaves
Ashes	Inorganic inerts from combustion	Coal and wood burning; solid waste incineration
Street sweepings	Mixed mess; high in paper, grit and dust	Litter, abrasion, spillage, dogs
Oversized discards	Combustible and noncombustible; some parts can be salvaged	Used furniture, home appliances, motor vehicles

in soil spans several decades, plastic disposal becomes an important environmental issue. In recent years, several techniques have been developed for treatment of plastic, including techniques that decompose plastic under natural conditions by using additives such as photosensitive agents in the process of production. These techniques include substitution with paper, starch, or vegetable fiber.

Most municipal solid waste systems do not allow chemical and other hazardous wastes so that they do not contaminate the solid waste stream. In the U.S., these hazardous wastes are required to be disposed of in a secure receiving site complying with Environmental Protection Agency (EPA) regulations. Even so, small amounts of domestic and commercial hazardous waste, such as discarded cans of insecticide or paint, may find its way into the trash stream.

The basic strategies for disposal of solid waste are as follows:

1. Reduction of waste sources: Disposal or treatment of solid waste costs billions of dollars every year in the U.S., and environmental problems continue to arise from the process of disposal or treatment. Source reduction is the first thing to consider in reducing pollution from solid waste.
2. Recycling and resource recovery: Hazardous chemical waste may contain materials that can be successfully recovered for reuse. For example, solvents collecting contaminants in a manufacturing process could be filtered of its contaminants and then be reused in the same or different manufacturing processes.
3. Incineration: Hazardous biologic and chemical waste can be successfully destroyed by high temperature (700° to 1,000°C) incineration. This method burns both garbage and rubbish, thus disposing of fly- and rodent-breeding material. Although this method is very efficient, it can also be very costly because of high operational, maintenance, and energy costs. Since ash, cans, and bottles still remain, there is further handling needed, a disadvantage of this system of disposal. There is also a problem of particulate, toxic substances, and odor emissions, which may result from a poorly operated incinerator. There are hundreds of organic chemicals generated from the process. Chlorinated organic compounds are found frequently in hazardous waste. Burned at temperatures that are too low, they may form persistent and toxic by-products, such as dioxins.
4. Sanitary landfill: The basic idea of the sanitary landfill is to confine the waste to a particular location, and control, collect, and treat the leachate that drains from the waste. In this method, a dike and liner confine the waste, and a system of internal drains concentrates the leachate in a collection basin from which it is pumped out and transported to a wastewater treatment plant. An anaerobic type of decomposition that occurs in landfill sites produces increased quantities of methane. The landfill site thus poses a potential fire hazard. This method of disposal can be advantageous because of its low capital investment and moderate operational cost. After closure of the landfill site, the land may be reclaimed for restricted use. Disadvantages result from the fact that there is leaching, stand-by fire control is required, and a specially selected soil is required for cover.

HAZARDOUS CHEMICALS

Although the total amount is less, the disposal of hazardous industrial waste has been a greater concern than of domestic waste because of the perceived hazard to health and the risk of environmental contamination.

Many kinds of hazardous waste are generated and emitted from industrial processes and commercial activities, and even generated by individuals in their own households. They include flammable waste with a burning point lower than 60°C, corrosive waste, and wastes capable of inducing a severe chemical reaction.

Hazardous waste is sometimes mixed with domestic waste and is dumped into landfills designed for domestic solid waste. This is prohibited in most developed countries, but it still occurs. In many developing countries, there may be no alternative system of disposal available. It is an unacceptable practice because chemicals may leach out of the waste and migrate through soil into groundwater, contaminating water supplies and the soil.

People come into contact with toxic substances in many ways. Exposure to a toxic substance may occur at several points in the use cycle of the substance. People may be exposed to heavy metals from ambient air, indoor air, drinking water, food, and cosmetics. They can bring hazardous chemicals from the workshop to the home via unchanged clothes or unwashed hands. They may be exposed to chemical pollutants emitted from a chemical plant nearby their home. Exposure may occur in the home as the result of mislabeled, poorly stored, and non-childproof consumer products.

In assessing the health risk of a hazardous chemical, the first step is always to determine whether there is a plausible *intact pathway of exposure,* that is, a means by which people actually come into contact with the agent. Ideally, this means that one should demonstrate that the chemical is emitted into and distributed in the environment, conveyed to the persons at risk, and that these persons come into direct physical contact with it. For example, before concluding that waterborne chemicals from a hazardous waste site affect human health, it is necessary to show that they are at the waste site, that they migrate off the site through contaminated groundwater or surface water, that this migration transports the chemical to local wells or ponds, and that the residents of a community actually consume the water or bathe in it. The most important routes of exposure to chemical substances are inhalation, ingestion, and absorption through skin. The toxic effects may vary depending on amount and route of exposure. Because adverse health effects are caused by total exposure to a chemical from all sources, total intake amount should be considered. However, if there is no intact pathway of exposure, a hazardous effect of the chemical is impossible, regardless of its intrinsic toxicity.

A major unresolved issue in municipal solid waste handling is contamination by hazardous waste disposed of intentionally or by accident. This can be minimized by diverting disposal into a separate waste stream. In the U.S., people are willing to drive up to 5 miles to dispose of household toxic wastes safely. Some decentralized system for collecting such hazardous waste from consumers is needed before it is poured on the ground, flushed down the drain, or burned and released into the air. Such a system has been introduced in many urban areas, involving home or convenient pickup of small quantities of toxic substances to be discarded.

Other means can be used to control release of the remaining hazardous substances from a landfill site not constructed to receive such materials. Some communities have organized periodic pickup drives to collect household hazardous wastes in order to prevent contamination of sanitary landfills.

Well-designed hazardous waste disposal facilities, using the best available technologies of recycling, dehalogenation, and containment, are urgently needed and have been built in many locations. However, when waste is hauled a tremendous distance at great expense, it may expose drivers and residents along the way to the risk of accidents and leakage. More often, the waste may mysteriously "disappear" by the side of the road, causing exposure of residents and uncontrolled contamination.

Incineration at high temperatures is an effective means of disposing of much hazardous waste, but is very expensive. Because of population distribution, land use restrictions, transportation costs, and concerns about environmental effects, there is intense pressure to find an economical solution to the problem of hazardous waste disposal. This has led to increased interest in proven methods such as source reduction, recycling, chemical neutralization, and secure hazardous waste disposal sites.

New disposal sites are not a perfect solution because someone, inevitably, has to live near one. The NIMBY ("not in my backyard") syndrome makes it very difficult for governments to find new sites for undesirable developments such as hazardous waste disposal sites. Without such sites, however, society may lose control of the situation entirely. What happens when a hazardous waste disposal site is not available is often worse than the presence of a poorly managed disposal site. Sometimes, hazardous waste is disposed of illegally and in an even more dangerous manner because the owner cannot find a cheap way to get rid of it.

Surface water contamination may occur by runoff from the site, if the top layer of soil is contaminated, or by groundwater. When the groundwater feeds into a local body of water, such as a river or lake, the contamination is carried into this body of water. Some chemicals tend to deposit in the bottom sediment and others are carried along by the flow.

Hazardous Properties of Chemicals

This section discusses the problem of hazardous materials management in general terms. Toxicology and the properties of hazardous substances are discussed in Chapters 37 and 39.

Hazardous substances are compounds and mixtures that pose a threat to health and property because of their toxicity, flammability, explosive potential, radiation, or other dangerous characteristics. Public attention tends to focus on carcinogens, industrial wastes, pesticides, and radiation hazards, to name a few. However, innumerable compounds that do not fall into these categories can pose a threat to the public's safety and health.

Hazardous chemicals may present physical hazards, although this is more common in transportation and industrial incidents. Hydrocarbons may catch fire and even explode. Fires and explosions may generate their own toxic hazards depending on the chemicals that were initially present. Fires involving pesticide storage areas are a particularly dangerous situation, as the pesticide compounds may be converted into even more highly toxic combustion products (such as paraoxons in the case of organophosphates), and substantial amounts of environmentally damaging dioxins and furans may be generated from combustion in the presence of chlorine compounds.

Toxicity, however, is the principal concern of most people with respect to hazardous waste. Chemicals may be toxic to human beings and they may also be damaging to the environment through toxicity to animal and plant species. They may be concentrated in the food chain. The number and hazardous nature of toxic substances in common use has changed dramatically. In the last generation, research and development in organic chemistry and chemical engineering introduced thousands of new compounds into widespread commercial use, including persistent compounds such as the polychlorinated biphenyls (PCBs), more potent pesticides, accelerators, and plasticizers with unusual and poorly understood effects. Most of these have been withdrawn from production by now, but they persist in the environment. Many compounds in common use today underwent little testing prior to their introduction, and are not well understood.

Groundwater Contamination

In well-designed hazardous waste disposal facilities, there is an effectively impermeable seal to prevent hazardous chemicals from migrating out of the site and into the underlying soil. A well-designed hazardous waste disposal site also has facilities to treat those chemicals that can be neutralized or transformed and to reduce the volume of waste that goes into the site. Those chemicals that cannot be so treated are contained in impermeable containers.

Permeability is relative. It is a property of the material, described in terms of the resistance of the material to a liquid or gas penetration under given conditions of pressure and temperature. Although it may take years and even centuries, even the least permeable barrier, such as plastic liners or packed clay, will eventually allow the passage of some liquid chemical. Once breakthrough occurs, the flow becomes continuous, although it may occur at a very slow rate. This means that groundwater immediately below a hazardous waste disposal site is always at some risk of contamination, even if it is very small. Once groundwater is contaminated, it is very difficult and often impossible to decontaminate.

Chemicals may escape by leaking if the container is compromised, leaching if water gets in, or spilling during handling or after the site is disturbed. Once they permeate the liner of a site, or the liner is broken, or if there is no liner, the chemicals enter the ground and migrate downward due to the effect of gravity. This migration is much more rapid through porous soil and is slow through clay and bedrock. Even underground, water flows downhill and will take the path of least resistance. If there is a water table under the ground, the chemicals eventually reach it. Lighter chemicals tend to float on the groundwater and form an upper layer. Heavier chemicals and water-soluble compounds tend to dissolve or be carried along by the groundwater as it flows slowly underground through porous rock or gravel. The region of contamination can be mapped by drilling test wells, or *bore holes,* and is called the *plume*. The plume slowly expands and moves in the direction of groundwater movement.

Groundwater contamination may take centuries to clear by itself. If shallow wells are used as a water source by local residents, there is a possibility of exposure by ingestion of, and skin contact with, contaminated ground water.

GLOBAL ECOLOGIC CHANGE

Global ecologic change (the greenhouse effect, stratospheric ozone depletion, interregional transport of pollution, large-scale resource depletion, deforestation, desertification, erosion of cultivable land) has been of greater concern to the public in recent years.

Enhanced Greenhouse Effect

This is an international issue and must be solved by the combined efforts of countries all over the world. In the last century rapid increase in world energy production and world food production has caused heat-trapping "greenhouse gases" to accumulate in the lower atmosphere (troposphere), which has changed the world's climate. Establishment by the United Nations of the Framework Convention on Climate Change (FCCC) is one of the actions taken by countries to mitigate these problems. The goal of the FCCC is to work within a time frame enabling ecologic systems to naturally adapt to climate changes and to let the greenhouse gases in the atmosphere stabilize. The ultimate hope is to prevent further risk of climate change and to ensure the protection of food supplies from endangerment in the face of sustainable economic development. The much-disputed Kyoto agreement was the basic instrument of the FCCC.

Projections of health implications are made difficult by both the absence of key data and uncertainty in the predictions by various "general circulation models" used by climatologists. The magnitude and timing of the changes (although not their existence) are a matter of controversy, but scientific consensus suggests the strong probability of significant changes occurring over the next two or three decades. Major changes in climate have occurred before in human history, but the rate of change predicted by some models for the next few decades would exceed historical experience.

The greenhouse effect results from the accumulation of heat stored as radiant energy and retained predominantly in the oceans. It is the direct result of accumulation of carbon dioxide and some other gases in the atmosphere. Carbon dioxide effectively traps or absorbs long-wave radiation emitted from the earth's surface, and this trapped radiation heats the atmosphere. Thus, as the amount of carbon dioxide in the atmosphere increases, the atmosphere has a corresponding increase in temperature.

It was estimated that the rate of increase of carbon dioxide in the atmosphere is 0.5% annually. This increase is a result of the combustion of fossil fuels as well as significant deforestation. The greenhouse effect is necessary for there to be a temperature suitable for life on Earth, but the expected exaggeration of the effect from emissions of carbon dioxide from human activity is expected to lead to numerous adverse consequences. These include chaotic weather conditions, rising ocean levels due to ice cap melting, and regional weather disturbances, possibly including local cooling in some areas. It has been predicted that mean global sea level will rise by around one-third to one-half meter by 2100. Health implications may include heat-related illness and deaths; physical and psychological trauma due to disasters; vector-borne diseases due directly to higher temperatures and indirectly to changes in vector distribution by flooding; decreased food availability and hunger; respiratory effects due to weather disturbances, and related air pollutants and pollens; population displacement; and social disruption. Morbidity and mortality resulting from the greenhouse effect can only be estimated, but not predicted with any certainty. The speed of CO_2 increase can be modified by emission controls and by protection and regrowth of forest lands. The ultimate consequences and the effect on health are difficult to predict.

Stratospheric Ozone Depletion

Depletion of the stratospheric ozone layer by released chlorofluorocarbons (CFCs) (including those contained in medical products), bromofluorocarbons, and some other chemicals such as nitrogen dioxide will result in increased ultraviolet radiation reaching the earth's surface. The predominant health effects associated with depletion of the stratospheric ozone layer are caused by ultraviolet B (UVB) (289–320 nm) radiation. One of the results of this depletion is skin cancer (including malignant melanoma). According to estimates by the EPA, with each percentage point of ozone depletion, the incidence of nonmelanoma skin cancer will increase by 2% to 3% (12). Other health implications include cataracts, accelerated actinic changes (skin aging), and possible immunologic responses.

The principal strategy for controlling depletion of the stratospheric ozone layer is to reduce or restrict the production and use of CFCs. Viable substitutes have been found for most CFCs in industrial and pharmaceutical applications. Unfortunately, some CFCs have half-lives as long as 75 years or more, so the effect will continue for many years.

To date, there has been more progress in reducing emissions of CFCs than in any other intervention for controlling global ecologic change. This is because of the Montreal Protocol, an international treaty negotiated in 1987.

Other Global and Regional Environmental Problems

Distant transport of air pollution, as in "acid rain," may result in relocation of direct effects away from the point of emission, to "touch down" on distant sites. A direct effect suggested by recent epidemiologic evidence is increased frequency and severity of asthma episodes. Some authorities suggest possible toxicologic implications of metals leached from soil.

Depletion of primary resources, reduction of cultivatable land, and disruption of economic activity may lead to social disruptions resulting in civil unrest and large-scale migration ("ecorefugees"). This is particularly likely in developing countries. Other effects mentioned above are likely to be especially severe in developing countries, as well.

FURTHER PREPARATION

Occupational physicians are often assigned responsibilities for environmental issues because of the common body of knowledge in toxicology and health risk. Increasingly, medical directors in large organizations are recruited to positions that combine these functions. In practice, these environmental health functions may include the following:

- Management of traditional public health problems, such as air and water quality
- Management of new or novel products or technologies in which there is a potential or feared future risk, such as genetically modified foods
- Management of emergencies involving release to a community, such as emissions from a chemical plant
- Disturbances to an ecosystem in which secondary human health effects are possible, such as the risk of vector-borne disease from dams and irrigation canals
- Provision of environmental health services to employees, such as food safety practices in eating facilities, and sanitation in residential areas where workers live
- Litigation support, in the case of lawsuits for damages or criminal prosecutions over infractions of laws for environmental protection
- Environmental health and protection in the context of economic development in developing countries.

Standard textbooks of environmental health rarely cover all of these areas. Occupational medicine training tends to emphasize risk management and toxics litigation. Deeper preparation will generally be required for these responsibilities than this chapter can provide. The textbooks listed in the Further Information section at the end of this chapter are recommended for broader preparation in environmental health.

REFERENCES

1. Botkin DB, Keller EA. *The waters, environmental studies,* 2nd ed. Shanghai: Merrill, 1987:373.
2. Craun GF. Surface water supplies and health. *J American Water Works Assoc* 1988;8(1):40–52.
3. De-Kun G, Zi-Shi W. Summary for investigation of water-borne diseases in whole country. *J Environ Health* 1990;7(3):128–129 [in Chinese].
4. Yu-lin L, Liang-Ming L, et al. A survey on diarrhea of children under five years old in China during 1991–1995. *J Chinese Children Health* 1998;6(3): 166–169 [in Chinese].
5. Rudo KM. Methyl tertiary butyl ether (MTBE)—evaluation of MTBE carcinogenicity studies. *Toxicol Ind Health* 1995;11(2):167.
6. Pirastu R, Lavarone I, Comba P. Bladder cancer: a selected review of the epidemiological literature. *Ann Ist Super Sanita* 1996;32(1):3–20.
7. International Agency for Research on Cancer. *Chlorinated drinking-water; chlorination by products; some other halogenated compound; cobalt and cobalt compound.* IARC monographs on the evaluation of carcinogenic risks to humans, vol 52. Lyon, France: IARC, 1991:45-359.
8. World Health Organization. *Guidelines for drinking-water quality: disinfectants and disinfectant by-products.* Geneva: WHO, 1996:788–903.
9. Ueno Y, Nagata S, Chen G, et al. Detection of microcystins, a blue-green algal tumor promoter, in drinking water sampled in Haimen and Fusui, endemic areas of primary liver cancer in China, by highly sensitive immunoassay. *Carcinogenesis* 1996;17(6):1317–1321.
10. Tayor D. Talking trash: the economic and environmental issues of landfills. *Environ Health Perspect* 1999;107 (8):A404–A409.
11. Aihua W, Yanping S. The current statues of white color pollution and the strategies for control. *Sources Saving and Comprehensive Utilization* 2000;9(3):15–17 [in Chinese].
12. Hong-Dao C. *Modern environmental health.* Beijing: People's Medical Publishing House, 1995:34 [in Chinese].

FURTHER INFORMATION

Wallace RB, et al., eds. *Maxcy-Rosenau-Last public health and preventive medicine,* 14th ed. Stamford, CT: Appleton & Lange, 1998.

Yassi A, Kjellström T, de Kok T, et al. *Basic environmental health.* New York: Oxford University Press, 2001.

50

Environmental Medicine: The Regulatory Issues

William B. Bunn, Claudia O'Brien, and Jack Shih

Environmental protection policies and laws create an expansive set of regulations to control pollution and an excellent database on the types and quantities of pollutants, some of which may result in environmental illnesses. These statutory requirements and resulting exposure data generate an abundance of useful scientific information. Multiple reporting requirements under the Environmental Protection Agency (EPA) may arise when environmental illnesses are diagnosed (1–5).

The primary prevention of environmental exposure and disease is implemented by a combination of local, state, and federal regulations. In contrast to human risk-based occupational standards, many environmental regulations are oriented to minimize exposure by controlling emissions of categories of pollutants according to the medium of exposure. However, environmental regulations are being carefully scrutinized to determine their impact on human health risk, an area of expertise for occupational and environmental physicians.

To comprehend the current approach to the prevention of environmental disease, one must understand the regulatory framework as well as the science that supports these rules. These prevention-based regulations serve as the bases for the control of hazardous exposure and, ultimately, prevention of disease. In fact, exposure control strategies must be recommended with clear knowledge of applicable regulations.

FRAMEWORK OF ENVIRONMENTAL REGULATIONS

Before environmental regulations can be established, a bill must be passed by Congress and signed into law. The statute enables an appropriate agency, usually the EPA, to develop and promulgate regulations, which are first published in the *Federal Register* in draft (or "proposed" form) to allow interested persons to comment. These regulations become part of the Code of Federal Regulation (CFR) and serve as the legal framework for implementing environmental policy and reducing environmental exposures. If they are not followed, the federal government, states, or private individuals can bring suits in the civil courts to ensure enforcement or to press for damages. The federal government or a state may also seek criminal charges. Alternatively, regulations may be challenged as inconsistent with legal intent or agency jurisdiction. Suits may be introduced in local, state, or federal courts. Case law, however, will help define the interpretation of the regulations promulgated in the instant jurisdiction.

Thus, both regulations and case law may be important in a particular case. In almost every environmental exposure/disease situation, multiple regulations may be involved (1,2).

CHRONOLOGY OF ENVIRONMENTAL LAWS IN THE UNITED STATES

Environmental regulations mirror public concern and its reflection of actual risk. As a result, regulations in the United States and other countries have been driven by a series of environmental issues, many of which arose from catastrophic situations. The EPA was established by Congress one year after a major oil spill off the coast of California. The formation of the EPA unified federal regulation of environment under one federal agency. The EPA's charter included all media: air, water, and solid and hazardous waste (including liquid waste). The EPA began a sequential review and tightening of federal environmental protection regulation in the early 1970s (1,2,4).

The creation of the EPA was concurrent with other major legislative initiatives. For example, in January 1970, the National Environmental Policy Act (NEPA) was passed. This act established a statement of national environmental policy that promoted concern for the environment by all federal agencies and established a Council of Environmental Quality (CEQ).

The Clean Air Act (CAA), passed in 1970 and amended in 1987 and 1990, is designed to prevent further air quality deterioration, improve air quality in areas where it was already degraded, and reduce emissions from industrial sources and mobile sources (e.g., cars and trucks). Legislative regulation of water followed in 1972 with the Federal Water Pollution Control Act (Clean Water Act, CWA).

To summarize, in response to growing public concern, early congressional actions created a unified agency for environmental policy development and enforcement (EPA) and addressed two major public issues with passage of the Clean Air Act and Clean Water Act. These early actions were followed by an expansion of federal authority into other areas of the environment.

Originally a recommendation of the CEQ founded under NEPA, the Toxic Substances Control Act (TSCA) was passed in 1976. TSCA responded to growing public concerns about the hazards of certain chemicals such as polychlorinated biphenyls (PCBs) and insecticides, such as kepone, and it requires that scientific data be submitted to the EPA to evaluate the potential hazards of new or existing products. The EPA has the authority to interpret these data and to regulate production, use, distribution, and disposal of the substance or product.

Also in 1976, the Resource Conservation and Recovery Act (RCRA) was passed to regulate the disposal of solid and liquid hazardous waste. It established the concept of "cradle to grave" management of hazardous waste. The passage of the TSCA and RCRA in the mid-1970s emphasized federal interest in comprehensively addressing environmental pollution and not simply cleaning up polluted air and water.

In 1980, the Comprehensive Environmental Response, Compensation, and Liability Act (CERCLA) was passed. CERCLA addresses existing hazardous waste sites in the U.S. Like other environmental regulations, it followed the national concern that focused on the health implications of a hazardous waste site in Love Canal, New York, and created a "superfund" to pay for cleanup of abandoned hazardous waste sites. CERCLA established retrospective responsibility and liability, unique for regulatory statutes. In 1986, CERCLA was amended to extend the scope of environmental oversight with the Emergency Planning and Community Right to Know Act (EPCRA). In the aftermath of Bhopal, India, accident, EPCRA requires industries to notify governmental authorities of the hazardous substances located on a site, and to provide information on chemicals released at the site. For manufacturing sites, specific information must be submitted on the materials and the quantities used. CERCLA and EPCRA extended environmental protection retrospectively and incorporated the requirement to provide information to the public as well as to the EPA (see Chapter 60).

Although this overview of major environmental actions does not cover the full scope of regulation or the subsequent amendments, it demonstrates a legislative pattern. First, a national policy was developed and an agency established for its enforcement. Second, the most obvious pollution problems of air and water pollution were addressed. Third, an act was passed to establish a comprehensive "cradle to grave" concept for pollution control. Later acts followed that addressed removal of existing hazardous waste and mandatory public communication (Table 50.1).

ENVIRONMENTAL REGULATION AND ITS INTERFACE WITH ENVIRONMENTAL MEDICINE

There are a myriad of potential interfaces of environmental medicine with environmental regulations. The most important issues are (a) recognition of the database for correlating an exposure to disease, (b) reporting requirements generated by environmental exposures, (c) knowledge of the regulatory system for environmental pollution, and (d) intervention strategies in environmentally induced disease or risk of disease (5–7).

Air Pollution Control

Air pollution control is accomplished primarily through the CAA, which addresses primary and hazardous pollutants. "Criteria" pollutants—ubiquitous pollutants with diverse sources and significant human health impacts—include sulfur dioxide, particulate matter, ozone, carbon dioxide, nitrogen oxides, and lead. These substances are regulated through federally

TABLE 50.1. *Major U.S. environmental regulatory statutes*

Clean Water Act (USC §1251 et seq.)	Restore and maintain the quality of the nation's surface waters by regulating the discharge of pollutants
Clean Air Act (42 USC §7401 et seq.)	Control and abate air pollution by regulating air emission from stationary and mobile sources
Resource Conservation Recovery Act (RCRA) (42 USC §6901 et seq.)	Minimize threats to human health and the environment by regulating the treatment, storage, and disposal of waste, including releases to air, ground water, and land
Toxic Substances Control Act (TSCA) (7 USC §136 et seq.)	Regulate the introduction of new and existing chemical substances into the environment by requiring testing and reporting, and restricting use as necessary
Comprehensive Environmental Response, Compensation and Liability Act (CERCLA) (42 USC §9601 et seq.)	Provide funding and enforcement authority for cleaning up thousands of hazardous waste sites and for responding to hazardous substance spills
Emergency Planning and Community Right to Know Act (EPCRA) (Title III, Public Law 94-499)	Require state and local governments to develop plans for responding to emergency releases of environmentally hazardous substances, and require businesses to notify local emergency planning groups of the presence of such substances at facilities, to do emergency planning, and to report on releases of designated chemicals
Federal Insecticide, Fungicide and Rodenticide Act (FIFRA) (7 USC §136 et seq.)	Protect human health and the environment from hazards associated with pesticides and herbicides by requiring registration, testing, and reporting, and regulating distribution, sale, and use
Safe Drinking Water Act (SDWA) (42 USC §300f et seq.)	Regulate public drinking water systems, set national standards for contaminants in drinking water, regulate underground injection wells, and protect sole source aquifers

created health-based standards called National Ambient Air Quality Standards (NAAQS). The states, however, have primary responsibility for regulating sources within their jurisdiction—through state implementation plans (SIPs)—to ensure the NAAQS are met. Specifically designated toxic emissions [called "hazardous air pollutants" (HAPs)] are regulated through federally mandated technology-based standards (called National Emissions Standards for Hazardous Air Pollutants or NESHAPs) that are specified for individual industry sectors (such as chemical manufacturing or automobile painting). Specific requirements also exist for newly constructed sources of pollution, new or modified sources in areas with better air quality, and factories in "non-attainment" areas where air quality is poor. In addition, the CAA has specific programs to address acid rain and to reduce emissions of substances that deplete the stratospheric ozone layer, such as chlorofluorocarbons (CFCs).

Site implementation of the CAA is based on obtaining a permit from the state or local agency, or in some cases from the EPA, to allow facility operation. The permit specifies the amount of pollutants that may be generated. It must be renewed (typically every 5 years) and may require regular and specific monitoring for renewal. In the interim period, any excursions beyond permitted levels must be reported; EPA inspections and required testing (e.g., stack testing) may also be performed. The control of air pollution is frequently achieved by scrubbers, incinerators, and filtering devices. Recently, more focus has been placed on process modification and pollution prevention. For example, the reduction of the use of hazardous substances is encouraged through the Superfund Amendments and Reauthorization Act (SARA) Title III by reporting specific amounts of chemicals used and by the EPA's efforts to encourage voluntary reductions in emissions allowable by permit.

For the physician evaluating a person exposed to many chemicals, these regulations provide data on both the types and quantity of chemicals emitted into the air. In many situations, a calculation of the exposure that a person may receive from a "plume" from a stack may have already been performed and thus may be obtained from the industry or the EPA. Moreover, exceedences and unusual emissions must be reported under CAA and Emergency Right to Know provisions. These publicly available reports can provide excellent exposure data in evaluating an individual case or a cluster of cases (1–4).

Clean Water Standards

The federal CWA, officially titled the Federal Water Pollution Control Act, was passed in 1972, refocused on toxic pollutants in 1977, and amended again in 1987 to address issues such as overall water quality and storm-water runoff. The CWA has the following six major components: (a) a system of minimum national "effluent guidelines," technology-based standards for specific industrial sectors; (b) water quality standards; (c) discharge permit programs; (d) provisions for special issues such as toxics; (e) a grant program for publicly owned treatment works (POTWs); and (f) provisions to protect wetlands. The most important change from the prior system of water regulation was the institution of an "end of the pipe" approach as a supplement to state ambient water standards. Under this approach, every facility seeking to discharge wastewater must obtain a permit under the National Pollutant Discharge Elimination Program (NPDES) or else send its wastewater to a POTW, which also must obtain a similar permit for the disposal of wastewater. Either type of permit sets allowable limits of biologic and chemical constituents and specifies methods for measuring water quality to ensure compliance. These specific requirements and measurements are available for regulatory or health risk analysis (1–4).

Storm water runoff is also regulated by the CWA. Although it is more difficult to know the exact chemical constituents of storm water, there are monitoring requirements in many industrial situations. Failures to meet discharge requirements for effluent or storm water must be reported to the EPA, normally at the state level. Records of all measurements will be available and reviewed in the event of an exceedence. The CWA also regulates spills of potentially hazardous substances. The programs developed are prevention oriented. Significant storage tank regulations also exist (see RCRA, below).

Regulation of Storage and Disposal of Toxics

The Resource Conservation and Recovery Act

RCRA addresses the management of solid and liquid hazardous waste and is designed to minimize hazardous waste by regulation of its storage, treatment, and disposal. It establishes a "cradle to grave" approach for management. RCRA also addresses underground storage tanks (USTs), by establishing design, monitoring, reporting, and removal requirements.

RCRA requires each regulated industry to monitor all RCRA-listed chemicals from delivery to the facility until they are properly disposed. Chemical waste from specific industrial processes, with significant potential risk, are similarly regulated. The lists of regulated substances and processes are determined by risk assessment and rule-making procedures (see Chapter 58). Organic solvents, particularly chlorinated compounds and heavy metals, are among the most commonly listed substances requiring special disposal.

Regulations also apply to contaminated nonhazardous waste such as soil and to discarded products and waste chemicals. If a waste is not on a specific RCRA list, it is still regulated if it is ignitable, corrosive, reactive, or toxic. After determination that the substance is a solid waste, the substance's toxicity is determined by specific testing techniques defined by the regulations.

RCRA requires a regular inventory of all hazardous chemicals at a site in a "cradle to grave" process. That is, all use and discharge of a chemical at a plant must be accounted for from a public policy and individual health risk assessment perspective. This database provides excellent information to assess potential health risk.

The RCRA also regulates the transportation, storage, and disposal of hazardous wastes. Waste carriers must know the exact composition of the materials and the corresponding potential hazard of those materials. Disposal is regulated both in terms of process (e.g., incineration, burial) and the type and amount of chemical at each site. Recycling is encouraged by RCRA and is a growing area of regulation. Incentives for recycling solid and liquid hazardous waste have been instituted, along with special requirements to encourage purchase of products incorporating nonhazardous solid waste. RCRA has recently placed emphasis on biologic and medical wastes as well as chemical waste. The biologic waste control programs are not as developed as chemical programs, but regulation is growing.

Superfund: Comprehensive Environmental Response, Compensation and Liability Act (CERCLA)

Congress enacted CERCLA (the Superfund) in 1980 to supplement RCRA, which covers current hazardous waste disposal. CERCLA is designed to cover past hazardous waste disposal activities. It also has reporting requirements for spills or other releases. In 1986, CERCLA was amended by SARA, which substantially expanded its scope.

CERCLA gives the federal government broad authority over polluters and the substances regulated. For example, CERCLA jurisdiction is triggered by the release of any amount of a substance without threshold, while other environmental statutes include a threshold before regulation.

CERCLA is also unique from the legal perspective. It is retrospective; that is, it applies to historic pollution, even if the disposal of the waste was legal, or the waste was not considered hazardous at the time. Further, CERCLA is "joint and several," in that any contributor to a waste site may be responsible for the entirety of the cost of the cleanup if other responsible parties cannot be found.

CERCLA may mandate cleanups of several types. Although the general mandate is for removal or remediation, or both, removal is rarely the total solution for large sites. Sites specifically regulated by CERCLA are maintained on the National Priority List (NPL). By mid-2002, thousands of remediation plans have been submitted, reviewed by the EPA, and cleanup begun—and over 800 cleanups have been completed. The decision on the procedure for cleanup begins with a remedial investigation (RI) and feasibility study (FS) to characterize the site and the pollution. The RI stage addresses the contamination on the site and the FS notes the techniques for cleanup. The RI/FS package for a site is then submitted to EPA for a decision. The EPA's review and decision are published as a record of decision (ROD) and are available for public comment. The key issues for the ROD involve how clean the site should be and how far the contamination extends.

The decision on how clean the site should be is based on appropriate or relevant and appropriate requirements (ARARs). The ARARs are determined on a case-by-case basis and may be based on EPA regulations, a guidance document, or other applicable state/local regulations. Consideration is given to a number of other factors, including the health risks of removal and disposal of the contamination. The determinations made under CERCLA must take RCRA guidelines into consideration in the decision-making process for a waste site. The cost of the investigation and cleanup is commonly in the millions to hundreds of millions of dollars.

The costs are borne not only by the owner of the waste site, but also by every hauler of waste to the site, or by any manufacturer or company whose hazardous materials were disposed at the site. The law requires contribution from each party up to the total cost of the remediation (e.g., joint and several liability). The EPA may also sue for damages to flora and fauna away from the remediation site, where applicable.

An important impact of CERCLA/Superfund has been in acquisitions and divestitures of property and businesses. In purchasing property or a business, the buyer typically assumes the environmental liability of the purchase (although the seller may retain liability in some cases). Since the environmental cleanup costs may be excessive, a major portion of due diligence investigations of potential purchases is an assessment of environmental liability (monetary/civil, administrative, and criminal). Due diligence teams will include a wide variety of health professionals to assess legal, monetary, and human health risks.

CERCLA also includes requirements for reporting of releases. If a certain quantity of any hazardous substance is released, immediate reporting is required to the National Response Center (NRC). There are stiff civil and criminal penalties for failures to report. Reporting does not include releases that are within the levels stated in the industry's permit. EPA has issued tables that will determine which substances require reporting when released and at what level (as expressed in the amount released during a 24-hour period).

The RI/FS/ROD site assessment and release reporting are excellent sources of data on potential environmental exposure. These reports are commonly used in tort actions to determine potential health risks. The information is also publicly available for use in evaluations of environmentally induced injury and illness. In addition, the parties responsible for exposures may be determined from EPA records and exposure information sought from that party for the chemical disposed or released. Information on toxicity developed by the manufacturers of the pollutants may also be obtained.

Superfund Amendments and Reauthorization Act: Emergency Planning and Community Right to Know Act (EPCRA)

EPCRA is a free-standing provision of SARA. It is designed to make emergency planning entities aware of the presence of potentially hazardous substances through reporting requirements to state and local authorities. It also requires reporting of releases and inventories (i.e., utilization rates) of regulated substances. These reports are available to any interested persons and are commonly published by local and national media. This reporting of cumulative results is designed to encourage reduction in the use and disposal of potentially hazardous chemicals.

EPCRA has three subtitles. Subtitle A sets the framework for emergency planning and release notification. Subtitle B requires two types of reports of inventories of hazardous chemicals. The first section requires facilities to maintain and provide to local authorities data on listed hazardous substances. Material Safety Data Sheets (MSDSs) must be prepared and provided to local authorities and the workforce in accordance with Occupational Safety and Health Administration (OSHA) regulations. Subtitle B also requires special reporting for certain larger manufacturers (SIC codes 20-39). These reports require reporting of the quantities of the listed substances at the facility (the chemicals are listed by governmental authorities), how these substances are disposed of or treated, and how much of each chemical enters the environment by each medium. Subtitle C creates substantial civil, criminal, and administrative penalties for violations of the reporting requirements. Enforcement actions may be brought by citizens as well as by the state. Therefore, EPCRA requires the preparation and submission of substantial information that may be relevant to health risk assessment. These data will be available for assessment of potential environmentally related disease. In addition, quantification (by media) of releases is required. Results are available to the public.

The Toxic Substances Control Act

Before 1976, there were no federal regulations for testing of chemicals entering commerce and the environment. In the late 1960s and early 1970s, concerns arose about multiple chemical products, including organic mercury, PCBs, vinyl chloride, and kepone. In addition, NEPA and the CEQ had expressed an interest in preventing toxic pollution as well as setting standards for emission or remediation. TSCA addresses the need to fully evaluate the potential toxicity and environmental impact of many existing and all new chemicals. It also includes some specific regulations on PCBs and asbestos.

Premanufacture Notification

The heart of the TSCA is the requirement for premanufacture notification (PMN) of new substances introduced into commerce. A manufacturer (or importer) must notify the Office of Pollution Prevention and Toxics (OPPT) 90 days before producing (or importing) a new chemical substance. Most companies approach the EPA well before the 90-day period preceding production. After notification, the EPA must publish in the *Federal Register* an item on the chemical, its intended use, its potential toxicity, and indicated testing. The EPA must be satisfied that there is no "unreasonable risk to human health or the environment." If these requirements are not met, the EPA may either prohibit or limit production or distribution, or both, or require specific additional tests at the expense of the manufacturer.

For existing chemicals, the act requires reporting of any significant adverse effects from animal or human studies or clinical cases that are not already known or reported.

To expedite the approval of testing of health effects, TSCA has issued testing guidelines (5). There are specific exemptions for chemicals in the stages of research and development. To determine whether a chemical is "new," the TSCA has developed an inventory of existing chemicals (section 8b). The list was designed to cover all chemicals produced during a 3-year period, before the time of TSCA regulation. At that time, companies submitted chemicals to be placed on the list, which is updated by the EPA as chemicals are added to the inventory.

The TSCA also regulates new uses of existing chemicals through significant new-use regulations (SNURs). Relevant issues as to whether existing chemicals come under the SNURs include changes in volume, type of exposure to humans or environment, duration of exposures, and life cycle of the chemical.

Reporting Requirements

In addition to the testing of new or existing chemicals, TSCA has a series of reporting requirements. First, under section 8b, an inventory of potentially toxic substances is compiled by OPPT. Section 8b also requires information from manufacturers that may lead to updating of the inventory. The inventory list is used in section 8 and other reporting requirements under the TSCA.

Section 8a requires submission of information on the listed chemical, the amount produced and distributed, and how it is manufactured. It applies to manufacturers, importers, and processors, although, as in most reporting requirements, exemptions are made for small quantities, research and development, and small industries. Section 8c is especially important for the occupational and environmental physician. This section requires recording and record maintenance for "significant adverse effects" alleged by any employee or user of the product/chemical. Employee allegations must be maintained for 30 years (nonemployee, 5 years). A significant adverse effect is described as "long-lasting irreversible damage to health or environment," but effects that indicate that such an ultimate effect could occur are also recordable. While all recorded allegations are not reportable unless requested, health effects are reportable (under section 8e) to the EPA if they meet the criteria of "substantial risk." If an effect is previously known, it is neither recordable nor reportable.

Section 8d requires submission to the EPA of all pertinent health and safety studies known to the manufacturer, importer, processor, or distributor on listed chemicals. Health and safety studies include those related to exposure (e.g., industrial hygiene studies) as well as toxicology and epidemiology. Unpublished studies are included; the requirement is retroactive for 10 years.

Section 8e requires submission of information "that reasonably supports the conclusion that such substance or mixture presents a substantial risk of injury to health or the environment." Reporting is required by manufacturers, processors, or distributors, but not by others receiving the information (e.g., testing laboratories). The EPA will often accept information that may not meet the "substantial risk" definition. The corporation, including corporate management and officers, may be assumed to have knowledge of the information, if anyone "capable of appreciating the information" obtains it. Civil fines may be substantial; criminal fines and sanctions also apply. If the finding has been previously reported or is a known effect, reporting is unnecessary. The reports must be received within 15 working days and will be available for public scrutiny.

Reporting responsibilities for TSCA 8c and 8e are significant. In fact, committees are commonly formed at the corporate level to evaluate 8c and 8e information and to determine the reportability and the wording of the report. These committees may include occupational and environmental physicians, industrial hygienists, toxicologists, operation managers, and environmental attorneys. Implementation of TSCA responsibilities may be coordinated through a product stewardship or member of the legal group, or both. Potential civil and criminal penalties, along with the public scrutiny of these reports, make the TSCA activities a highly sensitive area.

Furthermore, since occupational and environmental studies must be reported under the TSCA, an extensive database for the assessment of the potential toxicity of a chemical is available. In environmental medical cases, TSCA requirements are a source of reports regarding adverse health effects in people and in animals.

Testing Requirements and Regulation of Existing Chemicals

Premanufacture notification or reporting of potential health effects may prompt the need for additional testing under the TSCA. Testing requirements apply to situations in which more data are needed before a final decision may be made. Data may include those related to human exposures, potential toxicity, and/or environmental fate/impact. The cost of the testing is borne by the manufacturer.

If the data submitted are deemed not sufficient to meet the requirements of the act, TSCA has several alternatives. First, it can mandate additional testing before the chemical is sold. Second, TSCA may limit the amount of a chemical produced, or prohibit or limit certain uses that increase exposures. Third, TSCA may require specific warnings or labels, or extensive data on production or disposal of the substance. TSCA also has the option of referring the issue to other regulatory bodies. For example, OSHA may be a more appropriate agency to review the material if only a workplace potential health hazard exists. Finally, if an "imminent and unreasonable risk" is present, TSCA may actually ban the use of a chemical. The EPA has not chosen to use the total ban approach under section 7, but has focused on limitation of exposure by restriction of markets for such substances as PCBs. EPA's regulations to phase out asbestos use were overturned by the courts.

TSCA is of special importance for occupational and environmental physicians. Through the reporting of toxicologic and epidemiologic studies and "clinical adverse reactions," it mandates the establishment of a health risk database. It also includes several medical reporting requirements for manufacturers and importers. An awareness of these reports will be significant in any evaluation of environmentally based disease. OPPT, which administers TSCA, can be an extremely useful reference in assessing risks, especially when there is an ongoing scientific and regulatory debate concerning a chemical.

THE OCCUPATIONAL AND ENVIRONMENTAL PHYSICIAN'S ROLE

Environmental statutes require the creation of a massive database that can be used by the occupational and environmental physician (OEP) in clinical cases, and in assessing the risks of working groups and the community. Access to the data will be as challenging as its interpretation and integration into the decision-making process. Access will be determined by the position of the OEP. For example, if the physician is employed by the industry generating the data, it is generally accessible. The data needed, however, should be carefully defined in a specific request to the corporate office or site environmental manager. A clear description of the intended use of the information is recommended. If the OEP needs data on a clinical case and is not employed by the industry, a request can be made through the employee or directly to management of the industry. Environmental recordkeeping responsibilities are massive; as a result, a request for general data will not be acceptable. If the information is not made available, some of it may be accessed through environmental regulatory agencies. Local officials will usually be helpful; however, the physician may choose to call the regional EPA offices. Often, there is litigation and the records may be part of the discovery process. If special testing is needed and has not yet been performed, it may be requested by the industry or the EPA. Environmental testing services can be directly accessed. (The American Industrial Hygiene Association maintains a list of contractors specializing in environmental testing.)

Just as industrial hygiene data may be difficult to access, environmental exposure data may present similar challenges, especially for physicians who evaluate workers and who are not OEP specialists. If data access or interpretation is particularly difficult, subspecialists in environmental medicine can be contacted. Physicians in occupational and environmental residency training programs are an excellent resource when difficulties arise, since they commonly work with both industry and government and are often perceived as unbiased.

SUMMARY

The system of environmental regulation in the United States can serve as a framework for understanding common environmental problems, as well as a reference source for the practice of environmental medicine. Regulations that were well planned in the late 1960s have matured over time. While most regulations have been oriented to exposure control rather than actual health risk, the data generated by these requirements are vital to assessing the potential relationship between exposure and disease.

Although environmental laws developed based on the medium, a comprehensive and preventive approach to environmental pollution is evolving. A new emphasis has been placed on risk assessment both for new regulations and for implementation of existing regulations. The ultimate product of this process is the assessment of risk to people. These assessments mirror the exposure/disease determination in a clinical case in a more formal fashion. The use of preventive approaches and human risk assessment makes the occupational and environmental physician a key participant in future regulations and their implementation.

In assessing a person with an illness potentially related to an environmental exposure, a determination of causation must include the most comprehensive exposure measurements available. Commonly, these measurements are the product of regulatory requirements.

Whether data are requirements of permits or monitoring secondary to a release, they serve as a primary source of exposure information. In the occupational setting, personal monitoring data may be available. With environmental exposures, however, data require significant extrapolation and interpretation.

While the interpretation of data may be problematic, EPA officials and experts in occupational and environmental medicine can support these efforts. Although somewhat different from occupational health regulations, environmental statutes result in the generation of data that must be evaluated according to similar principles in exposure/disease/prevention assessments. Illness resulting from exposure to an environmental hazard is not different from that due to occupational exposure of similar concentration and route of entry. The medical approach requires similar diligence to evaluate each piece of the clinical puzzle to formulate a diagnosis and to propose treatment and preventive strategies.

REFERENCES

1. Sullivan TF, et al. *Environmental law handbook,* 16th ed. Rockville, MD: Government Institutes, 2001.
2. Findley RW, Farber DA. *Environmental law,* 4th ed. St. Paul: West Publishing, 1996.
3. Rodgers WH. *Environmental law.* St. Paul: West Publishing, 1992 (with updates).
4. O'Grady MJ, ed. *Environmental law deskbook.* Washington, DC: Environmental Law Institute, 2002.
5. Brown EC, et al. *TSCA deskbook.* Washington, DC: Environmental Law Institute, 2001.
6. Tarcher AB. *Principles and practice of environmental medicine.* New York: Plenum, 1992.
7. Sullivan JB, Krieger GR. *Hazardous materials toxicology.* Baltimore: Williams & Wilkins, 1992.

FURTHER INFORMATION

The environmental regulations and field of environmental laws are changing so rapidly that the most appropriate reading may be the *Federal Register* and a number of newsletters (e.g., *BNA Environmental Reporter, Inside EPA*) that contain the more recent information. The texts listed above all contain good summary information, but details may not affect the current regulations. The *Environmental Law Handbook* is comprehensive and relatively easy to read, and the *TSCA Deskbook* provides good detailed TSCA information.

In addition, a wealth of useful information can be accessed through EPA's Web site *(www.epa.gov),* including health assessments of individual chemicals, exposure information, EPCRA reporting data, and updates on current regulations and programs. While not always well organized, the Web site can be enormously useful to those involved in the practice of environmental medicine. Practitioners may find particularly helpful the OPPT Web site, the National Center for Environmental Assessment Web site, and the Integrated Risk Information System (IRIS) Web site (which contains typically conservative and sometimes outdated, but rather informative, health assessments of chemicals)—all of which can be accessed through the general EPA Web site listed above.

51

International Environmental Health

William B. Bunn and Jessica Herzstein

The public health impact of the environment is a global issue of increasing concern. Local and national regulations will not successfully protect the health of the public if international pollution continues to increase. In addition, industrial globalization has forced multinational corporations and governmental and nongovernmental organizations to think with a world perspective. Although environmental exposure has become a growing concern for international travelers, this issue is typically not addressed in the travel health literature or databases.

The regulatory structure of most countries is based on overlapping local, state, and federal regulations that are based on the medium of pollution—air, water, and solid and hazardous waste. Although the environmental health risks to an individual will result from a combination of exposures, an approach based on the pollution medium helps clarify these global environmental challenges.

GLOBAL AIR POLLUTION

The effects of air pollution have been recognized since the 13th century, but they became a prominent global issue with industrialization and with the use of motor vehicles in the 20th century. The risks in the earlier 20th century were primarily related to stationary sources, particularly the use of soft coal. Mobile sources (on-road and off-road) became the primary contributors to air pollution during the latter part of the 20th century. In addition, wind-blown dust remains an issue in many countries (Sahara Desert, Harmattan; Gobi Desert, Lugesse).

Globally, the World Health Organization (WHO) has played a major role in reporting air pollution, and in providing guidelines for acceptable exposure levels. The WHO publications are an important source of international data on a range of pollutants.

The "Great Smog" in London in 1952 was the first clear demonstration of the health effects of air pollution. Although there were earlier reports (Meuse, France; Donora, United States), the London episode focused international attention on air pollution. In the London smog episode, 4,000 to 8,000 deaths were attributed to atmospheric pollutants, including particulate matter (PM) and oxides of sulfur (SOx). Indoor as well as outdoor air pollution became a focus of environmental research and regulation in the 1970s.

SOURCES OF POLLUTION

In Western industrialized countries, the use of lignite (brown coal) is primarily of historical interest; however, on a global basis, lignite is still a significant pollutant. China is an example of a nation where the use of lignite (or similar sulfur-containing fuel sources) remains significant.

Electric power generation has been a significant source of atmospheric air pollution. The primary pollutants from power plants have been SOx and PM such as fly ash. Nitrogen oxide (NOx) is a major issue currently. There is also continued concern about the emission of air toxics (e.g., mercury).

Motor vehicle emissions are a major source of air pollution, and have replaced coal smoke as the chief concern in developed countries. The increase in motor vehicle traffic (on-road) and construction (off-road) has traditionally indicated an expanding economy; but despite measurable growth, until a significant level of air pollution has been recorded, actions may not be taken to address the issue. The first method of control is to limit vehicle use. This approach is common in large Asian cities, but is also practiced in Europe, the U.S., and in Mexico City, Mexico. A second approach has been the utilization of postcombustion control technologies (tailpipe controls). The elimination of lead in gasoline, for example, has prompted the use of catalytic converters. Similarly, low-sulfur diesel allows the use of continuously regenerating traps (CRTs) that effectively limit PM and volatile organic compounds (VOCs). Lead continues to be a pollutant in many countries, and carbon monoxide is also a major pollutant. In addition to primary pollutants from motor vehicles, there are secondary pollutants from atmospheric reactions like NOx, an ozone precursor.

Indoor air pollutants include combustion sources, and off-gassing of chemicals, dust, allergens, and many other compounds. In many societies, individuals spend 90% of their time indoors, and indoor air is a primary consideration. Indoor air concerns usually come from heating and cooking in developing countries, and from off-gassing in developed countries.

GLOBAL MONITORING OF AIR POLLUTION

Air pollution is commonly divided into primary pollutants (e.g., PM, SOx, NOx, CO) and air toxics. Although measured individually, combinations of pollutants must be considered as well as the level of the independent contaminants. Commonly, ambient target levels are set for primary pollutants, while point-source permitting (for smokestacks and tailpipes) or engine certification processes regulate air toxics. Currently, a regular government-based testing program is required for primary pollutants, and a network of monitoring stations and mobile monitoring stations is utilized with limited tailpipe testing after certification.

HEALTH EFFECTS OF PRIMARY POLLUTANTS: SOX, NOX, CO, PM

Historically the effects of SOx are related to the formation of acid and the secondary formation of sulfur-containing particles. Acid rain is primarily a product of sulfur-based acid formation.

NOx can also form nitric/nitrous acid and acidic fogs, but it is regulated due to its ability to produce ozone through a photochemical reaction. Ozone can have acute effects on the upper and lower airways, and has been associated with fibrosis in animal models. The acute effects of carbon monoxide are well known, although chronic effects from environmental levels are controversial.

The potential health effects of PM are highly debated and the science continues to develop. Daily increases in PM concentration have been associated with several indices of ill health including daily death rates, hospital admissions, emergency room visits, antiasthma drug use, and lung function measures. Confounding variables such as temperature, ozone, SOx, NOx, and other coexposures are still being carefully evaluated, but have not yet provided an adequate explanation for the effects. For example, the increased risk from fine particles less than 2.5 μm in diameter is under study. Some researchers suggest that $PM_{2.5}$ is a better marker than PM_{10}, while this effect is not evident in other studies. In addition, studies in animals/cells suggest that ultrafine particles (50–100 nm) could pose the greatest risk.

In addition to these reports, cross-sectional studies (e.g., Harvard Six Cities Study) have shown similar risk increases. The impact of particles at ambient levels on chronic lung disease is not clear, although in some studies (e.g., China) increased risk is shown with extremely high indoor and outdoor total-particulate levels.

AIR POLLUTION IN MAJOR CITIES

The exposure levels to pollutants are highest in the major cities of Asia, Mexico, and South America. Mexico City has had the highest environmental exposure levels for 15 years. The combination of high altitude (2,240 m), motor vehicle use, and industrial pollution makes Mexico City a challenging environment from a health risk perspective. Ground-level ozone has been a major challenge due to high photoreactivity. Ozone levels regularly exceed standards (90% of the time from 1991 to 1994). Particulate levels are also high due to combustion and natural sources. Warnings are regularly issued for individuals with underlying lung disease. Similar ozone pollution is seen in other South American cities such as Lima and Santiago.

In Asian cities like Beijing, pollution is a combination of many agents. In Beijing, particulate levels commonly exceed 1,000 $\mu m/m^3$, and $PM_{2.5}$ levels commonly exceed 100 $\mu m/m^3$ (U.S. maximum is 15 $\mu m/m^3$ as a yearly average). Sulfur oxide levels are significant due to the continued use of coal for heating, and nitrogen oxide levels are rising due to motor vehicle use. Carbon monoxide and air toxics have increased, and recent studies show significant increases in organic carbon particles from home cooking/heating sources. A similar mix is seen in several Asian cities including Delhi, Bombay, and Kathmandu (Katmandu). In Asia, special pollution issues such as land-clearing fires in Indonesia and blowing sand from the Gobi desert also exist.

In Eastern Europe there are significant particulate emissions from unregulated stationary sources and from mobile sources. In Athens, NOx is a problem, particularly in the spring. In North America, Los Angeles, Atlanta, and Denver have been noted for smog formation during thermal inversions. Houston has recently emerged as the most polluted city in the U.S.

There are significant levels of motor vehicle–related pollution in most major African cities (Cairo, Alexandria, Lagos). In addition, there is significant natural particulate pollution from the Sahara sands.

These cities exemplify air pollution patterns, but patterns are unique in each major city and country. Individuals traveling to or relocating to a new city or country should review the atmospheric pollution at that location.

ASTHMA AND AIR POLLUTION

Recent increases in asthma in Europe and the U.S. have led to careful study of the potential relationship between atmospheric air pollution and airways disease. Although the asthma incidence is increasing in industrialized countries, the atmospheric levels of pollutants have been decreasing since the 1980s. In addition, the incidence of asthma has not increased in several of the most polluted cities. However, the mix of pollutants and properties of pollutants (e.g., smaller particles) have changed and will differ between locations. This variance area offers a possible explanation for the increase in asthma due to air pollution.

ATMOSPHERIC POLLUTION

Although levels of atmospheric pollution are improving in the U.S. and in many developed countries, the levels of pollution have rapidly increased in many cities and regions on a global basis. An understanding of atmospheric pollution is essential to establish an occupational and environmental health program for national residents, expatriates, short-term assignees, and travelers.

GLOBAL WATER POLLUTION

Water pollution can generally be divided into ensuring safe drinking water and good sanitation. The causes of water pollution can be divided further into biologic and chemical agents, and source of pollution into runoff water versus treated sewage.

Throughout history, people settled in areas where water was available. As communities formed, sanitation practices became important because water contamination increased as the demand for drinking water increased.

The cities of industrializing countries have been and are currently the areas with the highest risk of waterborne infectious contamination. The pollution from upstream industrial and nonindustrial sites has had a major public-health impact on downstream communities. A classic example of contamination was the London cholera epidemic in the mid-19th century. Such epidemics have been eliminated largely by the introduction of filtration and chlorination, beginning at the turn of the 20th century. Although chlorination has been highly effective at reducing waterborne infectious diseases, many rapidly industrializing countries still suffer from waterborne and water-related diseases. Of special concern are the estimated 4 million children who die each year from infantile diarrhea.

In the latter half of the 20th century chemical pollution became a major issue for industrialized countries. Particular concern developed around contamination with potentially carcinogenic chemicals, and the formation of mutagenic compounds from the interactions of chlorine with organic materials. This chlorine interaction issue has led to ongoing debate, but chlorine's protection against infection outweighs the potential risk.

Water and Disease

Health concerns from water pollution go beyond ingestion. There are specific water-related diseases (waterborne, water contact, water hygiene, and water habitat), particularly in developing countries. Waterborne diseases include diseases caused by ingestion of human or animal wastes such as typhoid, cholera, giardiasis, cryptosporidiosis, amebiasis, and a wide range of bacterial diseases. Although rare in industrialized countries, these diseases are more common in developing countries. Water-contact diseases are similar, except the vectors usually penetrate the skin during contact with water or with moist, contaminated soil (e.g., schistosomiasis, ascariasis, hookworm). Water hygiene diseases are caused by lack of water for personal hygiene (e.g., lice-borne disease). Water-habitat diseases are caused by standing water, which allows breeding of insects (e.g., mosquito-borne diseases such as malaria, dengue, and yellow fever).

Water Supply and Quality Standards

Both water supply and sanitation (WSS) interventions are required to protect public health. However, due to convenience, water supply is a much more common focus in developing countries than sanitation.

In developing countries when WSS is not available, oral rehydration therapy (ORT) has been a cost-effective intervention for some water-borne diseases. ORT does not prevent future episodes because supplied water may continue to be contaminated, particularly in areas with poor sanitation.

Despite major international intervention, significant problems exist in much of the developing world. Many major cities do not supply water 24 hours a day. Although treatment plants may be effective, the water commonly becomes contaminated in transit. For example, water pipes are often poorly maintained and seepage occurs in the pipes during "off" periods. Distribution is also a major problem. Often the water system will supply only the center city and wealthy suburbs. Therefore, the poorest areas will use standposts or water vendors that charge large amounts for water.

The quantity of water required varies directly with the size of the community, its location and climate, and its economic status. For example, the water usage varies twofold or more between a poor community served by standposts and a community with indoor plumbing and several taps in households.

In developed countries, the quality of drinking water is assessed by biologic contaminates (e.g., coliform bacterial counts), chemical analysis, radionucleotides, and turbidity. Guidelines are issued by the WHO and by specific countries. Regulated chemical substances include volatile organics, pesticides, and heavy metals. The quality of water is maintained in developed countries by monitoring runoff water and treated water (from industries and publicly operated treatment works). Each permitted industrial or public facility has specific standards that must be met, and each has a permitted schedule of monitoring. The control of chemical and biological emissions from industrial and community facilities is usually accomplished through point-source regulations. Previous regulations focused on assuring safe levels in water sources (e.g., rivers, lakes), ground water, and point sources, and on permitting better control of emissions by prohibiting contaminants from entering industrial and community facilities or by diverting contaminants away from them. A remaining challenge for industrialized countries is the successful regulation of runoff water (water from non-point sources). Runoff water from industrial agriculture and mining creates significant pollution if it is not held (e.g., in holding ponds) and treated before discharge.

SANITATION

The introduction of flush toilets and sewers in the late 19th century moved contaminated water away from the domicile and into streams. The contamination of the receiving waters became a significant issue as the water supply of downstream communities became contaminated. This situation forced the introduction of open, and then closed, sewers, as well as the effective treatment of drinking water. As a further barrier to infection, wastewater treatment was also instituted in developed countries.

Sanitation is highly variable in developing countries. Often water is supplied without a sanitation system, which may exacerbate the spread of disease. In addition, sewers in more affluent areas may be discharged into the open drainage systems of less affluent areas. Where wastewater is untreated, it may be used for watering and fertilizing crops. Wastewater treatment is often ineffective, or only includes primary (sedimentation), and not secondary (biologic) treatment. Treatment facilities are often poorly maintained.

The major global environmental challenge for water quality remains the adequate provision of water supply and sanitation—particularly sanitation. A promising technology may be simulated wetlands in developing areas. However, the key to establishing sanitation in developing areas is to develop facilities as the community grows; another component is the ability of the community (often receiving outside funding) to plan, design, construct, operate, and manage sanitation facilities. Nevertheless, point-source controls must also continue, and better runoff control should be attained in industrialized countries.

Global Solid and Hazardous Waste

Solid waste is the nonhazardous waste produced by homes, industries, institutions, markets, and commercial establishments. Both developed and developing countries have significant challenges. Countries with greater gross national product (GNP) produce more waste per capita, and the waste contains less vegetable matter and more packaging, making recycling necessary. The waste in lower-income countries contains little packaging and is not recyclable. It requires fuel for burning due to moisture content. In less developed countries there is greater recycling at the source (e.g., homes).

Hazardous waste is defined by each country's regulation, and this waste is controlled by a series of laws designed to prevent more toxic substances from being produced, to improve management of toxics, and to remove buried hazardous wastes.

In developed countries, hazardous and sanitary waste are handled and regulated separately. However, in developing countries, a separate hazardous waste management system is not commonly established, or is poorly maintained. In developing countries, biologic wastes (e.g., medical waste) are commonly mixed with sanitary waste. Human fecal material is disposed in landfills or in open dumps.

WASTE DISPOSAL SYSTEMS

In developed countries' sanitary landfills, the processes of materials recovery and incineration dominate. In sanitary landfills, waste is placed on soils that protect groundwater and is lined with plastic membranes equipped with drainage systems (the water is then treated). An intermediate approach is a controlled landfill that has daily soil cover and perimeter drainage. Developing countries burn solid waste, use home or neighborhood landfills, or transport waste to local landfills. Waste management costs in developing countries are approximately one-tenth the cost of high-income generating countries, but it consumes much more of the personal income.

SPECIAL PROGRAMS FOR CHEMICAL/HAZARDOUS WASTES

Developing countries have limited management programs for chemical waste (and often have limited generation of hazardous waste). However, the country of generation is often not the country of disposal, and transportation of hazardous waste from developed to developing countries for disposal is a global health risk.

There are three primary systems of toxic waste management in developed countries. First, chemicals are required to be evaluated for toxicity by regulations, such as the U.S. Toxic Substances Control Act. These regulations require evaluation of the risks of a chemical before its sale and distribution; it also requires reporting of significant adverse effects when these results come to the attention of the manufacturer. Second, regulation-listed chemicals must be tracked from the manufacturing process through the storage, transportation, and disposal or recycling processes. Third, in some countries such as Germany and the U.S., there are active programs to clean up hazardous waste buried in past years (e.g., the Superfund). In addition, releases of hazardous chemicals into the air, water, and soil must be immediately reported. For environmental releases in developed countries, significant fines may be levied and criminal charges filed. Internationally, some countries do not have comprehensive laws for hazardous waste management, and if there are laws, they may not be enforced.

Developing countries face unique challenges such as preventing the transportation of hazardous or sanitary waste from more affluent to less affluent countries. A difficult problem is the safe disposal of persistent, bio-accumulative, toxic (organic and inorganic) compounds and radioactive substances (with prior informed consent). Knowledge of the chemical and physical nature of the substance, and appropriate transportation treatment and disposal are not always available.

GLOBAL ENVIRONMENTAL ISSUES

There are several global environmental issues that warrant special attention and require global environmental management. Air pollution is a global problem. The migration between countries and continents of acid rains, particulate matter (stationary- and mobile-source emissions, desert dust, forest burning), and ozone is a global issue. Greenhouse gas and climate change is a global environmental issue with major public health and political impact for all countries. Stratospheric ozone depletion can only be managed globally. In the area of water pollution, ocean pollution, biodiversity, and transportation of pollutants, particularly runoff waters, are global challenges. The disposal of hazardous pollutants is a global problem unless rigorous regulations are enforced nationally and internationally. Despite these issues, international environmental law has slowly developed and faces significant challenges, particularly enforcement of agreements such as the Kyoto and Montreal protocols.

52

Clinical Environmental Medicine

Alan M. Ducatman

The distinction between occupational and environmental exposure is artificial. It follows social rather than medical constructs. If there is a difference, it is that workers generally have higher exposures and greater anticipation that they will be exposed. Physiologically, exposures are exposures whether inside or outside of workplaces.

Occupational and environmental physicians possess a unique mix of skills, including clinical care, epidemiology, and toxicology, that are essential for patients with environmental needs. This chapter identifies an approach to environmental stressors from "beyond factory walls" and suggests clinical and public health guidelines for occupational and environmental physicians. The example of childhood lead poisoning is discussed, as are other pertinent topics.

The following definitions describe environmental medicine, its clinical application, and its role as a public health discipline. *Environmental medicine* is "the study of effects upon human beings of external physical, chemical, and biologic factors in the general environment" (1). *Clinical environmental medicine* is "the study of detectable human disease or adverse health outcomes from exposure to these environmental factors" (1). The *discipline* of environmental medicine "combines clinical epidemiologic, and toxicologic approaches. It uniquely seeks to understand external causation and then to adopt policy, engineering, or human factor interventions to prevent or mitigate the caused outcomes" (1).

Environmental medicine shares the public health paradox with its twin, occupational medicine. In either case, prevention of disease by reducing exposure is much more effective than treatment. And, in either case, the more effective the public health intervention, the smaller the clinical profile. Just as the effective intervention in obesity relates to caloric balance, the effective treatment for toxicity is to stop exposure. Physicians who are trained in occupational and environmental medicine interact with engineering, government, and policy organizations to diminish exposure. Physicians without this training are more likely to address exposure by writing a prescription, although pharmaceutical interventions are not usually effective. This generality holds even for those few environmental diseases for which we have well-established treatment regimens, such as lead poisoning.

The definitions state that the disease must be detectable. The increasingly marginal discussion about clinical ecology/multiple chemical sensitivity, along with unsubstantiated diagnosis and treatment of chronic Lyme disease and some other symptom-based syndromes, prompts reiteration of several clinical principles in the context of environmental health. Clinical or laboratory findings are considered compelling when they are repeatedly demonstrated, objectively present, and consistently related to outcomes. Physicians who treat symptom-based syndromes attributed to environmental causes must recognize that neither environmental nor any other type of medicine is based on the application of untested diagnostic and therapeutic regimens. Those who support new tests and procedures are obligated to prove their effectiveness in appropriate scientific testing (1–3). On the other hand, physicians alarmed by unsupported assertions must recognize that the patient's symptoms and suffering are important, even when the physiologic basis is unclear and the attribution to an environmental cause is unsupported by objective data. Care of patients with symptom-based syndromes that are attributed to the environment is best accomplished with frequent supportive clinician–patient contact, and minimal other intervention.

Table 52.1 lists office encounters common to office-based practice of environmental medicine.

TABLE 52.1. *Examples of office encounters in environmental medicine*[a]

Issue	Population
Lead exposure	Children, home renovators, hobbyists, rifle-range users, painters, workers
Building-related complaint	Schoolchildren and their parents, home renovators, and tenants
Allergy or asthma attributed to buildings	Mold or damp-home environments
Puzzling symptoms attributed to chemicals	Multiple Chemical Sensitivity
Environmental cancer concerns	Residents near power lines, older (asbestos-containing) buildings, waste or incineration sites, areas with radon problems; residents with contaminated water; dwellers in proximity to pesticides or superfund sites; proximity to golf courses; and many others
Reproductive concerns	See also Lead, hobbies, environmental cancer, endocrine disruptors
Pulmonary disease (asthma, colds, bronchitis)	Residents near power plants or industries, damp homes, animal and plant allergies
Restrictions on exercise	Air pollution days
Dietary concerns and advice	Fish (metals, natural toxins), meat, hormones in meat, endocrine disruptors, irradiated food, genetically modified crops, dietary supplements
Personal hygiene concerns	Tooth capping, fillings (replace mercury or not), deodorant (safety), use of cookware and food storage, type of water source
Reinterpret lab test results	Patients or populations referred with inappropriate or misinterpreted lab tests

[a]As in the rest of medicine, causation is a decision, not a certain implication of any encounter.

TABLE 52.2. *Examples of community-based public health activities of environmental physicians*[a]

Decisions	Activities
Siting an energy source (i.e., electric power generator, hospital incinerator, assisting neighbors of existing industrial stack)	Predicted pulmonary decrements for modeled ground-level emissions for fossil-fuel sources
Siting and mode of waste disposal for a former chemical drum cleanup facility, with heavily contaminated soil, upwind of one community and above the ground water of another	Consideration of neoplastic and reproductive hazards of ingestion, other potential outcomes for environmental emissions, focus on special populations of concern (school with a large education population) Description of epidemiologic nonatmospheric issues surrounding exposures, ranging from ingested doses, to noise and vehicular injury (coal trains/trucks) to electromagnetic fields
Advising industry concerning disease outbreaks	Evaluation and follow-up surveillance
Planning state programs for childhood lead exposure, chronic disease cluster	Planning, protocol development, telephone and television consultation to clinicians and municipalities
Assisting creation of state-wide dietary alerts for fish consumption based on mercury data	Planning, document development, patient help line
Planning regional response to toxic or biologic disasters	Selecting best uses of scarce resources for population and environmental surveillance, working in interdisciplinary groups to create exposure response, training programs and resources, distance continuing education courses for responder groups, simulations, working in interdisciplinary teams to safely reopen facilities

[a]Examples taken from actual environmental questions facing communities.

Table 52.2 lists community-based public health activities. Physicians from other areas of medicine have been slow to appreciate the importance of providing public health counseling to communities, local governments, and industries on such issues as air, water, and food quality. Patients and affected local government officials may be dissatisfied with "risk assessment" as provided by current mathematical models, and will seek decision-making alternatives to numerical constructs, especially when threats are perceived as immediate. Table 52.3 lists possible future roles for physicians with clinical, epidemiologic, and toxicologic skills. Occupational and environmental physicians-in-training will likely spend significant time performing the types of activities listed in the table, perhaps as much as occupational physicians have devoted to workplace surveillance in the past.

An example is the substantial need that government agencies, labor groups, and especially employers have for both rapid and long-term access to clinicians who understand surveillance, following September 11, 2001. Occupational and environmental clinicians, along with related disciplines (e.g., industrial hygienists and epidemiologists) figured prominently in the follow-up of disaster-response workforces and nearby populations in the aftermath of the terrorist attacks. This includes, but is not limited to, airway symptoms and signs, as well as responses to workforce and community stress reactions (4). The future economic implications of this need have not yet been calculated, nor have the many opportunities for service been completely integrated into medical practice. Some clinicians with environmental health public health expertise will fill this niche. It would now be an unusual planning effort that did not feature a link to occupational and environmental health.

EXAMPLE OF OFFICE-BASED PRACTICE OF ENVIRONMENTAL MEDICINE: LEAD POISONING

Heavy metal exposure is a common clinical and environmental issue. Childhood lead poisoning can serve to illustrate the multifaceted nature of office practice when the disease is caused by the environment. Childhood lead poisoning differs from lead poisoning in adults in that it is more common, much less likely to occur because of work (although parents' work or nearby workplaces may play a role), and of greater medical and social importance. It remains the best example among clinical environmental health outcomes to feature repeatable abnormal lab values and, sometimes, the need for pharmacologic intervention. But since the first edition of this volume appeared, evidence for proven efficacy of clinical chelation therapy now points to a narrower set of appropriate circumstances. Even for lead poisoning, the most clinical of common examples, the key to successful treatment is to minimize future exposure.

In urban areas, childhood lead poisoning referrals go to pediatric clinics accustomed to handling this specific need. In rural areas, a variety of clinical settings may fill this niche. Public health departments or nurse-run clinics refer patients, families, or groups of affected patients. Families self-refer when they face concerns about the future of affected children or the available means of preventing ongoing exposures. Their tenacity in identifying a physician who recognizes the environmental aspects of lead exposure is

TABLE 52.3. *Growing roles for occupational/environmental physicians*

Product/work	Clients
Product labeling, Material Safety Data Sheet reviews	Corporations, labeling contractors
New product liability reviews	Corporate planners and attorneys, citizen groups, regulatory agencies
Disaster planning/response	Corporations, labor organizations, government agencies
Continuing education for disaster response	Physicians and other professionals
Health policy decisions concerning facility sitings and rights-of-way	Governments (all levels), citizen groups, public utilities
Health policy decisions concerning hazard abatement	Governments, public health agencies, citizen groups

often impressive. The physician's ability to arrange for appropriate public health interventions depends on available programs and resources. Some states have relatively sophisticated and legally mandated programs for family education, lead detection, and lead exposure abatement. Other states have developed or may be developing childhood lead surveillance programs for children, but they may lack the infrastructure for reliably testing dwellings for the presence of lead at reasonable cost to the homeowner, or, when the presence of lead is confirmed, a consistent mechanism for accessing affordable lead abatement, or some other means to ensure children do not move back into the lead poisoning environment. In international settings, where lead dust exposure may be very substantial following the use of leaded gasoline or ceramics, resources and policy options may be limited in the face of substantial needs. As with differences among states, some clinicians put much more energy into mustering the large network of available resources for protecting poisoned patients. Treatment of lead poisoning works only when an interdisciplinary public health model is used.

Office referrals are generally made when a child's lead levels exceed 10 μg/100 mL of whole blood. This referral level from the Centers for Disease Control (CDC) recommendations is based on a strong and steadily growing body of evidence that low-level lead intoxication causes significant intellectual deficit in the developing fetus and young child. Children who are exposed are less likely to obtain an education and more likely to commit crimes than children with similar social indicators (5–8). Abnormal neuropsychological measures of lead poisoned children persist in adulthood (9), but these are not the only clinical outcomes. Renal damage, hearing loss, and hypertension are also potential consequences of lead exposure. A significant concern is reproductive toxicity, affecting a second generation of indirectly lead-poisoned children. Lead is mobilized from bone during pregnancy (10), or during lactation (11), and easily passes into the fetal circulation.

The key to treating lead poisoning is good public health, not medication. Nevertheless, the initial determinations to make concerning lead-poisoned children are (a) the present level of lead in the blood and (b) the need for chelation therapy. Because childhood lead poisoning clearly affects lifelong functioning, we need a pharmacologic intervention that works. Unfortunately, it is not clear that chelation treatment substantially reverses losses in functioning (12). Currently, chelation treatment is no longer recommended for blood lead levels below 45 μg/dL, unless the child is clearly symptomatic.

Dietary interventions, including mineral supplementation, can prove modestly helpful. Iron deficiency is both a cause (because it increases lead absorption) and an outcome (because lead disrupts the formation of hemoglobin) of lead poisoning. Therefore, an early step in treatment, supported by evidence, is determination of iron stores and iron supplementation if low or even borderline. Several cautions are needed concerning iron supplementation. It is inappropriate to give iron during chelation therapy (the chelation agent cannot distinguish between iron and lead). Parents will not tolerate black-tarry stools indefinitely, and at high doses iron becomes a toxin. Therefore, iron should be used only until blood stores are normal. There is less evidence for other potentially helpful dietary interventions. Calcium inhibits lead absorption, and calcium deficiency increases lead absorption. It is possible that a high-calcium diet will have a protective benefit. There is also some physiologic evidence for a protective role for vitamin C. A balanced diet is always appropriate, with some untested potential for benefit and low risk of harm if calcium and vitamin C are added.

The primary goal is to prevent exposures. Prevention requires understanding of the environmental source. In the overwhelming majority of childhood lead poisoning cases in the United States, the source of exposure is lead paint. (Countries that still permit lead in gasoline have an alternative and ubiquitous source in their environment.) Paint protects surfaces in part by slowly "dusting off." Lead paint in poor condition (peeling, chipping) is common, but not required to cause toxic effects. Normal aging of paint, home renovations, and other sources of dust provide toddlers with invisible but adequate hand-to-mouth sources of lead poisoning. Children who mouth and swallow non-food items (pica) are at greater risk, although pica is not required for lead poisoning. The most commonly implicated exposure areas of homes include windows (high lead levels, weathering, lots of friction), painted doorways (friction), porches (high lead levels, weathering), and even old radiators. Although older houses have higher lead levels, even homes built after the U.S. lead paint prohibition of the 1970s may have older paint applied within them. In fact, modern studies of "non-lead" paint may turn up surprising lead levels in some samples, particularly for outdoor and metal paints.

Outdoor soil is a secondary source of lead exposure. As a practical matter, young children have the most soil exposure near the home, often in the yard and as a result of peeled outdoor paint. Thus, paint from the home is the most important cause of accessible soil contamination. Playing near renovation jobs and child care in other people's lead-contaminated homes represent similar risks for lead paint and soil exposure outside of the child's own home. In other countries where leaded gasoline has been used, urban soil and soil near highways may contain enough lead so that simply playing on the soil represents a risk.

Water is a third source of lead exposure. Municipal supplies, municipal plumbing, or personal wells are occasionally implicated; most lead in drinking water comes from solder contained in the last few feet of plumbing. Lead in water has a large impact on population mean values, yet is an uncommon source of outright lead poisoning in most developed countries. [In cities where the Environmental Protection Agency (EPA) has discovered undesirable levels of lead in tap water, lead-poisoned children are still overwhelmingly characterized by their exposure to lead paint.] Another contributor to waterborne lead ingestion is boiling of babies' formula water, which may concentrate existing lead in water and lead from defective cookware. Still less common childhood ingestion sources include folk medicines and lead-based cosmetics, used by some ethnic groups, and lead candlewicks. The most startling source in my experience was intoxication from an inappropriate lead-contaminated dye in pool-cue chalk, a product made to be powdered indoors. Other environmental clinicians can provide equally strange tales of unanticipated lead sources. This is particularly true in other countries where lead solder may still be used in canning or lead glazes in pottery. Pottery from Mexico has historically contained lead glaze.

Lead smelting operations are another important source. Living near a dangerous industry is common in newly industrialized countries. Inhalation exposures more typically characterize workplace exposures, and may involve secondary ingestion. Workplace exposures also include paint. For example, bridge repair, junkyard workers, home renovators, and other construction workers face the same environmental risks from lead paint.

Why is determining the source important? The environmental clinician must recognize sources of exposure in order to provide families with a second, critical piece of information. Which of many possible steps should families take to prevent further childhood exposures? The "easy fixes" include removal of contaminated soil, growing ground covers such as grass, cessation of the practice of boiling water for baby's bottle (which may concentrate lead from water or utensil sources), and reconfiguring the last few feet of plumbing with nonleaded solder. Unfortunately, these easy measures are usually irrelevant to the underlying source of childhood lead poisoning in the U.S.—house paint. Furthermore, the offending paint source is rarely just in one area. Getting rid of the paint can be difficult and expensive, which leaves parents with unsatisfactory choices. They can more closely supervise their child at home, and the home can be regularly cleaned. But historically, these temporizing activities have had little impact on the blood lead levels. A more proactive approach is to move from the offending environment. This advice works, and is most attractive to renters, provided that alternative housing is available. The only medical requirement of "geographic removal protection" is that the new home not be another source of lead exposure.

A compromise between these positions is lead abatement in the existing home. This option is most attractive to homeowners, who feel the home is an economic anchor; but they also want to protect their children from unsafe conditions. Growing grass and removing outdoor topsoil address outdoor sources but rarely address the problem. Simply cleaning up indoor lead dust is not adequate abatement (13). It is also necessary to physically remove (or, in some cases, cover) the old paint that provides the common source of the lead. As a public health measure, parents can be advised that abatement works best if it is done by certified contractors with expert reputations and if it is done before the family moves in. However, abatement of already-existing lead that has already caused lead poisoning does not adequately protect these children (13), although it is not clear why. Furthermore, abatements performed while the family still lives in the house are a source of substantial additional risk. It is necessary to move out during the abatement.

Several interventions are recommended for children who have lead levels of 20 μg/100 mL or above. Neurologic and neuropsychological evaluations are appropriate at the time lead intoxication is discovered, after environmental removal, and at periodic intervals thereafter to assess the educational deficits associated with childhood lead toxicity. Deficits may become apparent by age 4 to 5 and be well characterized by age 7 to 8. Neuropsychological examinations are advantageously combined with frequent school evaluations, beginning in the preschool years. Recognition of the need for special educational services can save families frustration. Educational performance of children whose disabilities would otherwise predict rapid failure in school systems can be supported by early and specialized interventions. Obtaining these services often requires firm insistence; the environmental physician can facilitate the process by explaining the nature of the population data to the families, educators, and school system administrators.

Table 52.4 lists some of the issues in chelation therapy. Dosing instructions are not given; a physician knowledgeable about chelation should be consulted. Succimer (dimercaptosuccinic acid, a dimercaprol analogue) is gradually supplanting ethylenediaminetetraacetic acid (EDTA) as the chelating agent of choice. EDTA is a slightly but significantly better chelator in controlled clinical trials, but succimer is increasingly used because of lower toxicity and ease of oral administration. Succimer may also mobilize mercury and arsenic, but it appears to mobilize essential trace metals far less than EDTA. The choice between these agents is influenced by the home environment. If parental supervision is reliable, succimer therapy has several advantages. It is an oral medication, does not require a hospital setting, and therefore reduces expense. Blood lead levels do not need to be checked during treatment; they should be checked several weeks after treatment.

For any chelation, clinicians must address the appropriateness of prescribing medication when the real issue is continued exposure. We want to prevent lead poisoning more than we want to treat it, and we want to detect it as early as possible where it exists. For this reason, the CDC has long funded state and local health departments to conduct childhood lead poisoning surveillance (14). An interesting observation is how much the environmental health model of product substitution, removal control, engineering protection, medical surveillance, and sometimes treatment resembles the occupational model. The similarity is not coincidental; there is no physiologic reason to make distinctions.

Children are usually surveyed with capillary sticks or venous blood samples at age 9 months to 1 year (or so) for their first blood lead level. Capillary sticks are popular because of the difficulty of obtaining venous samples from young children. The time of the first sample is based on when lead poisoning usually begins in that population, and corresponds to infant mobility. When infants start crawling, exposure to dust increases, and when they can pull themselves up to a standing position, exposure to the sills and other parts of windows increases. Hence, the first test is around age 1 year. It is very important to thoroughly clean the skin before blood is obtained, as surface dust on digits or palms can give artificially high results, especially for a capillary sample. For this reason, elevated lab values from capillary samples are often repeated with venous samples for confirmation. Whether this repeat testing is necessary is questionable, as capillary samples have proved reliable under quality assurance conditions (15).

Interpretation of lab values requires knowledge of population data and CDC recommendations. The recommended action level for considering the child's environment is 10 μg/dL; this is not a "safe" or desirable level (14). Lead has no physiologic function, and less is better. The present population geometric mean is less than 3 μg/dL, and has decreased in the last three decades as a result of public health, public policy, and surveillance efforts. Unfortunately, this improving population mean still leaves behind many thousands of lead-poisoned children including new cases every year. Predictors of lead poisoning are older dwellings, the presence of children, and poverty (a likely covariable with older housing and poor home maintenance).

Ideally, most children, or at least most children who live in older homes, would receive a second test at around age 2, as initially recommended by the CDC. In practice, this level of surveillance follow-up occurs most often for children who have actually been lead poisoned and those who live in very high-risk housing areas. One of the barriers associated with CDC recommendations is that providers who are not supported by specific grants and contracts receive inadequate reimbursement for lead testing services. Another barrier is parents' natural responsiveness to their children's normal aversion to taking blood tests; new technology may someday address this barrier.

An interesting philosophical problem of medical surveillance is that it uses humans as biologic monitors of their own personal exposure, and this problem is more poignant in children. Primary prevention, first actively identifying housing that might in the future poison children and then actively abating such dwellings, would be a logical approach to our knowledge that lead exposure robs children of intellectual capability. In practice, our society has chosen to wait for the clear demonstration of exposure before seeking engineering or renewal protection. Mortgage and rental laws requiring disclosure have softened this harsh picture, but they are unevenly applied, not effectively proactive, require knowledgeable consumers, and are not fully effective as a preventive measure. As with so much else in environmental

TABLE 52.4. *Chelation agents and information*

Product	Generic name	Chemical name	Abbreviation
Calcium disodium versenate	Edetate disodium calcium	Calcium disodium ethylenediamine tetraacetate	$CaNa_2$ EDTA
BAL in oil	Dimercaprol	2,3-dimercapto-1-propanol	BAL
Chemet	Succimer	Meso 2,3-dimercaptosuccinic acid	DMSA

Proactive chelation testing is not usually indicated.

Drug	Available form	Special administration instructions	Monitoring parameters	Adverse effects
$CaNa_2$ EDTA	00 mg/mL (5 mL vials)	*do not use sodium If administering by IM injection, give in site separate from the BAL administration site. 1 mL of 1% procaine hydrochloride may be added to each mL of calcium disodium EDTA (final concentration 0.5% procaine) to minimize pain at the injection site Administer only after adequate urine flow is established	Daily urinalysis and urine output, SCr every 48 hrs, LFTs	Hypotension, arrhythmia, fever, hypercalcemia, numbness, tingling, headache, chills, GI upset, lacrimation, nasal congestion, diarrhea, transient marrow suppression, sneezing Zinc and iron depletion may occur; replace only after therapy is completed
BAL	100 mg/mL (3 mL vials) in peanut oil	Contraindicated in: patients allergic to peanuts, patients receiving iron therapy, and patients with G6PD deficiency Administer deep IM only	LFTs	Fever, increased LFT's N/V, headache, conjunctivitis, lacrimation, sneezing, nasal congestion
DMSA	100 mg	Can mix capsule contents with small amount of food immediately prior to administration	LFTs, CBC with differential, and platelet count weekly	Increased LFTs, rash, pruritus, N/V/D, drowsiness, paresthesia, sore throat, rhinorrhea, sulfur odor on breath

Adapted from the West Virginia Poison Center.

health, public policy represents a compromise based on perceptions of available resources.

OTHER ISSUES OF CLINICAL IMPORTANCE

We have used childhood lead poisoning as a model of office-based environmental practice because it is relatively common and has a rich literature with good population data; it features both environmental intervention and specific pharmacologic therapies (although they are less helpful than environmental/public health manipulations). Similar health problems occur in other countries (see Chapter 51), such as arsenic intoxication in parts of China and Bangladesh and air pollution in many countries. Other common home health issues are associated with water damage and mold in dwellings, which have much the same public health dynamic as lead poisoning. Provided that the home can be dried, the key to treatment is removal of the moldy materials. If wet or damp, the areas cannot be eliminated. The families' alternatives to suffering are symptomatic treatments, major reengineering projects, or moving. Clinical advice to patients taking defensive actions against mold or other established or perceived environmental hazards, ranging from bioterrorism to low-quality water supplies, requires an understanding of the level of threat, the utility of proposed actions, and the patients' mind set. A related activity is advising patients about inappropriate, non–evidence-based environmental treatments, such as chelation for heavy metals in the absence of poisoning, or chelation for the prevention of heart disease. A future edition of this volume could contain a compendium chapter on the pitfalls of confusing or ill-advised laboratory analyses and of non–evidence-based treatments of real or perceived environmental threats.

Our most challenging patients describe disabling symptoms, which sound as though they come from multiple organ systems. These severe disabilities persist in the absence of impairing physical findings, or significant, persistent laboratory abnormality, and in the setting of strong beliefs that the symptoms are due to exposures. Because of these strong beliefs that the symptoms are due to either specific classes of exposure or exposures in general, even in the face of nonverifiable physical or laboratory data, the clinical care of these patients warrants some attention.

It is helpful to identify the patient's stated and actual goals in an effort to understand if the clinician can help. Many, perhaps most, patients with these beliefs seek primarily contact, reassurance, and empathy. While they may seek to convert the clinician to their pattern of beliefs, they need and will accept frequent scheduled contact with their primary doctor, and, eventually, gentle challenges to be as well and functional as they can be. Interventions should be subtly "environmental" in that they are based on the patient's mastering the perceived stressors. The challenges to be well should be launched only after rapport has been firmly established, and they should come gradually and deliberately. Goals may include gradual, modest increases in exercise, or alternative things to do when challenged by an odor (carry a pleasant odor for needed reference). These simple interventions work in some, but not all, patients. Empirical focus on how not to create new problems is essential. The clinician should never advise avoidance of the perceived stressor, as this advice can result in the patient's increasingly severe social isolation. The patient should be advised to avoid falling into the hands of unscrupulous marketers of expensive, non–evidence-based, or potentially harmful remedies. If possible, the clinician should not prescribe medications or herbal supplements and should not refer the patient to specialists, as these steps might lead to the patient's displaying additional symptoms or relying on harmful remedies.

Patients with many environmental symptoms and no physiologic findings will seek affirmation rather than support. The perceived need may be for nonstandard treatment, insurance support for interventions not based on evidence, or endorsement for etiologic hypotheses that are, at best, "nondisprovable." The clinician's role with these patients is a matter partly of art and partly of ethics. It is important that clinicians try to support patients emotionally, while emphasizing the need for medical evidence. Often, the issues involve generalized symptoms triggered by odors. In this setting, it is useful to know what respiratory exposures are known to do. In contrast, most patients with discernible physical findings such as asthma following exposures are not alerted by odors, and offer less certain explanations for their health problems. Good environmental history taking is essential in both circumstances, yet we must recognize we are more likely to make a clinical difference when there are clear physical findings.

Table 52.5 addresses some of the clinical issues related to air pollution, such as exercising on air pollution alert days, the seriousness of mold overgrowth following flooding, clinical approaches to diagnoses and treatment of potentially related symptoms, and diagnosis of chronic sequelae of single or multiple episodes of carbon monoxide intoxication, including impairment and work placement issues. Each of the issues in Table 52.1 or 52.5 could be its own chapter in a text on respiratory aspects of environmental health.

Occupational and environmental physicians are also involved in clinical evaluation of exposure to marine toxins, evaluation of performance and safety in harsh physical environments, and travel medicine in a rapidly changing landscape of infectious diseases, which is in turn influenced by issues such as climate change. In each case, skills in clinical diagnosis, toxicology (or in some cases physiology of physical environmental hazards), and epidemiology are relevant. The medical surveillance disease outbreak literature can be clinically useful. In most cases, the intervention requires further knowledge of the public health aspects of the problem. Who else might be exposed? Who else is sick? What resources/agencies/individuals need to be involved? How are we going to prevent further exposure? Too often, we prescribe medication; this happens when we have failed in our prevention role.

TABLE 52.5. *Examples of clinical office questions regarding air pollution*

Question	Key data	Pitfalls
Exercise during air pollution alerts	Nature of pollution, time of day, existing or new clinical diagnoses: asthma, heart disease	Patient motivation; uncertain quality of indoor air
Indoor mold growth	Existing or new clinical diagnoses: allergy, asthma, allergic alveolitis	Distinguishing harmful environments from clinical problems
Chronic sequelae of CO intoxication, and secondary job issues	Exposure data, lab values, clinical presentation and course, preexisting disease, neuroimaging	Some data usually missing Existing clinical diagnoses
Alternative fuel use by patient, family, neighbors	Existing or new clinical diagnoses: patient perspective	Exposure data difficult and expensive to obtain
Infectious respiratory disease (often Legionnaires): attributed illness to a specific environmental source	Local epidemiologic findings	Attributions of population outcomes without documentation
Industrial sources: stacks, waste and mulch, sewage	Exposure data, existing or new clinical conditions, local epidemiology	Absent and difficult to obtain exposure data, difficult to verify attributions of population illness
Spills and catastrophic releases	Exposure data, existing or new clinical conditions, local epidemiology	Absent or difficult to obtain exposure data
Environmental tobacco smoke	Policies	

REFERENCES

1. Ducatman AM, et al. What is environmental medicine? *J Occup Med* 1990;32:1130–1132.
2. American College of Occupational and Environmental Medicine. Multiple Chemical Sensitivities: idiopathic environmental intolerance, June 8, 1999. On-line: *www.acoem.orgpositionposition.asp*.
3. Ducatman AM. Multiple chemical sensitivity. In: Rom WR, ed. *Environmental and occupational medicine,* 3rd ed. Philadelphia: Lippincott-Raven, 1998:891–904.
4. American College of Occupational and Environmental Medicine. ACOEM resources/response guidelines for occupational physicians who may deal with psychological trauma in the workplace as a result of the September 11 terrorist attacks. On-line: *www.acoem.orgdpguide.asp*.
5. Needleman HL, Gatsonis CA. Low-level lead exposure and the IQ of children. *JAMA* 1990;263:673–678.
6. Tong S, Baghurst PA, Sawyer MG, et al. Declining blood lead levels and changes in cognitive function during childhood. *JAMA* 1998;280:1915–1919.
7. Wasserman GA, Staghezza-Jaramillo B, Shrout P, et al. The effect of lead exposure on behavior problems in preschool children. *Am J Public Health* 1998;88: 481–486.
8. Needleman HA, Riess JA, Tobin M, et al. Bone lead levels and delinquent behavior. *JAMA* 1996;275: 363–369.
9. Stokes L, Letz R, Gerr F, et al. Neurotoxicity in young adults 20 years after childhood exposure to lead: the Bunker Hill experience. *Occup Environ Med* 1998;55: 507–516.
10. U.S. Department of Health and Human Services/Public Health Service/Agency for Toxic Substances and Disease Registry. Toxicological Profile for Lead (update). July, 1999.
11. Tellez-Rojo MM, Hernandez-Avila M, Gonzalez-Cossio T, et al. Impact of breastfeeding on the mobilization of lead from bone. *Am J Epidemiol* 2002;155:420–428.
12. Rogan WJ, Dietrich KN, Ware JH, et al. The effect of chelation therapy with succimer on neuropsychologic development in children exposed to lead. *N Engl J Med* 2001;344:1421–1426.
13. Aschengrau A, Beiser A, Bellinger D, et al. Residential lead-based paint hazard remediation and soil lead abatement: their impact among children with mildly elevated blood lead levels. *Am J Public Health* 1997;87:1698–1702.
14. Centers for Disease Control. *About lead.* On-line: *www.cdc.govncehaboutabout.htm*.
15. Schlenker TL, Johnson Fritz C, Mark D, et al. Screening for pediatric lead poisoning: comparability of simultaneously drawn capillary and venous blood samples. *JAMA* 1994;271:1346–1348.

53

Indoor Environmental Quality

Robert K. McLellan

Problems with indoor environmental quality (IEQ) did not begin with modern, energy-efficient office buildings. Open fire in primitive dwellings exposed our ancestors to a wide range of hazardous combustion products. People living in remote areas with the cleanest outdoor air imaginable still cook and heat indoors with poorly vented fires. These traditional practices potentially render the air in their drafty shelters more contaminated than the tightest of contemporary, sealed office towers. Though high-level exposures to toxicants such as combustion products occur in indoor settings, low-level exposures present the biggest and most common challenge to the occupational and environmental health practitioner. Despite overlap, the indoor environmental quality problems, regulation, and solutions for large, commercial and small, low-rise residential buildings differ.

HISTORICAL PERSPECTIVE

From the beginning of human history, buildings have sheltered people from the dangers and discomforts of the outdoors. With the burgeoning urban slums of the industrial age, the health hazards of inadequate housing became apparent. In 1892, Osler's (1) *Principles and Practice of Medicine* noted the association of tuberculosis with overcrowded living conditions. Globally, inadequate housing remains a major determinant of public health (2,3).

Complacency about the safety of modern, indoor settings in the Western world was shaken by a number of events beginning in the late 1970s. Newspaper headlines announced mysterious epidemics of health complaints in office buildings. Early investigators named the complaints "tight building syndrome" because of their association with energy-conserving building construction and ventilation measures. Industrial hygienists often found low ventilation rates and contaminants considerably less than permissible exposure limits (PELs). In the absence of toxic exposure levels approaching PELs, some investigators ascribed office worker complaints to mass hysteria.

A series of widely publicized building-related incidents in the 1970s and 1980s demonstrated the potential seriousness of indoor environmental exposures. In 1976, members of the American Legion convening in a Philadelphia hotel were struck by a pneumonia epidemic resulting in 182 cases and 29 deaths (4). Epidemiologic investigation linked the deaths to the contamination of a ventilation system with *Legionella pneumophila*. A fire in an office building in Binghamton, New York, resulted in widespread contamination of the interior with polychlorinated biphenyls released from electrical equipment. Acting on recognition of endemic lead poisoning, the United States Environmental Protection Agency (EPA) banned lead in interior paint in 1978. Concern about the hazards of the indoor environment was further piqued when an investigation of a radioactively contaminated nuclear power worker identified his home as an intense source of radon. After initial radon surveys revealed widespread residential contamination, the surgeon general's office and the EPA released a joint statement in September 1988 recommending nearly universal radon testing of the residential environment (5).

As research progressed through the late 1980s, the federal government recognized indoor air pollution (IAP) as a significant and expensive health concern. Investigators found the following (6):

- Poor indoor air quality (IAQ) was not simply a matter of comfort, but was associated with illness and death.
- Many toxicants were present at higher levels indoors than outdoors.

- Changes in lifestyle over the last century had led U.S. citizens to spend 90% of their lives indoors.
- The most vulnerable segments of our population, the infirm, the very young, and the very old, were the most exposed.

These revelations led the EPA to place IAP among the top environmental priorities.

Events during the 1990s have confirmed the potential seriousness and ubiquity of IAP and broadened concern to other aspects of the indoor environment that affect occupant comfort and productivity (7). This broader scope of concern reflects the fact that many indoor pollutants can be absorbed through dermal contact and ingestion as well as inhalation. A series of devastating floods in the 1990s prompted the EPA to post indoor cleanup instructions on its Web site to minimize otherwise inevitable widespread problems with bioaerosols (8). Hantavirus infection communicated by residential exposure to rodent feces led to pulmonary disease with high lethality (9). Aware of endemic, residential carbon monoxide poisonings, the Consumer Product Safety Commission advised all homeowners to install carbon monoxide alarms (10). Public health departments and clinicians reported deaths and neurotoxicity associated with residential contamination by metallic mercury (11). Television newsmagazines fanned public alarm about the hazards of *Stachybotrys*-contaminated houses (12). By the end of the 20th century, most national and international public health organizations joined the EPA in declaring environmental tobacco smoke a definite human carcinogen with multiple serious noncarcinogenic toxicities (13). Finally, the Food Quality Protection Act of 1996 spawned a far-reaching federal initiative to improve the protection of children from environmental hazards. Beyond health considerations, research has explored the impact of poor IAQ and other office environmental factors on productivity. Economic analysis supported the value of investment in facility design, construction, operation, and maintenance to achieve good IEQ (14). IEQ depends not only on the absence of hazardous environmental contaminants, but also on factors such as thermal comfort, odors, ergonomic workstations, lighting, noise, and work organization.

Many scientific questions remain regarding the etiology of nonspecific building-associated complaints. As well, uncertainties abound about the health effects of some specific indoor environmental contaminants. Nonetheless, accumulating building science has prompted federal agencies, state and local governments, trade organizations, and private businesses to mount a series of practical initiatives that have the potential to reduce the risks associated with poor IEQ. As a result, in the year 2001, considerable guidance is available to the building professions, building maintenance personnel, and facility managers to optimize IEQ. Unfortunately, newspaper headlines as well as formal surveys document the extent to which existing indoor environmental knowledge and technologies have yet to be widely applied.

THE INDOOR ENVIRONMENT

Five sources contribute to indoor environmental contamination: external surroundings, building structure, furnishings and finishings, mechanical systems, and occupant activities. Table 53.1 identifies sources and types of common indoor contaminants and routes of occupant exposure.

Sources of Indoor Environmental Contamination

External Sources

Without mechanical intervention, occupied buildings are usually under negative pressure with respect to the external environment. Temperature gradients, combustion devices, and wind contribute to this pressure differential, which allows contaminants to infiltrate a building. Not even the most aggressive attempts to seal a building can make it completely airtight.

In contrast to residential settings, mechanical ventilation positively pressurizes most modern, large office buildings. Theoretically, positive pressure prevents passive infiltration; however, uneven pressurization may lead to sporadic passive infiltration through inadvertent cracks in the building envelope or reentrainment through chimneys, open windows, and exhaust stacks. More importantly, ventilation systems purposely draw air into a building. The placement of outdoor intakes determines the cleanliness of the air entering the building. Investigations of problem buildings have often identified these intakes in polluted locations such as parking garages or in proximity to exhaust stacks.

Pollutants may also contaminate the indoor environment when carried on the shoes and clothing of people entering the building. Workers may inadvertently expose their families by bringing home on their clothes industrial toxicants like lead, mercury, or asbestos. People or pets may track outdoor environmental hazards, such as pollens and lead or pesticide contaminated soil, into the home.

TABLE 53.1. *Common sources and types of indoor contaminants*

Types and routes of exposure[a]	External	Building structure	Furnishings and finishings	Mechanical systems	Occupant activities
Asbestos (I/O)	Hazardous waste sites Abrasion of brake linings Building demolition Asbestos cement water pipe	Sprayed on fireproofing Roofing and siding Thermal insulation	Ceiling and floor tiles Textured wall and ceiling finishing	Gaskets Pipe and furnace insulation	Selected consumer products Take-home occupational contamination
Biologicals (I/O)	Pollens Molds Epidermoids Insects and their detritus Animals Flooding Contaminated tap water	Water damaged materials Poor site drainage Inadequate vapor barriers, ventilation, and insulation	Water damaged materials Fleecy materials Allergenic materials	Inadequately maintained and operated heating, ventilation, and air-conditioning systems Contaminated duct work Sewage overflow	Indoor pets Vacuuming and other cleaning practices Failure to use bathroom and kitchen exhaust fans Drying clothes outside when pollen counts highs Using firewood Respiratory droplet Fomite contamination
Combustion products (I)	Fossil fuel and firewood combustion Incinerators Forest fires	Building fires	Building fires	Malfunctioning and poorly vented heating and cooking devices	Environmental tobacco smoke
Lead (O,I)	Hazardous and mining waste Industrial emissions Exterior paint Demolition and paint removal Lead municipal water pipes		Lead paint	Lead plumbing fixtures and solder	Hobbies Folk Remedies Remodeling Consumer products Take-home occupational contamination
Ozone (I)	Ground level ozone			Office machines Ozone generators Malfunctioning electrostatic precipitators	

Pesticides and biocides (O,I,D)	Spray drift Foundation extermination Contaminated soil Hazardous waste Contaminated tapwater	Treated building materials	Carpets Wall coverings Shower curtains Paints	Contaminated ductwork Biocides in humidifiers and air conditioners	Professional extermination Consumer products Residues in food Take home occupational contamination
Radon (I,O)	Soil gas Well water Natural gas	Stone Brick Cement block Breaches in integrity of building envelope contacting soil		Mechanical devices that increase indoor negative pressure Emissions from radon mitigation systems	Areas of house occupied
Respirable particulates (I)	Wind-blown soil Industrial emissions Fossil fuel combustion Forest and brush fires Volcanic eruptions		Fleecy furnishings	Poorly vented and malfunctioning heating and cooking devices Humidifiers Degrading fiberglass ductwork	Environmental tobacco smoke Remodeling Hobbies Cleaning
Volatile organic chemicals (I,O,D)	Leaking underground storage tanks Hazardous waste Industrial emissions Tap water pollution Inadequately aired dry cleaning	Combustion board Adhesives Caulks Additives to fiberglass insulation Plastics	Spackling compound Paints and other surface coatings Cabinetry Carpets Soft plastics	Leaking fuel tanks Combustion products Office machines Furniture Lubricants Duct sealants and cleaners	Use and storage consumer products Personal care products Hobbies Environmental tobacco smoke Human metabolism

[a]Routes of exposure codes: **D,** dermal; **I,** inhalational; **O,** oral; listed for each contaminant in usual order of importance.
Modified from McLellan RK. Identification and control of selected residential hazards. *Dis Mon* 2000;46:590–616.

No single outdoor agent wreaks more havoc with IEQ than water. Rain, rising water tables, and floodwaters commonly breach poorly sited and constructed buildings. Not only can water incursion carry biologic and other contaminants indoors, but also residual moisture amplifies microbial multiplication and can release toxicants through hydrolysis.

Finally, water and natural gas pipelines may bring contaminants indoors. For example, water sources may carry particulates such as asbestos or dissolved gasses such as radon or volatile organic chemicals (VOCs) that come out of solution when taps are turned on.

Building Structure and Interior Furnishings

The building structure and interior furnishings may contribute to indoor air contamination through the emission of volatile components or physical degradation of products. A myriad of building products and finishes, ranging from composition board to new carpets to adhesives to paints, emit VOCs. The abrasion of products such as asbestos-containing floor coverings and pipe lagging can also pollute indoor air.

Floods, high humidity, smoking, and consumer chemical use may contaminate building structure elements and furnishings. With moisture, room temperature and the inevitable shower of organic debris from people and pets, absorbent materials like rugs or fiberglass ventilation duct liners serve as culture media for biologic contaminants such as dust mites and fungi. Physical agitation of these materials by vacuuming or human traffic can result in sprays of biologic aerosols. Absorbent materials may also serve as sinks for VOCs, pesticides, and other chemicals generated in the environment. These sinks will then slowly reemit the contaminants.

Mechanical Systems

Mechanical devices such as heating, ventilation, and air conditioning (HVAC) systems; humidifiers; dehumidifiers; wiring configurations; and lighting constitute the operating infrastructure of a building. When not properly designed, operated, or maintained, HVAC systems may lead to excursions beyond accepted indoor comfort parameters such as temperature, humidity, or air velocity. They may also contribute to the distribution of hazardous contaminants. Humidifiers and cooling towers may contribute to biologic and particulate contamination of indoor air. Lighting characteristics such as flicker, spectral range, and luminance are important environmental influences. Wiring configurations and mechanicals also add vibration and electromagnetic fields.

Occupant-generated Pollution

The habits, hobbies, business, and metabolism of buildings' occupants affect IEQ. Though increasingly restricted in public buildings, environmental tobacco smoke remains an important indoor pollutant. Personal products such as perfumes and deodorants can generate VOCs. Copiers, laser printers, and fax machines may produce pollutants. Carbonless copy paper, eraser fluids, marking pens, and adhesives contribute to the contaminant load. Pesticide residues, from trace to toxic concentrations, burden virtually every indoor space (15). When buildings mix functions, adjoining laboratories or industries may pollute office air when their hazardous processes are improperly contained.

Characterizing the Indoor Environment

Broadly categorized, the key factors in IEQ are biologic agents, combustion products, ozone, particulates, pesticides, radon, VOCs, and physical factors such as temperature, humidity, and air velocity. Though the potency of contaminant sources is a key determinant of indoor pollutant concentrations, other variables are codeterminants, including air exchange, ventilation mixing efficiency, building volume, and contaminant removal.

Biologic Agents

The metabolism and decay of large and microbial organisms produce gaseous pollution. Animals and humans shed hair, dander, epidermal scales, and allergens. Animal handling and changing of cage litter may result in exposures to saliva, urine, and feces. Animals nesting in ventilation systems can lead to wide dissemination of their products. Decaying carcasses of small animals lead to characteristic putrid odors.

Microbial contaminants include viruses, bacteria, protozoa, fungi, pollens, insect parts, and arachnid excrement. Microbes may produce toxins and VOCs that contribute to the degradation of IEQ. Humans transmit a variety of infectious diseases by respiratory droplet, some of which may be disseminated in indoor air.

Indoor microbial concentrations become more hazardous when amplified by favorable temperature, humidity, and nutrition. Hospitable microbial reservoirs include bedding, rugs, humidifiers, cooling towers, and condensate pans. Dissemination may occur through the actions of ventilation systems and machines, or agitation by occupant activities.

Combustion Products

Combustion generates gaseous and particulate products, some of which are prominent outdoor air pollutants: nitrogen oxides, sulfur dioxide, carbon monoxide, and respirable suspended particulates (RSPs). Environmental tobacco smoke (ETS) alone adds to indoor air at least 250 compounds known to be toxic or carcinogenic (16).

Indoor exposures to combustion products vary seasonally, with outdoor pollution, with the operation of combustion devices and with the presence of smokers. In addition to fires, malfunctioning or unvented combustion devices in poorly ventilated areas can create short-term, hazardous excursions above the Occupational Safety and Health Administration (OSHA) PEL for carbon monoxide (17). In large buildings, vehicle exhaust entrained by ventilation systems or passive infiltration causes complaints. Carbon monoxide may reach intoxicating levels in structures with parking garages.

Ozone

In addition to combustion products, other inorganic gasses may contaminate indoor spaces. As a commonly exceeded criterion outdoor air pollutant and an intended product of ozone-generating air cleaners, ozone has achieved notoriety. When used as directed, ozone generators sold as air cleaners may cause public health standards to be exceeded. To counter aggressive marketing of ozone-based indoor air cleaners, the EPA has published public alerts about both the ineffectiveness of these devices and associated adverse health effects (18). Ozone may also result from improperly functioning electrical machines such as electrostatic precipitators, photocopiers, laser printers, and fax machines.

Particulates

Indoor particulates are characterized by their chemical composition and physical conformation. Gaseous air pollutants, such as radon daughters or formaldehyde, may adhere to respirable, suspended particulates.

Indoor sources usually are the preeminent contributors to RSPs. Tobacco smoke and unvented combustion devices lead the list of important generators of RSPs; however, activities like vacuuming, sanding, sweeping, demolition, and unprofessional asbestos or lead abatement projects may generate short-term intense particulate exposures. Unfiltered ultrasonic humidifiers using tap water are capable of raising RSPs above the National Ambient Air Quality Standard (NAAQS) in a closed room. Although the building envelope typically excludes most large outdoor particulates, fine RSPs penetrate most buildings and contribute to indoor concentrations that can exceed the NAAQS.

The opportunity for indoor, nonindustrial exposure to asbestos fibers has been intensely scrutinized. Chrysotile asbestos was used extensively in building materials until 1978, when the EPA proscribed most construction and insulation uses. In 1991, the U.S. Fifth Circuit Court of Appeals set aside a 1989 broader EPA initiative to curtail the U.S. manufacturing, importation, processing, and commercial distribution of many more asbestos-containing products (19). The EPA has estimated that 20% of public buildings (733,000) have some asbestos-containing materials (20). This estimate excludes residential and school structures. A 1992 survey conducted in New York City found that 68% of the public buildings contained asbestos materials (21).

Alarm about potential exposures to asbestos led to widespread asbestos abatement projects in schools and houses. Several studies indicate, however, that steady-state indoor fiber counts are at least two orders of magnitude less than the current OSHA PEL of 0.2 fibers/cc (22–24). Further, the vast majority of indoor fibers tend to be less toxic, short fibers (less than 5 μm). On the other hand, poorly conducted asbestos abatement projects and activities that re-suspend settled fibers, such as dry sweeping or vacuuming, can generate short-term exposures well over 100 fibers/cc (25). As a result, the current EPA policy recommends identification of indoor sources of asbestos, alerting persons potentially exposed about measures to minimize exposure, and in-place management. If asbestos-containing materials are at risk of being substantially disturbed through such actions as remodeling, full precautions are recommended, including asbestos removal. OSHA's asbestos health standard mandates notification and protection of building service staff who may disrupt asbestos during maintenance activities. Investigations have shown that these new EPA and OSHA policies protect building occupants and facility workers from substantive exposures (26).

Despite a ban of lead in interior paint in 1978, lead poisoning persists as a major pediatric environmental health threat. According to U.S. Department of Housing and Urban Development estimates, lead paint burdens nearly 60% of all housing stock in the U.S. (27). Ingestion of lead particulates from degrading paint remains the largest contributor to children's lead body burdens. Although most of these particulates are nonrespirable, remodeling efforts and unprofessional lead abatement projects that involve heating, scraping, and sanding can produce respirable lead particulates that becomes a hazard to workers and adult occupants, as well as to children.

Pesticides

Almost all indoor environments contain pesticides (28). Health effects may include acute systemic intoxication, irritating and immunopathic effects, and chronic effects such as neurobehavioral disorders and increased cancer risk. Although concentrations are generally in the microgram range, reentering recently treated environments may result in exposures in the milligram range. As environmentally persistent products such as chlordane have been removed from the market because of chronic toxicities unacceptable to the EPA, they have been replaced with more acutely toxic substances such as the carbamates and organophosphates. Chlorpyrifos, an organophosphate, became one of the most commonly used alternative termiticides. As part of a risk review of pesticides in current use mandated by the 1996 Food Quality Protection Act, the EPA has recently eliminated certain uses of chlorpyrifos in the home because they do not provide an adequate margin of safety for children (29). Hundreds of chemicals classified as "inert ingredients" are included in pesticide formulations, many of which are of immediate toxicologic concern. Several are suspected carcinogens. Little toxicologic information is available to characterize the vast majority. Chemicals banned for use as an active ingredient in pesticides may be used as an inert component.

Radon

Radon 222, an inert gas, is the by-product of the radioactive decay of uranium 238. With a half-life of 3.8 days, radon decays into several short-lived chemically reactive, and radioactive progeny: polonium 218, lead 214, bismuth 214, and polonium 214. The carcinogenic effects of radon are ascribed to these short-lived progeny, which, in contrast to radon, adhere to respiratory tissue.

Indoor radon levels combine with building factors such as ventilation rates and structural characteristics to determine radon daughter concentrations. Though the technology exists to measure radon daughters directly, it is far cheaper to measure radon gas.

Radon exposures outdoors average less than 0.2 picocuries per liter (pCi/L). Indoor levels almost always are higher, averaging about 1.5 pCi/L in homes, but ranging as high as 2,700 pCi/L (30). The best estimates suggest that average annual radon levels exceed 8 pCi/L in 1% to 3% of U.S. houses. By way of comparison, uranium miners' exposures are limited to less than 16 pCi/L today, with historic levels thought to be between 24 and 1,380 pCi/L.

The bulk of radon enters low-rise buildings as a soil gas, though other sources include tap water from private wells, building products, and, minimally, natural gas. As a soil gas, radon primarily affects the lower levels of a building; concentrations of radon tend to decrease in higher levels. Unlike houses, the main source of indoor radon in high-rise buildings is the building material (31).

Volatile Organic Chemicals

A wide range of building products, furnishings, and consumer products emit VOCs. About two dozen of those substances are definite or probable human carcinogens (32). On average, the range of VOCs in new buildings (0.5 to 19 mg/m^3) exceeds by an order of magnitude the range present in older buildings (0.01–1.7 mg/m^3) (33). Emission rates typically drop dramatically within the first days to months of product application or installation. Many components of the indoor environment serve as sinks, which absorb and then reemit VOCs under certain environmental conditions. Months after the commissioning of a new building or remodeling, consumer products such as deodorizers (decane, methyl chloroform), mothballs (*p*-dichlorobenzene), and dry cleaned clothing (perchloroethylene) serve as the chief sources of indoor VOC levels. In houses, other important predictors of elevated VOCs include attached garages, forced air furnaces, air conditioner use, and frequently closed windows.

In most indoor environments, single VOCs rarely approach one tenth of OSHA PELs. When the total weight of indoor VOCs is considered, however, levels can reach concentrations in milligrams per cubic meter, sufficient to generate occupant complaints. Unfortunately, the complexity of VOC mixtures and of their measurement has foiled a simple definition of total VOCs (TVOCs). The total exposure assessment methodology (TEAM) studies conducted by the EPA found that time-weighted average indoor air level of

VOCs can be two to ten times that of outdoor levels (34). Peak exposures may exceed by 100 to 1,000 times the ambient concentrations. Freshly printed materials, various consumer products, and renovations involving application of adhesives, wall coverings, paints, and floor finishes produce some of the highest VOC air concentrations. Using gas chromatography–mass spectrometry (GCMS), VOC emissions sources can be "fingerprinted" to identify specific contaminants.

Some VOCs have achieved particular notoriety. Formaldehyde is an omnipresent indoor contaminant emitted by myriad products and processes, including occupant metabolism. Though regulations and litigation have resulted in decreased emissions from building products, indoor levels of formaldehyde may still exceed 0.2 parts per million (ppm) as the result of multiple emission sources. With low air exchange rates, small enclosed areas, and liberal use of composition board, new mobile homes tend toward the highest formaldehyde air concentrations (35).

Although new carpets emit a myriad of VOCs, 4-phenylcyclohexene (4-PC) has been identified as a preeminent peak in GCMS analysis. Levels have been measured in the range of 0.3 to 40 parts per billion (ppb). Airborne concentrations exceeding 5 ppb are very odiferous. Although little is known about the toxicology of 4-PC, levels greater than 1 ppb have been associated with the installation of new carpet and with outbreaks of health complaints, most famously at the EPA headquarters (36). In the context of these concerns, carpet manufactures voluntarily initiated a "green label" program that identifies carpets that reduce VOC emissions below established standards. However, a review of data from several studies concluded that under normal environmental circumstances, VOC emissions from new carpets are sufficiently low that they should not adversely affect IAQ or cause significant health effects in people (37).

Physical Factors

Several physical attributes of the indoor environment affect human comfort and are associated with health complaints. Temperature, relative humidity, and air velocity are the key factors affecting thermal comfort. The American Society of Heating, Refrigeration, and Air-Conditioning Engineers (ASHRAE) publishes guidelines that outline an envelope of thermal comfort that satisfies about 80% of the occupants of an interior space (38). Relative humidity and temperature also influence concentrations of pollutants. Increasing these parameters leads to higher rates of microbial growth, and emissions of some VOCs, such as formaldehyde. As relative humidity falls below 30%, mucous membranes become more susceptible to irritants, and electrostatic fields increase. Optimal humidification can reduce perception of dry air with lower reports of dry throat, but does not necessarily decrease the total score of building-associated symptoms (39). Temperature exceedences appear to have a much more predictable correlation with occupant complaints. Temperatures in excess of 24°C (75.2°F) routinely increase dissatisfaction with IAQ (40). Ergonomic analysis has identified optimal lighting characteristics for tasks ranging from living room conversation to work at a computer terminal (41). Glare, reflections, flickers, contrasts, and spectral distribution of light are as important as luminance and contribute to building-associated complaints. Florescent lighting has played a role in creating indoor smog through the photooxidation of VOCs and combustion products (42).

Rarely do indoor environments expose occupants to noise levels that induce hearing loss. But ambient noise levels may interfere with normal conversation and concentration. Levels of noise below 40 dBA (A-weighted decibels) are considered comfortable. The average residence without music or appliances running has a noise level of about 30 dBA, whereas the average office has a level of about 50 dBA. Proximity to vehicle traffic and jetports leads to noise exposures that are usually uncontrollable by building occupants. Community standards for ambient noise have been established by the EPA with reference to its annoying characteristics (see Chapter 26).

The relevance of other physical factors such as negative ion deficiency or electromagnetic fields to environmental quality remains controversial. Many indoor polluted environments have negative ion deficiencies when compared to settings such as waterfalls or ocean beachfronts. Nonetheless, no consensus exists regarding the role of negative and positive ion ratios in building-related health complaints. Indoor environments are awash in electromagnetic fields (EMFs) generated by electrical transmission equipment, wiring configurations, video display terminals, and household appliances. Dosimetry reveals widely fluctuating exposures related to the operation of these devices. Although the epidemiology has largely been reassuring, uncertainties linger about the health effects of EMF (43,44).

The Problem Building

Buildings can be categorized by both the complaint rates of their occupants and environmental factors. Only the rare building environment satisfies all occupants. By convention, a *problem building* is one in which either greater than 20% of the occupants have building-related health complaints or specific environmental contaminants have been linked with building-related illnesses. A building may be considered at risk for occupant complaints if an audit reveals one or more environmental problems that are commonly associated with health problems. A *crisis building* is one in which complaints and public concerns have reached the point that normal activities have been severely disrupted. A *healthy building* is one that is designed, maintained, and operated to minimize environmental risk factors and maximize comfort, well-being, and productivity.

A considerable body of literature points to several building characteristics that increase the likelihood of occupant complaints (45,46). A metaanalysis of several epidemiologic studies indicated that sealed, mechanically ventilated, humidified, and air-conditioned buildings are more likely to generate complaints than naturally ventilated buildings (47). Another systematic study noted the following building factors directly related to complaint rates: (a) the total weight and potential allergenic component of the floor dust; (b) the area of fleecy material (soft, absorbent fabric) per cubic meter of air; (c) the length of open shelving per cubic meter of air; (d) the number of workstations; and (e) the air temperature. Other investigators have identified engineering, operational, and maintenance deficiencies commonly found in problem buildings, including inadequate outside air ventilation, inadequate air distribution, insufficient air filtration to remove outdoor pollutants, malfunctioning humidifiers, standing water, visible mold contamination of porous materials, inadequate maintenance programs, and facility personnel ignorance of IAP control strategies. Occupants who use photocopiers, carbonless copy paper, and video display terminals more frequently report building-related symptoms. Complaint rates are more closely related to the intensity of pollution sources than to ventilation rates (48).

Environmental risk factors abound in both large and low-rise buildings. According to a 1995 General Accounting Office study, over 50% of U.S. schools have poor ventilation and significant sources of pollution (49). In OSHA's 1994 proposed IAQ standard, they noted that of 4.5 million commercial buildings in the U.S., only 6% had a computerized energy management and control system, and that 30% had notable indoor air quality problems. OSHA estimated that there are 1.4 million problem ("sick") buildings in the U.S. with 21.2 million exposed employees (50). Surveys for asbestos-containing materials, combustion gas exposures, lead paint, pesticide residues, radon, RSPs, VOCs, and water damage suggest that an even higher percentage of residential buildings present environmental concerns (51).

Health Effects of Indoor Pollution

Adverse health effects from indoor pollution (IP) have been broadly interpreted to include discomfort and decreased productivity along with frank disease (52). This spans the spectrum of biologic response from psychophysical symptoms, to reversible functional impairments, to irreversible biologic effects (53). The occupational physician is likely to be asked for assistance with IEQ prevention, control, and risk communication, as well as clinical management of associated health problems. The health problems arising from IP in nonindustrial environments are summarized by the term *building-associated illnesses,* which historically were categorized as either building-related illnesses (BRI) or the sick building syndrome (SBS). To avoid confusion between whether the building or the individual is sick, many indoor environmental practitioners have advocated that the term SBS be abandoned in favor of another such as *nonspecific BRI* or *building-related occupant complaint syndrome* (BROCS), which will be the preferred term in this chapter. *Specific BRIs* have a defined pathophysiology attributable to a specific building contaminant. In contrast, BROCS describes a group of transient symptoms, affected by entering and leaving a particular building. Substantial laboratory and field research contributions over the last two decades support an environmental basis for BROCS. Nonetheless, the case definition of BROCS remains vague and its causes speculative (54). Usually the attack rate of BRI in a building is relatively low, but it is commonly accompanied by an epidemic of BROCS.

Acute Building-related Illnesses

Hypersensitivity Diseases

Allergies

About 25% of Americans have asthma or other allergic diseases. The most common diseases related to indoor pollution are allergic syndromes affecting the eyes, upper airways, lungs, and skin. Symptoms are usually caused by exposure to biologic or chemical agents to which an individual has been sensitized. Though aeroallergens are ubiquitous, sensitizing or precipitating exposures may be linked to a specific building where exposure occurs to particularly high levels. After sensitization, trace amounts of the allergen may provoke episodes of illness in some individuals. The clinical presentation, skin testing or the radioallergoabsorbent test (RAST), and provocative challenges confirm the diagnosis. Symptom and peak flow diaries, pre- and postshift spirometry, and serial methacholine challenge tests can be used to implicate a specific environment's role in precipitating asthma. Both immediate and late-onset asthma are observed.

Uncommonly, allergic or pseudoallergic phenomena have been linked to indoor chemical contaminants. For example, a component of carbonless copy paper, alkyl–phenol novalac resin, has been found to be responsible for anaphylactoid reactions in a small number of users (55). Immunoglobulin E (IgE) antibodies to the substance can be measured. Challenge with the chemical re-creates the syndrome. Both urticaria and allergic dermatitis from contact with carbonless copy paper has also been described (56,57). Formaldehyde has been linked with allergic and pseudoallergic phenomena affecting the eyes, nose, skin, and lungs.

Hypersensitivity Pneumonitis

Hypersensitivity pneumonitis may result in fever, chest tightness, cough, shortness of breath, malaise, and myalgia. Laboratory findings may include restrictive patterns on pulmonary function tests, pulmonary infiltrates, leukocytosis, and elevated serum precipitins to biologic agents found in the culpable building. Pulmonary diffusion capacity and pulmonary exercise tolerance tests are the most sensitive indicators of the disease. T-lymphocyte–predominant alveolitis is noted on bronchial alveolar lavage, and lung biopsy usually reveals granulomatous changes. Precipitation of the illness by bronchial challenge with suspected antigens remains the gold standard for diagnosis, but the responsible antigen is often never identified. Smokers seem to be relatively protected from this disease, and atopy is not a predisposing factor.

Symptoms and signs usually resolve spontaneously with cessation of exposure to the offending agent. Because continued exposure to even a small amount of the responsible antigen can lead to a chronic, progressive interstitial lung disease, permanent removal from the precipitating environment may be necessary *even after remediation*. Though hypersensitivity pneumonitis usually affects only a small number of building occupants, the severity of this illness demands thorough environmental investigation and remediation.

Humidifier Fever

Humidifier fever presents as a flu-like syndrome similar to hypersensitivity pneumonitis but without objective pulmonary findings or the risk for chronic sequelae. Symptoms usually begin within 4 to 8 hours and resolve spontaneously within 24 hours after cessation of exposure to microbiologically contaminated aerosols. In contrast to hypersensitivity pneumonitis, the attack rate is high—between 25% and 40%. The syndrome develops abruptly, usually after a period of removal from exposure, hence the synonym "Monday morning fever." Recovery can occur despite continued exposure. Experimental challenges of symptomatic workers with humidifier antigens re-creates the syndrome, but only in previously exposed workers. Though biologic aerosols are the sine qua non of humidifier fever, the self-limited and benign nature of the illness has obstructed investigation of its pathophysiology. Too narrowly entitled humidifier fever, this inhalation fever syndrome can develop after exposures to any intense bioaerosol, such as contaminated bath water, water in a sauna bucket, or moldy books. Unlike hypersensitivity pneumonitis, no specific organisms seem more prone to cause this condition.

Infectious Diseases

The bacterium *Legionella pneumophila* is associated with two clinically and epidemiologically distinct diseases: Legionnaire's disease, a potentially fatal pneumonia and multisystem disease; and Pontiac fever, a self-limited flu-like syndrome. After an incubation period of 2 to 10 days, infection with the bacterium causes Legionnaire's disease in a small percentage of exposed people, who are commonly elderly or immunocompromised. Historically, 15% to 20% of those infected die from Legionnaire's disease. Diagnosis is made by chest x-ray, isolation of the organism from body fluids, and immunoassays. Treatment with antibiotics decreases morbidity and mortality.

Legionnaire's disease is contracted by the inhalation of aerosolized *Legionella*-contaminated water. Person-to-person transmission has never been observed. Only about 20% of cases occur epidemically with respiratory exposure to common, intensely contaminated building reservoirs. Organisms may also originate from external sources such as excavation projects that liberate the organism from the soil. Despite the ubiquity of the Legionella organism, the disease occurs only sporadically in the community.

Pontiac fever presents as a benign flu-like illness of fever, chills, headache, and myalgia, but no pulmonary involvement. Attack rates are high, sometimes nearing 100%. Though serologic testing demonstrates exposure, the organism has never been isolated from infected hosts. Why the same microbe can lead to two illnesses of very different severity and prognosis is not known, but the size of the inoculum, the mode of transmission, and host factors probably play important roles.

Many infectious diseases are transmitted by respiratory droplet. Indoor crowding dramatically increases opportunities for person-to-person transmission of diseases such as bacterial pharyngitis, mumps, measles, whooping cough, chickenpox, and tuberculosis. Some epidemics of airborne respiratory illnesses can also be specifically linked to the mechanical systems of the indoor environment. Rare examples include histoplasmosis related to the disturbance of contaminated bird droppings concentrated near windows or air intakes. Opportunistic fungal pathogens, *Pseudomonas,* and *Acinetobacter* may contaminate therapeutic respiratory devices or humidifiers but pose a risk only to immunocompromised hosts. A few airborne outbreaks of tuberculosis have been linked to poorly ventilated environments (58,59). Some evidence, not yet conclusive, supports the theory that epidemics of common communicable viral respiratory diseases like influenza, the common cold, measles, rubella, and chickenpox may be associated with airborne transmission in an indoor environment building, due to inadequate ventilation (60). A classic outbreak of influenza occurred in an unventilated plane in which 100% of the occupants contracted the disease from a single index case (61). The multiplicity of opportunities for acquiring these illnesses in the community and by close personal contact makes linking an illness to a specific environment problematic.

Intoxication Diseases

Acute or subacute intoxication may occur from exposure to several indoor pollutants, including carbon monoxide, heavy metals, pesticides, and volatile organics. Mycotoxins probably do not cause disease in typical indoor environments.

Carbon Monoxide

Though carbon monoxide poisoning rarely occurs in office settings, it is a leading cause of poisoning at home. About 1,800 accidental deaths occur annually (62). Many of these are caused by poorly vented or malfunctioning combustion devices. Fatalities may be considerably higher in people with preexisting cardiovascular disease, since carboxyhemoglobin levels in the 5% range can precipitate acute cardiovascular events. More insidiously, low-level carbon monoxide poisoning may present as a persistent flu-like syndrome. About 4% to 5% of people presenting to the emergency room with these symptoms during the heating season suffer from subacute carbon monoxide poisoning (63).

Heavy Metals

Though environmental lead poisoning is largely the result of lead paint, contaminated water ingestion, and lead-glazed pottery, poisoning may also occur by inhalation of dusts and fumes generated by the abrasion, heating, or burning of lead-painted surfaces. Hobbies such as glazing pottery, stained glass work, and making lead shot or fishing sinkers are particularly hazardous sources of airborne lead.

Hundreds of cases of acute mercury intoxication, some leading to fatalities, have occurred in residential settings. These incidents generally result from children or parents bringing large quantities of elemental mercury home for play, but have also been associated with medical instrument breakage, art supplies, traditional facial beauty creams, and gold ore processing (64–66). Mercury exposure has also occurred when old industrial buildings or laboratories have been converted to residential use. Acrodynia associated with exposure to a home recently painted with a latex paint containing phenyl mercury raised the concern of widespread exposures. Subsequently, an investigation identified elevated levels of mercury in other persons exposed to homes freshly painted with latex paint containing the preservative phenyl-mercuric acetate (67). As a result, the EPA banned the manufacture of mercury compounds in all latex paints as of September 1991.

Pesticides

The Toxic Exposure Surveillance System maintained by the American Association of Poison Control Centers reflects the extent of acute pesticide poisoning from nonagricultural uses. In 1998, over 30,000 adults contacted poison control centers in the U.S. to report overexposure. In the same year, poison control centers answered calls about exposures of 45,000 children younger than 19 years old (68). Over 92% of these exposures occurred at residences (69). The ban of environmentally persistent pesticides like chlordane has led to their substitution by products more acutely toxic to humans. Historically registered uses of pesticides have not necessarily considered the increased susceptibility of children. The Food Quality Protection Act of 1996 precipitated a reassessment of the risks to children associated with pesticides and led to the phased ban of diazinon and chlorpyrifos, two ubiquitous pesticides found indoors (70). Nonoccupational symptoms attributed to pesticides include sensitivity reactions, especially to pyrethrin products, which are antigenically similar to ragweed. The toxicology of many of the inert ingredients of pesticides remains unknown, but organic solvent carriers probably precipitate many of the acute complaints attributed to pesticide use in buildings.

Volatile Organic Chemicals

Exposure to VOCs, such as xylene, toluene, methylene chloride, and mineral spirits, can occur at levels exceeding OSHA PELs during remodeling efforts, with the use of solvent cleaning products or with hobbies like furniture refinishing. These exposures most commonly cause acute and subacute neurobehavioral as well as mucosal irritation characteristic of the VOCs in general.

Mycotoxicosis

Many molds produce toxins (mycotoxins), which are established as ingested poisons from food contamination, but have recently been suspected of causing discomfort and disease when present in indoor air. The toxin-producing molds found most often in buildings in excess of outdoor concentrations include *Cladosporium, Penicillium, Aspergillus,* and *Stachybotrys* (71,72). Investigators have particularly targeted *Stachybotrys* because of its toxic biologic activity including modulation of inflammation and altered alveolar surfactant phospholipid concentrations. Epidemiologic investigations of moldy buildings have also associated *Stachybotrys* with symptoms of BROCS, changes in laboratory immune parameters, and pulmonary hemorrhage in infants (73–76). Detailed re-evaluation of the original data has refuted the original conclusion that pulmonary hemorrhage was associated with stachybotrys and other mold exposures (76a). Other than in agricultural or industrial settings where massive mold exposure can occur, substantial dispute exists about the relationship of mycotoxins and building-associated illnesses. Although some molds clearly produce potent toxins, it remains unproven whether they elicit serious disease in the indoor environment (76b).

Irritant Diseases

Rarely does a single indoor pollutant achieve sufficient levels to cause an acute, new-onset building-related illness like conjunctivitis, rhinitis, pharyngitis, or reactive airway dysfunction syndrome (RADS). Exceptions include the mixture of chlorine and ammonia-based cleaners or formaldehyde. Fibrous glass and carpet shampoo residues may provoke transient upper respiratory and dermatologic irritant syndromes. More commonly, many airborne irritants are present at low levels and together aggravate preexisting respiratory diseases such as asthma or rhinitis. The vapor and particulate mixture of ETS raises the risk of sudden infant death, childhood asthma, and pediatric respiratory infections and symptoms. It irritates the eyes, nose, throat, and lower respiratory tract of others. Though not firmly established, ETS probably also increases adult respiratory symptoms and exacerbates asthma. Other combustion products, including particulates, sulfur dioxide, and nitrogen oxides, have been linked with respiratory illnesses in vulnerable populations.

CHRONIC BUILDING-RELATED DISEASES

Indoor pollutants have the potential for causing chronic diseases. Those of chief concern are cancer, and neurobehavioral, cardiovascular, and pulmonary disorders.

Cancer

The presence of carcinogens in indoor air has prompted aggressive public health and regulatory actions. Asbestos, benzene, radon, and ETS are all class A (EPA) carcinogens. Though radon and ETS are of most concern, the risks of VOCs, pesticides, and more recently EMFs have all been targeted.

Radon

The increased risk of lung cancer has been well demonstrated among uranium miners working underground with exposures to high concentrations of radon progeny. Most epidemiologic data suggest at least an additive if not a synergistic effect between smoking and radon. Extrapolating from the experience of uranium miners, various organizations have estimated that from 9,000 to 16,000 excess lung cancer deaths annually are attributable to residential radon exposure (77). Using EPA models, 50% of excess cancers occur at less than the mean residential level of 1.5 pCi/L due to radon. Despite relatively robust data, questions persist about a possible exaggeration of the significance of low-level, domestic radon exposures.

ETS and Combustion Products

The International Agency for Research on Cancer, the EPA, the surgeon general's Office and the National

Research Council all consider ETS a human pulmonary carcinogen. OSHA may soon regulate ETS as an occupational carcinogen. Though the epidemiology has not yet been clarified, ETS probably interacts with other indoor carcinogenic pollutants such as radon.

Fossil fuel combustion also produces carcinogenic by-products, such as polynuclear aromatic hydrocarbons (PAHs) that have been associated with cancer in coke oven and coal gas workers. Studies of populations in the developing world that heat and cook with poorly vented fires have noted increased risks of nasopharyngeal cancer.

Particulates

EPA risk estimates of cancer associated with indoor exposures to asbestos generated a massive regulatory and abatement effort in the 1980s. The estimates were based on the health experience of asbestos workers and their spouses along with assumptions about indoor exposures that have since been revised. In 1985, the EPA published lifetime estimated risks as high as 2.7×10^{-3}/0.01 fibers/cc of contracting cancer from asbestos (78). At the time, the EPA calculated that school children were exposed to about 0.01 fibers/cc. Subsequent environmental hygiene surveys have demonstrated that typical indoor exposures are several orders of magnitude lower than occupational exposures except when asbestos-containing materials (ACMs) are disturbed (79). Consequently, although case reports exist that attribute mesothelioma to indoor asbestos exposure (80), cancer risks from occupying buildings with ACMs are probably minimal. On the other hand, cancer associated with paraoccupational exposure of family members to asbestos is well documented.

Volatile Organic Chemicals and Pesticides

Individual risk estimates for the carcinogenic effects of VOCs and pesticides in indoor air have been generated. These estimates have led to the withdrawal of several pesticides, such as chlordane, from commercial use, and stricter regulation of some VOCs, such as formaldehyde and benzene. Six of the most prevalent and well-established carcinogenic VOCs may be responsible for 1,000 to 5,000 excess cancer cases annually.

Electromagnetic Fields

In the early 1980s, some reports raised concern that very low and extra low frequency EMFs emanating from video display units were associated with reproductive effects. Since then, careful epidemiology, which for the first time included actual measurements of fields, refuted these concerns (81). EMFs have also been implicated in increasing the risks of childhood leukemia and of cancers in occupationally exposed workers. Great uncertainties remain, however, regarding dose relationships of EMF to the studied health outcomes. Disagreement persists about the impact of these fields on human health (82–84). Indeed, because of a current lack of biologic plausibility, the question remains as to whether EMF is a confounding variable.

Cardiovascular Disease

Growing evidence points to a role of indoor pollution in cardiovascular disease. Environmental tobacco smoke is associated with heart disease mortality and morbidity. Exposure to indoor coal fumes has been identified as a risk factor for stroke (85). Further, a substantial literature has repeatedly found associations between atmospheric pollution episodes and the precipitation of cardiovascular events (86).

Neurobehavioral Disorders

Several indoor pollutants have the capability of causing chronic neurobehavioral disorders. Lead- and elemental mercury–related neurotoxicity have been best publicized, but these disorders include carbon monoxide, pesticide, and solvent encephalopathies resulting from high-dose acute intoxications. Whether chronic low-dose exposures to these agents as found in typical indoor settings can cause chronic encephalopathies remains controversial. Though the potential for persistent neurologic sequelae from chronic elemental mercury exposure is well described, no one knows the extent to which phenyl mercuric acetate emitted from latex paints may have caused similar problems.

Cognitive effects of lead have been identified at blood lead levels as low as 10 μg/dL (87). The most recent national data indicates that nearly one million children have blood lead levels higher than 15 μg/dL (88). Robust evidence indicates that these children have persistent measurable cognitive and behavioral problems with substantial social consequences (89,90).

Pulmonary Disorders

Several classes of indoor pollutants can cause chronic pulmonary disorders. Unremitting exposures to sensitizing chemical or biologic agents, such as dust mites, can lead to chronic asthma. Persistent exposures to immunogenic agents may also provoke hypersensitivity pneumonitis to progress to interstitial fibrosis. Historically, paraoccupational exposures to asbestos in family members of asbestos workers have been linked with pleural plaques, but typical indoor exposures to asbestos are not sufficient to cause fibrotic pulmonary diseases.

Building-related Occupant Complaint Syndrome

BROCS is a constellation of nonspecific symptoms related to occupation of a specific building environment. Molhave (91) has grouped the symptoms in five classes, with the possibility that BROCS may represent several pathophysiologic mechanisms: sensory irritation, neurologic or general health symptoms, skin irritation, nonspecific hypersensitivity reactions, and odor and taste problems. An individual typically suffers from BROCS in the context of an epidemic of occupant complaints. Although the identification of a single case of BROCS in a building remains contentious, the wide range in individual susceptibility to airborne irritants provides the physiologic basis for this diagnosis (92,93).

Though no single environmental condition or contaminant has been identified as causative of BROCS, numerous hypotheses have been advanced and supported with plausible data. An early theory attributed high complaint rates to inadequate dilution of building contaminants with ventilation. Blind manipulations of ventilation have been shown to affect complaints and productivity in some buildings (94). Substantial reduction of occupant complaints after ventilation improvements have been found to persist up to 3 years after the intervention (95). A review of 20 studies revealed that, almost uniformly, symptoms were more common in buildings with ventilation rates of less than 10 L/s [20 cubic feet per minute (cfm)] of outdoor air per person. Increasing ventilation rates up to 20 L/s (40 cfm) brought statistically significant reductions in complaints (96,97).

Substantial evidence has accrued that inadequate ventilation is only one component of the variance in complaints among buildings. The utility of increasing ventilation rates reaches an asymptote. In fact, increasing ventilation rates in some buildings heightens dissatisfaction. Both field and laboratory studies indicate that specific categories and sources of pollution influence the incidence of BROCS. One theory proposes that irritant and neurologic symptoms result from exposures to a large number of VOCs whose total weight (TVOC) reaches toxicologic significance. Though controlled laboratory evidence concerning the neurotoxic effects of low-level VOCs remain inconclusive, data clearly indicate dose-response relationships of mucous membrane irritation to VOC levels greater than 5 mg/m^3 (98,99). Other credible theories have implicated respirable suspended particulates and aberrant relative humidity (100). Much research currently points to an important role of microbiologic contamination, organic debris, and associated microbial volatile organic chemicals and endotoxins. As with ventilation, blinded manipulation of pollution loads in an office setting affects both symptoms and productivity (101).

Robust laboratory and field evidence has identified environmental contributors to BROCS, but organizational, psychosocial, and personal variables play a role as well (102–104). As an example of psychosocial contributors to the syndrome, women and those in clerical jobs report more symptoms than men, professionals, and managers. Organizational conflict and occupational stress have also been linked with higher complaint rates, but much of the research has been of a cross-sectional nature. This research cannot resolve the question of whether stress is an active precipitator or an outcome of BROCS (105). Some investigators have misinterpreted findings of psychosocial distress and invoked them as sole explanations for BROCS when building investigations have failed to reveal clear environmental etiologies. The importance of social dynamics, even in crisis buildings, should not be confused with mass psychogenic illness. Surely, the basis for BROCS is multifactorial and best fits a biopsychosocial model.

Whatever their cause, nonspecific building-related health complaints are common. Systematic surveys of occupants of buildings where environmental problems had not been previously identified consistently reveal complaint rates higher than 20% (106). At the extreme, a British study of 4,373 office workers in 42 office buildings found that 80% of the workers had at least one work-related symptom (107). BROCS is not necessarily work related; 25% to 50% of respondents to indoor air quality surveys ascribe BROCS to their home.

MASS PSYCHOGENIC ILLNESS

Mass psychogenic illness (MPI) presents with symptoms compatible with hyperventilation, features not readily explained by organic mechanisms, a visual or verbal chain of transmission, and higher incidence in women. Onset is usually explosive, and new cases correlate with person-to-person transmission rather than a common source outbreak. Chronic building-related health complaints, though influenced by psychosocial dynamics, are unlikely to be caused by MPI. MPI should not be diagnosed merely because of an absence of an environmental explanation for occupant complaints.

IDIOPATHIC ENVIRONMENTAL ILLNESS (MULTIPLE CHEMICAL SENSITIVITIES)

Practitioners interested in IEQ will invariably encounter the clinical problem of multiple chemical sensitivities (MCS), now more appropriately called idiopathic environmental illness (IEI). Controversy persists as to whether IEI represents a distinct diagnostic entity and whether it can be attributed to environmental exposures. Nonetheless, IEI exists as a clinically recognizable syndrome (108). Several working case definitions and plausible pathophysiologic mechanisms have been proposed (109). Though the etiology of IEI has yet to be ascertained, many sufferers report the onset and recurrence of nonspecific symptoms referable to multiple organ systems after perceived exposure to low levels of chemical, biologic, or physical agents. No consistent physical findings or laboratory abnormalities have yet been found to differentiate IEI patients from the remainder of the population.

In a position statement on IEI, the American College of Occupational and Environmental Medicine has concluded, "No scientific basis currently exists for investigating, regulating or managing the environment with the goal of minimizing the incidence or severity of MCS." Nonetheless, the social trend has been to consider IEI as a bona fide handicap deserving of Social Security Disability Insurance and reasonable accommodations under provisions of the Fair Housing Act and the Americans with Disabilities Act. Further, reasonable medical practice includes individualizing reasonable environmental approaches to accommodating the individual IEI patient with a goal of maintaining vocational and social functioning (110).

CLINICAL EVALUATION OF BUILDING-ASSOCIATED ILLNESS

Patients may present with health complaints or with anxiety about future health effects caused by indoor environmental contaminants. Most building-associated illnesses resemble common clinical problems seen by primary care physicians. On the one hand, in the context of a crisis building, clinicians must be wary of too readily accepting their patients' self-assessment of the building-relatedness of their problems. On the other hand, in the absence of a well-identified problem building, the clinician must be armed with a high index of suspicion to identify occult environmental contributors to a patient's illness. The clinical evaluation seeks to accomplish the following goals: (a) ascertain a diagnosis or complaint syndrome, (b) characterize exposure, (c) assess causation, and (d) establish a therapeutic plan.

The clinical evaluation begins with an interview aimed at eliciting symptoms and the temporal sequence of those symptoms in relationship to specific environments and activities. The practitioner compares complaints to expected symptoms for particular building contaminants. During the interview, the clinician should inquire about complaints of other building occupants. Individual and building psychosocial dynamics should be explored. All underlying, known medical problems should be identified. Detailed occupational and environmental histories constitute the first step of the exposure characterization (111–113). Environmental data that have been collected by formal investigation should be reviewed.

Physical examination of patients with BROCS is usually unrevealing. Slit-lamp examinations of BROCS patients often reveal tear film instability and diminished foam in the inner canthus (114,115). Dry eyes may be readily diagnosed with Schirmer's test. Examination findings with BRIs such as asthma are characteristic of the illness.

Laboratory investigations are unhelpful in the assessment of BROCS, but can be diagnostic of BRI. The evaluation of hypersensitivity syndromes can be assisted with skin tests, total and specific IgE, immunoglobulin G (IgG) panels, and precipitating antibodies with specific reference to biologic agents identified in the suspect building. Standard reference laboratory hypersensitivity panels, however, may not include the offending agents. When critical for clinical or forensic purposes, samples from the building may be used to develop antigen preparations for *in vitro* tests and *in vivo* bronchial challenges. Positive antibody tests confirm exposure but by themselves do not establish etiology of complaints. Though helpful, appropriately timed chest radiography is not a sensitive tool in the diagnosis of hypersensitivity pneumonitis. Serial spirometry, peak flow measurement, and methacholine challenge are particularly useful in evaluating lower respiratory complaints. Diffusion capacities are particularly sensitive in assessing hypersensitivity pneumonitis when timed to coincide with natural experiments of exposure to and avoidance of the suspected environment. Bronchial alveolar lavage and biopsy add confirmatory pathologic information when clinical diagnostic confusion persists about the possibility of hypersensitivity pneumonitis or bronchopulmonary aspergillosis.

The building-relatedness of upper airway diseases and complaints, whether irritant or allergic in origin, is particularly difficult to confirm with laboratory tests. Timed with environmental challenges, clinical tools include rhinometry (a measure of nasal resistance), rhinoscopy, laryngoscopy, and computerized analysis of voice quality (available from many speech pathologists). Nasal smears and lavage help define the pathophysiology of rhinitis (116).

Occasionally, laboratory examination can be helpful in the evaluation of building-associated dermatologic complaints. Probably the most common example is fiberglass dermatitis. Scotch tape applied to actively pruritic skin before washing can be examined microscopically for fiberglass fibers. Patch testing can document sensitivity to specific agents such as are found in carbonless copy paper.

An important clinical and legal responsibility of the physician is the decision about the relationship of a specific environment to an individual's symptoms. Medical diagnosis and appropriate therapeutic interventions may not be possible without an objective understanding of environmental exposures.

Practitioners may reach one of five possible causation conclusions when evaluating patients with building-associated complaints: (a) The person has a disease caused by a specific environmental agent; for example, a child with neurobehavioral abnormalities has lead poisoning. (b) The person has a disease to which multiple factors contribute, including an indoor environment. A sample case could be lung cancer diagnosed in a smoker who has lived his life in a house contaminated with high levels of radon. (c) The individual may have a preexisting problem originally unrelated to a specific environment, such as asthma, that is provoked by indoor air exposures to low-level irritants. (d) An individual is diagnosed with a problem, such as chronic fatigue syndrome, that has no known environmental etiology. (e) The individual is found to have a problem, such as systemic sclerosis, in which environmental etiologies remain speculative.

As with all occupational and environmental illness, the most specific treatment of a building illness always begins with minimizing exposure to the offending agent(s). Unfortunately, even for objectifiable illnesses with a suspected relationship to the environment, causative environmental agents may not be identified.

Healthy building occupants may also ask occupational physicians to evaluate future health risks associated with current exposures. Standard clinical toxicologic methods can be used with reference to published IEQ guidelines to communicate risks.

Litigation in the area of IP is increasing rapidly. The range of these legal issues is reviewed elsewhere (117–119).

EVALUATION OF PROBLEM BUILDINGS

Building evaluation protocols share a common theme. Investigations should be staged. Details of each of these phases for large and residential buildings have been reviewed elsewhere (120,121). The most useful tools in the early phases of investigation are the senses and experience of the investigator. Detailed measurement of specific contaminants is seldom necessary. Sophisticated measurements should be performed only late in an investigation when attempting to confirm environmental or medical hypotheses. When assessments proceed beyond the initial phases, a multidisciplinary team including engineers, industrial hygienists, physicians, epidemiologists, and microbiologists becomes essential to a satisfactory outcome.

Analysis of the psychosocial dynamics of building complaints is best begun early in an investigation. Too often, psychosocial issues are invoked as an explanation for symptoms when environmental factors are not readily identified. The investigators' activities are likely to affect social dynamics. Confrontation can result when investigators and facility managers dichotomize environmental and psychologic explanations. Organizational crisis may result, with decreased productivity and even evacuation, while occupants clamor for repeated investigations for ephemeral odorants and phantom toxicants. As part of a strategy to minimize opportunity for anxious speculation and distrust, building occupants should be kept informed of the progress and conclusions of the investigation. A task force that includes representatives of different job categories in a building serves this purpose well. The task force plays an equally important role of informing investigators and building managers about building occupants' concerns and their hypotheses about causation.

The first phase of an investigation begins with the collection of general information about the building and about the occupants' complaints. The use of semistructured questionnaires for the collection of data by interview and walk-around facilitates this process. In fact, protocols have been sufficiently refined so that many building managers are able to conduct the first phase of investigation and remediation without resorting to outside consultation (52). Occupants, facility managers, maintenance engineers, and custodial supervisors should be interviewed; appropriate representatives should accompany the investigator on the walk-around. Special attention should be focused on the age and general condition of the building, HVAC system, extent of fleecy material, areas of moisture and water intrusion, open combustion appliances, smoking policies, occupant activities, remodeling efforts, maintenance procedures, pesticide use, cleaning products and practices, office machines, chemical storage, and occupancy density. Measurements of temperature, relative humidity, and carbon dioxide are conveniently and cheaply included in this phase. Carbon dioxide concentrations are useful indicators of how effectively a space is ventilated for human occupation. Carbon dioxide levels above 800 ppm indicate inadequate ventilation. However, carbon dioxide levels do not reflect the adequacy of the ventilation in dealing with nonphysiologic sources of contamination, such as ETS or VOCs (48).

This general environmental assessment, in combination with a basic understanding of the epidemiology of building complaints, often suffices to identify environmental risk factors warranting intervention. Cluster analysis may help identify syndromes that can be tied to specific contaminants or areas of a building (123). If investigators identify individuals with suspected medical illness, especially pulmonary disorders, they should recommend medical evaluation.

The second phase of an investigation should proceed only with specific environmental or medical hypotheses in mind. In some cases, detailed epidemiology may be necessary to generate these hypotheses. Though seldom possible in practice, every attempt should be made to conduct such epidemiology with use of control buildings. Shotgun attempts to measure every possible pollutant should be avoided. One example of a specific hypothesis is a pattern of building-related headaches in people served by a ventilation system whose outdoor air intake is in a parking garage. This problem should lead to measurement of carbon monoxide. In another example, a history of extensive flooding of a carpet in an area of epidemic complaints or pulmonary disease might lead to biologic sampling of the carpet and nearby air. The results of these environmental analyses would then be correlated with clinical data.

Industrial hygienists must be careful to use sampling methods appropriate for IEQ investigations (124,125). The sensitivity and expense of industrial methods may not be appropriate (121,122). Timing of measurements will critically affect results. Climatic conditions, the operating state of HVAC systems, and building activities often impact contaminant levels. Establishing worst- case environmental scenarios is usually appropriate. For example, brief but intense showers of mold spores may be the event of interest in precipitating medical symptoms. This event may best be reproduced by actions such as banging a ventilation duct or jumping on a carpet. Research has also documented that personal breathing zone exposures may vary considerably from area samples in indoor settings (126). Biomonitoring for indoor contaminants has proven extremely useful in assessing exposure to such contaminants as ETS and carbon monoxide.

Seldom will contaminant levels exceed industrial guidelines. In addition, many contaminants, particularly the bioaerosols, cannot be simply and meaningfully compared to a recommended limit. As a possible clue to the significance of a contaminant level, the investigator should compare concentrations measured in different locations in a building with outdoor concentrations. These contaminant variations may become meaningful when compared to the spatial distribution of health complaints in a building.

Particularly when environmental causation is elusive, biologic assays may be used to assess perceived pollution. Human panels have the greatest utility. A panel of people can be trained to reliably rate their dissatisfaction with air quality (127). Though toxicology relies on animal, plant, and cellular systems, their use for building assessment remains investigational.

When an individual is affected in the absence of recognized or readily corrected environmental hazards, medical removal is usually the action of choice. In other cases, environmental interventions may be recommended. In discussion with the building's IAQ task force, investigators should devise written and oral methods for notifying all building occupants about the study conclusions and action plans. Follow-up environmental and medical assessments of the impact of abatement should be made. In cases of BROCS, building occupants and management must be informed that resolution of all building-related complaints is unlikely. Complaint rates are not likely to fall much below 20%.

IMPROVING IEQ

Concerns about productivity, costs, and litigation have prompted concerted efforts from diverse business, professional, and governmental sectors to devise strategies for preventing IEQ problems. If building investigation protocols can be considered as tertiary prevention, then additional approaches may be categorized as secondary and primary prevention.

Secondary Prevention

Secondary prevention of poor IEQ involves the identification of environmental risk factors and occupant concerns before they become problems. Routine preventive maintenance schedules are advised, with particular focus on the HVAC system and known potential sources of IP such as water incursion. Facility managers should conduct periodic environmental audits using published check sheets. Guidelines for audits of residential buildings also exist. Some audits are mandated in certain buildings, such as asbestos and lead hazard identification. Many states have laws about ETS in public buildings that require internal policies and monitoring. Radon levels should be measured according to current EPA recommendations.

Building managers are wise to devise a mechanism for soliciting and responding to occupant environmental concerns and comfort complaints. Notifying occupants about building audit activities is also recommended.

Primary Prevention

Steps to optimize IEQ can be can be taken in conjunction with other goals such as minimizing ecologic impact and optimizing energy efficiency, structural integrity, safety, spatial utility, and aesthetics. Primary prevention necessitates consideration of every stage of a building's life cycle from its siting and design to its construction, commissioning, operation, maintenance, and remodeling (128–132).

Building, furnishing, and consumer product choices represent important opportunities for minimizing IP. As the result of regulatory actions, some of the most prevalent indoor contaminants, such as asbestos, lead paint, and chlordane, are not found in new buildings. Ironically, in each case their substitutes, manmade mineral fibers, mercury contaminated latex paint, and organophosphate pesticides, have raised concerns of their own. Though desirable, substituting less hazardous products is unfortunately not always straightforward. Considerable controversy exists regarding the toxicity of many common building products and furnishings. Not only are there large gaps in basic toxicology for the thousands of chemicals used indoors, but also other important questions remain. For example, products with highly volatile organic chemicals may have very high emission rates for the first week of installation that then dramatically fall off. Are these items more or less hazardous than products with lower rates but considerably longer periods of emission? Standardized methods for evaluating the emissions of building products and furnishings have been developed. Product choice schemes based on emission rates, known health effects, quantity used, and other considerations have been developed to assist construction and design managers in the midst of uncertainty (133).

Many administrative measures may also be taken to minimize IP; these begin with the process of commissioning a building for its first use. Occupation should not occur until construction is finished and environmental controls are operating as designed. With the knowledge that new product emission rates are often high, some authorities have recommended that products be aged before installation. Renovations, maintenance activities, cleaning, exterminations, and other activities known to generate high levels of pollutants should always be scheduled and organized to minimize occupant exposures.

Finally, any comprehensive and successful attempt to manage air quality requires the training and education of all individuals managing the indoor environment. Specific OSHA standards mandate this communication for specific hazards such as asbestos. For more than a decade, several governmental and voluntary agencies have alerted facility managers and the general community about lead, radon, asbestos, and a variety of other indoor environmental hazards. Despite the wealth of practical building science useful in preventing poor IEQ, critical deficiencies persist in the education and practice of facility managers and building contractors.

CONCLUSION

IP has become a chief priority in the control of environmental threats to human health. Though our understanding of low-level air pollutants is hardly complete, known health effects range from discomfort, to illness, to death. Estimates of the associated economic impact are staggering. Those concerned with IEQ now have available considerable information to assist in the investigation, treatment, and prevention of building-associated illnesses.

REFERENCES

1. Osler W. *The principles and practice of medicine.* New York: D. Appleton, 1892:185.
2. Matte TD. Housing and health—current issues and implications for research and programs. *J Urban Health* 2000;77(1):7–25.
3. Bruce N. Indoor air pollution in developing countries:

a major environmental and public health challenge. *Bull World Health Organ* 2000;78:1078–1092.
4. Kreiss K. The epidemiology of building-related complaints and illness. In: Cone JE, Hodgson MJ, eds. Problem buildings: building-associated illness and the sick building syndrome. *Occup Med State of the Art Rev* 1989;4:575–592.
5. *New York Times* 1988 Sept 11:1.
6. EPA. Inside IAQ—EPA's indoor air quality research update. 600/N-98/002, Summer 1998: *http://www.epa.gov/appcdwww/crbiemb/insideiaqss98.pdf.*
7. United States General Accounting Office. Indoor pollution—status of federal research activities. Washington, DC: GAO/RCED-99-254; August 1999.
8. Office of Radiation and Indoor Air. Flood clean-up: avoiding indoor air quality problems. (6607J),402-F-93-005, August 1993: *URL:http://www.epa.gov/iaq/pubs/flood.html.*
9. Update: outbreak of hantavirus infection—southwestern United States [editorial]. *MMWR* 1993;42:441–443.
10. Consumer Products Safety Commission. Carbon monoxide detectors can save lives. CPSC Document 5010: *http://63.74.109.9/cpscpub/pubs/5010.html.*
11. Elemental mercury poisoning in a household [editorial]. *MMWR* 1990;39:424–425.
12. American Academy of Pediatrics. Committee on Environmental Health. Toxic effects of indoor molds. *Pediatrics* 1998;101[pt 1]:712–714.
13. Ducatman AM, McLellan RK. The epidemiological basis for an occupational and environmental policy on environmental tobacco smoke. *J Occup Environ Med* 2000;42:1137–1141.
14. Woods JE. Cost avoidance and productivity in owning and operating buildings. In: Cone JE, Hodgson MJ, eds. Problem buildings: building-associated illness and the sick building syndrome. *Occup Med State of the Art Rev* 1989;4:753–760.
15. Whitmore RW, Kelly JE, Reading PL. National home and garden pesticide survey: final report, 1992; (1). Research Triangle Park, NC: Research Triangle Institute, RTI\5100.121F.
16. U.S. Department of Health and Human Services, Public Health Service, National Toxicology Program Environmental Health Information Service. 9th report on Carcinogens; Revised January 2001: *http://ehis.niehs.nih.gov/roc/ninth/known/ets.pdf.*
17. Bizovi KE. Night of the sirens: analysis of carbon monoxide-detector experience in suburban Chicago. *Ann Emerg Med* 1998;31:737–740.
18. United States Environmental Protection Agency. Ozone generators that are sold as air cleaners: an assessment of effectiveness and health consequences. November 8, 2000: *http://www.epa.gov/iedweb00/pubs/ozonegen.html#TOC.*
19. United States Environmental Protection Agency. Information on asbestos: *URL:http://www.epa.gov/opptintr/asbestos/inforev.txt.*
20. U.S. Environmental Protection Agency, EPA study of asbestos containing materials in public buildings—a report to congress. Washington, DC: EPA, 1988.
21. Lundy P, Barer M. Asbestos-containing materials in New York City buildings. *Environ Res* 1992;58(1): 15–24.
22. Corn M. Airborne concentrations of asbestos in non-occupational environments. *Ann Occup Hyg* 1994;38: 495–502.
23. Lee RJ, Van Orden DR, Corn M, et al. Exposure to airborne asbestos in buildings. *Regul Toxicol Pharmacol* 1992;16(1):93–107.
24. Price B, Crump KS, Baird EC III. Airborne asbestos levels in buildings: maintenance worker and occupant exposures. *J Expo Anal Environ Epidemiol* 1992;2(3): 357–374.
25. Balmes JR, DaPonte A, Cone JE. Asbestos related disease in custodial and building maintenance workers from a large municipal school district. In: Landrigan PJ, Kazemi H, eds. The third wave of asbestos disease: exposure to asbestos in place. *Ann NY Acad Sci* 1991; 643:540–549.
26. Mlynarek S, Corn M, Blake C. Asbestos exposure of building maintenance personnel. *Regul Toxicol Pharmacol* 1996;23(3):213–224.
27. U.S. Department of Housing & Urban Development. Moving toward a lead-safe America: a report to the congress of the United States, Washington, DC, February 1997; Comprehensive and workable plan for the abatement of lead paint in privately owned housing: report to congress, Washington, DC, 1990.
28. U.S. Environmental Protection Agency. Nonoccupational pesticide exposure study (Nopes), final report. Ohio: National Service Center for Environmental Publications, 1990: *http://www.epa.gov/ncepihom/Catalog/EPA600390003.html.*
29. United States Environmental Protection Agency. Chlorpyrifos revised risk assessment and risk mitigation measures. Office of Pesticide Programs: *http://www.epa.gov/pesticides/op/chlorpyrifos/consumerqs.htm.*
30. Nero AV, et al. Distribution of airborne radon-222 concentrations in U.S. homes. *Science* 1986;234: 992–997.
31. Leung JK. Behavior of 222Rn and its progeny in high-rise buildings. *Health Phys* 1998;75(3):303–312.
32. Stolwijk JA. Assessment of population exposure and carcinogenic risk posed by volatile organic compounds in indoor air. *Risk Anal* 1990;10(1):49–57.
33. Cone J, Bush D, Stair S, et al. Indoor environmental quality. California Public Health Foundation and Hazard Evaluation System and Information Service, Department of Health Services, State of California, 1996.
34. Wallace LA. Volatile organic chemicals. In: Samet JM, Spengler JD, eds. *Indoor air pollution: a health perspective.* Baltimore: Johns Hopkins University Press, 1991:252–272.
35. Spengler JD. Sources and concentrations of indoor air pollution. In: Samet JM, Spengler JD, eds. *Indoor air pollution: a health perspective.* Baltimore: Johns Hopkins University Press, 1991:51–55.
36. Sullivan JB, Van Ert M, Krieger GR. Indoor air quality and human health. In: Sullivan JB Jr, Krieger GR, eds. *Hazardous materials toxicology: clinical principles of environmental health hazardous materials toxicology.* Baltimore: Williams & Wilkins, 1992:679.
37. Dietert RR, Hedge A. Toxicological considerations in evaluating indoor air quality and human health: impact of new carpet emissions. *Crit Rev Toxicol* 1996(26): 633–707.
38. American Society of Heating Refrigerating and Air-Conditioning Engineers. Standard 55 1981. Thermal environmental conditions for human occupancy. ASHRAE, 1981.
39. Nordstrom K, Norback D, Akselsson R. Effect of air humidification on the sick building syndrome and per-

ceived indoor air quality in hospitals: a four-month longitudinal study. *Occup Environ Med* 1994(51):683–688.
40. Levin H. Physical factors in the indoor environment. In: Selzer JM, ed. Effects of the indoor environment on health. *Occup Environ Med State of the Art Rev* 1995; 10:59–94.
41. U.S. Environmental Protection Agency. United States Public Health Service, National Environmental Health Association. Introduction to indoor air quality: a self-paced learning module. EPA/400/3-91/002, July 1991.
42. Sterling E, Sterling T. The impact of different ventilation levels and fluorescent lighting types on building illness: an experimental study. *Can J Public Health* 1983;74:385.
43. Repacholi MH. Interaction of static and extremely low frequency electric and magnetic fields with living systems: health effects and research needs. *Bioelectromagnetics* 1999;20:133–160.
44. Valberg PA. Electric and magnetic fields (EMF): what do we know about the health effects? *Int Arch Occup Environ Health* 1996;68(6):448–454.
45. Hodgson M. The sick-building syndrome. In: Seltzer JM, ed. *Effects of the indoor environment on health. Occup Med State of the Art Rev* 1995;10:167–175.
46. Menzies R, Bourbeau J. Building-related illness. *N Engl J Med* 1997;337:1524–1531.
47. Mendell MJ, Smith AB. Consistent pattern of elevated symptoms in air-conditioned office buildings: a reanalysis of epidemiologic studies. *Am J Public Health* 1990;80:1193–1199.
48. Menzies R. The effect of varying levels of outdoor air supply on the symptoms of sick building syndrome. *N Engl J Med* 1993;328:821–827.
49. General Accounting Office. School facilities: condition of America's schools. HEHS 95-61. Washington, DC: February 1, 1995.
50. Occupational Safety and Health Administration. Indoor air quality. *Fed Reg* 1994;59:15968–16039.
51. McLellan RK. Assessing residential environmental hazards. *OEM Rep* 1991;5:77–80.
52. U.S. Environmental Protection Agency, United States Public Health Service, National Environmental Health Association, Introduction to indoor air quality a reference manual. EPA/400/3-91/003, July 1991.
53. Rogers RE, Guidotti TL. Indoor air quality and building associated outbreaks. In: Dordasco EM, Demeter SL, Zenz C, eds. *Environmental respiratory diseases.* New York: Van Nostrand Reinhold, 179–207.
54. Hodgson M. Sick building syndrome. *Occup Med* 2000;15:571–585.
55. Lamarte FP, Merchant JA, Casale TB. Acute systemic reactions to carbonless copy paper associated with histamine release. *JAMA* 1988;260:242.
56. Marks JG Jr. Contact urticaria and airway obstruction from carbonless copy paper. *JAMA* 1984;252(8): 1038–1040.
57. Kanerva L. Occupational allergic contact dermatitis caused by diethylenetriamine in carbonless copy paper. *Contact Dermatitis* 1993;29(3):147–151.
58. Burge HA. Indoor air and infectious disease. In: Cone JE, Hodgson MJ, eds. Problem buildings: building-associated illness and the sick building syndrome. *Occup Med State of the Art Revs* 1989;4(4): 713–721.
59. Nardell EA, Keegan J, Cheney SA, et al. Airborne infection: theoretical limits of protection achievable by building ventilation. *Am Rev Respir Dis* 1991;144: 302–306.
60. Brundage JF, Scott RM, Lednar WM, et al. Building-associated risk of febrile acute respiratory diseases in army trainees. *JAMA* 1988;259:2108–2112.
61. Moser MR, Bender TR, Margolis HS, et al. An outbreak of influenza aboard a commercial airliner. *Am J Epidemiol* 1979;110:1.
62. Coultas DJ, Lambert WE. Carbon monoxide. In: Samet JM, Spengler JD, eds. *Indoor air pollution: a health perspective.* Baltimore: Johns Hopkins University Press, 1991:187–208.
63. Heckerling PS. Screening admissions from the emergency department for occult carbon monoxide poisoning. *Am J Emerg Med* 1990;8:301.
64. Lowry LK. The Texarcana mercury incident. *Tex Med* 1999;95(10):65–70.
65. ATSDR. National alert—a warning about continuing patterns of metallic mercury exposure. Agency for Toxic Substances and Diseases Registry: *http://www.atsdr.cdc.gov/alerts/970626.html.*
66. Solis MT. Family poisoned by mercury vapor inhalation. *Am J Emerg Med* 2000;18:599–602.
67. Agocs MM, Etzel RA, et al. Mercury exposure from interior latex paint. *N Engl J Med* 1990;323: 1096–1101.
68. Litovitz TL, Klein-Schwarz W, Caravati EM, et al. 1998 annual report of the American association of poison control centers toxic exposure surveillance system. *Am J Emerg Med* 1999;17:435–487: *http://www.aapcc.org Annual%20Reports/98Report/98%20anl%20rpt%2022 a%20and%2022b.PDF.*
69. Office of Pesticide Programs of the U.S. Environmental Protection Agency and the National Environmental Education and Training Foundation, Pesticides and National Strategies for Health Care Providers. Draft implementation plan, July 2000.
70. EPA announces elimination of all indoor uses of widely-used pesticide diazinon: begins phase-out of lawn and garden uses. December 5, 2000: *http://yosemite.epa.gov/opa/admpress.nsf/b1ab9f485b09897 2852562e7004dc686/c8cdc9ea7d5ff585852569ac007 7bd31?OpenDocument.*
71. World Health Organization. Indoor air quality: biological contaminants. WHO Regional Publications, 1988 European Series No. 31.
72. Cooley JD, Wong WC, Jumper CA, et al. Correlation between the prevalence of certain fungi and sick building syndrome. *Occup Environ Med* 1998;55(9):579–584.
73. Mahmoudi M. Sick building syndrome, III. Stachybotrys Chartarum. *J Asthma* 2000;37(2):191–198.
74. Johanning E, Biagini R, Hull D, et al. Health and immunology study following exposure to toxigenic fungi (Stachybotrys chartarum) in a water-damaged office environment. *Int Arch Occup Environ Health* 1996;68: 207–218.
75. Ammann HM. IAQ and human toxicosis: empirical evidence and theory. In: Johanning E, ed. *Bioaerosols, fungi, and mycotoxins: health effects, assessment, prevention, and control.* New York: Eastern New York Occupational and Environmental Health Center, 1999: 84–93.
76. Etzel RA, Darborn DG. Pulmonary hemorrhage among infants with exposure to toxigenic molds: an update. In: Johanning E, ed. *Bioaerosols, fungi, and mycotoxins: health effects, assessment, prevention,*

and control. New York: Eastern New York Occupational and Environmental Health Center, 1999:79–83.

76a. Centers for Disease Control and Prevention (CDC). Update: pulmonary hemorrhage/hemosiderosis among infants—Cleveland, Ohio, 1993–1996. *MMWR Morb Mortal Wkly Rep* 2000;49:180–184.

76b. American College of Occupational and Environmental Medicine. Adverse human health effects associated with molds in the indoor environment. Evidence-based position statement: http://www.acoem.org/guidelines/article.asp? ID=52.

77. Samet JM. Radon. In: Samet JM, Spengler JD, eds. *Indoor air pollution: a health perspective.* Baltimore: Johns Hopkins University Press, 1991:323–351.

78. U.S. Environmental Protection Agency. Airborne asbestos health update. EPA-600/8-84-003F. U.S. EPA Office of Health and Environmental Assessment: Research Triangle Park, NC, 1985.

79. Wilson R, Langer AM, Nolan RP, et al. Asbestos in New York City public school buildings-public policy: is there a scientific basis? *Regul Toxicol Pharmacol* 1994;20(2):161–169.

80. Schneider J, Rodelsperger K, Bruckel B, et al. Pleural mesothelioma associated with indoor pollution of asbestos. *J Cancer Res Clin Oncol* 2001;127(2):123–127.

81. Schnorr TM, Grajewskf BA, Hornung RW, et al. Video display terminals and the risk of spontaneous abortion. *N Engl J Med* 1991;3214:727–733.

82. Angelillo IF. Residential exposure to electromagnetic fields and childhood leukaemia: a meta-analysis. *Bull WHO* 1999;77(11):906–915.

83. Beers GJ. Biologic effects of low-level electromagnetic fields: current issues and controversies. *Magn Reson Imaging Clin North Am* 1998;6(4):749–774.

84. Ahlbom A. A pooled analysis of magnetic fields and childhood leukaemia. *Br J Cancer* 2000;83(5):692–698.

85. Zhang ZF, Yu SZ, Zhou GD. Indoor air pollution of coal fumes as a risk factor of stroke, Shanghai. *Am J Public Health* 1988;78(8):975–977.

86. Frampton MW, Samet JM, Utell MJ. Environmental factors and atmospheric pollutants. *Semin Respir Infect* 1991;6(4):185–193.

87. U.S. Department of Health and Human Services, Public Health Service, Centers for Disease Control. Preventing lead poisoning in young children—a statement by the centers for disease control, October 1991.

88. Centers for Disease Control and Prevention. Update: blood lead levels—United States 1991–1994. U.S. Department of Health and Human Services/Public Health Service. *MMWR* 1997 Feb 21;46(7):141–146 [published erratum appears in *MMWR* 1997 July 4;46(26):607].

89. U.S. Department of Health and Human Services, Public Health Service, Agency for Toxic Substances and Disease Registry. Case studies in environmental medicine: lead toxicity. ATSDR, 1995: *http://www.atsdr.cdc.gov HECcaselead.html.*

90. Needleman HL, Schell A, Bellinger D, et al. The long-term effects of exposure to lead in childhood: an 11-year follow-up report. *N Engl J Med* 1990;322:83–88.

91. Molhave L. Controlled experiments for studies of the sick building syndrome. In: Tucker WG, Leaderer BP, Molhave L, et al., eds. Sources of indoor air contaminants: characterizing emissions and health impacts. *Ann NY Acad Sci* 1992;641:46–54.

92. Bascom R. Differential responsiveness to irritant mixtures. In: Tucker WG, Leaderer BP, Molhave L, et al., eds. Sources of indoor air contaminants: characterizing emissions and health impacts. *Ann NY Acad Sci* 1992:641:225–247.

93. Bascom R, Kesavanathan J, Swift DL. Human susceptibility to indoor contaminants. *Occup Med* 1995;10:119–132.

94. Wargocki P, Wyon DP, Sundell J, et al. The effects of outdoor air supply rate in an office on perceived air quality, sick building syndrome (SBS) symptoms and productivity. *Indoor Air* 2000;10(4):222–236.

95. Bourbeau J. Prevalence of the sick building syndrome symptoms in office workers before and six months and three years after being exposed to a building with an improved ventilation system. *Occup Environ Med* 1997;54:49–53.

96. Seppanen OA, Fisk WJ, Mendell MJ. Association of ventilation rates and CO2 concentrations with health and other responses in commercial and institutional buildings. *Indoor Air* 1999;9:226–252.

97. Mendell MJ. Non-specific symptoms in office workers: a review and summary of the literature. *Indoor Air* 1993;4:227–236.

98. Molhave L, Bach B, Pedersen OF. Human reactions to low concentrations of volatile organic compounds. *Environ Int* 1986;12:167–175.

99. Otto D. Assessment of neurobehavioral response in humans to low-level volatile organic compound sources. *Ann NY Acad Sci* 1992;641:248–260.

100. Harrison J, Pickering CA, Faragher EB, et al. An investigation of the relationship between microbial and particulate indoor air pollution and the sick building syndrome. *Respir Med* 1992;86:225–235.

101. Wargocki P, Wyon DP, Baik YK, et al. Perceived air quality, sick building syndrome (SBS) symptoms and productivity in an office with two different pollution loads. *Indoor Air* 1999;9(3):165–179.

102. Norback D. Indoor air quality and personal factors related to the sick building syndrome. *Scand J Work Environ Health* 1990;16(2):121–128.

103. Thorn A. The sick building syndrome: a diagnostic dilemma. *Soc Sci Med* 1998;47(9):1307–1312.

104. Baker DB. Social and organizational factors in office building-associated illness. In: Cone JE, Hodgson MJ, eds. Problem buildings: building-associated illness and the sick building syndrome. *Occup Med State of the Art Rev* 1989;4(4):607–624.

105. Crawford JO. Sick building syndrome, work factors, and occupational stress. *Scand J Work Environ Health* 1996;22:243–250.

106. Hodgson MJ, Frohligher J, Permar E, et al. Symptoms and microenvironmental measures in nonproblem buildings. *J Occup Med* 1991;33:575–592.

107. Burge S, Hedge A, Wilson S, et al. Sick building syndrome: a study of 4,373 office workers. *Ann Occup Hyg* 1987;(31):493–504.

108. American College of Occupational and Environmental Medicine. Multiple chemical sensitivities: idiopathic environmental intolerance. Position statement: *http://www.acoem.org/paprguid/papersmcs.htm.*

109. Sparks PJ. Idiopathic environmental intolerances: overview. *Occup Med* 2000;15:497–510.

110. McLellan RK. Responding to chemical sensitivity in the workplace. *Indoor Air Quality Update* 1991;(4):8.

111. National Institute of Occupational Safety and Health. *Building air-quality: a guide for building owners and facility managers.* EPA/400/1-91/033. NIOSH publication No. 91-114. Washington, DC: Department of Health and Human Services, December 1991.
112. Quinlan P, Macher JM, Alevantis LE, et al. Protocol for the comprehensive evaluation of building-associated illness. In: Cone JE, Hodgson MJ, eds. Problem buildings: building-associated illness and the sick building syndrome. *Occup Med State of the Art Rev* 1989;4(4):771–797.
113. Frank AL. ATSDR case studies in environmental medicine, No. 26. Taking an environmental exposure history. U.S. Department of Health and Human Services, Public Health Service, Agency for Toxic Substances and Disease Registry, October 1992.
114. Kjaergaard S. Assessment of eye irritation in humans. In: Tucker WG, Loiterer BP, Molhave L, et al., eds. Sources of indoor air contaminants: characterizing emissions and health impacts. *Ann NY Acad Sci* 1992;641:187–198.
115. Wieslander G, Norback D, Nordstrom K, et al. Nasal and ocular symptoms, tear film stability and biomarkers in nasal lavage, in relation to building-dampness and building design in hospitals. *Int Arch Occup Environ Health* 1999;72(7):451–461.
116. Koren HS, Devlin RB. Human upper respiratory tract responses to inhaled pollutants with emphasis on nasal lavage. In: Tucker WG, et al., eds. Sources of indoor air contaminants: characterizing emissions and health impacts. *Ann NY Acad Sci* 1992;641:215–224.
117. Kitsch LS. Legal aspects of indoor air pollution. In: Samet JM, Spengler JD, eds. *Indoor air pollution: a health perspective.* Baltimore: Johns Hopkins University Press, 1991:378–397.
118. Brennan T. Untangling causation issues in law and medicine: hazardous substance litigation. *Ann Intern Med* 1987;(107):741–747.
119. Sweda EL. *Summary of legal cases regarding smoking in the workplace and other places.* Boston: Tobacco Control Resource Center, June 2000.
120. National Institute for Occupational Safety and Health. *Guidance for indoor air quality investigations.* Cincinnati: Hazard Evaluation and Technical Assistance Branch, Division of Surveillance, Hazard Evaluations and Field Studies, NIOSH, 1987.
121. McLellan RK. Identification and control of selected residential hazards. *Dis Month* 2000;46(pt 8):590–616.
122. Samimi BS. The environmental evaluation: commercial and home. *Occup Med* 1995;10:95–118.
123. Linz DH. Cluster analysis applied to building-related illness. *J Occup Environ Med* 1998;40(2):165–171.
124. Nagda NL, Rector HE, Kountz, MD. *Guidelines for monitoring indoor air quality.* New York: Hemisphere, 1987.
125. Cox CS, Wathes CM, eds. *Bioaerosols handbook.* Boca Raton, FL: CRC Lewis, 1995.
126. Hodgson MJ, Frohliger J, Permar E, et al. Symptoms and microenvironmental measures in non-problem buildings. *J Occup Med* 1991;33:527–533.
127. Odor evaluation as an investigative tool. *Indoor Air Quality Update* 1991;4:10.
128. Ventilation for acceptable indoor air quality. Atlanta: American Society of Heating, Refrigerating, and Air-Conditioning Engineers, ANSI/ASHRAE Standard 62-1999, 1999.
129. National Institute of Occupational Safety and Health. *Building air-quality: a guide for building owners and facility managers.* EPA/400/1-91/033. NIOSH publication No. 91-114. Washington, DC: Department of Health and Human Services, December 1991.
130. The American Institute of Architects. *Designing healthy buildings: indoor air quality.* Washington, DC: AIA, 1993.
131. New Hampshire Minimum Impact Development Bibliography: *http://www.nhmid.org/index.htm.*
132. Loftness V, Hartkopf V. The effects of building design and use on air quality. In: Cone JE, Hodgson MJ, eds. Problem buildings: building-associated illness and the sick building syndrome. *Occup Med State of the Art Rev* 1989;4(4):643–665.
133. Levin H. Building materials and indoor air quality. In: Cone JE, Hodgson MJ, eds. Problem buildings: building-associated illness and the sick building syndrome. *Occup Med State of the Art Rev* 1989;4(4):667–693.

FURTHER INFORMATION

National Institute of Occupational Safety and Health. *Building air-quality: a guide for building owners and facility managers.* EPA/400/1-91/033. NIOSH publication No. 91-114. Washington, DC: Department of Health and Human Services, December 1991.

An off-the-shelf, comprehensive guide for facility managers, maintenance personnel, and building investigators involved in preventing and correcting indoor air pollution problems.

Seltzer JM, ed. Effects of the indoor environment on health. *Occup Med* 1995;10:1–254.

A multidisciplinary review of what is known, not known, and needs to be known to better understand and solve the problem of adverse health effects caused by indoor environments.

Tucker WG, Leaderer BP, Molhave L, et al., eds. Sources of indoor air contaminants: characterizing emissions and health impacts. *Ann NY Acad Sci* 1992;641:1–329.

This volume of proceedings from a conference of international experts is a seminal compilation of the science of characterizing indoor air contaminants and their acute effects on humans.

United States Environmental Protection Agency. IAQ tools for schools kit. EPA document number 402-C-00-002, August 2000.

The kit shows schools how to carry out a practical plan of action to prevent and solve indoor air problems at little or no cost using straightforward activities and in-house staff.

United States Environmental Protection Agency Indoor Air Quality Information Clearinghouse.

The clearinghouse is an easily accessible, central source of information on indoor air quality, created and supported by the U.S. Environmental Protection Agency (EPA). Information is available about the following topics: indoor air pollutants and their sources; health effects of indoor air pollution; testing and measuring indoor air pollutants; controlling indoor air pollutants; constructing and maintaining homes and buildings to minimize indoor air quality problems; existing standards and guidelines related to indoor air quality; and general information on federal and state legislation. The clearinghouse can be accessed by phone at 1-(800)-438-4318 or by e-mail at *iaqinfo@aol.com.*

54

Medical Aspects of Environmental Emergencies

Jonathan B. Borak

There is a wide range of potential environmental emergencies. Some result from forces and processes that are wholly natural, such as storms (e.g., hurricanes and tornados and blizzards), geologic disturbances (e.g., earthquakes and volcanoes), and epidemics. Others are more closely tied to human activities. Among the most relevant and common of such manmade emergencies are industrial accidents, which are the focus of this chapter.

Emergency response planning is required at most work sites under a variety of federal and state regulations. Traditionally, occupational physicians have not been central to such planning. However, recent requirements contain specific medical components and involvement, and, as a result, occupational physicians are likely to be increasingly involved in the development and implementation of work-site emergency response plans. For that reason, physicians should be knowledgeable about the various emergency planning requirements that may affect their facilities. Also, as residents of the communities that house such facilities, physicians should understand the implications for community residents of accidents occurring at neighboring industrial facilities.

For the most part, work-site emergency planning requirements are found in the standards and regulations of the Occupational Safety and Health Administration (OSHA) and the Environmental Protection Agency (EPA). The focus of those two agencies is fundamentally different. Because OSHA is primarily concerned with the health and safety of workers, its emergency focus is on protecting employees, including emergency response personnel. By contrast, the EPA's concern is primarily protection of the "outside" world, that is, people, other living things, and the environment surrounding work sites.

Despite differing perspectives of OSHA and the EPA, their actual emergency planning requirements overlap and cross-reference one another. As a result, it is of only limited usefulness to categorize requirements according to the issuing agency. Likewise, there is little practical benefit in distinguishing "work-site emergencies" from "environmental emergencies" because many incidents simultaneously involve both employees and the environment.

A more practical approach is to consider the regulatory requirements in light of the response functions and activities that are actually mandated in the event of an emergency. This chapter takes such an approach. Work-site emergency response requirements of relevance to occupational physicians are grouped and discussed according to the following types of response functions and activities:

1. First aid and emergency medical care
2. Protection of emergency response personnel
3. Provision of emergency medical information
4. Medical surveillance
5. Coordination with community health care providers
6. Emergency response planning guidelines for chemical releases

FIRST AID AND EMERGENCY MEDICAL CARE

The most basic requirement for work-site emergency planning is OSHA's requirement that there be ready access to first aid for all injured employees. If there is no infirmary, clinic, or hospital near the workplace that is used for the treatment of all injured employees, then a staff person should be adequately trained to render first aid. First aid supplies approved by the consulting physician should be readily available [29 CFR 1019.151 (b)].

Although subject to interpretation, it is generally understood that "first aid" includes at least care for victims of trauma, response to corrosive and thermal injuries, and cardiopulmonary resuscitation (CPR). Many work sites meet this requirement by providing certification training to designated employees in first aid and CPR according to guidelines of the American Red Cross or the National Safety Council.

The need for training and the number of individuals to be trained is determined in part by the proximity of the work site to other sources of emergency care. As a rule of thumb, first aid and CPR must be available to employees within 5 minutes. Because even the most effective community emergency medical service (EMS) often takes longer than 5 minutes to respond to an emergency, most work sites must plan to provide first aid and CPR. In large facilities, it may be necessary to station trained individuals in multiple sites to ensure a prompt response for all employees.

The role of the consulting occupational physician in this setting is clear. At a minimum, the physician must approve the equipment and supplies used by first-aid providers. More logically, the physician would also oversee the training of emergency responders and ensure that their training and the number of responders meet OSHA requirements. In addition, special requirements for protection from blood-borne pathogens for first responders necessitate medical oversight.

Similar but somewhat broader requirements are found in OSHA's Hazardous Waste Operations and Emergency Response Standard (29 CFR 1910.120), which deals with the health and safety of hazardous waste site workers and response personnel at hazardous materials emergencies. The EPA has issued identical rules (Worker Protection Standards for Hazardous Waste Operations and Emergency Response, 40 CPR 311), which apply to all workers and emergency response volunteers otherwise exempted from the OSHA standard.

OSHA and EPA require that an emergency response plan be developed and implemented before the start of hazardous waste and emergency response operations at a facility: "The employer shall develop an emergency response plan for emergencies which shall address, as a minimum...emergency medical treatment and first aid" [29 CFR 1910.120(1)]. These concerns relate to the effects of exposure to hazardous materials and the consequences of hazardous materials emergencies, but such concerns are broad and far-reaching. The toxic effects of hazardous materials exposure can affect most of the body's organ systems. Thermal injuries and burns are common consequences of these incidents because nearly 65% of all hazardous materials are flammable. Explosions and trauma are also common outcomes. Accordingly, emergency response plans should include relatively comprehensive medial policies, protocols, and procedures for providing emergency care at the work site under a variety of conditions.

PROTECTION OF EMERGENCY RESPONSE PERSONNEL

Emergency response personnel are exposed to greater variety and severity of health risks than are most other employees. For example, fire fighters regularly risk thermal injuries, toxic exposures, and trauma. Likewise, emergency medical technicians (EMTs) and emergency physicians are at greater risk of blood-borne diseases than are most other health care workers. Employers are obliged by OSHA (and, in some cases, by the EPA) to provide acceptable levels of protection to those personnel. The occupational physician plays an important role in ensuring that adequate protection is available to response personnel.

Use of respirators is one example. OSHA requires that self-contained breathing apparatus (SCBA) be provided to and used by members of industrial fire brigades (29 CFR 1910.156) and emergency personnel responding to hazardous materials releases (29 CFR 1910.120). That latter requirement is also found in the EPA's Worker Protection Standards (40 CFR 311). Employers must ensure that response personnel are physically able to use the provided equipment, a process requiring the professional involvement of a physician.

Persons should not be assigned to tasks requiring use of respirators unless it has been determined that they are physically able to perform the work and use the equipment. The local physician should determine what health and physical conditions are pertinent. The respirator user's medical status should be reviewed periodically (for instance, annually) [29 CFR 1910.134 (b)].

These requirements are commonly guided by consensus standard designed by organizations such as the National Fire Protection Association (see Further Information, below).

Medical concerns also arise when emergency responders wear personal protective equipment (PPE), especially impervious clothing and encapsulating suits. By design, such PPE are impermeable to water, and therefore the wearer quickly loses the temperature control benefits normally derived from sweating. The higher the ambient temperature and the longer the suits are worn, the greater is the risk of dehydration and heat stress. A protocol to monitor response personnel, including at least some measure of vital signs before donning of PPE and after PPE removal, should be developed, along with criteria for referral for medical evaluation.

A third example of protection for emergency response personnel is OSHA's Bloodborne Pathogens Standard (29 CFR 1910.1030), which requires employers to develop an exposure control plan, including training and the availability of hepatitis B vaccination for employees who, as a result of performing their duties, risk contact exposure of skin, eye, and mucous membranes or parenteral exposure to blood and other potentially infectious materials.

Employees who provide first aid are specifically included in this requirement. Training and vaccination must be provided in advance of exposure to employees who staff first-aid stations, health care workers, and those who are members of emergency response and public safety organizations. For employees who provide first aid only as a collateral duty to other routine work assignments, training must be provided in advance of exposure, but vaccination may be provided within 24 hours of exposure to blood or other infectious materials.

Provision of vaccinations and postexposure follow-up are medical functions for which the occupational physician should be responsible. The employer should ensure that all medical evaluations and procedures including the hepatitis B vaccination series and postexposure evaluation and follow-up, including prophylaxis, are performed by or under the supervision of a licensed physician or by or under the supervision of another licensed health care professional [29 CFR 1910.1030 (f)].

PROVISION OF EMERGENCY MEDICAL INFORMATION

Work sites at which hazardous substances are processed or stored should have detailed medical information available on the specific health effects of exposure to those substances. Facility emergency response plans should include protocols and procedures for medical treatment of exposure victims. Facility managers should be prepared to promptly provide detailed medical information, including treatment recommendations, to community response organizations in the event of a hazardous materials emergency. The quantity and type of information required exceed those commonly found on Material Safety Data Sheets.

The most explicit example of the need for such detailed information is the Emergency Notification requirement in Title III of EPA's Superfund Amendments and Reauthorization Act (Title III). That requirement applies to spills or releases of hazardous substance in excess of their "reporting quantities." ("Reporting quantity" is defined for extremely hazardous substances in Title I and for hazardous substances in EPA's Comprehensive Environmental Response, Compensation, and Liability Act, CERCLA.)

In the event of such a spill or release exceeding the reporting quantity, the facility must immediately notify local and state emergency response officials of all local areas and states "likely to be affected by the release." Along with information identifying the released substance and the quantity released, the emergency notification must contain detailed medical information such as "any known or anticipated acute or chronic health risks associated with the emergency, and, where appropriate, advice regarding medical attention necessary for exposed individuals" [40 CFR 355.40 (b)].

Initially, the required notification may be provided orally, but written notice must be given "as soon as practicable." Facilities that use or store quantities of hazardous substances should anticipate the possible need for such information and arrange for its preparation before, rather than following, emergencies. Occupational physicians should be involved in compiling and preparing the appropriate emergency medical information for those facilities at which they work or provide services.

Provision of emergency medical information is also required by OSHA (29 CFR 1910.120) and the EPA (40 CFR 311) in their parallel rules for hazardous waste and emergency response operations. Both agencies require emergency response plans that address "emergency medical treatment" of hazardous materials exposure victims. In turn, the emergency plans are an important component of employee training that is also required. Occupational physicians working at or consulting facilities that must comply with these regulations should be aware of the health-related information contained in those training programs. Physicians should also review and approve any emergency treatment protocols developed for implementation at the site and included in facility training programs.

MEDICAL SURVEILLANCE

OSHA (29 CFR 1910.120) and the EPA (40 CFR 311) require employers to develop medical surveillance programs for emergency response personnel and other employees involved in hazardous materials emergencies. Members of "organized and designated

HAZMAT teams" and others trained to the OSHA/EPA level of hazardous materials specialist must receive baseline medical examinations, follow-up examinations at least every 12 to 24 months and at termination of employment, or reassignment if the previous examination was more that 6 months before. Medical consultation must also be provided to any emergency response personnel who "exhibit signs or symptoms which may have resulted" from exposure to hazardous substance during an emergency.

Medical examinations and consultations required by the regulations should include medical and work history (or updated history if one is in the employee's file) with special emphasis on symptoms related to the handling of hazardous substances and health hazards, and to fitness for duty including the ability to wear any required PPE under conditions (i.e., temperature extremes) that may be expected at the work site. "The content of medical examinations or consultations...shall be determined by the attending physician" [29 CFR 1910.120(f)].

The employer must provide to the attending physician a copy of the relevant OSHA or EPA standard, a description of the employee's duties (that is, the emergency response duties of the individual), known or anticipated exposure levels, a description of the PPE available to the employee, and past medical history.

The physician must render a written opinion as to whether the employee has suffered a condition that increases the risk of "material impairment of the employee's health" from emergency response work or from use of respirators. It seems apparent that physicians cannot accomplish this specific task without an adequate understanding of the component roles and functions of the facility's emergency response program, the hazards and risks of the PPE available at an emergency, and the potential hazards to be encountered during emergencies at the facility.

COORDINATION WITH COMMUNITY HEALTH CARE PROVIDERS

Important components of facility emergency response plans are explicit agreements between the facility and the surrounding community's emergency response organizations, including EMS organizations and hospitals. Such agreements are required under the EPA's Resource Conservation and Recovery Act (RCRA) (40 CFR 265 Subpart D), which mandates a contingency plan at facilities that generate, store, or process hazardous wastes. The facility contingency plan must contain actual letters of agreement signed by those organizations. If a community organization is unwilling to assist the facility, the facts of that refusal must be included in the plan.

Occupational physicians serve an important function by assisting the managers of industrial facilities to determine the community health care providers with which those facilities should develop agreements and by defining the parameters of those agreements. In communities with multiple hospitals, for example, it is often best to select and favor only one or a few for purposes of emergency planning and response.

The selection of such a hospital may reflect proximity to the facility, but other considerations should include the availability of specialized emergency care, such as trauma specialists, burn specialists, and toxicologists. In many communities, specific hospitals have been designated as providers of specialty care (e.g., trauma centers, burn centers, poison control centers) and, where appropriate, those hospitals should be recognized and included as part of the emergency planning conducted at local industrial facilities.

It is important that occupational physicians correctly understand the abilities and limitations of the hospitals and of the EMS that serve the facilities at which they work or to which they provide medical services. For example, many hospital emergency departments lack the equipment, knowledge, and experience to care for patients with toxic chemical exposures. In general, emergency physicians have only limited knowledge of industrial toxicology, and most poison control centers have relatively limited experience in responding to industrial emergencies. Facilities that manufacture or use large quantities of toxic chemicals should determine which local hospital is most capable of managing acute exposure victims and should develop agreements with that hospital to care for exposed workers. In some locations, it may be appropriate to designate one hospital for the care of exposed workers, a second for workers suffering significant burns, and another for trauma care. These items should be clearly stated in the contingency plan.

There can also be large differences among EMSs. Advanced services staffed with paramedics employ medications, endotracheal intubation, and cardiac monitoring, but basic services offer little more than first aid. Most EMSs, both advanced and basic, are not prepared to manage victims of toxic chemical exposures. Most EMT training courses devote little or no time to hazardous materials. Most EMSs lack decontamination protocols, carry no decontamination materials, and do not provide chemical protective equipment to the personnel. Although the National Fire Protection Association (NFPA) has established minimum competencies for EMS personnel responding to hazardous materials emergencies (NFPA standard no. 473], that standard is voluntary and currently ignored by many services and states. OSHA has shown little enthusiasm for extending the protection of its Hazardous Waste Operations and Emergency Response Standard (29 CFR 1910.120) to EMS personnel.

Physicians should determine that local EMSs can provide the scope emergency response support that might be required by the industrial facilities at which they work or to which they provide services. In many cases, those facilities can encourage and assist their EMS neighbors to develop necessary protocols and procedures. For example, industrial facilities using quantities of hydrofluoric acid should provide calcium gluconate gel to local EMSs along with appropriate training in its use for decontamination and burn care. Likewise, facilities that use or manufacture quantities of phenol should provide an appropriate skin cleanser such as polyethylene glycol 300 and training in its use.

EMERGENCY RESPONSE PLANNING GUIDELINES FOR CHEMICAL RELEASES

The accidental release of industrial chemicals can pose emergency hazards far beyond the point of release, most notably when the chemicals become airborne. Both industry- and community-based emergency planners must anticipate such releases, including consideration of the quantities that might be released, the direction of prevailing winds likely to blow the chemical plume, and the proximity of vulnerable populations and institutions. By means of computerized dispersion models, which estimate the likely path, migration rate, and dispersion behavior of chemical plumes, it is possible to estimate the expected levels and duration of exposures that will result at various locations downwind. That type of information is the first step in deciding whether it is necessary to evacuate or shelter community residents and if so, whom.

For such response planning, however, it is also necessary to determine the particular levels and durations of exposure likely to prove harmful. Unlike dispersion modeling, which is the primary domain of engineers and meteorologists, the setting of appropriate exposure levels is an activity dependent on medical and toxicological expertise. The American Industrial Hygiene Association developed the first generation of such exposure limits as Emergency Response Planning Guidelines. More recently, an international program has been developed under the leadership of the EPA to develop acute exposure guideline levels (AEGLs). The U.S. National Advisory Committee that develops AEGLs includes physicians representing the American College of Occupational and Environmental Medicine (ACOEM) and the American Association of Poison Control Centers and the actual exposure limits are peer reviewed by the National Research Council.

For each chemical considered, AEGLs are developed for exposure durations of 30 minutes, 1 hour, 4 hours, and 8 hours, and for each of three levels of toxicity. AEGL-1 is the airborne concentration of a substance above which it is predicted that there might be transient discomfort or irritation, but no disabling or persistent effects. AEGL-2 is the airborne concentration of a substance above which it is predicted that there might be disabling effects or impaired ability to escape. AEGL-3 is the airborne concentration of a substance above which life-threatening effects may occur.

Physicians can play an important role in facility and community emergency response planning by familiarizing themselves with these exposure limits and helping managers and community planners to better understand which chemical releases require extraordinary precautions. They can also provide an important and often reassuring perspective for community residents to understand which releases do and which do not pose meaningful health hazards.

FURTHER INFORMATION

Borak J, Callan M, Abbott W. *Hazardous materials exposure: emergency response and patient care.* Englewood Cliffs, NJ: Prentice Hall, 1991.

A concise overview of planning issues for hazardous materials emergencies that can serve as a manual for OSHA-mandated training.

Dynes RR. *Community emergency planning: false assumptions and inappropriate analogies.* Newark, DE: Disaster Research Center, University of Delaware, 1990.

A critical review of planning methodologies and models for community emergency planning.

Feldstein BD, et al. Disaster training for emergency physicians in the United States: a systems approach. *Ann Emerg Med* 1985;14:36.

A review of existing training systems for emergency physicians and a proposed approach to enhance capabilities for response to disasters of all sorts.

Leonard RB, et al. SARA (Superfund Amendments and Reauthorization Act) Title III: implications for emergency physicians. *Ann Emerg Med* 1989;18:1212.

An overview of the SARA legislation with particular emphasis on those components of relevance to physicians and hospital emergency departments.

National Research Council. *Standing operating procedures for developing acute exposure guidelines for hazardous chemicals.* Washington, DC: National Academy Press, 2001.

National Research Council. *Acute exposure guideline levels for selected airborne chemicals: vol 1.* Washington, DC: National Academy Press, 2000.
The rationale and process for development of AEGL exposure limits and the first volume of compiled AEGL values along with background and justification for each.

NFPA. *Competencies for EMS personnel responding to hazardous materials incidents: NFPA standard No. 473.* Quincy, MA: National Fire Protection Association, 2002.
Recommended training and performance standards for EMTs and paramedics involved in emergency medical response to victims of chemical exposure.

55

Emergency Response to Environmental Incidents

L. Kristian Arnold

The emergency response to environmental incidents combines the principles of occupational medicine (OM) and emergency medicine (EM). Considering the scope and purpose of this handbook, this chapter uses the knowledge bases of both disciplines to provide a practical resource for the OM practitioner. Since many practitioners of OM do not have formal training or are new to the field, this chapter focuses on their needs, although it is also a useful review for the specialist. This chapter also presents EM concepts and resources.

The field of environmental medicine continues to develop in scope. In fact, the definition of the environment has become increasingly global in relation to the activities of OM physicians. No longer does this term refer only to the physical and psychological milieu of the worker or to the confines of the property of the employer. As the geographic sphere of business responsibility has expanded, so have the responsibilities of the OM specialist. This responsibility extends into the local and regional community, especially regarding adverse effects from "incidents" involving hazardous materials (HazMats). This additional role includes reducing liability, especially if operations involve handling of hazardous substances. Government agencies and community residents have filed successful suits against corporate officials, some of whom have been sentenced to prison terms. This expanded scope and liability place a burden on the OM practitioner to encourage and assist in the development of safe operating policies and procedures, including emergency response plans (ERPs), to minimize the impact of adverse events involving hazardous substances. With passage of the Superfund Amendments and Reauthorization Act (SARA) of 1986, among others, Congress established requirements regarding accidental releases of HazMats.

As the concept of the environment continues to expand, so do the lists of substances that represent a potential threat to human health and the ecosystem. Under certain circumstances, substances that are ordinarily considered benign may become a threat. For example, a tank car of cooking oil overturned and burst in Colorado, spilling the oil into a local reservoir. Secondary to such incidents, the federal agencies with appropriate oversight continue to revise designated lists and measures regarding toxic materials. There are multiple listings of regulated hazardous substances and wastes that frequently cross-reference each other (Table 55.1).

Since the mid-1970s, emergency medical services (EMS) throughout the United States have developed plans to cope with the medical aspects of disasters and unexpected events that overwhelm the routine capabilities of local and regional emergency medical response systems. Once there are victims, such situations, known as mass casualty incidents (MCIs), are classified into three categories (Table 55.2). Preparation for MCIs necessitates cooperation of multiple agencies from the local and regional levels, including treatment facilities. Increasing attention has been turned to dealing with disasters that have as a principal component exposure to HazMats.

The potential for mishaps is underscored by the extent of HazMats in use. Government data gathered to support the Hazardous Materials Uniform Safety Act of 1990 indicated that around 4 billion tons of regulated materials are transported annually and that approximately 500,000 movements of such materials occur daily (1). In 1999, there were 17,069 transportation incidents involving HazMats reported to the Department of Transportation (DOT) on the Hazardous Materials Incident Report Form 5800 (1). From 1990 through 1997, the Agency for Toxic

TABLE 55.1. *Listings of U.S. Government designated toxic and hazardous substances and wastes*

Department of transportation	
Hazardous substances	49 CFR 172.101 and appendices
Hazardous wastes	49 CFR 171.8
Environmental Protection Agency	
Characteristics of hazardous waste	40 CFR 261.20–24
Lists of hazardous wastes	40 CFR 261.30–33
Designation of hazardous substances	40 CFR 302.4
Extremely hazardous substances and their threshold planning quantities	40 CFR 355, Appendices A and B
Occupational Safety and Health Administration	
Hazardous substances	29 CFR 1910.120.(a).(3).(A)–(D)
Toxic and hazardous substances	29 CFR 1910, Subpart Z

Online reference: Code of Federal Regulations. National Archives and Records Administration. *http://www.access.gpo.gov/nara/acfr.*

Substances and Disease Registry (ATSDR) logged over 27,000 events of HazMats releases with over 31,000 substances released resulting in 122 deaths and over 11,000 victims (2). Although these figures are enormous by any standard, relatively routine efforts such as moving a 55-gallon drum across a plant with a forklift are tabulated as well as driving a 10,000-gallon tank truck through a town. To regulate interstate transportation, DOT uses nine major classifications of regulated materials, including nearly 3,000 individual substances (Table 55.3) (3). The final DOT category, "Other," contains many seemingly innocuous substances that represent hazards on the ecosystem level, as in the cooking oil incident cited above.

As governmental bodies enact stricter measures regarding the disposition of chemical wastes, the clandestine transport, storage, and dumping of such products is likely to increase. Transportation of HazMats has local as well as international implications. Border regions between countries with different levels of regulation present a particular problem. Children along the Rio Grande river, for example, have been known to get "high" by sniffing glowing green chunks of solidified solvents found along the river border (4). In El Paso, Texas, an anonymous tip led to the discovery of four abandoned tractor-trailer rigs loaded with 175 55-gallon drums of polychlorinated biphenyls.

Incidents related to unauthorized transport of HazMats may also be due to ignorance of the shipper as exemplified in the following incident. A passenger checked, without declaring the contents, an ice chest containing two 1-gallon plastic bottles of 35% hydrogen peroxide on a Northwest Airlines flight. During flight the solution leaked, spilling into the cargo bay and onto other luggage and sacks of U.S. mail. At the flight destination, baggage handlers, thinking the wet luggage had water on it, were contaminated with resultant hand burns. Then some of the secondarily contaminated luggage and the leaking containers were transferred to 13 other flights. Prior to takeoff of the flight destined to receive the ice chest, the ramp employees had begun to complain of tingling and whiteness of their hands. The ice chest was identified as the source and off-loaded from the connecting flight prior to takeoff. All destinations of flights with potentially contaminated luggage were notified so that baggage handlers would wear gloves. Despite a notice of concern regarding the fire hazard of concentrated hydrogen peroxide by one of the airport fire department responders at the airport of initial identification of the incident, no fire hazard warning was

TABLE 55.2. *Classification of mass casualty incidents*

Level I	Manageable with resources available within the locality with alterations in normal operations
Level II	Significant numbers of casualties that exceed normal medical response capability of local community
Level III	Medical disaster—overwhelms capabilities of local and regional resources, exceeds capacity of available multijurisdictional medical, mutual aid—state/federal support

TABLE 55.3. *Department of transportation regulated substances classification*

Explosives
Gases (flammable and nonflammable)
Flammable liquids
Flammable solids
Oxidizers and organic peroxides
Poisons and infectious agents
Radioactive materials
Corrosives
Other regulated materials

transmitted to either the pilots in flight or the receiving airports. At Seattle airport, on initially opening the baggage compartment, baggage handlers noted smoke. They backed away and an equipment service employee, without any protective equipment, entered the compartment, retrieving two smoldering suitcases. Shortly thereafter he was nauseated, necessitating hospital evaluation with no apparent lasting ill effects (5). Although the clandestine transport of HazMats may not seem to involve the occupational physician, the expertise of the specialty is valuable in preparing transportation employees to respond appropriately in face of an emergency release.

The threat of intentional release of toxic or infectious substances has assumed a prominent position in the discussion of potential HazMats incidents. Although OM specialists, when considering events such as the release of sarin gas in the Tokyo subway in 1995, may initially wonder how they may be involved in a deliberate release, the evidence is clear that work sites are targets of violent attacks. At the time of this writing, most violent attacks at work sites in the U.S. have been carried out with firearms. It is totally conceivable, however, that an attacker might employ a biologic or chemical weapon with or without an explosive charge. In January 2001, detectives in London uncovered a plot to produce sarin and release it in the subway (6). Additionally, intentional releases at work sites may not be initially noted as such, increasing the difficulty in identifying the actual dangers to employees. A group of teenagers released pepper gas in several stores in a 3-mile radius in San Jose, California, during Christmas holiday shopping in 2000. The source of the store occupants' complaints of eye irritation was not identified until surveillance videotapes were reviewed, which showed three youths releasing a spray canister (7). Once again, the role of the OM physician is largely in preparing unsuspecting employees to respond appropriately to potential hazardous material emergencies. In cases such as this, the intentional release of pepper gas in a public space, the appropriate employee ERP should be to execute a predetermined evacuation and 911-notification plan in an orderly fashion that is safe for the employees as well as for visitors or customers in their location. In situations of such apparent intentional releases, first responders as well as professional emergency responders must always be attentive to the possibility of secondary devices. Explosive ordnance disposal (EOD) personnel trained to deal with biologic and chemical weapons should be included in emergency response teams (ERTs) responding to suspected intentional releases. In response to the National Defense Authorization Act for 1997, Title XIV, Defense Against Weapons of Mass Destruction, Subtitle A, Section 1417 (8), the Federal Emergency Management Agency (FEMA) has established the Rapid Response Information System (RRIS) as an Internet-accessible resource for response to the intentional release of chemical, biologic, or radioactive materials (9).

A number of well-known catastrophes have occurred due to the release of HazMats. In December 1984, water entry into a storage tank containing methyl isocyanate (MIC) in Bhopal, India, resulted in release of a cloud of toxic gases. Controversy still exists about whether the MIC or various reaction products such as hydrogen cyanide actually resulted in the deaths and injuries. Even the number of deaths directly related to the event remains uncertain; official government figures estimate about 1,800 deaths, but other sources estimate between 2,500 and 5,000 deaths. Despite the mortality uncertainties, within 24 hours following the release 90,000 people were evaluated by health care personnel. Due to uncertainty regarding the agent responsible for the toxic effects, most patients received only symptomatic management (10). In this case, a complete lack of either a plant or regional response plan, coupled with an inadequate understanding of the potential toxicity of the release, resulted in the susceptible populations not being notified about precautionary measures.

In Springfield, Massachusetts, during a heavy rainstorm, water leaked through the ceiling of a warehouse onto fiber drums storing defective swimming pool chlorination crystals. The resultant heat released from the reaction ignited the paper drums and other warehouse materials, causing a fire. A cloud of chlorine gas was released. That night, during another rainstorm, the same series of events occurred with a second release of chlorine gas! About 25,000 people were evacuated from the surrounding area. Several firemen suffered inhalation injuries and skin damage, but no civilian injuries occurred. Because the com-

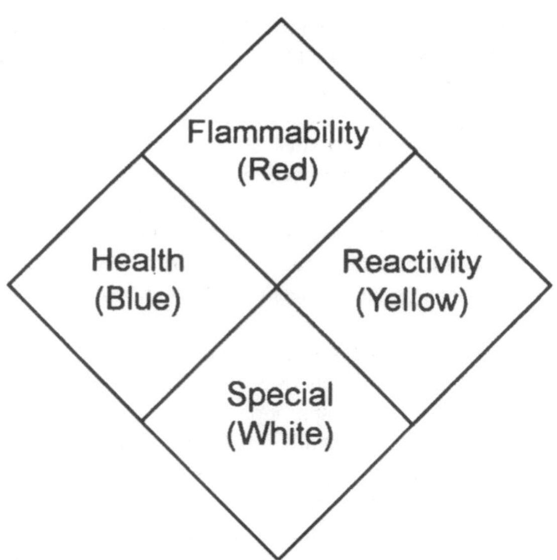

FIG. 55.1. National Fire Protection Association 704 Diamond. Each field except "Special" has a number to indicate the relative degree of danger, with 1 indicating the least and 4 indicating the most dangerous. The "Special" field has modification indicators, for example, OX = oxidizer. A full color version with the rating key is available for viewing on the Internet at *www.orcbs.msu.edu,* under "Chemical Safety."

pany failed to report the release to the National Response Center (NRC) and the local emergency planning committee (LEPC),[1] it was eventually sued by the federal government and fined $89,840 in civil penalties. The Environmental Protection Agency (EPA) has delineated levels of penalties for failure to report releases. Failure to report may result in fines of as much as $25,000 per day. If guilty parties are found to have "knowingly and willfully" not complied with the reporting guidelines, they may be subject to a prison term of up to 2 years (5 years on repeat conviction)! (11).

Frequently such incidents have multiple components. For example, in February 1989, a runaway 48-car railroad train crashed into a three-unit engine in a rail yard on the outskirts of Helena, Montana, after going 12 miles downhill from the continental divide. On impact, a car filled with hydrogen peroxide exploded, which led to other explosions when derailed cars struck propane tanks placed along the track to fuel switch heaters. The resulting explosions caused extensive property damage, loss of electricity to 37,000 people, and resulted in evacuation of 2,000 people at 4:30 a.m. in frigid temperatures (−53°F, with −85°F wind chill!). The fire was so intense that response personnel were unable to approach close enough to the tank cars to read any of the identifying placards (Fig. 55.1)[2]. In addition, there was significant concern about the potential for further danger from other rail cars in the yard due to their proximity to the fire. Again, there was no loss of life or serious injury, a fortuitous outcome, since a major manufacturer in the area uses thousands of gallons of sulfuric acid daily with shipments arriving by rail. Hence the possibility of the fire affecting tank cars loaded with sulfuric acid in the rail yard was also feared.

Although many incidents involve primarily one worker, the events may contaminate other workers or rescue personnel. Hydrofluoric (HF) acid, an etching agent used in the manufacture of computer chips, is highly corrosive and binds calcium. A worker was splashed with the agent on his upper body while working at a chip manufacturer in Massachusetts. Decontamination was an issue because of the risk of HF on the victim's clothing and in the surrounding area affecting others. Unfortunately, the worker died within 4 hours of arrival at the hospital despite appropriate treatment by massive calcium infusion.

[1]Section 103 of the Comprehensive Environmental Response, Compensation, and Liability Act (CERCLA) requires immediate reporting of releases of hazardous substances to the NRC. Section 304 of SARA Title III requires reporting in writing to the LEPC.

[2]Identification of contents of transportation vehicles is done through systems of placards and labels combined with the waybill carried on the carrier at the time of transport. The National Fire Protection Association (NFPA) has developed a system using a diamond divided into four smaller diamonds with each field representing different characteristics (Fig. 55.1). DOT has a system of specific labels and placards for different classes of HazMats. The United Nations has developed a system of numerical classification.

The above examples point out many of the settings dealing with HazMats, including (a) an in-house worker trained to respond to errors or mishaps or assist co-workers while maintaining their own safety; (b) cooperative planning between community representatives and facilities that pose risks to the community and residents; (c) cooperative planning among a manufacturing site, a transport system/facility, and community agencies; and (d) preparation of employees for unexpected accidental or intentional releases of HazMats. In each situation, the OM physician has a significant contribution to make. It is essential that the physician have a firm understanding of the toxicity of materials used at various sites to properly advise the planning for such emergencies. A well-developed and rehearsed plan, however, is essential for responding appropriately to the types of incidents that may occur, including accidental exposures at a fixed site, or in the transportation and storage of HazMats.

REGULATORY AUTHORITY

Since the mid-1970s, a number of federal statutes have been enacted that have direct relevance to dealing with the management of HazMat incidents. The most encompassing, in relation to employees at a work site with potential exposure to HazMats, is Title III of SARA, Title M (12). SARA was enacted as an amendment to the Comprehensive Environmental Response, Compensation, and Liability Act of 1980 (CERCLA), the original Superfund Act (13). Title III is commonly known as the Emergency Planning and Community Right-to-Know Act (EPCRA). This legislation mandated the Occupational Safety and Health Administration (OSHA) to develop regulations regarding HazMats handling, which appears as OSHA's final rule for Hazardous Waste Operations and Emergency Response (HAZWOPER) published as regulations in 29 CFR 1910.120 (14). The majority of the regulations in this section are directed at operations conducted at hazardous waste sites, particularly Superfund sites. Subsection (q) addresses non–waste sites. It covers all "emergency response operations for releases of, or substantial threats of releases of, hazardous substances without regard to the location of the hazard" (15). The foundations for paragraph (q) are in section 303 of SARA Title III (16).

SARA Title III, section 311, requires filing Material Safety Data Sheets (MSDSs) or a chemical information list with the appropriate LEPC, the state emergency response commission (SERC), and the local fire department (17). This section aids in planning for community response and promoting public awareness of HazMats present in the community.

Section 304 of SARA Title III (EPCRA) requires immediate reporting of accidental spills or releases of hazardous substances to a designated community emergency coordinator for the LEPC and to the SERC for any areas likely to be affected by the release. Additional reporting requirements can be found in several regulatory statutes including the Resource Conservation and Recovery Act (RCRA), CERCLA, and the Clean Water Act. These requirements are codified by the EPA in Title 40 of the Code of Federal Regulations (Table 55.4). All releases equal to or greater than the designated reportable quantity, whether into water, air, or ground are to be reported to the NRC per these EPA regulations.[3]

[3]The NRC is a division of DOT managed by the Coast Guard. Its jurisdiction covers the 50 states, the Virgin Islands, Puerto Rico, Guam, and the Pacific Island Governments (Samoa and Northern Mariana). The telephone number for reporting is 800-424-8802, or *www.nrc.uscg.mil.*

TABLE 55.4. *Hazardous substance release reporting regulations*[a]

Hazardous waste[b]	
Generators	40 CFR 262.34(d)(5)(iv)(C)
Transport	40 CFR 263.30(c)
TSD facilities	40 CFR 264.56(d)(2)
TSD facilities	40 CFR 265.56(d)(2)
Hazardous substances[c]	
Increase in continuous release	40 CFR 302.6
Noncontinuous release	40 CFR 302.6

[a]As codified by the Environmental Protection Agency.
[b]Mandated by the Solid Waste Disposal Act as amended by the Resource Conservation and Recovery Act of 1976, 42 USC 6901 et seq.
[c]As mandated by the Comprehensive Environmental Response, Compensation, and Liability Act of 1980 and the Clean Water Act.

Regulation of transportation of HazMats is addressed largely through Public Law 101-615 (PL 101-615) entitled "Hazardous Material Transportation Uniform Safety Act of 1990." This law was passed as an amendment to the Hazardous Materials Transportation Act of 1975 since the original law did not address a number of issues such as precedence of jurisdiction and training of response personnel. The regulations generated by PL 101-615 appear in volume 49 of the Code of Federal Regulations (CFR) in various sections. Section 172.604 of Title 49 CFR, for example, requires that any company shipping HazMats, whether intra- or interstate, provide a 24-hour emergency contact number on the shipping papers. Internet access to the CFR volumes via the Government Printing Office (18) and the DOT (19) allows easy access to review the various codes.

International standards vary greatly. The European Union (EU), for example, has worked hard to establish pan-European standards. This has led to heated political discussions. At the time of this writing European standards are not as well codified as corresponding regulations in the U.S. Most of the newly independent states and developing countries have not yet addressed these issues. The International Maritime Organization (IMO) has generated a set of codes for ocean shipping of HazMats that are subscribed to by over 150 countries, accounting for 98% of gross world tonnage. The DOT Web site offers several links to international regulatory agencies (20).

The right-to-know sections of SARA Title III are a starting point for guidelines for the training of workers in handling HazMats. These same sections also address community awareness as they refer to the filing of MSDSs and hazardous substance inventories with the LEPCs where they will be accessible to members of the community (21). As noted above, paragraph (q) of OSHA regulations 1910.120 addresses guidelines for workers involved in the emergency response to HazMats mishaps.

DEVELOPMENT OF AN EMERGENCY RESPONSE PLAN

Any facility or work site that handles HazMats is required to develop an ERP consistent with the same regulations that govern reporting of releases as well as other EPA and OSHA regulations. The first decision to be made for any organization using HazMats is whether their own employees should participate in responses to releases, since OSHA regulations allow reliance on outside responders (22). For small installations with good community support, the best course of action may be to simply have an OSHA-compliant emergency action plan in place that refers all but the smallest of releases to outside agencies (23). The cost of outside contractors is a consideration to management, but the costs of inappropriate or inadequate responses to releases in terms of fines and legal fees can quickly outpace the cost of contracted responses as demonstrated in the aforementioned example of the chlorine-generated fire. The OM specialist may sense pressure, explicit or implicit, to minimize the involvement of outside agencies in an attempt by management to minimize reporting of releases. Should management manifest an attitude such as this, it creates an opportune time for the OM specialist to encourage development of less release-prone processes at the work site while at the same time encouraging appropriate response plans.

ANTICIPATION OF SITUATIONS AND LOCATIONS OF NEED

By conducting a facility survey of materials used and their respective processes, a *risk inventory* can be developed. As well as addressing means to avoid untoward events, this analysis allows event-directed emergency response planning and the development of realistic drills.

To deal effectively with unexpected releases of HazMats, an ERP should take into account the following issues:

1. Exposures may affect the single worker or result in MCIs. A single worker exposure may escalate if not properly addressed.
2. Necessary contacts and information sources need to be identified and cataloged for easy access.
3. Guidelines should be prepared for grading the response (much like the concept of single versus multialarm fire responses). This will allow for objective decisions regarding invocation of increasingly complex responses.

Many variations of the above may occur depending on the site's location, geography, number of personnel, and types of substances present. A number of basic concepts, however, are applicable in virtually any setting. As the plan is developed, though, the complexities become readily apparent. It is imperative that the authors of any plan pay particular attention to clarity and succinctness in the final version. OSHA delineates minimum elements for an ERP (Table 55.5) (24).

TABLE 55.5. *Minimum elements of an emergency response plan*[a]

Preemergency planning
Personnel roles, lines of authority, and communications
Emergency recognition and prevention
Safe distances and places of refuge
Site security and control
Evacuation routes and procedures
Decontamination procedures not covered by the site safety and health plan
Emergency medical treatment and first aid
Emergency alerting and response procedures

[a]As proposed by the Occupational Safety and Health Administration (29 CFR 1910.120(1)(2)).

TABLE 55.6. *Resources for information on toxicity and hazards*[a]

TOXNET	Toxicology Data Network, a service of the National Library of Medicine *(http://toxnet.nlm.nih.gov/)*
	Several databases from different agencies addressing various aspects of toxicity, carcinogenicity
	Hazardous Substances Data Bank
	Toxline—reference database
	Chemical Carcinogenesis Research Information System (NCI)
	Integrated Risk Information System (EPA)
NFPA	National Fire Protection Association[b]
	Codes on a number of categories of substances that include information on flammability, volatility, explosivity
NIOSH	Occupational Health Guidelines for Chemical Hazards
	Original guidelines published in 1981, but many with revised information *(http://www.cdc.gov/niosh/chem-inx.html)*
	Immediately dangerous to life of health Concentrations (IDLHs)
	Originally published in the mid-1970s, updated in 1994 *(http://www.cdc.gov/niosh/idlh/intridl4.html)*
	NIOSH Pocket Guide to Chemical Hazards
	Chemical properties, IDLHs, permissible exposure limits (PELs), respirator recommendation, health hazards *(http://www.cdc.gov/niosh/npg/pgintrod.html)*

[a]See also references listed in the chapters on medical surveillance and toxicology in this text.

[b]See annotated bibliography and resources at end of this chapter for address.

Lewis, RJ. *Sax's Dangerous Properties of Industrial Materials,* 10th ed. New York: John Wiley & Sons, 1999 (a comprehensive treatise).

Hathaway GJ, Proctor NH, Hughes JP, Fischman ML. *Proctor and Hughes' chemical hazards in the workplace,* 4th ed. New York: John Wiley & Sons, 1996.

DETERMINATION OF SCOPE OF PLAN

For companies that install their own response plans, the following should be addressed: (a) the type of events that will trigger an ERP, and the corresponding level of response; (b) the responsibilities of the internal ERT; (c) the relationship with neighboring businesses through mutual aid agreements; and (d) the role and contact mechanisms for local, state, and federal agencies. In determining the events that trigger a response, a thorough review of the toxicity of the materials of concern is critical (Table 55.6).

EMERGENCY RESPONSE TEAM

Designating people or agencies that will respond to an incident as a team helps in planning for different levels of response. The membership of the on-site ERT will depend on the company's decisions regarding level of self-contained response. The ERP should specify on-site responders and outside agencies, such as the fire department, EMS, the Coast Guard, and consultants. After defining off-site team members, agreements should be formalized *before* an incident. The composition of the ERT will vary according to the type and severity of an incident. ERTs for incidents involving hazardous substances are usually referred to as *HazMat teams,* the members of which all should have clearly defined roles. OSHA defines four levels of responders and sets forth duty limitations and training guidelines for each level (Table 55.7) (25). In addition to these team members who will be trained to deal with the HazMats themselves, the team should have members designated to deal with casualties, scene control, and structural safety. These last components effectively correspond to the standard services of EMS, and the police and fire departments. Personnel serving in these roles, although not expected to enter the "hot" zone, should be equipped with and trained in the use of various levels of personal protective equipment (PPE). Members of the medical response component of the team particularly need to be outfitted with PPE as they may be quickly presented with severely injured casualties that are minimally decontaminated (26). Discussion of the details of medical response to HazMats incidents is beyond the scope of this chapter. An introductory overview can be found in the ATSDR publication *Managing Hazardous Materials Incidents.* Though published in 1992, this three-volume document covers most aspects of first response as well as initial hospital response (27).

All members of ERTs must have appropriate training for their roles, followed by repeated drills to

TABLE 55.7. *Responder levels and minimum training time (29 CFR 1910.120(q)(6)(i)–(iv))*

Responder level	Summary of activities	Training
First responder: awareness	Know what hazardous substances are, potential risks, how to recognize a release, how to activate emergency response plan (ERP)	To cover material, time not specified; may be experience
First responder: operations	Respond to a release to protect nearby persons, property, attempt to contain from a distance, "defensive" posture	Awareness level + at least 8 hours
Hazardous materials technician	Actively attempting to stop release	24 hours equal to operations + personal protective equipment (PPE), decontamination
Hazardous materials specialist	Similar to technician but with more specialist knowledge of various substances	24 hours equal to technician + specialized PPE, control, decontamination
On-scene incident commander	Able to take control of all the operations but would typically relinquish control to a fire department incident commander on arrival	24 hours equal to operations + understand issues of PPE, decontamination, local/regional emergency response plans/contacts

maintain and update skills. Numerous private agencies have developed both training materials and complete courses. Since a number of psychomotor skills are involved in the response to such incidents, active participation courses would be expected to produce a more effective team than classroom-only training. FEMA has also developed training courses.

PERSONAL PROTECTIVE EQUIPMENT

HazMat team members, starting at the technician level, must be familiarized with the proper use and care of PPE. The OM physician responsible for the medical aspects of the program must verify the physical capability of the person to use the designated type of PPE (28). The term *PPE* is used primarily in the realm of protection of members of response teams. The term *chemical protective clothing* (CPC) is used more commonly in referring to protective garments for routine handling of chemicals. In selecting either PPE or CPC, the substance to which the garment will be exposed and the duration of exposure must be known. In conjunction with understanding the risk associated with *penetration* (bulk flow of liq-

TABLE 55.8. *Regulations and standards governing personal protective equipment (PPE)*

OSHA (29 CFR)	
General (requirements for application, selection and use)	1910.132, 1910.1000, subpart E, part 1926
Noise	1910.95
Eye and face	1910.133
Respiratory	1910.134
Head and foot	1910.135 and 1910.136
Electrical protection	1910.137
American National Standards Institute (ANSI)	
General	Z37
Eye and face	Z87.1
Respiratory	Z88.2
Head	Z89.1
Footwear	Z41.1
Electrical	Z9.4
National Fire Protection Association (NFPA)[a]	
NFPA 1991	Standard on vapor-protective suits for hazardous chemical emergencies
NFPA 1992	Standard on liquid splash–protective suits for chemical emergencies
NFPA 1993	Standard on support function protective garments for hazardous chemical operations

[a]Available from NFPA at www.nfpa.org.

uid through material, seams, zippers, etc.) or *permeation* (passage through material on molecular level) of the material, one can critically evaluate various products (29,30). Garments should be certified as having been tested in accordance with standardized methods. The American Society of Testing Materials (ASTM) methods, for example, are frequently used as standards for testing both penetration (31) and permeation (32). The NFPA also has standards for testing protective garments; those that meet their standards are allowed to carry a certification tag (33). Different chemicals also require an appropriate respirator (34). A number of OSHA regulations address standards for different components of protective garments (Table 55.8). The OSHA regulations often refer to both NFPA and American National Standards Institute (ANSI) statements on standards of protection (Table 55.8). PPE is classified into levels A, B, C, or D depending on the degree of protection afforded (Table 55.9). Table 55.10 outlines factors relevant to the choice of level of protection. Specialized equipment, despite being initially impervious to hazardous fluids and vapors, can be degraded such that the protective lifetime may be reduced to as short as several hours or less of continuous exposure. It is important to know the composition of all components of totally encapsulating suits used for maximum protection, as witnessed by the experience of Captain Gerald Grey of the San Francisco Fire Department. A totally encapsulating suit that he was wearing suffered severe damage to the faceplate due to exposure to anhydrous dimethylamine. Compatibility tables indicated that the suit, made of butyl rubber, was appropriate for the situation; however, the integrated faceplate, made of polycarbonate, was not considered (35). Tolerances of various PPE materials to potential hazards have been tabulated (36).

TABLE 55.9. *Personal protective equipment grades*[a]

Level A	Totally encapsulating chemical-resistant suit Self-contained breathing apparatus (SCBA)
Level B	Splash protection with chemical-resistant clothing Positive pressure, full face-piece SCBA
Level C	Splash protection with chemical-resistant clothing Chemical-resistant full face-piece, air purifying, canister type respirator
Level D	Standard work uniform with no special chemical resistant properties and no respiratory protection

[a]These are partial descriptions to give an indication of the grades of protection. For a full description of required and optional gear at each level refer to 29 CFR 1910.120 appendix B, part A.

TABLE 55.10. *Selection of level of PPE*[a]

Level A	Maximum skin and respiratory protection from liquids, vapors, gases, and particulates; confined, poorly ventilated areas with unknown substances
Level B	Maximum respiratory protection; ambient O_2 <19.5%; lesser skin protection
Level C	Known substance and concentration meets specifications for air-purifying respirators; low skin toxicity
Level D	No anticipation of respiratory, skin, or mucous membrane toxicity

[a]29 CFR 1910.120 appendix B, part B.

Employees required to use PPE must be evaluated regarding "fitness for...the ability to wear any required PPE under conditions...that might be experienced at the work site" (37). These guidelines attempt to ensure that employees who need to use PPE are physically fit to wear the PPE in actual conditions. The most exacting of physical conditions in PPE are temperature extremes. Level A, which requires a totally encapsulating suit without ventilation, creates a potentially dangerous microclimate even at relatively cool ambient temperatures, especially if the wearer is engaged in heavy physical activity. Each worker required to use level A equipment needs to be evaluated for tolerance to heat stress. The NFPA has outlined a heat stress monitoring plan for persons using enclosed protective garments (38).

LEVELS OF RESPONSE

A number of factors should be considered in delineating the level of response appropriate for categories of incidents, including (a) level of technical expertise necessary to control the material(s) in question; (b) presence of fire or explosion hazard; and (c) potential radius of risk, i.e., contained in a small room or over an entire city. Levels of response delineated for a site might be:

Individual or buddy system of worker teams
Divisional ERT
Facility ERT
Mutual aid ERT
Outside EMS/ERT

These levels could be activated in a sequential fashion or, based on information at the time of an incident, a higher level of response may be initiated at the outset. In all emergency situations involving HazMats, a buddy system is essential wherein paired workers have protocols for checking the operations of each other and for providing immediate assistance to each other. As a part of the protocols for rendering assistance, early notification of senior officials is essential to enable them to summon medical assistance or activate a more comprehensive ERP. First responders must perform an immediate assessment of the potential risk for released substances to lead to other emergencies such as fire or explosion from reaction with either other products on site or spontaneously. Additionally, all designated responders should be trained to at least question the possibility of the release being intentional and the attendant risk for secondary devices in such situations.

Depending on the size and nature of the installation, the divisional and facility ERTs may be composed of persons trained only at the HazMat technician level. These personnel may be responsible for containing releases from a distance as well as alerting other employees to the potential risk without endangering themselves or others while they await the outside team that is summoned for definitive action. Alternatively, the response teams of facilities such as large chemical manufacturing installations may be comprehensive and include their own fire control, medical, and decontamination capabilities. This situation is most common when the community response systems may not be politically or financially able to support such services as, for example, in some foreign installations.

ACTIVATION OF ERP

Much like any fire alarm system, the system for activation of the ERP must be treated with respect and yet not feared. Every employee should be empowered to activate the ERP and should not be discouraged to do so if they have an honest concern. A protocol for internal verification that is not so cumbersome as to delay necessary response should be in place. Although risk is involved simply in the response (for example, EMS and fire personnel driving at high speed to respond), it is preferable to respond in the early stages of an incident rather than after the situation has deteriorated.

Evacuation

Once an incident has been identified and the ERP activated, an initial component of the plan must be orderly, safe evacuation of at-risk personnel. Each work area should have a designated "evacuation warden" responsible for no more than 20 co-workers. A designated employee must establish a roll-call check of employees (39).

Designation of Chain of Command

In the event of an incident, a clear chain of command is critical to prevent confusion. Authority needs to be designated at each level of response, including when authority will be relinquished to another designated incident commander (IC), for example, a shift foreman deferring command to a fire department official. The IC must coordinate the activities of uninjured workers remaining on-site and ensure that volunteers without specific training and roles are not allowed to participate in any activities within restricted areas. Initial reaction is often to designate a supervisory person as IC. It may actually be wiser to recruit members of the work group to undergo specific training as ICs. In this manner, the supervisory personnel can remain focused on more corporate operational issues. In an emergency department, for example, the role of IC for internal disasters and response to external disasters is frequently filled by a nurse with particular interest who has undergone specific training. In such cases the attending physician on duty when a disaster is declared must relinquish the usual doctor–nurse chain of command to the IC regarding disaster issues.

Decontamination

Decontamination of exposed personnel needs to be accomplished with strict adherence to guidelines that address four components:

1. Location of decontamination station, e.g., at the site of the spill, within the "warm" zone, or at the hospital. The site depends on the substances and injuries involved.
2. Removal of the substance from contaminated personnel in a way that will not cause further harm to them.
3. Avoidance of exposure of decontaminating personnel who should be members of the ERT with specific decontamination training.
4. Containment of offending agent in rinse solution, clothing, rescue material, etc.

It is often best to set up the decontamination zone in a corridor with progressive stations that move from fully contaminated to fully clean. Possible stations could include:

Initial shower/cleansing of victims or exterior of PPE
Removal of victim clothing or PPE
Removal of any undergarments possibly contaminated due to leakage of the outer PPE
Personal shower/cleansing
Medical station for any immediate minor treatment or monitoring needs

In addition to personnel, the entire site, including equipment, must be considered for decontamination. The emphasis in decontamination procedures should be on thoroughness rather than speed unless the victim(s) need emergency medical attention. Adequately protected personnel should decontaminate victims or injured response personnel with serious injuries in conjunction with instituting lifesaving interventions, since medical treatment may need to commence prior to the arrival of outside EMS personnel. Since the outside agency personnel are unlikely to have as detailed an understanding of the HazMats potentially involved in the incident, it is imperative that some of the internal response personnel be trained in emergency medical response under HazMat conditions.

Decontamination procedures should always be performed at the most stringent levels appropriate for substances that may be present at the site. Procedures should be downgraded only when specific information regarding actual exposure becomes available. This point is particularly important for ERT members as they approach or enter the "hot zone." Although the means of decontamination is substance dependent, most hazardous substances do not react in a water-detergent environment and, hence, water is an appropriate emergency starting point for liquid contaminants. If the water reactivity of the contaminating substance is unclear or in the case of dry contaminants, removal of clothing and brushing or vacuuming the victims should be carried out initially. Chemical-containing decontamination solutions should be used only when the offending agent is verified and an appropriate solution can be chosen.

Approaches for containment of decontamination waste range from using children's wading pools to collect flushing solutions to specially constructed trailers with self-contained air handling and waste water containers. More complete guidelines for decontamination exist in several of the resources listed below (see Further Information.)

CONTAINMENT OF INCIDENT

Containment should start at the first indication that a HazMat has been released; it may involve routine acts such as simply turning a switch or more complicated efforts such as dike building. All workers should be acquainted with how to shut down the processes on which they are working. The emergency shutdown procedure should include instructions for stopping the flow of any reagents that are supplied to the process.

Once a response has been initiated, graded restricted zones should be established to prevent further injury and to allow containment and rescue operations to proceed unimpeded. Typically, three zones are designated—hot, warm, and cold—based on older plans designed for dealing with radioactive substances. Only fully trained and properly attired HazMat specialists should enter the hot zone, if at all! Only the most fundamental lifesaving treatment such as opening a compromised airway should occur in the hot area, with most energy spent on evacuation to the decontamination/treatment area.

Additional zones may be designated if topography and weather conditions warrant. Weather must be constantly monitored because changes, such as shifting wind direction, may require redesignation of safe areas as "hot."

A decontamination area or areas should be designated as well. This is frequently placed at the inner margin of the "warm" zone. Staged decontamination areas may be necessary if multiple severely injured victims need immediate care following initial removal of clothing and offending agents. In this case, all personnel involved in the care of these victims prior to full decontamination need to be outfitted with appropriate PPE. Once the victim is stabilized adequately, more complete decontamination may be accomplished with further evacuation to the "cool" zone and on to a hospital. Progressive decontamination such as this is thought of as occurring along a corridor. This may be set up as successive separate stations or in a single unit such as a truck trailer with separate isolated compartments.

EVACUATION AND SITE SECURITY

Like fire escape plans, HazMats evacuation plans should be established. Plans should be posted and reviewed as part of the right-to-know (RTK) orientation. Regional evacuation plans should be filed with the local government agency responsible for coordinating the responses of other services.

Plans for community evacuations must have contingencies for weather, explosions, and fires. Computerized links to the National Weather Service for local and regional monitoring can assist in predicting evacuation needs. Computer programs are available that aid a sophisticated command center to make predictions regarding dispersion of any particular substance in light of local climate conditions. The OM specialist should consult with engineers regarding reliability of any such programs, as they are all subject to degrees of error based on assumptions made in the mathematical models.

Numerous factor are involved in securing the area of a release to allow for unimpeded rescue and containment activities as well as to prevent undue exposure of personnel not on the HazMat team. Not least among the issues is traffic control and rerouting. Designation of perimeters and plans for patrolling and securing them may be necessary. It is also important that public safety and security personnel be outfitted with appropriate emergency PPE should they suddenly be at risk for exposure, as, for example, should a sudden wind shift occur. These personnel need to be in constant communication with the command post regarding any shift in perimeter. They must not only restrict entry into the danger areas, but also ensure that potentially contaminated individuals do not leave the incident scene prior to appropriate decontamination.

SYSTEMS OF OUTSIDE NOTIFICATION

Cooperation agreements with neighboring facilities and community and regional support systems should be drawn up with attention to a simplified notification process. A central agency, similar to an emergency services dispatch unit, will reduce confusion and chances of omitting a critical respondent. SARA Title III requires that facilities with designated quantities of extremely hazardous substances in excess of EPAs threshold planning quantities must notify the LEPC with site/substance information (40).

Emergency notification procedures should include a checklist of information to be provided at the time of contacting respondents. This checklist should be prominently posted next to each telephone that might be used for notification and include the following information that should be given in this order:

Telephone number from which the call is coming
Name and location of the caller and facility/site
Time and location of the incident
Nature of incident (e.g., spill, explosion, confined space)
Material involved
Number of victims and extent of injuries
Condition and/or signs and symptoms of the victims
Name and phone number of safety officer responsible for the area of operations involved in the incident

If a community HazMat ERP does not exist, the responsible company will take the lead in establishing such a plan. A detailed discussion of community HazMat ERPs is beyond the scope of this chapter; however, excellent resources are described below (see Further Information). Planners should use a few resources to ensure that essential agencies are not omitted from the notification plan.

SITE COMMUNICATIONS

Effective communication among members of the ERT can be facilitated by using a dedicated radio frequency and by ensuring that all members of the team have radios. An analysis of a petroleum plant incident in Los Angeles in which hospital-based response teams participated indicated that some of the teams did not bring their hospital emergency administration radio (HEAR), which operates on VHF frequencies and is prone to electrical static, known as feedback, if too many are operated in close proximity. Apparently they felt there was too much feedback during drills due to the large number of radios operating on the same frequency (41). A secondary system of communication should be in place, such as hand signals for crew members wearing PPE that have face masks. All members of the ERT should wear some form of external identification easily seen from a distance that is specific for their agency or division.

ROLE OF OUTSIDE AGENCIES

The role of the municipal, county, state, federal, trade, and private consulting bodies that might be involved in an incident should be clearly defined. Many government agency roles will be obvious, but they should be stated in the ERP to avoid confusion and to reinforce their role and contact method.

Public Relations (PR)

A plan to notify and cooperate with local media to disseminate necessary information is essential. This plan should be conceived in a spirit of understanding the role of the media both in providing advice and information to those affected by the incident and in presenting a favorable image of the agencies and corporations involved in the response.

At the scene, the PR director acts as the funnel and filter for transfer of information from the operations technicians to the media. The PR director may also be responsible for maintaining the incident log for use in debriefing. The PR director's role can be expanded to include creating links of acquaintance prior to any incidents. Previously established relationships with the media and community agencies will reduce adverse reactions and offer an opportunity for the company to present itself as responsible and prepared.

Postincident Debriefing

After an activation of the ERP, debriefings should occur at several levels. ERP planners/managers should confer with in-house personnel including workers on site at the location of the incident as well as members of the ERT. Evaluation of the events leading up to the incident, with attention to preventing similar series of events, should be the basic philosophy of the debriefings.

Actions of workers present at the time of the incident should be evaluated to enhance response performance and prevent additional personnel from becoming victims in future incidents. A study of a plant explosion in Norway, for example, revealed a number of correlates to appropriate disaster response behavior (42). Among the correlates were experience in previous disasters, amount of training, and previous maritime employment (where there is a high attention to discipline regarding crisis situations as well as regular drills). Debriefings should be undertaken with partners in mutual aid agreements as well as local and regional public safety agencies. These debriefings should have a representative from the LEPC or at least share relevant conclusions and issues with the LEPC.

Critical Incident Stress Debriefing

When an incident occurs that involves either actual or significant potential risk of harm to persons, a system should be in place to provide critical incident stress debriefing (CISD). The effects of perceived as well as actual risk of injury on survivors can be debilitating. Even off-duty personnel may be appropriate candidates for CISD since they may manifest dysfunctional behavior patterns following a work-site disaster (43). For the OM specialist concerned with the overall health of the employee pool, this aspect of disaster response should be of paramount importance since it specifically addresses the future functionality of "survivors." Virtually all professional disaster response systems have CISD teams as a component of their services for their responders. For an overview comment regarding the value of preparedness and effective delivery of such services, the reader is referred to an article by one of the organizers of the CISD response invoked in Oklahoma City when a large bomb demolished part of a federal building including the day-care center, resulting in numerous child casualties (44).

Training

OSHA has specified general minimum parameters for training of HazMats incident emergency responders (45). Activity and scenario-based training are the preferred methods for training ERTs. Federal agencies supply training information and sponsor some training programs. Specialist contractors provide the majority of ERT training, either on-site or at their training facilities. Regardless of the original training, repeated drilling is the most important factor in ensuring a high-quality response. A significant correlation between drilling experience and appropriate behavior in a stressful situation has been documented (46).

ROLE OF THE OCCUPATIONAL MEDICINE PHYSICIAN

The OM physician has an integral role in addressing emergencies surrounding HazMats. At the outset, OM physicians should be aware of their company's potential HazMats. Materials used on site for manufacturing, service, or maintenance should be addressed. If outside contractors come on site, the physician should be aware of products used by the contractors that might affect employees. The physician should not rely solely on MSDSs for medical treatment guidelines, since the quality of these forms varies considerably. Once physicians are familiar with substances used, in conjunction with the safety officer(s), they can propose guidelines for safe handling and an ERP. They should also address the appropriate response to the possibility of an intentional release of HazMats that may not normally be on site.

Depending on the degree of interest and expertise of the physician, involvement in ERP development may range from review of and commentary on a plan, to development of the plan itself. The physician should not limit attention to the individual business, but should be aware of potential ramifications of HazMat incidents on surrounding facilities and the local community. Thus, it is well within the physician's purview to verify that the company has addressed regional problems, such as ground water contamination, that might arise in the event of a release. Meeting with local and regional EMS as well as EPA officials and participating in formation of mutual aid agreements will strengthen the OM physician's position in both planning and response phases. Corporate membership on LEPCs is encouraged and the OM physician would be an ideal candidate.

OSHA guidelines specify the role of the OM physician in relation to medical surveillance as well as pre- and postactivity assessments. In OSHA's regulations governing HazMats operations, virtually all workers who might be exposed to such materials are covered whether they work at a waste site; at a treatment, storage, disposal (TSD) facility; at a manufacturer, transporter, or professional emergency response organization; or at any other setting in which they might be exposed to HazMats (47). For all of these employees, OSHA requires medical surveillance programs (see Chapter 41) (48). Additionally, any workers, whether on site at a facility with HazMats or members of HazMats response teams, who must wear respirators or encapsulating personal protective clothing must be evaluated and followed in surveillance programs.

An OM physician may perform required physical exams or treat injured employees. Armed with information from the site survey and research on the effects of substances involved, the OM physician can either advise and treat directly or make informed choices of appropriate referrals.

SUMMARY

At the time of this writing, most work on ERPs has been directed at larger operations such as petroleum and chemical manufacturing facilities as well as the bulk transportation industry. Relatively little has been done to assist smaller businesses and the service sector in this arena. Additionally, the OM physician's role in developing response plans to intentional releases of chemical or biologic agents has just begun to develop.

This chapter was written to aid the OM professional, whether physician, nurse, physician assistant, or safety officer, in dealing with appropriate response to HazMats releases. Since many of the courses offered by either government agencies or private organizations designed for familiarization and training last 2 to 5 days, this chapter should be considered an introduction to the topic and a guide to further, more detailed resources.

REFERENCES

1. Hazardous Material Transportation Uniform Safety Act (1990), Public Law 101.615, Section 2 ("Findings").
2. Hazardous Substances Emergency Events Surveillance (HSEES). Agency for Toxic Substances and Disease Registry. Division of Health Studies. Epidemiology and Surveillance Branch. U.S. Department of Health and Human Services, Annual Report, 1997. *http://www.atsdr.cdc.gov/HS/HSEES/annual97.html.*
3. Code of Federal Regulations, Title 49, Part 172, Section 101. (Commonly referred to as 49 CFR 172.101 This notation method will be used throughout for references to sections of the Code of Federal Regulations.)
4. Tomsho R. Environmental posse fights a lonely war along the Rio Grande. *Wall Street Journal* 1992:Nov 10,B1.
5. Incident brief: spill of an undeclared shipment of hazardous materials in a cargo compartment of an aircraft Northwest Airlines Flight 957 10/28/98. National Transportation Safety Board. Accident: DCA-99-MZ-001. Report Adopted 17 May, 2000. *http://www.ntsb.gov/publictn/2000/hzb000l.htm.*
6. Hastings C. Police foil terror plot to use sarin gas in London. *London Telegraph* (electronic version) 2001 Feb 18; issue 2095. *www.telegraph.co.uk.*
7. Holiday shoppers get pepper-sprayed. Haz-Mat Archive. EmergencyNet. *http://www.emergency.com/hzmtlpage.htm.*
8. Public Law 104-201:Title XIV:Subtitle A: Sec. 1417. *http://thomas.loc.gov.*
9. *http://www.rris.fema.gov.*
10. Mehta PS, et al. Bhopal tragedy's health effects. *JAMA* 1990;264(21):2781–2787.
11. 40 CFR 355.50(a–c).
12. Enacted October 17, 1986, as Public Law 99-499 and published in v. 42 U.S.C., Sections 11001–11050. Relevant OSHA rulings are published in 29 CFR 1910.120.
13. Public Law 96-510, found at 40 CFR 300. *www.access.gpo.gov/nara/cfr/.*
14. 29 CFR 1910.120.
15. 29 CFR 1910.120.(a).(1).(v).
16. 42 U.S.C. 11003.
17. 42 U.S.C. 11021(a), EPA regulations covering this are in 40 CFR part 370.
18. Central site for Internet access to United States federal regulations and other documents: *http://www.gpo.gov/nara/cfr/index.html.*
19. *http://hazmat.dot.gov.*
20. *http://hazmat.dot.gov/intstandards.htm.*
21. 40 CFR 370.
22. 29 CFR 1910.120 (1)(1)(ii).
23. 29 CFR 1910.38(a).
24. 29 CFR 1910.120(1)(2).
25. 29 CFR 1910.120.(q).(6).
26. *Managing hazardous materials incidents: vol I, emergency medical services; vol II, hospital emergency departments; vol III, medical management guidelines for acute chemical exposures.* Agency for Toxic Substance and Disease Registry. Atlanta: Centers for Disease Control, 1992. *http://www.atsdr.cdc.gov/prevent.html.*
27. This document is available from the Agency for Toxic Substance and Disease Registry in Atlanta or via the Internet at *http://www.atsdr.cdc.gov/prevent.html.*
28. 29 CFR 1910.120(f)(4)(i).
29. Forsberg K, Mansdorf SZ. *Quick selection guide to chemical protective clothing,* 3rd ed. New York: John Wiley & Sons, 1997.
30. Recommendations for chemical protective clothing: a companion to the NIOSH pocket guide to chemical hazards. *NIOSH* 1998. *http://www.cdc.gov/niosh/ncpc1.html.*
31. Standard test method for resistance of protective clothing materials to permeation by liquids or gases under

conditions of continuous contact. American Society for Testing and Materials, F739-99a.
32. Standard test method for resistance of materials used in protective clothing to penetration by liquids. American Society for Testing and Materials, F903-99a.
33. NFPA 1991, Standard on vapor-protective suits for hazardous chemicals emergencies; NFPA 1992, standard on liquid splash-protective suits for hazardous chemical emergencies; and NFPA 1993, standard on support function protective garments for hazardous chemical operations.
34. NIOSH Respirator Decision Logic. DHHS (NIOSH) publication No. 87-116. May, 1987 *http://www.cdc.gov/niosh/87-116.html.*
35. Grey GL. Supplement VII–Quick reference chemical compatibility chart for protective clothing. In: Henry MF, ed. *Hazardous materials response handbook.* Quincy, MA: National Fire Protection Association, 1989. This section, which includes an extensive listing based on a number of sources does not appear in the latest (1997) edition. Readers are currently referred by the handbook to manufacturer information.
36. Johnson JS, Anderson KJ. *Chemical protective clothing.* Product and performance information. Akron, OH: American Industrial Hygiene Association, 1990.
37. 29 CFR 1910.120(f)(4)(i).
38. Tokle G, ed. Heat stress monitoring in level C. In: *Hazardous materials response handbook.* Quincy, MA: NFPA, 1992:494–500.
39. 29 CFR 1910.38.a.2.
40. 40 CFR 370.
41. Haynes BE, Emmel AC. Role of a hospital team at an industrial explosion. Department of Emergency Medicine, Harbor/UCLA Medical Center, Torrance, California. *Am J Emerg Med* 1988;6(3):260–265.
42. Weisaeth L. A study of behavioral responses to an industrial disaster. *Acta Psychiatr Scand Suppl* 1989;355: 13–24.
43. Weisaeth L. The stressors and the post-traumatic stress syndrome after an industrial disaster. *Acta Psychiatr Scand Suppl* 1989;355:25–37.
44. Tassey J. Personal impressions of the Federal Building bombing in Oklahoma City. National Center for PTSD (Veterans Administration) Clinical Quarterly 1995 (Fall);5(4). *http://www.ncptsd.org.*
45. 29 CFR 1910.120(q)(6)(i)–(iv).
46. Weisaeth L. A study of behavioral responses to an industrial disaster. *Acta Psychiatr Scand Suppl* 1989;355: 13–24.
47. 29 CFR 1910.120(a)(1)(i–iv).
48. 29 CFR 1910.120(f)(3–8).

FURTHER INFORMATION

Agency for Toxic Substances and Disease Registry (ATSDR)

This federal agency is an agency of the U.S. Department of Health and Human Services created by Superfund legislation in 1980 to "prevent or mitigate adverse human health effects and diminished quality of life resulting from exposure to hazardous substances in the environment." The headquarters address is 1600 Clifton Rd., Atlanta, GA 30333. Information on training, current research, as well as many of the agency's publications are available at the agency's Web site: *http://www.atsdr.cdc.gov*. The Science Corner section of the Web site is set up as a "resource gateway" to environmental health information. Although the entry pages were, at the time of this writing (2001), last updated in 1998, the links often had more recent dates. *http://www.atsdr.cdc.gov/cx.html.*

Managing Hazardous Materials Incidents, 1992.

A three-volume set covering various aspects of the emergency medical response to hazardous materials exposures: *httl2://www.atsdr.cdc.gov/prevent.html.*

Emergency medical systems: a planning guide for the management of contaminated patients.

This volume addresses issues relevant to the prehospital setting. Emergency medical services personnel are the primary targeted audience; however, much of the information would be useful in developing an on-site ERT.

Hospital emergency departments: a planning guide for the management of contaminated patients.

This volume focuses on issues in dealing with hazardous materials incident victims in the emergency department setting. It is a good introduction to the topic and to relevant issues such as labeling and MSDSs. It is a good resource for the on-site health center in addressing issues of treatment and self-protection.

Medical management guidelines for acute chemical exposure.

This volume provides basic guidelines for medical treatment, though it should be cross-referenced since it was published in 1992.

National Institute for Occupational Safety and Health (NIOSH)

Numerous guidelines and databases regarding exposure, protection, and immediate first aid. Most available via the Internet: *http://www.cdc.gov/niosh/.*

Immediately dangerous to life or health concentrations (IDLHs): *http://www.cdc.gov/niosh/idlh/idlh-1.html.*

NIOSH pocket guide to chemical hazards

Information for all substances for which NIOSH has recommended exposure limits (RELs) and those with permissible exposure limits (PELs) as found in the OSHA General Industry Air Contaminants Standard. It also contains information to aid in recognition and control of chemical hazards: *www.cdc.gov/niosh*

Recommendations for chemical protective clothing: a companion to the NIOSH pocket guide to chemical hazards: http://www.cdc.gov/niosh/87-108.html

NIOSH pocket guide to chemical hazards and other databases (CD-ROM). NIOSH publication 99-115.

CD-ROM (Windows and Macintosh versions on same CD) containing IDLHs, international chemical safety cards, recommendations for chemical protective clothing, medical tests for OSHA regulated substances, toxicologic reviews of selected chemicals, NIOSH manual of analytical methods, NIOSH pocket guide, and DOT's North American emergency response guidebook (1996 version).

Chemical Transportation Emergency Center (CHEMTREC)

A service of the American Chemical Council (formerly the Chemical Manufacturers Association) that provides assistance in transportation incidents received 48,000 calls in HazMat emergencies from 1986 through 1991: 1300 Wilson Boulevard, Arlington, VA 22209-2307.

American Society for Testing and Materials

Standard testing procedures and other standards. ASTM, 100 Barr Harbor Drive West, Conshohocken, PA 19428-2959; *http://www.astm.org/*.

U.S. Department of Defense Chemical and Biologic Weapons/Terrorist Threats Resources

U.S. Army Soldier and Biologic Chemical Command (SBCCOM)
Domestic Preparedness

The home Web site for a federal interagency program formed under the Nunn-Lugar-Domenici bill (Defense Authorization Bill FY 1997; PL 104-201) directed toward information on preparation for possible chemical and biologic weapons attacks. Information is useful in helping employers develop emergency plans for possible intentional releases of such agents. The Web site provides links to a large amount of information on protective equipment and other aspects of dealing with chemical and biologic weapons: *http://dip.sbccom.army.mil/au.html*.

First Responders Chemical/Biological Hotline (1-800-424-8802).

National Domestic Preparedness Office

A clearinghouse for state, local, and federal weapons of mass destruction (WMD) information and assistance. It also has the compendium for all WMD/nuclear, biologic, and chemical (NBC) training at or sponsored by the federal government: *http://www.ndpo.gov*.

The Office of the Surgeon General for Nuclear Biologic and Chemical Issues

Information on the management of chemical, biologic, and radiologic exposure casualties: *www.nbc-med.org*.

The U.S. Army Medical Research Institute of Chemical Defense (USAMRICD)

On-line textbook on chemical and biologic weapons including appropriate countermeasures such as decontamination, PPE, medical management: *http://chemdef.apgea.army.mil*.

Casualty Care Research Center (Crisis Management)

Training programs in Chem/Bio Hazards for providers, first responders, and managers: *http://www.usuhs.mil/ccr/wmdtp1.htm*.

Department of Transportation

Hazardous materials information available via the Internet at *http:hazmat.dot.gov*.

The National Response Center: central reporting agency for any qualifying releases: *http://www.nrc.uscg.mil/index.htm*.

Federal Emergency Management Agency (FEMA)

U.S. Fire Administration. Entity of FEMA. Training Division

Training of fire and EMS personnel.

USFA Hazardous Materials Guide for First Responders: *http://www.usfa.fema.gov/hazmat/*.

Community Awareness and Emergency Response Program Handbook.

Reference listing of related HazMat sites: *http://www.fema.gov/emi/hmep/hmlinks.htm*.

National Fire Protection Association

Many federal standards cross-reference to standards put forward by the NFPA. It will provide a catalogue on request. One Battery Park, Quincy, MA 02269; *http://www.nfpa.org*.

The National Library of Medicine

Several relevant databases available via the Specialized Information Services: *http://sis.nlm.nih.gov/Chem/ChemMain.html* or *http://sis.nlm.nih.gov/tehip.cfm*.

TOXNET

The Hazardous Substances Data Bank: *http://chem.sis.nlm.nih.gov/hsdb*.
The Registry of Toxic Effects of Chemical Substances
The Chemical Carcinogenesis Research Information System

Safety Information Resources. Inc. (SIRI)

Chemical safety resources Internet site sponsored by the University of Vermont: *http://hazard.com*. A large database of MSDSs: *http://siri.uvm.edu/msds*.

The SIRI editors note one particular company as having exemplary MSDSs in terms of providing detailed, useful information.

Cornell University: Planning, Design, and Construction Department

Maintains a very complete MSDS database: *http://msds.pdc.cornell.edu/ msdssrch.asp*.

Books

Smeby LC. *Hazardous materials response handbook,* 3rd ed. Quincy, MA: National Fire Protection Association, 1997.
Forsberg K, Mansdorf SZ. *Quick selection guide to chemical protective clothing,* 3rd ed. New York: John Wiley & Sons, 1997.
The industry standard found as the reference resource throughout government and other sources.
Lewis RJ. *Sax's dangerous properties of industrial materials,* 10th ed. New York: John Wiley & Sons, 1999.
A comprehensive treatise.

56

Occupational Medicine Aspects of Terrorism

L. Kristian Arnold

WHOM CAN WE TRUST?

"First of all, based on my former experience...I think the U.S. has sound counter-terrorism policies and a very resourceful and effective counter-terrorism program" (January 25, 2000) (1). This statement was made to a congressional committee by a former coordinator for counterterrorism at the U.S. Department of State in a presentation in which he addressed the need for funding of programs to get at the social and political root causes of terrorism. Analyses following jetliner attacks on the World Trade Center on September 11, 2001, brought into discussion the difficulty for the international intelligence community to forewarn potential targets of specific events.

Thus, it behooves each corporation or organization to perform some of their own intelligence gathering to assess their risk in order to develop their own strategy to decrease the risk of attack where possible and to mitigate the effects of an attack should one occur.

The official Department of State operational definition of terrorism states: "The term 'terrorism' means premeditated, politically motivated violence perpetrated against noncombatant targets by subnational groups or clandestine agents; and the term 'terrorist group' means any group practicing, or which has significant subgroups which practice, international terrorism" (1). Although this definition is limiting in its reference to international terrorism, Title 18 of the U.S. Code, which addresses crimes, defines a terrorist act as a "violent act or an act dangerous to human life that is a violation of criminal laws of the United States or of any State, or that would be a criminal violation if committed within the jurisdiction of the United States or of any State; and appears to be intended to intimidate or coerce a civilian population; to influence the policy of a government by intimidation or coercion; or to affect the conduct of a government by assassination or kidnapping" (2).

Attacks on businesses and their employees represent an area of increasing concern to employers and employees alike.

Intentional, aggressive, indiscriminate attacks on corporate entities, their real properties, or employees have all escalated over the last years of the 20th century. Some have been highly targeted, politically motivated attacks by individuals such as the Unabomber (Theodore Kaczynski), who sent letter and package bombs to corporate and university personnel whom he had determined were deserving of injury or death in his paradigm. Others have been more property oriented, such as bombings of an oil pipeline in Colombia by rebels. Attacks have occurred at central corporate headquarters and remote field establishments. Since the 1994 breakup of the Soviet Union, the number of armed militant groups with various agendas looking for a convenient target that represents their opposition has significantly increased. It is also no longer easy to predict the likelihood of an organization's becoming a target, as victims have ranged from oil and mining companies to international humanitarian aid organizations.

The apparent level of violence and the indiscriminate nature of such violence both increased significantly in the last 20 years of the 20th century. An increasing number of attacks have been carried out that, though directed at a specific target, were executed without regard to minimizing collateral casualties and, seemingly, with attention to actually maximizing such casualties (Fig. 56.1). The Department of State statistics for 2000 revealed 200 attacks directed at U.S. interests out of a total of 423 international attacks.

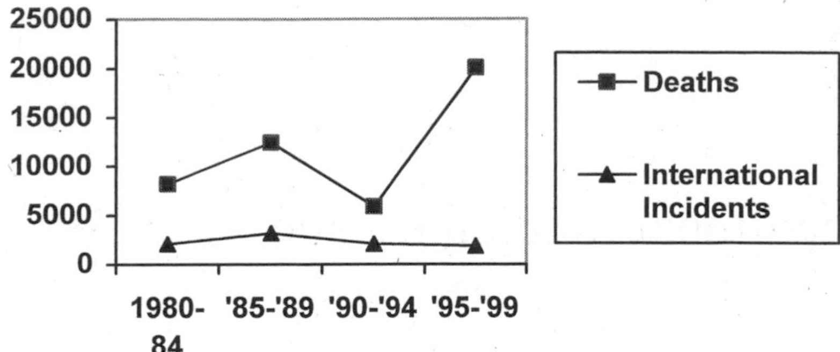

FIG. 56.1. Lethality of terrorist attacks. (Adapted from FBI and CIA statistics. Presented as part of a course on CD-ROM offered by Palladium Media, Inc. *http://www.bombsecurity.com/typerisk.html.*)

Although the vast majority of multicasualty aggressions have involved simple explosive devices, increasing attention has been directed at the possibility of aggressive acts involving what have come to be know as weapons of mass destruction (WMD). The agents typically covered by this classification include nuclear, biological and chemical (NBC) agents that have been specifically developed or altered to serve as weapons.

A number of international sociopolitical events have led to an international network of groups with a variety of agendas that, in one way or another, have been shown to have a potential for a violent interaction with businesses. These relations are as varied as the interconnections among mainstream businesses. They range from international drug cartels, to ethnic or religious groups that feel they are fighting for the rights of some oppressed peoples, to agents of governments with an interest in destabilizing another government. Sometimes business interests or employees are the specific target. Other times they are either a convenient target or simply "collaterally involved."

Although some practitioners of occupational medicine (OM), particularly in the international domain, have had to deal with aspects of terrorism for many years, events in 2001 brought the concern of terrorist attacks to a higher level of consciousness throughout the OM world.

As the events of September 11, 2001, demonstrated, when dealing with fanatics with nothing to lose, the rules of engagement have changed. In a later incident in which a passenger stormed the cockpit of a United Airlines flight, the quick, and seemingly very violent, response of the co-pilot to strike the man in the head with a fire ax may well have saved the entire flight from disaster (3).

For businesses in general, trying to provide total safety against all potential terrorist attacks can prove to be a costly and elusive goal, as the U.S. airline industry is discovering with attempts to effectively screen passengers and luggage.

This chapter discusses threat/risk assessment, types of threats, and critical elements of response plans. This is not a complete manual for establishing a victim mitigation response. At the end of the chapter a number of resources are presented, primarily from the Internet.

PHILOSOPHICAL POSITION OF THE OCCUPATIONAL MEDICINE PHYSICIAN

OM practitioners working with corporations have typically been involved in development of emergency safety plans. Most commonly this has been in relation to processes and products that are a part of the work-site and production process. Although the emergency safety response plans for unexpected natural or man-made disasters share many characteristics in common with responses to terrorist attacks, there are significant differences, particularly in the pre-event risk assessment and protection planning. Although many of the elements important in the planning phase, such as site security and architectural design for safety, would be outside the expertise of OM practitioners consulting with business, they should be involved in the discussions from a systems level. In some settings, it may be the informed OM physician who will help a company realize a potential threat.

Corporate strategic decisions affect the potential health and well-being of the employees and of the corporation as an entity in and of itself. Much as weak management structure may adversely affect employees in a number of ways, some corporate policy decisions may have relatively more or less influence on the risk of terrorist attack. Ideally, for example, when a corporation would be designing a new manufacturing facility, OM specialists would be consulted to create a facility with a minimal risk to the employees. Attack risk analysis should be an added aspect of the corporate strategic planning process. The OM practitioner with an interest and knowledge in this domain can provide a valuable, potentially lifesaving service.

Much like planning for mitigating the effect of natural disasters accepts the fact that events such as earthquakes, major storms, or other natural disasters cannot be stopped, part of the approach to decreasing the risk of injury and death from terrorist attacks assumes a degree of expectation that such events will occur.

RISK ASSESSMENT

An increasing number of corporations and agencies are recognizing the need to develop terrorism action plans. The foundation of any well-developed response plan is a risk assessment analysis. North Carolina requires all state government agencies to perform a terrorist attack risk assessment and has provided a 19-question assessment form for that purpose (4). Some insurance carriers offer terrorist risk assessment in conjunction with the purchase of insurance products (5).

The OM physician advising an organization regarding the development of a terrorism mitigation plan will find useful information in a number of resources outside the traditional medical information reference set, effectively the equivalent of obtaining the social history of a patient to assist with framing preventive health advice.

The increased awareness of risk of terrorist attack has put into a new light some incidents that may have been previously viewed as isolated pranks. For example, youths set off irritant gas canisters in several stores in California during a busy shopping season. Although the act itself would not be classified as a terrorist attack, because of the heightened concern level of the American public, the likelihood for panic among public and personnel underscores the need for well-thought-out plans and training. Thus, terrorism emergency response plans (TERPs) should be developed and maintained with an understanding that employees and the general public may be affected by terrorist attacks. The National Safety Council has published a list of the ten most common errors found in instituting Occupational Safety and Health Administration (OSHA)-mandated emergency response plans (ERPs) (6) (Table 56.1). Overall, they reflect a lack of commitment on the part of management to take seriously the possibility of needing to activate the plan.

Since terrorist actions, as opposed to vandalism, are based on an agenda, the more that organizations can understand about how they may fit the agenda as a target the better can be the risk assessment. In addition to the Department of State, a number of foundations specialize in gathering and disseminating information to assist corporations, government agencies, and other organizations with risk assessment in this domain (7). The Department of State and the Central Intelligence Agency (CIA) host Internet sites with country reports as well as reports on different known terrorist groups (see Further Information, below).

Cyber attack is an increasingly important potential form of corporate terrorism. Disruption of critical computer-dependent industrial processes may lead to injury or death. A survey by Price Waterhouse Cooper of 1,600 high-ranking information officers found that 79% had experienced a security breach in the preceding year; 58% of these breaches were attributable to employees (8). It is imperative for the responsible OM professionals to understand how the information systems operations of their corporations may be linked to issues of employee safety.

Risk assessment information on the Internet may become a casualty of terrorism. Increasing concern has been voiced regarding the availability of data from vulnerability assessments. The Department of

TABLE 56.1. *National safety council list of errors in emergency response plans*

Ten most common errors found with emergency response plans:

1. No upper management support
2. Lack of employee buy-in
3. Poor or no planning
4. Lack of training and practice
5. No designated leader
6. Failure to keep the plan up to date
7. No method of communication to alert employees
8. OSHA regulations are not a part of the plan
9. No procedures for shutting down critical equipment
10. Employees are not told what actions to take in an emergency

From (6).

Justice has issued a report on the risks of terrorist use of on-line information regarding the vulnerability of chemical manufacturing sites in the U.S. and abroad (9). Public access to a variety of information sources on the Internet has suffered as some sites have been closed. At the time of this writing, the Department of Energy had temporarily closed their Internet site to revamp it to offer less potentially strategic information.

Types of Threats and Relevant Responses

One can divide terrorist aggressions into two distinct classes: immediately apparent and insidious. Immediately apparent aggressions would include incidents wherein the attack is relatively immediately apparent, such as bombs and most chemical agents. Insidious aggressions would include most biologic agents and chemicals that do not have an immediately apparent effect on life or health. This section provides a brief synopsis of information on a variety of threats that have been or could be used on a small or large scale.

Several resources oriented to health care personnel have published overview information regarding NBC threats. Although the Centers for Disease Control (CDC) generally has the most up-to-date versions, emergency planners should cross-reference other sites such as the American College of Occupational and Environmental Medicine, the American Medical Association (AMA), and the American College of Emergency Physicians. Information may vary between different products generated by the same organization. For example, the AMA distributed a CD-ROM titled *Bioterrorism Awareness* that contains a table listing potential biologic agents of terrorism (10). A similar listing on the AMA Web site did not have the same set of organisms (11).

This chapter does not present detailed information regarding the various agents, as this is well presented in several resources such as those of the CDC. This chapter does, however, correlate to the OM setting some of the information related in a number of sites.

As with all attempts to mitigate the effect of potentially seemingly unpreventable adverse events, the application of the Haddon matrix (Fig. 56.2) to the problem will likely greatly facilitate "brainstorming" and cataloging of issues that could be addressed to minimize the overall potential death and disability from terrorist attacks.

Explosive Blast

Explosive devices remain the most common of all terrorist attack tools. Explosive ordnance devices (EODs) come in a vast array of sizes, shapes, and strengths, and are delivered through various means (Table 56.2). Unfortunately, the materials necessary to manufacture an explosive device are readily available on the open market.

In 1996, the Department of Treasury's Bureau of Alcohol, Tobacco, and Firearms (ATF) registry reported 1,212 bombings in the U.S. with 180 people injured, 11 killed, and over $2 million in damage. It recorded an additional 473 attempted bombings, resulting in 13 deaths (12). Targeted organizations ranged from abortion clinics to religious organizations. Outside the U.S., State Department figures for 1999 report a general decrease in the number of deaths despite a 43% increase in the number of attacks versus 1998. The decrease in deaths was attributed to not having any mass casualty incidents; 169 of the attacks were directed at American interests, with five Americans killed.

Since explosions are events that arrive rapidly and usually without any chance for assuming a defensive posture, to minimize the number and severity of injuries anticipatory planning is imperative. At the time of an event, employees must react rapidly and effectively, which requires a well-developed and rehearsed response plan.

	Human	Agent*	Environment*
Pre-Event			
Event			
Post-Event			

FIG. 56.2. The Haddon matrix. *These items may be defined in various ways in regard to such events. For example, the agent may be seen as the actual offending material (biologic, chemical, bomb, etc.) or as the operator of the event.

TABLE 56.2. *Delivery mechanisms used by terrorists*

Mail delivered
Courier delivered
Vehicle bombs
Proximity devices
Projected devices

The effect of a blast on structural stability may extend well beyond the region of obvious damage. The ATF has developed a table of blast effects to be used as an evacuation indicator (Fig. 56.3). Private vendors also offer tools for assessing potential damage through computer simulation (13).

Although the majority of announced bomb threats have not been associated with finding an actual device, the risk remains. Receptionists/switchboard operators should have specific training in handling bomb threats. The Royal Canadian Mounted Police have published a downloadable checklist for receiving a bomb threat (14). There are three potential organizational responses to bomb threats: no action, full evacuation, or search followed by evacuation if a device is found. There is no consensus regarding the correct response, though some sources suggest a staged response of initial evacuation, gauged to the character of the threat, while simultaneously conducting a search.

Biologic Agents

Without knowing of the existence of bacteria, armies have employed biologic agents as weapons for many centuries. Corpses of soldiers or animals killed in battle have been used to contaminate water supplies. Corpses of persons dying of the plague have been catapulted into cities under siege. In the French and Indian War, British soldiers gave blankets from smallpox patients to Native American tribes, anticipating the recipients would become ill (15). Biologic warfare divisions of several militaries have explored "weaponizing" a number of different microorganisms, with varying degrees of success. The most extensive view of such a system has come from the former associate director of the Soviet Union's biologic weapons development program, Ken Alibek, M.D., after he defected in 1992. Although other countries have developed and continue to develop biologic weapons, there is very little unclassified information directly available. A much longer list of agents has been employed in small-scale attacks than the classic list largely drawn from state-sponsored programs that generally seek organisms amenable to large-scale dispersal against troops as opposed to in terrorist operations (16,17).

Some of these agents require very sophisticated laboratory and production facilities to render them appropriate for military weapon use, historically

Vehicle Description	Maximum Explosives Capacity	Lethal Air Blast Range	Minimum Evacuation Distance	Falling Glass Hazard
COMPACT SEDAN	500 Pounds 227 Kilos *(In Trunk)*	100 Feet 30 Meters	1,500 Feet 457 Meters	1, 250 Feet 381 Meters
FULL SIZE SEDAN	1,000 Pounds 455 Kilos *(In Trunk)*	125 Feet 38 Meters	1,750 Feet 534 Meters	1,750 Feet 534 Meters
PASSENGER VAN OR CARGO VAN	4,000 Pounds 1,818 Kilos	200 Feet 61 Meters	2,750 Feet 838 Meters	2,750 Feet 838 Meters
SMALL BOX VAN *(14 FT BOX)*	10,000 Pounds 4,545 Kilos	300 Feet 91 Meters	3,750 Feet 1,143 Meters	3,750 Feet 1,143 Meters
BOX VAN OR WATER/FUEL TRUCK	30,000 Pounds 13,636 Kilos	450 Feet 137 Meters	6,500 Feet 1,982 Meters	6,500 Feet 1,982 Meters
SEMI-TRAILER	60,000 Pounds 27,273 Kilos	600 Feet 183 Meters	7,000 Feet 2,134 Meters	7,000 Feet 2,134 Meters

FIG. 56.3. Vehicle bomb explosion hazard evacuation distance table. (From the Bureau of Alcohol, Tobacco, and Firearms, Department of the Treasury. *http://www.atf.treas.gov.*)

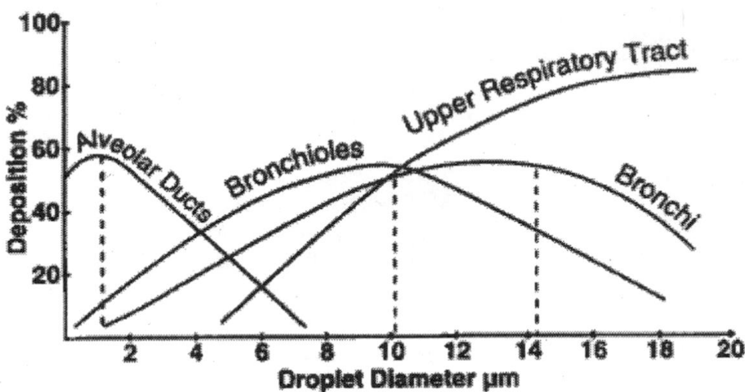

FIG. 56.4. Departments of the Army, Navy, and Air Force. Part II Ch 1 Sec III para. 106. a (1). NATO Handbook on the Medical Aspects of NBC Defensive Operations. Washington, DC: Department of Defense, 1996. *http://www.fas.org/nuke/guide/usa/doctrine/dod/fm8-9/toc.htm* and *http://www.fas.org/nuke/guide/usa/doctrine/dod/fm8-92ch1.htm#s2pl.*

making it less likely that they would be procured by substate groups or individuals. Some factors such as potential purchasing of knowledge or skills from scientists and changes in access to former biologic production sites have changed this. For example, recent drying of the Aral Sea has created a land bridge to Vozrozhdeniye Island, site of a former Soviet biowarfare production and testing facility with large amounts of agents stored in disposal sites. Additionally, access now by rodents increases the risk of unintentional migration of agents such as plague (18).

Most of the biologic organisms considered by governments for weaponization depend on dispersal through the air. For effective air dispersion with adequate respiratory tree penetration, particles must generally be in the range of 5 μm or less (Fig. 56.4). The standard hospital guidelines for prevention of airborne transmission of diseases are most commonly used as the reference for bioweapon protection levels. Hospital guidelines consider two levels of transmission (Table 56.3). Respirator choice is related to the type of exposure and whether the agent is a dry powder or a vapor (Table 56.4).

Substate groups have used non-airborne biologic agents as weapons, as when a religious sect in Oregon introduced *Salmonella typhi* into a public salad bar in an attempt to influence local elections that would impact their activities (19).

TABLE 56.3. *Airborne infectious disease transmission protection*

Level of transmission	Particle size/character	Protection
Droplet	>5 μm Droplets produced by cough, sneeze, talking	>3 feet separation Standard surgical mask[a] with face shield to prevent conjunctival exposure
Airborne	>5 μm Droplet nuclei (evaporated droplets) containing microorganisms that remain suspended in the air for long periods of time or dust particles containing the infectious agent	N95 (95% efficiency particulate filter) High-efficiency particulate air filtration (HEPA)

[a]From CDC. Guideline for isolation precautions in hospitals; part II. Recommendations for isolation precautions in hospitals, 1997 *(http://www.cdc.gov/ncidod/hip/ISOLAT/isopart2.htm).*

TABLE 56.4A. *Respirator protection levels classifications*

Designation	Explanation	Protection	Comments
SCBA	Self-contained breathing apparatus	Immediate Dangerous to life and health or inadequate oxygen	Bottled compressed air worn by worker Delivery by demand valve
Line feed	Positive pressure from base via hose	Immediate Dangerous to life and health or inadequate oxygen	Delivery may be by demand valve or continuous flow
PAPR	Powered air-purifying respirator	100× threshold limit value (TLV)	Full hood with fan-driven forced air circulation
Full face mask Dual cartridge Cannister	Negative pressure	50× threshold limit value (TLV) Longer duration during dual cartridge	Choose cartridge for application Standard "gas mask" used with appropriate cannister/cartridge
Half face mask cartridge Cartridge and particulate disposable	Negative pressure	10× threshold limit value (TLV)	Typical of Tb protection mask for short exposures to particulates of >0.5 μm (e.g., N95)
HEPA	High-efficiency particulate air	>0.3 μm	Old designation—considered equivalent to 100 series in efficiency

TABLE 56.4B. *Nonpowered, air-purifying particulate filter respirator categories*

Filter efficiency	Oil resistance		
	N-series particulate filters Not resistant to oil No time limitations solid particulate or liquid particulate hazards	R-series particulate filters Oil resistant Time limitation[a]: 8 hours or manufacturer recommendation Solid and liquid particulate hazards	P-series filters Oil-proof Time limitation: manufacturer recommendation, usually more than 8 hours
95%	N95	R95	P95
99%	N99	R99	P99
100% (99.7%)	N100	R100	P100

[a]Time limitation refers to the maximum time the filter will retain its efficiency in the face of oils. Filters depend on electrostatic charges on the fibers to trap particles. Oil coats the fibers and eliminates the charge, thus reducing the efficiency. Not applicable to N series since they should not be exposed to any oil.

TABLE 56.4C. *Respirator chemical cartridge coding*

Color	Application
White	Acid
Black	Organic
Green	Ammonia
Yellow	Acid gas and organic vapor
Olive	Multi gas and vapor
Magenta	Particulate (HEPA = P100)

Anthrax

Historically anthrax has been recognized in its relation to animal skins as a medical condition through the tannery and leather working trades. The name comes from Greek for coal, referring to the coal-black eschar that forms in cutaneous anthrax. The agent *Bacillus anthracis* grows as gram-positive non-motile rods in blood culture. It is the capability of creating a storage mode as a spore that gives this

TABLE 56.5. *Clinical syndromes produced by Bacillus anthracis*

Pulmonary	Prodrome of flu-like symptoms Nonminimally productive cough May have nausea/vomiting 2–4 days later—rapidly progressing respiratory failure Specific hallmark of widened mediastinum Hemorrhagic mediastinitis Lymphadenopathy Septicemia Multiorgan failure Toxin mediated Incubation—2–60 days Depends on activation of spores to active bacillus
Cutaneous	Localized itching, followed by a papular lesion that turns vesicular, and within 2–6 days develops into a depressed black eschar Commonly on hands, forearms, or head Still frequent in West Texas among ranchers Incubation 1–7 days
Gastrointestinal	Abdominal pain, nausea, vomiting, and fever Bloody diarrhea, hematemesis Commonly fatal Incubation average 1–7 days

bacillus the potential to be used as a weapon. The spores are between 0.4 to 0.6 μm in diameter. When produced in a culture medium and encouraged to form spores, the resultant material, when dried, creates clumps of spores. To produce a "weapon-grade" material, among other treatments, this material must be milled to a small enough size that it will easily penetrate the pulmonary tree to the bronchiolar level to have the greatest likelihood of producing disease.

Anthrax infection presents as three relatively distinct clinical syndromes: cutaneous, gastrointestinal, and pulmonary. Table 56.5 presents some of the characteristics of each of these syndromes.

At the time of this writing, an inactivated cell-free vaccine has been developed. It is, however, only recommended for military personnel being deployed on a high-risk operation. As improvements are made and depending on the particular situation, vaccination of nonmilitary personnel with a high risk of exposure may be recommended. Current CDC recommendations should be followed.

Postrelease Procedures

Prevention of Inoculation

Respiratory tract and cutaneous protection are the primary means of protection during an active release, though food should be suspect, especially if there is any chance it was vulnerable to aerosolized spores settling on it and it will not be cooked prior to consumption. Intact adult skin is reportedly fairly resistant to active infection even with direct exposure.

Regardless, skin protection along with respiratory protection should be used in any moderate to high risk-of-exposure situations such as mailroom personnel in high-risk targets during a known incident. During the 2001 anthrax mailings in the U.S., there was an evolution in the understanding of the potential for mail-delivered spores to disperse. Considering the ease with which any powder in a package apparently could be dispersed with very little effort, a safe, reasonable approach to use of personal protective equipment during a known mail delivery event would be for high-risk mailroom personnel to wear light full-body protection with gloves and an N95 respirator. Despite such protections and having mailroom personnel that screen incoming mail, there would still remain a chance of contaminated mail being delivered to an individual. Following the 2001 incidents in the U.S., a great deal of discussion has ensued regarding decontamination systems, with mention of ultraviolet, x-ray, or other radiation techniques as possible solutions.

Decontamination of Exposed Persons

In the event of an aerosolization exposure, each person exposed becomes a potential vector and must be considered for decontamination. Since there is no risk of immediate disease, decontamination should be undertaken as quickly as possible, with one of the goals being containment of the exposed personnel so that they do not disperse, spreading spores even more widely. Any decontamination must be undertaken with attention to the risk of generating aerosols of spores. Formal decontamination should take place in an airtight designated space with an air-lock type of entry and egress system following standard decontamination principles of having the entry to the decontamination unit located in the contaminated zone and the exit in a clean zone (see the discussion of hot, warm, and cool zones in Chapter 55). Personnel performing the decontamination should be wearing National Institute of Occupational Safety and Health (NIOSH)-approved personal protective equipment. Level B and possibly even level C protection may be adequate (see Chapter 55, Table 55.9). Contaminated persons who undress themselves should immediately place clothing in sealable plastic bags for either decontamination or disposal.

OSHA has not developed standards for employees exposed to biologic agents. The International Association of Fire Fighters requested NIOSH to offer guidance on respirator use in the aftermath to the anthrax situations during the fall of 2001. Their response is summarized in Table 56.6.

Much was learned from the experiences at the U.S. Capitol in terms of how far spores were found from

TABLE 56.6A. *National Institute for Occupational Safety and Health (NIOSH) interim recommendations for the selection and use of protective clothing and respirators against biologic agents*

Organic airborne particles share the same physical characteristics in air or on surfaces as inorganic particles from hazardous dusts. Because biologic weapons are particles, they will not penetrate the materials of properly assembled and fitted respirators or protective clothing. Existing recommendations for protecting workers from biologic hazards require the use of full face-piece air-purifying respirators with particulate filter efficiencies ranging from N95 (for half-mask or hazards such as pulmonary tuberculosis) to P100 (for hazards such as hantavirus) as a minimum level of protection. Some devices used for intentional biologic terrorism may have the capacity to disseminate large quantities of biologic materials in aerosols.	Emergency first responders typically use self-contained breathing apparatus (SCBA) respirators with a full face-piece operated in the most protective, positive pressure (pressure demand) mode during emergency responses. This type of SCBA provides the highest level of protection against airborne hazards when properly fitted to the user's face and properly used. NIOSH respirator policies state that, under those conditions, SCBA reduces the user's exposure to hazard by a factor of at least 10,000.This reduction is true whether the hazard is from airborne particles, a chemical vapor, or a gas. SCBA respirators are used when hazards and airborne concentrations are either unknown or expected to be high. Respirators providing lower levels of protection are generally allowed once conditions are understood and exposures are determined to be at lower levels.

From Interim recommendations for the selection and use of protective clothing and respirators against biological agents. NIOSH, Centers for Disease Control, October 25, 2001. *http://ww.cdc.gov/niosh/unp-intrecppe.htm.*

TABLE 56.6B. *NIOSH interim recommendations for the selection and use of protective clothing and respirators against biologic measures*

Responders should use a NIOSH-approved, pressure-demand SCBA in conjunction with a level A protective suit in responding to a suspected biologic incident where any of the following information is unknown or the event is uncontrolled: Type(s) of airborne agent(s) Dissemination method If dissemination via an aerosol-generating device is still occurring or it has stopped but there is no information on the duration of dissemination, or what the exposure concentration might be Responders may use a level B protective suit with an exposed or enclosed NIOSH-approved pressure-demand SCBA if the situation can be defined in which:	The suspected biologic aerosol is no longer being generated Other conditions may present a splash hazard Responders may use a full face-piece respirator with a P100 filter or powered air-purifying respirator (PAPR) with high-efficiency particulate air (HEPA) filters when it can be determined that: An aerosol-generating device was not used to create high airborne concentration Dissemination was by a letter or package that can be easily bagged These types of respirators reduce the user's exposure by a factor of 50 if the user has been properly fit tested.

From Interim recommendations for the selection and use of protective clothing and respirators against biological agents.
NIOSH, Centers for Disease Control, October 25, 2001. *http://www.cdc.gov/niosh/unp-intrecppe.htm.*

the actual delivery vehicle. Some spores were found over 75 feet from the room where an envelope was actually opened.

Rehabilitation of Facilities

Prior to October 2001, most sources recommended dilute household bleach (0.5% hypochlorite) for decontaminating areas and clothing contaminated with anthrax. Attempts to rid the U.S. Senate Office Building of spores proved quite difficult. Chlorine dioxide gas was used, but the humidity turned out to be critical. It was necessary to get the humidity above 75%.

Prophylaxis of Persons Likely Exposed

Recommendations for prophylaxis are subject to change. Up-to-date recommendations should be obtained in consultation with local and state health departments and CDC. Prophylaxis should be initiated upon confirmation of an anthrax exposure (Table 56.7).

Prophylaxis should continue until *B. anthracis* exposure has been excluded. If exposure is confirmed, prophylaxis should continue for 8 weeks. Based on one study in 60 monkeys and a very small margin of difference, the Medical Letter recommends ideally treating with an antibiotic and the vaccine (21). If available, postexposure vaccination consists of three doses of vaccine at 0, 2, and 4 weeks after exposure. With vaccination, postexposure antimicrobial prophylaxis may be able to be reduced to 4 weeks as per the Medical Letter. CDC recommendations at the time of this writing do not support the general use of anthrax vaccine.

From October 8 through November 9, 2001, approximately 32,000 persons with potential exposure to *B. anthracis* in Florida, New Jersey, New York City, and Washington, DC, initiated antimicrobial prophylaxis to prevent anthrax infection. For approximately 5,000 persons, a 60-day course of antibiotics was recommended (21). Immunization was not employed in these incidents.

Smallpox

Most authorities consider smallpox the next most likely agent after anthrax to be used for terrorist attacks on larger population groups. The variola virus causes smallpox. Following 2 to 4 days of fever and myalgia, a papular rash appears that then breaks down to ulcerations. The rash may look like varicella; however, the onset is synchronous as opposed to the sequential appearance of crops of papules with varicella (Table 56.8). Once patients develop skin lesions, they are infectious until all scabs drop off. Transmission occurs via both droplet and airborne mechanisms. Smallpox is relatively easily weaponized since it does not lose virulence on drying. No cases of smallpox have been recorded in over 20 years. Since the organism retains infectious capability after drying, any contaminated clothing, equipment, and environments need to be cleaned carefully and thoroughly. Although millions of people have been vaccinated against smallpox, it is unclear how many have actually retained any immunity.

Brucellosis

Brucellosis generally has a relatively high morbidity with relatively low mortality. It is caused by one of four species of *Brucellae* that are pathogenic in humans. It is transmitted usually from animals via

TABLE 56.7. *Recommended postexposure prophylaxis for exposure to bacillus anthracis*

Antimicrobial agent	Adults	Children
Oral fluoroquinolones		
One of the following:		
Ciprofloxacin	500 mg twice daily	20–30 mg per kg of body mass daily, divided into two doses[a]
Levofloxacin	500 mg twice daily	Not recommended
Ofloxacin	400 mg twice daily	Not recommended
If fluoroquinolones not available or contraindicated		
Doxycycline	100 mg twice daily	5 mg per kg of body mass per day divided into two doses[b]

[a]Use of fluoroquinolones in children discouraged unless absolutely necessary. Concern re: arthropathy demonstrated in juvenile lab animals. From Schaad UB. Pediatric use of quinolones. *Pediatric Infect Dis J* 1999;18(5):469–470.

[b]Tetracyclines can lead to staining of teeth in children still laying down calcium. If *B. anthracis* exposure is confirmed by obtaining a sample of the exposure material, penicillin sensitivity testing should be done with children changed to amoxicillin (40 mg/kg/d divided every 8 hours).

TABLE 56.8. *Differentiation of smallpox and chickenpox*

Smallpox	Chickenpox
Synchronous lesion development	Asynchronous lesions development
Centrifugal lesion development	Centripetal lesion development

aerosol. Doxycycline and rifampin are used in combination for 6 weeks to prevent recurring infection. Recovery may take a few weeks to several months. Some listings do not include it as a potential bioweapon due to the low mortality and technical difficulties in weaponizing it.

Response issues would be similar to those outlined for anthrax.

Plague

The plague manifests in several forms: bubonic, septicemic and pneumonic. The agent responsible in each case is *Yersinia pestis*. Bubonic and septicemic plague result from transmission by infected fleas. Pneumonic plague is usually transmitted by aerosolized germs, though it may develop as advancement of bubonic plague. Most commonly, naturally occurring pneumonic plague is found in densely populated areas. It is easily treated when found early. If treatment is delayed at all, however, the mortality is very high. Most recent natural outbreaks have been in impoverished regions of the world. A summary of the clinical syndrome is presented in Table 56.9.

No effective vaccine currently exists against pneumonic plague. The only real prevention is avoidance.

TABLE 56.9. *Pneumonic plague clinical syndrome*

Pneumonic plague	Fever, cough, chest pain Hemoptysis Mucopurulent or watery sputum with gram-negative rods Radiographic evidence of bronchopneumonia
Incubation period	Normally 2–8 days if due to flea-borne transmission; shorter for pulmonary exposure (1–3 days)
Prevention of transmission	Droplet precautions for patients with pneumatic form
Period of communicability	Until on antibiotics for 72 hours

Once people become symptomatic with the pneumonic form, they become contagious through droplet transmission. Thus, in terms of risk assessment for co-workers or health care workers, anyone who came no closer than approximately 3 feet to a contagious individual should be considered at low risk. Since the initial symptoms are nonspecific, however, the infected patient may not necessarily be recognized as a threat.

Although several countries have tried to develop *Y. pestis* as a bioweapon, the only effective method of dissemination used to date has been via deploying infected fleas.

The risk for reaerosolization of *Y. pestis* from the contaminated clothing of exposed persons is low. It is not very hardy outside the host, and, according to the Working Group on Civilian Biodefense, there is very little risk of infection from an environment exposed to a cloud of intentionally released *Y. pestis*. Contaminated bodily materials, however, may present a risk for handlers to develop cutaneous or bubonic plague (22).

Postexposure prophylaxis should be initiated following confirmed or suspected bioterrorism *Y. pestis* exposure, and for health care workers and others who had unprotected close contact with symptomatic patients. Prophylaxis should continue for 7 days after the last known or suspected *Y. pestis* exposure, or until exposure has been excluded (Table 56.10).

TABLE 56.10. *Recommended mass casualty postexposure prophylaxis for exposure to Yersinia pestis*

Antimicrobial agent	Agent	Children[a]
First choice: doxycycline	100 mg twice daily	5 mg per kg of body mass per day divided into two doses
Second choice: ciprofloxacin	500 mg twice daily	20 mg per kg of body mass per day divided into two doses

[a]<45 kg. Pediatric use of tetracyclines and fluoroquinolones is associated with adverse effects that must be weighed against the risk of developing a lethal disease. From Ingelsby TV, Dennis DT, Henderson DA. Plague as a biological weapon. *JAMA* 2000;283: 2281–2290. *http://jama.ama-assn.org/issues/v283n17/figtab/jst90013 t2.html.*

From APIC Bioterrorism Task Force, CDC Hospital Infections Program. Bioterrorism Working Group. Bioterrorism readiness plan: a template for healthcare facilities. April 13, 1999.

Other Biologic Agents

A number of other agents appear on various listings of potential biologic agents of terrorism. These include glanders and Q fever, which were researched heavily by the Soviet Union. Other agents with potential for smaller scale attacks include cholera, *Salmonella,* and other gastrointestinal agents. Various viruses have also been identified as having a possible potential for use. These include the hemorrhagic fever agents such as Lassa fever, Crimean Congo hemorrhagic fever, Ebola, and others (23).

Chemical/Toxic

A variety of chemical agents have been used as weapons throughout the ages. Some of the earliest known Western historical references refer to the use of substances such as quicklime and smoke from burning various noxious substances. In his *History of the Peloponnesian War,* Thucydides described the use of smoke from a fire of pitch and sulfur to route the Athenians from their fortress at Delium around 420 B.C. (24).

Although some use of chemical agents, primarily chlorine, was contemplated in the American Civil War, the modern era of chemical warfare really began with World War I. The attendees at the Hague Convention of 1899 agreed to "abstain from the use of projectiles the object of which is the diffusion of asphyxiating or deleterious gases" (25). The 1907 convention officially outlawed the use of "poison or poisoned weapons" and "arms, projectiles, or material calculated to cause unnecessary suffering" (26). Despite this, WWI became a major testing ground for various chemical weapons from tear gas grenades employed by the French to the famous and effective use of mustard gas by the Germans.

Following WWI, there were several developments. On the positive side, the Geneva Convention of 1928 declared the prohibition against the use of chemical and biologic weapons (27). Unfortunately, various governments continued to use such agents, from the British dropping mustard bombs on Afghani tribesmen at the Khyber Pass to the Italians dropping them on Egyptian forces and saturating the roadside with mustard agent since the Egyptians were barefoot.

World War II was effectively free of any chemical warfare. The greatest known casualties came from the German bombing of an American munitions ship secretly carrying mustard bombs while in the Italian port of Bari. Some reports indicate the gas released in the explosion of the ship killed 83 U.S. servicemen and nearly 1,000 civilians.

Since WWII, there have been several documented instances in which chemical weapons have been used. The Egyptians used mustard bombs against Yemini royalists. The U.S. used chemical defoliants and tear gas in Vietnam. The Iraqis used mustard, cyanide, and probably nerve agents in their war against Iran and against the Kurdish population in Northern Iraq (28).

Despite initial reluctance, the U.S. Senate in 1997 voted to join other United Nations member countries in signing the Convention on the Prohibition of the Production, Stockpiling, and Use of Chemical Weapons and on Their Destruction, which had taken over 20 years to negotiate. As of 2002, 145 countries have ratified their adhesion to this convention that, in addition to proscribing the use of chemical agents on humans, also contains a proscription against the use of herbicides.

Of greater concern to most occupational health practitioners is the increasing use of chemical weapons by individuals or extremist organizations over the last 20 years of the 20th century. A few of the publicly documented events of recent times include several releases of sarin gas by the Japanese Aum Shinrikyo cult, most notably in 1995 in the Tokyo subway and the intentional release of a toxic gas in a nightclub in Lisbon, Portugal, in April 2000, resulting in several deaths (29). In such terrorist attacks, it may be difficult to accurately determine the exact number of injuries and deaths directly attributable to the agent versus other factors such as being crushed in the stampede of panic.

THE AGENTS

Chemical weapon agents are generally divided into several classes (Table 56.11). The vesicants, which cause vesicle formation and burns to the mucosa and skin, have been the most widely used in actual warfare as the mustard compounds. The most publicized terrorist use of one of the organophosphate nerve agents was the release of sarin gas in the Tokyo subway in 1995. Table 56.11 contains a list of the classic military agents along with antidotes when they exist. A number of other chemicals could be used as terrorist weapons since the limitations of deployment on a large scale that makes them problematic for the military would not necessarily apply. One such agent is cyanide in its various toxic forms that could be deployed from short range, as it was when the Nazis used it to kill concentration camp prisoners.

Botulinum Toxin

Though a biologic product, botulinum toxin is classed here as a chemical agent since, as a weapon,

TABLE 56.11. *Chemical warfare agents*

Class	Agents	Antidotes
Historical vesicants	Chlorine	
	Nitrogen mustard	None
	Sulfur mustard	None
	Lewisite	BAL
	Phosgene oxime (CX)	
Nerve agents (cholinesterase inhibitors)	Tabun (GA)	Atropine
	Sarin (GB)	
	Soman (GD)	
	GF (Cyclohexyl-methylphosphonofluoridate)	
	VX (*o*-Ethyl*S*-[2-(diisopropylamino)ethyl] methylphosphonothiolate)	
Smoke and other substances	Zinc oxide (HC)	
	Phosphorous smokes	
	Sulfur trioxide-chlorosulfonic acid	
	Titanium tetrachloride	
	Nitrogen oxides	
	Organofluoride polymers: Teflon and perfluoroisobutylene	
Incapacitating agents	Anticholinergics	Physostigmine
	BZ (3-Quinuclidinyl benzilate (QNB))	
	Atropine	
	Scopolamine	
Riot control agents	Lacrimators	
	CS (Pepper spray) (2-Chlorobenzalmalononitrile)	
	CN (Mace) (2-Chloro-1-phenylethanone)	
	Vomiting agents	
	DM (Adamsite) (10-Chloro-5,10-dihydrophenarsazine)	
	CA (Bromobenzylcyanide)	

it would be used as the isolated chemical. The Japanese Aum Shinrikyo cult made three attempts to release botulinum toxin as a weapon during the early 1990s without any apparent success.

Clostridium botulinum, an anaerobic gram-positive bacillus, is present throughout nature. It produces a toxin that inhibits the release of acetylcholine, leading to a dose-related flaccid paralysis. People are affected most commonly from eating inadequately sterilized, hermetically sealed foods. The toxin is heat labile, but stable in the open once produced. It can be dried as well. Thus, it could be introduced into foods in a variety of settings or potentially dispersed as an aerosol.

If recognized early, botulinum toxoid injection may lessen the full impact of an exposure. The mainstay of treatment of exposed persons is supportive care up to and including prolonged mechanical ventilation and subsequent rehabilitation.

Nuclear Agents

With technologic advances and the presumed migration of some nuclear weapons programs scientists from the former Soviet Union to more profitable post–Cold War employment, various sources have speculated that they may have developed smaller devices that could be deployed clandestinely. Contrary to the popular conception of nuclear explosions as the Cold War image of the large mushroom cloud, these smaller devices would likely have a greater strategic value if multiple small devices were deployed to take maximum advantage of the radioactive contamination effect rather than the blast effect itself.

Additional nuclear threat comes from the possible aerosol dispersal of radioactive material generated at a distant site, thus affording no warning as the explosion of a device would do.

Much speculation regarding terrorist group intents was given credence when, following the flight of the Taliban regime from Kandahar, Afghanistan, troops found drums with uranium 238 stored in underground tunnel complexes. Although it was unlikely that the group that had likely procured this stock had the means to produce a true nuclear bomb, the uranium 238 could have been used to create a "dirty bomb" in which the radioactive material is wrapped around a conventional bomb and simply dispersed over an area with explosion of the conventional bomb (30).

In either case, beyond the immediate blast effects of the explosion and immediate radiation burns, the effects of radioactive particle exposure would be much more insidious.

Unfortunately, considering current trends of terrorist motives and operations, attempts at slow destruction of the health of a target population over as much as several generations are comprehensibly within the logic of some terrorist groups. The Department of Energy has developed nuclear emergency search teams to be deployed to sites of questionable nuclear releases (31).

Hostage Situations

It is beyond the scope of this chapter to function as an employee training manual for response to kidnapping and hostage situations. These situation must be individually assessed. Employees in businesses or business sites with any apparent risk should be briefed about the specific relative risks and the fundamentals of assessment of such situations. As much as corporate regional and headquarters teams, in conjunction with appropriate authorities and consultants, will likely institute operations to minimize the risk of injury or death to the victims, at times the victims themselves have the best assessment of the situation.

In recent years the character of hostage situations has changed. Hostage takers have seemed to become more brutal and less concerned about world opinion in regards to the production of casualties. Additionally, in a growing number of such attacks the hostage takers have demonstrated a willingness to accept their own death as inevitable. Old advice to remain calm, cooperative, and quiet may not always be the in the best interest of kidnappees or hostages.

PSYCHOLOGICAL IMPACT

The psychological impact of terrorist attacks is a major goal of any such action. The psychological effects of any attack or even of a threat are pervasive. The bombing of the Murrah federal building in Oklahoma City, the airliner attacks on the World Trade Center in New York, and the mailing of anthrax-laden letters in the eastern U.S. all provoked fears of similar attacks world wide, resulting in disruption of normal operating procedures throughout society. As with many crises, persons who were not directly involved were, at times, more disabled from the psychological impact than people who were directly involved. The perceived risks conjured in the imagination are generally much harder to process than fears rooted in concrete experiences.

In the event of any attack that is either direct or well publicized, psychological support services are likely to mitigate the dysfunctional responses. Acknowledging the potential for impact may be all that is necessary for employees to begin processing their reactions. Supervisory staff should be briefed to be aware of dysfunctional behaviors as well as being informed of the likely impact on their own supervisory behaviors.

PREPARATION

The medical aspects of planning for and responding to intentional attacks on a business should be viewed as an integral part of the overall business continuity plan. As with natural disasters and inadvertent industrial disasters, planning for responses to terrorist actions should follow the guidelines put forth in Chapter 55. Responses are viewed as occurring in stages of responders, with larger and larger domains of responsibility and greater training (Table 56.12).

As the potential impact of the event spreads beyond the designated sphere of responsibility of any responding group, that group relinquishes responsibility and command to the next higher authority for certain aspects of the response. In the interface between a corporate response team and the local public service response teams, the corporate response team should subject itself to the authority of the public agencies for those activities within the scope of activity of the public agency. Thus, the corporate response plan would ideally have built in it a plan for allied and supplemental response activities that would be carried out by the corporate response team even following the arrival of the public responders, but not designated as in the command domain of the public responders. The delineation of the domains of responsibility must be established and agreed upon by corporate and public bodies prior to any need to activate the plan in order to avoid potentially disastrous outcomes.

Planners should be well apprised that such setting of guidelines for domains of responsibility is, at all levels, one of the most time-consuming of the planning activities as it involves many issues of "turf" and ego. In some corporate installation settings, local public service response capabilities may not be capable of providing a level of service appropriate for a full-scale response. In such situations, the corporate entity must make a decision as to whether to assist the local services to improve to an appropriate level or to develop internal response plans to the level of capability necessary to deliver an adequate response.

As discussed in Chapter 55, responders to terrorist events should be designated at several advancing lev-

TABLE 56.12. *Examples of typical responsibilities and training at different levels of employee responders*

Responder level	Typical activities/level of responsibility	Training (examples)
Individual employee	Minor first aid Knowledge of evacuation plan and local emergency response plan Knowledge of who to contact locally and who to contact in the event the first level of contact is incapacitated	General education regarding risks and safety of actions for evacuation
Work group leader	Responsibility for local readiness including local employee Training and practice of responses Evacuation plan Worker education Some simple decontamination Principles and practices	Advanced first aid Crowd management (to aid orderly evacuation)
Response team	Members with specific response training and training in use of safety equipment Containment of threat—would include preventing contaminated employees from spreading the threat	Simple risk containment techniques Crowd control techniques

els of capability. The first level should be each individual employee through an education program on both the risks involved with different threats and the corporate response plan. Individual employees should be encouraged to participate with suggestions and discussion, particularly regarding the immediate local response at each workstation, as this participation will improve the sense of ownership and, hence, comprehension of and participation in the final version of the response plan. Additionally, education of workers regarding the reality of risk and appropriate response in various events will likely decrease the incidence of "collateral disability," which refers to the effect of an event on persons with no direct risk of injury, but with a fear of potential harm based on ignorance of the realities related to an event. This may be manifest either acutely by persons with little or no risk of injury seeking emergency medical attention or chronically, by varying degrees of disability due to fear of potential effects.

Depending on the corporate risk profile, preparation may be as simple as developing an evacuation and family notification plan for general emergencies as required by OSHA. Alternatively, in a high-risk setting, extensive planning and use of many outside consultants may be necessary to seek security for the staff.

With the number of threats and the variety of methods that attackers could use, total defense is relatively impossible. Thus, a reasonable program for dealing with the possibility of terrorist attack begins with the assurance of safety of the work site.

Prevention of Site Compromise

Ensuring a safe work environment involves planning for potential routes of entry of an attack as well as ensuring that the structure is constructed in such a way as to offer maximum protection to the occupants. In certain circumstances this may extend to the vehicles used by personnel to travel to various field sites and to the level of armed security presence necessary.

Secure Perimeter

Bombing of buildings in Lebanon and Oklahoma City demonstrate the importance of a secure perimeter. Stand-off distances, barriers, and security control stations should all be used as means to prevent unauthorized vehicles from gaining close proximity to potential targets. In the bombing of the U.S. embassy in Kenya, more people would have been killed if the pickup truck carrying the bomb had not been stopped by an alert guard.

Ideally, any organization planning either for the construction of a new facility or the purchase of a physical site for operations would consider security pursuant to a corporate risk assessment. The OM physician would not necessarily be considered an expert regarding the actual plans. However, just as OM physicians should have input into choices of new machinery or operational procedures in terms of projected injury risk, it is equally logical that they would have a voice in the site development process.

The perimeter of a building should be considered in relation to the classic approaches above ground.

A plot was uncovered in Italy in which a several men were arrested with potassium ferrocyanide, a relatively nontoxic substance, and water line plans detailing the area supplying the U.S. Embassy in Rome (32).

Mail Handling

Virtually all of the threats outlined in this chapter could arrive via the mail. Mail bombs have been a part of terrorist campaigns for many years. Although law enforcement personnel have vastly increased their understanding of characteristics of mail bombs, as is too often the case the perpetrators constantly look for better ways to disguise bombs.

A letter bomb campaign in 1996 against several offices of Al-Hayat, a progressive Islamic newspaper, and Leavenworth Prison utilized musical Christmas card circuitry to detonate Czech Semtec (33).

Mail screening training is essential for any large organization. Despite the best training in the mailroom, some items may get through and some techniques of attack may not be covered in the training. Full protection at all times against all possible threats is prohibitively cumbersome and expensive. As in many terrorist situations, again, early recognition of an active situation should initiate an escalation of screening efforts.

Since the mailroom screening process may not be fully secure, certain key personnel should also be trained to recognize suspicious letters and packages depending on an organization's initial risk assessment. The U.S. Postal Service (USPS) published guidelines for mail evaluation. Numerous private security consulting firms also would address this in any consultation. Some have published information on the Internet (34). Cross-referencing several sources and verifying that the information, particularly on Internet sites, is the most up-to-date is critical. The USPS guidelines developed in conjunction with the CDC for screening for anthrax underwent modification during the 2001 situation. In the updated version the USPS removed the initial recommendation to cover any powder that may have spilled out of an envelope, since this would have been more likely to create air currents that would aerosolize the particles.

The USPS Postal Customer Council has published guidelines for overall security of the mail center (35). These are variably applicable to different size operations. The USPS Inspection Service has, in conjunction with the FBI, published guidelines for identification of mail bombs (Table 56.13). Although some of these characteristics could apply to many innocuous mail items, they are generally based on historical cases, thus having some degree of specificity.

TABLE 56.13. *Clues to potential mail bombs*

Construction	Markings
Rigidity	Incorrect addressing
Irregular shape	Foreign handwriting
Unbalanced weight	Poorly typed or handwritten
Oily stains	No return address
Sloshing sound or shifting weight	False or fictitious sender
Feel of wires or foil	Restrictive markings
Feel of cylindrical tube	Place of origin
Soft spots	Excessive postage
Excessive tape	
Signs of reassembly	
Strange odors	

From Bombs by Mail: Notice 71. United States Postal Service. *http://new.ups.com/cpim/ftp/notices/not71.pdf.*

Ensuring Integrity of Essential Services

Provision of secure, safe essential services from water to fuel to electricity should be addressed. Planners should ensure the continuation of service in the event of a critical incident.

Policy and Procedural Preparation

Unlike preparation of a workforce for response to a potential uncontrolled release of industrial substances with which they are working on a regular basis, preparation for the potential events covered in this chapter applies to many new and rarely encountered substances. Education of the workforce regarding offending agents is a critical part of response training and response policy development. Initial education sessions coupled with handouts for reference would likely form the core of an employee preparation program. Front-line workers who are familiar with everyday work habits and personnel movements will likely be able to provide significant input to generic response plans developed by managers or outside consultants.

"Live" drills in addition to tabletop exercises are essential to identifying and eliminating potential problems in response plans.

Special Considerations in International Domain

Business operations in foreign domains have a number of additional factors that must be considered when planning for responses. Local medical support services may not be at a level capable of providing support in the event of even a simple bomb attack with blunt trauma victims. In such a case the medical direction team would need to make appropriate contractural arrangements with an international medical evacuation service. Additionally, in such remote settings that may have a more hostile general environment, employee protection during off-hours must be addressed through provision of appropriate housing and transportation possibilities as well as education regarding indigenous risks. This last component should be done prior to relocation to give the employee the opportunity to request alternate posting.

Psychological Preparation

Psychological preparation of the entire workforce is an essential feature of terrorist event response in order to minimize the risks for panic as well as to minimize the amount of collateral disability among personnel not directly impacted by an event. Presentation of reality-based information regarding the risk of an event occurring and of potential types of events along with active participation in development of response plans will generally provide the workers with a greater sense of control over their destiny. Such knowledge will mitigate the feelings of helplessness that are frequently identified among workers who experience psychological disability with fear of, but no actual direct exposure to, threats to personal safety.

Response

Regardless of the relative risk of various potential events for any one work site or business operation, once an event occurs many of the response activities are generic. Almost all responses involve multiple internal and external services. Recognizing the multiple difficulties in coordinating responses to open land fires, in the 1970s an interagency task force, FIRESCOPE (Firefighting Resources of California Organized for Potential Emergencies), developed an Incident Command System (ICS). This system provides an overall organizational plan to be agreed to pre-event by all responding agencies as well as a common language and coordination of activities and resources. ICS structures are meant to be scalable and interlocking as various responders become involved in an incident. Further development of the original ICS plan was undertaken in the 1980s by the National Interagency Incident Management System (NIIMS), associated with the U.S. Forest Service. Information and downloadable forms are available through several government and private sites since the information is in the public domain. OSHA has mandated that businesses with hazardous materials incident potential should adopt ICS principles in planning responses. The San Mateo County Emergency Medical Services Agency in conjunction with the California Emergency Medical Services Authority developed a spin-off hospital-based emergency incident command system (HEICS).

ICS management has been adopted by most public emergency response agencies in the U.S. Because it is a scalable system with interlocking units, if it is employed in a corporate setting, as the situation escalates to involve outside agencies the management structure will be compatible, minimizing confusion in transfer of information and designation of command. Links are provided below (see Further Information) for more in-depth discussion and on-line forms.

Regulations

OSHA has put forth a number of regulations governing emergency response (Table 56.14). According to the National Safety Council, the ten most common faults in emergency response plans are direct reflections of management's not taking seriously the possibility of a critical incident (36). A number of the issues relevant to emergency response have been addressed in Chapter 55.

As stated at the outset, risk assessment should be the foundation for development of an emergency response plan. From an OSHA perspective, any responders to chemical/biologic situations would fall under the regulations of 29 CFR 1910.120, which covers hazardous materials emergency response workers. This would include any persons trained as internal safety wardens for

TABLE 56.14. *OSHA regulations pertaining to emergency response plans*

All are found in Code of Federal Regulations (CFR) Title 29
Subpart E—Means of Egress
1910-37 Means of Egress
1910-38 Employee Emergency Plans
Appendix to Subpart E—Means of Egress
Subpart H—Hazardous Materials
1910.120 Hazardous Waste Operations and Response
Subpart K—Medical and First Aid
1910.151 Medical Services and First Aid
Subpart L—Fire Protection
1910.155 through 1910.165
Subpart Z—Toxic and Hazardous Substances
1910.1200 Hazardous Communications

responses. OSHA publishes a booklet, "How to Respond to Workplace Emergencies and Evacuations," that is available on the Internet (37).

General Protective Measures

Although each of the possible biologic or chemical threats has associated protective measures, it is impractical to practice these behaviors full time. Regarding corporate practices, it is far more practical to look at the union of two variables: generic types of exposure mechanisms and corporate risk. Procedures should also be established for upgrading the level of protection in the event of an actual event. General protective measures for various routes and types of exposures/events are summarized in Table 56.15.

Internal/Corporate

In the corporate setting, particularly in medically remote settings, it may be necessary for a facility health center to manage the initial phase of any response. It is imperative in the pre-event planning to identify sources of antibiotics and to develop a system of coordination with local health care facilities and follow-up for exposed employees.

Protocols should be installed to deal with the medical–public safety official interface that will develop in the event of a chemical or biologic attack. Though it is important to collect evidence to facilitate the apprehension and conviction of attackers, it is arguably of greater public health importance to gain medical information regarding the nature of any of the biologic or chemical agents potentially used. The CDC has established a phone number to provide up-to-date information: Bioterrorism Emergency Number at the CDC Emergency Response Office, 1-770-488-7100.

Policies

Evacuation

In the immediate moments following any of the events that involve known compromise of the quality of the local environment, evacuation of the living becomes a first priority. Orderly, safe evacuation requires preplanning and running drills. Ideally, team leaders should be designated from different work sites. A unique work site may be considered to be even different sections of a single building. The evacuation groupings should be set based on commonality of expected routes as well as existing work groups.

TABLE 56.15. *General protective measures*

Route of exposure	General preparedness protective measures	Event level response
Regional atmospheric release	Risk assessment-based level of restrictions of normal day-to-day activities	Shut down HVAC air exchange systems Close windows/doors
Chemical vapors/gas	Building with door, window seals, and HVAC controls	Apply any available personal protective device Stay inside
Large droplet	Risk assessment-based level of restriction of normal day-to-day activities	Surgical masks considered adequate for temporary exposure Large droplets considered to not transmit greater than 3 feet
Small droplet (<0.5 μm)	Risk assessment-based level of restriction of normal day-to-day activities	Airborne protection: N95, HEPA filters required as minimal and then only for brief exposure Longer or higher dose exposure should have level A protection (fully encapsulated with purified air either by SCBA or line feed with HEPA filter from outside hot zone)
Contact	Be attentive to liquids and powders that are not normally present	Avoid any contact If necessary use latex or nitrile gloves with at least a Tyvek level 1 suit
Ingestion	Risk assessment–based level of restriction of activities of eating in uncontrolled environments	Do not eat at any site that is not secure; preferably preparing own food

HVAC, heating, ventilation, and air-conditioning systems.

Designated team leaders are not necessarily organizational managers.

Regardless of assurances from structural engineers and builders, the integrity of the structure may be damaged by a blast or ensuing fires. As a part of planning for any necessitated rapid evacuation, multiple routes that ideally interconnect should be available. Special provisions should be made for employees with special needs to be able to be evacuated in a timely manner.

Kidnap/Hostage

The historic advice in the event of kidnapping and hostage situations has been to remain calm since the kidnappers or hostage takers typically wanted either money or publicity more than some form of revenge, which seems to be more the case recently. The U.S. State Department offers a number of points of advice for traveling abroad on how to decrease the risk of violent attack and on how to respond in a hostage situation. Each situation is individual; however, since the attacks on the World Trade Center in New York with hijacked airliners, there is a general realization that hostage situations have taken on a higher level of concern for an ultimate safe resolution.

Physical Plant

Physical plant issues to be considered in the event of a terrorist attack include the entire structure and all connections to the outside world. The U.S. government has developed a "shadow government" site to address this issue. This unit consists of a complete redundancy of what have been determined to be critical functional components to maintain operations. As the destruction of the World Trade Center well demonstrated, a terrorist attack may have a major effect not only on the direct target, but, through disruption of infrastructure, on the operations of many more organizations. The American Hospital Association has prepared a checklist for chemical and bioterrorism preparedness that has many elements that can be modified to be applicable to any organization (38).

Psychological Support

Immediate psychological support should be arranged for survivors of any lethal attacks. Family members should be involved as well. One frequently overlooked aspect is early notification of immediate family of the status of employees. Additionally, if the attack is one that has any community-wide implications that have led to restricting employees from leaving the work site, establishing contact with families is critical to ensuring the optimum functioning of employees unable to go to check on them. As a part of the emergency response plan for earthquakes in California, virtually all fire departments have agreements such that each firefighter is registered with the nearest fire-fighting facility. One of the first duties of a local fire station is to check on the families of colleagues and relay notification to the firefighter's base station. Historically, firefighters had had problems with being so concerned about their own family's safety that they had trouble maintaining focus on their duties. During the 1994 Northridge earthquake, these problems were significantly reduced by the new policy.

The psychological impact of any disaster may manifest well after the actual events. Such posttraumatic stress–based dysfunction can persist for prolonged periods. The best prevention of dysfunction from posttraumatic stress disorder (PTSD) is through early detection of vulnerable populations and addressing the likely fears that may become unrealistic if not addressed early (39).

Training

In addition to training of designated safety personnel and "wardens" for responses, any employees anticipated to be in higher risk situations, such as travel to higher risk areas, should receive specific training to decrease risk. Training can be developed in-house for larger organizations; however, it is often more desirable to contract it out. Considering the variability in recommendations from different government agencies and private organizations as well as the changes related to experience with more recent events, any vendor-proposed training program should be scrutinized for content validity. This is a clear role for the OM physician in conjunction with selected content experts.

Drills

The best way to ensure an optimal response in such situations is through repeated practice. Public safety agencies have found that a combination of tabletop strategic drills, mock event drills, and subsequent debriefing produces the best results. A well-drafted ERP that addresses all possible contingencies and that has been placed in a binder on a shelf is useless in the time of crisis.

CONCLUSION

Although statistically a small part of the overall occupational health field, consideration for worker safety in the face of increased general societal risk of terrorist attacks has brought this topic to the forefront of many discussions. As the professional with responsibility for the safety of all employees of an enterprise, whether with 10 or 10,000 employees, the OM physician has a critical role to play in ensuring a safe work environment.

REFERENCES

1. United States Code Title 22 Chapter 38 Section 2656f(d) paragraphs 2 and 3. *http://www4.law.cornell.edu/uscode/22/2656f.html.*
2. United States Code: Title 18 Part II Chapter 204 Sec. 3077. *http://www4.law.cornell.edu/uscode/18/3077.html.*
3. Passenger storms U.S. jet cockpit. *Guardian Unlimited* 2002 Feb 8. *http://www.guardian.co.uk/airlines/story/0,1371,646778,00.html.*
4. Terrorism vulnerability self-assessment. North Carolina Department of Crime Control and Public Safety. *http://www.nccrimecontrol.org/forms/terrorismselfassessment.htm.*
5. Series of articles on risk assessment. Kingsley Technologies (PTY) LTD. *http://www.terrorism.uk.com/default.asp?Page=riskMang.asp.*
6. Griffith C, Vulpitta R. Effective emergency response plans: anticipate the worst, prepare for the best results. National Safety Council, 2001. http://www.nsc.org/issues/emerg/99esc.htm#SIDEBAR2.
7. Smithson AE, Levy LA. Stimson Center report No. 35: ataxia: the chemical and biological terrorism threat and the U.S. response. Washington, DC: The Henry L. Stimson Center, October 2000. *http://www.stimson.org/cbw/pubs.cfm?ID=12.*
8. Smith JD, Murray K. White paper: developing a corporate security policy. *TNC Engineering* 2000 Jan 1. *http://www.tnc.com/assets/information/TNCDevelopPolicy.pdf.*
9. Department of Justice assessment of the increased risk of terrorist and other criminal activity associated with posting off-site consequence analysis information on the Internet. Washington, DC: DOJ, April 18, 2000. *http://www.usdoj.gov/criminal/april18final.pdf.*
10. AMA quick reference guide to biological weapons. Resources for physicians. *Bioterrorism Awareness* (CD-ROM). Chicago: American Medical Association, 2001.
11. Vogt F. Resources on bioterrorism. Physician resources. Disaster preparedness and medical response. Public Health. *American Medical Association*. Dec 17, 2001 (last updated). *http://www.ama-assn.org/ama/pub/category/6215.html.*
12. Arson and Explosives Incidents System. Bureau of Alcohol, Tobacco and Firearms, Treasury Department. *http: // www.atf.treas.gov / aexis2 / type_files / f_aexis_report 1.html.*
13. One of many: Applied Research Associates, Inc. *http://www.ara.com/at_planner.htm.*
14. Bomb Threat Telephone Procedures. Canadian Bomb Data Centre. Royal Canadian Mounted Police. *http://www.cbdc-ccdb.org/english/cbdc_eng.htm.*
15. d'Errico P. Jeffrey Amherst and smallpox blankets: Lord Jeffrey Amherst's letters discussing germ warfare against American Indians. *http://www.nativeweb.org/pages/legal/amherst/lord_jeff.html.*
16. Kortepeter MG, Parker GW. Potential biological weapons threats. Emerging infectious diseases. Last updated July 1, 1999. *http://www.cdc.gov/ncidod/EID/vol5no4/kortepeter.htm.*
17. Departments of the Army, Navy, and Air Force. NATO Handbook on the Medical Aspects of NBC Defensive Operations. Washington, DC: Department of Defense, 1996. *http://www.fas.org/nuke/guide/usa/doctrine/dod/fm8-9toc.htm.*
18. Center for Non-proliferation Studies. Russia announces plans to participate in research on Vozrozhdeniye Island. March 19, 2002. *http://cns.miis.edu/pubs/week/020318.htm.*
19. Science News Update. The American Medical Association. 6 August, 1997. *http://www.ama-assn.org/sci-pubs/sci-news/1997/snr0806.htm.*
20. *Medical Letter* 2001 Oct 29; 43.
21. CDC. Update: investigation of bioterrorism-related anthrax and adverse events from antimicrobial prophylaxis. *MMWR* 2001;50(44):973–976.
22. Inglesby TV, et al. Plague as a biological weapon: medical and public health management. *JAMA* 2000;283:2281–2290. *www.bt.cdc.gov/Agent/Plague/Consensus.pdf.*
23. Kortepeter MG, Parker GW. Potential biological weapons threats. *Emerging Infectious Diseases* CDC 1999;5(4). *http://www.cdc.gov/ncidod/EID/vol5no4/kortepeter.htm.*
24. Thucydides (trans. by R. Crawley). *The history of the Peloponnesian War*. Great Books of the Western World. Chicago: Encyclopedia Britannica, 1952.
25. Laws of war: declaration on the use of projectiles the object of which is the diffusion of asphyxiating or deleterious gases; international peace conference at The Hague. The Avalon Project at the Yale Law School, July 29, 1899. *http://www.yale.edu/lawweb/avalon/lawofwar/dec99-02.htm.*
26. Art 21. Ch. I. Sec. II. *Laws of War: Laws and Customs of War on Land. Hague Convention IV*. The Avalon Project at the Yale Law School, October 18, 1907. *http://www.yale.edu/lawweb/avalon/lawofwar/hague04.htm.*
27. Protocol for the Prohibition of the Use in War of Asphyxiating Gas, and of Bacteriologic Methods of Warfare. Geneva: The Avalon Project at the Yale Law School, February 8, 1928.
28. Joy RJ. Historical aspects of medical defense against chemical warfare. In: *Textbook of military medicine*. Chapter 3.
29. BBC. Seven die in gas attack at Portuguese nightclub. International Policy Institute for Counter-Terrorism. *http://www.ict.org.il/spotlight/det.cfm?id=420.*
30. Dutter B, Fenton B. Uranium and cyanide found in drums at bin Laden base. News Online. *London Telegraph* 2001 Dec 24. *http://www.telegraph.co.uk/news/main.jhtml?xml=%2Fnews%2F2001%2F12%2F24%2Fwbin24.xml.*
31. Nuclear Emergency Search Team. DOE O 5530.2. U.S. Department of Energy Directive. September 20, 1991. *http://www.directives.doe.gov/serieslist.html.*

32. Croddy E, Osborne M, McCloud K. Chemical terrorist plot in Rome. Center for Non-proliferation Studies. Monterey Institute of International Studies. March 11, 2002. *http://cns.miis.edu/pubs/week/020311.htm.*
33. Roth R, Lowrie M. Third letter bomb found at U.N.: ties to London explosion at newspaper office suspected. *CNN Interactive.* January 13, 1997. *http://www.cnn.com/US/97011/13/un.bomb.update.*
34. Bomb Countermeasures CD-ROM Demo. Bombsecurity.com. Palladium Media Group. *http://www.bombsecurity.com/demo.html.*
35. Best practices for mail center security: incoming and outgoing operations. USPS. *http://www.usps.com/nationalpcc/security.html.*
36. Griffith C, Vulpitta R. Effective emergency response plans: anticipate the worst, prepare for the best results. Every Second Counts magazine. National Safety Council. Fall 1999. *http://www.nsc.org/issues/emerg/99esc.htm.*
37. How to respond to workplace emergencies and evacuations. OSHA, 2001. *http://www.osha-slc.gov/SLTC/emergencyresponse/index.html.*
38. Chemical and bioterrorism preparedness checklist. Resources hospital readiness, response, and recovery resources. American Hospital Association. *www.hospitalconnect.com/aha/key_issues/disaster_readiness/resources/HospitalReady.html.*
39. Lange JT, Lange CL, Cabaltica RBG. Primary care treatment of post-traumatic stress disorder. *Am Fam Physician* 2000;62:1035–1040,1046.

FURTHER INFORMATION

The Internet sites provided here as potential resources were all available as of March 2002. For sites that are not official government agency sites, I have followed source links as much as possible to verify at least some of the information presented in these sites, but I do not maintain these sites.

General Terrorist Risk/Vulnerability

North Carolina Department of Crime Control and Public Safety.

http://www.nccrimecontrol.org/forms/terrorismselfassessment.htm.

Kingsley Technologies (PTY) Ltd.

A Cape Town, South Africa, computer security company that has published a series of articles on risk assessment. *http://security:kingsley.co.za/articles/article3.htm.*

U.S. Department of State travel warnings and public announcements. *http://travel.state.gov.*

Overseas Security Advisory Council. U.S. Department of State. Cooperation to share security-related information between the State Department and U.S. corporations operating outside the U.S. *http://www.ds-osac.org.*

International Information Programs. This site has a variety of information from security reports to assessments regarding terrorist risk and health risks. There is also political policy analysis. *http://usinfo.state.gov/topical/pol/terror.*

The National Security Institute (NSI) provides a variety of professional information and security awareness services. It publishes newsletters and special reports, and conducts seminars electronically via its Internet site. *http://www.nsi.org.*

The World Factbook. Central Intelligence Agency.

http://www./cia.gov/cia/publications/factbook/index.html.

The United States Federal Bureau of Investigation (FBI). *http://www.fbi.gov.*

Jane's Intel Web.

This site is a part of Jane's diverse products of military and foreign policy services. It requires either free login for limited access or a subscription for full access. *http://intelweb.janes.com/.*

The Henry L. Stimson Center

Located in Washington, D.C., the center conducts research on national and international security and publishes a number of white papers, some of which are available on the Internet. *http://www.stimson.org/?SN=TI200110174.*

Center for Non-proliferation Studies. Monterey Institute of International Studies.

The world's largest NGO devoted to combating the spread of weapons of mass destruction. Study of international affairs and publications. Analyses of news items. *http://cns.miis.edu/index.htm.*

Oklahoma City National Institute for the Prevention of Terrorism.

Many links to topics related to terrorism. The institute puts up a number of links specifically directed at businesses on a subpage. *http://www.mipt.org/bussecurity-rpt.html,http://www.mipt.org.*

Bomb Threats and Assessment

Department of the Treasury, Bureau of Alcohol, Tobacco, Firearms.

Phone number to report suspicious potential or real bombs or bomb supplies. 1-800-ATF-BOMB 1-(800)-283-2662.

ATF Arson and Explosives National Repository

Established by congressional mandate in 1996 as a national collection center for information on arson and explosives-related incidents throughout the U.S. The databases incorporate information from various sources such as the Bureau of Alcohol, Tobacco, and Firearms; the Federal Bureau of Investigation; and the United States Fire Administration. *http://www.atf.treas.gov/aexis2.*

Applied Research Associates, Inc

Downloadable blast effect calculator: *http://www.bombsecurity.com/downloads2/atblast.zip.*

Bioterrorism

Bioterrorism Emergency Number at the CDC Emergency Response Office: 1-(770)-488-7100.

Trivalent botulinum antitoxin is available by contacting state health departments or by contacting CDC (1-(404)-639-2206 during office hours, 1-(404)-639-2888 after hours).

Alibek K. *Biohazard.* New York: Random House, 1999.

This is the first hand account of the Soviet biological warfare program from Ken Alibek, M.D., who was deputy director of the research arm of this program when he defected to the U.S. shortly before the collapse of the Soviet Union.

AMA Index of Bioterrorism Resources
http://www.amaassn.org/ama/pub/category/6671.html#Top.
The American Academy of Family Physicians
The Web site has a number of references to articles regarding primary care issues in relation to terrorism and specific threats. *http://www.aafp.org/btresponse/index.xml.*
Johns Hopkins University Center for Civilian Biodefense Studies
A center associated with the School of Public Health. Excellent resource for information on the overview of biologic warfare risks. The information on individual agents is limited to fact sheets with relatively little specifics.
http://www.hopkins-biodefense.org.

Chemical Terrorism

U.S. Army Medical Research Unit of Chemical Defense (USAMRICD)
U.S. Army center for study of chemical warfare agents. Excellent overview with historical as well practical information. *http://chemdef.apgea.army.mil/.*
The Defense Threat Reduction Agency
An agency of the Department of Defense charged with "safeguarding America and its friends from weapons of mass destruction." The site has various discussions of threats and mitigating threats. *http://www.dtra.mil/.*

Response Planning

OSHA Respiratory Protection Advisor.
This site is a fairly comprehensive discussion of developing a respirator program geared largely to situations needing regular use of respirators. The principles still apply for the emergency use.
http://www.osha-slc.gov/SLTC/respiratory_advisor/mainpage.html.
How to respond to workplace emergencies and evacuations. Publication 3088. OSHA, 2001.
This brochure reviews the general issues involved in creating emergency action and evacuation plans. It is built on the various OSHA regulations and provides comprehensive lists of relevant regulations. *http://www.osha-slc.gov/SLTC/emergencyresponse/index.html.*
San Mateo County Emergency Medical Services Agency
Originators of the Hospital Emergency Incident Command System modification of the fire fighting incident command system. Information and forms are available through its Web site.
http://www.emsa.ca.gov/dms2/heics3.htm.
Department of Energy (DOE)
At the time of this writing much of the DOE Web site had been removed for revision in the aftermath of terrorist attacks of 2001 and concern regarding misuse of information posted.
The United States Coast Guard
In developing a national response system for hazardous materials incidents that may affect waterways and cross state boundaries, the U.S. Coast Guard adopted the National Interagency Incident Management System (NIIMS)-based Incident Command System structure. The Coast Guard "Field Operations Manual for Oil Spills" has a discussion of establishing the structure for managing an emergency incident. The system is adaptable to any emergency situation. The manual and Incident Command System forms are available via the U.S. Coast Guard Web site. *http://www.uscg.mil/hq/gm/mor/articles/ics.htm.*
The National Oceanic and Atmospheric Administration provides downloadable electronic Incident Command System forms. *http://response.restoration.noaa.gov/oilaids/ICS/intro.html.*
The National Safety Council
Several useful pages on emergency response plans and worker safety
http://www.nsc.org/index.htm.
National Wildfire Coordinating Group
Additional information on Incident Command Systems including training materials and downloadable forms is available in its publications.
http://www.nwcg.gov/pms/pubs/pubs/.htm.
United States Forest Service Fire and Aviation
Examples of organizational charts for wildland fires that may be adjusted and applied to other situations can be found at the Web page. *http://www.fs.fed.us/fire/operations/niims.shtml.*

57

The Environmental, Health, and Safety Audit

Ridgway M. Hall, Jr., William B. Bunn, and Thomas J. Slavin

The environmental, health, and safety audit serves an increasingly important role in compliance assurance both in the United States and internationally. Primarily companies that seek to identify and correct existing and potential compliance problems, or to identify areas where health, safety, and environmental performance can be improved, conduct these audits. The audit process reduces the risk of legal liability for current and past activities, and identifies future issues that may need attention not only for compliance purposes but also for cost-effective strategic planning.

The phrase *environmental, health, and safety audit* (EH&S audit) describes a process that includes the gathering of information on the activities at a facility that may impact the environment, safety, or human health, especially any activity subject to legal or regulatory requirements. Examples of the information obtained include releases to the air and water; hazardous and solid waste management and disposal practices; compliance with permit requirements; compliance with safety and health standards; environmental, health, and safety management practices; and numerous other activities that are regulated at the federal, state, and local level. The data are then measured against the regulatory requirements to determine a facility's compliance profile.

Typically, areas of noncompliance are noted, along with activities that, though not illegal, could expose the company to liability. At the conclusion of this process, an action plan is developed, which sets forth all findings that need a response. The action plan includes the proposed action, a timetable for completion, and a designation of the person or persons responsible.

The audit may be conducted by skilled personnel from within the organization, but independent of the entity being audited, or from other outside organizations, such as environmental engineering, safety, or law firms. The qualifications of auditors vary depending on the situation, but knowledge of the relevant regulations, and skills and training in the audit process, are essential. Environmental engineers, safety engineers, environmental lawyers, process engineers, industrial hygienists, occupational physicians and nurses, and other qualified professionals may serve as auditors or as part of the audit team. The key areas of expertise are an understanding of pertinent regulations and the ability to carefully analyze the industrial or commercial processes and related activities, which are subject to regulation. Auditors must understand the implications for the audit site and the parent company of their findings and recommendations on legal liability. The document produced by an environmental audit is usually comprehensive and contains substantial information on processes and programs as well as a list of findings and action items for management's consideration. Some audits, more commonly health and safety (H&S) audits, may also use a scoring system designed to focus on nonregulatory issues that may reduce injuries and illnesses.

In the last 5 years increasing emphasis has been placed on what is sometimes called an environmental management system (EMS), or in its expanded form, an EH&S management system. This is a broader program committed to ensuring compliance with applicable legal and regulatory requirements, and an evaluation of everything a company or facility does that may affect the environment, public health, or safety. It often includes a commitment to activities that go beyond compliance, including pollution prevention, waste minimization, recycling, reduction of loss-time accidents, injuries and illnesses, community outreach, energy conservation, and the like.

Internationally, the adoption of EH&S management systems got a boost in 1996 with publication by the International Organization for Standardization (ISO) of its 14000 series of standards for environmental management systems and related auditing. The EMS or EH&S management system is getting widespread use as a management tool. Increased public concern over environmental, health, and safety issues is likely to continue to spur the interest in and use of these management systems.

Health and safety lacks a well-recognized international standard such as ISO 14001, but within the U.S., the Occupational Safety and Health Administration's (OSHA) Voluntary Protection Program (VPP) certification has been a credible recognition of a well-functioning H&S management system (as of December 2000 there were only 543 VPP sites). In the United Kingdom, the British Standards Institute (BSI) has published OHSA's 18001:1999—occupational H&S management systems—specification, and OHSA's 18002:2000—guidelines for implementation, in response to urgent customer demand for a recognizable standard against which management systems can be assessed and certified.

THE ROLE OF THE ENVIRONMENTAL, HEALTH, AND SAFETY AUDIT

The most important role of the EH&S audit is to ensure regulatory compliance and prevent violations, fines and penalties, and public relations problems. Under most of the major federal environmental statutes, penalties can be imposed at up to $25,000 per day for civil violations. In addition, corporations and corporate officers, and in some cases "responsible individuals" may be fined up to $50,000 per day for criminal charges and face jail sentences as well. Some environmental laws, such as the Clean Water Act, authorize criminal sanctions for mere negligence, as well as for its more traditional "knowing" or "deliberate" violations. Furthermore, any person who claims personal injury or property damage, based on common law remedies such as nuisance, negligence, trespass, or strict liability, may then file civil suits. OSHA fines can be assessed up to $70,000 for willful or repeated violations, but most violations are assessed fines of less than $7,000. Although OSHA fines are often less significant than environmental fines, violations are more common, resulting in sizable proposed penalties. Although a regulatory violation is a significant part of the evidence for any litigation, liability can be imposed even without a violation. Compliance with a permit or regulation may not be a defense to a common law "toxic tort" if the business activities in question cause injuries. But the audit is a good tool for senior management to show good-faith efforts at responsible corporate governance.

Avoiding fines and litigation is not the only financial reason for establishing EH&S audit programs. Cost-effective planning that anticipates changing regulations or enforcement practices can yield competitive advantage. Moreover, the capital used for pollution control or ergonomics may increase efficiency and product quality. In addition, EH&S audits may identify strategies for waste minimization that will improve efficiency and decrease disposal costs and risks of liability. Environmental audits may be combined with energy audits, resulting in significant savings on energy costs. H&S audits may identify process improvements, such as ergonomic changes, that increase quality and productivity. In evaluating potential environmental or occupational diseases or clusters in assessing potential risk, the EH&S audit can provide a wealth of information to the occupational physician. It can also help assess the potential health risks of the facility's operations to the workforce and surrounding community. Finally, once risks are identified and assessed, strategies can be implemented to manage or avoid them.

Injury and illness prevention in the workplace is the appropriate focus of safety audits. Legal compliance is an important baseline, but legal compliance without a program that reduces injuries, lost time, workers' compensation costs, and absenteeism is not a successful audit program. Therefore, audit programs should focus on the specific risks of each facility/process in addition to addressing compliance. A challenge of auditing for compliance is to ensure and document the formation of an action plan to address findings rather than reengineering the job during the audit. Ensuring safe human behavior in the workplace is another audit challenge. Noncompliance with safety policies must be examined carefully. In some cases a policy change may be called for to modify an impractical rule; in other cases enforcement must be strengthened. In either case, practice should match policy. Another major challenge for the safety audit is to serve as a scorecard for the safety program that not only addresses regulatory compliance but also facilitates goal setting, benchmarking, and improvement. The audit score can provide a leading or predicting indicator of safety performance and also help set priorities for improvement efforts based on scoring opportunities.

The Legal Foundation for the Audit

The EH&S audit addresses federal, state, and local regulations. Typically, audit inspection checklists or protocols are created for each of the major statutory regimes or to match a company's policies and procedures. These in turn relate to the specific activities of a company, which are subject to regulation. For example, effluent discharges to water bodies or sewer systems are regulated under the federal Clean Water Act; typically a separate checklist is created for that statute. Air emissions are addressed using a separate checklist, as are such subjects as hazardous waste management and compliance with relevant provisions of the Toxic Substances Control Act and the Emergency Planning and Community Right to Know Act.

Safety and health audits may include OSHA standards, such as those for asbestos, confined spaces, and hazard communication. H&S audits also include voluntary consensus standards, including National Fire Protection Association (NFPA) fire codes and American National Standards Institute (ANSI) machine guarding standards. Voluntary consensus standards can be enforced by OSHA under the general duty clause of the Occupational Safety and Health Act or used to interpret generally worded regulations. For example, the OSHA machine guarding regulation (29 CFR 1910.212) requires protecting the point of operation of machines but does not specify what is appropriate. OSHA uses ANSI standards to determine that.

Audits may use separate checklists that address institutional programs or management systems, including corporate policies on training and education and other mechanisms to enhance compliance. Thus, audits focus on regulatory issues that may be subject to fines, legal issues that may involve the risk of toxic tort litigation, and matters of insurance or safety concern that may cause injury of property loss.

The Timing of the Audit

Normally audits should be conducted at facilities with sufficient frequency to ensure compliance and reduce risk. While some companies conduct the audits every 2 or 3 years, increasingly companies are determining the frequency of audits based on the risk posed by a facility. For example, a facility with large and complex operations, a large number of employees, or with very substantial air and water emissions or hazardous waste management issues should be audited more frequently than a small facility that has few if any emissions to the environment. Similarly, a facility that has had a prior history of noncompliance problems, or that is a recent acquisition and its compliance profile is unknown, should generally receive a prompt audit initially, and possibly more frequent audits than facilities that do not have these conditions. In addition, interim audits that focus on particular areas of concern can be conducted at more frequent intervals as needed. An incident, such as an explosion, that reveals a previously unknown problem may trigger interim audits focused on that particular problem area at other facilities.

Most importantly, companies should place a high premium on putting in place measures and management systems to ensure compliance with applicable requirements between major audits. This includes providing the plants with trained personnel as well as regular training and education to be sure that the personnel at the plant responsible for compliance have the tools they need to do the job.

Mergers and acquisitions (M&A) are special occasions that may trigger an audit. A site assessment and a compliance audit are typically done to identify potential problems and liabilities at the plants or facilities to be acquired. This is sometimes referred to as "environmental, health and safety due diligence." In addition, if a company is considering investing in new or upgraded facilities, this may be an appropriate occasion for an audit.

Conducting the Environmental Audit

The environmental audit itself is divided into several steps. The first step is information gathering, which usually precedes the actual visit to the site. This step involves an extensive questionnaire on the environmental programs at the site. A request for copies of key documents may accompany the questionnaire. For example, plant layouts and flow diagrams, process and product information, permits and applications, notifications, monitoring reports, spill control plans, emergency response plans, training programs, shipping manifests, manuals, inspection reports, complaints or legal proceedings, and product safety data are often reviewed in advance, or conveniently assembled at the plant. Permits and documentation of discussions with regulatory agencies are of particular interest. Applicable federal, state, and local laws and regulations are reviewed before the visit.

During the site visit, the checklist serves as a useful tool for information gathering and facility inspection. Site inspection focuses on emissions sources, such as pipes and stacks, storage areas for wastes, and processing areas. As noted above, specific checklists are usually developed for major areas (e.g., air, water, hazardous waste) or may simply address areas of focused concern, such as spill control. These are keyed to the applicable legal requirements. The site review focuses on the entire process from the raw materials to the final product and waste disposal. The physical layout of the operating facility, industrial processes, sampling and analysis program, waste and by-products handling, disposal practices, and environmental releases are reviewed. Samples of soil, air, or water are taken when indicated. The ultimate objective of this activity is to develop a "compliance profile"—in short, a picture of the extent to which a plant is or is not in compliance with regulatory requirements. Areas not in compliance or areas of potential liability are written up as findings in the audit report.

Interviews with plant personnel are an essential part of the on-site audit process. The site visit typically begins with a kickoff meeting with the plant manager, the environmental and/or safety coordinator, and any other staff with major operational or compliance responsibilities. People who know the manufacturing process and its problems, along with operations and maintenance workers, can provide valuable insights for understanding potential environmental risks. It may also be desirable to conduct interviews with the regional Environmental Protection Agency (EPA) or state agency personnel.

At the conclusion of the site visit, an exit interview is usually held to discuss the auditors' findings. Any apparent violations and other significant problems are highlighted. It even may be possible to begin discussing corrective measures and to draft an action plan depending on the circumstances.

The audit team then prepares a report. It may or may not be subject to "privilege and confidentiality" based on the attorney–client or attorney's work product privilege, or on state audit privilege laws (24 states have such laws). While some reports are extensive, it is often preferable to keep the report short and put key supporting material into appendices. A typical report includes an executive summary and a succinct list of findings. It also may include corrective measures and a description of items that could become violations in the future. Often the audit includes a root-cause analysis that identifies the underlying cause of one or more violations. This may help address multiple violations and prevent future similar violations. For example, if the cause of a noncompliance is lack of personnel training, lack of knowledge of the requisite regulations, inadequacy of control technology, or some other underlying cause, it is important for management to know that and have the opportunity to address not only the "symptom" of noncompliance but the underlying cause to avoid repetition.

For some companies, the corrective action plan may be embodied in a report that follows and is separate from the audit findings. The corrective action plan addresses each finding of apparent noncompliance or other problem, and sets forth the steps to correct the problem, with an anticipated timeline for a finishing point. Action plans are often prioritized, based on the seriousness of the findings. Notes of the auditors and other materials used to prepare the audit report are usually maintained for a certain duration depending on company policies, but the draft is usually destroyed. The action plan is often entered into a computer database to enhance management efforts.

This database can be used to track compliance and to plan for the future. For example, environmental audits might reveal patterns of increasing air (or water) emissions such as volatile organic compounds (VOCs) that will exceed permit requirements in the future (1 to 2 years). This finding prompts consideration of at least three options: a new permit or variance, new emissions control equipment, or a process change. Since in most industrial areas permitted emissions are decreasing, the choice is narrowed to expensive new pollution abatement equipment (often tens to hundreds of millions of dollars) or a process change. A process change may require significant lead time. A change to an aqueous-based rather than solvent-based process that eliminates use of VOCs requires not only research to ensure that the process works but also the development of new equipment since components will be different (aqueous systems can cause rust).

The EH&S audit can be designed to identify potential health risks. Thus, if a person has an illness that may be related to an environmental or workplace exposure, the audit may indicate a correlation with a specific release and exposure. Through its response, a company may not only achieve a safer and healthier work environment, but also demonstrate a commitment to health and safety, which will enhance employee morale, productivity, and community relations.

Conducting the Health and Safety Audit

Health and safety audits require a significant time commitment from site safety personnel, engineers, labor, insurance/workers' compensation personnel, and the medical staff. Unlike the environmental audit, every portion of the facility and every machine in every manufacturing process is a concern—which leads to a longer audit period. For example, it is has not been unusual for an OSHA wall-to-wall inspection audit to take more than 1 to 3 months for an industrial site. Internal compliance audits are not commonly as detailed and time-consuming, but 1 to 2 weeks is not uncommon. Therefore, early scheduling is important; however, unscheduled audits may take place if needed.

A typical audit team may include (a) outside safety professionals, (b) internal safety auditors (audit only), (b) internal safety professionals who audit as a part of their corporate responsibility (and provide safety support), or (d) management and union safety auditors who provide cross-plant audits. Safety audits require special knowledge of the manufacturing process and regulations. Hence, the safety audit team tends to be larger than the environmental team and may be structured quite differently depending on the resources, culture, and focus of the company. General safety audit team members or occupational physicians and nurses or safety auditors with special medical training (e.g., emergency medical teams) may perform the occupational health portion of the audit.

Like the environmental audit, safety auditing involves several steps. The first step is pre-audit information gathering. This step may involve a detailed questionnaire like the environmental audit or be a more general questionnaire where the focus is on regulatory compliance. Pre-audit information may include site-specific policies and procedures, OSHA reportable incidents, workers' compensation costs and medical records, results of previous internal and/or external audits, and plant records of any safety or health problems or OSHA inspections.

On the first day of the audit, an opening meeting is held to review the purpose of the audit, the personnel, and resources needed, and schedule for the closing conference. If a schedule has not already been set up during pre-audit discussions, this is a good time to schedule interviews with key people such as the maintenance supervisor, senior managers, and medical professionals.

Next the audit team divides the audit areas according to the individual expertise of the auditors. Also if possible, an individual from the plant is chosen to accompany the auditor, verifying findings and making timely corrections of audit findings. After audit area assignments, an initial walkthrough or quick tour of the facility by the audit team is conducted to familiarize new auditors with the plant or make note of changes in the facility since the last audit. To keep the tour moving, auditors make notes on observations for later investigation.

A complete on-site review of all policies, procedures, training records, and other required documentation is then made with the facility safety management. Verification of the correction of previous findings—policies, procedures, and physical changes—is conducted. Any outstanding OSHA violations are reviewed in detail.

An in-depth audit of each target area then begins, including extensive site reviews and personal interviews. Personal interviews are key aspects of the audit and are conducted with workers, line managers, plant management, safety professionals, engineers, and on-site personnel of contractors to verify that written programs and policies are being followed in practice. If resulting observations are not of significance, e.g., a missing sign, blocked access or exit, etc., these can be managed at the time of observation through immediate correction or work orders. Typically, at the end of each day a meeting is held with the site safety management to discuss the day's findings and concerns.

Exposure measurement records for chemical and physical agents (noise, heat, radiation) are reviewed. Exposure measurements may be taken at the time of audit using direct reading instruments to verify measurements on record or identify new areas for investigation.

At the end of the audit process the observations may be classified as compliance issues or preferred practices. These findings are presented to site management at a closing conference. Any questions about the findings can be answered at that time. Photographs are often taken and reviewed at the closing conference or included in the written report. For preferred practices, benchmarking information is often presented at the closing conference.

A written report is then generated of key compliance and preferred practice findings. The audit team's report may be a letter with observations, or a prioritized list of findings in conjunction with a scorecard. This report is sometimes combined with other audit reports (environmental, financial, operations audit). The report should be coordinated with the legal department (for applicable privilege issues) before copies are sent to site safety management, site manager, and senior corporate management.

It is important to present findings carefully to avoid creating undue liability. Findings are stated simply and factually, focusing on future improvement or correction. It is usually unnecessary to speculate on possible consequences of an uncorrected observation. For example, "replace guard on drive motor" is preferred to "Someone may lose an arm if drive motor is not guarded." A response and action plan for correction by the facility is required for each finding. Certain observations or findings that require a long-term plan or industrial hygiene samples, or results that may not be available by the time of the closing conference, become a part of the follow-up.

After the response, a time-specific correction action plan is jointly developed. Compliance issues require a response to ensure correction. For more complex issues an action plan is needed to investigate root causes and establish progress toward correction. Action plans specify who has accountability and when milestones must be achieved. Even if compliance cannot be achieved right away, an action plan with significant progress may establish good faith.

Follow-up is typically conducted by written request at 90-day intervals to include corrective actions taken and to update the list of observations. A timely follow-up is necessary to ensure that findings are addressed with action plans. On site follow-up may be provided by safety professionals or as part of the overall audit process.

Preferred practices and other observations that do not involve compliance or exposure to hazards may be advisory or presented as discussion points. These may or may not require mandatory action depending on company policy and practice.

To facilitate improvement through H&S audits, one approach is to use a quantitative scoring system that enables a company to document improvement from year to year, and allows clear (quantitative) goals to be set. For example, each policy and procedure may be assigned a weighted numeric value and the score tracked from year to year. This approach assures that plants with outstanding programs that exceed regulatory requirements receive recognition for their management practices.

A quantitative audit is a leading performance indicator that provides a roadmap for improvement. Management can easily tell what areas are strong or weak and what will be the effect of various improvement options on the overall audit score. Many organizations with aggressive programs commonly report safety performance indicators to senior management and the board of directors regularly. Audit scores fit well with other traditional safety performance indicators to provide a balanced scorecard.

Although the H&S audit parallels the environmental audit in many areas, the H&S audit is more focused on nonregulatory measures, commonly takes longer time, and involves more audit and site personnel. Like the environmental audit, records (e.g., injury data, training records) and measurements of exposure levels (e.g., noise levels, solvent exposures) are a key part of the audit process.

COMPARISON OF ENVIRONMENTAL AND H&S AUDITS

In the 1980s and early 1990s, the civil and criminal penalties imposed in environmental cases created an impetus for companies to conduct environmental/EH&S audits. The safety audit actually precedes the environmental audit process for many large corporations and has been routinely performed since 1910. With the introduction of workers' compensation, some insurance companies began to promote loss control/safety audits. During the late 1980s, OSHA's wall-to-wall inspections, targeting industries for inspection, and increased fines resulting in multimillion dollar initial penalties, brought more attention and focus to the safety audit.

In many instances, separate audits are conducted for safety, industrial hygiene, and environmental, financial, and other functions. It is becoming increasingly common to combine several of these audit areas, or at least to perform them at the same time. In particular, the integration of the environmental and H&S audits is a common consideration in larger corporations. On the one hand, significant synergies exist. On the other hand, there are significant procedural, cultural, and institutional challenges. Two major considerations are the different skill sets of the audit groups, the challenge for site personnel to accommodate both audits in one time period, and the differences in audit focus. A world-class environmental audit ensures regulatory compliance and proactive pollution prevention, whereas a world-class safety audit ensures regulatory compliance and prevention and reduction of injuries and illnesses.

However, the ultimate goal—protection of human health and the environment—suggests that these audit processes can be coordinated or integrated. The result may be a group of auditors with specialized skills in both environmental and H&S auditing. Otherwise, a joint audit using professionals from each group or an audit by professional auditors (traditional corporate auditors) without EH&S skills will result in larger teams. This can lead to difficulties at the site related to resources and scheduling, without any significant gain in efficiency or effectiveness. The decision to integrate audits is often a function of both corporate policy and the practicality of dual auditors at sites. EH&S organizational and reporting structure may pose another challenge.

ENVIRONMENTAL, HEALTH, AND SAFETY MANAGEMENT SYSTEMS

As noted at the outset, there is increasing interest among corporate management in adoption of EH&S management systems. As of this writing, many thousands of facilities in Europe have become ISO 14000 certified. A smaller number have become certified in the U.S., where public and commercial pressures to do so have been less strong so far. However, this appears to be changing in response to pressures from the global market place.

The principal relevant ISO 14000 standard at this time is ISO 14001, "Environmental Management Systems—Specification with Guidance for Use" (1996). Numerous countries around the world have adopted this standard. It is a voluntary performance standard. It has been approved and recognized by ANSI, the American Society of Testing Materials (ASTM), and the American Society for Quality Control, and is subject to copyright. It is widely regarded as the definitive international benchmark for environmental management systems. Significantly, it does not explicitly apply to health and safety, though its processes can be easily adapted so as to include those elements.

Most importantly, the ISO 14001 standard is a framework for the development of management systems designed to achieve environmental objectives. These include compliance with not only applicable laws and regulations, but also other environmentally protective goals, including pollution prevention, waste minimization, corrective action, recycling, energy reduction, toxics reduction, and related goals. To become ISO 14001 certified, a facility must also be committed to a process of continuous improvement as well as community outreach. A planning process is required to identify those activities that affect the environment and/or are subject to regulation. A high priority is placed on training, awareness, and competence. Emergency preparedness and response as well as documentation and effective communication are vital components of the program.

Regular monitoring and measurement through an effective environmental management system audit is required, including identification of any nonconformance and the taking of appropriate corrective and preventive action. The program must receive regular review and evaluation by senior management. ISO 14004, entitled "Environmental Management Systems—General Guidelines on Principles, Systems, and Supporting Techniques," also adopted in 1996, is a companion piece that provides more detailed guidance on compliance.

There are a number of environmental management systems in place besides those that comply with ISO 14000. Many companies in the U.S., for example, have decided to adopt a program that is the functional equivalent of ISO 14000 without incurring the paperwork burdens and expenses of becoming certified. Many trade associations have promoted the use of the functional equivalent of environmental management systems among their members and have broadened the focus beyond environmental systems to include health and safety, product stewardship, and community relations. For example, the American Chemistry Council has adopted its Responsible Care program, which is based on published guiding principles regarding the protection of the environment, health, and safety, and consists of seven codes addressing community awareness and emergency response, pollution prevention, process safety, employee health and safety, product stewardship, security and matters arising out of the distribution and handling of chemicals. The American Petroleum Institute and the American Forest and Paper Association have similar programs and guidance.

Other professional organizations as well have published principles for environmental management. The International Chamber of Commerce has published *Principles for Environmental Management.* These principles have in turn been endorsed by the Global Environmental Management Initiative (GEMI), a membership organization that produces guidance documents on a variety of aspects of EH&S management systems and methods to achieve sustainable development and environmental protection. The Coalition for Environmentally Responsible Economies (CERES), based in Boston, developed in 1992 a series of principles that have been adopted by a number of companies. These focus on responsible environmental stewardship, safe products and services, regulatory compliance, and sustainable use of resources.

No international health and safety equivalent to ISO 14000 has yet been adopted, although standards-setting bodies of several countries are working on such a standard. For example, the BSI published BS8800 in 1996: Guide to Occupational Health and Safety Management Systems. The consulting arm of BSI has a companion auditable version [OHSAS 18001: Occupational Health and Management Systems—Specification (1999)]. These are widely used in the U.K. and several other countries. Other countries that have developed draft standards for H&S management systems include Australia/New Zealand (AS/NZ 4801) and Spain (UNE 81900). In the U.S. an ANSI standards committee (Z10 Occupational Health and Safety Systems) has been formed under the secretariat of the American Industrial Hygiene Association (AIHA).

Several professional organizations are developing occupational safety and health management system guidance documents. AIHA published a document in 1996, "Occupational Safety and

Health Management Systems: an AIHA guidance document." The Japan Industrial Safety and hygiene Association also published guidelines in 1997 and revised them in 2000. Other guidelines are under development by the International Labour Organization and the Industry Cooperation on Standards and Conformity Assessment. In short, there are many guidelines for the adoption of EH&S management systems depending on the needs of the entity or the organization involved.

THE ROLE OF STANDARDS AND GUIDELINES

Over the past 15 years the EPA, OSHA, ANSI, the Justice Department, and other organizations have published guidelines and standards with respect to the environment, H&S auditing practices and procedures, and the elements of effective auditing programs. In addition, various nongovernment organizations have published such standards. These are often useful to organizations and businesses in designing their own programs or in evaluating their existing programs to determine whether changes should be made. The more important guidelines issued by government agencies are as follows:

- EPA's Environmental Auditing Policy Statement, 51 *Fed Reg* 25003 (July 9, 1986): This statement encourages the development of effective and comprehensive auditing programs and includes EPA's seven basic elements of an effective environmental auditing program.
- U.S. Justice Department's "Factors in Decisions on Criminal Prosecutions for Environmental Violations in the Context of Significant Voluntary Compliance or Disclosure Efforts by the Violator" (July 1, 1991): This important document sets forth the Justice Department's policy of encouraging self-auditing and voluntary disclosure of environmental violations. Of particular relevance to the design of an effective environmental auditing program are the Preventive Measures and Compliance Programs, the existence of which will result in significant mitigation of penalties.
- EPA's Code of Environmental Management Principles, 61 *Fed Reg* 54062 (October 16, 1996).
- EPA's Incentives for Self-Policing, Discovery, Disclosure, Correction and Prevention of Violations, 65 *Fed Reg* 19618 (April 11, 2000).
- EPA's "Compliance-Focused Environmental Management System—Enforcement Agreement Guidance" (revised January 2000).
- OSHA's Voluntary Protection Programs, 53 *Fed Reg* 26339 (July 12, 1988).
- OSHA's Safety and Health Program Management Guidelines, 54 *Fed Reg* 3904 (January 26, 1989).

There are others, but these are the principal guidelines utilized. In addition, a number of practitioners make use of the "Draft Corporate Sentencing Guidelines For Environmental Violations;" the guidelines were proposed on November 16, 1993, by the U.S. sentencing commission but were never finalized. This document contains a number of factors relating to environmental management processes and systems, which if adopted by a company will result in substantial mitigation of penalties and sanctions. There are substantial overlaps among all of these guidelines.

In addition to the guidelines adopted by government agencies, a number of professional organizations, such as ASTM, the Board of Environmental Health and Safety Auditor Certifications (BEAC), and the Environmental Health and Safety Auditing Roundtable (EAR), now known simply as The Auditing Roundtable, have adopted relevant auditing standards. Citations to these materials are provided below (see Further Information).

One of the dilemmas posed for the practitioner by the proliferation of guidance documents is which one to choose in designing or benchmarking an auditing program. The answer is that no one set of guidelines guarantees success or is best for all organizations. A number of paths can be taken to achieve the desired goals. If compliance and penalty mitigation is a primary objective, we recommend use of the EPA and the Justice Department guidance documents as very helpful in making sure that an auditing program contains all of the elements that will satisfy those agencies. Where guidance is sought with respect to auditing procedures as well as elements of a sound program, the ASTM, BEAC, and EAR standards are useful (see Further Information).

THE ROLE OF THE OCCUPATIONAL AND ENVIRONMENTAL PHYSICIAN

Occupational and environmental medicine (OEM) physicians may be a part of the environmental audit team, review the audit report, or be informed users of it. Environmental or chemical engineers commonly perform environmental audits. The OEM physician has a unique understanding of the relationship between human health and environmental exposure. Although the environmental audit commonly focuses on regulatory compliance, protection of human health is the ultimate goal of regulations. In fact, many regulations essentially require an assessment of health risk. As a result, the OEM physician may increasingly become a part of the audit team and participate in report preparation.

A second role for the OEM physician is to review the environmental audit. This activity may focus on the accuracy of the observations and conclusions, especially the implications of the audit on the health of the workforce or community, or both, and the need for preventive actions. Although the environmental audit does not usually include an initial action plan, a plan is commonly generated for each major observation noted in the audit. Implementing and integrating the substance of this plan with ongoing health programs is an important activity that may require the knowledge of an OEM physician. For example, particularly in acquisition audits, representative sampling of soils and final products will be conducted. The product may be contaminated with substances that may present a health risk for the public or require product labeling under OSHA's Hazard Communication Standard. The OEM physician's multidisciplinary skills are valuable in interpreting audit results. For example, many raw products from mines often contain crystalline silica or some form of asbestos. When the substance is used in consumer products, in particular food or beverages, a clear assessment of both public health risk and labeling and other regulatory requirements is critical. The recognition of route of exposure for crystalline silica (inhalation versus ingestion) and the potential difference in toxicity (and significant difference in regulation) of cleavage fragment tremolite asbestos are risk-determining issues that require knowledge of pathophysiology and toxicology as well as regulatory requirements. In both instances, the future of the company or product may turn on the OEM physician's appropriate interpretation and communication of audit results.

A third interface of the OEM physician with environmental auditing is using the data, especially exposure sampling findings, modeling results, and risk assessment reports. This information may prove useful in evaluating a clinical case or an illness among groups of individuals, or in communicating risk to members of the community. Reliable data should be preferentially used, especially those that document exposure, biologic dose, and potential health effect.

OEM physicians may also play a role in H&S audits. Safety professionals, often with special expertise in industrial hygiene or ergonomics, most commonly perform H&S audits. The qualifications of audit team members and the choice of internal versus external auditors varies with the size of the industry, the internal staff, and the complexity of the potential H&S risks. Larger employers commonly use internal staff, adding special expertise when needed, while smaller employers are more likely to use external consultants. Organizations with internal audit processes commonly utilize an external audit to ensure quality on an ad hoc or less frequent basis.

Besides safety programs such as right-to-know, hazardous materials communication, or emergency response, safety audits typically review OSHA-reportable injuries and illnesses, first-aid and near-miss cases, and workers' compensation data. Therefore, it is common to include occupational health and medical department audits with safety audits. These audits ensure appropriate on-site medical care and regulatory compliance. Audits have also begun to address health promotion programs, travel, international diseases, and many other medical issues.

Although the H&S audit team may primarily consist of safety professionals, the occupational physician and occupational health nurse have significant roles that vary with the capacity in which they serve—EH&S director, manager, auditor, consultant, etc. Occupational physicians or nurses are often members of the audit team when there is an occupational health unit, or special health-related issues have been reported. While safety professionals commonly are familiar with OSHA reporting, medical personnel are also able to evaluate record keeping as well as medical staffing, clinical issues, and medical surveillance requirements. Therefore, the occupational health physician or occupational health nurse may be a participant in the medical portion of the audit or the entirety of the audit process. For example, reporting of musculoskeletal injuries due to cumulative trauma is a commonly reported health outcome requiring special expertise to determine what is reported or recorded. Similarly, occupational health expertise helps ensure that workers' compensation records match the OSHA recordables. Lastly, individuals with an occupational health background are best suited to audit a health promotion and disease prevention program, which is becoming a common part of H&S programs.

The occupational physician or occupational health nurse may also serve as a consultant to the audit team. In this capacity, the occupational health professional may be asked to review specific records, answer clinical or occupational medical questions, or conduct a selected portion of the audit such as review case management records or ensure appropriate treatment for selected cases.

For EH&S audits, the occupational health professional (e.g., medical director) may also serve as the overall coordinator for the audit or have oversight responsibility for the audit process. The medical director's role is to design the overall environmental H&S program, develop comprehensive policies and procedures, and design an effective audit program. The medical director should also determine the appropriate H&S and environmental measures (number/severity of findings, OSHA violations, work-related injuries, and illnesses) that reflect the quality of the audit and may be used for annual goals for improvement. Since the audit is designed to integrate the EH&S components and protect public health and environment, the OEM physician is an excellent manager/coordinator for integrated audit functions.

FURTHER INFORMATION

American Industrial Hygiene Association, 2700 Prosperity Avenue, Fairfax, VA 22031. *www.aiha.org*.

American Society For Testing and Materials, 100 Barr Harbor Drive, West Conshohocken, PA 19428.

Association of Groundwater Scientists and Engineers (a division of the National Groundwater Association). Guidance to Environmental Site Assessments. September 1992. (Explains and discusses the numerous tasks involved in conducting an environmental site assessment, including working checklists and suggestions for the content of an environmental audit report.)

The Auditing Roundtable (formerly Environmental Health and Safety Auditing Roundtable), 15111 North Hayden Road, Suite 160355, Scottsdale, AZ 85260-2555. *www.auditear.org*.

Board of Environmental, Health and Safety Auditor Certifications, 249 Maitland Avenue, Altamonte Springs, FL 32701-4201. *www.beac.edu*.

British Standards Institute, 389 Chiswick High Road, London W4 4AL.

Global Environmental Management Initiative, 2000 L Street, N.W., Suite 710, Washington, DC 20036.

Guidance Documents

AIHA. Occupational health and safety management system: an AIHA guidance document (AIHA OHSMS 96/3/26) (1996).

ANSI. Standard guide for development and implementation of a pollution prevention program (E 1609-94, September 15, 1994).

ANSI. Standard practice for environmental regulatory compliance audits (E 2107-00, December 2000).

ANSI. Standard practice for environmental site assessments: phase 1 environmental site assessment process (E 1527-97) (1997).

ANSI. Standard practice for environmental site assessments: transaction screen process (E 1528-96) (1996).

BEAC. Standards for the professional practice of environmental, health, and safety auditing (1999).

BSI. Occupational health and safety management systems (BS 8800) (1996).

BSI. Occupational health and management systems—specification (OHSAS 18001) (1999).

The Auditing Roundtable. Standard for the design and implementation of an environmental, health, and safety audit program (January 1997).

The Auditing Roundtable. Standards for performance of environmental, health, and safety audits (February 1993).

Texts

Allenby BR. *Industrial ecology: policy framework and implementation*. Upper Saddle River, NJ: Prentice Hall, 1999.

Epstein MJ. *Measuring corporate environmental performance: best practices for costing and managing an effective environmental strategy.* Chicago: Institute of Management Accountants and Irwin Professional Publishing, 1996.

Friedman F. *Practical guide to environmental management*, 8th ed. Washington, DC: Environmental Law Institute, 2000.

Hall RM Jr, Case DR. *All about environmental auditing,* 2nd ed. Washington, DC: Federal Publications, 1992.

National Academy of Engineering. *Industrial environmental performance metrics: challenges and opportunities*. Washington, DC: National Academy Press, 1999.

Nattrass B, Altomare M. *The natural step for business: wealth, ecology, and the evolutionary corporation.* Gabriola Island, British Columbia, Canada: New Society Publishers, 1999.

Voorhees J, Woellner RA. *International environmental risk management: ISO-14000 and the Systems Approach.* New York: Lewis, 1997.

58

Environmental Risk Assessment

Roger O. McClellan and William B. Bunn

The clinical approach to environmental illness is described in Chapter 49. Although there is always a spectrum of approaches to evaluating any disease, low-level exposures that may produce chronic diseases, particularly neoplasms, are often managed through the process of risk assessment, which has both qualitative and quantitative elements. This approach is particularly desirable where large numbers of individuals may be exposed, the exposures vary, and clinical, biologic, or physiologic markers are unavailable or not practical. Risk assessments are also used for policy decisions at local, state, and federal levels, and in multiple regulatory settings, such as site and water permitting, Superfund cleanup, and Toxic Substances Control Act (TSCA) decision making. Although risk assessment mirrors clinical analysis of an environmental medicine clinical case, it is of necessity a more formal process because public policy is often formulated based on the results.

Qualitative risk assessment is commonly performed by authoritative bodies, including the International Agency for Research on Cancer (IARC), American Conference of Governmental Industry Hygienists (ACGIH), Environmental Protection Agency (EPA), National Toxicology Program (NTP), Agency for Toxic Substances and Disease Registry (ATSDR), National Institute for Occupational Safety and Health (NIOSH), Occupational Safety and Health Administration (OSHA), and other agencies. These organizations weigh available evidence and classify agents or occupations as to their potential for causing cancer or determine guidance levels for exposure to toxicants based on traditional noncancer end points such as respiratory diseases. In addition, the EPA and NTP in recent years have begun characterizing chemicals as to their endocrine-disrupting properties.

Historically, quantitative risk assessments have typically been developed for carcinogens. For example, the EPA has frequently calculated the lifetime exposure level (in air or water) that would result in a lifetime cancer risk of one in a million individuals. The results of such calculations are used to prioritize risk reduction strategies. Quantitative analysis often involves the use of default options (to be described) in the absence of specific scientific knowledge. In recent years, quantitative estimates of risk have also been developed for some of the criteria air pollutants, especially particulate matter.

Since environmental regulation is driven by specific and quantitative assessments, this chapter provides a detailed review of risk analysis in the environmental setting. Chapter 42 addresses risk assessment in the clinical setting using a general approach, and an example is given.

THE RISK ASSESSMENT PROCESS

A risk assessment (Fig. 58.1) (1–3) provides a structured process for integrating and synthesizing the available scientific information for risk management purposes. As may be noted in the figure, the process aids in identification of research needs that will create new information to reduce uncertainties in subsequent assessments. It is critical that the total risk paradigm be communicated to all the stakeholders.

The risk assessment process, as codified by the National Research Council, involves four steps (1). The first, *hazard identification,* is qualitative; that is, it assesses the likelihood that a toxicant can cause health effects. The second, *exposure dose–response assessment,* establishes a quantitative relationship between exposure and response. Both of these steps use human data if available. In the absence of comprehensive human data (which is usually the case), information from studies with laboratory animals, cells, and/or tissues from animals and people must be used.

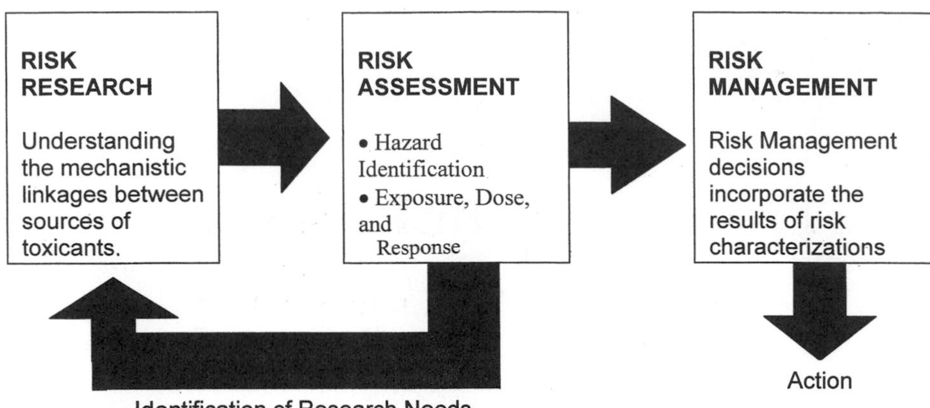

FIG. 58.1. Expanded risk paradigm developed from recommendations of the National Research Council (1,2).

This step is frequently referred to as exposure-response. We have included a dose component because knowledge of tissue aids in understanding exposure response relations. Knowledge of exposure-dose relationships is especially useful in making extrapolations from laboratory animals to humans. The third step, *exposure assessment,* may use actual measurements or, more frequently, results obtained by modeling. The fourth step, *risk characterization,* involves integration of results from steps 2 and 3 to assess risk for the specific exposure scenario under consideration. A fifth step, the identification of research needs as a feedback loop to guide future research, was recommended in the 1994 report of a National Research Council committee (2). An historical overview of the risk assessment process is available (3).

Approaches to Acquiring Information

A number of risk assessments for specified chemicals and various occupations have been conducted by the various agencies identified above. A search of the agency Web sites usually provides access to the risk assessments done by the agency. Increasingly, summaries of these have been used in the development of Material Safety Data Sheets. However, the occupational and environmental health specialist is always encouraged to review the complete documentation for the assessment to gain a comprehensive understanding of the sources of information used to develop the assessment and the strengths and weaknesses of the assessment. If an assessment has not been developed by one of the government bodies, it may be necessary to develop independently an assessment using the same approach as the bodies.

Multiple sources of information are used in developing guidance and standards for limiting human risk from toxicants (Fig. 58.2). Each approach has advantages and disadvantages, as is discussed briefly below (3). Clinical and epidemiologic studies are especially useful in that the data are obtained on people. Clinical studies with exposures carried out under carefully controlled laboratory conditions allow the test atmosphere to be precisely defined and the exposure concentration and duration of exposure to be experimentally controlled. A drawback in such studies is the extent to which the range of exposure conditions must be limited to those that the clinician feels confident will not produce irreversible effects; to study higher exposure conditions would be unethical. If occupational limits exist for a chemical, some investigators use such limits to define their exposure levels in controlled exposure clinical studies. A wide range of procedures can be used to evaluate biologic changes related to the exposure conditions. The resulting data can be readily evaluated to qualitatively or quantitatively define exposure–response relationships.

It is possible to study people under natural exposure conditions rather than to use carefully controlled conditions of the laboratory. In these studies, comparisons may be made between responses evaluated under low- and high-pollutant conditions. The exposure gradients and the quality of the exposure characterization are likely to be best for short-term (days) rather than long-term (months) observations. Although usually conducted in the field, a broad range

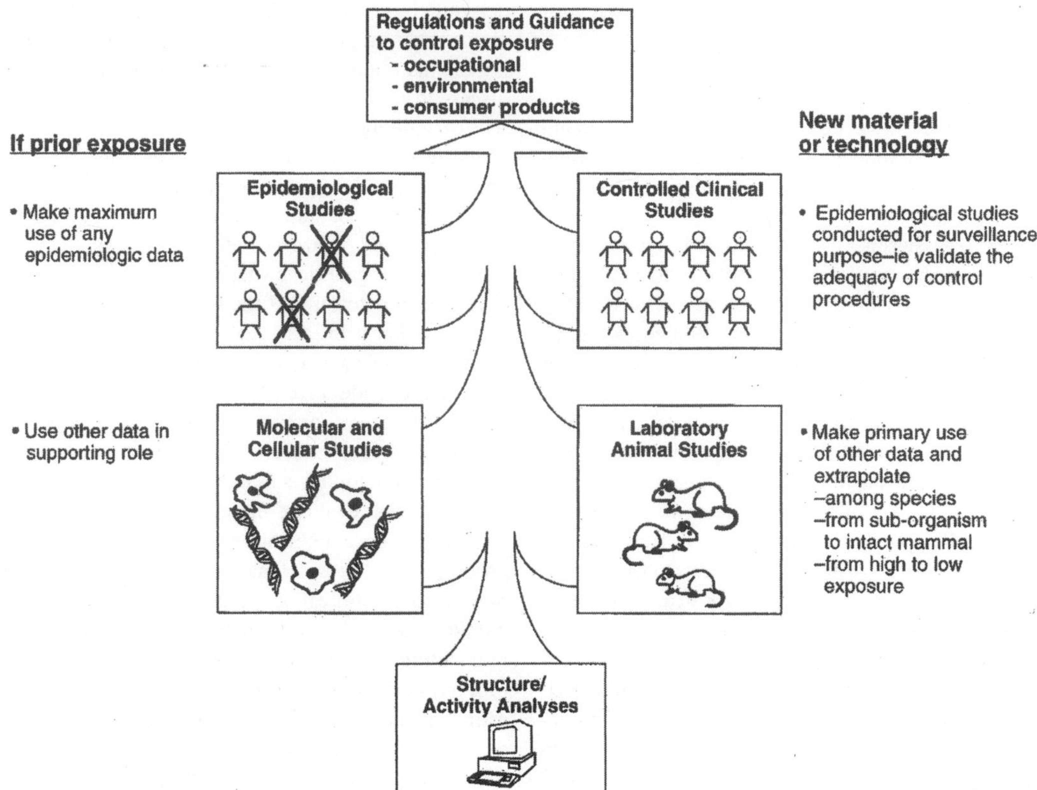

FIG. 58.2. Sources of information for developing guidance and standards for limiting risks for toxicants.

of procedures can be conducted to evaluate the functional status of the individuals being studied. The results of such studies can be evaluated to provide a semiquantitative or, perhaps in some cases, a quantitative relationship between exposure and response. The relevance of the exposure is not open to debate, since it occurred naturally.

Epidemiologic studies, beyond their advantage of directly studying humans, also have the advantage of involving real-world conditions. However, a related major difficulty is that the exposure conditions cannot be controlled as in an experimental setting; one must study the exposure conditions available. The range of procedures that can be used to evaluate the health status of individuals and changes related to exposure are substantial and range from symptom questionnaires to sophisticated pulmonary function evaluations to mortality records. Because the exposure conditions in the epidemiologic studies may not be precisely defined, especially for long periods of observation, the exposure–response relationship tends to be more qualitative than quantitative. It is especially difficult to establish even semiquantitative relationships between exposure and response for chronic diseases, such as emphysema and bronchitis and also for cancer, when the outcome is presumably related to exposures that occurred much earlier and frequently were of long duration.

Laboratory animal studies, like controlled human exposure studies, have the advantage of using carefully defined conditions matched to the experimental needs. Moreover, the range of procedures used to evaluate the dose of pollutant received by the experimental subjects can include invasive procedures as well as end-of-life observations that could not be used with people. The study of intact mammals is advantageous in that all of the body functions are subject to the complex integrated physiology and pathobiology that occurs in people. Because exposure conditions and evaluation procedures can be rigorously controlled, it is possible to develop quantitative assessments of exposure-response relationships. Approaches to the conducting of animal bioassays with inhaled or ingested chemicals, however, must be carefully scrutinized. Standard protocols are commonly used. Laboratory animal studies have the major disadvantage of requiring extrapolation of results to people. However, we are rapidly approaching the point where such extrapolations can be facilitated by using species characteristics including genomic information in the process.

In vitro studies that use cells and tissues from people and laboratory animals represent the ultimate "reductionist" approach of defining pollutant effects. They have the advantage in that exposure conditions can be precisely controlled and a wide range of procedures of varying complexity can be used to evaluate responses. Observations can be made at a level of detail that cannot be readily made in intact laboratory animals or people. For example, the influence of pollutants on the production and release of specific cellular mediators from defined cell populations can be assessed. The disadvantage is that the observations must be extrapolated to the intact mammal, which has a complex array of feedback mechanisms that modulate interactions.

In the final analysis, a risk assessment for a substance, such as an air pollutant, should be based on available data regardless of the methods used to acquire them. Maximum use should be made of human data, with results from other systems employed to complement and extend the value of the human data, frequently by giving insight into the mechanisms that may be operative in people. In the absence of human data, priorities should be given to data obtained in controlled studies of laboratory animals, preferably those that include life span assessments. If concern exists for the material as an air pollutant with inhalation as the primary route of entry to people, then it is appropriate to conduct laboratory animal studies using inhalation exposures. This approach obviates the need for making extrapolations between routes of exposure, such as from oral intake to inhalation intake. Studies with isolated cells or tissues can be used as "screening" systems to identify and rank potential toxicants and give insight into mechanisms of action. Finally, in the absence of data from biologic systems, insight into the potential toxicity of new materials can be gained from evaluating structure-activity relationships for the new material relative to materials that have been extensively studied in biologic systems (3,4).

Approaches to Conducting Risk Assessment

The use of formal qualitative and quantitative risk assessment in occupational and environmental cases will vary depending on the situation. Authoritative determinations of the IARC, EPA, NTP, OSHA, and others must be given significant weight in determining the likelihood that a given exposure can cause the disease. Although newer literature may be available, it will very likely not be accepted until it has been subjected to the scrutiny of world experts and been endorsed by regulatory agencies. In each case, a consensus opinion of authoritative bodies is preferred. Most agencies, however, identify and characterize hazards on a generic basis; that is, they assess the chemical to determine if there is any evidence in the literature that a hazard, such as the potential for an agent causing cancer, has been identified. The fact that the preponderance of the literature has not found the adverse effect, or that exposure levels associated with the effect do not exist in occupational or environmental situations, is not considered. The clinician, however, must evaluate the context of the exposure, estimate the dose to the target organ, and correlate exposure with disease. Quantitative risk assessments may support clinical judgment in evaluating cases, but these determinations are best used as part of communicating risk to individuals or groups. Regardless of a physician's frequent preference to avoid numeric estimates, quantitative determinations and regulatory definitions of safe or acceptable levels may be useful in assessing a clinical case. Since quantitative analyses are usually designed to overstate rather than understate risks, these risk assessments may also serve to reassure individual clinicians of their judgment in settings with multiple and complex factors.

A range of approaches to conducting risk assessments, and especially exposure dose–response assessments, has evolved for both noncancer and cancer health end points. Because of differences in the approaches for the two end points, they are discussed separately.

Noncancer End Points

The approach used by the ACGIH and EPA for noncancer end points makes use of safety factors (or "uncertainty factors," the term used most recently by the EPA) in establishing reference doses for noncancer end points (Fig. 58.3) (Table 58.1). In both cases, the starting point is the use of human data, if available. Otherwise, laboratory animal data must be used. A series of safety factors is employed to extrapolate from levels of observed effect or absence of effect to levels of exposure that may be viewed as acceptable limits. This acceptable level of exposure is believed to provide a margin of safety below a threshold at which no effect has been found (5,6). The de-

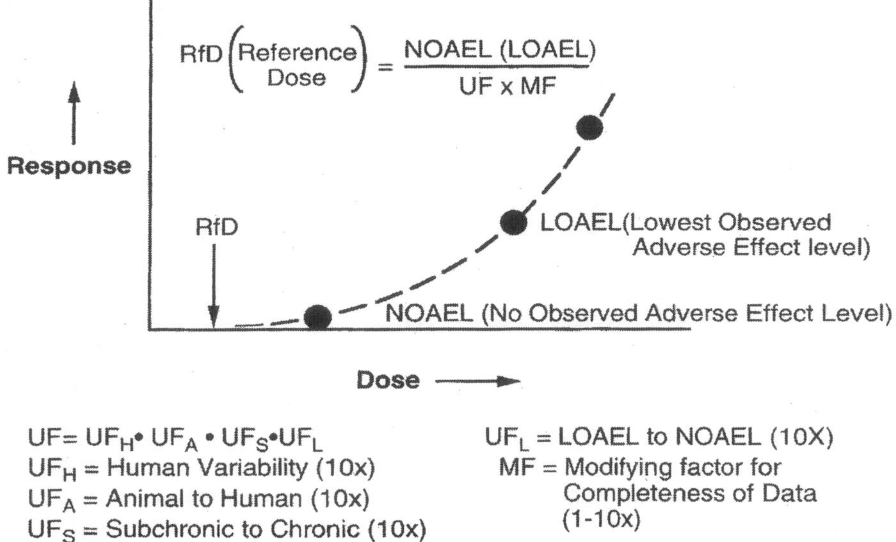

FIG. 58.3. Schematic representation of a threshold relationship between dose and response and key information for establishing a reference dose.

TABLE 58.1. *Use of uncertainty factors in deriving reference dose (5,6)*

	Standard uncertainty factor
H—Human to sensitive human	Use a tenfold factor when extrapolating from valid experimental results from studies using prolonged exposure to average healthy humans. This factor is intended to account for the variation in sensitivity among the members of the human population.
A—Animal to human	Use a tenfold factor when extrapolating from valid results of long-term studies on experimental animals when results of studies of human exposure are not available or are inadequate. This factor is intended to account for the uncertainty in extrapolating animal data to the case of average healthy humans.
S—Subchronic to chronic	Use up to a tenfold factor when extrapolating from less than chronic exposure results on experimental animals or humans when there are no useful long-term human data. This factor is intended to account for the uncertainty in extrapolating from less than chronic NOAELs to chronic NOAELs.
L—LOAEL to NOAEL	Use up to a tenfold factor when deriving an RIC from an LOAEL, instead of an NOAEL. This factor is intended to amount for the uncertainty in extrapolating from LOAELs to NOAELs.
D—Incomplete to complete data	Use up to a tenfold factor when extrapolating from valid results in experimental animals when the data are incomplete. This factor is intended to account for the inability of any single animal study to adequately address all possible adverse outcomes in humans.
	Modifying factor (MF)
	Use professional judgment to determine another uncertainty factor (MF) that is ≤10. The magnitude of the MF depends on the professional assessment of scientific uncertainties of the study and database not explicitly treated above, e.g., the number of animals tested. The default value for the MF is 1.

LOAEL, lowest observed adverse effect level; NOAEL, no observable adverse effect level; RIC, reference concentration.

From Jarabek AM, et al. The U.S. Environmental Protection Agency's inhalation RFD methodology: risk assessment for air toxics. *Toxicol Ind Health* 1990;6:279.

rivation of a reference dose (RFD) for noncancer end points is illustrated in Fig. 58.3 using information presented in Table 58.1.

The EPA uses a similar but less rigorously quantitative approach in assessing exposure–response relationships for criteria pollutants (sulfur dioxide, particulate matter, ozone, carbon dioxide, nitrogen oxides, and lead) (4–6). With criteria pollutants such as ozone, a substantial amount of human exposure–response data is available from controlled exposure studies, especially for short-term exposures. With significant human data available on short-term exposures, the primary extrapolation is from levels of observable effects to lower levels of acceptable exposure. This extrapolation involves the critical issue of determining an adequate margin of safety that may lead to differences of opinion regarding the methods used to ensure the protection of the public or sensitive individuals (7). A recent challenge in environmental epidemiology has been the use of time-series studies where various morbidity indices, e.g., emergency room visits or mortality, are correlated with low levels of pollution, taking into account various lag times (e.g., 1 to 2 days) between exposure and health outcome. It is a major statistical challenge to separate the potential effects of multiple pollutants over different lag times and adequately consider multiple other factors (such as temperature and barometric pressure changes) that may influence health. Testing of ambient pollution in animal models is also very challenging.

Cancer

Authoritative risk assessments for cancer were initially limited to determinations of whether a compound was a carcinogen, based on evidence from epidemiologic studies. Later, such assessments were broadened to include consideration of results from animal experimentation. This change gave rise to use of formal criteria for evaluating the likelihood that an agent (such as a specific chemical or microbe) or occupation could pose a carcinogenic hazard to humans (7,8). In 1969, IARC initiated a program to evaluate the human carcinogenic hazard of exposure to various chemicals and employment in various occupations. These evaluations are routinely published in IARC monographs. This program has had substantial impact on cancer risk assessment because the IARC monographs are widely viewed as authoritative and serve as the basis for action by other groups, including state and federal regulatory agencies as well as other countries. Each monograph contains a review of the monograph development process (9).

The IARC conducts a formal review of the literature that leads to a qualitative classification of carcinogenic hazard, i.e., the likelihood of exposure to an agent or employment in an occupation producing cancer. The IARC does not generally provide quantitative evaluations of the carcinogenic potency of specific chemicals.

The IARC approach provides an excellent model of a formal hazard classification process. It uses international working groups of experts with contributions from the IARC staff to carry out five tasks: (a) ascertain that all appropriate references have been collected; (b) select the data relevant for the evaluation on the basis of scientific merit; (c) prepare accurate summaries of the data to enable the reader to follow the reasoning of the working group; (d) evaluate the results of experimental and epidemiologic studies; and (e) make an overall evaluation of the carcinogenic potential of the agent to humans (8,9).

In the monographs, the term *carcinogen* denotes an agent that is capable of increasing the incidence of malignant neoplasms. Traditionally, the IARC has evaluated the evidence for carcinogenicity independent of the underlying mechanisms involved. In 1991, it convened a group of experts to consider how mechanistic data could be used in the classification process. This group suggested a greater use of mechanistic data including information relevant to extrapolation between laboratory animals and humans (10).

The evaluation process considers three types of evidence: human carcinogenicity data, animal carcinogenicity data, and supporting evidence of carcinogenicity.

The epidemiologic evidence is classified into four categories: (a) sufficient evidence of carcinogenicity is used when a causal relationship has been established between exposure to the agent and human cancer; (b) limited evidence of carcinogenicity is used when a positive association between exposure to an agent and human cancer is considered to be credible, but change, bias, or confounding could not be ruled out with reasonable confidence; (c) inadequate evidence of carcinogenicity is used when available studies are of insufficient quality, consistency, or statistical power to permit a conclusion regarding the presence or absence of a causal association; (d) evidence suggesting lack of carcinogenicity is used when there are several adequate studies covering the full range of doses to which humans are known to be exposed, which are mutually consistent in showing no positive association between exposure and any studied cancer at any observed level of exposure.

The IARC evaluation process gives substantial weight to carcinogenicity data from laboratory animals. The IARC concluded that "in the absence of adequate data in humans, it is biologically plausible and prudent to regard agents for which there is sufficient evidence of carcinogenicity in experimental animals as if they presented a carcinogenic risk to humans" (10).

Thus, the IARC classifies the strength of the evidence of carcinogenicity in experimental animals in a fashion analogous to that used for the human data. In the past, the IARC has not commented on the extent of carcinogenic potency or on the mechanisms involved. Based on the recommendations of the 1991 Working Group on Use of Mechanistic Data, such data are increasingly being considered in the evaluation process. This approach should be especially useful in classifying agents that may cause species-specific effects such as those associated with end points such as α_{2u}-globulin–mediated renal toxicity and neoplasia in the male rat. The evidence of carcinogenicity is classified into four categories: (a) Sufficient evidence of carcinogenicity: A working group considers that a causal relationship has been established between the agent and an increased incidence of malignant neoplasms or an appropriate combination of benign and malignant neoplasms in two or more species of animals or in two or more independent studies in one species carried out at different times, in different laboratories, or under different protocols. A single study in one species might be considered under exceptional circumstances to provide sufficient evidence when malignant neoplasms occur to an unusual degree with regard to incidence, site, type of tumor, or age at onset. (b) Limited evidence of carcinogenicity: The data suggest a carcinogenic effect but are limited for making a definitive evaluation. (c) Inadequate evidence of carcinogenicity: Studies cannot be interpreted as showing either the presence or absence of a carcinogenic effect because of major qualitative or quantitative limitations. (d) Evidence suggesting lack of carcinogenicity: Adequate studies involving at least two species are available that show that, within the limits of the tests used, the agent is not carcinogenic (Table 58.2) (see Appendix E). Such a conclusion is inevitably limited to the species, tumors, and doses of exposure studied.

Supporting evidence for the classification includes a range of information, such as structure-activity correlations, toxicologic information, and data on kinetics, metabolism, and genotoxicity. Data from laboratory animals, humans, and lower levels of biologic organization such as tissues and cells are included. In short, any information that may provide a clue as to the cancer-causing potential of an agent will be reviewed and presented.

TABLE 58.2. *International Agency for Research on Cancer (IARC) cancer classification*

Group 1: The agent is carcinogenic to humans. This category is used only when there is sufficient evidence of carcinogenicity in humans.

Group 2: This category is used for a range of agents; from those for which the human evidence of carcinogenicity is almost sufficient to those for which no human data are available but for which there is experimental evidence of carcinogenicity.

Group 2A: The agent is probably carcinogenic to humans. The category is typically used when there is limited evidence of carcinogenicity in humans and sufficient evidence of carcinogenicity in experimental animals.

Group 2B: The agent is possibly carcinogenic to humans. This category is typically used when there is limited evidence in humans in the absence of sufficient evidence in experimental animals or when there is sufficient evidence of carcinogenicity in experimental animals in the face of inadequate evidence or no data in humans.

Group 3: The agent is not classifiable as to carcinogenicity in humans. This category is used when agents do not fall into any other group.

Group 4: The agent is probably not carcinogenic to humans. This category is typically used for agents for which there is evidence suggesting lack of carcinogenicity in humans, together with evidence suggesting lack of carcinogenicity in experimental animals.

Finally, all relevant data are integrated and the agent categorized on the basis of the strength of the evidence derived from humans and animals and from other studies as shown in Table 58.2 (8,9).

The IARC categorization scheme does not address the potency of carcinogens, which poses constraints on the use of the IARC classification scheme beyond hazard identification. In short, a carcinogen is a carcinogen irrespective of potency. This "lumping" of carcinogens regardless of potency can be misleading to the nonspecialist including policy makers and the public. Another office within the World Health Organization, the International Program for Chemical Safety (IPCS), addresses potency through an assessment of actual occupational and environmental risk. The IPCS reviews substances studied by the IARC and produces documents that go further than identification of potential risk. Unfortunately, IPCS documents do not receive the same attention as IARC documents, and they are not incorporated in policy making even though they parallel IARC documents.

In 1986, the EPA issued guidelines for cancer risk assessment to codify the agency's practices (7–11), which built on a policy document prepared by the United States Office of Science and Technology Policy (12) on chemical carcinogens. The 1986 EPA guidelines use an approach similar to that of the IARC in categorizing agents based on the weight of the evidence of carcinogenicity, except ending up with an alphabetic rather than a numeric notation for the categories (Table 58.3) For quantitative risk assessment, regulatory agencies commonly use a multistage model that is linear at low doses to determine risk, and then use the upper confidence limit of that model to provide a greater level of certainty. From these calculations, a lifetime risk acceptable to the agency must be met, typically one in a million for an individual (9–11).

In the quantitative analysis of carcinogens, the 1986 EPA guidelines go beyond the IARC approach in offering guidance for developing quantitative estimates of carcinogen potency, that is, cancer risk per unit exposure. Because the information base for individual chemicals varies markedly and is rarely complete, the guidelines include a number of default options that are used in the assessment process in the absence of specific relevant scientific data. Some of the key default assumptions are (a) humans are as sensitive as the most sensitive laboratory animal species, strain, or sex evaluated; (b) chemicals act like radiation at low doses in inducing cancer with a linearized multistage model appropriate for estimating dose–response relationships below the range of experimental observations; (c) the biology of humans and laboratory animals, including the rate of metabolism of chemicals, is a function of body surface area; (d) a given unit of intake of chemical has the same effect irrespective of the intake time or duration; and (e) laboratory animals are a surrogate for humans in assessing cancer risks, with positive cancer bioassay results in laboratory animals taken as evidence of the chemical's potential to cause cancer in people. All of the default assumptions have been vigorously debated as to their validity (2).

The EPA has been in the process of revising the 1986 cancer risk assessment guidelines almost since they were developed. An early draft was discussed extensively in the 1994 National Academy of Sciences report, "Sciences and Judgment in Risk Assessment." As of this writing in 2002, the revised guidelines (13) have not been formally promulgated. The draft guidelines give increased emphasis to consideration of mechanistic data, especially when it can be used to describe an agent's mode of action, the key obligatory steps that link the agent to the disease of concern. It is anticipated that the revised formal guidance will adopt the view that an agent's mode of action can be considered in both the classification of agents as to their potential carcinogenicity and in developing a quantitative estimate of risk. An example would be the recognition that chloroform causes cancer in rodents at high dose levels through cell killing, and furthermore that such a process is unlikely to occur in humans exposed to low levels of chloroform as occurs from drinking water; hence, chloroform at such levels is unlikely to be a human carcinogen.

It is also anticipated that the revised guidelines will allow for more flexibility in estimating risks at low levels of exposure rather than defaulting to the use of a linear multistage model. A schematic rendering of

TABLE 58.3. *EPA and IARC carcinogenicity groupings*

EPA group	IARC group	Evaluation		Evidence in humans	Evidence in animals
A	1	Carcinogenic to humans		Sufficient	
	2A	Probably carcinogenic to humans		Limited	Sufficient
B1		Probable human carcinogen		Limited	Sufficient
B2		Probable human carcinogen		Inadequate	Sufficient
	2B	Possibly carcinogenic to humans			Absence of sufficient evidence
			or	Inadequate	Sufficient
			or	Inadequate	Limited
C		Possible human carcinogen		Absent	Limited
	3	Not classifiable as to carcinogenicity to humans		No data	No data
D		Not classified as to human carcinogenicity		Inadequate	Inadequate
			or	No data	No data
	4	Probably not carcinogenic to humans		Evidence in humans and animals suggests lack of carcinogenicity	
E		Evidence of noncarcinogenicity for humans		No evidence of carcinogenicity in at least two adequate animal tests in different species or in both adequate epidemiologic and animal studies.	

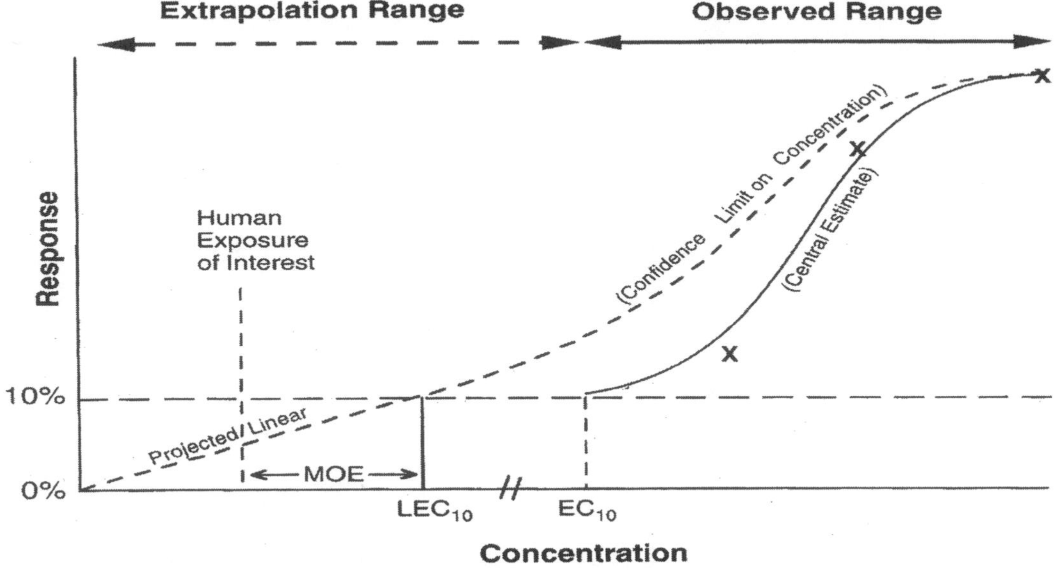

FIG. 58.4. Schematic rendering of concentration-cancer response relationship and approaches to extrapolation from observations. [Adapted from U.S. EPA (1998).]

the extrapolation process is shown in Fig. 58.4. The process illustrated emphasizes identifying the lower limits of what can typically be observed, i.e., a 10% response and an associated effective concentration, as a starting point for extrapolation to lower levels of concern. The figure also introduces the concept of "margin of exposure" for relating levels known to have produced effects (from other studies) to the current exposure levels of concern.

Similar analytic processes are used by other authoritative and regulatory bodies. The NTP conducts a similar, although less formal, assessment and categorization (6–8). The NTP process uses only two categorizes for agents: category 1 for human carcinogens, and category 2 for agents reasonably anticipated to be a human carcinogen. The NTP following the action of the IARC has also revised its process to allow greater use of mechanistic information. With this change an agent can be placed in category 1 in the absence of human carcinogenic evidence, based on strong evidence of carcinogenic activity from laboratory animal studies and mechanistic evidence that the agent is likely to cause cancer in humans. Likewise, strong mechanistic data on an agent's potential carcinogenicity, even in the absence of positive carcinogenicity findings in laboratory animals, can result in an agent being placed in category 2.

USE OF A SOURCE–RESPONSE PARADIGM

In evaluating particular situations as to potential human health risks, it is frequently useful to attempt to summarize the available information within a dose–response paradigm as shown in Fig. 58.5. This paradigm has provision for the use of all the available scientific information extending from the source to health responses using various mechanistic linkages. The stronger the evidence for causal linkages from the source through the intermediate steps to response, the higher the level of confidence of a causality linkage rather than merely a statistical association between source and response. Conversely, a failure to establish the linkages may provide a basis for more thorough investigations of alternative explanations for the observed disease in a patient or population. While this figure emphasizes airborne materials and intake via inhalation, it can be readily appreciated that the same approach can be taken with food and water and oral intake or materials gaining access to skin.

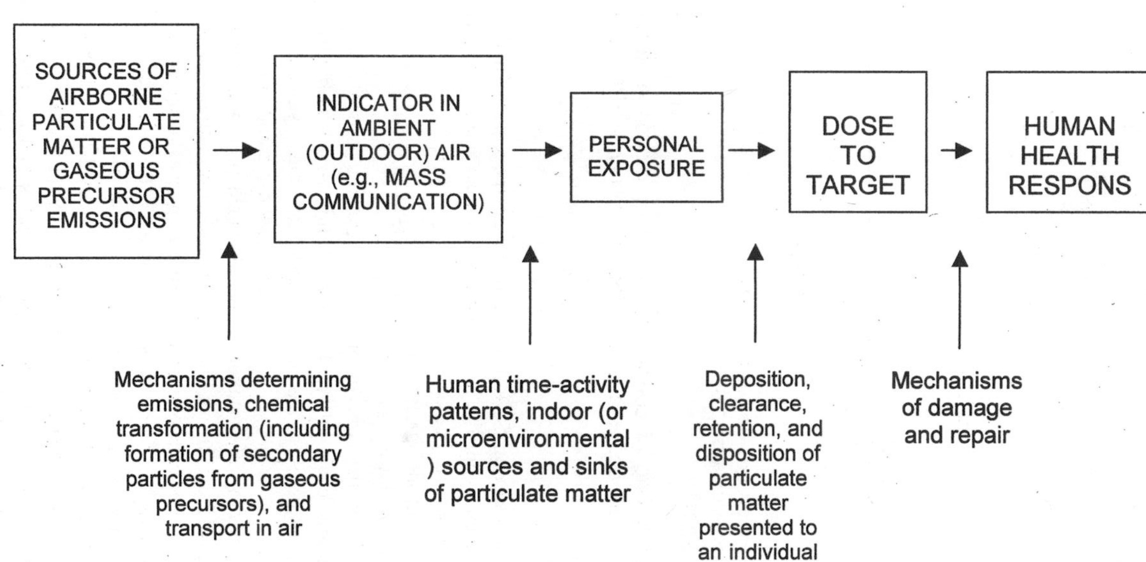

FIG. 58.5. Integrative framework for evaluating risks extending from sources of toxicants to responses (14).

The Occupational and Environmental Medicine Physician

The results of qualitative and quantitative risk assessments performed by governmental or authoritative bodies or by the occupational and environmental medicine (OEM) physician should be an integral part of the evaluation of a disease potentially related to the environment. Hazard identification processes (such as performed by the IARC) and the listing of potentially hazardous agents help the OEM physician determine if a potential association between exposure and disease is plausible. Quantitation of the risk at specific exposure levels allows a more refined evaluation and can be used to communicate information to individuals or groups.

Risk assessments specific to an exposure situation may also be available. For example, an important determination is the potential risk from a site where hazardous wastes have been improperly disposed, a potential Superfund site. The risk is initially defined during the remedial investigation feasibility study (RI/FS) of the site. The assessed risk will be quantitated, and the quantitation will determine priority. If the priority is high, the site may become a part of the National Priority List (NPL) established by the EPA, and cleanup mandated. In addition to the initial risk assessment of the site, each NPL site will also be evaluated by the Agency for Toxic Substances and Disease Registry (ATSDR). These assessments are available for public use. The data from the RI/FS and ATSDR studies and detailed risk assessments can be very useful in answering questions raised by individual cases or by community groups. While generic dispersion models and default values must be examined, it is important that OEM physicians use all the data available in each exposure/disease situation.

In addition to utilizing risk assessments in clinical practice, the physician knowledgeable in occupational and environmental medicine can play a valuable role in evaluating and refining default options associated with risk assessment. There may be physiologic reasons that humans are not equivalent to rodents when studies report excesses of cancer that are sex and strain specific. One may also offer judgment as to whether a threshold or linearized multistage model of exposure–response relationships should be applied, particularly when exposure levels approximate background levels. The problems of extrapolating results from maximum tolerated doses in animals (which by definition overwhelm normal defense mechanisms) to low doses in humans must be scrutinized carefully. For example, the metabolism of humans can often differ from that of animals, a difference that may be significant when high-dose animal responses are compared to those observed following low-dose exposure of humans.

Specific knowledge of the actual occupational and environmental exposure situation may be most important. The extent to which the agent is respirable must be considered in evaluating exposure to fibers and particles. The likelihood of a particular route of exposure actually occurring as well as the comparative level of occupational or environmental exposure is of crucial importance in determining the actual human risk. Consideration of the source–response paradigm in Fig. 58.5 will aid in these evaluations.

Further, the OEM physician has a role both in the standard-setting process through risk assessment and in interpreting the standards based on knowledge of the specific situation. When regulations are proposed, it is not always possible to analyze each integral element of the risk assessment process. Key questions should be posed and default assumptions and risk characterizations challenged, when appropriate, by OEM physicians. Risk assessments based on regulatory guidelines always need to be considered as candidates for refinement based on regulatory guidelines knowledge.

SUMMARY

Risk assessment, qualitative and quantitative, has an important role in OEM. This approach must be carefully integrated with clinical assessments. Furthermore, the clinician should take an active part in the conduct of risk assessments when appropriate and in the examination of qualitative or quantitative risk assessments that are used in formulating regulatory policies or enforcement proceedings.

ACKNOWLEDGMENTS

The word-processing assistance of Yolanda M. Talley is gratefully acknowledged.

REFERENCES

1. National Research Council. *Risk assessment in the federal government: managing the process.* Washington, DC: National Academy Press, 1983.
2. National Research Council. *Science and judgment in risk assessment.* Washington, DC: National Academy Press, 1994.
3. McClellan RO. Human health risk assessment: a historical overview and alternative paths forward. *Inhalation Toxicol* 1999;11:477–518.
4. Barnes DG, Dourson M. Reference dose (RfD): description and use in health risk assessments. *Reg Toxicol Pharmacol* 1988;8:471.
5. Jarabek AM, et al. The U.S. Environmental Protection Agency's inhalation RFD methodology: risk assessment for air toxics. *Toxicol Ind Health* 1990;6:279.

6. Jarabek AM. Inhalation RFC methodology: dosimetric adjustments and dose-response estimation of noncancer toxicity in the upper respiratory tract. In: Miller F, ed. *Nasal toxicity and dosimetric of inhaled xenobiotics: implications for human health.* Washington, DC: Taylor, France, 1995:301–325.
7. Albert RE. Carcinogen risk assessment in the U.S. EPA. *Crit Rev Toxicol* 1994;24:70–85.
8. Higginson J. The International Agency for Research on Cancer. A brief review of its history, mission, and program. *Toxicol Sci* 1998;43:79–85.
9. International Agency for Research on Cancer. *IARC monographs on the evaluation of carcinogenic risks to humans, vol 73. Some chemicals that cause cancer tumors of the kidney or urinary bladder in rodents and some other substances.* Taylor, France: IARC, 1999.
10. International Agency for Research on Cancer. *A consensus report of an IARC monograph working group on the use of mechanisms of carcinogenesis in risk identification.* IARC internal technical report No. 91/002). Taylor, France: IARC, 1991.
11. United States Environmental Protection Agency. Guidelines for carcinogenic risk assessment. *Fed Reg* 1986; 51:33992.
12. Office of Science and Technology Policy (OSTP). *Chemical carcinogens: a review of the science and its associated principles.* OSTP, 1985.
13. U.S. Environmental Protection Agency proposed guidelines for carcinogen risk assessment. Notice. *Fed Reg* 1996;61(79):19760–18011.
14. National Research Council. *Research priorities for airborne particulate matter I. Immediate priorities and a long-range research portfolio.* Washington, DC: National Academy Press, 1998.

FURTHER INFORMATION

Breslow NE, Day NE. *Statistical methods in cancer research: the analysis of case control studies.* Lyon, France: International Agency for Research on Cancer, 1980, part 1.

Breslow NE, Day NE. *Statistical methods in cancer research: the design and analysis of cohort studies.* Lyon, France: International Agency for Research on Cancer, 1987, part 2.

Butterworth BE, Conolly RB, Morgan KT. A strategy for establishing mode of action of chemical carcinogens as a guide for approaches to risk assessments. *Cancer Lett* 1995;93:129–146.

Felman AJ, Fitzhugh. 100-fold margin of safety. *Q Bull Assoc Food Drug Office* 1954;18:33–35, 1954.

Lippmann M. Effective strategies for population studies as acute air pollution health effects. *Environ Health Perspect* 1989;81:115.

Lippmann M, ed. *Environmental toxicants,* 2nd ed. New York: Wiley-Interscience, 2000.

National Academy of Sciences/National Research Council. *Human exposure assessment for airborne pollutants: advances and opportunities.* Washington, DC: National Academy Press, 1990.

National Toxicology Program, U.S. Department of Health and Human Services. *Biennial report on carcinogens,* 9th ed. Rockville, MD: Technical Services, 2000.

Rodricks JV. *Calculated risks.* Cambridge: Cambridge University Press, 1992.

Rozenkranz HS, Klopmen G. Structural implications of the ICPEMEC method for quantifying genotoxicity. *Date Mutal Res* 1994;305:99–116.

Stayner L, Smith RJ, Gilbert S, et al. Epidemiological approaches to risk assessment. *Inhal Toxicol* 1999;11: 593–601.

United States Environmental Protection Agency. Guidelines for the health assessment of suspect developmental toxicants. *Fed Reg* 1989;54:9386.

United States Environmental Protection Agency. *Alpha globulin association with chemically induced renal toxicity and neoplasia in the male rat.* EPA report No. 625-3-91/019P. Washington, DC: EPA, 1991.

United States Environmental Protection Agency. *Interim methods for development of inhalation reference concentrations.* EPA report No. /600/8, 90/006A. Washington, DC: EPA, 1990.

United States Environmental Protection Agency. *National air quality and emissions trends report, 1999.* EPA report No. 454/R-01-004. Research Triangle Park, NC: EPA, 2001.

Vianio H, et al. Working group on mechanisms of carcinogenesis and evaluation of carcinogenic risks. *Cancer Res* 1991;52:2357.

Wilbourn J, et al. Response of experimental animals to human carcinogens: an analysis based upon the IARC monograph programme. *Carcinogenesis* 1986;7:1853.

59

Ambient Particulates and Health Effects

Peter A. Valberg

AIRBORNE PARTICULATE MATTER

Serious health effects can result from chronic inhalation of elevated levels of certain classes of particulate matter (PM), as demonstrated by health statistics for cigarette smokers, for workers exposed to elevated levels of specific types of airborne PM, and for populations that have experienced elevated air-pollution episodes. Over the years, standards and guidelines have been developed, aimed at protecting the health both of workers exposed occupationally and of the general public exposed to outdoor, ambient PM.

Over the past decade, increasing interest has focused on correlations detected between low, ambient PM concentrations and population health statistics, notably mortality. These findings have sparked controversy, because associations with health outcomes are reported for ambient PM concentrations (10–30 μg/m³) that are 100-fold below those typical of occupations in which workers are exposed to dusty conditions (1,000–3,000 μg/m³). If mortality rates are truly increased by ½% over baseline for every 1 μg/m³ increment in PM (1,2), and if the effect is linear with PM concentration, then worker health statistics should reflect a doubling of mortality risk at PM exposures above 200 μg/m³. But the statistics do not show such an effect. Perhaps the PM effect is limited to sensitive populations, but then the effect in these populations is vastly larger than the ½% per μg/m³ observed in the general population. Yet we have no reports of serious impacts in, for example, intensive care unit (ICU) populations due to dust episodes, random smoking, or ventilation malfunctions.

What lines of investigation do (or do not) support health effects from exposure to low PM levels, and if the reported PM associations are not causal, what factors might be responsible? If it should turn out that the epidemiologic correlations between mortality and ambient levels of PM (at microgram per cubic meter levels) truly reflect a causal process, then there are profound implications for workers exposed at milligram per cubic meter levels.

Agencies that Identify PM Levels Protective of Health

Some work environments have the potential for elevated PM exposures. Occupational studies have provided health data on workers in "dusty trades." Additional data have come from laboratory experiments and clinical experiences with accidental exposures (such as spills, eruptions, fires). On the basis of these data, limits for workplace exposure to PM are set on a chemical- or substance-specific basis. Guidelines for health-protective levels in the United States are available from both the American Conference of Governmental Industrial Hygienists (ACGIH) for threshold limit values (TLVs) (3) and the Occupational Health and Safety Administration (OSHA) for permissible exposure levels (PELs). For generic particulates not otherwise classified as to specific toxicity, Table 59.1 lists the levels, representing concentrations averaged over an 8-hour workday, that have been developed to protect worker health.

For the ambient environment, the 1967 Clean Air Act (modified by the 1970, 1977, and 1990 Clean Air Act Amendments) requires the U.S. Environmental Protection Agency (EPA) to set the National Ambient Air Quality Standards (NAAQSs) for sulfur dioxide, carbon monoxide, nitrogen dioxide, lead, photochemical oxidants (later was changed to ozone), and PM. The EPA is directed to prepare criteria documents summarizing the science with regard to health effects of PM and other pollutants. As a result of the 1977 Clean Air Act Amendments, the EPA Clean Air Sci-

TABLE 59.1. *Occupational standards for PM not otherwise specified (PNOS), and PM not otherwise regulated (PNOR)*

Agency[a]	Averaging period	Concentration	Particle size range
ACGIH, PNOS	8-hour, occupational	10,000 μg/m^3	"inhalable"
ACGIH, PNOS	8-hour, occupational	3,000 μg/m^3	"respirable"
OSHA, PNOR	8-hour, occupational	15,000 μg/m^3	"total dust"
OSHA, PNOR	8-hour, occupational	5,000 μg/m^3	"respirable dust"

[a]10,000 μg/m^3 is also the occupational standard for total inhalable dust in Australia, Sweden, and the United Kingdom. Germany's occupational standard is 6,000 μg/m^3 for "fine dust."

entific Advisory Committee (CASAC) was created and charged with evaluating the scientific basis for the NAAQSs every 5 years.

The original NAAQS for PM, was set for total suspended particulates (TSPs), which included particles with diameters less than about 40 μm. Subsequently, it was determined that little of the PM with aerodynamic diameter greater than 10 μm was inhaled, so in 1987 the standards were changed to particles with diameters of 10 μm or less (PM-10). More recently it became appreciated that penetration to the lung alveoli is primarily limited to particles less than 2.5 μm aerodynamic diameter (PM-2.5). Consequently, the EPA reviewed PM again in 1994 to 1996, partially due to a legal suit brought against the agency by the American Lung Association. In 1997, the approved NAAQS for PM retained (reaffirmed) the existing annual and 24-hour standards for PM-10 and established new annual-average and 24-hour standards for PM-2.5. The new PM-2.5 standards (and the ozone standards) were challenged in federal court on the basis that the EPA had exceeded its authority under the Clean Air Act, but the Supreme Court rejected the challenge and affirmed EPA's ability to set PM standards over time. Table 59.2 gives the numerical values of the various PM standards over time. The TSP standard is no longer enforced.

The EPA's PM criteria document (4) describes the data, assumptions, interpretations, and conclusions behind the PM standards, with particular focus on the new PM-2.5 data. In addition, a new PM criteria document is underway (5). There continues to be controversy regarding the interpretation of the data on which the EPA based the new PM-2.5 standard, and the public accessibility of these data. The controversy surrounds the epidemiologic studies, which show correlations between ambient levels of PM and mortality and morbidity statistics. Although such associations have been reported in many studies worldwide, the interpretation of these correlations remains open to question, because other lines of toxicology evidence do not adequately support the hypothesis that the associations are due to a causal link.

Ideally, the validity of ambient PM standards would be tested by the results of natural experiments in which improvement of air quality at or near the levels in question have produced measurable improvements in a certain number of health statistics. However, such controlled experiments are rare. For example, the 1-year closure of a steel mill in Utah produced a 1-year reduction in air pollution (particularly PM). Declines in population morbidity and mortality were indeed reported in synchrony with the mill closure (6,7). However, an every-other-year periodicity of respiratory syncytial virus, with a low during mill closure, confounded a causal interpretation (8,9). Particles collected in the Utah Valley from all three periods (PM prior to closure of the steel mill, during

TABLE 59.2. *Evolution of ambient air quality standards for particulate matter*

Year promulgated	Averaging period	Concentration	Particle size range
USEPA, 1971	24-hour	260 μg/m^3	TSP (below 40 μm)
"	Annual average	75 μg/m^3	"
USEPA, 1987	24-hour	150 μg/m^3	PM - 10
"	Annual average	50 μg/m^3	"
USEPA, 1997	24-hour	65 μg/m^3	PM - 2.5
"	Annual average	15 μg/m^3	"

the closure, and after its reopening) were tested in toxicologic and human experiments. The Utah Valley particles from the years before and after the closure induced stronger short-term inflammatory responses in the lung than did particles collected during the year of the closure (10). The authors' conclusion was that "mass may not be the most appropriate metric to use in assessing health effects after PM exposure, but rather, specific components must be identified and assessed." The issue of specific PM characteristics is addressed in a subsequent section.

Approaches to Assessing the Toxicity of PM

Historically, certain short-term weather extremes caused population exposure to elevated levels of a mixture of air pollutants, for example, in the Meuse Valley, Belgium, in 1930, in Donora, Pennsylvania, in 1948, in London in 1952, and in New York City in the early 1960s. The health statistics recorded during these events show increased hospitalizations and mortality. For these historical episodes, it has not been possible, however, to separate out which pollutants were the primary or causal components, largely because of inadequate air monitoring data (11).

Studies of much lower levels of air pollution began with the pioneering work of Lave and Seskin (12–14). These studies and others reported mortality and chronic morbidity to be associated with short-term (daily) fluctuations or long-term (geographical) differences in one or several of the criteria air pollutants. The criteria air pollutants include air PM, sulfur dioxide, nitrogen dioxide, carbon monoxide, ozone, and lead. Typical measures of air pollution that have been consistently monitored over extended periods of time include the following:

Airborne particles [black smoke (BS), TSP, coefficient of haze (COH), PM-10, PM-2.5, ultrafines][1]
Sulfur dioxide (SO_2), and the secondary sulfates ($SO_4^{=}$) formed in the atmosphere
Nitrogen dioxide (NO_2), and the secondary nitrates (NO_3^-) formed in the atmosphere
Ozone (O_3)
Carbon monoxide (CO)
PM constituents, e.g., crustal, elemental carbon (EC), organic matter (OM), acids

A number of different health effects have been linked with the constituents of ambient air pollution, including PM (15–17). Recently, a World Health Organization (WHO) working group considering air pollution health impacts recommended a model of the natural history of diseases, in which physiologic changes precede the development of physical symptoms, followed by reduced function, and ultimately death (18). One of their recommendations was to include all scientific evidence in the analysis: "Health hazard characterization involves the identification of environmental hazards via the collection, evaluation, and interpretation of available evidence from epidemiology, and other scientific disciplines concerning the association between an environmental factor and human health."

Epidemiology of general populations is a crucial component of available evidence, because in these studies the response of sensitive subgroups is included. Yet, to protect these groups, it is essential to understand which PM emissions may be responsible, i.e., to elucidate the underlying mechanisms. Careful consideration must be given to whether the correlative studies mesh with other research approaches, such as chamber studies, experience from occupational exposures, animal exposures, experimental studies in genes, cells, organs, and autopsy studies, which all provide essential insight into mechanisms.

Extensive data on the toxicology of air pollution constituents have accumulated over many years. As is the case with any potentially toxic agent, researchers use four major avenues of investigation to identify and quantify health effects:

1. Experimental studies on human volunteers, including clinical data on chamber exposures.
2a. Epidemiology of highly exposed groups (e.g., smokers, workers in dusty trades).
2b. Population studies that exploit heterogeneity over time or space to investigate patterns between air pollution and health outcomes (e.g., cohort studies of residents of cities with different levels of air pollution, or time series studies of residents in the same city experiencing time patterns of air pollution).
3. Experimental studies using laboratory animals exposed over various periods of time to known, elevated concentrations of specific pollutants, mixtures, or concentrated ambient particulate.

[1]For particulate matter (PM), the most frequently examined measures are the following: black smoke (BS); coefficient of haze (COH); total suspended particulate (TSP) matter; particulate matter less than 10 μm in aerodynamic diameter (PM-10); particulate matter less than 2.5 μm in aerodynamic diameter (PM-2.5); sulfate ($SO_4^{=}$)-containing particles; nitrate (NO_3^-)-containing particles.

4. In vitro studies of tissues, cells, and molecules (e.g., proteins, DNA), probing and quantifying possible mechanisms of action.

Each of these lines of evidence has strengths and weaknesses. Approaches 1, 3, and 4 are experimental studies, and their results bear more directly on cause and effect, but approaches 3 and 4 require extrapolation to humans at ambient levels. Volunteer studies, approach 1, are limited to low-level, short-term exposures. Analysis of smoking populations and occupational studies, approach 2a, generally rely on reasonably accurate indices of individual exposure. The studies of disease patterns in the general population, approach 2b, utilize indirect measures of personal exposure and are difficult to interpret, because an individual's exposure to all the important factors (including potential confounders) cannot be accurately reconstructed. Animal experiments allow well-characterized air concentrations at elevated levels followed by careful assessment of pathology, but extrapolation of animal data to humans poses additional questions. Also, animal models cannot fully mimic the complex mixtures of ambient air pollution to which humans are exposed over a lifetime. Mechanistic and in vitro studies, approach 4, build on the solid principles of chemistry, biology, and toxicology, but interpretation of how the results apply to the intact, complex organism can be difficult.

Of these several lines of evidence, 2b, the epidemiologic studies of the general population, at present provide the most voluminous literature on health effects at ambient pollution levels near to and below the NAAQS. In spite of considerable effort, other lines of evidence, e.g., clinical exposures, analysis of smoking populations, occupational studies, studies in animals, and mechanistic toxicology, have not provided strong support for the existence of health effects at low levels of PM. Likewise, despite several thorough reanalyses (e.g., by applying different methodologic approaches to investigate the same hypotheses), it has not been possible to identify errors, bias, or confounding in the reported associations. More focused efforts on disproof through testing alternative hypotheses, however, have not been vigorously pursued. Due to significant increases in funding, the number of studies showing associations of ambient PM and various health outcomes has dramatically increased in recent years.

Understanding of the mechanistic basis for the PM associations has lagged behind the accumulating epidemiology. It remains possible that at least some of the many health outcome associations reported in the epidemiologic studies have a non–air-pollution basis. Such an interpretation is consistent with the finding that effects are generally of about the same magnitude, regardless of the specific pollutant, health end point, background levels, or median concentration levels. In fact, there is evidence that effect factors are larger at lower median concentration levels, and it is difficult to conceive of a pathophysiologic model that would be consistent with this finding.[2]

Epidemiologic Studies of Populations on Health Effects of Ambient PM

Population studies examine differences in mortality and morbidity across time or across different locations. Cross-sectional cohort studies correlate geographic differences in monitored air pollution levels over long periods of time with chronic disease rates or mortality rates. Time-series studies exploit short-term (e.g., day-by-day) time heterogeneity in air pollution levels measured at central monitors to look for correlations with day-by-day mortality or morbidity counts.

At the outset, it is important to realize that the population epidemiology used by the EPA in setting the 1997 PM NAAQS did not involve studies of individual PM exposures. In these studies, individual PM exposure is unknown. There is also limited information available on the health history of individuals being hospitalized or dying. The time-series studies use a weak design, called "ecologic," albeit the population acts as its own control. An ecologic study relies on aggregate, group-level measures of exposure and outcome. The cohort studies are "semi-ecologic" in that they have data on individual health outcomes, but use aggregate data on exposure. Typically, occupational epidemiology (or cigarette-smoker epidemiology)

[2]An example of the difficulties in knowing what the epidemiologic associations mean was provided in the Netherlands review of the current literature (Netherlands Aerosol Program, 2001). The Dutch National Institute of Public Health and the Environment (RIVM in Bilthoven) noted: "The causal factor for the PM associated health effects is still unknown. PM10, PM2.5 and other PM metrics such as Black Smoke or a foreign metric as Coefficient of Haze all seem to be a proxy for the causal factor(s).... More than one third of the PM10 in the Netherlands seems to be toxicologically inert at the current concentrations: water, sea salt, ammonium sulphate, ammonium nitrate and probably the non-crystalline crustal material too.... Decreasing the levels of inert components will not reduce the health risk of the population."

uses a stronger design that compares health outcomes in known individuals whose level of exposure to a specific agent is known with greater accuracy than in the air pollution studies.

In essence, almost all the air pollution correlative studies are opportunistic (meaning they use existing, observational data as opposed to data generated specifically for the study). The statistical regression analysis consists of examining the following correlation, in a wide variety of settings, and with a wide variety of corrections and smoothing:

[Outdoor PM concentrations measured routinely at central locations by monitoring programs]

versus

[Daily morbidity and/or mortality statistics routinely collected by health agencies]

The statistical correlations can arise for a variety of reasons aside from cause and effect, and are susceptible to artifactual factors such as coincidence, measurement error, confounding, and bias. Understanding such statistical associations calls for considerable after-the-fact examination in the light of alternative statistical models as well as other lines of evidence (e.g., animal toxicology, voluntary human exposures, occupational data). The statistical validity has been probed (19,20), and alternatives to a causal interpretation have been proposed (21–25).

For PM, analyses of cohorts living in multiple cities have reported relative risks for a variety of health outcomes in relation to air pollution levels as monitored over a number of years (5). For mortality, four major cohort studies have been published. These include the six-cities study (26), the American Cancer Society (ACS) study (also referred to as the Pope study or the Krewski reanalysis) (19,27), the Adventist Health Study of Smog (AHSMOG) (28), and the veterans' study (29). In these studies, mortality rates were accumulated for cohorts of individuals living in different cities over many years. Air pollution data (measured at central monitors within the study cities) were obtained over a corresponding, or sometimes longer, time period. As is also the case with the time-series studies, the cohort studies rely heavily on data obtained originally for other purposes.

In the ACS study, the cohort involved about 500,000 adults who were mostly self-selected to be part of the ACS Cancer Prevention Study II (CPS-II). The individuals were generally acquaintances of volunteers for the ACS, and were at least 30 years of age at the time of enrollment. The cohort was followed from 1982 to 1989, and the air pollution exposure measure consisted of the mean concentration for each metropolitan area calculated over the year or two prior to the beginning of the study period. Although the air pollution data were taken to be characteristic of the population for a given city, individual exposures were likely substantially different from concentrations measured at central monitors. The data for this cohort study were reanalyzed by the Health Effects Institute (HEI) (19), and the result for the PM correlation with mortality is about a 5% increase in premature mortality per 10 $\mu g/m^3$ increase in annual PM-2.5. A subsequent reanalysis increased the follow-up time to 1998 (16 years total), and separated the premature mortality into several components (58). Each 10 $\mu g/m^3$ increase in PM-2.5 was associated with a 4% increase in all-cause mortality, a 6% increase in cardiopulmonary mortality, and an 8% increase in lung cancer mortality. (As discussed in a later section, this degree of PM lethality seems implausible. The reported results would predict that all-cause, cardiopulmonary, and lung cancer mortality would be doubled by long-term average PM concentrations of 250 $\mu g/m^3$, 170 $\mu g/m^3$, and 125 $\mu g/m^3$, respectively.)

Time-series studies or panel studies examine the correlation between daily changes in air pollution levels and short-term (daily) changes in health outcomes (symptoms, respiratory function, morbidity or mortality rates, etc.). Available health statistics are "smoothed" to remove day-of-the-week, weekly, seasonal, weather, and influenza trends from the data to the extent possible, and the remaining, short-term fluctuations are correlated with short-term deviations of pollutant levels away from the average concentration. With reasonable confidence, weak but somewhat consistent associations exist between increments in various health outcomes and increments in available measures of air pollution. As with the cohort studies, the measures of air pollution have generally been opportunistic; that is, the only chemicals entered into the models have been those available from monitoring for general levels of air pollution.

The time-series relative risks are quite small (e.g., ~0.5% increase in daily mortality for a 10 $\mu g/m^3$ increase in PM-10). Extracting such small effect coefficients requires both implementing a complex statistical analysis and making assumptions regarding periodicity in mortality rates (20). That is, long-term trends (weekly, monthly, seasonal) are assumed to result from nonpollution factors (such as weather), while short-term (daily) trends in health (with a lag of 0 to 3 days or sometimes longer) are assumed to result from air pollution increments (e.g., PM). Because of the use of "smoothing," the health end point results apply to changes in pollution concentrations, and not to the absolute level itself. As before, areas of concern include the absence of well-documented biologic mechanisms of action and the similarity of coefficients of effects regardless of study, pollutant end point, or method, and the general lack of validation.

Health Effects of Inhaled PM as Revealed by the Other Lines of Investigation

Data on Humans (Including Asthmatics) Exposed to Elevated Levels of PM

Other lines of human evidence with better characterization of individual exposure and individual sensitivity/outcome include (a) exposure of normal and asthmatic volunteers to controlled atmospheres, and (b) health data on smokers (a population heavily exposed to "combustion" particulate).

Chamber Studies on Volunteers

Research results in a number of laboratories (30–38) have provided data on the pulmonary response of both normal subjects and asthmatics to air pollution. These are "chamber studies," in which volunteers are exposed to controlled, low concentrations of various airborne substances (e.g., carbon particles, sulfate aerosols) (32). Although asthmatics were found to be more sensitive to high levels of acid aerosols than normal subjects, neither asthmatics nor normal subjects exhibited decrements in pulmonary function after exposure to PM at levels in the 100 to 200 μg/m^3 range. Low levels of exposure, typical of the outdoor environment, did not produce a response.

A combustion particulate with an extensive human health effects database is cigarette smoke, which can lead to a variety of adverse health effects in humans. The dose–response curves for these effects have been the subject of extensive investigation and have been carefully characterized. Extrapolation from the lowest levels of smoking and the equivalent particulate levels that correspond to smoking exposure confirm that outdoor concentrations of PM are vastly smaller than even low levels of smoking (23). Linear extrapolation of studies on the health effects of tobacco smoke in smokers does not provide support for the idea that low levels of ambient PM, with fewer potentially toxic compounds, can induce significant morbidity and mortality.

A 40 m/wk occupational exposure to, for example, 5,000 μg/m^3 generic PM would translate into about a 1,000 μg/m^3 continuous lifetime exposure. If the health effect function derived from the population cohort studies is assumed (e.g., 5% increase in mortality per 10 μg/m^3 PM), workers exposed at this level should be dying at 500% of (five times) the rate of unexposed workers. Such increments in mortality (or morbidity) would not be missed by occupational physicians, and nothing approaching such a level of effect has been reported in PM-exposed workers. For example, three major mortality studies have been conducted on carbon black workers (39–41). In spite of the elevated PM exposure levels that have historically characterized this cohort of workers (42), the epidemiology does not reveal increased risk of death from any illness, including cancer, among carbon black workers. In fact, the carbon black workers show a deficit of deaths from all causes (approximately 15%) and a deficit from circulatory and nonmalignant respiratory deaths. Thus, data available from workers exposed to elevated PM levels contradict the idea that PM causes morbidity and mortality at low outdoor levels.

Data from Animal and Laboratory Toxicology

Laboratory animals have been exposed in inhalation chambers under controlled conditions to a variety of particulate atmospheres. These studies were analyzed in the EPA criteria document on particulate (4). The strengths of animal studies include the following factors:

- Multiple animal species can be studied, and the most sensitive species can be identified.
- Elevated concentrations not possible with human volunteers can be used.
- Exposure over the whole animal lifetime is possible.
- Young, aged, and diseased animals can be tested.
- Comprehensive pathologic follow-up is possible.

Laboratory animals have been exposed to PM at levels many-fold greater than outdoor PM levels with little in the way of adverse effects to lung tissues or to systemic functions. In this regard, the laboratory rat appears to be the most sensitive species (43). Even with rats, continuous lifetime exposure concentration of 100 to 200 μg/m^3 must be exceeded before adverse health effects become manifest (4,44). Other laboratory species (such as mice and hamsters) can be exposed to such levels without equivalent adverse effects.

Toxicology researchers are attempting to narrow the possibilities. For example, some studies evaluate insoluble ultrafine particles (45). Researchers at the EPA

(10,46) are focusing on specific transition metals. Still others quantify various immunologically active fractions of fine PM (47), or focus on PM rich in specific sets of organic chemicals, such as polycyclic aromatic hydrocarbons (PAHs) (48). Finally, Long et al. (49) have suggested that endotoxin may be an important component of PM toxicity. In contrast, the toxicity of ambient levels of sulfate, a PM component that is frequently implicated by the epidemiologic studies, is not supported by experimental studies (50,51).

Currently, there is considerable research underway in which laboratory animals are exposed to concentrated ambient air particulates (CAPs) (i.e., increasing the outdoor air particulate concentration, say, by a 30-fold factor). Some of the CAPs experiments involve animals that have been treated to mimic humans with respiratory disease. Although some of these experiments have reported biologic effects at the concentrated air particulate levels (52), others have not (53). Whether this approach to animal toxicology will provide support for the statistical associations remains to be seen.

Overall, other lines of research do not adequately support the statistical associations reported in the populations studies. In fact, the other lines of evidence appear to be in opposition to causal links between low levels of PM and health effects. PM does cause health effects at sufficiently high concentrations, but the disagreement between the epidemiologic associations and direct-exposure data is substantial, and should give risk–benefit analysts pause. These contradictions cannot be legitimately dismissed by merely noting that, at the present time, a mechanistic understanding is lacking. The current situation is one where solid and direct lines of evidence provide data that contradict the statistical associations.

Attribution of Health Effects to Undifferentiated, "Generic" PM

If the associations are suggesting that any form of generic, undifferentiated ambient PM[3] causes a wide, undifferentiated range of health outcomes, then our ability to conclude that a causal link exists is compromised.

[3]For mortality, a dependence on particle size has been noted. An analysis of 21 published studies found that the PM-10 mortality relationship was stronger in locations where the PM-2.5 to PM-10 ratio was larger (53a).

Epidemiology studies that make distinctions among PM constituents are in the early stages (54–56). Different studies have reached divergent conclusions as to which measure of airborne PM best correlates with the health outcomes. Conversely, given the mix of ambient pollutants, a useful approach (not yet implemented) would be to identify which constituents/characteristics can be dropped without losing significant explanatory power of the overall health-outcome correlations. The ones left would be representative of the constituents needed in the effects model for that particular health effect.

PM Differs in Physical, Biologic, and Chemical Nature

Just as one would not attribute health effects to "generic gases" in the air, whether a given systemic, respiratory, or cardiovascular health outcome can arise from PM depends on the nature of the PM, i.e., its form and concentration. Some physical, biologic, and chemical forms of PM may initiate or exacerbate adverse health effects at certain concentrations, while other forms and lower concentrations of PM may not. A hallmark for causality is consistently finding a specific chemical species linked to a specific health effect. If health-outcome associations consistently arise with undifferentiated PM, particularly at concentrations below toxicologic plausibility, then one might suspect that the association reflects bias (23,57). If so, the likelihood of causality is in question, or may be diminished.

EPA's Integrated Risk Information System (IRIS) lists potency factors and threshold concentrations for a large number of chemical substances. However, the IRIS information does not identify any chemicals with effect levels as low as would be required for the PM associations. For example, the recent expanded analysis of the ACS cohort study (58) reported that each 10 $\mu g/m^3$ of fine PM resulted in an 8% increased risk of cancer mortality. This could be interpreted as a lifetime cancer risk of 0.008 per 1 $\mu g/m^3$ lifetime exposure, which means that PM has a carcinogenic potency twice as great as arsenic (0.0043 per 1 $\mu g/m^3$), ten times greater than coke oven emissions (0.00062 per 1 $\mu g/m^3$), and a thousand times greater than vinyl chloride (0.0000088 per 1 $\mu g/m^3$). Thus, PM, which surely contains a large fraction of relatively inert substances such as elemental carbon, sulfate, nitrate, and silicate, is portrayed by the epidemiology as being more carcinogenic per unit weight than specific chemicals known to be human carcinogens.

TABLE 59.3. *Concentration-response functions are unknown for the many separate characteristics of ambient PM*

	Examples of health effects that have been studied					
PM characteristics	Cardiovascular disease	Acute respiratory infections	Chronic obstructive pulmonary disease	Asthma	Mortality	Morbidity
Coarse PM mass						
Fine PM mass						
Ultrafine PM						
PM surface area						
PM number concentration						
Acidity (pH)						
Aldehydes						
Metals						
Allergens						
Sulfates						
Nitrates						
Peroxides						
Elemental carbon						
Organic carbon						
Wood smoke						
Oil fly ash						
Tire wear dust						
Allergens, pollen, spores						
Diesel exhaust						
Crustal dust						
Hazardous air pollutants						
Pathogens						
Gaseous co-pollutants						
Endotoxins						

The concentration-response functions, for the diseases listed across the top of the table, as a function of the PM characteristics listed down the side of the table, are presently UNKNOWN.

Laboratory toxicology and animal exposures have not as yet provided a mechanistic basis for the health-effect associations with low, ambient PM levels. Moreover, if PM produces different adverse health effects at low levels, each effect likely depends on distinctly different, yet presently unknown, aspects of PM. Table 59.3 illustrates a matrix of characteristics and effects. The exposure–response functions that need to be entered in each cell are presently unknown at the low PM concentrations examined by the population studies.

An additional significant problem with interpreting the PM associations is that the list of airborne contaminants tested so far in the epidemiologic studies is extremely short, omitting many vapors and gases that may also be associated with general air pollution. For example, formaldehyde (HCHO) gas is formed by the oxidation of many organic materials in air, and sampling programs have monitored its presence in ambient air. Formaldehyde also produces physiologic effects at high levels in experimental situations that might be extrapolated to indicate the possibility of morbidity and/or mortality of the nature seen in epidemiologic studies. However, formaldehyde is not (and cannot be) included in any of the epidemiologic analyses because no general monitoring program exists for it. That is, there are no good databases of past HCHO measurements. The same is true for many chemicals that may be identified in general air pollution.

Aside from the long list of hazardous air pollutants that in all likelihood co-vary with particulate levels, the PM associations have not identified which component of PM is key to health effects at low levels. As indicated by Table 59.3, particulate material has many sources, for example, geologic (crustal dust, salt nuclei, geothermal emissions), biologic (spores, pollen, bacteria), or anthropogenic (fuel combustion, ore smelting, manufacturing). The epidemiology studies have not as yet ruled out any of the potentially causal components, e.g., benzene, aldehydes, oxidants, acidity, allergens, metals, organics, polycyclic aromatic hydrocarbons (PAHs), sulfates, nitrates, spores, crustal dust, ultrafine particles, chlorinated organics, hydrocarbons, elemental carbon, fly ash, fibers.

Sulfate as an Example of Fine PM

For the eastern region of the U.S., the majority of PM-2.5 is due to secondary particulate formed from sulfur dioxide that reacts in the atmosphere to produce ammonium sulfate [$(NH_4)_2SO_4$]. Ammonium sulfate is a common substance that is soluble in water, and any sulfate particles landing on lung surfaces will immediately dissolve in body fluids. Ammonium sulfate has widespread application as a fabric flameproofing ingredient and as a fertilizer. It is also used for preparing an inert powder called alum (aluminum ammonium sulfate), which is used in baking powder and other consumer products.

In spite of the widespread potential for human contact with ammonium sulfate (and ammonium nitrate), comprehensive databases on the human health effects of chemicals do not identify ammonium sulfate as an important chemical of health concern. That is, in spite of available toxicologic data, the databases that describe inhalation exposure standards for hundreds of chemical compounds do not list ammonium sulfate and ammonium nitrate as hazardous compounds (e.g., Integrated Risk Information System of the EPA; toxicologic profiles of the Agency for Toxic Substances and Disease Registry; TLVs of the ACGIH; time-weighted average exposure limits of the National Institute for Occupational Safety and Health and OSHA). Neither ammonium sulfate nor ammonium nitrate are on rhe EPA's list of hazardous air pollutants (HAPs).

In fact, both the ammonium ion [NH_4^+] and the sulfate ion [$SO_4^=$] are normal ingredients of human blood and other body fluids, and are constantly cycling through the body. For example, a portion of the sulfur content in food is excreted from the body as inorganic sulfate ion. The normal quantity of (inorganic) sulfate dissolved in the water in our bodies is 4 g. The additional quantity of sulfate bound to proteins is higher.

How much sulfate could a person inhale daily if the ambient airborne $(NH_4)_2SO_4$ concentration was equal to the PM-2.5 NAAQS (15 $\mu g/m^3$)? An upper bound estimate of the air breathed by an adult per day is 24 m^3 of air. Hence the daily intake by inhalation (assuming 100% of sulfate penetrates indoors) will be 0.3 mg of sulfate.[4] This amount of sulfate is insignificant in comparison to the body content of sulfate, but also, over that same 1-day period, a person will normally excrete 1,400 mg of sulfate in urine, or nearly 5,000 times more than the estimated amount of sulfate intake from ambient PM.

Studies in many laboratories describe inhalation of sulfate aerosol by volunteers under controlled conditions. The pulmonary effects of sulfate have been studied in both normal and asthmatic subjects at concentrations up to 1,000 $\mu g/m^3$ (32). Most of the studies identify 100 $\mu g/m^3$ as a "no effect level" in exercising asthmatics (30,31,33,59). These data on controlled human exposures are contrary to predictions of adverse health effects from ambient levels (e.g., 15 $\mu g/m^3$ sulfate).

Sources of Personal PM Exposure

A major fraction of an individual's exposure to PM comes from indoor, nearby sources and personal activities, not general, outdoor PM.

For almost all of us, the majority of our time is spent indoors rather than outdoors. During a 24-hour day, Americans spend approximately 21 hours indoors (88%), 1½ hours in (or near) a vehicle, and 1½ hours outdoors (60). Estimates by Spengler and Sexton (61) suggest that Americans spend closer to 93% of their time indoors and only 2% of their time outdoors. Even Californians spend 90% of their time indoors (62). Elderly individuals with preexisting respiratory or cardiovascular disease are likely to spend an even greater fraction of their day indoors.

Also, from information collected by the EPA in the Criteria Document for Particulate Matter (4) and by others (63–65), it is clear that indoor sources generally dominate PM concentrations in the indoor environment. Sources of indoor PM include home heating, air conditioning, cooking, smoking, other combustion sources, dusting, vacuuming, spraying, cleaning, and resuspension of settled dust by human activity.

The EPA reviewed three large-scale studies characterizing the levels and sources of indoor PM—(a) the Harvard six-city study, (b) the New York State Energy Research and Development Administration (NYSERDA) study, and (c) the EPA particle total exposure assessment methodology (PTEAM) study—as well numerous smaller-scale studies. A further refinement for assessing PM exposure is to measure personal exposure by means of monitors carried around during daily activities. The results show that

[4] 15 $\mu g/m^3$ of [$(NH_4)_2SO_4$] would be about 12 $\mu g/m^3$ of the sulfate [SO_4] part of the molecule. Then, 12 $\mu g/m^3$ times 24 m^3 is 288 μg, which is approximately 0.3 mg.

personal exposure to respirable PM is higher than predicted by either outdoor or indoor PM levels, and is poorly correlated with outdoor PM concentrations (63). High personal PM exposures are attributed to a "personal cloud" effect. Although not completely understood, reentrainment of household dust and localized sources of high air particulate levels (outdoor grilling, garden work, grass mowing, proximity to operating vehicles, etc.) have been suggested as the basis for the personal cloud effect.

In areas where smoking is allowed, environmental tobacco smoke is the major contributor to indoor PM. Cooking also represents a large indoor source. For the EPA PTEAM study, cooking added 10 to 20 $\mu g/m^3$ PM to a 12-hour average. During periods of cooking, levels can be much higher. Brauer et al. (66) reported that the mean level of PM-2.5 (15 to 30 minutes prior, during, and up to 30 minutes after cooking) in residential kitchens was 75 $\mu g/m^3$. In both restaurants and residential kitchens, 5-minute average peaks above 400 $\mu g/m^3$ were observed. Even aside from identified sources, data from the EPA PTEAM study showed that as much as 14% (PM-2.5) to 26% (PM-10) of indoor PM came from unknown sources.

In summary, an individual's total dose, whether of PM-10 or of PM-2.5, will be dominated by sources other than regional outdoor PM concentrations. This result poses another difficulty for correctly interpreting the epidemiologic associations.

Asthma and Ambient PM

Asthma is a chronic respiratory disease characterized by episodic narrowing of the lumen of lung airways. Asthma prevalence (the percentage of people susceptible to asthma attacks) should be distinguished from asthma attacks. For asthmatics, sufficiently high levels of some chemicals or physical agents can initiate lung responses leading to airway constriction.

The American Lung Association (2002) lists significant triggers of asthma attacks as the following: colds and chest infections; insect and animal allergens (e.g., dust mite and cockroach allergen, pet dander, bird droppings, rodent feces); plant and fungal bioaerosols [e.g., alternaria (mold), pollen (ragweed), mildew, flowers, grass, trees]; indoor air contaminants (ozone, tobacco smoke, grain dust, cooking fumes, carpet organics); prescription drugs; cold air inhalation; exercise; and stress/excitement (67).

A number of lines of reasoning suggest outdoor PM levels are not significant contributors to present-day asthma problems. Four are discussed in the following subsections.

Variations in Asthma Hospitalizations by Location

Geographic variations in asthma hospitalization rates do not mirror differences in air pollution. In a Massachusetts study, it was found that Merrimack Valley communities have widely disparate asthma hospitalization rates, even though they are in the same air-quality airshed (68). For example, asthma hospitalizations in Lawrence were 7.5-fold greater than in Andover, even though these are bordering towns. Such differences could not be attributed to differences in outdoor air quality. Generally, more affluent communities have much lower asthma hospitalization rates than the poorer sections of large cities, and this may be due to the greater presence of substances capable of triggering asthma attacks in deteriorating housing stock.

Asthma hospitalizations across communities in Boston were examined by researchers at Boston University's School of Public Health (69). Among the neighborhoods of Boston, dramatic differences in asthma hospitalizations were evident. Some areas had hospitalization rates as high as 10 per 1,000. The more affluent downtown and Back Bay areas were in the lowest group, with rates of about 1.3 per 1,000. Dorchester had a much greater asthma hospitalization rate than West Roxbury, despite the fact that these two nearby neighborhoods share similar outdoor air quality.

In New York City, several groups have analyzed the distribution and factors affecting asthma hospitalizations and mortality (70–72). Asthma prevalence in New York City correlates strongly with socioeconomic status, and several factors link asthma with poverty. Factors that related to asthma risk in low-income areas were the number of occupants per apartment (related to bacterial and viral exposures), water leaks (related to fungal exposures), moist basements (related to fungal exposures), deteriorating building materials (related to fungal and mite exposures), and house dust exposure (containing insect parts, animal dander, and rodent excreta).

Variations in Asthma Prevalence by Location

Aside from the triggering of asthma attacks, ambient PM concentrations seem not to increase the incidence of the asthmatic condition. Studies around the world report low prevalence of asthma in countries with air pollution problems such as Mexico, Eastern Europe, China, and Greece, whereas asthma rates are nearly 10 times higher in countries that have better air quality, for example, New Zealand, Australia, and

Canada (73,74). In the United Kingdom, regional differences in outdoor air pollution do not correlate with asthma prevalence (75). In Europe, asthma rates are lower in more polluted regions than in regions with cleaner air (76–79).

In summary, available information on the geographic distribution of asthma suggests that variations in PM concentrations are not likely a factor in the prevalence of asthma.

Time Trends in Asthma and in Ambient PM Levels

In the U.S. and other developed countries, over the past two or three decades both the prevalence of asthma and asthma hospitalizations have increased. Air pollution has been decreasing over the same period of time (80) during which asthma diagnoses have been on the rise (75). Moreover, clinicians feel that indoor air components are more likely triggers of asthma episodes than outdoor air (17). People spend over 90% of their time indoors. Some of the most potent allergens (such as cockroach, rodent, pet, fungal, and dust mite allergens) are found indoors, especially in deteriorating housing stock.

The reasons for the rise in asthma are not understood, but suspected factors include changing patterns of childhood illnesses, changing diet, changing exercise patterns, changing housing, changing body mass index, increased vaccinations against childhood respiratory disease, and increased exposure to indoor-air allergens (81–84). Whatever the reasons, the ambient PM time trends and time trends for reported asthma problems (a combination of asthma prevalence and asthma attacks) are in opposition.

A community-based study of asthma incidence in Rochester, Minnesota, found that asthma episodes in children increased about 1.6-fold over the 20-year time period from 1964 to 1983 (85). The authors concluded that this increase was "not likely to be caused by outdoor air pollution" but rather may be linked to "energy conservation, which has resulted in increased exposure to indoor allergens."

Time trends for asthma in East versus West Germany show that the proportion of East Germans with atopy (a predisposition to allergic reactions) is increasing as the population becomes Westernized and industrial air pollution problems are cleaned up (86).

In summary, time trends in outdoor PM levels are opposite to time trends in asthma diagnoses, and this lack of concordance suggests PM is not playing a causal role in the prevalence of asthma.

Clinical Evidence on Environmental Factors in Asthma Prevalence

The clinical literature on asthma in children does not identify outdoor PM as a key element in asthma prevalence or asthma attacks. A recent commentary on the increase in asthma prevalence (87) gives the following ordered list of possible environmental factors, with no mention of a factor having to do with outdoor PM:

1. improved hygiene (reduced early-life exposure to soil bacteria, fungi, and parasites is hypothesized to increase asthma risk);
2. changes in diet;
3. increased use of antibiotics;
4. altered patterns of infant feeding;
5. greater exposure to allergens;
6. increased obesity in children;
7. reduced physical activity in children;
8. changes in the prenatal environment.

Genetic differences are also a key factor, at least with respect to the predominant allergic type of asthma. Familial risk factors and racial risk factors have been identified (88,89). These findings suggests that some children may be predisposed to more severe asthma than others.

Cookson and Moffatt (90) have hypothesized that the increase in asthma is related to the decline of certain types of respiratory infections in modern societies. The reduction in respiratory infections shifts the balance of the immune system in favor of factors that predispose persons to asthma and allergy. For example, in some less-modernized societies, the population is exposed to certain pathogens that "compete" with allergens for the saturation of inflammatory cell sites by different antibodies. In industrial societies, the protective effect of infectious diseases may have been significantly reduced by the use of antibiotics and immunization programs.

In summary, several lines of evidence suggest that outdoor PM levels are not significant contributors to asthma. Clinicians who deal with asthma patients on a day-by-day basis look for causes of asthma prevalence and asthma hospitalizations other than PM.

Exposure of Asthmatic Volunteers to PM

Asthmatics show little symptomatic response during voluntary exposure to much higher levels of air particulate than are characteristic of the outdoor environment. Studies in a number of laboratories (33,50, 91,92) have compared pulmonary function tests of asthmatics to those of normal subjects in chamber studies. In chamber studies volunteers are exposed to measured, controlled concentrations of various airborne substances. Although respiratory function tests of asthmatics showed more response to elevated concentrations of acid aerosols than for normal subjects, neither asthmatics nor normal subjects exhibited decrements in pulmonary function after exposure to nonacidic airborne particulates. The concentrations used ranged from 100 to 1,000 $\mu g/m^3$—many-fold higher than the levels found in outdoor environments, yet no asthma attacks were reported in the volunteers.

In summary, clinical data, time-trend data, and prevalence data do not support a causal basis for correlations between outdoor PM levels and frequency or severity of asthma.

Examining the Hypothesis Behind the Time-Series PM Associations

The current literature is dominated by repeated application of the same methodology (93). But reporting yet another generally consistent correlation does not constitute strong support. For most of the health outcomes, the potential role of alternative causal pathways has not been carefully investigated. Outdoor air pollution levels are potentially measures of other factors, e.g., changes in indoor air pollution exposure (24), increased traffic, and increased industrial activity. If traffic and other social stresses are causing anger or psychosomatic effects that are increasing people's risk of asthma attacks, hospitalization, or sudden death, then lowering ambient pollution per se may have no health benefit. An effective test of whether PM is the direct causal basis of the correlations is through vigorous efforts at disproof. If the PM hypothesis survives such a challenge, then it will be strengthened.

Tests of Causality

Problems with causality in the PM associations are suggested by several studies. Wyzga (94) conducted a preliminary analysis in which he demonstrated that ambient PM levels in one city correlated with health outcomes in a completely different city. A more recent study (95) also found that mortality correlations with PM were often stronger with more distant ambient monitors than with local monitors. Because just as many distant correlations were significant as local correlations, these authors caution "against considering any of these associations to be causal." These types of analyses probe the plausibility of causation. It would be worthwhile to test a number of toxicologically implausible models such as cross-city effects using the National Morbidity, Mortality, and Air Pollution Study (NMMAPS) database (the 90 cities study) to conduct a similar cross-city analysis (93).

In fact, the very ubiquity of the PM associations with mortality and morbidity suggests the importance of social factors that co-vary with PM levels. That is, the correlations arise in different locations, for different populations, in different settings, with different chemicals being the predominant contributors, and showing no clear threshold. The one common factor worldwide, in fact, is that human industry and activity are predominant sources of PM emissions. If social factors were driving both PM levels and mortality/morbidity rates, then no threshold would be expected. The correlations would appear in different cities and countries, and the precise chemical nature of the anthropogenic emissions would not be of importance.

Another test for causality is to run the time-lag models backward, that is, how often does the model detect an increase in mortality rates prior to an elevation in pollutant levels? This possibility has not been consistently tested, but one study that evaluated this possibility did not find such a reverse association (96). Another approach is to enter nonpollution factors, e.g., atmospheric pressure or daily electricity consumption, into the models in place of pollutant concentrations. One study found that an increase in barometric pressure of 10 millibar (mb) (out of a total atmospheric pressure of ~1,000 mb) was associated with a 12% increase in risk of sudden infant death syndrome (SIDS) (97). Another validation approach is to determine if a control health outcome, such as accidental deaths, is affected by air pollution. Such an association is not seen; however, accidental deaths are a small fraction of all deaths, and accidents are not affected by the myriad factors that modify a leading cause of death such as cardiovascular disease. Thus, in the absence of vigorous efforts at validation (i.e., disproof) the time-series correlative results must be interpreted with caution.

Alternative Causal Pathways

The association of low levels of PM with small changes in mortality/morbidity rates is toxicologically implausible, but if real, confidence in the causal role of PM can be improved by demonstrating that other, implausible variables do not correlate with mortality/morbidity end points. For example, if daily electricity use were entered as the independent variable instead of daily PM, what degree of association will be found? In the absence of any effort at disproof, the actual basis of the reported associations will remain unclear and unsuitable for promulgation of air quality standards.

Thus, more analyses are needed to determine what, if any, implausible variables will also give a generally consistent correlation when the same degree of modeling effort is focused on producing an association as has been focused on developing models that produce associations with PM.

Many of the analyses and reanalyses focus on the statistical parameters in the association (19) without examining alternative hypotheses. The plausibility of a hypothesis can be tested only by vigorous efforts devoted to disproving it. The hypothesis is strengthened if these efforts at disproof fail. Various lines of investigation have been suggested in this regard (24), but serious tests of alternative hypotheses have not been implemented.

Available data are suggestive of alternative causal pathways. Increased levels of PM are in general caused by increased societal activity, such as increased driving of cars and trucks, increased emissions from factories and power plants, resuspension of dust, plowing of fields, construction, and various other kinds of dust-generating endeavors. Many things that correlate with these activities—increases in cars and trucks on the road, for example, or increases in people working overtime—are themselves strongly correlated with daily rates of death. Epidemiologic studies have shown, for example, that psychological stresses of various kinds, such as anger, are strongly associated with increased risk of deaths due to heart attacks. Moller et al. (98) reported that one's risk of having a heart attack is increased by 900% within an hour of an episode of anger. Other studies show mortality rates have small but highly significant correlations with calendar date (99–103), which clearly is a societal construct and not an environmental toxin. In terms of the symptoms and severity of asthma and respiratory episodes, psychological stress has been shown to have significant effects (104,105).

Although the PM associations may be due to alternative pathways, the biologic plausibility of PM as a cause of airways disease, or the existence of some toxicologic characteristic of PM as causal, cannot be totally excluded. But if PM levels are surrogates for something else, like traffic and increased industrial activity, and if traffic and other social stresses are causing anger or psychosomatic effects that are increasing people's risk of asthma attacks, hospitalization, or sudden death, then lowering ambient PM levels would have no health benefit. Moreover, the potentially causal toxicologic characteristic of PM is unknown. The physical and chemical characters of PM emissions or PM precursors from particular sources are well known, but widespread monitoring systems that attempt to distinguish the measurably different characteristics of ambient PM are in the early stages of deployment.

Changes in personal exposure to a variety of agents may result from behavioral changes that accompany changes in ambient PM. In addition to societal factors that may vary in step with PM emissions, the reporting of PM levels themselves can be responsible for behavioral changes. Because of the perceived hazard of air pollution, it is often true that during pollution episodes, elderly and health-compromised persons are encouraged to remain indoors and turn on their air-conditioners. If this occurs during heat waves, heat stress would be relieved. However, the use of air conditioners, fans, or dehumidifiers can re-suspend deposited indoor PM, generate mold suspensions, and otherwise increase personal exposure to elevated levels of biologically potent PM. Infection is the most common cause of respiratory hospitalizations (106). Heat waves also increase energy consumption, which would be coupled to increased emissions of PM from local electricity generating plants. Thus, we are left with the scenario of a potentially sensitive person being affected by increased levels of indoor PM, even though from the regulator's viewpoint they are being protected from ambient PM. Moreover, despite the fact that the person remained indoors, changes in health (mortality, hospitalization) due to increased exposure to indoor particulate would, in this scenario, appear to be linked to increased ambient PM.

CONCLUSION

At the present time, the meaning of the PM associations is an open question. The PM associations appear not to be specific to any particular chemical or physical form of PM. The associations crop up in a wide variety of settings, regardless of the locale, geography, or particle composition. A toxicologic role for ambient PM cannot be ruled out, but neither can we rule out the possibility that monitored PM levels are acting as a surrogate measure for fluctuating societal factors linked to mortality/morbidity risk. The role of gaseous criteria pollutants remains unclear, and analyses yield a variety of results as to which pollutant is the key one (107). Of all pollutant substances present at low concentrations in ambient air, only a small number have been tested for associations with health end points. None of the 189 hazardous air pollutants have been examined by this technique. Finally, available occupational, laboratory animal, and toxicology data for PM effects at elevated levels are not able to adequately support the reported associations with PM at low concentrations. Drawing the conclusion that "generic" PM alone is the causal factor in the associations may lead to the true cause(s) being missed and left unaddressed.

REFERENCES

1. Abt Associates. Particulate-related health impacts of eight electric utility systems. 2002. Abt Associates, 4800 Montgomery Lane, Bethesda, MD 20814-5341.
2. Levy JI, Spengler JD. Modeling the benefits of power plant emission controls in Massachusetts. *J Air Waste Manage Assoc* 2002;52:5–18.
3. American Conference of Governmental Industrial Hygienists (ACGIH). Threshold limit values for chemical substances and physical agents. Biological exposure indices. 2002. ACGIH, 1330 Kemper Meadow Drive, Cincinnati, OH 45240.
4. U.S. Environmental Protection Agency (USEPA). 1996. Air quality criteria for particulate matter, vols I–III. Tables 13.3, 13.4, and 13.5. EPA/600/P95/001aF-cF. Research Triangle Park, NC: Office of Health and Environmental Assessment, Office of Research and Development, 1996.
5. United States Environmental Protection Agency. Third external review draft of air quality criteria for particulate matter (April 2002): vol I and II. EPA/600/P-99/002aC. *www.epa.govnceapdfspartmattVOL_I_AQCD_PM_3rd_Review_Draft.pdf.*
6. Pope CA. Respiratory disease associated with community air pollution and a steel mill, Utah Valley. *Am J Public Health* 1989;79(5):623–628.
7. Pope CA. Particulate pollution and health: a review of the Utah Valley experience. *J Exp Anal Environ Epidemiol* 1996;6(1):23–34.
8. Lyon JL, Stoddard G, Ferguson D, et al. An every other year cyclic epidemic of infants hospitalized with respiratory syncytial virus. *Pediatrics* 1996;97(1):152–153.
9. Lamm SH, Hall TA, Engel A, et al. PM10 particulates: are they the major determinant of pediatric respiratory admissions in Utah County, Utah? *Ann Occup Hyg* 1994;38[suppl 1]:969–972.
10. Ghio AJ, Costa DL. Acute pulmonary toxicity of particulate matter filter extracts in rats: coherence with epidemiologic studies in Utah Valley Residents. *Environ Health Perspect* 2001;109[suppl 3]:395–404.
11. Ito K, Thurston GD, Hayes C, et al. Associations of London, England, daily mortality with particulate matter, sulfur dioxide, and acidic aerosol pollution. *Arch Environ Health* 1993;48(4):213–220.
12. Lave LB, Seskin EP. Air pollution and human health. *Science* 1970;169:723–733.
13. Lave LB, Seskin EP. Air pollution, climate, and home heating: their effects on U.S. mortality rates. *Am J Public Health* 1972;62(7):909–916.
14. Lave LB, Seskin EP. Epidemiology, causality, and public policy. *Am Sci* 1979;67:178–185.
15. American Thoracic Society (ATS). American Thoracic Society Guidelines as to what constitutes an adverse respiratory health effect, with special reference to epidemiologic studies of air pollution. *Am Rev Respir Dis* 1985;131:666–669.
16. Bascom R, Bromberg PA, Costa DA, et al. Health effects of outdoor air pollution. Part 1. Committee of the Environmental and Occupational Health Assembly of the American Thoracic Society. *Am J Respir Crit Care Med* 1996;153(1):3–50.
17. American Thoracic Society (ATS). What constitutes an adverse health effect of air pollution? Official statement of the American Thoracic Society. *Am J Respir Crit Care Med* 2000;161(2 pt 1):665–673.
18. World Health Organization (WHO). WHO Working Group. Evaluation and use of epidemiological evidence for environmental health risk assessment: WHO Guideline Document. *Environ Health Perspect* 2000; 108:997–1002.
19. Health Effects Institute (HEI). Reanalysis of the Harvard Six Cities Study and the American Cancer Society Study of Particulate Air Pollution and Mortality. Part I: replication and validation, and part II: sensitivity analyses. HEI special report. Cambridge, MA: HEI, 2000.
20. Health Effects Institute (HEI). The National Morbidity, Mortality, and Air Pollution Study. Part II: morbidity, mortality, and air pollution in the United States. HEI report No. 94, part II. Cambridge, MA: HEI, 2000.
21. Gamble JF, Lewis RJ. Health and respirable particulate (PM10) air pollution: a causal or statistical association? *Environ Health Perspect* 1996;104:838–850.
22. Phalen RF. Uncertainties relating to the health effects of particulate air pollution: the US EPA's particle standard. *Toxicol Lett* 1998;96–97:263–267.
23. Gamble JF. PM-2.5 and mortality in long-term prospective cohort studies: cause-effect or statistical associations? *Environ Health Perspect* 1998;106:535–549.
24. Valberg PA, Watson AY. Alternative hypotheses for PM associations with daily mortality and morbidity. *Inhalation Toxicol* 1998;10:641–662.
25. Gamble JF, Nicolich MJ. Comparison of ambient PM risk with risks estimated from PM components of smoking and occupational exposures. *J Air Waste Manage Assoc* 2000;50(8):1514–1531.
26. Dockery DW, Pope CA III, Xu X, et al. An association between air pollution and mortality in six U.S. cities. *N Engl J Med* 1993;329:1753–1759.
27. Pope CA, Thun MJ, Namboodiri MM, et al. Particulate air pollution as a predictor of mortality in a prospective study of U.S. adults. *Am J Respir Crit Care Med* 1995;151(3 pt 1):669–674.
28. Abbey DE, Nishino N, McDonnell WF, et al. Long-term inhalable particles and other air pollutants related to mortality in nonsmokers. *Am J Respir Crit Care Med* 1999;159(2):373–382.
29. Lipfert FW, Perry HM, Miller JP, et al. The Washington University—EPRI Veterans' cohort mortality study: preliminary results. *Inhalation Toxicol* 2000; 12[suppl 4]:41–73.
30. Utell MJ, Morrow PE, Speers DM, et al. Airway responses to sulfate and sulfuric acid aerosols in asthmatics: an exposure-response relationship. *Am Rev Respir Dis* 1983;128:444–450.
31. Utell MJ, Morrow PE, Hyde RE. Airway reactivity to sulfate and sulfuric acid aerosols in normal and asthmatic subjects. *J Air Pollution Control Assoc* 1984;34: 931–935.
32. Utell MJ. Effects of inhaled acid aerosols on lung mechanics: an analysis of human exposure studies. *Environ Health Perspect* 1985;63:39–44.
33. Avol EL, Linn WS, Shamoo DA, et al. Respiratory responses of young asthmatic volunteers in controlled exposures to sulfuric acid aerosol. *Am Rev Respir Dis* 1990;142:343–348.
34. Aris R, Christian D, Sheppard D, et al. Lack of bronchoconstrictor response to sulfuric acid aerosols and fogs. *Am Rev Respir Dis* 1991;143(4 pt 1):744–750.
35. Kulle TJ, Kerr HD, Farrell BP, et al. Pulmonary function and bronchial reactivity in human subjects with exposure to ozone and respirable sulfuric acid aerosol. *Am Rev Respir Dis* 1982;126:996–1000.

36. Kulle TJ, Sauder LR, Hebel JR, et al. Pulmonary effects of sulfur dioxide and respirable carbon aerosol. *Environ Res* 1986;41:239–250.
37. Menon P, Rando RJ, Stankus RP, et al. Passive cigarette smoke-challenge studies: increase in bronchial hyperreactivity. *J Allergy Clin Immunol* 1992;89:560–566.
38. Menon PK, Stankus RP, Rando RJ, et al. Asthmatic responses to passive cigarette smoke: persistence of reactivity and effect of medications. *J Allergy Clin Immunol* 1991;88:861–869.
39. Robertson JM, Inman KJ. Mortality in carbon black workers in the United States. Brief communication. *J Occup Environ Med* 1996;38:569–570.
40. Hodgson JT, Jones RD. A mortality study of carbon black workers employed at five United Kingdom factories between 1947–1980. *Arch Environ Health* 1985; 40:261–268.
41. Sorahan T, Hamilton L, Van Tongeren M, et al. A cohort mortality study of UK carbon black workers 1951–96. *Am J Ind Med* 2001;39:158–170.
42. Valberg PA, Watson AY. Lung cancer rates in carbon-black workers are discordant with predictions from rat bioassay data. *Regul Toxicol Pharmacol* 1996;24: 155–170.
43. International Life Sciences Institute (ILSI). Risk Science Institute Workshop: the relevance of the rat lung response to particle overload for human risk assessment. *Inhalation Toxicol* 2000;12:1–17.
44. Stöber W, Miller FJ, McClellan RO. Requirements for a credible extrapolation model derived from health effects in rats exposed to particulate air pollution: a way to minimize the risks of human risk assessment? *Appl Occup Environ Hyg* 1998;13:421–431.
45. Oberdörster G. Pulmonary effects of inhaled ultrafine particles. *Int Arch Occup Environ Health* 2001;74(1):1–8.
46. Dye JA, et al. Acute pulmonary toxicity of particulate matter filter extracts in rats: coherence with epidemiologic studies in Utah Valley residents. Environ Health Perspect 2001;109[suppl 3]:395-404.
47. Miguel AG, Cass GR, Weiss J, et al. Latex allergens in tire dust and airborne particles. *Environ Health Perspect* 1996;104(11):1180–1186.
48. Hannigan MP, Cass GR, Lafleur AL, et al. Seasonal and spatial variation of the bacterial mutagenicity of fine organic aerosol in Southern California. *Environ Health Perspect* 1996;104(4):428–436.
49. Long CM, Suh HH, Kobzik L, et al. A pilot investigation of the relative toxicity of indoor and outdoor fine particles: in-vitro effects of endotoxin and other particulate properties. *Environ Health Perspect* 2001;109: 1019–1026.
50. Frampton MW, Morrow PE, Cox C, et al. Sulfuric acid aerosol followed by ozone exposure in healthy and asthmatic subjects. *Environ Res* 1995;69(1):1–14.
51. Heyder J, Beck-Speier I, Busch B, et al. Health effects of sulfur-related environmental air pollution. I. Executive summary. *Inhalation Toxicol* 1999;11(5):343–359.
52. Godleski JJ, et al. Mechanisms of morbidity and mortality from exposure to ambient air particles. Res Rep Health Eff Inst 2000;91:5-88; discussion 89-103.
53. Gordon T, et al. Effects of concentrated ambient particles in rats and hamsters: an exploratory study. Res Rep Health Eff Inst 2000;93:5-34; discussion 35-42.
53a. Levy JI, et al. Estimating the mortality aspects of particulate matter: what can be learned from between-study variability? *Environ Health Perspect* 2000;108: 109–117.
54. Tolbert PE, Klein M, Metzger KB, et al. Interim results of the study of particulates and health in Atlanta (SOPHIA). *J Exp Anal Environ Epidemiol* 2000;10(5): 446–460.
55. Laden F, Neas LM, Dockery DW, et al. Association of fine particulate matter from different sources with daily mortality in six U.S. cities. *Environ Health Perspect* 2000;108(10):941–947.
56. Katsouyanni K, Touloumi G, Samoli E, et al. Confounding and effect modification in the short-term effects of ambient particles on total mortality: results from 29 European cities within the APHEA2 project. *Epidemiology* 2001;12:521–531.
57. Choi CK, Noseworthy AL. Classification, direction, and prevention of bias in epidemiologic research. *J Occup Med* 1992;34:265–271.
58. Pope CA, Burnett RT, Thun MJ, et al. Lung cancer, cardiopulmonary mortality, and long-term exposure to fine particulate air pollution. *JAMA* 2002;287:1132–1141.
59. Linn WS, Anderson KR, Shamoo DA, et al. Controlled exposures of young asthmatics to mixed oxidant gases and acid aerosol. *Am J Respir Crit Care Med* 1995; 152:885–891.
60. Robinson J, Nelson WC. *National human activity pattern survey data base.* Research Triangle Park, NC: EPA, 1995.
61. Spengler JD, Sexton K. Indoor air pollution: a public health perspective. *Science* 1983;221:9–17.
62. Jenkins PL, Phillips TJ, Mulberg EJ, et al. Activity patterns of Californians: use of and proximity to indoor pollutant sources. *Atmos Environ* 1992;26(A): 2142–2148.
63. Spengler JD, Treitman RD, Tosteson TD, et al. Personal exposures to respirable particulates and implications for air pollution epidemiology. *Environ Sci Technol* 1985;19:700–707.
64. Wallace L. Indoor particles: a review. *J Air Waste Manage Assoc* 1996;46:98–126.
65. Long CM, Suh HH, Koutrakis P. Characterization of indoor particle sources using continuous mass and size monitors. *J Air Waste Manage Assoc* 2000;50: 1236–1250.
66. Brauer M, Mannetje A, Lang B. Continuous assessment of indoor fine particles with a portable nephelometer. Proceedings of the Second Colloquium on Particulate Air Pollution and Human Health, 1996:4-55–4-62.
67. American Lung Association. 2002. http://www.lungusa.org/asthma/astastrig.html.
68. Declercq E. 1998. *The Health of the Merrimack Valley.* Report to the Massachusetts Prevention Center, Greater Lawrence Family Health Center, 101 Amesbury Street, Lawrence, MA.
69. Gottlieb DJ, Beiser AS, O'Connor GT. Poverty, race, and medication use are correlates of asthma hospitalization rates: a small area analysis in Boston. *Chest* 1995;108:28–35.
70. Carr W, Zeitel L, Weiss K. Variations in asthma hospitalization and deaths in New York City. *Am J Public Health* 1992;82:59–65.
71. De Palo VA, Mayo PH, Friedman P, et al. Demographic influences on asthma hospital admission rates in New York City. *Chest* 1994;106:447–451.
72. Claudio L, Tulton L, Doucette J, et al. Socioeconomic factors and asthma hospitalization rates in New York City. *J Asthma* 1999;36:343–350.
73. Peat JK, Li J. Reversing the trend: reducing the preva-

lence of asthma. *J Allergy Clin Immunol* 1999;103 (1):1–10.

74. International Study of Asthma and Allergies in Childhood (ISAAC) Steering Committee. Worldwide variation in prevalence of symptoms of asthma, allergic rhinoconjunctivitis, and atopic eczema: ISAAC. *Lancet* 1998;351:1225–1232.
75. Anderson HR. Air pollution and trends in asthma. In: Chadwick D, Cardew G. *The rising trends in asthma.* Ciba Foundation Symposium 206. New York: John Wiley & Sons, 1997:190–207.
76. von Mutius E, Martinez FD, Fritzsch C, et al. Prevalence of asthma and atopy in two areas of West and East Germany. *Am J Respir Crit Care Med* 1994;149(2 pt 1):358–364.
77. Nowak D, Heinrich J, Jorres R, et al. Prevalence of respiratory symptoms, bronchial hyperresponsiveness and atopy among adults: West and East Germany. *Eur Respir J* 1996;9:2541–2552.
78. Bjorksten B. Epidemiology of pollution-induced airway disease in Scandinavia and Eastern Europe. *Allergy* 1997;52[suppl 38]:23–25.
79. Nicolai NT. Epidemiology of pollution-induced airway disease: urban/rural differences in East and West Germany. *Allergy* 1997;52[suppl 38]:26–29.
80. United States Environmental Protection Agency. National Air Quality and Emission Trends Report. EPA 454/R-01-004, 2001.
81. Burge H. Bioaerosols: prevalence and health effects in the indoor environment. *J Allergy Clin Immunol* 1990; 86:687–701.
82. Sporik R, Holgate ST, Platts-Mills TAE, et al. Exposure to house-mite antigen and the development of asthma in childhood. *N Engl J Med* 1990;323:502–507.
83. Platts-Mills TAE, Sporik RB, Chapman MD, et al. The role of domestic allergens. In: Chadwick D, Cardew G, eds. *The rising trends in asthma.* Ciba Foundation Symposium 206. New York: John Wiley & Sons, 1997: 173–189.
84. Crater S, Platts-Mills T. Searching for the cause of the increase in asthma. *Curr Opin Pediatr* 1998;10:594–599.
85. Yunginger JW, Reed CE, O'Connell EJ, et al. A community-based study of the epidemiology of asthma: incidence rates, 1964–1983. *Am Rev Respir Dis* 1992; 146:888–894.
86. Heinrich J, et al. Trends in prevalence of atopic diseases and allergic sensitization in children in Eastern Germany. Eur Respir J 2002;19(6):1040-1046.
87. Gern JE, Weiss ST. Protection against atopic diseases by measles—a rash conclusion? *JAMA* 2000;283:394-395.
88. Bleecker ER, Postma DS, Meyers DA. Genetic susceptibility to asthma in a changing environment. In: Chadwick D, Cardew G, eds. *The rising trends in asthma.* Ciba Foundation Symposium 206. New York: John Wiley & Sons, 1997:90–105.
89. Joseph LM, Ownby DR, Peterson EL, et al. Racial differences in physiologic parameters related to asthma among middle-class children. *Chest* 2000;117: 1336–1344.
90. Cookson WOCM, Moffatt MF. Asthma: an epidemic in the absence of infection? *Science* 1997;275:41–42.
91. Frampton MW, Voter KZ, Morrow PE, et al. Sulfuric acid aerosol exposure in humans assessed by bronchoalveolar lavage. *Am Rev Respir Dis* 1992;146:626–632.
92. Hanley QS, Koenig JQ, Larson TV, et al. Response of young asthmatic patients to inhaled sulfuric acid. *Am Rev Respir Dis* 1992;145:326–331.
93. Samet JM, Zeger SL, Dominici F, et al. The National Morbidity, Mortality, and Air Pollution Study (NMMAPS). Parts I: methods and methodologic issues. Part II: morbidity and mortality from air pollution in the United States. *Res Rep Health Eff Inst* 2000; 94(94 pt 1):5–14; discussion 75–84(94 pt 2):5–70; discussion 71–79.
94. Wyzga RE. Statement to the Clear Air, Wetlands, Private Property and Nuclear Safety Subcommittee of the Committee of Environment and Public Works, United States Senate. February 5, 1997.
95. Lipfert FW, Morris SC, Wyzga RE. Daily mortality in the Philadelphia metropolitan area and size-classified particulate matter. *J Air Waste Manage Assoc* 2000;50 (8):1501–1513.
96. Campbell MJ, Tobias A. Causality and temporality in the study of short-term effects of air pollution on health. *Int J Epidemiol* 2000;29(2):271–273.
97. Campbell MJ, Julious SA, Peterson CK, et al. Atmospheric pressure and sudden infant death syndrome in Cook County, Chicago. *Paediatr Perinat Epidemiol* 2001;15(3):287–289.
98. Moller J, Hallqvist J, Diderichsen F, et al. Do episodes of anger trigger myocardial infarction? A case-crossover analysis in the Stockholm Heart Epidemiology Program (SHEEP). *Psychosom Med* 1999;61:842–849.
99. Phillips DP, King EW. Death takes a holiday: mortality surrounding major social occasions. *Lancet* 1988;2 (8613):728–732.
100. Phillips DP, Smith DG. Postponement of death until symbolically meaningful occasions. *JAMA* 1990;263 (14):1947–1951.
101. Phillips DP, Van Voorhees CA, Ruth TE. The birthday: lifeline or deadline? *Psychosom Med* 1992;54(5): 532–542
102. Phillips DP, Christenfeld N, Ryan NM. An increase in the number of deaths in the United States in the first week of the month—an association with substance abuse and other causes of death. *N Engl J Med* 1999; 341(2):93–98.
103. Phillips DP, Liu GC, Kwok K, et al. The Hound of the Baskervilles effect: natural experiment on the influence of psychological stress on timing of death. *Br Med J* 2001;323:1443–1446.
104. Smyth JM, Soefer MH, Hurewitz A, et al. Daily psychosocial factors predict levels and diurnal cycles of asthma symptomatology and peak flow. *J Behav Med* 1999;22(2):179–193.
105. Rietveld S, van Beest I, Everaerd W. Stress-induced breathlessness in asthma. *Psychol Med* 1999;29(6): 1359–1366.
106. Stieb DM, Beveridge RC, Smith-Doiron M, et al. Beyond administrative data: characterizing cardiorespiratory disease episodes among patients visiting the emergency department. *Can J Public Health* 2000;91: 107–112.
107. Stieb DM, Judek S, Burnett RT. Meta-analysis of time-series studies of air pollution and mortality: effects of gases and particles and the influence of cause of death, age, and season. *J Air Waste Manage Assoc* 2002;52: 470–484.

60

Accessing Environmental Data

David M. Gute

This chapter reviews the utility of ambient environmental information for the clinical management of putative environmental disease. Knowledge of environmental agents can facilitate the diagnosis and control of conditions of possible environmental origin.

Data sources for environmental information are growing rapidly as the influence of the World Wide Web continues to expand. But these databases generally were collected for purposes other than clinical medicine, so in most cases only exposure data are available, not clinically relevant dose parameters. Thus it is important for the clinician to know how to use these proliferating databases and how to assess the quality of the data.

The etiologic contribution of the ambient environment to the development of human disease is a matter of controversy. This chapter does not enter into this debate; suffice it to say that there is increasing acknowledgment of the intricate relationship between the environment and human health. This chapter discusses the available environmental information, how to access environmental exposure databases, the sources and the legal mandates for the collection of such databases, the types of environmental information available from government agencies, and the possible applications of environmental exposure databases in the practice of clinical medicine.

Ambient environmental information of relevance to the practicing clinician can take many forms. Information includes data collected as a result of statute, such as air pollution monitoring as mandated by the Clean Air Act to other burgeoning environmental exposure databases. Environmental information is collected by all levels of government—local, county, state, and federal—and by private corporations. These data are also collected for different time periods and vastly different geographic units. Accessing environmental data systems may be of clinical interest, to improve diagnosis and treatment and to formulate prevention strategies (1). The benefits of integrating environmental data within the sister discipline of occupational medicine were recently presented (2).

Another reason for accessing such data is to respond to patient queries on environmental health. Survey research indicates that the physician is highly regarded by the public as a source of objective information on the environment but is usually ill prepared for addressing occupational/environmental health issues (3).

Physicians have been urged to become knowledgeable about environmental health because of their special responsibilities in their advocacy role and in their role as actors in fostering preventive actions by governments, corporations, and communities (4). These responsibilities are likely to increase as the knowledge base documenting links between human health and the environment increases.

Environmental exposure databases were reviewed in a workshop hosted by the U.S. Environmental Protection Agency (EPA), the Agency for Toxic Substances and Diseases Registry (ATSDR), and the National Center for Health Statistics (NCHS) (5). This workshop considered the uses of environmental exposure databases collected by the federal government. In general, these databases report on exposure data, in contrast to the more clinically useful parameter of dose. Of the 67 federally sponsored data systems reviewed, 13 (19%) contained human tissue results.

The importance of maintaining current and complete information on environmental health was the focus of a major assessment conducted by the Institute of Medicine as requested by the National Library of Medicine (NLM). This assessment was published in 1997 and entailed a review of the 16 on-line databases maintained by the NLM as part of the Toxicology and Environmental Health Information Program (TEHIP) (6).

TABLE 60.1. *Parameters of interest for environmental data*

Parameter	Comments
Temporal period of data collection	Sufficient length of time to capture seasonal effects?
Collection *frequency*	Annual, monthly, daily
Smallest *unit* of geographic aggregation	City/town, census tract
Type of media	Soil, water, air

Before reviewing available data, it is helpful to describe the manner in which databases are arrayed to consider which parameters are of potential clinical interest (Table 60.1). Information is presented on the data sources available for air, water, soil, and hazardous waste that can be useful in medical practice.

DATA QUALITY ISSUES

Environmental data and information will benefit the practicing physician in the diagnosis, treatment, and prevention of disease. What distinguishes data from information? *Data* are raw measurements of the concentration, distribution, and environmental fate of a given agent or contaminant. *Information* represents data that is interpretable and useful for decision making. The products of any data system should be viewed through the lens of *statistics,* which are key parameters of a given population used to describe the natural world.

For example, with sufficient resources it is possible to measure the blood leads of all 6-year-olds in the United States. The mean value, or other measures of central tendency such as mode or median, would constitute a parameter of this population. The usual approach is to draw a sample of subjects from a population and then calculate statistics resulting from this sample. A key hurdle is ensuring that the sample accurately represents the underlying population from which it was drawn. The following attributes of the data must be assessed:

- Validity: Do the data truly measure the desired attribute? For example, if you are measuring contaminant levels in a stream, are the sampling stations up- or downstream of a point source generator?
- Accuracy: Is the method representative of the true value? That is, can the method adequately approach the true result? Note that data can be accurate but not necessarily valid.
- Reliability: Can the method demonstrate consistency in the generation of values? For instance, a method may be highly reliable by generating consistent results in multiple tests. Reliability, however, should not be confused with accuracy. A technique can be very consistent, or reliable, without being accurate.

These are generic constraints in employing statistics to increase the understanding of any problem. Practitioners in occupational and environmental medicine in particular are well aware of the vagaries that can plague indices of health, especially clinical laboratory results. A critical eye should also be cast on environmental data. Table 60.2 lists the questions to ask in evaluating environmental databases. The practitioner should become a sophisticated consumer of environmental data. This sophistication can result from familiarity with the sources of these data and from an intelligent appreciation of their use in the practice of medicine.

TABLE 60.2. *Key questions to ask in evaluating environmental data*

1. How representative is the sample of the affected area?
2. Were standard laboratory methods used?
3. Were the samples handled, transported, and stored properly?
4. What were the quality assurance procedures?
5. How were the samples obtained?
6. What was the level of detection of the procedure? (What was the smallest amount of the substance that could be detected?)
7. If latency is a factor of interest, do retrospective exposure data exist?

TYPES OF ENVIRONMENTAL DATA

There are a variety of environmental data collection systems in the United States. (This chapter focuses largely on U.S. sources, but this does not imply that environmental health problems benefit from such insularity. It is simply a matter of space limitations.) Some of these systems exist because of regulatory requirements and fulfill either monitoring or surveillance requirements of statutes or regulations. These data may be collected at the federal or state level. Many of these data systems are collected for reasons other than human health concerns.

The potential for human exposure to a specific contaminant is of primary clinical interest in diagnosis and treatment. A compilation of federal environmental exposure data systems reflects the profusion and variety of these sources (7). This listing includes 67 data systems for data obtained from three distinct sources: (a) passive sensors located in an enclosed environment (e.g., radon sampling device); (b) personal monitoring equipment actually worn by volunteers or workers (e.g., radiation badge); and (c) biologic media for laboratory analysis (e.g., the quantitation of blood lead levels).

For a true picture of human exposure to emerge, the practitioner must address the cumulative nature of exposure from multiple pathways, including routes of exposure such as dermal, respiratory, and ingestion. Any such consideration must include the impact of food-chain exposures especially for substances readily stored (lead) or concentrated selectively in certain tissues such as polychlorinated biphenyls (PCBs) in fat. There are other factors to consider in relation to a patient's health:

- Magnitude of exposure: What is the effective concentration in biologic media? Measures of magnitude are more likely expressed in a volume of environmental media such as air or water.
- Duration of exposure: How long was the actual exposure? Was it acute or chronic? A particular concern is whether sharp spikes in concentration for short periods may be relevant.
- Frequency of exposure: How often does this exposure occur? Does it vary seasonally or temporally?

Data are also generated as a result of requirements of regulatory agencies and can be thought of as constituting three specific functions: (a) monitoring, (b) surveillance, and (c) special studies tied to a geographic site. For instance, in the above-mentioned 67 data collection systems, 36 performed monitoring functions, 19 primarily supported regulatory activities, and 29 shaped research needs.

Monitoring data are routinely collected by federal, state, and sometimes local governments to measure environmental media (air, water, soil) for selected contaminants as specified either by statute (criteria pollutants as defined by the Clean Air Act) or special interest. Surveillance connotes a more encompassing and ambitious research plan for the visualization of a specific environmental agent. For example, the National Health and Nutrition Examination Survey (NHANES) characterizes, among other things, food chain exposure to selected environmental agents including lead.

Special studies are performed for a variety of purposes, most notably in the area of hazardous waste, including the cleanup and discovery process surrounding specific Superfund sites.

Agent-specific information concerning the toxicologic characteristics may be of use to practitioners in assessing the potential for health effects in a specific case. Two on-line data systems, which can provide the practitioner with general information regarding an agent are the Toxicology Information Online (TOXLINE) and Toxicology Data Network (TOXNET). Both are supported by the Medical Literature Analysis and Retrieval System (MEDLARS) of the National Library of Medicine. TOXLINE is composed of 16 subfiles and TOXNET I of 10 files, many of which are of interest to the practitioner. TOXNET includes the following files:

- Registry of Toxic Effects of Chemical Substances (RTECS) as maintained by the National Institute for Occupational Safety and Health: This file contains information on agent-specific characteristics, such as toxicity in both humans and animals, that are of importance to clinicians.
- Integrated Risk Information System (IRIS) from the EPA is an electronic on-line database of summary health risk assessment and regulatory information on chemical substances. Its primary purpose is to provide guidance risk values to EPA risk assessors and decision makers for use in EPA risk assessments. IRIS is not an exhaustive toxicologic database, but rather presents a summary of information on hazard and dose–response assessments. The heart of the IRIS system is its collection of computer files covering individual chemicals. These chemical files contain descriptive and quantitative information in the following categories: (a) oral reference doses and inhalation reference concentrations (RfDs and RfCs, respectively) for chronic noncarcinogenic health effects; and (b) hazard identification, oral slope factors, and oral and inhalation unit risks for carcinogenic effects (8) (see Chapter 39 for a review of relevant concepts).
- Toxic Release Inventory (TRI): This file is a compilation of information on the release of toxic substances by manufacturing facilities. These data are available in an annual report as well as by accessing an EPA database via microcomputer telephone modem (9). The federal statute which created TRI, the Emergency Planning and Community Right-To-Know Act of 1986, specifically required the EPA to provide public access to this file via an on-line format. This law is one of the first instances where the

mode of dissemination of a database, in contrast to its content, was stipulated.

COMMONLY ASKED QUESTIONS THAT TRIGGER ENVIRONMENTAL DATA SEARCHES

Many analysts of medical practice in the U.S. note the rise in the public's interest in environmental health questions and the growing role of the physician in serving as an expert and opinion leader for such answering questions posed by patients (10). Many of these questions are generated and fueled by patients' concerns surrounding news media coverage of environmental "pressure points." Examples include the possible health effects of a given agent, the environmental and health effects attributable to a hazardous waste site, and the unknown consequences of a newly emerging technology (release of engineered microbes) or the possible health effects in mature technologies (electromagnetic fields).

Beyond helping patients interpret news events in environmental health, the practitioner must distill information of critical importance in the differential diagnosis and treatment of a patient. Such investigations can be enhanced with data concerning a hazardous agent. Inquiries may be started through data sources that contain agent-specific information (refer back to the toxicologic databases previously described). In addition, the clinician must verify the exposure pathways in relation to a particular environmental agent. In performing such an analysis, the central tenets of exposure assessment (previously discussed) must be addressed.

Workers may be exposed to substances on the job that can affect their health. Transport of these same occupational agents to family members via the workers' clothes is widely acknowledged. Hobbies and recreational activities also must be critically evaluated for a comprehensive picture of all sources of potential exposure. In a similar manner, community residents may suffer complaints and health problems attributable to industrial facilities and/or hazardous waste sites or other facilities associated with solid waste streams such as landfills, incinerators, and transfer stations.

Physicians are increasingly presented with environmental medicine complaints. Pivotal community environmental health cases in Times Beach, Missouri; Love Canal, New York; and Woburn, Massachusetts, among others, and have forced local, state, and federal government to develop and augment resources to address environmental disease.

This transition has not been easy. Public health authorities have been upbraided for a variety of faults including lack of compassion, deficiencies in the scope and focus of epidemiologic studies, and the general inability to include community representatives in the drafting and dissemination of community-based scientific protocols (11). The questions posed to public health authorities regarding the linkages between site-specific contaminants and the relationship to somatic disease highlight some of the limits of epidemiology. These limits have been demonstrated in stark relief in celebrated cases and have resulted in thoughtful commentary concerning the feasibility of conducting such "reactive" epidemiology (12).

AGENCY RESOURCES

Many federal and state agencies are responsible for the collection and dissemination of environmental data. The agencies listed here are of singular importance to environmental health. (For further discussion of relevant regulatory agencies, see Chapter 3.)

Agency for Toxic Substances and Disease Registry (ATSDR)

This agency in the Department of Health and Human Services was created by the Comprehensive Environmental Response, Compensation, and Liability Act of 1980 (CERCLA). Under CERCLA, commonly known as the Superfund, and the Superfund Amendments and Reauthorization Act of 1986, ATSDR's mission is to prevent or mitigate human health problems and diminished quality of life resulting from exposure to hazardous substances. ATSDR is also mandated to develop information and educational programs to help health professionals evaluate, diagnose, treat, and conduct surveillance on patients exposed to hazardous substances.

In 1984, amendments to the Resource Conservation and Recovery Act of 1976 (RCRA), which provides for the management of legitimate hazardous waste storage or destruction facilities, charged the ATSDR to conduct health assessments at these sites, when requested by the EPA, states, or individuals, and to assist the EPA in determining which substances should be regulated and the levels at which they may pose a threat to human health.

In 1986, amendments to CERCLA, known as the Superfund Amendments and Reauthorization Act of 1986 (SARA), broadened ATSDR's responsibilities in the areas of health assessments, toxicologic data bases, information dissemination, and medical education.

Environmental Protection Agency (EPA)

The EPA was formed in 1970 and acquired regulatory responsibility, under the Clean Air Act Amendments of 1970 and the Clean Water Act of 1972, to set national air and water standards for selected contaminants. As the EPA has developed and matured, it has placed greater reliance on the activity of its ten regional offices throughout the country to maintain oversight. Added burdens imposed on the agency include the Toxic Substances Act of 1976 (TSCA), CERCLA, and SARA (the Superfund). The Superfund is grappling with an estimated 23,000 potential hazardous-waste sites in the U.S. The EPA initially weathered severe criticism for the perceived lack of speed and responsiveness to the identification, control, and abatement on these sites. Performance has improved as methods and resources were developed and deployed. Given the complexity of achieving compliance and oversight of these statutes, many states have assumed delegated authority to enforce EPA mandates in these areas.

The EPA, in concert with state and local environmental agencies, has also become more active in assisting in the development of "Brownfields." Estimates of the number of such sites within the U.S. vary, but it is likely that there are more than 300,000. Although Brownfields have lower levels of toxic material than do Superfund sites, the perception of contamination and possible human health threats needs to be addressed and understood as well as communicated to constituencies. The need for physician input on these sites may increase as the surrounding communities are being vested with greater amounts of decision-making capacity regarding the specification of reuse options for these properties.

State and Local Health and Environmental Departments

Because of the trend toward delegation, state and local health and environmental agencies can represent useful resources for data, technical assistance, and information pertaining to the environment. State agencies are generally responsible for administering pollution control programs and environmental monitoring programs for air and water, and, in conjunction with local officials, administering an array of environmental protection activities. This close coordination is particularly true in implementing the reuse of brown fields.

OTHER RESOURCES

Poison control centers, through the dispensing of critical clinical information for practitioners and patients alike, have become well established in the medical landscape. The proportion of inquiries that have some connection to the environment has continued to increase (13). This reality, coupled with suggestions from organizations such as the Institute of Medicine that advocate "single access" sources of information for clinicians, has led certain poison control centers to provide environmental health information. One of the first of these enhanced poison control centers has been established and staffed by the faculty of the Division of Occupational and Environmental Health of the Duke University Medical School (14).

The physician can also search for environmental data on Internet sites, such as MEDLINE. Reviews of how to access and utilize this technology began in the early 1990s and are growing and improving in sophistication (15). See Appendices A to C at the end of this chapter for current assessments of Web-based resources and compact disc (CD) information in the areas of occupational health.

CASE STUDIES IN ENVIRONMENTAL MEDICINE

The following two cases are concrete examples of how environmental data may be used by practitioners in ascertaining and evaluating putative environmental disease, and provide practical advice on how to approach two distinct classes of problems. The first case focuses on a particular disease and its relationship to a population at risk. The second case focuses not on the disease end point but rather on the pathways of exposure.

Case 1: Adult Diagnosed with Acute Leukemia

A 28-year-old white man has been diagnosed with acute nonlymphocytic leukemia (ANLL), a category of leukemia that accounts for over 50% of all leukemia cases in adults. The patient and his family express the belief that other neighborhood residents have also recently suffered leukemia and other cancers. You are asked for your assessment of whether there is a possible environmental factor that might explain this situation. [For an in-depth review of the etiology and epidemiology of leukemia, see Linet (16).]

Your first steps should consist of the following. Respond to what the patient and his family are feeling and saying. It is critically important to listen and then give counsel. The astute clinician can represent the first line of intelligence about the etiology of human carcinogens. One of the best examples of this occurrence is found in the association of vinyl chloride with angiosarcoma of the liver, which began in the practice of a single physician (17). All too often, however, it is difficult to link the occurrence of community clusters of cancer with any specific etiologic agent.

In the case of leukemia, specifically ANLL, it is prudent to review with the patient the known causes of this disease. The two most important causes are benzene exposure and ionizing radiation. Such exposures could come from a variety of sources including both occupational and environmental, and, in the case of ionizing radiation, through medical therapy. In pursuing any evaluation of the patient's leukemia, it is important to seek information on the combined histopathologic and clinical classification scheme of the leukemia under study. Unfortunately, many epidemiologic studies simply lump all leukemia together, thus frustrating the attempt to improve upon existing etiologic information for the major subtypes. A relatively new agent of some concern with reference to childhood leukemia is the proximity of cases to electromagnetic fields. These studies have found relative risks in the 0.8 to 2.0 range for this disease outcome. These studies, however, are plagued by poor ascertainment of retrospective or historical exposure to the agent (18). This lack of retrospective environmental data is a continuing problem for most investigations of occupational and environmental agents and is a particular concern for those health problems exhibiting long latency.

With regard to concerns about the existence of a community cluster or raised level of incidence in the immediate area, there are a number of possible sources of information. First, contact the local board of health or the state health department to inquire if there is a tumor or cancer registry in existence. Statewide rates can be compared to the community of interest to yield some relative assessment of the magnitude of the problem. Ask for data that are aggregated over at least 3- to 5-year intervals, particularly for towns of small population size, so that the values for the area of interest are a little more stable. In addition, try to ascertain the incidence instead of the mortality. If the state or local health agency does not maintain a registry, inquire at the regional tertiary cancer hospital and see if an institution-specific registry is maintained. The American Cancer Society maintains annual estimates of the number of cancer cases occurring in each state. These estimates are largely driven by mortality information, but they might be helpful in providing some information.

The most important subject to pursue with the patient's family is determining the types of exposures that the patient may have suffered in his lifetime, from occupational or environmental exposures or from hobbies or crafts. The goal of such an evaluation is to confront directly the fears that the disease resulted from some known agent that the patient could have avoided or reduced exposure to if the information had been available. A structural problem to be discussed early is that the science of epidemiology attempts to discern etiology for groups of people who exhibit certain characteristics. The generalizations gained from such analysis do not translate well into making statements about where individual cases of a particular disease arise.

Patients and families may want information about the number of cases of the cancer that have been found within the community. They may even supply you with lists of people who have been diagnosed with cancer. These lists should be passed on to the appropriate public health authority for verification and evaluation. Important parameters to check on such lists include the actual diagnosis, the date of diagnosis, and, if available, the length of residence in the neighborhood if the concern centers on a community risk of specific cancers. This level of detail is usually missing from community-generated lists but is critical in order to support further epidemiologic evaluation. Such community-generated lists can suffer from a variety of problems including inaccurate information and various forms of information biases (see Chapter 40).

Another factor to consider in any suspected environmental disease is the relative contribution of personal risk factors such as tobacco, drug, and alcohol use. In the case of ANLL, tobacco and alcohol do not demonstrate consistent patterns as major risk factors.

In summary, listen to the patient and family in their quest to understand why this disease happened. Be aware that the investigations may shed some light on etiology but be prepared for the much more likely result that you will not be able to ascertain a cause to the satisfaction for all concerned parties.

Case 2: Patient Concern over Proximity to Superfund Hazardous Waste Site

A 34-year-old woman presents to an occupational physician with concerns about her proximity (1 mile) to a Superfund hazardous waste site, and the possibility of air pollution and water pollution from this site causing a variety of nonspecific symptoms that she is experiencing.

Given the nonspecific nature of the patient's symptoms, your first goal should be to obtain information about the point source of interest. There are a variety of data sources that can be consulted. As a first step, contact the local health authorities concerning the existence of a public health assessment of the Superfund site. SARA set a 1-year deadline for the characterizing of sites after they are proposed for inclusion as a Superfund site and listing on the National Priorities List (NPL). Listing on the NPL qualifies the site for cleanup under CERCLA or Superfund authority. Sites that are not listed on the NPL are abated subject to state or private action (19). ATSDR has determined that hazardous substances had been released at 85% of the sites and that about 15% of these sites merited further public health investigation (20).

SARA requires that the public health assessments be based on such factors as the nature and extent of site contamination, the size and susceptibility of the community, and the effects of exposure. SARA sets two goals for such assessments: (a) deciding whether the exposure to a site's hazardous substances should be reduced, and (b) stating whether additional health studies should be conducted at the site. The law requires ATSDR to provide its health assessments to the EPA and to the states. ATSDR's role at Superfund sites is mostly advisory; the EPA is in charge of the actual cleanup (19).

What are the likely pathways of exposure emanating from a hazardous waste site? There are three principal routes: airborne exposure, runoff to ground and surface waters, and dermal contact with contaminated soils and agents. The routine monitoring of air concentrations of volatiles on the site is usually not feasible, and the study of this pathway is made difficult by the generally small number of exposed cases.

Water contamination is not just confined to ingestion but also should include airborne exposures from materials that can outgas during showering, bathing, or cooking or can be absorbed through the skin. Where can water data be obtained? It depends on the source of the water. Private wells are generally tested at the initiative of the owner. Most regulatory agencies have been loath to accept responsibility for the regulation of this drinking water source. If the sources of drinking water are surface or ground waters distributed as part of a municipal or regional system, information on quality may be obtained from the relevant water board or company. Most existing protocols in the U.S. are in place to guard against bacteriologic contamination and other threats that could affect gross water quality such as turbidity and biologic oxygen demand (BOD). Special studies to characterize waterborne concentrations of hazardous materials such as lead have been implemented periodically by agencies such as the EPA or state environmental and health departments. The testing of residential water for organics, heavy metals, and other agents can usually be accomplished through commercial laboratories or in conjunction with special testing protocols provided by local authorities for residents. Some states are launching certification programs aimed at improving the accuracy and validity of data obtained from such commercial laboratories.

Under the federal Safe Drinking Water Act of 1974, the EPA is required to prepare and promulgate regulations and standards concerning public water supplies. Two different standards are required: the recommended maximum contaminant levels (RMCLs) and the maximum contaminant levels (MCLs). The RMCLs are not enforceable but exist for advisory purposes; in contrast, the MCLs are enforceable, and if an MCL is exceeded, corrective action must be taken by the supplier to ensure compliance with the standard. Where no guidance exists from the EPA, states are left to their own devices in promulgating regulatory standards, particularly in the area of organic contaminants.

The rethinking of approaches to regulatory decision making in the area of drinking water extends to how risks are assessed, particularly for non–point-source contaminants (urban runoff, nutrients from the intensive practice of agriculture, airborne deposition) and for emerging or new classes of contaminants. Physicians need to be knowledgeable about these issues in order to address patients' questions and concerns (21).

An associated problem is establishing acceptable levels for soils through which groundwater may percolate. Soil levels are also of concern in attempting to answer questions such as, How clean is clean? This question is regularly encountered in monitoring any abatement project. It poses the questions of what level of cleanliness should a source attain before the site is returned to a more general pattern of use.

In general, the caveats that physicians are aware of in reference to the interpretation of clinical laboratory results hold for the interpretation of environmental data. Keep in mind some of the central questions that should inform the assessment of these data (Table 60.2).

The third possible route of exposure is through the medium of soil. Soil can be ingested by young children, and can serve as a means of uptake (along with airborne deposition) and as a means of increasing the load on crops eaten for human consumption.

It is important to discuss with the patient all possible routes of exposure for the point source of interest. Often, if the possibility of exposure can be rigorously pursued, the level of fear and concern can either be substantiated or placed in an appropriate context. This is in contrast with case 1, in which a specific health end point forms the basis of the investigation and the dialogue between patient and physician. The presence of a Superfund site can galvanize public concern. This public dimension of the problem complicates an understanding of the levels of risk posed to the patient. Perception of risk from the perspective of the patient turns on issues with which the physician must be acquainted, such as the perceived benefit and attendant risks, the severity of the health end point associated with the risk, the certainty of the association, the ability of the individual to exercise some control of the risk, the newness of the risk, and whether the risk is limited to the individual or is also conferred on other family members and/or future generations.

EMERGING AND REEMERGING DISEASE

Part of the burden of incorporating accurate environmental information into clinical practice is simply remaining aware of leading-edge applications for such information. This is especially true in the area of emerging and reemerging disease. The recent expression of focal epidemics of vector-borne infectious disease such as West Nile Virus throughout much of the U.S. and the spread of raccoon rabies are examples of how patterns of human disease may by influenced by changes in global climate. Other outcomes that reflect the increasing recognition of the environment and human health are such pandemics as new-variant Creutzfeldt-Jakob disease. The surveillance and control of this risk will turn on the effectiveness of concerted global cooperation and action.

Brief mention must be made of the Human Genome Project and its potential for both clinical gains and ethically troubling applications. The results of this work have clear implications for the practice of environmental and occupational medicine (22).

SUMMARY

As in all professions, the skill of practitioners can be improved by investing in training and education to enhance skills and competence. It is prudent to remain aware of developments in other professions that can contribute to the enhancement of clinical medicine. The comprehensiveness of community assessment evident in a review of the nursing profession serves as one possible example of such utility (23). This chapter has provided an overall framework for transforming data into the more clinically useful commodity of information. This transformation rests on the acumen and integrative abilities of the practitioner more than it does on a mastery of the hardware or software involved in the storage and dissemination of environmental data. There is greater depth and sophistication in continuing education and training programs directed at the physician community and targeting environmental health concerns. This change has ranged from the creation of environmental medicine residencies to a panoply of other formats and models (24). It is also reflected concretely in the specification of core competencies for the full spectrum of medical specialties in 14 clinical areas as promulgated by the American College of Occupational and Environmental Medicine. The vast increase in the number of sources and density of information at the intersection of human health and the environment have only increased the need for physicians to be adept in integrating this material into clinical and advocacy applications.

REFERENCES

1. Goldman R, Peters J. The occupational and environmental health history. *JAMA* 1981;246:2831–2836.
2. Herbert R, London M, Nagin D, et al. The diagnosis and treatment of occupational diseases: integrating clinical practice with prevention. *Am J Ind Med* 2000;37:1–5.
3. Burstein JM, Levy BS. The teaching of occupational health in U.S. medical schools: little improvement in 9 years. *Am J Public Health* 1994;84:846–849.
4. McCally M, Cassel CK. Medical responsibility and global environmental change. *Ann Intern Med* 1990; 113:467–473.
5. Sexton K, Selevan SG, Wagener DK, et al. Estimating human exposures to environmental pollutants: availability and utility of existing databases. *Arch Environ Health* 1992;47:6:398–407.
6. Liverman CT, Ingalls CE, Fulco CE, et al., eds. *Toxicology and environmental health information resources: the role of the National Library of Medicine.* Washington, DC: National Academy Press, 1997.
7. U.S. Environmental Protection Agency. National Center for Health Statistics, Agency or Toxic Substances and Disease Registry. Inventory of exposure-related data systems sponsored by federal agencies. EPA/600/R-92/078. May 1992.
8. Anonymous. Health and environment digest. Navarre, MN: Freshwater Foundation, 1993;7:8.
9. U.S. Environmental Protection Agency. *The toxics release inventory: a national perspective.* EPA 560/4-89-005. Washington, DC: U.S. Government Printing Office, 1989.

10. Kilbourne EM, Weiner J. Occupational and environmental medicine: the internist's role. *Ann Intern Med* 1990;113:974–982.
11. Ozonoff D, Boden LI. Truth and consequences: health agency responses to environmental health problems. *Sci Technol Human Values* 1987;12:70–77.
12. Anderson HA. Evolution of environmental epidemiologic risk assessment. *Environ Health Perspect* 1985; 62:389–392.
13. Litovitz TL, White JD. Occupational and environmental illness and the poison center. *West J Med* 1990;152: 178–179.
14. Darcey DJ, Greenberg GN, Jackson GW. Resource center for occupational and environmental medicine. *Ann Intern Med* 1991;114:607.
15. Alston PG. ENVIRONTENTONLINE: the greening of Databases-Part 2. Scientific and technical databases. DATABASE October 1991, 34–52.
16. Linet MS. *The leukemias-epidemiologic aspects*. New York: Oxford University Press, 1985.
17. U.S. Department of Health and Human Services. Agency for Toxic Substances and Disease Registry. *Vinyl chloride toxicity. Case studies in environmental medicine,* vol 2. Washington, DC: DHHS, 1990.
18. Tenforde TS. Health effects of low-frequency electric and magnetic fields. *Environ Sci Technol* 1992;27: 56–58.
19. U.S. General Accounting Office. *SUPERFUND—public health assessments: incomplete and of questionable value.* GAO/RCED-91-178. Washington, DC: U.S. Government Printing Office, August 1991.
20. National Research Council. *Environmental epidemiology. Public health and hazardous waste.* Washington, DC: National Academy Press, 1991.
21. Committee to Assess the Scientific Basis of the Total Maximum Daily Load Approach to Water Pollution Reduction, Water Science and Technology Board, National Research. Assessing the TMDL approach to water quality management, 2001.
22. Rawbone RG. Future impact of genetic screening in occupational and environmental medicine. *Occup Environ Med* 1999;56:721–724.
23. Institute of Medicine. *Nursing, health and the environment: strengthening the relationship to improve the public's health.* Washington, DC: National Academy Press, 1995.
24. Byrns G, Spahr J, Knapp A. Emerging issues in health care: the role of the environmental health residency. *J Environ Health* 1992;July/August:31–35.

FURTHER INFORMATION

Chivian E, McCally M, Hu H, et al., eds. *Critical condition: Human health and the environment.* Cambridge, MA: MIT Press, 1993.

This volume provides a comprehensive yet brief account of what is known medically about the effects of environmental degradation. It is accessible to a lay readership, and provides valuable and current information to practitioners. The volume also addresses occupational health problems.

Am J Epidemiol 1990;132[suppl 1].

An entire issue of this journal was devoted to papers associated with the National Conference on Clustering of Health Events. This meeting was jointly sponsored by the Centers for Disease Control, the ATSDR, and the Association of State and Territorial Health Officials. The issue describes state responses to hazardous waste sites, discusses protocols for the conducting of cluster studies, and provides details on appropriate analytic software and on the history of such inquiries. This discussion provides the practitioner with both conceptual and applied information regarding environmental health surveillance as well as the conducting of cluster studies.

Hazardous substances and public health. Atlanta, GA: ATSDR.

This bimonthly publication discusses current developments at the ATSDR. Subscription information (free publication): ATSDR, 1600 Clifton Road, NE, Mailstop E33, Atlanta, GA 30333, Tel. 1-404-639-6206, Fax 1-404-639-6208.

Aldrich T, Griffith J. *Environmental epidemiology and risk assessment.* New York: Van Nostrand Reinhold, 1993.

A comprehensive and systematic work that examines exposure to contamination by hazardous materials in the ambient environment and the potential adverse effects on human health.

National Research Council. *Environmental epidemiology—public health and hazardous wastes,* vol 1. Washington, DC: National Academy Press and National Research Council, 1991. *Environmental epidemiology—use of the gray literature and other data in environmental epidemiology,* vol 2. Washington, DC: National Academy Press, 1997.

These reports provide an in-depth discussion of the intersection between human health and the distribution of hazardous wastes in the U.S. Volume 1 identifies research gaps in our present level of knowledge concerning this relationship. Volume 2 discusses in some detail the strengths and weaknesses of data sources, particularly in the domain of public agencies as well as prescriptions about how to improve environmental epidemiology.

ADDITIONAL RESOURCES

American Medical Association Department of Preventive Medicine and Public Health, 515 North State Street, Chicago, Illinois, 60610.

Reports on environmental topics as issued by the AMA Council on Scientific Affairs.

Agency for Toxic Substances and Disease Registry Division of Health Education, 1600 Clifton Road, NE, Atlanta, GA 30333, Tel. 1-404-639-6205.

ATSDR offers continuing medical education (CME) credit for environmental case studies on toxic substances ranging from arsenic to vinyl chloride, and provides medical management guidelines for acute chemical exposures. Many other physician-oriented educational activities are offered in cooperation with state health departments.

The ATSDR Information Center, e-mail: *ATSDRIC@cdc.gov,* 1-404-498-0110, Fax 1-404-498-0057, toll-free tel. 1-888-42-ATSDR or 1-888-422-8737.

Washington Physicians for Social Responsibility, 4554 12th Avenue NE, Seattle, WA 98105, Tel. 1-206-547-2630, Fax 1-206-547-2631, *wpsr@wpsr.org*.

This national membership organization has expanded its campaign against the proliferation of nuclear weapons to include environmental issues. One focus is to further educate the medical community on the linkages between environmental exposures and health as well as to activate the medical community to protect the environment and public health. There are chapters in Boston, Los Angeles, San Francisco, Oregon, Madison, Atlanta, and Philadelphia.

APPENDIX A: INVENTORIES OF WEB AND COMPACT DISC ENVIRONMENTAL/OCCUPATIONAL INFORMATION

Agency for Toxic Substances and Disease Registry. www.atsdr.cdc.gov.

Kumar R, Kumar A, Shah N. A guide to workplace environmental health and safety: Internet sites and databases on CDs. *Environ Prog* 1999;18 W7–W12.

Kumar A, Vashisth S, D'Souza F. Introduction to WWW. *Environmental_Health_& Safety.Com*. *Environ Prog* 1996; 15 W13–W16.

Patel I, Kumar A. A guide to information on pollution prevention on the World Wide Web. *Environ Prog* 2000;19 W9–W14.

Kumar R, Kumar A. A directory of environmental health, safety, and management related software. *Environ Prog* 1998;17 S13–S17.

These inventories are annotated by the authors to reflect both content and utility, and are quite useful for planning search strategies.

APPENDIX B: OTHER NON-WEB INVENTORIES OF ENVIRONMENTAL OR HEALTH DATABASES

Abramowitz JN, Baker DS, Turnstall DB. *Guide of key environmental statistics in the U.S. government.* World Resources Institute, 1990.

Frisch JD, Shaw GM, Harris JA. Epidemiologic research using existing databases of environmental measures. *Arch Environ Health* 1990;45:303–307.

HHS Data Inventories. U.S. Department of Health and Human Services. Washington, DC: U.S. Government Printing Office, various years of issue.

Environmental Protection Agency. *Information resources directory.* Office of Information and Resources Management, 1989.

U.S. Public Health Service. Some publicly available sources of computerized information on environmental health and toxicology.

Centers for Disease Control and Prevention. National Center for Environmental Health. National Report on Human Exposure to Environmental Chemicals. NCEH Pub. No. 01-0164, March 2001.

National Center for Health statistics. U.S. Department of Health and Human Services. *Environmental health: a plan for collecting and coordinating statistical and epidemiologic data.* DHSS publication No. (PHS) 80-1248. Washington, DC: U.S. Government Printing Office, 1980.

National Center for Health Statistics. U.S. Department of Health and Human Services. *Environmental health: a study of the issues in locating, assessing and treating individuals exposed to hazardous substances.* DHHS publication No. (PHS) 81-1275. Washington, DC: U.S. Government Printing Office, 1981.

The potential for linking environmental and health data. Washington, DC: National Governors' Association, 1989.

Task Force on Environmental Cancer and Heart and Lung Disease. *Directory of exposure-related data bases,* 1981.

APPENDIX C: SELECTED GENERAL BIOMEDICAL RESOURCES FOR ACCESSING ENVIRONMENTAL INFORMATION: WEB PAGES

The World Wide Web Virtual Library: Epidemiology *http://chanane.ucsf.edu/epidem/epidem.html.*

University of Wisconsin at Milwaukee environmental health, safety and risk management home page: *www.uvm.edu/Dept/EHSRM/EHSLINKS.*

Organizing Medical Networked Information (OMNI): A gateway to evaluated, quality Internet resources in health and medicine, aimed at students, researchers, academics, and practitioners in the health and medical sciences. OMNI is created by a core team of information specialists and subject experts at the University of Nottingham Greenfield Medical Library. *http://omni.ac.uk/about/*

Also consult the hub from which it comes: *http://biome.ac.uk* has vet, biology, natural science and agricultural areas.

Karolinska Institute Disorders of Environmental Origin: *http://www.mic.ki.se/Diseases/c21.html.*

Hardin MD. Preventive medicine and public health—University of Iowa: *http://www.lib.uiowa.edu/hardin/md/publ.html.*

Department of Environmental Health, School of Public Health and Community Medicine, University of Washington. Environmental health library: *http://staff.washington.edu/ehlib/outlinks/ref2.html.*

National Environmental Health Association: *www.neha.orglinks.html.*

Appendix A
First Aid Supplies in the Occupational Setting

Larry M. Starr

When sudden injury or illness present in the occupational setting, the appropriate procedure is to provide immediate care. To do this effectively, definitions and methods of performance and supplies must be understood and available.

The 88-year-old National Safety Council (1) has differentiated the meaning of "first aid" from "medical treatment" as follows: "First aid is immediate care given to an injured or suddenly ill person. First aid does not take the place of proper medical treatment. Rather it furnishes temporary assistance until the victim receives competent medical care, if needed, or until the chance for recovery without medical care is assured."

The Occupational Safety and Health Administration (OSHA) (2), which regulates occupational health and safety, states, "Employers are required to provide medical and first aid personnel and supplies commensurate with the hazards of the workplace." To provide guidance to "institutions teaching first aid courses, consumers of these courses, and OSHA personnel who review courses," a formal guideline (OSHA CPL 2-2.53) (3) was issued to define "the essential elements of what OSHA considers a basic first aid program." Included are topics to be covered and, in some instances, supplies to be used (Table A.1).

TABLE A.1. *Occupational Safety and Health Administration (OSHA) first-aid training guidelines*

Basic adult cardiopulmonary resuscitation (CPR)
Basic first aid intervention
Bandaging of the head, chest, shoulder, arm, leg, wrist, elbow, foot, ankle, fingers, toes, and knee
Splinting of the arm, elbow, clavicle, fingers, hand, forearm, ribs, hip, femur, lower leg, ankle, knee, foot, and toes
Moving and rescuing victims including one- and two-person lifts, ankle and shoulder pulls, and the blanket pull
Specific training elements
Shock
Bleeding
Poisoning
Burns
Temperature extremes
Musculoskeletal injuries
Bites and stings
Medical emergencies (heart attack, stroke, asthma, diabetes, seizures, pregnancy)
Confined spaces
Universal precautions
Need for and use of universal precautions
Necessity for keeping gloves and other protective equipment readily available and their appropriate use
Appropriate tagging and disposal of any sharp item or instrument requiring special disposal measures such as blood-soaked material
If corrosive materials are used, eyewash and body flush facilities must be provided; the water source must be pressure controlled and clearly identified; portable eyewash stations must contain a minimum of 1 gallon of water

CATEGORIES OF FIRST AID RESPONDERS

The following categories of employees may provide first aid at the occupational site. A *good samaritan* is a nonmedical person who, by chance and voluntarily, happens to be nearby when a workplace injury or illness presents itself. According to OSHA (4), a good samaritan is not notified or designated to respond, but rather "renders first aid voluntarily at the worksite (and)...no expectation exists that the person render first aid." The person may attend a company-sponsored first aid class, but does so only for one's own benefit. A good samaritan may or may not hold a recognized or current first aid course completion card.

A *first aid responder* is a nonmedical person who completes a program of first aid training and is notified when a workplace emergency or first aid event occurs. In some cases the trained person holds a formal expectation, even if the person has another primary job, because it is written in the job description that first aid will be required. In other cases, OSHA (5) has written, "There may be instances when the expectation to provide first aid/CPR is clear even though it is not in writing." The training content provided to first aid responders may be delivered by agents of national agencies or by private vendors; the curriculum may be fixed and standardized, or customized to the needs of the site; the procedures may be oriented to applications in the community or to the workplace; and course time may range from brief (1–2 hour) awareness training to advanced classes lasting several days. Some first aid courses meet national agency or OSHA training guidelines; others meet neither.

A *first responder* completes the U. S. Department of Transportation (DOT) National Highway Traffic Safety Administration (NHTSA) first responder curriculum (6). The first responder is the highest level of first aid responder because completion is also recognized as an entry level for the emergency medical services (EMS) system (followed by EMT and paramedic). The curriculum covers at least seven modules and takes at least 40 hours to complete. Most occupational sites with infrequent injuries and illnesses do not bring their nonmedical responders to this level of preparation.

CATEGORIES OF FIRST AID SUPPLIES

First aid supplies may be categorized according to the degree of required medical control and access. *Individual first aid (IFA)* supplies may be issued directly to and routinely carried by trained first aid responders who anticipate or are expected to respond to immediately life-threatening events. These supplies, applied immediately upon arrival, may include barrier gloves/resuscitation masks and compact trauma dressings/supplies. *Portable first aid (PFA)* supplies are placed into a portable container (case or bag). When a medical emergency is identified, these supplies are accessed and transported to the emergency scene. PFA supplies are appropriate for immediately life-threatening and serious, but not life-threatening events. *Stationary first aid (SFA)* supplies are stored in a permanent container or cabinet. These supplies are used only when an injured or ill person is in the vicinity of the cabinet. *Occupational health (OH)* supplies include medically controlled (Rx) medications and devices. These are usually stored in an occupational health office or where an occupational health practitioner controls access and use.

REGULATORY RECOMMENDATIONS OR REQUIREMENTS FOR FIRST AID SUPPLIES

The OSHA guideline for first aid supplies has been described in an amendment to the General First Aid Standard (29 CFR 1910.151) published June 18, 1998 (7). Previously, a consulting physician was required to review and approve all first aid supplies. The amended standard continues to require that first aid supplies be readily available. However, rather than physician approval, OSHA considers a commercial kit acceptable. If an employer has unique or changing first aid needs, OSHA advises, "Consultation from the local fire/rescue department, appropriate medical professional, or local emergency room may be helpful."

To help a workplace decide among commercial kits, OSHA suggested reviewing a 1978 list published by the American National Standard Institute (ANSI). Coincident with the publication of the OSHA amendment, ANSI released an updated list of supplies in document ANSI Z308.1-1998 (8). The Federal Aviation Administration (FAA) has also identified a list of supplies required immediately and after April 2004 (9) for commercial airlines with at least one flight attendant. Washington State Department of Labor and Industries provides first aid guidance to employers by listing sample and optional first aid kit contents (10). As with OSHA documents, the items listed were noted to be performance based.

PEER-REVIEWED AND AGENCY RECOMMENDATIONS FOR SUPPLIES

A peer-reviewed list of supplies is available from the American Society for Testing and Materials (ASTM) (11). ASTM committee F30.01.10 applied comments from ANSI and OSHA (12) for a proposed national standard, "First Aid Kits in Occupational Health." The proposed standard is also linked to another proposed ASTM document, "Standard Guideline Defining the Performance of First Aid Providers in the Occupational Setting." This coordination of documents is designed to ensure that the workplace first aid curriculum includes use of a minimum set of first aid supplies.

The American College of Emergency Physicians (ACEP) has suggested supplies for cruise and maritime applications (13). The ACEP list includes portable and stationary equipment as well as medications. The Occupational and Environmental Medical Practice Committee of the American College of Occupational and Environmental Medicine (ACOEM) has suggested supplies for an occupational setting without an on-site medical department (14). While not an official ACOEM position, the committee suggested that its list is a starting point for consideration.

The National Safety Council (NSC) has provided a list of supplies that are appropriate for the general workplace (15). Its list is included in the 2001 NSC basic and standard first aid textbooks. The American Red Cross has also published "Anatomy of a First Aid Kit," containing suggestions for contents (16).

SUMMARY TABLES OF RECOMMENDED FIRST AID SUPPLIES

Tables A.2 to A.9 present supplies recommended by the federal and state training agencies and national organizations described above. The lists are for basic and advanced kits and emergency devices. Quantities of items are noted when provided by the agencies. Table A.10 summarizes the recommendations for a basic first aid kit. Items agreed to by the majority of the agencies for inclusion in a basic first aid kit are indicated.

TABLE A.2. *National Safety Council first-aid supplies*

Item	Quantity
Adhesive strip bandages (1″ × 3″)	20
Triangular bandages (muslin, 30″–40″ × 36″–40″ × 52″–56″	4
Sterile eye pads (2″ × 2⅝″)	2
Sterile gauze pads (4″ × 4″)	6
Sterile nonstick pads (3″ × 4″)	6
Sterile trauma pads (5″ × 9″)	2
Sterile trauma pads (8″ × 10″)	1
Sterile conforming roller gauze (2′ wide)	3 rolls
Sterile conforming roller gauze (4.5″ wide)	3 rolls
Waterproof tape (1″ × 5 yards)	1 roll
Porous adhesive tape (2″ × 5 yards)	1 roll
Elastic roller bandages (4″ and 6″ wide)	1 each
Antiseptic skin wipes, individually wrapped	10
Medical-grade exam gloves (medium, large, extra large) conforming to Food and Drug Administration (FDA) requirements	2 pairs per size
Mouth-to-barrier device, either a face mask with a one-way valve or a disposable face shield	1
Disposable instant-activating cold packs	2
Resealable plastic bags (quart size)	2
Padded malleable splint (SAM splint, 4″ × 36″)	1
Emergency blanket, Mylar	1
Paramedic shears (with one serrated edge)	1
Splinter tweezers (about 3″ long)	1
Biohazard waste bag (3.5-gallon capacity)	2
First-aid and cardiopulmonary resuscitation (CPR) manual and list of emergency telephone numbers	1

TABLE A.3. *American Red Cross first-aid supplies*

Item	Quantity
Activated charcoal (use only if instructed by Poison Control Center)	
Syrup of ipecac (use only if instructed by Poison Control Center)	
Adhesive tape	
Antiseptic ointment	
Band-Aids (assorted sizes)	
Blanket	
Cold pack	
Disposable gloves	
Gauze pads (assorted sizes)	
Roller gauze (assorted sizes)	
Hand cleaner	
Plastic bags	
Scissors	
Tweezers	
Small flashlight and extra batteries	
Triangular bandage	

TABLE A.4. *American Society for Testing and Materials first-aid supplies*

Item	Quantity
A. Basic supplies (proposed)	
Adhesive bandage, 1″ × 3″ strip	1
Triangular bandage, 40″ × 40″ × 56″ minimum size	16
Sterile pad, 4″ × 4″	5
Sterile pad, 4″ × 8″ or 5″ × 9″	1
Sterile conforming gauze, 3″ × 6′ minimum length	1 roll
Antiseptic application, individually packaged	10 packs
Waterproof tape, 1″ × 5 yards or 1″ × 2.5 yards	1 or 2 units
Medical-grade gloves, small, medium, large, or extra-large size, meeting FDA guidelines	2 pair of each size
CPR barrier device with one-way valve	1
Utility scissors/shears to cut first-aid supplies	1
Instant cold package, 4″ × 5″	1
Blood-borne pathogens personal responder kit	1
Blood-borne pathogens clean up kit	1
Instructions to describe BLS CPR and first aid, including use of items in this kit	1
B. Enhanced (Proposed)[a]	
Portable emergency oxygen device	1
Oral glucose paste	2
Trauma dressing, 10″ × 30″	2
Burn sheet (sterile), 500" square minimum size	1
Waterproof tape, 2″ × 5 yards minimum size	1
Conforming gauze, 4″ × 6′ minimum length	2
Triangular bandage, 40″ × 40″ × 56″ minimum size	2
Sealing plastic bag, ½ gallon	1
Splint, 24″ × 3¾″	1
Rescue blanket, 4,300"-square minimum size	1
Pencil	1
Permanent marking pen	1
First-aid patient information report form	1
Instructions to describe use of items in this kit	1

[a]Also includes all supplies listed in the basic first-aid kit.

TABLE A.5. *American National Standards Institute (ANSI) Z308.1–1998 first-aid supplies*

Item	Quantity
A. Basic	
Absorbent compress, 32″ sq (81.3 sq cm), no side smaller than 4″ (10 cm)	1
Adhesive bandage, 1″ × 3″ (2.5 × 7.5 cm)	16
Adhesive tape, 5 yards (457.2 cm) total	1
Antiseptic, 0.5 g (0.14 fl oz) application	10
Burn treatment, 0.5 g (0.14 fl oz) application	6
Medical exam gloves	2 pair
Sterile pad, 3″ × 3″ (7.5 × 7.5 cm)	4
Triangular bandage, 40″ × 40″ × 56″ (101 × 101 × 142 cm)	1
B. Augmented	
Absorbent compress, 24″ sq (60 sq cm)	1
Adhesive bandage, 1″ × 3″ (2.5 × 7.5 cm)	16
Adhesive tape, 5 yards (457.2 cm) total	1 or 2
Antiseptic swab, 0.5 g (0.14 fl oz) application	10
Antiseptic wipe, 1″ × 1″ (2.5 × 2.5 cm)	10
Antiseptic towelette, 24″ sq (60 sq cm)	10
Bandage compress, 2″ × 36″ (5 × 91 cm)	4
Bandage compress, 3″ × 60″ (7.5 × 152 cm)	2
Bandage compress, 4″ × 72″ (10 × 183 cm)	1
Burn treatment, 0.5 g (0.14 fl oz) application	6
Cold pack, 4″ × 5″ (10 × 12.5 cm)	1
Eye covering, with means of attachment	1
Eye wash, 1 fl oz (30 mL) total	1
Eye wash and covering with means of attachment	1
Medical exam gloves	2 pair
Roller bandage, 4″ × 6 yards (10 × 550 cm)	1
Roller bandage, 2″ × 6 yards (5 × 550 cm)	1
Sterile pad, 3″ × 3″ (7.5 × 7.5 cm)	4
Triangular bandage, 40″ × 40″ × 56″ (101 × 101 × 142 cm)	1

TABLE A.6. *Washington Department of Labor and Industries first-aid supplies*

Item	Quantity
A. Sample kit	
Absorbent compress, 4″ × 8″	1
Adhesive bandages, 1″ × 3″	16
Adhesive tape, 5 yards	1
Antiseptic single-use packages, 0.5 g application	10
Burn treatment, single-use packages, 0.5 g application	6
Eye covering for two eyes	1
Eye wash, 1 fl oz	1
Sterile pads, 3″ × 3″	4
Medical exam gloves	2 pair
Triangular bandage, 30″ × 39″ × 55″	1
B. Optional contents	
Bandage compress, 2″ × 2″	1
Bandage compress, 3″ × 3″	1
Bandage compress, 5″ × 5″	1
Self-activating cold pack, 4″ × 5″	1
Roller bandage, 6 yards	1
Mouth-to-mouth barrier for CPR	1

TABLE A.7. *Federal Aviation Administration first-aid supplies*

Item	Quantity
A. First-aid kit	
Adhesive bandage compresses, 1″	16
Antiseptic swabs	20
Ammonia inhalants	10
Bandage compresses, 4″	8
Triangular bandage compresses, 40″	5
Arm splint, noninflatable	1
Leg splint, noninflatable	1
Roller bandage, 4″	4
Adhesive tape, 1″ standard roll	2
Bandage scissors	1
B. Emergency medical kit (until 4/12/04)	
Sphygmomanometer	1
Stethoscope	1
Airways, oropharyngeal (three sizes)	3
Syringes (sizes necessary to administer medications)	4
Self-inflating manual bag mask with three masks: pediatric, small adult, large adult	1–3 masks
Needles (sizes to administer medications)	6
Protective nonpermeable gloves	1 pair
Medications	
50% dextrose injection, 50 cc	1
Epinephrine 1:1,000, single dose ampule	2
Diphenhydramine HCl injection, single-dose ampule	2
Nitroglycerine tablets	10
Basic instructions for use of the drugs in the kit	1
C. Emergency device (after 4/12/04)	
Automated external defibrillator	1
D. Emergency medical kit (after 4/12/04)	
Sphygmomanometer	1
Stethoscope	1
Airways, oropharyngeal (three sizes): pediatric, small adult, large adult	3
Self-inflating manual bag mask with three masks: pediatric, small adult, large adult	1–3 masks
CPR mask (three sizes): pediatric, small adult, large adult	3
IV administration set: Tubing w/2 Y connectors	1
Alcohol sponges	2
Adhesive tape, 1″ standard roll	1
Tape scissors	1 pair
Tourniquet	1
Saline solution, 500 cc	1
Protective nonpermeable gloves	1 pair
Needles (2-18, 2-20, 2-22 gauges, or sizes to administer medications	6
Syringes (1–5 cc, 2–10 cc, or sizes necessary to administer medications)	4
Medications (OTC and Rx)	
Analgesic, nonnarcotic tablets, 325 mg	4
Antihistamine tablets, 25 mg	4
Antihistamine injectable, 50 mg (single-dose ampule)	2
Atropine, 0.5 g, 5 cc (single-dose ampule)	2
Aspirin tablets, 325 mg	4
Bronchodilator, inhaled (metered-dose inhaler)	1
Dextrose, 50%/50 cc injectable (single-dose ampule)	1
Epinephrine 1:1,000, 1 cc injectable (single-dose ampule)	2
Epinephrine 1:10,000, 2 cc injectable (single-dose ampule)	2
Lidocaine, 5 cc, 20 mg/mL, injectable (single-dose ampule)	2
Nitroglycerine tablets, 0.4 mg	10
Basic instructions for use of the drugs in the kit	1

TABLE A.8. *American College of Emergency Physicians health care guidelines for cruise ship medical facilities*

Item	Quantity
A. Portable medical equipment and supplies	
Medical waste and personal protective equipment	
Airway equipment, oxygen, and supplies	
IV fluids and supplies	
Immobilization equipment and supplies	
Diagnostic and laboratory supplies	
Dressings	
Treatment medications and supplies	
Defibrillator and supplies	
Documentation and planning materials	
B. Emergency medical equipment	
Airway equipment—bag mask, endotracheal tubes, stylet, lubricant vasoconstrictor, portable suction equipment	
Cardiac monitor and backup monitor	2
Defibrillators, portable, one of which may be semiautomatic	2
External cardiac pacing capability	
Electrocardiograph	
Infusion pump	
Pulse oximeter	
Nebulizer	
Automatic or manual respiratory support equipment	
Oxygen, including portable oxygen	
Wheelchair	
Stair chair and stretcher	
Refrigerator/freezer	
Long and short back boards, cervical spine immobilization capability	
Trauma cart supplies	
C. Medications	
Thrombolytics and sufficient quantities of advanced life support (ALS) medications in accordance with international ALS guidelines for the management of two complex cardiac arrests	
Gastrointestinal system medications	
Cardiovascular system medications	
Respiratory system medications	
Center nervous system medications	
Infectious disease medications	
Endocrine system medications	
Obstetrics, gynecology, and urinary tract disorder medications	
Musculoskeletal and joint disease medications	
Eye medications	
Ear, nose, and oropharynx medications	
Skin disease medications	
Immunologic products and vaccines	
Anesthesia medications	

TABLE A.9. *American College of Occupational and Environmental Medicine (ACOEM) (unofficial) Occupational and Environmental Medical Practice Committee recommendations for first-aid supplies without an on-site medical department*

Item	Quantity
Sterile gauze pads—assorted sizes	
Adhesive tape	
Sterile adhesive bandages	
Elastic bandages—assorted sizes	
Disposable medical-grade gloves	
Cotton-tip applicators	
Antibacterial ointment	
Antiseptic wipes	
Cold packs	
Tweezers	
Scissors	
Soap	
Pen and paper	
Flashlight	
First-aid instructions	
Biohazard infectious waste bag	

TABLE A.10. *Summary of supplies recommended for a basic first-aid kit*[a]

	NSC	ARC	ASTM	ANSI	WDLI	FAA	ACOEM
Adhesive strip bandages	√	√	√	√	√	√	√
Triangular bandages	√	√	√	√	√	√	
Sterile eye pads	√				√		
Sterile gauze pads	√	√	√	√	√		√
Sterile nonstick pads	√	√	√				√
Sterile trauma pads (compress)	√			√	√	√	
Sterile conforming roller gauze	√	√	√				√
Adhesive tape, waterproof	√		√				
Adhesive tape, unspecified (porous)	√	√		√	√	√	√
Elastic roller bandages	√					√	
Antiseptic skin wipes, individually wrapped	√	√	√		√	√	√
Medical-grade examination gloves	√	√	√	√	√		√
Mouth-to-barrier device	√		√				
Disposable instant-activating cold packs	√	√	√				√
Resealable plastic bags	√	√					
Padded malleable splints	√					√	
Emergency blanket	√	√					
Paramedic shears/scissors	√	√	√			√	√
Splinter tweezers	√	√					√
Biohazard waste bag	√						√
First aid/CPR manual/instructions	√		√				√
List of emergency telephone numbers							
Activated charcoals		√					
Syrup of ipecac		√					
Antiseptic ointment		√		√			√
Small flashlight with extra batteries		√					√
Blood-borne pathogens personal kit			√				
Blood-borne pathogens cleanup kit			√				
Burn treatment, individually wrapped				√	√		
Eye wash fluid					√		
Ammonia inhalants						√	
Cotton-tip applicators							√
Soap							√
Pen and paper							√

[a]Items in boldface denote recommendations by at least four groups.

NSC, National Safety Council (Table A.2); ARC, American Red Cross (Table A.3); ASTM, American Society for Testing and Materials (Table A.4, part A); ANSI, American National Standards Institute (Table A.5, part A); WDLI, Washington Department of Labor and Industries (Table A.6, part A); FAA, Federal Aviation Administration (Table A.7, part A); ACOEM, American College of Occupational and Environmental Medicine, unofficial (Table A.9).

REFERENCES

1. Alton T. *National Safety Council First Aid and CPR,* 4th ed. Boston: Jones and Bartlett, 2001.
2. Medical and first aid. U.S. Department of Labor Technical Links. *http://www.osha-slc.gov:80SLTCmedical-firstaidindex.html.*
3. Guidelines for basic first aid training programs. Directorate of Technical Support, OSHA Instruction CPL 2-2.53, Appendix A, 1991.
4. Personal communication from Kenneth W. Gerecke, Assistant Regional Administrator, Eastern Region, Occupational Safety and Health Administration, Philadelphia, November 10, 1998.
5. Personal communication from Linda R. Anku, Regional Administrator, Eastern Region, Occupational Safety and Health Administration, Philadelphia, April 6, 1992.
6. Department of Transportation. National Highway Traffic Administration first responder curriculum, 1995. *http://www.nhtsa.dot.gov/people/injury/ems/nsc.htm.*
7. OSHA 29 CFR Parts 1910 and 1926 standards improvement (miscellaneous changes) for general industry and construction standards. *Fed Reg* 1998(June 18);63: 33450–33469.
8. Minimum requirements for workplace first aid kits. ANSI Z308.1-1998. Arlington, VA: Industrial Safety Equipment Association, 1998.
9. Department of Transportation, Federal Aviation Administration. Emergency medical equipment; final rule. *Fed Reg* 2001;66(71):19028–19046.
10. Washington Department of Labor and Industries. Chapter 296-24 WAC, First Aid Kit Guidance, *http://www.lni.wa.gov/wisha/regs/wacindex.htm.*
11. Starr LM. A new first aid training curriculum. *Occup Health Safety* 1998;66(4):24–28, 38.
12. Personal communication from Steve F. Witt, Director, Directorate of Technical Support, U.S. Department of Labor/OSHA, Washington, DC, February 7, 1997.
13. American College of Emergency Physicians. Health care guidelines for cruise ship medical facilities (revised). October 2000. *http://www.acep.org/2,593, 0.html.*
14. Lerner P. Occupational medicine forum: what first aid supplies should be kept in an occupational setting without an on-site medical department? *J Occup Environ Med* 1997;39(9):825–826.
15. Thygerson A. *First aid and CPR basic.* Sudbury, MA: Jones and Bartlett, 2001.
16. American Red Cross. Anatomy of a first aid kit, 2001. *http://www.redcross.org/services/lifeline/fakit.html.*

Appendix B
Government and Regulatory Agencies

Nancy English

OCCUPATIONAL SAFETY AND HEALTH ADMINISTRATION

The Occupational Safety and Health Administration (OSHA), part of the Department of Labor, is charged with enforcing workplace health and safety standards. This federal agency also has responsibility for establishing safe exposure limits and other protective measures required of various workplaces. Although OSHA plays a fundamental role in the enforcement of workplace health standards, the agency can also be instrumental in providing consultative support to business and industry. For more information contact:

Occupational Safety and Health Administration (OSHA)
Headquarters Office
U.S. Department of Labor
3rd and Constitution Avenue, NW
Washington, DC 20210

There are ten regional OSHA offices where information, advice, and lists of currently available publications can be obtained. These offices can answer questions and can direct inquiries to appropriate local offices or specialized OSHA services. States may administer their own plans if these plans are at least as effective as federal requirements and are approved by OSHA. Currently, 25 states have state plans. Check with your regional office for more information.

Region I (CT, ME, MA, NH, RI, VT)

133 Portland Street, 1st floor
Boston, MA 02114
617-565-7164

Connecticut

Federal Office Bldg.
450 Main Street
Hartford, CT 06103
203-240-3152

Maine

U.S. Federal Bldg.
40 Western Avenue, Room 121
Augusta, ME 04330
207-622-8417

Massachusetts

1145 Main Street, Room 108
Springfield, MA 01103
413-785-0123
639 Granite Street, 4th floor
Braintree, MA 02184
617-565-6924

New Hampshire

Federal Bldg., Room 334
55 Pleasant Street
Concord, NH 03301
603-225-1629

Rhode Island

380 Westminster Mall
Room 243
Providence, RI 02903
401-528-4669

Region II (NJ, NY, PR, VI)

201 Varick Street, Room 670
New York, NY 10014
212-337-2378

New Jersey

Plaza 35, Suite 205
1030 Saint Georges Avenue
Avenel, NJ 07001
201-750-3270
2 East Blackwell Street
Dover, NJ 07801
201-361-4050
500 Route 17 South, 2nd floor
Hasbrouck Heights, NJ 07604
201-288-1700
Marlton Executive Park
701 Rte. 73, South Bldg. 2
Marlton, NJ 08053
609-957-5181

New York

Leo W. O'Brien Federal Bldg.
Clinton Ave. and N. Pearl St.
Rm. 132
Albany, NY 12207
518-472-6085
42-40 Bell Blvd., 5th Floor
Bayside, NY 11361
718-279-9060
5360 Genesee St.
Bowmansville, NY 14026
716-684-3891
90 Church St., Rm. 1407
New York, NY 10007
212-264-9840
100 S. Clinton St., Rm. 1267
Syracuse, NY 13260
315-423-5188
990 Westbury Rd.
Westbury, NY 11590
516-334-3344

Puerto Rico

U.S. Courthouse and FOB
Carlos Chardon St., Rm. 559
Hato Rey, PR 00918
809-766-5457

Region III (DC, DE, MD, PA, VA, WV)

Gateway Bldg., Suite 1200
3535 Market St.
Philadelphia, PA 19104
215-596-1201

Maryland

Federal Bldg., Rm. 1110
Charles Ctr., 31 Hopkins Plaza
Baltimore, MD 21201
301-962-2840

Pennsylvania

850 N. 5th St.
Allentown, PA 18102
215-776-4220
Rothrock Bldg., Rm. 408
121 West 10th St.
Erie, PA 16501
814-453-4351
Progress Plaza
49 N. Progress St.
Harrisburg, PA 17109
717-782-3902
U.S. Custom House, Rm. 242
Second and Chestnut St.
Philadelphia, PA 19106
215-597-4955
1000 Liberty Ave., Rm. 2236
Pittsburgh, PA 15222
412-644-2903
Penn Pl., Rm. 2005
20 N. Pennsylvania Ave.
Wilkes-Barre, PA 18701
717-826-6538

West Virginia

550 Eagan St., Rm. 206
Charleston, WV 25301
304-347-5937

Region IV (AL, FL, GA, KY, MS, NC, SC, TN)

Peachtree St., NE, Suite 587
Atlanta, GA 30367
404-347-3573

Alabama

2047 Canyon Rd., Todd Mall
Birmingham, AL 35216
205-731-1534

Florida

299 East Broward Blvd., Rm. 302
Fort Lauderdale, FL 33301
305-527-7292
3100 University Blvd. South
Jacksonville, FL 32216
904-791-2895
700 Twiggs St., Rm. 624
Tampa, FL 33602
813-228-2821

Georgia

Bldg. 7, Suite 110
La Vista Perimeter Office Park
Tucker, GA 30084
404-331-4767/0353

Kentucky

John C. Watts Federal Bldg., Rm. 108
330 W. Broadway
Frankfort, KY 40601
502-227-7024

Mississippi

Federal Bldg., Suite 1445
110 West Capitol St.
Jackson, MS 39269
601-965-4606

North Carolina

Century Station, Rm. 104
300 Fayetteville Street Mall
Raleigh, NC 27601
919-856-4770

South Carolina

1835 Assembly St., Rm. 1468
Columbia, SC 29201
803-765-5904

Tennessee

2002 Richard Jones Rd., Suite C-205
Nashville, TN 37215-2809
615-736-5313

Region V (IL, IN, MI, MN, OH, WI)

230 S. Dearborn St., Rm. 3244
Chicago, IL 60604
312-353-2220

Illinois

1600 167th St., Suite 12
Calumet City, IL 60409
312-891-3800
2360 E. Devon Ave., Suite 1010
Des Plaines, IL 60018
312-803-4800
344 Smoke Tree Business Park
North Aurora, IL 60542
312-869-8700
2001 W. Willow Knolls Rd. Suite 101
Peoria, IL 61614-1223
309-671-7033

Indiana

46 East Ohio St., Rm. 423
Indianapolis, IN 46204
317-269-7290

Michigan

300 E. Michigan Ave., Rm. 305
Lansing, MI 48993
517-377-1892

Minnesota

110 South 4th St., Rm. 425
Minneapolis, MN 55401
612-348-1994

Ohio

Federal Office Bldg., Rm. 4028
550 Main St.
Cincinnati, OH 45202
513-684-3784
Federal Office Bldg., Rm. 899
1240 East Ninth St.

Cleveland, OH 44199
216-522-3818
Federal Office Bldg., Rm. 620
200 N. High St.
Columbus, OH 43215
614-469-5582
Federal Office Bldg., Rm. 734
234 N. Summit St.
Toledo, OH 43604
419-259-7542

Wisconsin

2618 North Ballard Rd.
Appleton, WI 54915
414-734-4521
2934 Fish Hatchery Rd.
Suite 225
Madison, WI 53713
608-264-5388
Suite 1180
310 W. Wisconsin Ave.
Milwaukee, WI 53203
414-291-3315

Region VI (AR, LA, NM, OK, TX)

525 Griffin St., Rm. 602
Dallas, TX
214-767-4731

Arkansas

Savers Bldg., Suite 828
320 West Capitol Ave.
Little Rock, AR 72201
501-378-6291

Louisiana

2156 Wooddale Blvd.
Hoover Annex, Suite 200
Baton Rouge, LA 70806
504-389-0474

New Mexico

320 Central Ave., SW
Suite 13
Albuquerque, NM 87102
505-776-3411

Oklahoma

420 West Main Pl., Suite 725
Oklahoma City, OK 73102
405-231-5351

Texas

611 E. 6th Street, Rm. 303
Austin, TX 78701
512-482-5783
Government Plaza, Rm. 300
400 Mann St.
Corpus Christi, TX 78401
512-888-3257
North Star 2 Bldg., Suite 430
8713 Airport Freeway
Fort Worth, TX 76180-7604
817-885-7025
2320 La Branch St., Rm. 1103
Houston, TX 77004
713-750-1727
1425 W. Pioneer Dr.
Irving, TX 75061
214-767-5347
Federal Bldg., Rm. 421
1205 Texas Ave.
Lubbock, TX 79401
806-743-7681

Region VII (IA, KS, MO, NE)

911 Walnut St.
Kansas City, MO 64106
816-426-5861

Kansas

216 N. Waco, Suite B
Wichita, KS 67202
316-269-6644

Missouri

911 Walnut St., Rm. 2202
Kansas City, MO 64106
816-426-2756
4300 Goodfellow Blvd., Bldg. 105E
St. Louis, MO 63120
314-263-2749

Nebraska

Overland-Wolf Bldg., Rm. 100
6910 Pacific St.
Omaha, NE 68106
402-221-3182

Region VIII (CO, MT, ND, SD, UT, WY)

Federal Bldg., Rm. 1576
1961 Stout St.
Denver, CO 80294
303-844-3061

Colorado

1244 Speer Blvd.
Colonnade Ctr., Suite 360
Denver, CO 80204
303-844-5285

Montana

19 N. 25th St.
Billings, MT 59101
406-657-6649

North Dakota

Federal Bldg., Rm. 348
PO Box 2439
Bismarck, ND 58501
701-250-4521

Utah

1781 South 300 West
Salt Lake City, UT 84115
801-524-5080

Region IX (AZ, CA, HI, NV, American Samoa, Guam, Trust Territories of the Pacific)

71 Stevenson St., Rm. 415
San Francisco, CA 94105
415-744-6670

Arizona

3221 N. 16th St., Suite 100
Phoenix, AZ
602-640-2007

California

71 Stevenson St., Suite 415
San Francisco, CA 94105
415-744-6670

Hawaii

300 Ala Moana Blvd., Suite 5122
Honolulu, HI 96850
808-541-2685

Nevada

1413 N. Carson Blvd., 1st Floor
Carson City, NV 98701
702-885-6963

Region X (AK, ID, OR, WA)

1111 Third Ave., Suite 715
Seattle, WA 98174
206-442-5930

Alaska

Federal Bldg., USCH Rm. 211
222 West 7th Ave., #29
Anchorage, AK 99513-7571
907-271-5152

Idaho

Suite 134
3050 N. Lake Harbor Lane
Boise, ID 83903
208-334-1867

Oregon

1220 SW Third Ave., Rm. 640
Portland, OR 97204
503-326-2251

Washington

121 70th Ave., NE
Bellevue, WA 98004
206-442-7520

NATIONAL INSTITUTE FOR OCCUPATIONAL SAFETY AND HEALTH

The National Institute for Occupational Safety and Health (NIOSH) was established by the Occupational Safety and Health Act of 1970, which made NIOSH responsible for conducting research to make the nation's workplaces healthier and safer. NIOSH was part of the U.S. Public Health Service until 1973, when it became part of the Centers for Disease Control.

NIOSH may require employers to measure and report employee exposure to potentially hazardous materials and to provide medical examinations and tests to determine the incidence of occupational illness among employees. NIOSH is required by law to respond to urgent requests for assistance from employers, employees, and their representatives where imminent hazards are suspected. To identify hazards, NIOSH is authorized to conduct workplace inspections.

NIOSH conducts laboratory and epidemiologic research, publishes its findings, and makes recommendations for improved working conditions to regulatory agencies such as OSHA and the Mine Safety and Health Administration. NIOSH has completed and published many surveys and studies on hazards in the workplace, as well as recommendations for limits on certain workplace exposures. For more information or to obtain a list of publications contact:

Department of Health and Human Services
Public Health Service
Centers for Disease Control
National Institute for Occupational Safety and Health
Robert A. Taft Laboratories
4676 Columbia Pkwy.
Cincinnati, OH 45226

NIOSH technical information resources can be accessed at 1-800-35-NIOSH. NIOSH offers many services that may be requested by both employers and employees (reference CDD/NIOSH), and maintains extensive databases of occupational safety and health information from around the world. Databases: 513-533-8326. NIOSH supports educational resource centers at 14 U.S. universities to help ensure an adequate supply of trained occupational safety and health professionals. Educational Resource Centers: 513-533-8241.

NIOSH sponsors extramural research in priority areas and coordinates this with its intramural and contract research and that of other health and human services and U.S. departments. Extramural Grants: 404-639-3343.

NIOSH identifies risk factors for work-related fatalities and injuries through its Fatal Accident Circumstances and Epidemiology project. Fatal Accident Investigations: 304-291-4575.

Employers, employees, or their representatives who suspect a health problem in the workplace can request a NIOSH Health Hazard Evaluation (HHE) to assess the problem. Health Hazard Evaluation: 800-3.5-NIOSH.

NIOSH administers periodic chest x-rays to coal miners to facilitate early detection of coal worker's pneumoconiosis. Miners' x-rays: 304-291-4301.

NIOSH publishes and distributes a variety of publications related to occupational safety and health. Publications: 513-533-8287.

NIOSH tests and certifies respirators to ensure their compliance with federal requirements. Respirators: 304-291-4331.

NIOSH has offices in four locations:

NIOSH Headquarters
Bldg. 1, Rm. 3007
Centers for Disease Control
1600 Clifton Rd.
Atlanta, GA 30333
404-639-3061

NIOSH Washington Office
200 Independence Ave., SW
Washington, DC 20201
202-472-7134

Appalachian Laboratories
944 Chestnut Ridge Rd.
Morgantown, WV 26505-2888
Division of Respiratory Disease Studies: 304-291-4474
Division of Safety Research: 304-284-5100

Cincinnati Laboratories
4676 Columbia Pkwy.
Cincinnati, OH 45226-1998
Division of Biomedical and Behavioral Science: 513-533-8465
Division of Standards Development and Technology Transfer: 513-533-8302
Division of Training and Manpower Development: 513-533-8221
Division of Physical Sciences and Engineering: 513-841-4321
Division of Surveillance, Hazard Evaluation and Field Studies: 513-841-4428

ENVIRONMENTAL PROTECTION AGENCY

The U.S. Environmental Protection Agency (EPA), created in 1970, administers nine comprehensive environmental protection laws: the Clean Air Act (CAA); the Clean Water Act (CWA); the Safe Drinking Water Act (SDWA); the Comprehensive Environmental Response, Compensation, and Liability Act (CERCLA or Superfund) amended by the Superfund Amendments and Reauthorization Act (SARA); the Resource Conservation and Recovery Act (RCRA); the Federal Insecticide, Fungicide, and Rodenticide Act (FIFRA); the Toxic Substances Control Act (TSCA); the Marine Protection Research and Sanctuaries Act (MPRSA); and the Uranium Mill Tailings Radiation Control Act (UMTRCA). The EPA is responsible for implementing these federal laws and for conducting research relevant to environmental concerns.

The EPA has ten regional offices from which information and publications can be obtained.

Region 1 (CT, ME, MA, NH, RI, VT)

JFK Federal Bldg.
Boston, MA 02203
617-565-3420

Connecticut

Federal Office Bldg.
450 Main St.
Hartford, CT 06103
203-240-3152

Maine

U.S. Federal Bldg.
40 Western Ave., Rm. 121
Augusta, ME 04330
207-622-8417

Massachusetts

JFK Federal Bldg.
Boston, MA 02203
617-565-3420

New Hampshire

Federal Bldg., Rm. 334
55 Pleasant St.
Concord, NH 03301
603-225-1629

Rhode Island

380 Westminster Mall
Rm. 243
Providence, RI 02903
401-528-4669

Region 2 (NJ, NY, PR, VI)

Jacob K. Javits Federal Bldg. 26
Federal Plaza
New York, NY 10278
212-264-2515

New Jersey

Plaza 35, Suite 205
1030 Saint Georges Ave.
Avenel, NJ 07001
201-750-3270
2 E. Blackwell St.
Dover, NJ 07801
201-361-4050
500 Rte. 17 South, 2nd Floor
Hasbrouck Heights, NJ 07604
201-288-1700
Marlton Executive Park
701 Rte. 73, South Bldg. 2
Marlton, NJ 08053
609-757-5181

New York

Leo W. O'Brien Federal Bldg.
Clinton Ave. and N. Pearl St.
Rm. 132
Albany, NY 12207
518-472-6085
42-40 Bell Blvd., 5th Floor
Bayside, NY 11361
718-279-9060
5360 Genesee St.
Bowmansville, NY 14026
716-684-3891
90 Church St., Rm. 1407
New York, NY 10007
212-264-9840
100 S. Clinton St., Rm. 1267
Syracuse, NY 13260
315-423-5188
990 Westbury Rd.
Westbury, NY 11590
516-334-3344

Puerto Rico

U.S. Courthouse and FOB
Carlos Chardon St., Rm. 559
Hato Rey, PR 00918
809-766-5457

Region 3 (DC, DE, MD, PA, VA, WV)

841 Chestnut St.
Philadelphia, PA 19107
215-597-9370

Maryland

Federal Bldg., Rm. 1110
Charles Ctr., 31 Hopkins Plaza
Baltimore, MD 21201
301-962-2840

Pennsylvania

850 N. 5th St.
Allentown, PA 18102
215-776-4220
Rothrock Bldg., Rm. 408
121 West 10th St.
Erie, PA 16501
814-453-4351
Progress Plaza
49 N. Progress St.
Harrisburg, PA 17109
717-782-3902
U.S. Custom House, Rm. 242
Second and Chestnut St.
Philadelphia, PA 19106
215-597-4955
1000 Liberty Ave., Rm. 2236
Pittsburgh, PA 15222
412-644-2903
Penn Pl., Rm. 2005
20 N. Pennsylvania Ave.
Wilkes-Barre, PA 18701
717-826-6538

West Virginia

550 Eagan St., Rm. 206
Charleston, WV 25301
304-347-5937

Region 4 (AL, FL, GA, KY, MS, NC, SC, TN)

345 Courtland St., NE
Atlanta, GA 30365
404-347-3004

Alabama

2047 Canyon Rd., Todd Mall
Birmingham, AL 35216
205-731-1534

Florida

299 East Broward Blvd., Rm. 302
Fort Lauderdale, FL 33301
305-527-7292
3100 University Blvd. South
Jacksonville, FL 32216
904-791-2895
700 Twiggs St., Rm. 624
Tampa, FL 33602
813-228-2821

Georgia

Bldg. 7, Suite 110
La Vista Perimeter Office Park
Tucker, GA 30084
404-331-4767/0353

Kentucky

John C. Watts Federal Bldg., Rm. 108
330 W. Broadway
Frankfort, KY 40601
502-227-7024

Mississippi

Federal Bldg., Suite 1445
110 West Capitol St.
Jackson, MS 39269
601-965-4606

North Carolina

Century Station, Rm. 104
300 Fayetteville Street Mall
Raleigh, NC 27601
919-856-4770

South Carolina

1835 Assembly St., Rm. 1468
Columbia, SC 29201
803-765-5904

Tennessee

2002 Richard Jones Rd., Suite C-205
Nashville, TN 37215-2809
615-736-5313

Region 5 (IL, IN, MI, MN, OH, WI)

230 S. Dearborn St.
Chicago, IL 60604
312-353-2072

Illinois

1600 167th St., Suite 12
Calumet City, IL 60409
312-891-3800
2360 E. Devon Ave., Suite 1010
Des Plaines, IL 60018
312-803-4800
344 Smoke Tree Business Park
North Aurora, IL 60542
312-869-8700
2001 W. Willow Knolls Rd.
Suite 101
Peoria, IL 61614-1223
309-671-7033

Indiana

46 E. Ohio St., Rm. 423
Indianapolis, IN 46204
317-269-7290

Michigan

300 E. Michigan Ave., Rm. 305
Lansing, MI 48993
517-377-1892

Minnesota

110 South 4th St., Rm. 425
Minneapolis, MN 55401
612-348-1994

Ohio

Federal Office Bldg., Rm. 4028
550 Main St.
Cincinnati, OH 45202
513-684-3784
Federal Office Bldg., Rm. 899
1240 East Ninth St.
Cleveland, OH 44199
216-522-3818
Federal Office Bldg., Rm. 620
200 N. High St.
Columbus, OH 43215
614-469-5582
Federal Office Bldg., Rm. 734
234 N. Summit St.
Toledo, OH 43604
419-259-7542

Wisconsin

2618 North Ballard Rd.
Appleton, WI 54915
414-734-4521
2934 Fish Hatchery Rd.
Suite 225
Madison, WI 53713
608-264-5388
Suite 1180
310 W. Wisconsin Ave.
Milwaukee, WI 53203
414-291-3315

Region 6 (AR, LA, NM, OK, TX)

1445 Ross Ave.
Suite 1200
Dallas, TX 75202
214-655-2200

Arkansas

Savers Bldg., Suite 828
320 West Capitol Ave.
Little Rock, AR 72201
501-378-6291

Louisiana

2156 Wooddale Blvd.
Hoover Annex, Suite 200
Baton Rouge, LA 70806
504-389-0474

New Mexico

320 Central Ave., SW
Suite 13
Albuquerque, NM 87102
505-776-3411

Oklahoma

420 West Main Pl., Suite 725
Oklahoma City, OK 73102
405-231-5351

Texas

611 E. 6th Street, Rm. 303
Austin, TX 78701
512-482-5783
Government Plaza, Rm. 300
400 Mann St.
Corpus Christi, TX 78401
512-888-3257
North Star 2 Bldg., Suite 430
8713 Airport Freeway
Fort Worth, TX 76180-7604
817-885-7025
2320 La Branch St., Rm. 1103
Houston, TX 77004
713-750-1727
1425 W. Pioneer Dr.
Irving, TX 75061
214-767-5347
Federal Bldg., Rm. 421
1205 Texas Ave.
Lubbock, TX 79401
806-743-7681

Region 7 (IA, KS, MO, NE)

726 Minnesota Ave.
Kansas City, KS 66101
913-551-7003

Kansas

216 N. Waco, Suite B
Wichita, KS 67202
316-269-6644

Missouri

911 Walnut St., Rm. 2202
Kansas City, MO 64106
816-426-2756
4300 Goodfellow Blvd., Bldg. 105E
St. Louis, MO 63120
314-263-2749

Nebraska

Overland-Wolf Bldg., Rm. 100
6910 Pacific St.
Omaha, NE 68106
402-221-3182

Region 8 (CO, MT, ND, SD, UT, WY)

999 18th St., Suite 500
Denver, CO 80202
303-293-1692

Colorado

1244 Speer Blvd.
Colonnade Ctr., Suite 360
Denver, CO 80204
303-844-5285

Montana

19 N. 25th St.
Billings, MT 59101
406-657-6649

North Dakota

Federal Bldg., Rm. 348
PO Box 2439
Bismarck, ND 58501
701-250-4521

Utah

1781 South 300 West
Salt Lake City, UT 84115
801-524-5080

Region 9 (AZ, CA, HI, NV, American Samoa, Guam, Northern Mariana Islands)

1235 Mission St.
San Francisco, CA 94103
415-556-5145

Arizona

3221 N. 16th St., Suite 100
Phoenix, AZ
602-640-2007

California

71 Stevenson St., Suite 415
San Francisco, CA 94105
415-744-6670

Hawaii

300 Ala Moana Blvd., Suite 5122
Honolulu, HI 96850
808-541-2685

Nevada

1413 N. Carson Blvd., 1st Floor
Carson City, NV 98701
702-885-6963

Region 10 (AK, ID, OR, WA)

1200 Sixth Ave.
Seattle, WA 98101
206-442-1465

Alaska

Federal Bldg., USCH Rm. 211
222 West 7th Ave., #29
Anchorage, AK 99513-7571
907-271-5152

Idaho

Suite 134
3050 N. Lake Harbor Lane
Boise, ID 83903
208-334-1867

Oregon

1220 SW Third Ave., Rm. 640
Portland, OR 97204
503-326-2251

Washington

121 70th Ave., NE
Bellevue, WA 98004
206-442-7520

Appendix C

A History of the American College of Occupational and Environmental Medicine and the Growth of a Specialty

Jean Spencer Felton

> Not only in antiquity but in our own times also laws have been passed in well-ordered cities to secure good conditions for the workers; so it is only right that the art of medicine should contribute its portion for the benefit and relief of those for whom the law has shown such foresight; indeed we ought to show peculiar zeal, though so far we have neglected to do so, in taking precautions for their safety, so that as far as possible they may work at their chosen calling without loss of health.
>
> —Bernardino Ramazzini (1713)

Although physicians in the United States were knowledgeable about the existence of work-related illness and injury in the late 19th century, it was only at the century's turn that comprehensive texts began to appear in this country, with the emphasis on the trauma sustained by the worker (1–5). While there were practitioners in the field of the then-termed "industrial medicine," there was no formal organization for such physicians. Departments had been established at certain universities in the early years, and a few clinics for the study of occupational diseases were established, but were short lived (6). There was no activity in the United States at that time that matched the publications, dedicated hospitals, or morbidity studies emanating from European sources. A summation of the current status was well stated at an international conference in Brussels by a member of the Belgian Labor Department, who said, "It is well known that there is no industrial hygiene in the United States (*à* n'existe pas)" (7).

THE BIRTH OF A SOCIETY

With the initial passage of liability laws and the subsequent enactment of workers' compensation legislation, there was an awakening in several industries of the need for better standards in the burgeoning field of medical care for injured employees. With the creation of the National Safety Council in 1912, the health and safety movement began to grow and programs headed by physicians were found in such corporate entities as the Norton Grinding Company of Worcester, Massachusetts; the Cincinnati Milling Machine Company; People's Gas Company of Chicago; General Motors Corporation, Ford Motor Company; E. I. du Pont de Nemours and Company of Wilmington, Delaware; and Sears, Roebuck and Company of Chicago.

In an early conversation between Drs. Harry E. Mock of Sears and Andrew M. Harvey of the Crane Company, the thought of an association of physicians serving industry emerged. Eventually, in Detroit on June 12, 1916, the American Association of Industrial Physicians and Surgeons (AAIPS) was organized with over 100 members (6). The stated objective of the association was to "foster the study and discussion of the problems peculiar to the practice of industrial medicine and surgery; to develop methods adapted to the conservation of health among workmen in the industries; to promote a more general understanding of the purposes and results of the medical care of employees; and to unite into one organization members of the medical profession specializing in industrial medicine and surgery for their mutual advancement in the practice of their profession" (6). While the scope of the field has enlarged into research, education, and the involvement of bodies of workers outside of industry, the founding tenets still have validity.

Apart from the changes undergone by the specialty over the ensuing decades, interesting socioeconomic observations may be made about the founding of AAIPS. The dues were set at $2 per annum and the initial banquet held at the Cadillac Hotel carried a charge of $2 with no provision for the inclusion of cigars (6).

The mix of the officers elected at the initial gathering foretells, in a sense, the various affiliations of the membership to follow over the years. The president was Dr. Joseph W. Schereschewsky of the relatively new Office of Industrial Hygiene of the Public Health Service, seen today as the National Institute for Occupational Safety and Health (NIOSH). In the position of vice president was Dr. Robert T. Legge from the University of California, Berkeley. Dr. Francis D. Patterson served as second vice president; he was a member of the Pennsylvania Department of Labor. Dr. Harry E. Mock was elected secretary-treasurer and, as indicated earlier, was from industry (6).

Members of AAIPS became active during World War I, becoming involved with both the introduction of placement physical examinations and the identification, and possibly the control, of occupational health hazards. In 1917, Dr. Alice Hamilton published a list of 2,432 cases of work-related poisonings, of which 1,389 were caused by nitrous fumes, as were 28 of 58 deaths. Second in number were 660 relating to trinitrotoluene (TNT), of which 13 were deaths (7).

THE BOOST BY WAR

Little in the way of growth was seen in occupational medicine following World War I. Some research was conducted in academe, and the beginnings of epidemiologic studies were seen in some of the states' official agencies.

The period between the wars had seen the elimination of phosphorus as a hazard in the match industry (8) and the substitution of other carroting agents for mercury in the making of felt hats (9). Also, the causation of osteogenic sarcoma among radium dial painters was identified (10).

That there was growing recognition of the value of a medical service in industry was seen in the creation of the Knudsen Award in 1938, named after the General Motors president, that was to be given annually to "the industrial physician making the most outstanding contribution to industrial medicine" (6). The presentation of the award at the annual meeting of AAIPS and its successors has highlighted the honors ceremonies conducted during the American Occupational Health Conference.

In the early 1930s, an episode of great proportion was seen in the boring of the Hawk's Nest Tunnel through a vein of silica near the town of Gauley Bridge, West Virginia. The tunnel was cut in order to bring water from a river to a hydroelectric power plant. The engineering activity was undertaken during the early years of the depression, and workers came from all over the U.S. for the employment opportunity. About 5,000 men worked on the project, and 50% to 60% saw some service underground. There were three times as many blacks as whites in the labor force. Within 5 years following completion of the tunnel, over 700 deaths resulted from acute or chronic silicosis or other pneumoconioses (11). The toll of lives led to a congressional investigation in 1936 and the recognition of silicosis—despite doubt among industrial health professionals—as a definite occupational disease entity. Several conferences followed, and research efforts were begun. In the words of the epidemiologist who put the data together, "Not all was in vain, however. By the end of 1937, forty-six states had enacted laws covering workers afflicted with silicosis. Where the federal government had failed, the states, through the workers' compensation system, had recognized silicosis as the prototypical occupational disease" (11).

That industrial medicine had finally reached a point of recognition was seen in the creation of the Council on Industrial Health by the American Medical Association (AMA) in late 1937. The council continued to act until 1960, when its functions were absorbed by other segments of the AMA. The designation of the council, a standing committee of the AMA, was based on the objective of studying further work-related disease so that uniform workers' compensation laws might result (6). For many years, members of AAIPS served on the council.

It was the technology of World War II and the demand for workers, however, that led to medical staffing of the large war production plants. Physicians in uniform were assigned posts in armed services facilities, for the installations had taken on all of the characteristics of heavily staffed industries, and programs in occupational medicine were needed. In late 1942, it was determined that the Army alone owned and operated more than 160 plants, with an employee population of approximately 400,000 (12).

The first general directive concerning the Army industrial medical program was promulgated in early

1943, calling for the establishment of such programs in all Army-owned and operated plants, arsenals, depots, and ports of embarkation (13). Many of the young medical officers serving at military facilities remained in occupational medicine after the war and were added to the membership of AAIPS.

Almost in parallel with this augmentation of worker care was the development of the Manhattan Project and its various subprojects, all of which had as their objective the production of an atomic bomb that, it was hoped, would end World War II. As the effects of exposure to ionizing radiation were not known fully and since many of the workers had little idea of the materials with which they were in contact, there was "a need for physicians who were competent not only to distinguish the illnesses due to special hazards but who were also capable of seeing that all types of cases were treated properly" (14). During the developmental phase and until war's end, the physicians assigned industrial medical responsibilities were oncologists or radiologists, but in early 1946 they were replaced by practitioners experienced in the organization of plant programs.

CERTIFICATION AND EDUCATION

During these early years, many elder statesmen of AAIPS tried to obtain board certification for its members, but repeatedly the concept was rejected due to a lack of appropriate training in the specialty, if, indeed, it was one. One of the last remaining objections to the proposal was the absence of a period of hospital training, which was deemed essential by the AMA for the establishment of a board. It was believed at the time, and later proved to be true, that a year of in-plant training would be the equivalent of a hospital year, the latter not being a feasible site for a practicum in a specialty practiced at work sites. It was finally accepted that occupational medicine could be a subspecialty of the American Board of Preventive Medicine, and in June 1955, after a long and diligent effort, board certification became a reality. Of some 325 names that were submitted for initial diplomate status, 100 were chosen to form a "grandfather group" (6).

Board certification has subsequently been sought by graduates of the various residency training programs that followed. By 1993, 1,867 physicians had been certified by the American Board of Preventive Medicine in the subspecialty of occupational medicine. In 1992, 169 applications were filed by prospective examinees; in 1991, 195 applied, and in 1990, 166 sought examination, an increase over the 131 applicants of 1989. In 1992, 62% of those physicians applying passed the examination (15).

To substantiate board status, training programs were needed. Although the first intensified course in industrial medicine was offered by the Department of Industrial Hygiene of the University of Pittsburgh School of Medicine in 1938 in cooperation with the Allegheny County Medical Society (16), the longer in-residence programs were yet to be developed.

In 1950, for the first time, at a University of Pittsburgh convocation, the degree of Doctor of Industrial Medicine was conferred on three graduates who had completed the special course established by Dr. T. Lyle Hazlett. In the same year, the new graduate school of public health was created at the University of Pittsburgh, headed by the eminent Dr. Thomas Parran, former surgeon general of the U.S. Public Health Service, and the degrees to be granted became the Master and Doctor of Public Health, the degrees currently being granted at several approved graduate schools (6). Since 1984, graduates may be admitted to the board examination only after completing accredited training in preventive medicine, with no equivalency pathways available. The specialty examination today comprises material on the workplace, the worker, occupational medical services, occupational medical practice, clinical occupational medicine, industrial toxicology, physical hazards, and biologic hazards. All graduates must have completed courses for the core examination, including administration, biostatistics, clinical (medicine), epidemiology, behavioral (science), and environmental (science) (17).

The special requirements for residency education in preventive medicine and its subspecialties are laid down by the Accreditation Council for Graduate Medical Education (ACGME). The council is sponsored jointly by the American Board of Medical Specialties, the American Hospital Association, the AMA, the Association of American Medical Colleges, and the Council of Medical Specialty Societies. The ACGME is responsible for the evaluation and accreditation of programs in graduate medical education in keeping with established standards and mechanisms that are designed to ensure that acceptable graduate medical education is provided. Various residency review committees meet periodically to determine compliance of a residency program with both general and special requirements, and representatives of the occupational medical organization have served as the specialty society members (18,19).

Presently, there are 37 accredited residency programs in occupational medicine, based in schools of medicine, schools of public health, hospitals, and specialized health agencies, or in combinations of such organizations (20). Periodic reviews of the programs offered ensure currency of the programs and compliance with established requirements.

IN STEP WITH THE TIMES

While AAIPS was gaining members slowly, it was realized that the designation "AAIPS" was cumbersome and not necessarily representative of its constituency. While remnants of surgical practice remained in day-to-day clinic sessions, the focus of practice was more on medicine, particularly preventive medicine. In April 1951, the name of the organization became the Industrial Medical Association. That this designation was not to remain permanently was seen in the various work populations being covered by occupational health services. The term *industrial* had a connotation of corporate America, with its large manufacturing plants and thousands of employees. However, many occupations in the U.S. were not found in such installations though they presented health hazards unique to their work. Such groups as servicemen, students, beauticians, farmers, aircraft pilots, and retail sales personnel did not work in industry as such, yet required the same kind of preventive health programs offered to corporate workers.

With this realization, in 1974, the Industrial Medical Association became the American Occupational Medical Association, the new name implying that its members were concerned with the health of persons in all occupations, irrespective of size, service, end product, or locale of the operation or activity.

Other thought began to germinate with the ensuing years. In 1946, the American Academy of Occupational Medicine had been founded, its membership comprising full-time physicians in occupational medicine. Annual meetings were held and the program content was always scientifically solid. However, with the passage of the years, it was believed that some consolidation was needed, so that in late 1988, the American College of Occupational Medicine was created, combining the Academy and the Association, and thus avoiding immediate identification of either component body in the new name.

This newest designation was short lived, for attention was being given to the extension of occupational medicine to include environmental health as an area of activity (21,22). In keeping with this expansion of the professional's concern, a new name was given to the organization in 1992—the American College of Occupational and Environmental Medicine (ACOEM). That the latest title was truly representative of the college's interests has been seen in subsequent supportive writings (23,24), and the change now requires the college "to move forward and broaden its educational offerings, its scientific reporting, and its societal influence into the discipline of environmental medicine" (25).

ACOEM ACTIVITIES

The ACOEM consists of over 6,500 physicians worldwide. The organizational structure consists of an executive committee as well as a board of directors, whose function is to set policy, oversee committee activities and other related functions, and generally act in the best interest of the membership. Members of the board are elected to 3-year terms. Each year, approximately five new board members assume office. The executive committee consists of elected officers, such as the president, president elect, and first and second vice president, as well as the secretary, treasurer, and executive director.

In addition to the national organization, ACOEM consists of 29 chapters in the U.S. Each chapter has a range of members and is entitled to one representative in the House of Delegates per each 100 members of the chapter. Like the national organization, the local chapters function primarily in an educational and professional role by promoting scientific meetings and professional exchanges.

The majority of ACOEM activities are carried out by respective committees, which are overseen by councils. Numerous areas of professional practice in occupational medicine are addressed, including epidemiology, toxicology, publishing, and external affairs. In addition, a government affairs committee alerts the membership to various regulatory and legislative activities that may affect the practice of occupational medicine. The college owns and publishes the *Journal of Occupational Medicine,* the editor of which, although a member of ACOEM, functions independently of the organization with respect to editorial prerogative. The ACOEM's main activity is to sponsor two educational conferences a year. The spring meeting is the largest professional meeting in the world of occupational health professionals and annually attracts over 6,000 physicians, nurses, and various exhibitors. The ACOEM also publishes a monthly newsletter, sponsors standing courses in occupational medicine, and coordinates a basic curriculum in occupational medicine for those physicians new to the field. In the fall of 1993, a core curriculum in environmental medicine was introduced.

Within the past few years, the ACOEM has been successful in acquiring its own headquarters in Arlington Heights, north of Chicago. The ACOEM's activities are administrated by a variety of staff at the corporate headquarters, who assist in meeting planning and development and operational aspects, and also help to promote interchange with other medical disciplines.

A survey of the membership of the ACOEM was conducted in March 1993. Approximately 70% of over 1,500 people who completed a questionnaire practice full time in occupational medicine. The survey rate, which comprised 27% of those who received the ACOEM monthly report, indicated that half of those responding had been practicing occupational medicine for fewer than 10 years, and that only 30% were board certified. Topics in ergonomics and toxicology, especially risk assessment and occupational cancer, were highlighted as areas that were worthy of the ACOEM's formal attention.

The ACOEM is open to physicians and doctors of osteopathic medicine worldwide. Members are invited to participate in a variety of committees and educational and professional challenges assumed by the organization.

The ACOEM and Education

Education is one objective of the ACOEM and was seen early on, when in 1961 the first intensive refresher courses were offered as preliminary to the American Industrial Health Conference. The courses included cardiology in industry, treatment of radiation injuries, dermatology in industry, and hearing conservation in industry. Such courses have increased in number and precede the annual conference.

As a related organization, the Samuel Bacon Research and Education Fund Board, now the Bacon Foundation, was founded in 1976 "to promote educational, scientific and charitable work of ACOEM by accepting, holding, administering and investing such funds and property...as may...be given it; disburse...the income and principal...in the form of grants; promote and develop educational activities related to advanced training in occupational medicine, and promote and support scientific research in occupational medicine" (26). The foundation is active and continues to receive and disburse funds. Royalties from the sale of this text benefit the foundation.

The Occupational Health Institute was created in 1945 as a trust for educational purposes in connection with occupational medical research and education. While it functioned for several years, supporting certain courses and publishing activities, it ceased to exist in recent years as its functions were absorbed by the ACOEM.

Education took another form in the association of AAIPS with the journal *Industrial Medicine* (later *Industrial Medicine and Surgery*), first published in 1932. Apart from the *Journal of Industrial Hygiene,* initiated in 1919, there was no periodical devoted to the specialty. While it represented AAIPS and its successor designations, it was not the official publication of the association. In 1959, volume 1, number 1 of the *Journal of Occupational Medicine* appeared, under the dedicated editorship of Dr. Adolph G. Kammer. The journal is the official publication of the ACOEM and is currently edited by Dr. Paul W. Brandt-Rauf of Columbia University. Frequently, special issues are published that explore subjects in depth, for example, "Conference on Medical Screening and Biological Monitoring for the Effects of Exposure in the Workplace," a two-part, 1,126-page issue (27). The journal carries such departments as the Occupational Medicine Forum (answers to subscribers' questions), Selected Reviews from the Literature, Original Articles, Letters to the Editor, Committee Reports, Book Reviews, General Information for Authors, and People and Events, among others.

It is the publication of committee reports that brings guidelines to the readership in the practice of occupational medicine. The reports are approved by ACOEM's board of directors and represent a knowledgeable consensus regarding an issue at hand. Examples of such conclusive opinions are seen in "Scope of Occupational and Environmental Health Programs and Practice" (28) and "ACOEM Position Statement on Residential Radon Exposure" (29).

In 1978, the position of director of education was created at the ACOEM headquarters office to stimulate and oversee educational activities.

OCCUPATIONAL MEDICINE IN THE 1990S

The annual conferences have continued to reflect the changing concerns of the specialty. While recent clinical studies and research in toxicology share a primary post of interest with epidemiology at the workplace, program management, economics, ergonomics, health care, substance abuse, counseling, stress, and musculoskeletal problems continue to capture the attention of writers and investigators. Other organizations maintain their interest in the expansion of occupational medicine into their own specialty areas, such as the Institute of Medicine (30), the AMA (31), and the American

College of Physicians (32). A publishing house, established in 1987, OEM (Occupational and Environmental Medicine) Health Information, based in Beverly, Massachusetts, is the only publisher devoted to a single specialty—occupational and environmental medicine—and that carries some 300 related monographs in stock.

Graduates of the training programs are turning more to academic posts and consultant practices as industry continues to downsize. NIOSH and the Occupational Safety and Health Administration (OSHA) fluctuate in strength and effectiveness in keeping with the philosophic tenor of the administration in power. Legislative dicta such as the Occupational Safety and Health Act; the Federal Toxic Substances Control Act (TSCA); the Federal Mine Safety and Health Act (FMSHA); the Comprehensive Environmental Response, Compensation, and Liability Act of 1980 (CERCLA—Superfund); and the Americans with Disabilities Act (ADA) will continue to demand the attention of ACOEM members. Occupational safety and health is number 10 among 22 priority areas of the year 2000 national health objectives and Public Health Service–led agencies (33), and remains a concern of the Centers for Disease Control and Prevention, designated as the lead agency. Although all residency posts at various universities are not filled, federal funding has become stronger and the numbers of graduates and programs increase in comparison with related specialties (34). The 29 component societies of the ACOEM continue to gain new members.

It is anticipated that the ACOEM will return to a physician director in the years ahead, will begin to produce annual reports, and will develop upscale educational modalities whose use will carry continuing medical education credits.

The future bodes well for ongoing growth, for, as stated in a mid-1993 report, "The field of occupational and environmental medicine is not static. The demand for trained occupational and environmental physicians in private industry, education, and governmental agencies far exceeds the supply, and the need continues to grow" (35). To paraphrase *Occupational Health in America's* closing statement, it is safe to say that whatever the triumphs of chemical therapy, whatever miracles are wrought in the war on ailments that scourge society, and whatever feats man may perform in the conquest of space, organized occupational medicine, and the ACOEM with its 6,000 members, will play a vital role in their accomplishment (6).

REFERENCES

1. Eastman C. *Work-accidents and the law.* New York: Russell Sage Foundation, Charities Publication Committee, 1910.
2. Thompson WG. *The occupational diseases: their causation, symptoms, treatment, and prevention.* New York: D. Appleton, 1914.
3. Price GM. *The modern factory: safety, sanitation, and welfare.* New York: Wiley, 1914.
4. Kober GM, Hanson WC, eds. *Diseases of occupation and vocational hygiene.* Philadelphia: P. Blakiston's Son, 1916.
5. Mock HE. *Industrial medicine and surgery.* Philadelphia: Saunders, 1920.
6. Selleck HB, Whittaker AH. *Occupational health in America.* Detroit: Wayne State University Press, 1962.
7. Hamilton A. *Exploring the dangerous trades.* Boston: Little, Brown, 1943.
8. Felton JS. Phosphorus necrosis—a classical occupational disease. *Am J Ind Med* 1982;3:77.
9. Goldwater LJ. *Mercury—a history of quicksilver.* Baltimore: York Press, 1972:270.
10. Sharpe WD. The New Jersey radium dial painters: a classic in occupational carcinogenesis. *Bull Hist Med* 1978;52:560.
11. Cherniak, M. *The Hawk's Nest incident—America's worst industrial disaster.* New Haven: Yale University Press, 1986.
12. Medical Department, United States Army. *Preventive medicine in World War II,* vol 9, special fields. Washington, DC, 1969:110.
13. *Industrial medical program of the United States Army.* War Department Circular no. 59, February 24, 1943.
14. Stone RS, ed. *Industrial medicine on the plutonium project.* New York: McGraw-Hill, 1951:20.
15. Hyland, C. Personal communication.
16. Hazlett TL, Hummel WW. *Industrial medicine in Western Pennsylvania, 1850–1950.* Pittsburgh: University of Pittsburgh Press, 1957:174.
17. The American Board of Preventive Medicine. *Study guide materials, exam content outlines.* Schiller Park, IL: ABPM, 1993:1–4, 9–14.
18. Accreditation Council for Graduate Medical Education. *Manual of structure and functions for graduate medical education review committees.* Chicago: ACGME, 1993.
19. Accreditation Council for Graduate Medical Education. *An orientation to residency review committees.* Chicago: ACGME, 1993.
20. Accreditation Council for Graduate Medical Education. *Residency programs verification list-specialty: preventive medicine: occupational medicine).* Chicago: ACGME, 1993.
21. Goldstein BD, Gockfeld M. Role of the physician in environmental medicine. *Med Clin North Am* 1990; 74:245.
22. American College of Physicians. Occupational and environmental medicine: the internist's role. *Ann Intern Med* 1990;113:975.
23. Ducatman AM. Occupational physicians and environmental medicine. *J Occup Med* 1993;35:251.
24. Goldstein BD. Global issues in environmental medicine. *J Occup Med* 1993;35:260.

25. De Hart RL. Accepting the environmental medicine challenge. *J Occup Med* 1993;35:265.
26. *ACOEM executive manual.* July 1992:F-11.
27. Halperin WF, Schulte PA, Greathouse DG, eds. Conference on Medical Screening and Biological Monitoring for the Effects of Exposure in the Workplace, parts I and II. *J Occup Med* 1986;28:543, 913.
28. Occupational Medical Practice Committee, ACOEM. Scope of occupational and environmental health programs and practice. *J Occup Med* 1992;34:436.
29. Ad Hoc Committee on Residential Radon, ACOEM. ACOEM position statement on residential radon exposure. *J Occup Med* 1992;34:1028.
30. *Addressing the physician shortage in occupational and environmental medicine. Report of a study by the Institute of Medicine.* Washington, DC: National Academy of Sciences, 1991.
31. American Medical Association Council on Long Range Planning and Development. *The future of family practice.* Chicago: American Medical Association, 1988.
32. American College of Physicians. *Role of internist in occupational medicine.* Philadelphia: ACP, 1984.
33. Healthy People 2000: national health promotion, disease prevention objectives of the year 2000. *JAMA* 1990;264:2057.
34. Stoll DA. Personal communication, June 10, 1993.
35. Publications Committee of the American College of Occupational and Environmental Medicine (ACOEM). Careers in occupational and environmental medicine. *J Occup Med* 1993;35:628.

Appendix D

Lists of Carcinogens Rated by the International Agency for Research on Cancer (IARC)

In the first 80 volumes of monographs series, some 878 agents (chemicals, groups of chemicals, complex mixtures, occupational exposures, cultural habits, biologic or physical agents) have been evaluated.

In the following lists, the agents, mixtures, or exposures are classified as to their carcinogenic risk to humans in accordance with the procedures adopted as standard International Agency for Research on Cancer (IARC) practice:

- List of all agents, mixtures, and exposures evaluated to date
- Evaluations classified by group

Group 1—The agent (mixture) is carcinogenic to humans. The exposure circumstance entails exposures that are carcinogenic to humans.

Group 2 (two classifications):

Group 2A—The agent (mixture) is probably carcinogenic to humans. The exposure circumstance entails exposures that are probably carcinogenic to humans.

Group 2B—The agent (mixture) is possibly carcinogenic to humans. The exposure circumstance entails exposures that are possibly carcinogenic to humans.

Group 3—The agent (mixture or exposure circumstance) is not classifiable as to carcinogenicity in humans.

Group 4—The agent (mixture or exposure circumstance) is probably not carcinogenic to humans

These lists should be read only in conjunction with the IARC preamble, and it is strongly recommended to refer also to the individual monographs concerning the agents, mixtures, and exposures in which you may be interested. These lists are updated regularly.

Each monograph consists of a brief description, where appropriate, of the potential exposure to the agent or mixture, by providing data on chemical and physical properties, methods of analysis, methods and volumes of production, use, and occurrence. For exposure circumstances, a history and description of the exposure are given. Then, the relevant epidemiologic studies are summarized. Subsequent sections cover evidence for carcinogenicity obtained in experimental animals, and a brief description of other relevant data, such as toxicity and genetic effects. The IARC makes every effort to ensure that the factual material presented is reported without bias, and it is meticulously checked for accuracy.

The monographs are used widely by research scientists, public health authorities, and national and international regulatory authorities. These users apply the information contained in the monographs in different ways, but it is hoped that none uses the overall evaluations of carcinogenicity in isolation from the body of scientific evidence on which they are based.

OVERALL EVALUATIONS OF CARCINOGENICITY TO HUMANS

IARC Monographs volumes 1–80 (a total of 878 agents, mixtures, and exposures)

Group 1—Carcinogenic to Humans (87 Agents)

Agents and Groups of Agents

Aflatoxins, naturally occurring [1402-68-2] (Vol. 56; 1993)

4-Aminobiphenyl [92-67-1] (Vol. 1, Suppl. 7; 1987)

Arsenic [7440-38-2] and arsenic compounds (Vol. 23, Suppl. 7; 1987)

(NB: This evaluation applies to the group of compounds as a whole and not necessarily to all individual compounds within the group)

Asbestos [1332-21-4] (Vol. 14, Suppl. 7; 1987)
Azathioprine [446-86-6] (Vol. 26, Suppl. 7; 1987)
Benzene [71-43-2] (Vol. 29, Suppl. 7; 1987)
Benzidine [92-87-5] (Vol. 29, Suppl. 7; 1987)
Beryllium [7440-41-7] and beryllium compounds (Vol. 58; 1993) (NB: Evaluated as a group)
N,N-Bis(2-chloroethyl)-2-naphthylamine (chlornaphazine) [494-03-1] (Vol. 4, Suppl. 7; 1987)
Bis(chloromethyl)ether [542-88-1] and chloromethyl methyl ether [107-30-2] (technical-grade) (Vol. 4, Suppl. 7; 1987)
1,4-Butanediol dimethanesulfonate (Busulphan; Myleran) [55-98-1] (Vol. 4, Suppl. 7; 1987)
Cadmium [7440-43-9] and cadmium compounds (Vol. 58; 1993)
(NB: Evaluated as a group)
Chlorambucil [305-03-3] (Vol. 26, Suppl. 7; 1987)
1-(2-Chloroethyl)-3-(4-methylcyclohexyl)-1-nitrosourea (methyl-CCNU; Semustine) [13909-09-6] (Suppl. 7; 1987)
Chromium[VI] compounds (Vol. 49; 1990)
(NB: Evaluated as a group)
Cyclosporin [79217-60-0] (Vol. 50; 1990)
Cyclophosphamide [50-18-0] [6055-19-2] (Vol. 26, Suppl. 7; 1987)
Diethylstilboestrol [56-53-1] (Vol. 21, Suppl. 7; 1987)
Epstein-Barr virus (Vol. 70; 1997)
Erionite [66733-21-9] (Vol. 42, Suppl. 7; 1987)
Ethylene oxide [75-21-8] (Vol. 60; 1994)
(NB: Overall evaluation upgraded from 2A to 1 with supporting evidence from other data relevant to the evaluation of carcinogenicity and its mechanisms)
Etoposide [33419-42-0] in combination with cisplatin and bleomycin (Vol. 76; 2000)
[Gamma Radiation: see X- and Gamma (γ)-Radiation]
Helicobacter pylori (infection with) (Vol. 61; 1994)
Hepatitis B virus (chronic infection with) (Vol. 59; 1994)
Hepatitis C virus (chronic infection with) (Vol. 59; 1994)
Human immunodeficiency virus type 1 (infection with) (Vol. 67; 1996)
Human papillomavirus type 16 (Vol. 64; 1995)
Human papillomavirus type 18 (Vol. 64; 1995)
Human T-cell lymphotropic virus type I (Vol. 67; 1996)
Melphalan [148-82-3] (Vol. 9, Suppl. 7; 1987)
8-Methoxypsoralen (Methoxsalen) [298-81-7] plus ultraviolet A radiation (Vol. 24, Suppl. 7; 1987)
MOPP and other combined chemotherapy including alkylating agents (Suppl. 7; 1987)
Mustard gas (sulfur mustard) [505-60-2] (Vol. 9, Suppl. 7; 1987)
2-Naphthylamine [91-59-8] (Vol. 4, Suppl. 7; 1987)
Neutrons (Vol. 75; 2000)
(NB: Overall evaluation upgraded from 2B to 1 with supporting evidence from other data relevant to the evaluation of carcinogenicity and its mechanisms)
Nickel compounds (Vol. 49; 1990)
(NB: Evaluated as a group)
Oestrogen therapy, postmenopausal (Vol. 72; 1999)
Oestrogens, nonsteroidal (Suppl. 7; 1987)
(NB: This evaluation applies to the group of compounds as a whole and not necessarily to all individual compounds within the group)
Oestrogens, steroidal (Suppl. 7; 1987)
(NB: This evaluation applies to the group of compounds as a whole and not necessarily to all individual compounds within the group)
Opisthorchis viverrini (infection with) (Vol. 61; 1994)
Oral contraceptives, combined (Vol. 72; 1999)
(NB: There is also conclusive evidence that these agents have a protective effect against cancers of the ovary and endometrium)
Oral contraceptives, sequential (Suppl. 7; 1987)
Phosphorus-32, as phosphate (Vol. 78; 2001)
Plutonium-239 and its decay products (may contain plutonium-240 and other isotopes), as aerosols (Vol. 78; 2001)
Radioiodines, short-lived isotopes, including iodine-131, from atomic reactor accidents and nuclear weapons detonation (exposure during childhood) (Vol. 78; 2001)
Radionuclides, α-particle-emitting, internally deposited (Vol. 78; 2001)
(NB: Specific radionuclides for which there is sufficient evidence for carcinogenicity to humans are also listed individually as group 1 agents)
Radionuclides, β-particle-emitting, internally deposited (Vol. 78; 2001)
(NB: Specific radionuclides for which there is sufficient evidence for carcinogenicity to humans are also listed individually as group 1 agents)
Radium-224 and its decay products (Vol. 78; 2001)
Radium-226 and its decay products (Vol. 78; 2001)
Radium-228 and its decay products (Vol. 78; 2001)
Radon-222 [10043-92-2] and its decay products (Vol. 78; 2001)
Schistosoma haematobium (infection with) (Vol. 61; 1994)
Silica [14808-60-7], crystalline (inhaled in the form of quartz or cristobalite from occupational sources) (Vol. 68; 1997)

Solar radiation (Vol. 55; 1992)
Talc-containing asbestiform fibers (Vol. 42, Suppl. 7; 1987)
Tamoxifen [10540-29-1] (Vol. 66; 1996)
(NB: There is also conclusive evidence that this agent (tamoxifen) reduces the risk of contralateral breast cancer)
2,3,7,8-Tetrachlorodibenzo-*para*-dioxin [1746-01-6] (Vol. 69; 1997)
(NB: Overall evaluation upgraded from 2A to 1 with supporting evidence from other data relevant to the evaluation of carcinogenicity and its mechanisms)
Thiotepa [52-24-4] (Vol. 50; 1990)
Thorium-232 and its decay products, administered intravenously as a colloidal dispersion of thorium-232 dioxide (Vol. 78; 2001)
Treosulfan [299-75-2] (Vol. 26, Suppl. 7; 1987)
Vinyl chloride [75-01-4] (Vol. 19, Suppl. 7; 1987)
X- and Gamma (γ)-Radiation (Vol. 75; 2000)

Mixtures

Alcoholic beverages (Vol. 44; 1988)
Analgesic mixtures containing phenacetin (Suppl. 7; 1987)
Betel quid with tobacco (Vol. 37, Suppl. 7; 1987)
Coal-tar pitches [65996-93-2] (Vol. 35, Suppl. 7; 1987)
Coal-tars [8007-45-2] (Vol. 35, Suppl. 7; 1987)
Mineral oils, untreated and mildly treated (Vol. 33, Suppl. 7; 1987)
Salted fish (Chinese-style) (Vol. 56; 1993)
Shale-oils [68308-34-9] (Vol. 35, Suppl. 7; 1987)
Soots (Vol. 35, Suppl. 7; 1987)
Tobacco products, smokeless (Vol. 37, Suppl. 7; 1987)
Tobacco smoke (Vol. 38, Suppl. 7; 1987)
Wood dust (Vol. 62; 1995)

Exposure Circumstances

Aluminium production (Vol. 34, Suppl. 7; 1987)
Auramine, manufacture of (Suppl. 7; 1987)
Boot and shoe manufacture and repair (Vol. 25, Suppl. 7; 1987)
Coal gasification (Vol. 34, Suppl. 7; 1987)
Coke production (Vol. 34, Suppl. 7; 1987)
Furniture and cabinet making (Vol. 25, Suppl. 7; 1987)
Haematite mining (underground) with exposure to radon (Vol. 1, Suppl. 7; 1987)
Iron and steel founding (Vol. 34, Suppl. 7; 1987)
Isopropanol manufacture (strong-acid process) (Suppl. 7; 1987)
Magenta, manufacture of (Vol. 57; 1993)
Painter (occupational exposure as a) (Vol. 47; 1989)
Rubber industry (Vol. 28, Suppl. 7; 1987)
Strong-inorganic-acid mists containing sulfuric acid (occupational exposure to) (Vol. 54; 1992)

Group 2A—Probably Carcinogenic to Humans (63)

Agents and Groups of Agents

Acrylamide [79-06-1] (Vol. 60; 1994)
(NB: Overall evaluation upgraded from 2B to 2A with supporting evidence from other data relevant to the evaluation of carcinogenicity and its mechanisms)
Adriamycin [23214-92-8] (Vol. 10, Suppl. 7; 1987)
(NB: Overall evaluation upgraded from 2B to 2A with supporting evidence from other data relevant to the evaluation of carcinogenicity and its mechanisms)
Androgenic (anabolic) steroids (Suppl. 7; 1987)
Azacitidine [320-67-2] (Vol. 50; 1990)
(NB: Overall evaluation upgraded from 2B to 2A with supporting evidence from other data relevant to the evaluation of carcinogenicity and its mechanisms)
Benz[*a*]anthracene [56-55-3] (Vol. 32, Suppl. 7; 1987)
(NB: Overall evaluation upgraded from 2B to 2A with supporting evidence from other data relevant to the evaluation of carcinogenicity and its mechanisms)
Benzidine-based dyes (Suppl. 7; 1987)
(NB: Overall evaluation upgraded from 2B to 2A with supporting evidence from other data relevant to the evaluation of carcinogenicity and its mechanisms)
Benzo[*a*]pyrene [50-32-8] (Vol. 32, Suppl. 7; 1987)
(NB: Overall evaluation upgraded from 2B to 2A with supporting evidence from other data relevant to the evaluation of carcinogenicity and its mechanisms)
Bischloroethyl nitrosourea (BCNU) [154-93-8] (Vol. 26, Suppl. 7; 1987)
1,3-Butadiene [106-99-0] (Vol. 71; 1999)
Captafol [2425-06-1] (Vol. 53; 1991)
(NB: Overall evaluation upgraded from 2B to 2A with supporting evidence from other data relevant

to the evaluation of carcinogenicity and its mechanisms)

Chloramphenicol [56-75-7] (Vol. 50; 1990)

(NB: Overall evaluation upgraded from 2B to 2A with supporting evidence from other data relevant to the evaluation of carcinogenicity and its mechanisms)

α-Chlorinated toluenes (benzal chloride [98-87-3], benzotrichloride [98-07-7], benzyl chloride [100-44-7]) and benzoyl chloride [98-88-4] (combined exposures) (Vol. 29, Suppl. 7, Vol. 71; 1999)

1-(2-Chloroethyl)-3-cyclohexyl-1-nitrosourea (CCNU) [13010-47-4] (Vol. 26, Suppl. 7; 1987)

(NB: Overall evaluation upgraded from 2B to 2A with supporting evidence from other data relevant to the evaluation of carcinogenicity and its mechanisms)

4-Chloro-*ortho*-toluidine [95-69-2] (Vol. 77; 2000)

Chlorozotocin [54749-90-5] (Vol. 50; 1990)

(NB: Overall evaluation upgraded from 2B to 2A with supporting evidence from other data relevant to the evaluation of carcinogenicity and its mechanisms)

Cisplatin [15663-27-1] (Vol. 26, Suppl. 7; 1987)

(NB: Overall evaluation upgraded from 2B to 2A with supporting evidence from other data relevant to the evaluation of carcinogenicity and its mechanisms)

Clonorchis sinensis (infection with) (Vol. 61; 1994)

(NB: Overall evaluation upgraded from 2B to 2A with supporting evidence from other data relevant to the evaluation of carcinogenicity and its mechanisms)

Dibenz[*a,h*]anthracene [53-70-3] (Vol. 32, Suppl. 7; 1987)

(NB: Overall evaluation upgraded from 2B to 2A with supporting evidence from other data relevant to the evaluation of carcinogenicity and its mechanisms)

Diethyl sulfate [64-67-5] (Vol. 54, Vol. 71; 1999)

(NB: Overall evaluation upgraded from 2B to 2A with supporting evidence from other data relevant to the evaluation of carcinogenicity and its mechanisms)

Dimethylcarbamoyl chloride [79-44-7] (Vol. 12, Suppl. 7, Vol. 71; 1999)

(NB: Overall evaluation upgraded from 2B to 2A with supporting evidence from other data relevant to the evaluation of carcinogenicity and its mechanisms)

1,2-Dimethylhydrazine [540-73-8] (Vol. 4, Suppl. 7, Vol. 71; 1999)

(NB: Overall evaluation upgraded from 2B to 2A with supporting evidence from other data relevant to the evaluation of carcinogenicity and its mechanisms)

Dimethyl sulfate [77-78-1] (Vol. 4, Suppl. 7, Vol. 71; 1999)

(NB: Overall evaluation upgraded from 2B to 2A with supporting evidence from other data relevant to the evaluation of carcinogenicity and its mechanisms)

Epichlorohydrin [106-89-8] (Vol. 11, Suppl. 7, Vol. 71; 1999)

(NB: Overall evaluation upgraded from 2B to 2A with supporting evidence from other data relevant to the evaluation of carcinogenicity and its mechanisms)

Ethylene dibromide [106-93-4] (Vol. 15, Suppl. 7, Vol. 71; 1999)

(NB: Overall evaluation upgraded from 2B to 2A with supporting evidence from other data relevant to the evaluation of carcinogenicity and its mechanisms)

N-Ethyl-*N*-nitrosourea [759-73-9] (Vol. 17, Suppl. 7; 1987)

(NB: Overall evaluation upgraded from 2B to 2A with supporting evidence from other data relevant to the evaluation of carcinogenicity and its mechanisms)

Etoposide [33419-42-0] (Vol. 76; 2000)

(NB: Overall evaluation upgraded from 2B to 2A with supporting evidence from other data relevant to the evaluation of carcinogenicity and its mechanisms)

Formaldehyde [50-00-0] (Vol. 62; 1995)

Glycidol [556-52-5] (Vol. 77; 2000)

(NB: Overall evaluation upgraded from 2B to 2A with supporting evidence from other data relevant to the evaluation of carcinogenicity and its mechanisms)

Human papillomavirus type 31 (Vol. 64; 1995)

Human papillomavirus type 33 (Vol. 64; 1995)

IQ (2 - Amino - 3 - methylimidazo [4,5 - *f*]quinoline) [76180-96-6] (Vol. 56; 1993)

(NB: Overall evaluation upgraded from 2B to 2A with supporting evidence from other data relevant to the evaluation of carcinogenicity and its mechanisms)

Kaposi's sarcoma herpesvirus/human herpesvirus 8 (Vol. 70; 1997)

5-Methoxypsoralen [484-20-8] (Vol. 40, Suppl. 7; 1987)

(NB: Overall evaluation upgraded from 2B to 2A with supporting evidence from other data relevant to the evaluation of carcinogenicity and its mechanisms)

4,4′-Methylene bis(2-chloroaniline) (MOCA) [101-14-4] (Vol. 57; 1993)
(NB: Overall evaluation upgraded from 2B to 2A with supporting evidence from other data relevant to the evaluation of carcinogenicity and its mechanisms)
Methyl methanesulfonate [66-27-3] (Vol. 7, Suppl. 7, Vol. 71; 1999)
(NB: Overall evaluation upgraded from 2B to 2A with supporting evidence from other data relevant to the evaluation of carcinogenicity and its mechanisms)
N-Methyl-*N*′-nitro-*N*-nitrosoguanidine (MNNG) [70-25-7] (Vol. 4, Suppl. 7; 1987)
(NB: Overall evaluation upgraded from 2B to 2A with supporting evidence from other data relevant to the evaluation of carcinogenicity and its mechanisms)
N-Methyl-*N*-nitrosourea [684-93-5] (Vol. 17, Suppl. 7; 1987)
(NB: Overall evaluation upgraded from 2B to 2A with supporting evidence from other data relevant to the evaluation of carcinogenicity and its mechanisms)
Nitrogen mustard [51-75-2] (Vol. 9, Suppl. 7; 1987)
N-Nitrosodiethylamine [55-18-5] (Vol. 17, Suppl. 7; 1987)
(NB: Overall evaluation upgraded from 2B to 2A with supporting evidence from other data relevant to the evaluation of carcinogenicity and its mechanisms)
N-Nitrosodimethylamine [62-75-9] (Vol. 17, Suppl. 7; 1987)
(NB: Overall evaluation upgraded from 2B to 2A with supporting evidence from other data relevant to the evaluation of carcinogenicity and its mechanisms)
Phenacetin [62-44-2] (Vol. 24, Suppl. 7; 1987)
Procarbazine hydrochloride [366-70-1] (Vol. 26, Suppl. 7; 1987)
(NB: Overall evaluation upgraded from 2B to 2A with supporting evidence from other data relevant to the evaluation of carcinogenicity and its mechanisms)
Styrene-7,8-oxide [96-09-3] (Vol. 60; 1994)
(NB: Overall evaluation upgraded from 2B to 2A with supporting evidence from other data relevant to the evaluation of carcinogenicity and its mechanisms)
Teniposide [29767-20-2] (Vol. 76; 2000)
(NB: Overall evaluation upgraded from 2B to 2A with supporting evidence from other data relevant to the evaluation of carcinogenicity and its mechanisms)
Tetrachloroethylene [127-18-4] (Vol. 63; 1995)
ortho-Toluidine [95-53-4] (Vol. 77; 2000)
Trichloroethylene [79-01-6] (Vol. 63; 1995)
1,2,3-Trichloropropane [96-18-4] (Vol. 63; 1995)
Tris(2,3-dibromopropyl) phosphate [126-72-7] (Vol. 20, Suppl. 7, Vol. 71; 1999)
(NB: Overall evaluation upgraded from 2B to 2A with supporting evidence from other data relevant to the evaluation of carcinogenicity and its mechanisms)
Ultraviolet radiation A (Vol. 55; 1992)
(NB: Overall evaluation upgraded from 2B to 2A with supporting evidence from other data relevant to the evaluation of carcinogenicity and its mechanisms)
Ultraviolet radiation B (Vol. 55; 1992)
(NB: Overall evaluation upgraded from 2B to 2A with supporting evidence from other data relevant to the evaluation of carcinogenicity and its mechanisms)
Ultraviolet radiation C (Vol. 55; 1992)
(NB: Overall evaluation upgraded from 2B to 2A with supporting evidence from other data relevant to the evaluation of carcinogenicity and its mechanisms)
Vinyl bromide [593-60-2] (Vol. 39, Suppl. 7, Vol. 71; 1999)
(NB: Overall evaluation upgraded from 2B to 2A with supporting evidence from other data relevant to the evaluation of carcinogenicity and its mechanisms)
Vinyl fluoride [75-02-5] (Vol. 63; 1995)

Mixtures

Creosotes (from coal-tars) [8001-58-9] (Vol. 35, Suppl. 7; 1987)
Diesel engine exhaust (Vol. 46; 1989)
Hot mate (Vol. 51; 1991)
Non-arsenical insecticides (occupational exposures in spraying and application of) (Vol. 53; 1991)
Polychlorinated biphenyls [1336-36-3] (Vol. 18, Suppl. 7; 1987)

Exposure Circumstances

Art glass, glass containers, and pressed ware (manufacture of) (Vol. 58; 1993)

Hairdresser or barber (occupational exposure as a) (Vol. 57; 1993)
Petroleum refining (occupational exposures in) (Vol. 45; 1989)
Sunlamps and sun beds (use of) (Vol. 55; 1992)

Group 2B—Possibly Carcinogenic to Humans (234)

Agents and Groups of Agents

A-α-C (2-Amino-9*H*-pyrido[2,3-*b*]indole) [26148-68-5] (Vol. 40, Suppl. 7; 1987)
Acetaldehyde [75-07-0] (Vol. 36, Suppl. 7, Vol. 71; 1999)
Acetamide [60-35-5] (Vol. 7, Suppl. 7, Vol. 71; 1999)
Acrylonitrile [107-13-1] (Vol. 71; 1999)
AF-2 [2-(2-Furyl)-3-(5-nitro-2-furyl)acrylamide] [3688-53-7] (Vol. 31, Suppl. 7; 1987)
Aflatoxin M1 [6795-23-9] (Vol. 56; 1993)
para-Aminoazobenzene [60-09-3] (Vol. 8, Suppl. 7; 1987)
ortho-Aminoazotoluene [97-56-3] (Vol. 8, Suppl. 7; 1987)
2-Amino-5-(5-nitro-2-furyl)-1,3,4-thiadiazole [712-68-5] (Vol. 7, Suppl. 7; 1987)
Amsacrine [51264-14-3] (Vol. 76; 2000)
ortho-Anisidine [90-04-0] (Vol. 73; 1999)
Antimony trioxide [1309-64-4] (Vol. 47; 1989)
Aramite [140-57-8] (Vol. 5, Suppl. 7; 1987)
Auramine [492-80-8] (technical-grade) (Vol. 1, Suppl. 7; 1987)
Azaserine [115-02-6] (Vol. 10, Suppl. 7; 1987)
Aziridine [151-56-4] (Vol. 9, Suppl. 7, Vol. 71; 1999)
(NB: Overall evaluation upgraded from 3 to 2B with supporting evidence from other data relevant to the evaluation of carcinogenicity and its mechanisms)
Benzo[*b*]fluoranthene [205-99-2] (Vol. 32, Suppl. 7; 1987)
Benzo[*j*]fluoranthene [205-82-3] (Vol. 32, Suppl. 7; 1987)
Benzo[*k*]fluoranthene [207-08-9] (Vol. 32, Suppl. 7; 1987)
Benzofuran [271-89-6] (Vol. 63; 1995)
Benzyl violet 4B [1694-09-3] (Vol. 16, Suppl. 7; 1987)
2,2-Bis(bromomethyl)propane-1,3-diol [3296-90-0] (Vol. 77; 2000)
Bleomycins [11056-06-7] (Vol. 26, Suppl. 7; 1987)
(NB: Overall evaluation upgraded from 3 to 2B with supporting evidence from other data relevant to the evaluation of carcinogenicity and its mechanisms)
Bracken fern (Vol. 40, Suppl. 7; 1987)
Bromodichloromethane [75-27-4] (Vol. 52, Vol. 71; 1999)
Butylated hydroxyanisole (BHA) [25013-16-5] (Vol. 40, Suppl. 7; 1987)
β-Butyrolactone [3068-88-0] (Vol. 11, Suppl. 7, Vol. 71; 1999)
Caffeic acid [331-39-5] (Vol. 56; 1993)
Carbon black [1333-86-4] (Vol. 65; 1996)
Carbon tetrachloride [56-23-5] (Vol. 20, Suppl. 7, Vol. 71; 1999)
Catechol [120-80-9] (Vol. 15, Suppl. 7, Vol. 71; 1999)
Ceramic fibers (Vol. 43; 1988) [see new evaluation]
Chlordane [57-74-9] (Vol. 79; 2001)
Chlordecone (Kepone) [143-50-0] (Vol. 20, Suppl. 7; 1987)
Chlorendic acid [115-28-6] (Vol. 48; 1990)
para-Chloroaniline [106-47-8] (Vol. 57; 1993)
Chloroform [67-66-3] (Vol. 73; 1999)
1-Chloro-2-methylpropene [513-37-1] (Vol. 63; 1995)
Chlorophenoxy herbicides (Vol. 41, Suppl. 7; 1987)
4-Chloro-*ortho*-phenylenediamine [95-83-0] (Vol. 27, Suppl. 7; 1987)
Chloroprene [126-99-8] (Vol. 71; 1999)
Chlorothalonil [1897-45-6] (Vol. 73; 1999)
CI Acid Red 114 [6459-94-5] (Vol. 57; 1993)
CI Basic Red 9 [569-61-9] (Vol. 57; 1993)
CI Direct Blue 15 [2429-74-5] (Vol. 57; 1993)
Citrus Red No. 2 [6358-53-8] (Vol. 8, Suppl. 7; 1987)
Cobalt [7440-48-4] and cobalt compounds (Vol. 52; 1991)
(NB: Evaluated as a group)
para-Cresidine [120-71-8] (Vol. 27, Suppl. 7; 1987)
Cycasin [14901-08-7] (Vol. 10, Suppl. 7; 1987)
Dacarbazine [4342-03-4] (Vol. 26, Suppl. 7; 1987)
Dantron (Chrysazin; 1,8-Dihydroxyanthraquinone) [117-10-2] (Vol. 50; 1990)
Daunomycin [20830-81-3] (Vol. 10, Suppl. 7; 1987)
DDT [*p,p′*-DDT, 50-29-3] (Vol. 53; 1991)
N,N′-Diacetylbenzidine [613-35-4] (Vol. 16, Suppl. 7; 1987)
2,4-Diaminoanisole [615-05-4] (Vol. 79; 2001)
4,4′-Diaminodiphenyl ether [101-80-4] (Vol. 29, Suppl. 7; 1987)
2,4-Diaminotoluene [95-80-7] (Vol. 16, Suppl. 7; 1987)
Dibenz[*a,h*]acridine [226-36-8] (Vol. 32, Suppl. 7; 1987)
Dibenz[*a,j*]acridine [224-42-0] (Vol. 32, Suppl. 7; 1987)
7*H*-Dibenzo[*c,g*]carbazole [194-59-2] (Vol. 32, Suppl. 7; 1987)

Dibenzo[*a,e*]pyrene [192-65-4] (Vol. 32, Suppl. 7; 1987)
Dibenzo[*a,h*]pyrene [189-64-0] (Vol. 32, Suppl. 7; 1987)
Dibenzo[*a,i*]pyrene [189-55-9] (Vol. 32, Suppl. 7; 1987)
Dibenzo[*a,l*]pyrene [191-30-0] (Vol. 32, Suppl. 7; 1987)
1,2-Dibromo-3-chloropropane [96-12-8] (Vol. 20, Suppl. 7, Vol. 71; 1999)
2,3-Dibromopropan-1-ol [96-13-9] (Vol. 77; 2000)
para-Dichlorobenzene [106-46-7] (Vol. 73; 1999)
3,3′-Dichlorobenzidine [91-94-1] (Vol. 29, Suppl. 7; 1987)
3,3′-Dichloro-4,4′-diaminodiphenyl ether [28434-86-8] (Vol. 16, Suppl. 7; 1987)
1,2-Dichloroethane [107-06-2] (Vol. 20, Suppl. 7, Vol. 71; 1999)
Dichloromethane (methylene chloride) [75-09-2] (Vol. 71; 1999)
1,3-Dichloropropene [542-75-6] (technical-grade) (Vol. 41, Suppl. 7, Vol. 71; 1999)
Dichlorvos [62-73-7] (Vol. 53; 1991)
1,2-Diethylhydrazine [1615-80-1] (Vol. 4, Suppl. 7, Vol. 71; 1999)
Diglycidyl resorcinol ether [101-90-6] (Vol. 36, Suppl. 7, Vol. 71; 1999)
Dihydrosafrole [94-58-6] (Vol. 10, Suppl. 7; 1987)
Diisopropyl sulfate [2973-10-6] (Vol. 54, Vol. 71; 1999)
3,3′-Dimethoxybenzidine (*ortho*-Dianisidine) [119-90-4] (Vol. 4, Suppl. 7; 1987)
para-Dimethylaminoazobenzene [60-11-7] (Vol. 8, Suppl. 7; 1987)
trans-2-[(Dimethylamino)methylimino]-5-[2-(5-nitro-2-furyl)-vinyl]-1,3,4-oxadiazole [25962-77-0] (Vol. 7, Suppl. 7; 1987)
2,6-Dimethylaniline (2,6-Xylidine) [87-62-7] (Vol. 57; 1993)
3,3′-Dimethylbenzidine (*ortho*-Tolidine) [119-93-7] (Vol. 1, Suppl. 7; 1987)
1,1-Dimethylhydrazine [57-14-7] (Vol. 4, Suppl. 7, Vol. 71; 1999)
3,7-Dinitrofluoranthene [105735-71-5] (Vol. 65; 1996)
3,9-Dinitrofluoranthene [22506-53-2] (Vol. 65; 1996)
1,6-Dinitropyrene [42397-64-8] (Vol. 46; 1989)
1,8-Dinitropyrene [42397-65-9] (Vol. 46; 1989)
2,4-Dinitrotoluene [121-14-2] (Vol. 65; 1996)
2,6-Dinitrotoluene [606-20-2] (Vol. 65; 1996)
1,4-Dioxane [123-91-1] (Vol. 11, Suppl. 7, Vol. 71; 1999)
Disperse Blue 1 [2475-45-8] (Vol. 48; 1990)
1,2-Epoxybutane [106-88-7] (Vol. 47, Vol. 71; 1999)
(NB: Overall evaluation upgraded from 3 to 2B with supporting evidence from other data relevant to the evaluation of carcinogenicity and its mechanisms)
Ethyl acrylate [140-88-5] (Vol. 39, Suppl. 7, Vol. 71; 1999)
Ethylbenzene [100-41-4] (Vol. 77; 2000)
Ethyl methanesulfonate [62-50-0] (Vol. 7, Suppl. 7; 1987)
Foreign bodies, implanted in tissues (Vol. 74; 1999)
Polymeric, prepared as thin smooth films (with the exception of poly(glycolic acid))
Metallic, prepared as thin smooth films
Metallic cobalt, metallic nickel and an alloy powder containing 66–67% nickel, 13–16% chromium and 7% iron
2-(2-Formylhydrazino)-4-(5-nitro-2-furyl)thiazole [3570-75-0] (Vol. 7, Suppl. 7; 1987)
Furan [110-00-9] (Vol. 63; 1995)
Glasswool (Vol. 43; 1988) [see new evaluation]
Glu-P-1 (2-Amino-6-methyldipyrido[1,2-*a*:3′,2′-*d*]imidazole) [67730-11-4] (Vol. 40, Suppl. 7; 1987)
Glu-P-2 (2-Aminodipyrido[1,2-*a*:3′,2′-*d*]imidazole) [67730-10-3] (Vol. 40, Suppl. 7; 1987)
Glycidaldehyde [765-34-4] (Vol. 11, Suppl. 7, Vol. 71; 1999)
Griseofulvin [126-07-8] (Vol. 79; 2001)
HC Blue No. 1 [2784-94-3] (Vol. 57; 1993)
Heptachlor [76-44-8] (Vol. 79; 2001)
Hexachlorobenzene [118-74-1] (Vol. 79; 2001)
Hexachloroethane [67-72-1] (Vol. 73; 1999)
Hexachlorocyclohexanes (Vol. 20, Suppl. 7; 1987)
Hexamethylphosphoramide [680-31-9] (Vol. 15, Suppl. 7, Vol. 71; 1999)
Human immunodeficiency virus type 2 (infection with) (Vol. 67; 1996)
Human papillomaviruses: some types other than 16, 18, 31 and 33 (Vol. 64; 1995)
Hydrazine [302-01-2] (Vol. 4, Suppl. 7, Vol. 71; 1999)
Indeno[1,2,3-*cd*]pyrene [193-39-5] (Vol. 32, Suppl. 7; 1987)
Iron-dextran complex [9004-66-4] (Vol. 2, Suppl. 7; 1987)
Isoprene [78-79-5] (Vol. 60, Vol. 71; 1999)
Lasiocarpine [303-34-4] (Vol. 10, Suppl. 7; 1987)
Lead [7439-92-1] and lead compounds, inorganic (Vol. 23, Suppl. 7; 1987)
(NB: Evaluated as a group)
Magenta [632-99-5] (containing CI Basic Red 9) (Vol. 57; 1993)
Magnetic fields (extremely low-frequency) (Vol. 80; 2002)

MeA-*a*-C (2-Amino-3-methyl-9*H*-pyrido[2,3-*b*]indole) [68006-83-7] (Vol. 40, Suppl. 7; 1987)
Medroxyprogesterone acetate [71-58-9] (Vol. 21, Suppl. 7; 1987)
MeIQ (2-Amino-3,4-dimethylimidazo[4,5-*f*]quinoline) [77094-11-2] (Vol. 56; 1993)
MeIQx (2-Amino-3,8-dimethylimidazo[4,5-*f*]quinoxaline) [77500-04-0] (Vol. 56; 1993)
Merphalan [531-76-0] (Vol. 9, Suppl. 7; 1987)
2-Methylaziridine (Propyleneimine) [75-55-8] (Vol. 9, Suppl. 7, Vol. 71; 1999)
Methylazoxymethanol acetate [592-62-1] (Vol. 10, Suppl. 7; 1987)
5-Methylchrysene [3697-24-3] (Vol. 32, Suppl. 7; 1987)
4,4′-Methylene bis(2-methylaniline) [838-88-0] (Vol. 4, Suppl. 7; 1987)
4,4′-Methylenedianiline [101-77-9] (Vol. 39, Suppl. 7; 1987)
Methylmercury compounds (Vol. 58; 1993)
(NB: Evaluated as a group)
2-Methyl-1-nitroanthraquinone [129-15-7] (uncertain purity) (Vol. 27, Suppl. 7; 1987)
N-Methyl-*N*-nitrosourethane [615-53-2] (Vol. 4, Suppl. 7; 1987)
Methylthiouracil [56-04-2] (Vol. 79; 2001)
Metronidazole [443-48-1] (Vol. 13, Suppl. 7; 1987)
Mirex [2385-85-5] (Vol. 20, Suppl. 7; 1987)
Mitomycin C [50-07-7] (Vol. 10, Suppl. 7; 1987)
Mitoxantrone [65271-80-9] (Vol. 76; 2000)
Monocrotaline [315-22-0] (Vol. 10, Suppl. 7; 1987)
5-(Morpholinomethyl)-3-[(5-nitrofurfurylidene)amino]-2-oxazolidinone [3795-88-8] (Vol. 7, Suppl. 7; 1987)
Nafenopin [3771-19-5] (Vol. 24, Suppl. 7; 1987)
Nickel, metallic [7440-02-0] and alloys (Vol. 49; 1990)
Niridazole [61-57-4] (Vol. 13, Suppl. 7; 1987)
Nitrilotriacetic acid [139-13-9] and its salts (Vol. 73; 1999)
(NB: Evaluated as a group)
5-Nitroacenaphthene [602-87-9] (Vol. 16, Suppl. 7; 1987)
2-Nitroanisole [91-23-6] (Vol. 65; 1996)
Nitrobenzene [98-95-3] (Vol. 65; 1996)
6-Nitrochrysene [7496-02-8] (Vol. 46; 1989)
Nitrofen [1836-75-5] (technical-grade) (Vol. 30, Suppl. 7; 1987)
2-Nitrofluorene [607-57-8] (Vol. 46; 1989)
1-[(5-Nitrofurfurylidene)amino]-2-imidazolidinone [555-84-0] (Vol. 7, Suppl. 7; 1987)
N-[4-(5-Nitro-2-furyl)-2-thiazolyl]acetamide [531-82-8] (Vol. 7, Suppi. 7; 1987)
Nitrogen mustard *N*-oxide [126-85-2] (Vol. 9, Suppl. 7; 1987)
Nitromethane [75-52-5] (Vol. 77; 2000)
2-Nitropropane [79-46-9] (Vol. 29, Suppl. 7, Vol. 71; 1999)
1-Nitropyrene [5522-43-0] (Vol. 46; 1989)
4-Nitropyrene [57835-92-4] (Vol. 46; 1989)
N-Nitrosodi-*n*-butylamine [924-16-3] (Vol. 17, Suppl. 7; 1987)
N-Nitrosodiethanolamine [1116-54-7] (Vol. 17, Suppl. 7, Vol. 77; 2000)
N-Nitrosodi-*n*-propylamine [621-64-7] (Vol. 17, Suppl. 7; 1987)
3-(*N*-Nitrosomethylamino)propionitrile [60153-49-3] (Vol. 37, Suppl. 7; 1987)
4-(*N*-Nitrosomethylamino)-1-(3-pyridyl)-1-butanone (NNK) [64091-91-4] (Vol. 37, Suppl. 7; 1987)
N-Nitrosomethylethylamine [10595-95-6] (Vol. 17, Suppl. 7; 1987)
N-Nitrosomethylvinylamine [4549-40-0] (Vol. 17, Suppl. 7; 1987)
N-Nitrosomorpholine [59-89-2] (Vol. 17, Suppl. 7; 1987)
N′-Nitrosonornicotine [16543-55-8] (Vol. 37, Suppl. 7; 1987)
N-Nitrosopiperidine [100-75-4] (Vol. 17, Suppl. 7; 1987)
N-Nitrosopyrrolidine [930-55-2] (Vol. 17, Suppl. 7; 1987)
N-Nitrososarcosine [13256-22-9] (Vol. 17, Suppl. 7; 1987)
Ochratoxin A [303-47-9] (Vol. 56; 1993)
Oestrogen-progestogen therapy, postmenopausal (Vol. 72; 1999)
Oil orange SS [2646-17-5] (Vol. 8, Suppl. 7; 1987)
Oxazepam [604-75-1] (Vol. 66; 1996)
Palygorskite (attapulgite) [12174-11-7] (long fibers, >5 μm) (Vol. 68; 1997)
Panfuran S [794-93-4] (containing dihydroxymethylfuratrizine) (Vol. 24, Suppl. 7; 1987)
Phenazopyridine hydrochloride [136-40-3] (Vol. 24, Suppl. 7; 1987)
Phenobarbital [50-06-6] (Vol. 79; 2001)
Phenolphthalein [77-09-8] (Vol. 76; 2000)
Phenoxybenzamine hydrochloride [63-92-3] (Vol. 24, Suppl. 7; 1987)
Phenyl glycidyl ether [122-60-1] (Vol. 47, Vol. 71; 1999)
Phenytoin [57-41-0] (Vol. 66; 1996)
PhIP (2-Amino-1-methyl-6-phenylimidazo[4,5-*b*]pyridine) [105650-23-5] (Vol. 56; 1993)
Polychlorophenols and their sodium salts (mixed exposures) (Vol. 41, Suppl. 7, Vol. 53, Vol. 71; 1999)

Ponceau MX [3761-53-3] (Vol. 8, Suppl. 7; 1987)
Ponceau 3R [3564-09-8] (Vol. 8, Suppl. 7; 1987)
Potassium bromate [7758-01-2] (Vol. 73; 1999)
Progestins (Suppl. 7; 1987)
Progestogen-only contraceptives (Vol. 72; 1999)
1,3-Propane sultone [1120-71-4] (Vol. 4, Suppl. 7, Vol. 71; 1999)
b-Propiolactone [57-57-8] (Vol. 4, Suppl. 7, Vol. 71; 1999)
Propylene oxide [75-56-9] (Vol. 60; 1994)
Propylthiouracil [51-52-5] (Vol. 79; 2001)
Rockwool (Vol. 43; 1988) [see new evaluation]
Safrole [94-59-7] (Vol. 10, Suppl. 7; 1987)
Schistosoma japonicum (infection with) (Vol. 61; 1994)
Slagwool (Vol. 43; 1988) [see new evaluation]
Sodium *ortho*-phenylphenate [132-27-4] (Vol. 73; 1999)
Sterigmatocystin [10048-13-2] (Vol. 10, Suppl. 7; 1987)
Streptozotocin [18883-66-4] (Vol. 17, Suppl. 7; 1987)
Styrene [100-42-5] (Vol. 60; 1994)
(NB: Overall evaluation upgraded from 3 to 2B with supporting evidence from other data relevant to the evaluation of carcinogenicity and its mechanisms)
Sulfallate [95-06-7] (Vol. 30, Suppl. 7; 1987)
Tetrafluoroethylene [116-14-3] (Vol. 19, Suppl. 7, Vol. 71; 1999)
Tetranitromethane [509-14-8] (Vol. 65; 1996)
Thioacetamide [62-55-5] (Vol. 7, Suppl. 7; 1987)
4,4′-Thiodianiline [139-65-1] (Vol. 27, Suppl. 7; 1987)
Thiouracil [141-90-2] (Vol. 79; 2001)
Toluene diisocyanates [26471-62-5] (Vol. 39, Suppl. 7, Vol. 71; 1999)
Toxins derived from *Fusarium moniliforme* (Vol. 56; 1993)
Trichlormethine (Trimustine hydrochloride) [817-09-4] (Vol. 50; 1990)
Trp-P-1 (3-Amino-1,4-dimethyl-5*H*-pyrido[4,3-*b*]indole) [62450-06-0] (Vol. 31, Suppl. 7; 1987)
Trp-P-2 (3-Amino-1-methyl-5*H*-pyrido[4,3-*b*]indole) [62450-07-1] (Vol. 31, Suppl. 7; 1987)
Trypan blue [72-57-1] (Vol. 8, Suppl. 7; 1987)
Uracil mustard [66-75-1] (Vol. 9, Suppl. 7; 1987)
Urethane [51-79-6] (Vol. 7, Suppl. 7; 1987)
Vinyl acetate [108-05-4] (Vol. 63; 1995)
4-Vinylcyclohexene [100-40-3] (Vol. 60; 1994)
4-Vinylcyclohexene diepoxide [106-87-6] (Vol. 60; 1994)
Zalcitabine [7481-89-2] (Vol. 76; 2000)
Zidovudine (AZT) [30516-87-1] (Vol. 76; 2000)

Mixtures

Bitumens [8052-42-4], extracts of steam-refined and air-refined (Vol. 35, Suppl. 7; 1987)
Carrageenan [9000-07-1], degraded (Vol. 31, Suppl. 7; 1987)
Chlorinated paraffins of average carbon chain length C12 and average degree of chlorination approximately 60% (Vol. 48; 1990)
Coffee (urinary bladder) (Vol. 51; 1991)
(NB: There is some evidence of an inverse relationship between coffee drinking and cancer of the large bowel; coffee drinking could not be classified as to its carcinogenicity to other organs)
Diesel fuel, marine (Vol. 45; 1989)
(NB: Overall evaluation upgraded from 3 to 2B with supporting evidence from other data relevant to the evaluation of carcinogenicity and its mechanisms)
Engine exhaust, gasoline (Vol. 46; 1989)
Fuel oils, residual (heavy) (Vol. 45; 1989)
Gasoline (Vol. 45; 1989)
(NB: Overall evaluation upgraded from 3 to 2B with supporting evidence from other data relevant to the evaluation of carcinogenicity and its mechanisms)
Pickled vegetables (traditional in Asia) (Vol. 56; 1993)
Polybrominated biphenyls [Firemaster BP-6, 59536-65-1] (Vol. 41, Suppl. 7; 1987)
Toxaphene (polychlorinated camphenes) [8001-35-2] (Vol. 79; 2001)
Welding fumes (Vol. 49; 1990)

Exposure Circumstances

Carpentry and joinery (Vol. 25, Suppl. 7; 1987)
Dry cleaning (occupational exposures in) (Vol. 63; 1995)
Printing processes (occupational exposures in) (Vol. 65; 1996)
Textile manufacturing industry (work in) (Vol. 48; 1990)

Group 3—Unclassifiable as to Carcinogenicity to Humans (493 Agents)

Agents and Groups of Agents

Aciclovir [59277-89-3] (Vol. 76; 2000)
Acridine orange [494-38-2] (Vol. 16, Suppl. 7; 1987)
Acriflavinium chloride [8018-07-3] (Vol. 13, Suppl. 7; 1987)
Acrolein [107-02-8] (Vol. 63; 1995)

Acrylic acid [79-10-7] (Vol. 19, Suppl. 7, Vol. 71; 1999)
Acrylic fibers (Vol. 19, Suppl. 7; 1987)
Acrylonitrile-butadiene-styrene copolymers (Vol. 19, Suppl. 7; 1987)
Actinomycin D [50-76-0] (Vol. 10, Suppl. 7; 1987)
Agaritine [2757-90-6] (Vol. 31, Suppl. 7; 1987)
Aldicarb [116-06-3] (Vol. 53; 1991)
Aldrin [309-00-2] (Vol. 5, Suppl. 7; 1987)
Allyl chloride [107-05-1] (Vol. 36, Suppl. 7, Vol. 71; 1999)
Allyl isothiocyanate [57-06-7] (Vol. 73; 1999)
Allyl isovalerate [2835-39-4] (Vol. 36, Suppl. 7, Vol. 71; 1999)
Amaranth [915-67-3] (Vol. 8, Suppl. 7; 1987)
5-Aminoacenaphthene [4657-93-6] (Vol. 16, Suppl. 7; 1987)
2-Aminoanthraquinone [117-79-3] (Vol. 27, Suppl. 7; 1987)
para-Aminobenzoic acid [150-13-0] (Vol. 16, Suppl. 7; 1987)
1-Amino-2-methylanthraquinone [82-28-0] (Vol. 27, Suppl. 7; 1987)
2-Amino-4-nitrophenol [99-57-0] (Vol. 57; 1993)
2-Amino-5-nitrophenol [121-88-0] (Vol. 57; 1993)
4-Amino-2-nitrophenol [119-34-6] (Vol. 16, Suppl. 7; 1987)
2-Amino-5-nitrothiazole [121-66-4] (Vol. 31, Suppl. 7; 1987)
11-Aminoundecanoic acid [2432-99-7] (Vol. 39, Suppl. 7; 1987)
Amitrole [61-82-5] (Vol. 79; 2001)
(NB: Overall evaluation downgraded from 2B to 3 with supporting evidence from other data relevant to carcinogenicity and its mechanisms)
Ampicillin [69-53-4] (Vol. 50; 1990)
Anesthetics, volatile (Vol. 11, Suppl. 7; 1987)
Angelicin [523-50-2] plus ultraviolet A radiation (Vol. 40, Suppl. 7; 1987)
Aniline [62-53-3] (Vol. 27, Suppl. 7; 1987)
para-Anisidine [104-94-9] (Vol. 27, Suppl. 7; 1987)
Anthanthrene [191-26-4] (Vol. 32, Suppl. 7; 1987)
Anthracene [120-12-7] (Vol. 32, Suppl. 7; 1987)
Anthranilic acid [118-92-3] (Vol. 16, Suppl. 7; 1987)
Antimony trisulfide [1345-04-6] (Vol. 47; 1989)
Apholate [52-46-0] (Vol. 9, Suppl. 7; 1987)
para-Aramid fibrils [24938-64-5] (Vol. 68; 1997)
Atrazine [1912-24-9] (Vol. 73; 1999)
(NB: Overall evaluation downgraded from 2B to 3 with supporting evidence from other data relevant to carcinogenicity and its mechanisms)
Aurothioglucose [12192-57-3] (Vol. 13, Suppl. 7; 1987)
2-(1-Aziridinyl)ethanol [1072-52-2] (Vol. 9, Suppl. 7; 1987)
Aziridyl benzoquinone [800-24-8] (Vol. 9, Suppl. 7; 1987)
Azobenzene [103-33-3] (Vol. 8, Suppl. 7; 1987)
Benz[*a*]acridine [225-11-6] (Vol. 32, Suppl. 7; 1987)
Benz[*c*]acridine [225-51-4] (Vol. 32, Suppl. 7; 1987)
Benzo[*ghi*]fluoranthene [203-12-3] (Vol. 32, Suppl. 7; 1987)
Benzo[*a*]fluorene [238-84-6] (Vol. 32, Suppl. 7; 1987)
Benzo[*b*]fluorene [243-17-4] (Vol. 32, Suppl. 7; 1987)
Benzo[*c*]fluorene [205-12-9] (Vol. 32, Suppl. 7; 1987)
Benzo[*ghi*]perylene [191-24-2] (Vol. 32, Suppl. 7; 1987)
Benzo[*c*]phenanthrene [195-19-7] (Vol. 32, Suppl. 7; 1987)
Benzo[*e*]pyrene [192-97-2] (Vol. 32, Suppl. 7; 1987)
para-Benzoquinone dioxime [105-11-3] (Vol. 29, Suppl. 7, Vol. 71; 1999)
Benzoyl peroxide [94-36-0] (Vol. 36, Suppl. 7, Vol. 71; 1999)
Benzyl acetate [140-11-4] (Vol. 40, Suppl. 7, Vol. 71; 1999)
Bis(1-aziridinyl)morpholinophosphine sulfide [2168-68-5] (Vol. 9, Suppl. 7; 1987)
Bis(2-chloroethyl)ether [111-44-4] (Vol. 9, Suppl. 7, Vol. 71; 1999)
1,2-Bis(chloromethoxy)ethane [13483-18-6] (Vol. 15; Suppl. 7, Vol. 71; 1999)
1,4-Bis(chloromethoxymethyl)benzene [56894-91-8] (Vol. 15, Suppl. 7, Vol. 71; 1999)
Bis(2-chloro-1-methylethyl)ether [108-60-1] (Vol. 41, Suppl. 7, Vol. 71; 1999)
Bis(2,3-epoxycyclopentyl)ether [2386-90-5] (Vol. 47, Vol. 71; 1999)
Bisphenol A diglycidyl ether (Araldite[â]) [1675-54-3] (Vol. 47, Vol. 71; 1999)
Bisulfites (Vol. 54; 1992)
Blue VRS [129-17-9] (Vol. 16, Suppl. 7; 1987)
Brilliant Blue FCF, disodium salt [3844-45-9] (Vol. 16, Suppl. 7; 1987)
Bromochloroacetonitrile [83463-62-1] (Vol. 52, Vol. 71; 1999)
Bromoethane [74-96-4] (Vol. 52, Vol. 71; 1999)
Bromoform [75-25-2] (Vol. 52, Vol. 71; 1999)
n-Butyl acrylate [141-32-2] (Vol. 39, Suppl. 7, Vol. 71; 1999)
Butylated hydroxytoluene (BHT) [128-37-0] (Vol. 40, Suppl. 7; 1987)
Butyl benzyl phthalate [85-68-7] (Vol. 73; 1999)

g-Butyrolactone [96-48-0] (Vol. 11, Suppl. 7, Vol. 71; 1999)
Caffeine [58-08-2] (Vol. 51; 1991)
Cantharidin [56-25-7] (Vol. 10, Suppl. 7; 1987)
Captan [133-06-2] (Vol. 30, Suppl. 7; 1987)
Carbaryl [63-25-2] (Vol. 12, Suppl. 7; 1987)
Carbazole [86-74-8] (Vol. 32, Suppl. 7, Vol. 71; 1999)
3-Carbethoxypsoralen [20073-24-9] (Vol. 40, Suppl. 7; 1987)
Carmoisine [3567-69-9] (Vol. 8, Suppl. 7; 1987)
Carrageenan [9000-07-1], native (Vol. 31, Suppl. 7; 1987)
Chloral [75-87-6] (Vol. 63; 1995)
Chloral hydrate [302-17-0] (Vol. 63; 1995)
Chlordimeform [6164-98-3] (Vol. 30, Suppl. 7; 1987)
Chlorinated drinking water (Vol. 52; 1991)
Chloroacetonitrile [107-14-2] (Vol. 52, Vol. 71; 1999)
Chlorobenzilate [510-15-6] (Vol. 30, Suppl. 7; 1987)
Chlorodibromomethane [124-48-1] (Vol. 52, Vol. 71; 1999)
Chlorodifluoromethane [75-45-6] (Vol. 41, Suppl. 7, Vol. 71; 1999)
Chloroethane [75-00-3] (Vol. 52, Vol. 71; 1999)
Chlorofluoromethane [593-70-4] (Vol. 41, Suppl. 7, Vol. 71; 1999)
3-Chloro-2-methylpropene [563-47-3] (Vol. 63; 1995)
4-Chloro-*meta*-phenylenediamine [5131-60-2] (Vol. 27, Suppl. 7; 1987)
Chloronitrobenzenes [88-73-3; 121-73-3; 100-00-5] (Vol. 65; 1996)
Chloropropham [101-21-3] (Vol. 12, Suppl. 7; 1987)
Chloroquine [54-05-7] (Vol. 13, Suppl. 7; 1987)
5-Chloro-*ortho*-toluidine [95-79-4] (Vol. 77; 2000)
2-Chloro-1,1,1-trifluoroethane [75-88-7] (Vol. 41, Suppl. 7, Vol. 71; 1999)
Cholesterol [57-88-5] (Vol. 31, Suppl. 7; 1987)
Chromium[III] compounds (Vol. 49; 1990)
Chromium [7440-47-3], metallic (Vol. 49; 1990)
Chrysene [218-01-9] (Vol. 32, Suppl. 7; 1987)
Chrysoidine [532-82-1] (Vol. 8, Suppl. 7; 1987)
CI Acid Orange 3 [6373-74-6] (Vol. 57; 1993)
Cimetidine [51481-61-9] (Vol. 50; 1990)
Cinnamyl anthranilate [87-29-6] (Vol. 77; 2000)
CI Pigment Red 3 [2425-85-6] (Vol. 57; 1993)
Citrinin [518-75-2] (Vol. 40, Suppl. 7; 1987)
Clofibrate [637-07-0] (Vol. 66; 1996)
Clomiphene citrate [50-41-9] (Vol. 21, Suppl. 7; 1987)
Coal dust (Vol. 68; 1997)
Copper 8-hydroxyquinoline [10380-28-6] (Vol. 15, Suppl. 7; 1987)
Coronene [191-07-1] (Vol. 32, Suppl. 7; 1987)
Coumarin [91-64-5] (Vol. 77; 2000)
meta-Cresidine [102-50-1] (Vol. 27, Suppl. 7; 1987)
Crotonaldehyde [4170-30-3] (Vol. 63; 1995)
Cyclamates [sodium cyclamate, 139-05-9] (Vol. 73; 1999)
Cyclochlorotine [12663-46-6] (Vol. 10, Suppl. 7; 1987)
Cyclohexanone [108-94-1] (Vol. 47, Vol. 71; 1999)
Cyclopenta[*cd*]pyrene [27208-37-3] (Vol. 32, Suppl. 7; 1987)
D & C Red No. 9 [5160-02-1] (Vol. 57; 1993)
Dapsone [80-08-0] (Vol. 24, Suppl. 7; 1987)
Decabromodiphenyl oxide [1163-19-5] (Vol. 48, Vol. 71; 1999)
Deltamethrin [52918-63-5] (Vol. 53; 1991)
Diacetylaminoazotoluene [83-63-6] (Vol. 8, Suppl. 7; 1987)
Diallate [2303-16-4] (Vol. 30, Suppl. 7; 1987)
1,2-Diamino-4-nitrobenzene [99-56-9] (Vol. 16, Suppl. 7; 1987)
1,4-Diamino-2-nitrobenzene [5307-14-2] (Vol. 57; 1993)
2,5-Diaminotoluene [95-70-5] (Vol. 16, Suppl. 7; 1987)
Diazepam [439-14-5] (Vol. 66; 1996)
Diazomethane [334-88-3] (Vol. 7, Suppl. 7; 1987)
Dibenz[*a,c*]anthracene [215-58-7] (Vol. 32, Suppl. 7; 1987)
Dibenz[*a,j*]anthracene [224-41-9] (Vol. 32, Suppl. 7; 1987)
Dibenzo-*para*-dioxin (Vol. 69; 1997)
Dibenzo[*a,e*]fluoranthene [5385-75-1] (Vol. 32, Suppl. 7; 1987)
Dibenzo[*h,rst*]pentaphene [192-47-2] (Vol. 3, Suppl. 7; 1987)
Dibromoacetonitrile [3252-43-5] (Vol. 52, Vol. 71; 1999)
Dichloroacetic acid [79-43-6] (Vol. 63; 1995)
Dichloroacetonitrile [3018-12-0] (Vol. 52, Vol. 71; 1999)
Dichloroacetylene [7572-29-4] (Vol. 39, Suppl. 7, Vol. 71; 1999)
meta-Dichlorobenzene [541-73-1] (Vol. 73; 1999)
ortho-Dichlorobenzene [95-50-1] (Vol. 73; 1999)
trans-1,4-Dichlorobutene [110-57-6] (Vol. 15, Suppl. 7, Vol. 71; 1999)
2,6-Dichloro-*para*-phenylenediamine [609-20-1] (Vol. 39, Suppl. 7; 1987)
1,2-Dichloropropane [78-87-5] (Vol. 41, Suppl. 7, Vol. 71; 1999)
Dicofol [115-32-2] (Vol. 30, Suppl. 7; 1987)
Didanosine [69655-05-6] (Vol. 76; 2000)
Dieldrin [60-57-1] (Vol. 5, Suppl. 7; 1987)

Diethanolamine [111-42-2] (Vol. 77; 2000)
Di(2-ethylhexyl) adipate [103-23-1] (Vol. 77; 2000)
Di(2-ethylhexyl) phthalate [117-81-7] (Vol. 77; 2000) (NB: Overall evaluation downgraded from 2B to 3 with supporting evidence from other data relevant to carcinogenicity and its mechanisms)
N,N'-Diethylthiourea [105-55-5] (Vol. 79; 2001)
Dihydroxymethylfuratrizine [794-93-4] (Vol. 24, Suppl. 7; 1987)
Dimethoxane [828-00-2] (Vol. 15, Suppl. 7; 1987)
3,3'-Dimethoxybenzidine-4,4'-diisocyanate [91-93-0] (Vol. 39, Suppl. 7; 1987)
para-Dimethylaminoazobenzenediazo sodium sulfonate [140-56-7] (Vol. 8, Suppl. 7; 1987)
4,4'-Dimethylangelicin [22975-76-4] plus ultraviolet A radiation (Suppl. 7; 1987)
4,5'-Dimethylangelicin [4063-41-6] plus ultraviolet A radiation (Suppl. 7; 1987)
N,N-Dimethylaniline [121-69-7] (Vol. 57; 1993)
Dimethylformamide [68-12-2] (Vol. 47; Vol. 71; 1999)
Dimethyl hydrogen phosphite [868-85-9] (Vol. 48, Vol. 71; 1999)
1,4-Dimethylphenanthrene [22349-59-3] (Vol. 32, Suppl. 7; 1987)
1,3-Dinitropyrene [75321-20-9] (Vol. 46; 1989)
3,5-Dinitrotoluene [618-85-9] (Vol. 65; 1996)
Dinitrosopentamethylenetetramine [101-25-7] (Vol. 11, Suppl. 7; 1987)
2,4'-Diphenyldiamine [492-17-1] (Vol. 16, Suppl. 7; 1987)
Disperse Yellow 3 [2832-40-8] (Vol. 48; 1990)
Disulfiram [97-77-8] (Vol. 12, Suppl. 7; 1987)
Dithranol [1143-38-0] (Vol. 13; Suppl. 7; 1987)
Doxefazepam [40762-15-0] (Vol. 66; 1996)
Doxylamine succinate [562-10-7] (Vol. 79; 2001)
Droloxifene [82413-20-5] (Vol. 66; 1996)
Dulcin [150-69-6] (Vol. 12, Suppl. 7; 1987)
Electric fields (extremely low-frequency) (Vol. 80; 2002)
Electric fields (static) (Vol. 80; 2002)
Endrin [72-20-8] (Vol. 5, Suppl. 7; 1987)
Eosin [15086-94-9] (Vol. 15, Suppl. 7; 1987)
3,4-Epoxy-6-methylcyclohexylmethyl-3,4-epoxy-6-methylcyclo-hexane carboxylate [141-37-7] (Vol. 11, Suppl. 7, Vol. 71; 1999)
cis-9,10-Epoxystearic acid [2443-39-2] (Vol. 11, Suppl. 7, Vol. 71; 1999)
Estazolam [29975-16-4] (Vol. 66; 1996)
Ethionamide [536-33-4] (Vol. 13, Suppl. 7; 1987)
Ethylene [74-85-1] (Vol. 60; 1994)
Ethylene sulfide [420-12-2] (Vol. 11, Suppl. 7; 1987)
Ethylenethiourea [96-45-7] (Vol. 79; 2001) (NB: Overall evaluation downgraded from 2B to 3 with supporting evidence from other data relevant to carcinogenicity and its mechanisms)
2-Ethylhexyl acrylate [103-11-7] (Vol. 60; 1994)
Ethyl selenac [5456-28-0] (Vol. 12, Suppl. 7; 1987)
Ethyl tellurac [20941-65-5] (Vol. 12, Suppl. 7; 1987)
Eugenol [97-53-0] (Vol. 36, Suppl. 7; 1987)
Evans blue [314-13-6] (Vol. 8, Suppl. 7; 1987)
Fast Green FCF [2353-45-9] (Vol. 16, Suppl. 7; 1987)
Fenvalerate [51630-58-1] (Vol. 53; 1991)
Ferbam [14484-64-1] (Vol. 12, Suppl. 7; 1987)
Ferric oxide [1309-37-1] (Vol. 1, Suppl. 7; 1987)
Fluometuron [2164-17-2] (Vol. 30, Suppl. 7; 1987)
Fluoranthene [206-44-0] (Vol. 32, Suppl. 7; 1987)
Fluorene [86-73-7] (Vol. 32, Suppl. 7; 1987)
Fluorescent lighting (Vol. 55; 1992)
Fluorides (inorganic, used in drinking-water) (Vol. 27, Suppl. 7; 1987)
5-Fluorouracil [51-21-8] (Vol. 26, Suppl. 7; 1987)
Foreign bodies, implanted in tissues (Vol. 74; 1999)
Metallic chromium or titanium, cobalt-based, chromium-based and titanium-based alloys, stainless steel and depleted uranium
Furazolidone [67-45-8] (Vol. 31, Suppl. 7; 1987)
Furfural [98-01-1] (Vol. 63; 1995)
Furosemide (Frusemide) [54-31-9] (Vol. 50; 1990)
Gemfibrozil [25812-30-0] (Vol. 66; 1996)
Glass filaments (Vol. 43; 1988) [see new evaluation]
Glycidyl oleate [5431-33-4] (Vol. 11, Suppl. 7; 1987)
Glycidyl stearate [7460-84-6] (Vol. 11, Suppl. 7; 1987)
Guinea Green B [4680-78-8] (Vol. 16, Suppl. 7; 1987)
Gyromitrin [16568-02-8] (Vol. 31, Suppl. 7; 1987)
Haematite [1317-60-8] (Vol. 1, Suppl. 7; 1987)
HC Blue No. 2 [33229-34-4] (Vol. 57; 1993)
HC Red No. 3 [2871-01-4] (Vol. 57; 1993)
HC Yellow No. 4 [59820-43-8] (Vol. 57; 1993)
Hepatitis D virus (Vol. 59; 1994)
Hexachlorobutadiene [87-68-3] (Vol. 73; 1999)
Hexachlorophene [70-30-4] (Vol. 20, Suppl. 7; 1987)
Human T-cell lymphotropic virus type II (Vol. 67; 1996)
Hycanthone mesylate [23255-93-8] (Vol. 13, Suppl. 7; 1987)
Hydralazine [86-54-4] (Vol. 24, Suppl. 7; 1987)
Hydrochloric acid [7647-01-0] (Vol. 54; 1992)
Hydrochlorothiazide [58-93-5] (Vol. 50; 1990)
Hydrogen peroxide [7722-84-1] (Vol. 36, Suppl. 7, Vol. 71; 1999)
Hydroquinone [123-31-9] (Vol. 15, Suppl. 7, Vol. 71; 1999)
4-Hydroxyazobenzene [1689-82-3] (Vol. 8, Suppl. 7; 1987)

8-Hydroxyquinoline [148-24-3] (Vol. 13, Suppl. 7; 1987)
Hydroxysenkirkine [26782-43-4] (Vol. 10, Suppl. 7; 1987)
Hydroxyurea [127-07-1] (Vol. 76; 2000)
Hypochlorite salts (Vol. 52; 1991)
Iron-dextrin complex [9004-51-7] (Vol. 2, Suppl. 7; 1987)
Iron sorbitol-citric acid complex [1338-16-5] (Vol. 2, Suppl. 7; 1987)
Isatidine [15503-86-3] (Vol. 10, Suppl. 7; 1987)
Isonicotinic acid hydrazide (Isoniazid) [54-85-3] (Vol. 4, Suppl. 7; 1987)
Isophosphamide [3778-73-2] (Vol. 26, Suppl. 7; 1987)
Isopropanol [67-63-0] (Vol. 15, Suppl. 7, Vol. 71; 1999)
Isopropyl oils (Vol. 15, Suppl. 7, Vol. 71; 1999)
Isosafrole [120-58-1] (Vol. 10, Suppl. 7; 1987)
Jacobine [6870-67-3] (Vol. 10, Suppl. 7; 1987)
Kaempferol [520-18-3] (Vol. 31, Suppl. 7; 1987)
Kojic acid [501-30-4] (Vol. 79; 2001)
Lauroyl peroxide [105-74-8] (Vol. 36, Suppl. 7, Vol. 71; 1999)
Lead, organo [75-74-1], [78-00-2] (Vol. 23, Suppl. 7; 1987)
Light Green SF [5141-20-8] (Vol. 16, Suppl. 7; 1987)
d-Limonene [5989-27-5] (Vol. 73; 1999)
(NB: Overall evaluation downgraded from 2B to 3 with supporting evidence from other data relevant to carcinogenicity and its mechanisms)
Luteoskyrin [21884-44-6] (Vol. 10, Suppl. 7; 1987)
Magnetic fields (static) (Vol. 80; 2002)
Malathion [121-75-5] (Vol. 30, Suppl. 7; 1987)
Maleic hydrazide [123-33-1] (Vol. 4, Suppl. 7; 1987)
Malonaldehyde [542-78-9] (Vol. 36, Suppl. 7, Vol. 71; 1999)
Maneb [12427-38-2] (Vol. 12, Suppl. 7; 1987)
Mannomustine dihydrochloride [551-74-6] (Vol. 9, Suppl. 7; 1987)
Medphalan [13045-94-8] (Vol. 9, Suppl. 7; 1987)
Melamine [108-78-1] (Vol. 73; 1999)
(NB: Overall evaluation downgraded from 2B to 3 with supporting evidence from other data relevant to carcinogenicity and its mechanisms)
6-Mercaptopurine [50-44-2] (Vol. 26, Suppl. 7; 1987)
Mercury [7439-97-6] and inorganic mercury compounds (Vol. 58; 1993)
Metabisulfites (Vol. 54; 1992)
Methimazole [60-56-0] (Vol. 79; 2001)
Methotrexate [59-05-2] (Vol. 26, Suppl. 7; 1987)
Methoxychlor [72-43-5] (Vol. 20, Suppl. 7; 1987)
Methyl acrylate [96-33-3] (Vol. 39, Suppl. 7, Vol. 71; 1999)
5-Methylangelicin [73459-03-7] plus ultraviolet A radiation (Suppl. 7; 1987)
Methyl bromide [74-83-9] (Vol. 41, Suppl. 7, Vol. 71; 1999)
Methyl *tert*-butyl ether [1634-04-4] (Vol. 73; 1999)
Methyl carbamate [598-55-0] (Vol. 12, Suppl. 7; 1987)
Methyl chloride [74-87-3] (Vol. 41, Suppl. 7, Vol. 71; 1999)
1-Methylchrysene [3351-28-8] (Vol. 32, Suppl. 7; 1987)
2-Methylchrysene [3351-32-4] (Vol. 32, Suppl. 7; 1987)
3-Methylchrysene [3351-31-3] (Vol. 32, Suppl. 7; 1987)
4-Methylchrysene [3351-30-2] (Vol. 32, Suppl. 7; 1987)
6-Methylchrysene [1705-85-7] (Vol. 32, Suppl. 7; 1987)
N-Methyl-*N*,4-dinitrosoaniline [99-80-9] (Vol. 1, Suppl. 7; 1987)
4,4′-Methylene bis(*N*,*N*-dimethyl)benzenamine [101-61-1] (Vol. 27, Suppl. 7; 1987)
4,4′-Methylenediphenyl diisocyanate [101-68-8] (Vol. 19, Suppl. 7, Vol. 71; 1999)
2-Methylfluoranthene [33543-31-6] (Vol. 32, Suppl. 7; 1987)
3-Methylfluoranthene [1706-01-0] (Vol. 32, Suppl. 7; 1987)
Methylglyoxal [78-98-8] (Vol. 51; 1991)
Methyl iodide [74-88-4] (Vol. 41, Suppl. 7, Vol. 71; 1999)
Methyl methacrylate [80-62-6] (Vol. 60; 1994)
N-Methylolacrylamide [90456-67-0] (Vol. 60; 1994)
Methyl parathion [298-00-0] (Vol. 30, Suppl. 7; 1987)
1-Methylphenanthrene [832-69-9] (Vol. 32, Suppl. 7; 1987)
7-Methylpyrido[3,4-*c*]psoralen [85878-63-3] (Vol. 40, Suppl. 7; 1987)
Methyl red [493-52-7] (Vol. 8, Suppl. 7; 1987)
Methyl selenac [144-34-3] (Vol. 12, Suppl. 7; 1987)
Modacrylic fibers (Vol. 19, Suppl. 7; 1987)
Monuron [150-68-5] (Vol. 53; 1991)
Morpholine [110-91-8] (Vol. 47, Vol. 71; 1999)
Musk ambrette [83-66-9] (Vol. 65; 1996)
Musk xylene [81-15-2] (Vol. 65; 1996)
1,5-Naphthalenediamine [2243-62-1] (Vol. 27, Suppl. 7; 1987)
1,5-Naphthalene diisocyanate [3173-72-6] (Vol. 19, Suppl. 7, Vol. 71; 1999)

1-Naphthylamine [134-32-7] (Vol. 4, Suppl. 7; 1987)
1-Naphthylthiourea (ANTU) [86-88-4] (Vol. 30, Suppl. 7; 1987)
Nithiazide [139-94-6] (Vol. 31, Suppl. 7; 1987)
5-Nitro-*ortho*-anisidine [99-59-2] (Vol. 27, Suppl. 7; 1987)
9-Nitroanthracene [602-60-8] (Vol. 33, Suppl. 7; 1987)
7-Nitrobenz[*a*]anthracene [20268-51-3] (Vol. 46; 1989)
6-Nitrobenzo[*a*]pyrene [63041-90-7] (Vol. 46; 1989)
4-Nitrobiphenyl [92-93-3] (Vol. 4, Suppl. 7; 1987)
3-Nitrofluoranthene [892-21-7] (Vol. 33, Suppl. 7; 1987)
Nitrofural (Nitrofurazone) [59-87-0] (Vol. 50; 1990)
Nitrofurantoin [67-20-9] (Vol. 50; 1990)
1-Nitronaphthalene [86-57-7] (Vol. 46; 1989)
2-Nitronaphthalene [581-89-5] (Vol. 46; 1989)
3-Nitroperylene [20589-63-3] (Vol. 46; 1989)
2-Nitropyrene [789-07-1] (Vol. 46; 1989)
N′-Nitrosoanabasine [37620-20-5] (Vol. 37, Suppl. 7; 1987)
N′-Nitrosoanatabine [71267-22-6] (Vol. 37, Suppl. 7; 1987)
N-Nitrosodiphenylamine [86-30-6] (Vol. 27, Suppl. 7; 1987)
para-Nitrosodiphenylamine [156-10-5] (Vol. 27, Suppl. 7; 1987)
N-Nitrosofolic acid [29291-35-8] (Vol. 17, Suppl. 7; 1987)
N-Nitrosoguvacine [55557-01-2] (Vol. 37, Suppl. 7; 1987)
N-Nitrosoguvacoline [55557-02-3] (Vol. 37, Suppl. 7; 1987)
N-Nitrosohydroxyproline [30310-80-6] (Vol. 17, Suppl. 7; 1987)
3-(*N*-Nitrosomethylamino)propionaldehyde [85502-23-4] (Vol. 37, Suppl. 7; 1987)
4-(*N*-Nitrosomethylamino)-4-(3-pyridyl)-1-butanal (NNA) [64091-90-3] (Vol. 37, Suppl. 7; 1987)
N-Nitrosoproline [7519-36-0] (Vol. 17, Suppl. 7; 1987)
Nitrotoluenes [88-72-2; 99-08-1; 99-99-0] (Vol. 65; 1996)
5-Nitro-*ortho*-toluidine [99-55-8] (Vol. 48; 1990)
Nitrovin [804-36-4] (Vol. 31, Suppl. 7; 1987)
Nylon 6 [25038-54-4] (Vol. 19, Suppl. 7; 1987)
Oestradiol mustard [22966-79-6] (Vol. 9, Suppl. 7; 1987)
Opisthorchis felineus (infection with) (Vol. 61; 1994)
Orange I [523-44-4] (Vol. 8, Suppl. 7; 1987)
Orange G [1936-15-8] (Vol. 8, Suppl. 7; 1987)
Oxyphenbutazone [129-20-4] (Vol. 13, Suppl. 7; 1987)
Palygorskite (attapulgite) [12174-11-7] (short fibers, <5 μm) (Vol. 68; 1997)
Paracetamol (Acetaminophen) [103-90-2] (Vol. 73; 1999)
Parasorbic acid [10048-32-5] (Vol. 10, Suppl. 7; 1987)
Parathion [56-38-2] (Vol. 30, Suppl. 7; 1987)
Patulin [149-29-1] (Vol. 40, Suppl. 7; 1987)
Penicillic acid [90-65-3] (Vol. 10, Suppl. 7; 1987)
Pentachloroethane [76-01-7] (Vol. 41, Suppl. 7, Vol. 71; 1999)
Permethrin [52645-53-1] (Vol. 53; 1991)
Perylene [198-55-0] (Vol. 32, Suppl. 7; 1987)
Petasitenine [60102-37-6] (Vol. 31, Suppl. 7; 1987)
Phenanthrene [85-01-8] (Vol. 32, Suppl. 7; 1987)
Phenelzine sulfate [156-51-4] (Vol. 24, Suppl. 7; 1987)
Phenicarbazide [103-03-7] (Vol. 12, Suppl. 7; 1987)
Phenol [108-95-2] (Vol. 47, Vol. 71; 1999)
Phenylbutazone [50-33-9] (Vol. 13, Suppl. 7; 1987)
meta-Phenylenediamine [108-45-2] (Vol. 16, Suppl. 7; 1987)
para-Phenylenediamine [106-50-3] (Vol. 16, Suppl. 7; 1987)
N-Phenyl-2-naphthylamine [135-88-6] (Vol. 16, Suppl. 7; 1987)
ortho-Phenylphenol [90-43-7] (Vol. 73; 1999)
Picloram [1918-02-1] (Vol. 53; 1991)
Piperonyl butoxide [51-03-6] (Vol. 30, Suppl. 7; 1987)
Polyacrylic acid [9003-01-4] (Vol. 19, Suppl. 7; 1987)
Polychlorinated dibenzo-*para*-dioxins (other than 2,3,7,8-tetrachlorodibenzo-*para*-dioxin) (Vol. 69; 1997)
Polychlorinated dibenzofurans (Vol. 69; 1997)
Polychloroprene [9010-98-4] (Vol. 19, Suppl. 7; 1987)
Polyethylene [9002-88-4] (Vol. 19, Suppl. 7; 1987)
Polymethylene polyphenyl isocyanate [9016-87-9] (Vol. 19, Suppl. 7; 1987)
Polymethyl methacrylate [9011-14-7] (Vol. 19, Suppl. 7; 1987)
Polypropylene [9003-07-0] (Vol. 19, Suppl. 7; 1987)
Polystyrene [9003-53-6] (Vol. 19, Suppl. 7; 1987)
Polytetrafluoroethylene [9002-84-0] (Vol. 19, Suppl. 7; 1987)

Polyurethane foams [9009-54-5] (Vol. 19, Suppl. 7; 1987)
Polyvinyl acetate [9003-20-7] (Vol. 19, Suppl. 7; 1987)
Polyvinyl alcohol [9002-89-5] (Vol. 19, Suppl. 7; 1987)
Polyvinyl chloride [9002-86-2] (Vol. 19, Suppl. 7; 1987)
Polyvinyl pyrrolidone [9003-39-8] (Vol. 19, Suppl. 7, Vol. 71; 1999)
Ponceau SX [4548-53-2] (Vol. 8, Suppl. 7; 1987)
Potassium bis(2-hydroxyethyl)dithiocarbamate [23746-34-1] (Vol. 12, Suppl. 7; 1987)
Prazepam [2955-38-6] (Vol. 66; 1996)
Prednimustine [29069-24-7] (Vol. 50; 1990)
Prednisone [53-03-2] (Vol. 26, Suppl. 7; 1987)
Proflavine salts (Vol. 24, Suppl. 7; 1987)
Pronetalol hydrochloride [51-02-5] (Vol. 13, Suppl. 7; 1987)
Propham [122-42-9] (Vol. 12, Suppl. 7; 1987)
n-Propyl carbamate [627-12-3] (Vol. 12, Suppl. 7; 1987)
Propylene [115-07-1] (Vol. 60; 1994)
Ptaquiloside [87625-62-5] (Vol. 40, Suppl. 7; 1987)
Pyrene [129-00-0] (Vol. 32, Suppl. 7; 1987)
Pyridine [110-86-1] (Vol. 77; 2000)
Pyrido[3,4-*c*]psoralen [85878-62-2] (Vol. 40, Suppl. 7; 1987)
Pyrimethamine [58-14-0] (Vol. 13, Suppl. 7; 1987)
Quercetin [117-39-5] (Vol. 73; 1999)
para-Quinone [106-51-4] (Vol. 15, Suppl. 7, Vol. 71; 1999)
Quintozene (Pentachloronitrobenzene) [82-68-8] (Vol. 5, Suppl. 7; 1987)
Reserpine [50-55-5] (Vol. 24, Suppl. 7; 1987)
Resorcinol [108-46-3] (Vol. 15, Suppl. 7, Vol. 71, 1999)
Retrorsine [480-54-6] (Vol. 10, Suppl. 7; 1987)
Rhodamine B [81-88-9] (Vol. 16, Suppl. 7; 1987)
Rhodamine 6G [989-38-8] (Vol. 16, Suppl. 7; 1987)
Riddelliine [23246-96-0] (Vol. 10, Suppl. 7; 1987)
Rifampicin [13292-46-1] (Vol. 24, Suppl. 7; 1987)
Ripazepam [26308-28-1] (Vol. 66; 1996)
Rugulosin [23537-16-8] (Vol. 40, Suppl. 7; 1987)
Saccharated iron oxide [8047-67-4] (Vol. 2, Suppl. 7; 1987)
Saccharin [81-07-2] and its salts (Vol. 73; 1999)
(NB: Overall evaluation downgraded from 2B to 3 with supporting evidence from other data relevant to carcinogenicity and its mechanisms)
Scarlet Red [85-83-6] (Vol. 8, Suppl. 7; 1987)
Schistosoma mansoni (infection with) (Vol. 61; 1994)
Selenium [7782-49-2] and selenium compounds (Vol. 9, Suppl. 7; 1987)
Semicarbazide hydrochloride [563-41-7] (Vol. 12, Suppl. 7; 1987)
Seneciphylline [480-81-9] (Vol. 10, Suppl. 7; 1987)
Senkirkine [2318-18-5] (Vol. 31, Suppl. 7; 1987)
Sepiolite [15501-74-3] (Vol. 68; 1997)
Shikimic acid [138-59-0] (Vol. 40, Suppl. 7; 1987)
Silica [7631-86-9], amorphous (Vol. 68; 1997)
Simazine [122-34-9] (Vol. 73; 1999)
Sodium chlorite [7758-19-2] (Vol. 52; 1991)
Sodium diethyldithiocarbamate [148-18-5] (Vol. 12, Suppl. 7; 1987)
Spironolactone [52-01-7] (Vol. 79; 2001)
Styrene-acrylonitrile copolymers [9003-54-7] (Vol. 19, Suppl. 7; 1987)
Styrene-butadiene copolymers [9003-55-8] (Vol. 19, Suppl. 7; 1987)
Succinic anhydride [108-30-5] (Vol. 15, Suppl. 7; 1987)
Sudan I [842-07-9] (Vol. 8, Suppl. 7; 1987)
Sudan II [3118-97-6] (Vol. 8, Suppl. 7; 1987)
Sudan III [85-86-9] (Vol. 8, Suppl. 7; 1987)
Sudan Brown RR [6416-57-5] (Vol. 8, Suppl. 7; 1987)
Sudan Red 7B [6368-72-5] (Vol. 8, Suppl. 7; 1987)
Sulfafurazole (Sulfisoxazole) [127-69-5] (Vol. 24, Suppl. 7; 1987)
Sulfamethazine [57-68-1] (Vol. 79; 2001)
(NB: Overall evaluation downgraded from 2B to 3 with supporting evidence from other data relevant to carcinogenicity and its mechanisms)
Sulfamethoxazole [723-46-6] (Vol. 79; 2001)
Sulfites (Vol. 54; 1992)
Sulfur dioxide [7446-09-5] (Vol. 54; 1992)
Sunset Yellow FCF [2783-94-0] (Vol. 8, Suppl. 7; 1987)
Surgical implants (Vol. 74; 1999)
  Orthopaedic implants and devices, of complex composition
  Cardiac pacemakers
  Dental materials
  Ceramic materials
Surgical implants, female breast reconstruction, silicone (Vol. 74; 1999)
Symphytine [22571-95-5] (Vol. 31, Suppl. 7; 1987)
Talc [14807-96-6], not containing asbestiform fibers (Vol. 42, Suppl. 7; 1987)
Tannic acid [1401-55-4] and tannins (Vol. 10, Suppl. 7; 1987)
Temazepam [846-50-4] (Vol. 66; 1996)
2,2′,5,5′-Tetrachlorobenzidine [15721-02-5] (Vol. 27, Suppl. 7; 1987)

1,1,1,2-Tetrachloroethane [630-20-6] (Vol. 41, Suppl. 7, Vol. 71; 1999)
1,1,2,2-Tetrachloroethane [79-34-5] (Vol. 20, Suppl. 7, Vol. 71; 1999)
Tetrachlorvinphos [22248-79-9] (Vol. 30, Suppl. 7; 1987)
Tetrakis(hydroxymethyl)phosphonium salts (Vol. 48, Vol. 71; 1999)
Theobromine [83-67-0] (Vol. 51; 1991)
Theophylline [58-55-9] (Vol. 51; 1991)
Thiourea [62-56-6] (Vol. 79; 2001)
Thiram [137-26-8] (Vol. 53; 1991)
Titanium dioxide [13463-67-7] (Vol. 47; 1989)
Toluene [108-88-3] (Vol. 47, Vol. 71; 1999)
Toremifene [89778-26-7] (Vol. 66; 1996)
Toxins derived from *Fusarium graminearum*, *F. culmorum,* and *F. crookwellense* (Vol. 56; 1993)
Toxins derived from *Fusarium sporotrichioides* (Vol. 56; 1993)
Trichlorfon [52-68-6] (Vol. 30, Suppl. 7; 1987)
Trichloroacetic acid [76-03-9] (Vol. 63; 1995)
Trichloroacetonitrile [545-06-2] (Vol. 52, Vol. 71; 1999)
1,1,1-Trichloroethane [71-55-6] (Vol. 20, Suppl. 7, Vol. 71; 1999)
1,1,2-Trichloroethane [79-00-5] (Vol. 52, Vol. 71; 1999)
Triethanolamine [102-71-6] (Vol. 77; 2000)
Triethylene glycol diglycidyl ether [1954-28-5] (Vol. 11, Suppl. 7, Vol. 71; 1999)
Trifluralin [1582-09-8] (Vol. 53; 1991)
4,4′,6-Trimethylangelicin [90370-29-9] plus ultraviolet A radiation (Suppl. 7; 1987)
2,4,5-Trimethylaniline [137-17-7] (Vol. 27, Suppl. 7; 1987)
2,4,6-Trimethylaniline [88-05-1] (Vol. 27, Suppl. 7; 1987)
4,5′,8-Trimethylpsoralen [3902-71-4] (Vol. 40, Suppl. 7; 1987)
2,4,6-Trinitrotoluene [118-96-7] (Vol. 65; 1996)
Triphenylene [217-59-4] (Vol. 32, Suppl. 7; 1987)
Tris(aziridinyl)-*para*-benzoquinone (Triaziquone) [68-76-8] (Vol. 9, Suppl. 7; 1987)
Tris(1-aziridinyl)phosphine oxide [545-55-1] (Vol. 9, Suppl. 7; 1987)
2,4,6-Tris(1-aziridinyl)-*s*-triazine [51-18-3] (Vol. 9, Suppl. 7; 1987)
Tris(2-chloroethyl) phosphate [115-96-8] (Vol. 48, Vol. 71; 1999)
1,2,3-Tris(chloromethoxy)propane [38571-73-2] (Vol. 15, Suppl. 7, Vol. 71; 1999)
Tris(2-methyl-1-aziridinyl)phosphine oxide [57-39-6] (Vol. 9, Suppl. 7; 1987)
Vat Yellow 4 [128-66-5] (Vol. 48; 1990)
Vinblastine sulfate [143-67-9] (Vol. 26, Suppl. 7; 1987)
Vincristine sulfate [2068-78-2] (Vol. 26, Suppl. 7; 1987)
Vinyl chloride-vinyl acetate copolymers [9003-22-9] (Vol. 19, Suppl. 7; 1987)
Vinylidene chloride [75-35-4] (Vol. 39, Suppl. 7, Vol. 71; 1999)
Vinylidene chloride-vinyl chloride copolymers [9011-06-7] (Vol. 19, Suppl. 7; 1987)
Vinylidene fluoride [75-38-7] (Vol. 39, Suppl. 7, Vol. 71; 1999)
N-Vinyl-2-pyrrolidone [88-12-0] (Vol. 19, Suppl. 7, Vol. 71; 1999)
Vinyl toluene [25013-15-4] (Vol. 60; 1994)
Vitamin K [12001-79-5] substances (Vol. 76; 2000)
Wollastonite [13983-17-0] (Vol. 68; 1997)
Xylenes [1330-20-7] (Vol. 47, Vol. 71; 1999)
2,4-Xylidine [95-68-1] (Vol. 16, Suppl. 7; 1987)
2,5-Xylidine [95-78-3] (Vol. 16, Suppl. 7; 1987)
Yellow AB [85-84-7] (Vol. 8, Suppl. 7; 1987)
Yellow OB [131-79-3] (Vol. 8, Suppl. 7; 1987)
Zectran [315-18-4] (Vol. 12, Suppl. 7; 1987)
Zeolites [1318-02-1] other than erionite (clinoptilolite, phillipsite, mordenite, nonfibrous Japanese zeolite, synthetic zeolites) (Vol. 68; 1997)
Zineb [12122-67-7] (Vol. 12, Suppl. 7; 1987)
Ziram [137-30-4] (Vol. 53; 1991)

Mixtures

Betel quid, without tobacco (Vol. 37, Suppl. 7; 1987)
Bitumens [8052-42-4], steam-refined, cracking-residue, and air-refined (Vol. 35, Suppl. 7; 1987)
Crude oil [8002-05-9] (Vol. 45; 1989)
Diesel fuels, distillate (light) (Vol. 45; 1989)
Fuel oils, distillate (light) (Vol. 45; 1989)
Jet fuel (Vol. 45; 1989)
Mate (Vol. 51; 1991)
Mineral oils, highly-refined (Vol. 33, Suppl. 7; 1987)
Petroleum solvents (Vol. 47; 1989)
Printing inks (Vol. 65; 1996)
Tea (Vol. 51; 1991)
Terpene polychlorinates (Strobane) [8001-50-1] (Vol. 5, Suppl. 7; 1987)

Exposure Circumstances

Flat-glass and specialty glass (manufacture of) (Vol. 58; 1993)

Hair coloring products (personal use of) (Vol. 57; 1993)
Leather goods manufacture (Vol. 25, Suppl. 7; 1987)
Leather tanning and processing (Vol. 25, Suppl. 7; 1987)
Lumber and sawmill industries (including logging) (Vol. 25, Suppl. 7; 1987)
Paint manufacture (occupational exposure in) (Vol. 47; 1989)
Pulp and paper manufacture (Vol. 25, Suppl. 7; 1987)

Group 4—Probably Not Carcinogenic to Humans (One Agent)

Caprolactam [105-60-2] (Vol. 39, Suppl. 7, Vol. 71; 1998)

Source: Reprinted from World Health Organization International Agency for Research on Cancer. *IARC Monographs on the Evaluation of Carcinogenic Risks to Humans: Lists of IARC Evaluations*. Lyon, France: IARC, March 8, 2002.

Appendix E

Lists of Carcinogens of the National Toxicology Program (NTP)

Table E.1 lists the names and synonyms of carcinogens listed in the ninth National Toxicology Program (NTP) report.

For more information on the Ninth Report on Carcinogens, including how to order a hard copy of the report or access it on the Web, visit the NTP Report on Carcinogens Homepage at *http://ntp-server.niehs.nih.gov*.

TABLE E.1. *Names and synonyms of carcinogens listed in the 9th report on carcinogens*

CASRN	Name or synonym	Listing in the 9th RoC[a]	First listed[b]	Page No. III-
II.A. Known to be human carcinogens: This list includes agents, substances, mixtures, and exposure circumstances that are known to be carcinogenic in humans. These carcinogens are profiled in Section III.A.				
1402-68-2	Aflatoxins	K	1	1
	Alcoholic beverage consumption	**K**	**9**	**2**
92-67-1	4-Aminobiphenyl (4-aminodiphenyl)	K	1	3
91-59-8	2-Aminonaphthalene (see 2-naphthylamine)	K	1	41
	Analgesic mixtures containing phenacetin	K	4	4
	Arsenic compounds, inorganic	K	1	4
1332-21-4	Asbestos	K	1	6
446-86-6	Azathioprine	K	4	9
71-43-2	Benzene	K	1	10
92-87-5	Benzidine	K	1	11
542-88-1	bis(Chloromethyl) ether	K	1	13
55-98-1	Busulfan (see 1,4-butanediol dimethylsulfonate)	K	4	17
106-99-0	**1,3-Butadiene**	**K**	**5[c]** **9[d]**	**14**
55-98-1	1,4-Butanediol dimethylsulfonate (Myleran; busulfan)	K	4	17
7440-43-9	**Cadmium (under cadmium and cadmium compounds)**	**K**	**1[c]** **9[d]**	**17**
10108-64-2	**Cadmium chloride (under cadmium and cadmium compounds)**	**K**	**1[c]** **9[d]**	**17**
1306-19-0	**Cadmium oxide (under cadmium and cadmium compounds)**	**K**	**1[c]** **9[d]**	**17**
10124-36-4	**Cadmium sulfate (under cadmium and cadmium compounds)**	**K**	**1[c]** **9[d]**	**17**
1306-23-6	**Cadmium sulfide (under cadmium and cadmium compounds)**	**K**	**1[c]** **9[d]**	**17**
305-03-3	Chlorambucil	K	2	21
13909-09-6	1-(2-chloroethyl)-3-(4-methylcyclohexyl)-1-nitrosourea (MeCCNU)	K	6	22

CASRN, Chemical Abstracts Service Registry Number(s).

Continued on next page

TABLE E.1. *Continued*

CASRN	Name or synonym	Listing in the 9th RoC[a]	First listed[b]	Page No. III-
107-30-2	Chloromethyl methyl ether	K	1	13
	Chromium hexavalent compounds (under chromium hexavalent compounds)	K	1	22
8007-45-2	Coal tar (under tars and mineral oils)	K	1	54
	Coke oven emissions	K	1	24
8001-58-9	Creosote (coal) (under tars and mineral oils)	K	4	54
8021-39-4	Creosote (wood) (under tars and mineral oils)	K	4	54
14464-46-1	**Cristobalite [under silica, crystalline (respirable size)]**	**K**	**6[c]** **9[d]**	**43**
50-18-0	Cyclophosphamide	K	1	26
59865-13-3	Cyclosporin A (cyclosporine A; cyclosporin)	K	8	27
56-53-1	Diethylstilbestrol	K	1	28
1937-37-7	**Direct black 38**	**K**	**3[c]** **9[d]**	**31**
2602-46-2	**Direct blue 6**	**K**	**3[c]** **9[d]**	**32**
	Dyes that metabolize to benzidine	**K**	**9**	**29**
	Environmental tobacco smoke	**K**	**9**	**33**
66733-21-9	Erionite	K	1	34
75-21-8	**Ethylene oxide**	**K**	**2[c]** **9[d]**	**35**
7758-97-6	Lead chromate (under chromium hexavalent compounds)	K	1	22
13909-09-6	MeCCNU [see 1-(2-chloroethyl)-3-(4-methylhexyl)-1-nitrosourea]	K	6	22
148-82-3	Melphalan	K	1	39
298-81-7	Methoxsalen [under methoxsalen with ultraviolet A therapy (PUVA)] (methoxsalen not carcinogenic alone)	K	4	40
	Mineral oils	K	1	54
505-60-2	Mustard gas	K	1	41
55-98-1	Myleran (see 1,4-butanediol dimethylsulfonate)	K	4	17
91-59-8	2-Naphthylamine (β-naphthylamine; 2-aminonaphthalene)	K	1	41
7280-37-7	Piperazine estrone sulfate (under conjugated estrogens)	K	4	25
14808-60-7	**Quartz [under silica, crystalline (respirable size)]**	**K**	**6[c]** **9[d]**	**43**
10043-92-2	Radon	K	7	42
	Silica, crystalline (respirable size)	**K**	**6[c]** **9[d]**	**43**
	Smokeless tobacco	**K**	**9**	**46**
16680-47-0	Sodium equilin sulfate (under conjugated estrogens)	K	4	25
438-67-5	Sodium estrone sulfate (under conjugated estrogens)	K	5	25
	Solar radiation and exposure to sunlamps and sunbeds	**K**	**9**	**48**
	Soots	K	1	50
	Strong inorganic acid mists containing sulfuric acid	**K**	**9**	**51**
7789-06-2	Strontium chromate (under chromium hexavalent compounds)	K	1	22
10540-29-1	**Tamoxifen**	**K**	**9**	**53**
	Tars	K	1	54
52-24-4	Thiotepa [in 7th ARC as tris(1-aziridinyl)phosphine sulfide]	K	2[c] 8[d]	58
1314-20-1	Thorium dioxide	K	2	59
	Tobacco smoking	**K**	**9**	**60**
15468-32-3	**Tridymite [under silica, crystalline (respirable size)]**	**K**	**6[c]** **9[d]**	**43**
52-24-4	Tris(1-aziridinyl)phosphine sulfide (thiotepa)	K	2[c] 8[d]	58
75-01-4	Vinyl chloride	K	1	61
13530-65-9	Zinc chromate (under chromium hexavalent compounds)	K	1	22

TABLE E.1. *Continued*

II.B. Reasonably anticipated to be human carcinogens: This list includes agents, substances, mixtures, and exposure circumstances that are reasonably anticipated to be human carcinogens. Theses carcinogens are profiled in Section III.B.

CASRN	Name or synonym	Listing in the 9th RoC[a]	First listed[b]	Page No. III-
75-07-0	Acetaldehyde	R	6	65
53-96-3	2-Acetylaminofluorene	R	2	66
79-06-1	Acrylamide	R	6	67
107-13-1	Acrylonitrile	R	2	69
25316-40-9	Adriamycin (doxorubicin hydrochloride)	R	4	70
117-79-3	2-Aminoanthraquinone	R	3	71
97-56-3	*o*-Aminoazotoluene	R	5	72
82-28-0	1-Amino-2-methylanthraquinone	R	3	73
61-82-5	Amitrole	R	2	73
134-29-2	*o*-Anisidine hydrochloride	R	3	74
	Aroclor (under polychlorinated biphenyls)	R	2	186
11097-69-1	Aroclor 1254 (under polychlorinated biphenyls)	R	2	186
11096-82-5	Aroclor 1260 (under polychlorinated biphenyls)	R	3	186
320-67-2	Azacitidine (5-azacytidine)	R	8	75
154-93-8	BCNU [see bis(chloroethyl) nitrosourea]	R	4	78
56-55-3	Benz[*a*]anthracene (under polycyclic aromatic hydrocarbons, 15 listings)	R	2	187
205-99-2	Benzo[*b*]fluoranthene (under polycyclic aromatic hydrocarbons, 15 listings)	R	2	187
205-82-3	Benzo[*j*]fluoranthene (under polycyclic aromatic hydrocarbons, 15 listings)	R	2	187
207-08-9	Benzo[*k*]fluoranthene (under polycyclic aromatic hydrocarbons, 15 listings)	R	2	187
50-32-8	Benzo[*a*]pyrene (under polycyclic aromatic hydrocarbons, 15 listings)	R	2	187
98-07-7	Benzotrichloride	R	4	76
12770-50-2	Beryllium aluminum alloy (under beryllium and certain beryllium compounds)	R	2	76
7787-47-5	Beryllium chloride (under beryllium and certain beryllium compounds)	R	2	76
7787-49-7	Beryllium fluoride (under beryllium and certain beryllium compounds)	R	2	76
13327-32-7	Beryllium hydroxide (under beryllium and certain beryllium compounds)	R	2	76
1304-56-9	Beryllium oxide (under beryllium and certain beryllium compounds)	R	2	76
13598-15-7	Beryllium phosphate (under beryllium and certain beryllium compounds)	R	2	76
13510-49-1 7787-56-6	Beryllium sulfate and its tetrahydrate (under beryllium and certain beryllium compounds)	R	2	76
39413-47-3	Beryllium zinc silicate (under beryllium and certain beryllium compounds)	R	2	76
1302-52-9	Beryl ore (under beryllium and certain beryllium compounds)	R	2	76
154-93-8	bis(Chloroethyl) nitrosourea (BCNU)	R	4	78
90-94-8	bis(dimethylamino)benzophenone (see Michler's ketone)	R	3	153
117-81-7	bis(2-ethylhexyl) phthalate [see di(2-ethylhexyl) phthalate]	R	3	113
75-27-4	Bromodichloromethane	R	6	79
25013-16-5	Butylated hydroxyanisole (BHA)	R	6	80
56-23-5	Carbon tetrachloride	R	2	82
13010-47-4	CCNU [see 1-(2-chloroethyl)-3-cyclohexyl-1-nitrosourea]	R	4	86
	Ceramic fibers	R	7	83
143-50-0	Chlordecone (see Kepone)	R	2	144
115-28-6	Chlorendic acid	R	5	84

Continued on next page

TABLE E.1. *Continued*

CASRN	Name or synonym	Listing in the 9th RoC[a]	First listed[b]	Page No. III-
108171-26-2	Chlorinated paraffins (C_{12}, 60% chlorine)	R	5	85
13010-47-4	1-(2-chloroethyl)-3-cyclohexyl-1-nitrosourea (CCNU)	R	4	86
67-66-3	Chloroform	R	2	86
563-47-3	3-Chloro-2-methylpropene	R	5	88
95-83-0	4-Chloro-*o*-phenylenediamine	R	4	89
126-99-8	**Chloroprene**	**R**	**9**	**89**
95-69-2	*p*-Chloro-*o*-toluidine	R	8	90
3165-93-3	*p*-Chloro-*o*-toluidine hydrochloride	R	8	90
54749-90-5	Chlorozotocin	R	8	92
569-61-9	C.I. basic red 9 monohydrochloride	R	5	93
15663-27-1	Cisplatin	R	6	93
120-71-8	*p*-Cresidine	R	2	94
135-20-6	Cupferron	R	3	95
4342-03-4	Dacarbazine	R	4	95
117-10-2	Danthron (1,8-dihydroxyanthraquinone)	R	8	96
50-29-3	DDT (dichlorodiphenyltrichloroethane)	R	4	97
13654-09-6	Decabromobiphenyl (under polybrominated biphenyls)	R	3	185
117-81-7	DEHP [see di(2-ethylhexyl) phthalate]	R	3	113
55-18-5	DEN (See *N*-nitrosodiethylamine)	R	2	167
39156-41-7	2,4-diaminoanisole sulfate	R	3	98
101-80-4	Diaminodiphenyl ether (see 4,4′-oxydianilinc)	R	5	179
95-80-7	2,4-Diaminotoluene	R	2	99
226-36-8	Dibenz[*a,h*]acridine (under polycyclic aromatic hydrocarbons, 15 listings)	R	2	187
224-42-0	Dibenz[*a,j*]acridine (under polycyclic aromatic hydrocarbons, 15 listings)	R	2	187
53-70-3	Dibenz[*a,h*]anthracene (under polycyclic aromatic hydrocarbons, 15 listings)	R	2	187
194-59-2	7H-Dibenzo[*c,g*]carbazole (under polycyclic aromatic hydrocarbons)	R	2	187
192-65-4	Dibenzo[*a,e*]pyrene (under polycyclic aromatic hydrocarbons, 15 listings)	R	2	187
189-64-0	Dibenzo[*a,h*]pyrene (under polycyclic aromatic hydrocarbons, 15 listings)	R	2	187
189-55-9	Dibenzo[*a,i*]pyrene (under polycyclic aromatic hydrocarbons, 15 listings)	R	2	187
191-30-0	Dibenzo[*a,l*]pyrene (under polycyclic aromatic hydrocarbons, 15 listings)	R	2	187
96-12-8	1,2-Dibromo-3-chloropropane	R	2	100
106-93-4	1,2-Dibromoethane (ethylene dibromide; EDB)	R	2	102
106-46-7	1,4-Dichlorobenzene (*p*-dichlorobenzene)	R	5	103
91-94-1	3,3′-Dichlorobenzidine	R	2	105
612-83-9	3,3′-Dichlorobenzidine dihydrochloride	R	6	105
50-29-3	Dichlorodiphenyltrichloroethane (see DDT)	R	4	97
107-06-2	1,2-Dichloroethane (ethylene dichloride)	R	2	106
75-09-2	Dichloromethane (methylene chloride)	R	5	107
542-75-6	1,3-Dichloropropene (technical grade)	R	5	109
1464-53-5	Diepoxybutane	R	3	110
	Diesel exhaust particulates	**R**	**9**	**110**
95-06-7	*N,N*-Diethyldithiocarbamic acid 2-chloroallyl ester (see sulfallate)	R	3	115
117-81-7	di(2-ethylhexyl) phthalate [DEHP; bis(2-ethylhexyl phthalate)]	R	3	113
55-18-5	Diethylnitrosamine (see *N*-nitrosodiethylamine)	R	2	167
64-67-5	Diethyl sulfate	R	4	115
101-90-6	Diglycidyl resorcinol ether	R	5	116
117-10-2	1,8-Dihydroxyanthraquinone [see danthron]	R	8	96
119-90-4	3,3′-Dimethoxybenzidine	R	3	116
60-11-7	4-Dimethylaminoazobenzene	R	2	117
119-93-7	3,3′-Dimethylbenzidine	R	3	118
79-44-7	Dimethylcarbamoyl chloride	R	2	119

TABLE E.1. *Continued*

CASRN	Name or synonym	Listing in the 9th RoC[a]	First listed[b]	Page No. III-
57-14-7	1,1-Dimethylhydrazine (UDMH)	R	4	121
62-75-9	Dimethylnitrosamine (see *N*-nitrosodimethylamine)	R	2	168
77-78-1	Dimethyl sulfate	R	2	121
513-37-1	Dimethylvinyl chloride	R	6	122
42397-64-8	1,6-Dinitropyrene	R	8	159
42397-65-9	1,8-Dinitropyrene	R	8	160
123-91-1	1,4-Dioxane	R	2	122
2475-45-8	Disperse blue 1	R	8	124
62-75-9	DMN (See *N*-nitrosodimethylamine)	R	2	168
25316-40-9	Doxorubicin hydrochloride (see adriamycin)	R	4	70
759-73-9	ENU [see *N*-nitroso-*N*-ethylurea (*N*-ethyl-*N*-nitrosourea)]	R	2	171
106-89-8	Epichlorohydrin	R	4	125
50-28-2	Estradiol-17β (under estrogens [not conjugated])	R	4	126
53-16-7	Estrone (under estrogens [not conjugated])	R	4	127
57-63-6	Ethinylestradiol (under estrogens [not conjugated])	R	4	128
51-79-6	Ethyl carbamate (see urethane)	R	3	214
106-93-4	Ethylene dibromide [see 1,2-Dibromoethane (EDB)]	R	2	102
107-06-2	Ethylene dichloride (see 1,2-Dichloroethane)	R	2	106
96-45-7	Ethylene thiourea	R	3	129
62-50-0	Ethyl methanesulfonate	R	6	130
759-73-9	*N*-Ethyl-*N*-nitrosourea (see *N*-nitroso-*N*-ethylurea)	R	2	171
	FireMaster BP-6 (under polybrominated biphenyls)	R	3	185
67774-32-7	FireMaster FF-1 (hexabromobiphenyl; under polybrominated biphenyls)	R	3	185
50-00-0	Formaldehyde (gas)	R	2	131
110-00-9	Furan	R	8	133
	Glasswool	R	7	134
556-52-5	Glycidol	R	7	136
67774-32-7	Hexabromobiphenyl (FireMaster FF-1, under polybrominated biphenyls)	R	3	185
118-74-1	Hexachlorobenzene	R	3	137
319-84-6	α-Hexachlorocyclohexane (under lindane and other hexachlorocyclohexane)	R	2	146
319-85-7	β-Hexachlorocyclohexane (under lindane and other hexachlorocyclohexane)	R	2	146
58-89-9	γ-Hexachlorocyclohexane (under lindane and other hexachlorocyclohexane)	R	2	146
608-73-1	Hexachlorocyclohexane (under lindane and other hexachlorocyclohexane)	R	2	146
67-72-1	Hexachloroethane	R	7	138
680-31-9	Hexamethylphosphoramide	R	4	139
302-01-2	Hydrazine	R	3	140
10034-93-2	Hydrazine sulfate	R	3	140
122-66-7	Hydrazobenzene	R	2	141
193-39-5	Indeno[1,2,3-*cd*]pyrene (under polycyclic aromatic hydrocarbons, 15 listings)	R	2	187
9004-66-4	Iron dextran complex	R	2	142
78-79-5	**Isoprene**	**R**	**9**	**143**
37317-41-2	Kanechlor 500 (under polychlorinated biphenyls)	R	3	186
143-50-0	Kepone (chlordecone)	R	2	144
301-04-2	Lead acetate	R	2	145
7446-27-7	Lead phosphate	R	2	145
58-89-9	Lindane (under lindane and other hexachlorocyclohexane isomers)	R	2	146
101-14-4	MBOCA [see 4,4′-methylenebis(2-chloraniline)]	R	3	148
72-33-3	Mestranol (under estrogens [not conjugated])	R	4	129
75-55-8	2-Methylaziridine (propylenimine)	R	4	147
3697-24-3	5-Methylchrysene (under polycyclic aromatic hydrocarbons, 15 listings)	R	2	187

Continued on next page

TABLE E.1. *Continued*

CASRN	Name or synonym	Listing in the 9th RoC[a]	First listed[b]	Page No. III-
101-14-4	4,4′-Methylenebis(2-chloraniline) (MBOCA)	R	3	148
101-61-1	4,4′-Methylenebis(*N,N*-dimethylbenzenamine)	R	3	149
75-09-2	Methylene chloride (see dichloromethane)	R	5	107
101-77-9	4,4′-Methylenedianiline	R	4	150
13552-44-8	4,4′-Methylenedianiline dihydrochloride	R	4	150
66-27-3	Methyl methanesulfonate	R	6	151
70-25-7	*N*-methyl-*N*′-nitro-*N*-nitrosoguanidine	R	6	151
684-93-5	*N*-methyl-*N*-nitrosourea (see *N*-nitroso-*N*-methylurea)	R	2	171
443-48-1	Metronidazole	R	4	152
90-94-8	Michler's ketone [4,4′-(dimethylamino)benzophenone]	R	3	153
2385-85-5	Mirex	R	2	154
7440-02-0	Nickel (under nickel and certain nickel compounds)	R	1	155
373-02-4	Nickel acetate (under nickel and certain nickel compounds)	R	1	155
3333-67-3	Nickel carbonate (under nickel and certain nickel compounds)	R	1	155
13463-39-3	Nickel carbonyl (under nickel and certain nickel compounds)	R	1	155
12054-48-7	Nickel hydroxide (under nickel and certain nickel compounds)	R	1	155
11113-74-9	Nickel hydroxide (under nickel and certain nickel compounds)	R	1	155
1271-28-9	Nickelocene (under nickel and certain nickel compounds)	R	1	155
1313-99-1	Nickel oxide (under nickel and certain nickel compounds)	R	1	155
12035-72-2	Nickel subsulfide (under nickel and certain nickel compounds)	R	1	155
139-13-9	Nitrilotriacetic acid	R	3	157
91-23-6	*o*-Nitroanisole	R	8	158
7496-02-8	6-Nitrochrysene	R	8	161
1836-75-5	Nitrofen	R	3	163
55-86-7	Nitrogen mustard hydrochloride	R	4	163
79-46-9	2-Nitropropane	R	4	164
5522-43-0	1-Nitropyrene	R	8	161
57835-92-4	4-Nitropyrene	R	8	162
38252-74-3	*N*-nitroso-*n*-butyl-*N*-(3-carboxypropyl)amine (under *N*-nitrosodi-*n*-butylamine)	R	2	165
3817-11-6	*N*-nitroso-*n*-butyl-*N*-(4-hydroxybutyl)amine (under *N*-nitrosodi-*n*-butylamine)	R	2	165
924-16-3	*N*-nitrosodi-*n*-butylamine	R	2	165
1116-54-7	*N*-nitrosodiethanolamine	R	2	166
55-18-5	*N*-nitrosodiethylamine (diethylnitrosamine; DEN)	R	2	167
62-75-9	*N*-nitrosodimethylamine (dimethylnitrosamine; DMN)	R	2	168
621-64-7	*N*-nitrosodi-*n*-propylamine	R	2	170
759-73-9	*N*-nitroso-*N*-ethylurea (*N*-ethyl-*N*-nitrosourea; ENU)	R	2	171
64091-91-4	4-(*N*-nitrosomethylamino)-1-(3-pyridyl)-1-butanone (NNK)	R	6	171
684-93-5	*N*-nitroso-*N*-methylurea (*N*-methyl-*N*-nitrosourea)	R	2	172
4549-40-0	*N*-nitrosomethylvinylamine	R	2	173
59-89-2	*N*-nitrosomorpholine	R	2	174
16543-55-8	*N*-nitrosonornicotine	R	2	174
100-75-4	*N*-nitrosopiperidine	R	2	175
930-55-2	*N*-nitrosopyrrolidine	R	2	176
13256-22-9	*N*-nitrososarcosine	R	2	177
64091-91-4	NNK [see 4-(*N*-nitrosomethylamino)-1-(3-pyridyl)-1-butanone]	R	6	171
68-22-4	Norethisterone	R	4	177
303-47-9	Ochratoxin A	R	6	178
61288-13-9	Octabromobiphenyl (under polybrominated biphenyls)	R	3	185
101-80-4	4,4′-oxydianiline	R	5	179

TABLE E.1. *Continued*

CASRN	Name or synonym	Listing in the 9th RoC[a]	First listed[b]	Page No. III-
434-07-1	Oxymetholone	R	1	180
	PAHs (see polycyclic aromatic hydrocarbons)	R	5	187
	PBBs (see polybrominated biphenyls)	R	3	185
1336-36-3	PCBs (under polychlorinated biphenyls)	R	2	185
127-18-4	Perchloroethylene (see tetrachloroethylene)	R	5	199
62-44-2	Phenacetin (see also analgesic mixtures containing phenacetin)	R	1	180
136-40-3	Phenazopyridine hydrochloride	R	2	181
77-09-8	**Phenolphthalein**	**R**	**9**	**182**
63-92-3	Phenoxybenzamine hydrochloride	R	5	183
57-41-0	Phenytoin	R	1	184
	Polybrominated biphenyls (PBBs)	R	3	185
1336-36-3	Polychlorinated biphenyls (PCBs)	R	2	186
	Polycyclic aromatic hydrocarbons (PAHs)	R	5	187
366-70-1	Procarbazine hydrochloride	R	2	190
57-83-0	Progesterone	R	4	191
1120-71-4	1,3-Propane sultone	R	4	192
57-57-8	β-Propiolactone	R	2	192
75-56-9	Propylene oxide	R	6	193
75-55-8	Propylenimine (see 2-methylaziridine)	R	4	147
51-52-5	Propylthiouracil	R	4	195
50-55-5	Reserpine	R	2	195
94-59-7	Safrole	R	2	196
7446-34-6	Selenium sulfide	R	3	197
18883-66-4	Streptozotocin	R	2	198
95-06-7	Sulfallate	R	3	199
1746-01-6	**2,3,7,8-Tetrachlorodibenzo-*p*-dioxin (TCDD)[e]**	**R**	**2[c]**	
			9[d]	**199**
127-18-4	Tetrachloroethylene (perchloroethylene)	R	5	200
116-14-3	**Tetrafluoroethylene**	**R**	**9**	**202**
509-14-8	Tetranitromethane	R	7	203
62-55-5	Thioacetamide	R	3	204
62-56-6	Thiourea	R	3	204
26471-62-5	Toluene diisocyanate	R	4	205
95-53-4	*o*-Toluidine	R	3	207
636-21-5	*o*-Toluidine hydrochloride	R	2	207
8001-35-2	Toxaphene	R	2	208
79-01-6	**Trichloroethylene**	**R**	**9**	**209**
88-06-2	2,4,6-Trichlorophenol	R	3	211
96-18-4	1,2,3-Trichloropropane	R	8	212
126-72-7	tris(2,3-dibromopropyl) phosphate	R	2	213
57-14-7	UDMH (see 1,1-dimethylhydrazine)	R	4	120
51-79-6	Urethane (urethan; ethyl carbamate)	R	3	214
106-87-6	4-Vinyl-1-cyclohexene diepoxide	R	7	216

[a]Known (K), known to be a human carcinogen.
RAHC (R), reasonably anticipated to be a human carcinogen.
[b]Numbers designate the number of the report on carcinogens when first listed:
1 = first annual report on carcinogens, 1980;
2 = second annual report on carcinogens, 1981;
3 = third annual report on carcinogens, 1983;
4 = fourth annual report on carcinogens, 1985;
5 = fifth annual report on carcinogens, 1989;
6 = sixth annual report on carcinogens, 1991;
7 = seventh annual report on carcinogens, 1994;
8 = eighth report on carcinogens, 1998;
9 = ninth report on carcinogens, 2000.
[c]First listed as reasonably anticipated to be a human carcinogen.
[d]First listed as known to be a human carcinogen.
[e]This substance has been proposed for upgrade to the known to be a human carcinogen category. The proposed listing is currently in litigation. Depending on the outcome of the litigation an addendum may be published following the court's ruling.
Bold entries indicate new listing in the report on carcinogens, 9th edition.

Appendix F

Recommended Library for Occupational and Environmental Physicians

For additional updates to the library, visit *www.acoem.org*.

OCCUPATIONAL MEDICINE: BASIC CORE

Encyclopedia of occupational health and safety, 3rd ed. International Labor Office/Boyd Printing, 1991.

Hathaway GJ, Proctor NH, Hughes JP, et al. *Proctor and Hughes' chemical hazards in the workplace,* 4th ed. New York: John Wiley & Sons, 1996.

Last JM, Wallace RB, eds. *Maxcy-Rosenau-Last public health and preventive medicine,* 13th ed. Appleton & Lange, 1992.

Wald P, Stave G. *Physical and biological hazards in the workplace*. New York: John Wiley & Sons, 1994.

OCCUPATIONAL MEDICINE TEXTBOOKS: GENERAL

Harbison RD, ed. *Hamilton and Hardy's Industrial Toxicology,* 5th ed. Mosby, 1998.

Harris JS, ed. *ACOEM Occupational and Environmental Practice Guidelines: evaluation and management of common health problems and function recovery in workers.* OEM Press, 1997.

Harris JS, ed. *ACOEM Occupational and Environmental Practice Guidelines: a quick reference.* OEM Press, 1999.

Harris JS, Loeppke RR, eds. *Integrated health management: the key role of occupational medicine in managed care, disability management, productivity, and integrated delivery systems*. OEM Press, 1998.

The health care worker. In: McDiarmid MA, Kessler ER, eds. *Occup Med State of the Art Rev* 1997;12(4).

Jeyaratnam J, Koh D, eds. *Textbook of occupational medicine practice.* World Scientific Publishing, 1996.

LaDou J. *Occupational and environmental medicine,* 2nd ed. Appleton & Lange, 1996.

Levy BS, Wegman DH, eds. *Occupational health: recognizing and preventing work-related disease and injury,* 4th ed. Philadelphia: Lippincott Williams & Wilkins, 1999.

McCunney RJ, ed. *A practical approach to cccupational and environmental medicine,* 2nd ed. (formerly the *Handbook of occupational medicine*). Philadelphia: Lippincott Williams & Wilkins, 1994.

McCunney RJ, Rountree PP, eds. *Occupational and environmental medicine self-assessment review*. Philadelphia: Lippincott Williams & Wilkins, 1998.

Raffle PAB, Adams PH, Baxter PJ, et al., eds. *Hunter's diseases of occupations,* 8th ed. Oxford University Press, 1994.

Rom WN, ed. *Environmental and occupational medicine,* 3rd ed. Lippincott Williams & Wilkins, 1992.

Rosenstock L, Cullen MR, eds. *Textbook of clinical occupational and environmental medicine*. WB Saunders Co, 1994.

Zenz C, Dickerson OB, Horvath EP. *Occupational medicine,* 3rd ed. Mosby, 1994.

HISTORICAL TEXTS

Greaves WW, ed. *Occupational and environmental medicine: "pearls" of the specialty.* OEM Press, 1996.

Hamilton A. *Exploring the dangerous trades*. OEM Press, 1995.

Schilling R. *A challenging life: sixty years in occupational health*. Canning Press, a division of Drake International, 1998.

ENVIRONMENTAL MEDICINE: GENERAL

Auerbach PS, ed. *Wilderness medicine: management of wilderness and environmental emergencies,* 3rd ed. Mosby, 1995.

Brooks SM, Gochfeld M, Herzstein J, et al., eds. *Environmental medicine—principles and practice.* Mosby, 1995.

Etzel RA, Balk SJ. *The handbook of pediatric environmental health*. American Pediatric Association, 1999. Order at *Amazon.com*.

Introduction to indoor air quality: a reference manual. EPA/400/3-91/003. U.S. Environmental Protection Agency, U.S. Public Health Service, National Environmental Health Association , July 1991. National Environmental Health Association.

Introduction to indoor air quality: a self-paced learning module. EPA/400/391/002. U.S. Environmental Protection Agency, U.S. Public Health Service, National Environmental Health Association, July 1991. National Environmental Health Association.

Koren H, Bisesi M. *Handbook of environmental health and safety,* vol I & II: principles and practices, 3rd ed. CRC Press/Lewis Publishers, National Environmental Health Association, 1996.

Pope AM, Rall DP, eds. *Environmental medicine—integrating a missing element into medical education.* Institute of Medicine, National Academy Press, 1995 (Contains bound form of ATSDR Case Studies in Environmental Medicine.)

Samett JM, Spengler JD. *Indoor air pollution: a health perspective.* Johns Hopkins University Press, 1991.

Seltzer JM, ed. Effects of indoor environment on health. *Occup Med State of the Art Rev* 1995;10(1).

ADMINISTRATION

DiBenedetto DV, Harris JS, McCunney RJ. *OEM occupational health and safety manual,* version 2.0. OEM Press, 1995.

Goldenthal N. *Understanding the Americans with Disabilities Act: a compliance guide for health professionals and employers.* OEM Press, 1993.

Moser R. *Effective management of occupational and environmental health and safety programs: a practical guide.* OEM Press, 1992.

AEROSPACE MEDICINE

DeHart R. *Fundamentals of aerospace medicine,* 2nd ed. Philadelphia: Lippincott Williams & Wilkins, 1996.

COMMUNICABLE DISEASES AND TRAVEL MEDICINE

Benenson AS, ed. *Control of communicable diseases manual,* 16th ed. American Public Health Association, 1995. (Also available on CD-ROM.)

Gorbach SL, Bartlett JG, Blacklow NR. *Infectious diseases,* 2nd ed. WB Saunders, 1997.

Health information for international travel. Centers for Disease Control and Prevention. U.S. Government Printing Office, 1995.

Jong EC, McMullen R. *The travel and tropical medicine manual,* 2nd ed. WB Saunders, 1995.

Rose SR. *International travel health guide,* 11th ed. Travel Medicine, 2000.

DERMATOLOGY

Adams RM. *Occupational skin disease,* 2nd ed. WB Saunders, 1990.

Habif TP. *Clinical dermatology: a guide to diagnosis and therapy,* 3rd ed. Mosby, 1996.

Marks JG, DeLeo VA. *Contact and occupational dermatitis.* Mosby, 1992.

EAR, NOSE, AND THROAT

Morata TC, Dunn DE, eds. Occupational hearing loss. *Occup Med State of the Art Rev* 1995;10(3).

Sataloff RT, Sataloff J. *Occupational hearing loss,* 2nd ed. Marcel Dekker, 1993.

EPIDEMIOLOGY AND BIOSTATISTICS

Hennekens CH, Buring JE. *Epidemiology in medicine.* Philadelphia: Lippincott Williams & Wilkins, 1987.

Monson RR. *Occupational epidemiology,* 2nd ed. CRC Press, 1990.

Morton RF, Hebel JR, McCarter RJ. *A study guide to epidemiology and biostatistics,* 3rd ed. Aspen Publishers, 1990.

Schuman SS. *Environmental epidemiology for the busy clinician.* Harwood Academic Publishers, a division of the Gordon and Breach Publishing Group, 1997.

Selvin S. *Statistical analysis of epidemiologic data.* Oxford University Press, 1991.

ERGONOMICS

Chaffin DB, Andersson GBJ. *Occupational biomechanics,* 2nd ed. New York: John Wiley & Sons, 1991.

Dul J, Weerdmeester B. *Ergonomics for beginners: a quick reference guide.* Taylor & Francis Group, 1993.

Eastman Kodak. *Ergonomic design for people at work,* vols I and II. New York: John Wiley & Sons, 1986.

Erdil M, Dickerson OB, eds. *Cumulative trauma disorders: prevention, evaluation, and treatment.* New York: John Wiley & Sons, 1996.

Moon SD, Suater SL. *Beyond biomechanics—psychosocial aspects of musculoskeletal disorders in office work.* Taylor & Francis Group, 1995.

FITNESS FOR DUTY

Cox RAF, Edwards FC, Palmer K, eds. *Fitness for work: the medical aspects,* 3rd ed. Oxford University Press, 1995.

HEALTH PROMOTION AND SCREENING

Guide to clinical preventive services: an assessment of the effectiveness of 169 interventions report of the U.S. Preventive Services Task Force, 2nd ed. Philadelphia: Lippincott Williams & Wilkins, 1995.

O'Donnell MP, Harris JS, eds. *Health promotion in the workplace,* 2nd ed. Delmar Thomson Learning, 1994.

Peterson KW, Hyner GC, Foerster JJ, et al., eds. *The handbook of health assessment tools,* 4th ed. The Society of Prospective Medicine, 1999.

Woolf SH, Jonas S, Lawrence R, eds. *Health promotion and disease prevention in clinical practice.* Philadelphia: Lippincott Williams & Wilkins, 1995.

INDUSTRIAL HYGIENE

Burgess WA. *Recognition of health hazards in industries: a review of materials and processes,* 2nd ed. New York: John Wiley & Sons, 1995.

Clayton GD, Clayton FE, eds. *Patty's industrial hygiene and toxicology,* 4th rev. ed. Volume I, A & B; Volume II, A–F, 1995; Volume III A & B, 4th ed, Cralley LJ, Cralley LV, eds. New York: John Wiley & Sons, 1995.

Documentation of the threshold limit values and biological exposure indices, 6th ed. American Conference of Governmental Industrial Hygienists, 1993.

Forsberg K, Mansdorf SZ. *Quick selection guide to chemical protective clothing,* 3rd ed. New York: John Wiley & Sons, 1997.

NIOSH Pocket Guide to Chemical Hazards U.S. Department of Health and Human Services, Public Health and Service, Centers for Disease Control and Prevention, National Institute for Occupational Safety and Health, 1997.

Plog BA. *Fundamentals of industrial hygiene,* 4th ed. National Safety Council, 1996.

2000 threshold limit values and biological exposure indices. American Conference of Governmental Industrial Hygienists, 2000.

INTERNATIONAL ISSUES

Fleming LE, Herzstein J, Bunn WB, eds. *Issues in international occupational and environmental medicine.* OEM Press, 1997.

LEGAL ISSUES IN MEDICINE

Horsley JE, Carlova J. *Testifying in court: a guide for physicians,* 3rd ed. Practice Management Information, 1988.

MUSCULOSKELETAL MEDICINE

Anderson BC. *Office orthopedics for primary care: diagnosis and treatment,* 2nd ed. WB Saunders, 1998.

Herington TN, Morse LH, eds. *Occupational injuries: evaluation, management, and prevention.* Mosby, 1995.

Isernhagen SJ, ed. *The comprehensive guide to work injury management.* Aspen, 1995.

Kuorinka I, Hagberg M, Silverstein B, et al. *Work-related musculoskeletal disorders: a reference for prevention.* Taylor & Francis, 1995.

Magee DJ. *Orthopedic physical assessment,* 3rd ed. WB Saunders, 1997.

Nordin M, Andersson G, Pope M. *Musculoskeletal disorders in the workplace: principles and practice.* Mosby, 1996.

Pope MH, Andersson GBJ, Frymoyer JW, et al. *Occupational low back pain: assessment, treatment, and prevention.* Mosby, 1991.

PSYCHIATRY

Kahn JP. *Mental health in the workplace.* New York: John Wiley & Sons, 1992.

REPRODUCTIVE MEDICINE

Frazier L, Hage M. *Reproductive hazards of the workplace.* New York: John Wiley & Sons, 1998.

Gold EB, Lasley BL, Schenker MB. Reproductive hazards. *Occup Med State of the Art Rev* 1994;9(3).

Schardein JL. *Chemically induced birth defects,* 3rd ed. Marcel Dekker, 2000.

RESPIRATORY MEDICINE

Bernstein IL, Chan-Yeung M, Mallo JL, et al. *Asthma in the workplace.* Marcel Dekker, 1993.

Cordasco EM Sr, Zenz C, Demeter SL. *Environmental respiratory diseases.* New York: John Wiley & Sons, 1994.

Harber P, Schenker M, Balmes J, eds. *Occupational and environmental respiratory diseases.* Mosby, 1995.

Morgan WKC, Seaton A. *Occupational lung diseases,* 3rd ed. WB Saunders, 1995.

Parkes WR. *Occupational lung disorders,* 3rd ed. Oxford University Press, 1994.

SAFETY

Charney W. *Handbook of modern hospital safety.* CRC Press, 1999.

Kohn JP, ed. *Safety and health management planning.* Government Institutes, 1999.

Krause TR, Hidley JH, Stanley JH. *The behavior-based safety process: managing involvement for an injury-free culture,* 2nd ed. New York: John Wiley & Sons, 1996.

Krieger GR, Montgomery JF, eds. *Accident prevention manual for business and industry,* 12th ed. National Safety Council, 1996.

Langley RL, McLymore RL, Meggs WJ, et al. *Safety and health in agriculture, forestry, and fisheries.* Government Institutes, 1997.

Manuele FA. *On the practice of safety,* 2nd ed. New York: John Wiley & Sons, 1997.

McCunney RJ, Barbanel CS. *Medical center occupational health and safety.* Philadelphia: Lippincott Williams & Wilkins, 1999.

McSween TE. *The values-based safety process: improving your safety culture with a behavioral approach.* New York: John Wiley & Sons, 1995.

Vincoli J. *Basic guide to accident investigation and loss control.* New York: John Wiley & Sons, 1994.

Wilkinson CW. *Violence in the workplace: preventing, assessing, and managing threats at work.* Government Institutes, 1998.

SUBSTANCE ABUSE AND DRUG TESTING

Swotinsky RB. *The medical review officer's manual: MROCC's guide to drug testing.* OEM Press, 1999.

TOXICOLOGY

Amdur MO, Doull J, Klaessen CD, eds. *Casarett and Doull's toxicology: the basic science of poisons,* 5th ed. Organic substances. New York: McGraw-Hill, 1995.

ATSDR toxicological profiles. U.S. Department of Health and Human Services, Public Health Service, Centers for Disease Control and Prevention, Agency for Toxic Substances and Disease Registry. (Also available on CD-ROM.)

Goldfrank LR, Flomenbaum NE, Lewin NA, et al., eds. *Goldfrank's toxicological emergencies,* 5th ed. Appleton & Lange, 1998.

Haddad LM, Shannon MW, Winchester JM, eds. *Clinical management of poisoning and drug overdose,* 3rd ed. WB Saunders, 1997.

Lauwerys RR, Hoet P. *Industrial chemical exposure: guidelines for biologic monitoring,* 2nd ed. CRC Press, 1993.

Lewis RJ. *Hazardous chemicals desk reference,* 4th ed. New York: John Wiley & Sons, 1996.

Lewis RJ. *Sax's dangerous properties of industrial materials,* 9th ed. New York: John Wiley & Sons, 1996. (Also available on CD-ROM with Hawley's Condensed Chemical Dictionary by Lewis.)

Managing hazardous materials incidents, volume I, emergency medical services. U.S. Department of Health and Human Services, Public Health Service, Agency for Toxic Substances and Disease Registry.

Managing hazardous materials incidents, volume II, hospital emergency departments. U.S. Department of Health and Human Services, Public Health Service, Agency for Toxic Substances and Disease Registry.

Managing hazardous materials incidents, volume III, medical management guidelines for acute chemical exposures. U.S. Department of Health and Human Services, Public Health Service, Agency for Toxic Substances and Disease Registry.

Olson KR, Anderson IB, Blanc PD, et al., eds. *Poisoning & drug overdose,* 3rd ed. New York: McGraw Hill, 1999.

Reigart R, Roberts JR, eds. *Recognition and management of pesticide poisonings,* 5th ed. EPA's Office of Pesticide Programs, March 1999.

Ryan RP, Terry CE, eds. *Toxicology desk reference: the toxic exposure and medical monitoring index,* 3rd ed. Taylor & Francis, 1996. (Also available on CD-ROM.)

Sullivan JB Jr, Krieger GR, eds. *Hazardous materials toxicology: clinical principles of environmental health.* Philadelphia: Lippincott Williams & Wilkins, 1992.

TRANSPORTATION

Hartenbaum NP. *The DOT medical examination: a guide to commercial drivers medical certification,* 2nd ed. OEM Press, 2000.

WORKER'S COMPENSATION AND DISABILITY EVALUATION

Demeter SL, Anderson GBJ, Smith GM, eds. *Disability evaluation.* Mosby, 1996.

Guides to the evaluation of permanent impairment, 5th ed. American Medical Association, 2000.

Menzel NN. *Workers' comp management from A to Z: a "how to" guide with forms.* OEM Press, 1994.

Reed P. *The medical disability advisor: workplace guidelines for disability duration,* 3rd ed. Reed Group, 1997.

Smith GL. *How to write a winning workers' compensation report: a programmed text.* OEM Press, 1995.

PRIMARY PEER-REVIEWED JOURNALS

Journal of Occupational and Environmental Medicine (complimentary for ACOEM members) published by Lippincott Williams & Wilkins.

Occupational and Environmental Medicine (formerly *British Journal of Industrial Medicine*) published by BMJ Publishing Group.

ADVANCED JOURNALS

American Industrial Hygiene Journal published by the American Industrial Hygiene Association.

American Journal of Industrial Medicine published by John Wiley & Sons.

Annals of Occupational Hygiene published by Elsevier Science Publishers.

Archives of Environmental Health published by Heldref Publications.

International Archives of Occupational and Environmental Health published by Springer-Verlag.

Journal of Toxicology—Clinical Toxicology published by Marcel Dekker.

Scandinavian Journal of Work, Environment, and Health published by the Finnish Institute of Occupational Health.

ELECTRONIC MEDIA

Peterson KW, ed. *Handbook of occupational health and safety software,* Version 10.0. American College of Occupational and Environmental Medicine, 1997.

CD-ROM

BNA's Safety Library on CD. Bureau of National Affairs, 1994.

CCINFO. Canadian Centre for Occupational Health and Safety.

OSHA CD-ROM. U.S. Department of Labor, Occupational Safety and Health Administration, U.S. Government Printing Office, Quarterly updates.

Portable Medline for Occupational and Environmental Medicine (formerly Physicians' SilverPlatter by SilverPlatter Education, Inc.). HealthStream, Inc., Quarterly updates.

TOMES Plus. Micromedix, Inc.

The Recommended Library for Occupational and Environmental Physicians was compiled by the Publications Committee of the American College of Occupational and Environmental Medicine (ACOEM). Inclusion in the library does not signify endorsement by ACOEM. Recommendations regarding future editions are welcome and should be directed to Marianne Dreger, MA, Director of Publications, 1114 North Arlington Heights Road, Arlington Heights, IL 60004.

Source: Reprinted with permission from *J Occup Med* 1997;39(5).

Subject Index

Page numbers followed by *f* indicate figures; those followed by *t* indicate tabular material.

E

F

Q

Y

Z